PETERSON'S GUIDE TO NURSING PROGRAMS

BACCALAUREATE AND GRADUATE NURSING EDUCATION IN THE U.S. AND CANADA

Third Edition

Published in cooperation with the

American Association of Colleges of Nursing

Peterson's
Princeton, New Jersey

Visit Peterson's Education Center on the Internet
(World Wide Web) at http://www.petersons.com

Editorial inquiries concerning this book should be addressed to the editor at Peterson's, 202 Carnegie Center, P.O. Box 2123, Princeton, New Jersey 08543-2123 (609-243-9111).

ISSN 1073-7820
ISBN 1-56079-817-3

Printed in the United States of America

10 9 8 7 6 5 4 3 2 1

Contents

Foreword

The American Association of Colleges of Nursing again is proud to collaborate with Peterson's in the publishing of the third edition of *Peterson's Guide to Nursing Programs.* Now more than ever, it is vital for those seeking to enter or advance in a nursing career to find the appropriate nursing program. As registered nurses find employment outside of hospitals, in such areas as home care, community health, and long-term care, newly licensed RNs must have the specific education and training required to work in these settings. This guide allows prospective students to find the program that best fits their needs, whether they are starting their nursing career or attempting to advance it.

When the first edition of *Peterson's Guide to Nursing Programs* was published, it was our hope that there would be enough interest in it to warrant publication of a second edition. Indeed, interest in both the first and second editions has been so strong that Peterson's moved the publication date of the third edition ahead by a full year. Although nursing has seen tremendous change in its role within health care, it remains the largest health-care profession. This is an opportune time to pursue or further a career in nursing.

Higher education in nursing expands the gateway to a variety of career opportunities in the health-care field. Nurses with appropriate education can enjoy careers as nurse practitioners providing needed primary care to patients. They can work as case managers for the growing numbers of managed-care companies, or they can assume administrative or managerial roles in hospitals, clinics, insurance companies, and other diverse settings.

Though the health-care environment is complex and dynamic, there continues to be a significant demand for professional-level nurses. The primary route into professional-level nursing is the four-year baccalaureate degree. The professional nurse with a baccalaureate degree is the only basic nursing graduate prepared to practice in all health-care settings, including critical care, public health, primary care, and mental health. In addition, advanced practice nurses (APNs) deliver essential services as nurse practitioners, certified nurse-midwives, clinical nurse specialists, and nurse anesthetists. APNs typically are prepared in master's degree programs, and the demand for their services is expected to increase substantially.

"The Nursing School Adviser" section of this guide is instructive and valuable to read. Whether you are a high school student looking for a four-year program, an RN seeking to return to school, or a professional in another field contemplating a career change to nursing, this advisory section will address your concerns. This information presents various nursing perspectives to benefit students from diverse backgrounds.

Peterson's effort in making this guide well organized and convenient to read cannot be overstated. Peterson's has worked with AACN in producing a publication that is comprehensive as well as user-friendly. Like the previous two editions, this third edition is a genuine collaborative work. AACN provided its input from start to finish.

AACN's dedication and achievements in advancing the quality of baccalaureate and graduate nursing education are appreciated by Peterson's. We at AACN are fortunate to work with an organization that prides itself on being the leading publisher of education and career guides.

This publication would not be possible without the responses from those institutions included within. In particular, we acknowledge the time and effort of those individuals who undertook the task of completing and returning the questionnaires regarding their programs. We appreciate their contribution.

Peterson's Guide to Nursing Programs is the only comprehensive and concise guide to baccalaureate and graduate nursing education programs in the United States and Canada. We hope its contents will provide the impetus for those looking for a rewarding and satisfying career in health care. AACN is proud to present this publication to the nursing profession and to those who seek to enter it.

Carole A. Anderson, Ph.D., RN, FAAN
President, AACN

Geraldine D. Bednash, Ph.D., RN, FAAN
Executive Director, AACN

Introduction—How to Use Peterson's Guide to Nursing Programs

Peterson's Guide to Nursing Programs provides prospective nursing students with the most comprehensive information on baccalaureate and graduate nursing education in the United States and Canada. For those seeking to enter the nursing profession or to further their nursing careers, *Peterson's Guide to Nursing Programs* includes the exact help they need to make important college decisions and to approach the admissions process without fear.

The following includes an overview of the various components of the book, along with background information on the criteria used for including institutions and nursing programs in the guide, and explanatory material to help users interpret details presented within the guide.

How Schools and Programs Get into the Guide

Peterson's Guide to Nursing Programs covers accredited institutions in the United States, U.S. territories, and Canada that grant baccalaureate and graduate degrees. To be included in this guide, an institution must have full accreditation or candidate-for-accreditation status granted by an institutional or specialized accrediting body recognized by the U.S. Department of Education or the Commission on Recognition of Postsecondary Accreditation. A Canadian institution must be chartered and authorized to grant degrees by the provincial government, affiliated with a chartered institution, or accredited by a recognized accrediting body.

Baccalaureate-level and master's-level nursing programs represented by a profile within the guide are accredited by the National League for Nursing (NLN). Canadian nursing schools are accredited by the Canadian Association of University Schools of Nursing (CAUSN).

Doctoral, postdoctoral, continuing education, and other nursing programs included in profiles are offered by nursing schools or departments affiliated with colleges or universities that meet the criteria outlined above.

Research Procedures

The data contained in the preponderant number of nursing college profiles, as well as in the indexes to them, were collected through Peterson's Survey of Nursing Programs during winter 1996–97. Questionnaires were sent to almost 650 colleges and universities with baccalaureate and graduate programs in nursing. With minor exceptions, data for those colleges or schools of nursing that responded to the questionnaires were submitted by officials at the schools themselves. Whenever unusual figures or facts, discrepancies, anomalies, or missing data were discovered, Peterson's editorial staff contacted the schools to verify and clarify the information. All usable information received in time for publication has been included. For those few schools that failed to return questionnaires in time to meet Peterson's deadline, information was drawn from college catalogs and World Wide Web sites. The omission of a particular item from a profile means that it is either not applicable to that institution or not available or usable. In the handful of instances in which no information regarding an eligible nursing program was submitted and research of reliable secondary sources was unable to elicit the desired information, the name, location, and some general information regarding the nursing program appear in the profile section to indicate the existence of the program. Because of the extensive system of checks performed on the data collected by Peterson's, we believe that the information presented in this guide is accurate. Nonetheless, errors and omissions are possible in a data collection and processing endeavor of this scope. Also, facts and figures, such as tuition and fees, can suddenly change. Therefore, students should check at the time of application with a specific college or university to verify all pertinent information.

Organization of the Guide

Peterson's Guide to Nursing Programs is divided into four main sections:

- A Nursing Career and Educational Guidance Section includes useful articles, charts, and lists to help guide nursing education choices, with information on nursing careers today, how to select a nursing program, financing nursing education, going back to school, etc.
- The Nursing School Profiles Section contains detailed profiles of nursing schools and the programs they offer. This section is organized geographically; U.S. schools are listed alphabetically by state or territory, followed by Canadian schools listed alphabetically by province.
- The In-Depth Descriptions Section is an open forum for nursing schools to communicate, on a voluntary basis, their particular message to prospective students. The absence of any college or university from this section does not constitute an editorial decision on the part of Peterson's. Those who have chosen to write these inclusions are responsible for the accuracy of the content.

Statements regarding a school's objectives and accomplishments represent its own beliefs and are not the opinions of the editors. These articles are arranged alphabetically by the official institution name.

- Indexes at the back of the book provide references to profiles by institution name, type of program offered, and, for master's-level programs, by area of study or concentration.

Nursing School Profiles

The profiles contain basic information about the colleges and universities, along with details specific to the nursing school or department, the nursing student body, and the nursing programs offered.

An outline of the profile follows. The items of information found under each section heading are defined and displayed. Any item discussed below that is omitted from an individual profile either does not apply to that particular college or university or is one for which no information was supplied.

Heading

Each profile begins with a heading with the name of the institution (the college or university), the nursing school or unit, and the location of the nursing facilities. In most cases, this location is identical to the main campus of the institution; however, in a few instances, the nursing facilities are not located in the same city or state as the main campus of the college or university.

Programs

Nursing programs offered at the baccalaureate, graduate, postgraduate, and continuing education level are listed under this category. Programs are listed first and use bullets in place of standard punctuation marks. We have done this in order to facilitate scanning of the profiles to select the programs that relate to a prospective student's particular interests and needs.

For most programs listed in this section, application details, degree requirements, and other relevant data are enumerated further along in the profile under the large, boldface heading for the specific program. However, in instances where the nursing school did not furnish details regarding a specific program, we nevertheless list the program in this section to alert students to its availability.

Among the programs that may be listed are:

Generic baccalaureate—programs that admit students with no previous nursing education, require at least four academic years of full-time-equivalent college work, and award a baccalaureate degree in nursing. Included here, also, are baccalaureate programs of the few colleges that have not furnished sufficient information to permit a precise categorization.

RN baccalaureate—programs that admit registered nurses with associate degrees or diplomas in nursing and award a baccalaureate nursing degree.

Baccalaureate for second degree—programs that admit students with baccalaureate degrees in areas other than nursing and award a baccalaureate degree in nursing.

LPN to baccalaureate—programs that admit licensed practical nurses and award a baccalaureate nursing degree.

Accelerated pathways of the above baccalaureate programs are so indicated. These programs enable students to complete programs in less time than regularly required.

MS and *MSN*—programs that admit students with baccalaureate degrees in nursing and award a master's degree in nursing.

RN to Master's—master's programs that combine the baccalaureate and master's degree into one program for nurses who are graduates of associate or hospital diploma programs.

Master's for nurses with non-nursing degrees—programs that admit registered nurses with non-nursing baccalaureate degrees and award a master's degree in nursing.

Master's for non-nursing college graduates—programs that admit students with baccalaureate degrees in areas other than nursing and prepare them for entry into the profession and award a master's degree in nursing.

Master's for Second Degree—programs that admit nurses with a master's degree in nursing.

Master of Education—programs that award a master's degree in education with a nursing major.

Joint-degree programs—profiles and indexes specify which two degrees are given, e.g., *MSN/MBA, MS/MHA, MSN/MPH*, etc.—combine a master's degree (or doctorate) in nursing with the master's degree in another discipline, such as business administration, hospital administration, or public health.

Accelerated pathways of the above master's programs are indicated. These programs enable students to complete programs in less time than regularly required.

Post-master's—programs that admit students with master's degrees in nursing who wish to continue their studies in a specific clinical area, typically for certification in a specialty.

PhD, also called *Generic Doctorate*—programs that admit students with master's degrees in nursing and award a doctorate in nursing.

Postbaccalaureate doctorate—programs that admit students with a baccalaureate degree in nursing and award a doctorate in nursing.

Doctor of Education—programs that award a Doctor of Education degree with a major in nursing.

The College or University

Data from fall 1995 are used for non-nursing units of the institution. An institutional type is described as one of the following:

Four-year college: Awards baccalaureate degrees and may also award associate degrees; does not award graduate degrees.

Upper-level institution: Awards baccalaureate degrees, but entering students must have at least two years of previous college-level credit; may also offer graduate degrees.

Comprehensive institution: Awards baccalaureate degrees and may also award associate degrees; offers graduate degree programs primarily at the master's, specialist's, or professional level, although one or two doctoral programs may be offered.

University: Offers four-year undergraduate programs plus graduate degrees through the doctorate in more than two academic or professional fields.

Graduate institution: Awards only postbaccalaureate academic or professional degrees.

Any of the above types except university may be designated as *specialized*, indicating that degrees are offered in one field only. In this guide, those so designated are specialized in nursing.

Each college or university is also identified by its student body as either *women's, primarily women's, coed* (coeducational), or *coordinate* (having separate colleges or campuses for men and women but sharing facilities and courses). If applicable, an indication of affiliation with a government or religious entity is incorporated within the description of the college or university, as is the name of the group of institutions or single institution with which the college may be affiliated.

Other information provided about the institution includes:

Founding Date: This is the year in which the institution was chartered. If the year the institution was chartered differs from the year when instruction actually began, the earlier date is given.

Primary Accreditation: In most instances, this accreditation will be designated as *regional*, meaning that accreditation of the institution is granted through one of the six regional associations of schools and colleges (Middle States, New England, North Central, Northwest, Southern, and Western).

Campus Setting: The location of the campus is designated as *urban* (located within a major city), *suburban* (a residential area within commuting distance of a major city), *small-town*, or *rural* (a remote and sparsely populated area).

Total enrollment: The total number of matriculated full-time and part-time undergraduate and graduate students (if applicable) as of fall 1995 is given.

The Nursing School or Unit

The name of the nursing unit of the college or university is followed by the year in which the program of nursing education was started. Other information in this section includes:

Faculty: The total of full-time and part-time faculty members, followed by, if provided, the percentage of the faculty members holding doctoral degrees.

Off-campus sites: Locations (cities or towns) other than the main facilities of the nursing program where nursing classes can be attended. Off-campus classes generally are held in health-care facilities or other educational facilities that are part of or affiliated with the college or nursing school.

Noteworthy

"Noteworthy" items, which appear within some institutions' profiles, have been written by those colleges or universities that wished to supplement the profile data with timely or important information about their institutions or nursing programs. Some choose to mention degree programs that are not yet NLN accredited.

Academic Facilities

The following sections cover data that was collected regarding the facilities of the college and the nursing school that enrich the educational experience of the student.

Campus Library: Figures are provided for the total number of bound volumes held by the college or university, the number of those volumes in health-related subjects, and the number in nursing; the number of periodical subscriptions held and the number of those in health-related subjects.

Nursing School Resources: This section lists special learning resources available for nursing students within the nursing school's or unit's facilities.

Student Life

Information on campus life includes:

Student Services: Services on campus, which may include health clinics, child-care facilities, personal counseling, career counseling, work-study programs, job placement, campus safety programs, special assistance for disabled students, and other services.

International Student Services: Services that the college provides for international students, including counseling and support, ESL courses, special assistance for nonnative speakers of English, and other services.

Nursing Student Organizations: Organizations open only to nursing students, including nursing clubs, Sigma Theta Tau (the international honor society for nursing), recruiter clubs, and student nurses associations.

Calendar

Most colleges indicate one of the following: *semesters; trimesters; 3-3,* under which there are three courses for each of three terms; *quarters; 4-1-4, 4-4-1,* or a similar arrangement, which refers to two terms of equal length plus an abbreviated winter or spring term, with the numbers referring to months; *modular*, whereby the academic year is divided into small blocks of time.

Nursing Student Profile

This snapshot of the nursing student body indicates the number of matriculated students, both full-time and part-time, in undergraduate and graduate nursing programs. For both undergraduate and graduate enrollments, the school's estimate of the percentage of nursing students in each of the following categories is provided, if applicable: women, men, minority, international, and part-time.

Baccalaureate Programs—General

General information provided on baccalaureate programs includes:

Contact

The name, title, mailing address, telephone number, and, if available, fax number and e-mail address of the person to contact for admission information are given.

Expenses

In this section, figures are provided for tuition, mandatory and other fees, and room and board as well as an estimate of costs for books and supplies, based on the 1996–97 academic year. Unless indicated otherwise, tuition is for one full academic year. If applicable, distinct tuition figures are given for state residents and nonresidents. Part-time, summer, and evening tuition is expressed in terms of the per-unit rate (per credit, per semester hour, etc.) specified by the institution. The tuition structure at some institutions is very complex, with different rates for freshmen and sophomores than for juniors and seniors, or with part-time tuition prorated on a sliding scale according to the number of credit hours taken. In cases where a school has a variable tuition schedule, the minimum and maximum figures are given. Ranges are also given for other expense areas, where applicable. Mandatory fees include such items as activity fees, health insurance, and malpractice insurance.

Financial Aid

Information on college-administered aid for baccalaureate-level nursing students includes all types of aid offered, the percentage of undergraduate nursing students receiving financial aid, and application deadlines. Financial aid reported in this guide can include:

Scholarships and Grants: Awards for which the college uses funds under its control and usually chooses the recipient, broken down into *need-based* and *non-need-based* awards.

Loans: Specified as *Federal Direct Loans, Federal Nursing Student Loans, Federal Perkins Loans,* and low-interest *long-term loans* from college funds and external sources.

Federal Work-Study: A federal program that enables students to earn money by working on or off campus in public or private nonprofit organizations.

Federal Pell Grants and FSEOG (Federal Supplemental Educational Opportunity Grants): Federally funded need-based award programs administered through the colleges.

The information in this section is limited to financial aid channeled through the college and does not cover awards to help pay college costs that students might independently obtain from private and public sources.

Baccalaureate Programs—Specific

For each specific baccalaureate program, the following information is supplied:

Applying

In this section under "required," the tests for which the student must have scores submitted to the institution are listed, along with other admission requirements and credentials. Tests may include American College Testing's *ACT*, the College Board's *SAT I, SAT II: Writing Tests,* or *SAT II Subject Tests,* and the *Test of English as a Foreign Language (TOEFL)* for nonnative speakers of English. Other requirements may include a *written essay, a high school transcript, letters of recommendation, an interview,* and a *transcript of college record* for transfer students or those students entering completion programs. Credentials can include, depending upon the school and the specific program, a *minimum GPA* (grade point average) expressed on a scale of 0 to 4.0, a *high school class rank* expressed as a percentage of the top of the class, *three or four years in certain academic subject areas,* an *RN license,* and a *hospital diploma or A.D. in nursing.* Programs may also indicate a specific number of college credits that must be completed before admission into the nursing program. Under "Options," information regarding the availability of advanced placement, accelerated courses, and transfer of credits is provided. Finally, application deadlines and fees are given.

Degree Requirements

This section lists the total number of credit hours required for the degree that is awarded as a result of successful completion of the program. When different tracks or options are available within the program, the lowest and highest number of credit hours required by the program are listed. The specific number of hours, within the total credit hours, that must be in nursing are also listed, along with other degree requirements provided by the school.

Graduate Programs—General

General information provided on master's and doctoral programs includes:

Contact

The name, title, mailing address, telephone number, and, if available, fax number and e-mail address of the person to contact for admission information are given.

Areas of Study

In this section specific areas of study and concentrations that are offered by the school are provided.

For master's-level programs, areas of study can include *clinical nurse specialist* and *nurse practitioner* programs, in each of which the particular area of specialization is indicated. Areas of specialization in *nurse anesthesia, nurse midwifery, nurse administration,* and *nurse education* also are denoted.

For doctoral programs, areas of study include *clinical practice, nursing administration, nursing policy, information systems, nursing education,* and *nursing research.*

Expenses

In this section figures are provided for tuition, mandatory and other fees, and room and board as well as an estimated cost for books and supplies, based on the 1996–97 academic year. Unless indicated otherwise, tuition is for one full academic year. If applicable, distinct tuition figures are given for state residents and nonresidents. Part-time, summer, and evening tuition is expressed in terms of a per-unit rate (per credit, per semester hour, etc.) specified by the institution. The tuition structure at some institutions is very complex, with part-time tuition prorated on a sliding scale according to the number of credit hours taken. In cases where a school has a variable tuition schedule, the minimum and maximum figures are given. Ranges are also given for other expense areas, where applicable. Mandatory fees include such items as activity fees, health insurance, and malpractice insurance.

Financial Aid

Information on college-administered aid for graduate-level nursing students includes all types of aid offered, the percentage of master's-level nursing students receiving financial aid, and application deadlines.

Financial aid for master's-level nursing students may include *graduate assistantships, nurse traineeships, Federal Direct Loans, Federal Nursing Student Loans, institutionally sponsored loans, employment opportunities,* and *institutionally sponsored scholarships and/or grants.*

Financial aid for doctoral-level nursing students may include *graduate assistantships, nurse traineeships, fellowships, dissertation grants, Federal Direct Loans, Federal Nursing Student Loans, institutionally sponsored loans, employment opportunities,* and *institutionally sponsored scholarships and/or grants.*

Graduate Programs—Specific

For specific graduate programs the following information is provided:

Applying

In this section under "required," the tests for which the student must have scores submitted to the institution are listed, along with other admission requirements and credentials. Tests may include the *Graduate Record Examinations (GRE), Miller Analogies Test,* the *Test of English as a Foreign Language (TOEFL)* for nonnative speakers of English, and other specific testing instruments.

For master's programs, other requirements may include, depending upon the school and the specific program, *a bachelor's degree in nursing, a minimum college GPA, an RN license, a specific number of years of clinical experience, professional liability or malpractice insurance, a statistics course, a physical assessment course, a written essay, an interview, letters of recommendation, a vita,* and *a transcript of college record.*

For doctoral programs, other requirements may include *an MSN or equivalent master's degree, a specific number of years of clinical experience, a specific number of years of experience in the proposed area of specialization, a specific number of scholarly papers, a statistics course, an interview, letters of recommendation, a writing sample,* and *a competitive review by a faculty committee.*

Degree Requirements

This section lists the total number of credit hours required for the degree that is awarded as a result of successful completion of the program. When different tracks or options are available within the program, the lowest and highest number of credit hours required by the program are listed. Within the total credit hours, the specific number of hours that must be in nursing are also indicated. If a thesis or a dissertation is required or if there are other specific requirements for the awarding of the degree, these requirements are given.

Postdoctoral Programs

Under the heading "Postdoctoral Program," a description of the programs available is provided along with the name, title, mailing address, telephone, and, if available, fax number and e-mail address of the person to contact regarding the program.

Continuing Education Programs

The appearance of this heading indicates that the nursing school has a program of continuing education. If provided, the name, title, mailing address, telephone number, fax number, and e-mail address of the person to contact regarding the program are given.

NURSING 2000

Counselors of Care in the Modern Health-Care System

Geraldine Bednash, Ph.D., RN, FAAN
Executive Director, American Association of Colleges of Nursing

A Different Era

The nursing profession is alive, ever evolving and reshaping itself. The role of nurses as those who minister exclusively to a patient's basic care needs has changed. Much of the effectiveness and productivity of the future health-care industry will derive from the training and services provided by nurses.

Instead of a reactive position, nurses will take a proactive role in health care by addressing health issues before they develop into problems. They will oversee the continued care of patients who have left the health-care facility. Nurses will be expected to make complex decisions in areas ranging from patient screening to diagnosis and education. They will explore and document the effect of alternative therapies (e.g., guided imagery) and will address public health problems, such as teen pregnancy, at their social and economic sources. They will have to explore and understand new technology and how it relates both to patient care and to their own job performance. They will be asked to work in a variety of settings and will be held accountable for their decisions. The mandate for health-care administrators will be to recruit nurses with broad, well-rounded education and training.

Health-care providers must change the way care is given to the public. Instead of an industry focused on the treatment of illness, the emphasis will be on the promotion of wellness. Nurses will oversee patient treatment and medication and must understand the repercussions of these medical processes for the patient and his or her family.

Cost is the driving force behind this industry-wide transformation. Insurance companies, for the most part, have instigated changes in the way health-care benefits are paid. The old fee-for-service system is no longer the only option. The trend toward managed care, in which a fixed amount of money is allocated for the care of each patient, is changing the way care is provided. A number of legislative proposals, including the possible revamping of Medicare and the implementation of a voucher-based payment system, are currently being debated in the U.S. Congress. The medical community continues to wrestle with the ethics of doctor-controlled or doctor-owned medical services, such as testing laboratories. The outcome of these and other pending proposals during the upcoming year could have a significant impact on the responsibilities of the twenty-first-century nurse. At this time, it seems that employers of the future will recruit nurses who understand the overall structure of the health-care industry, who possess highly developed critical-thinking skills, and who bring to their positions a well-rounded understanding of the risks and benefits of every health-care decision.

Counselors of Care

Job prospects for graduates of nursing programs are positive. Although a majority of graduates receive two-year associate degrees as registered nurses (RNs), hospital administrators are looking for applicants with a four-year baccalaureate degree in nursing.

Health-care administrators realize that patients are becoming more sophisticated about the care they receive, requiring an explanation and understanding of their health needs. Nurses will have to be knowledgeable care providers, working in interdisciplinary relationships with physicians, pharmacists, and public health officials to satisfy these requirements.

Whereas the continuing education of a nurse used to be almost exclusively limited to a hospital setting, this restricted environment has now expanded to include the workplace, clinics, community centers, schools, and the home. Additional training enables graduates of baccalaureate programs to provide improved and more diverse care and ensures stability and security in an industry now noted for its instability.

Promising Opportunities

One of the rewards of baccalaureate education can be a salary competitive with that of other disciplines. Graduates of four-year degree programs can expect salaries starting at approximately $30,000 per year, a figure that might fluctuate depending on geographic area, and more specifically, by the demand in that area. Obviously, the greater the need, the higher the salary.

The baccalaureate degree also serves as a foundation for the pursuit of a master's degree in nursing, which prepares students for the role of advanced practice nurse (APN). Students can earn degrees as a clinical nurse specialist in neonatology, oncology, cardiology, and other specialties or as a nurse practitioner, nurse midwife, or nurse anesthetist. Master's-prepared nurses also can enjoy rewarding careers in nursing administration and education.

These programs generally span one to two years. Graduates can expect starting salaries of approximately $50,000 annually in APN settings, and demand for these graduates is expected to be high over the next fifteen years. In some localities, for example, the nurse practitioner may be the sole provider of health care to a family.

Overall Transformation

The nursing field must be transformed to be compatible with the overall changes in the health-care industry. The latest statistics put the average age of nurses at 43, with only 11 percent of nurses under the age of 30. It is projected that over the next ten years, much of the nursing population will be retiring. Employment figures for RNs will be about 2.2 million—a 23 percent increase over 1990 figures.

The traditional career path of nurses is expected to change. More nurses will enter master's programs directly from baccalaureate programs, sidestepping a traditional period of practice in a clinical or hospital setting. More master's degree graduates will pursue doctoral degrees at a younger age. Since nurses will play a critical role in providing health care, a four-year baccalaureate degree is a crucial first step in preparing nurses to assume increased patient responsibility within the health-care system.

THE NURSING SCHOOL ADVISER: Baccalaureate Programs

Linda K. Amos, Ed.D., FAAN
Dean, College of Nursing
University of Utah

The only constant in today's health-care industry is change. Almost every facet of health care is being analyzed: Are certain procedures necessary? Do they work? Who will provide them? Where and for how long? Everyone agrees, however, that nurses will play a vital role in the application and quality of health care in the future.

The scope of nursing will grow immensely as nurses by and large become the front-line providers of health care. They will be diagnosing health problems and offering solutions. They will be dealing with the effects of the patient's recovery. They will be responsible for coordinating and continuing the care outside the health facility. They will play a big role in educating the public and addressing the social and economic causes of health issues.

Worldwide Standards

The nursing student of the future will be given much more information and, thus, knowledge of the technology used to manage that information will be essential to tracking and assessing care. In this area, nurses will be able to provide care over great distances. In some cases it might not be inconceivable to provide care over the phone to patients 2,000 miles away. Use of the Internet and other computer-oriented systems will become an integral part of most nursing positions. Nurses of the future, therefore, will have to become aware of worldwide standards of care. Yet despite this growth of technology, the essential function of the nurse's role will remain that of making sure that the right person is providing the right care for the patient at the right cost.

This will be accomplished as the industry turns away from the hospital as the center of the operation. Nurses will work in a broad array of locations, such as clinics, outpatient facilities, community centers, schools, and even places of business. In the very near future, hospitals will be places only for the very sick, and the name itself may be changed to acute-care centers.

Much of the emphasis in health care will be shifted toward preventive care and the promotion of health. The nurse will be asked to take on a broader and more diverse role in this system.

Unlimited Opportunities, Expanded Responsibilities

First and foremost, the four-year programs in today's nursing colleges provide the training ground not only for entry-level professional practice, but they serve as the platform on which to build a career through graduate-level study for roles as advanced practice nurses, such as nurse practitioners, nurse midwives, clinical specialists, and nurse administrators and educators. Nurses at this level can be expected to specialize in oncology, pediatrics, neonatology, obstetrics and gynecology, critical care, infection control, psychiatry, women's health, and neuroscience. The potential at this level is great, but so are the responsibilities. In some urban and rural settings, families may use the nurse practitioner for all their health-care needs. In all but two states, the nurse practitioner can prescribe medication.

The health-care system will demand more from nurses. Their education will have to transcend the traditional areas, such as chemistry and anatomy, to enable them to gain a deeper understanding of health promotion, disease prevention, screening, and immunization. Nurses will have to understand how medical problems may have a social cause, such as poverty, as well as have insight into human psychology, behavior, cultural mores, and values.

The transformation of the health-care system offers unlimited opportunities for nurses at the baccalaureate and graduate levels as care in urban and rural settings becomes more accessible. This change accounts for the estimates that, by the year 2000, hospitals and outpatient clinics will be hiring 40 to 45 percent more nurses, according to the president of the National Association for Healthcare Recruitment. The U.S. Department of Labor estimates that nearly 2.5 million nurses will be employed by the turn of the century, nearly a 40 percent increase over 1990. It is an exciting era in nursing; one that holds exceptional promise for nurses with a baccalaureate nursing degree.

The compensation for nurses is quite favorable compared to other industries. Entry-level nurses with baccalaureate degrees in nursing can expect a salary range from about $23,000 to $32,000 per year, depending on geographic location and experience. Five years into their careers, the national average for nurses with four-year degrees is $38,000 per year, but some earn close to $45,000.

Applying to College

Meeting the school's general entrance requirements is the first step toward a university or college degree in nursing. Admission requirements may vary, but a high school diploma or equivalent is necessary. Most accredited colleges consider SAT I scores along with high school grade point average. A strong preparatory class load in science and mathematics is generally preferred among nursing schools. Specific admission information can be obtained by writing to the schools' nursing departments.

To apply to a nursing school, contact the admission office of the colleges or universities you are interested in and request the appropriate application forms. With limited spaces in nursing schools, programs are more competitive, so an early submission of the application is recommended.

Focusing Your Education

Academic performance, however, is not the sole basis of acceptance into the upper level of the nursing program. Admission officers also weigh such factors as student activities, employment, and references. Moreover, many require an interview and/or an essay in which the nursing candidate offers a "goal statement." This part of the admission process can be completed prior to a student's entrance into the college or university or prior to the student's entering the school of nursing itself, depending on the program.

In this interview or essay, students may list career preferences and reasons for their choices. This allows admission officers to assess the goals of students and gain insights into their values, integrity, and honesty. One would expect that a goal statement from a student who is just entering college would be more general than that of a student who has had two years of preprofessional nursing studies. The more experienced student would be likely to have a more focused idea of what is to be gained by an education in nursing; there would be more evidence of the student's values and the ways in which she or he relates them to the knowledge gained from preprofessional nursing classes.

Baccalaureate Curriculum

A traditional or generic baccalaureate program in nursing is a four-year college or university education that incorporates a variety of liberal arts courses with professional education and training. It is designed for high school graduates with no previous nursing experience.

Currently, there are 600 baccalaureate programs in the United States. Of the 514 programs that responded to a recent survey conducted by the American Association of Colleges of Nursing, there were approximately 124,000 students enrolled in the 1996–97 academic year.

The baccalaureate curriculum is designed to prepare students for work within the growing, changing health-care environment. With nurses taking more of an active role in all facets of health care, they are expected to develop critical thinking and communication skills in addition to receiving standard nurse training in clinics and hospitals. In a university or college setting, the first two years include classes in the humanities, social sciences, business, psychology, technology, sociology, ethics, and nutrition.

In some programs, the nursing classes start in the sophomore year, whereas others have students wait until they are juniors. Many schools require satisfactory grade point averages before students advance into professional nursing classes. On a 4.0 scale, admission into the last two years of the nursing program may require a minimum GPA of 2.5 to 3.0 in preprofessional nursing classes. The national average is about 2.8, but the cutoff level varies with each program.

In the junior and senior years, the curriculum focuses on the nursing sciences, and emphasis moves from the classroom to the health facility. This is where students are exposed to clinical skills, nursing theory, and the varied roles nurses play in the health-care system. Courses include nurse leadership, health promotion, family planning, mental health, environmental and occupational health, adult and pediatric care, medical and surgical care, psychiatric care, community health, and management.

This level of the education comes in a variety of settings: community hospitals, clinics, social service agencies, schools, and health maintenance organizations. Training in diverse settings is the best preparation for becoming a vital player in the growing health-care field.

Reentry Programs

Practicing nurses returning to school to complete the baccalaureate will have to meet requirements that may include possession of a valid RN or LPN license and an A.D. or hospital diploma from an accredited institution. Again, it's best to check with the school's admissions department to see what the criteria are.

Nurses returning to school will have to consider the rapid rate of change in health care and science in general. A nurse who passed an undergraduate-level chemistry class ten years ago would probably not receive credit for that class today, due to the growth of knowledge in that and all other scientific fields. The need to reeducate applies not only to practicing nurses returning to school but to all nurses throughout their careers.

In the same vein, nurses with diplomas from hospital programs who want to work toward a baccalaureate degree would find themselves in need of meeting the common requirement for more clinical practice as well as developing a deeper understanding of community-based nursing practices, such as health prevention and promotion.

There are colleges and universities available to the RN in search of a baccalaureate that give credit for previous nurse training. These programs are designed to accommodate the needs and career goals of the practicing nurse by providing flexible course schedules and credit for previous experience and education. Some programs lead to a master's-level degree, a process that can take up to three years. Licensed practical nurses (LPNs) can also continue their education through baccalaureate programs.

Nurses thinking of reentering school may also consider other specialized programs. For example, there are programs aimed at enabling a nurse with an ADN or an LPN/LVN degree to earn a B.S.N. Also, accelerated B.S.N. programs are available, as are accelerated B.S.N. programs for nurses with degrees in other fields. (Some of these programs can be found in the Program Index on page 591.)

Choosing a Program

With approximately 600 baccalaureate programs in the United States, some research will reveal which programs match your needs and career objectives.

If you have no health-care experience, it might be best to gain some insight into the field by volunteering or working part-time in a care facility, such as a hospital or outpatient clinic. Talking to nurse professionals about their work will also lend insight into how your best attributes may apply in the nursing field.

When considering a nursing education, consider your personal needs: Is it best for you to work in a heavily structured environment or one that offers more flexibility in terms of, say, integrating a part-time work schedule into studies? Do you need to stay close to home? Do you prefer to work in a large health-care system, such as a health maintenance organization, or do you prefer smaller, community-based operations?

As for nursing programs, it's best to ask the following: How involved is the faculty in developing students for today's health-care industry? In light of the industry's move away from hospitals, how strong is the school's affiliation with clinics? Is there any assurance a student will gain an up-to-date educational experience for the current job market? Are a variety of care settings available? How much time in clinics will be needed for graduation? What are the program's resources in terms of computer and science laboratories? How available is the faculty to oversee a student's curriculum? What kind of student support is available in terms of study groups and audiovisual aids? Moreover, what kind of counseling from faculty members and administrators is available to help students develop well-rounded, effective progress through the program?

Visiting a school and talking to the program's guidance counselors will give you a better understanding of how a particular program or school will fit your needs. You can get a closer look at the faculty, its members' credentials, and the focus of the program. It's also not too early to consider what each program can offer in terms of job placement.

Accreditation

Accreditation is very important, and it should be considered on two levels—the accreditation of the university or college and the accreditation of the nursing program. Accreditation is a voluntary process in which the school or the program asks for an external review of its programs, facilities, and faculty. For nursing programs, the review is performed by peers in nursing education to assure a comparable level of quality with other schools.

Nursing programs have two types of accreditation. The first is administered by a nationally recognized nursing accreditation organization that is approved by the U.S. Department of Education (DOE). The other is the state board accreditation, which ensures that the program matches the state's requirements.

Though accreditation is a voluntary process, most graduate schools will only accept students who have earned degrees from accredited schools. Canadian nursing school programs are accredited by the Canadian Association of University Schools of Nursing. Canadian programs listed must be accredited by the Canadian Association of University Schools of Nursing.

Master's Programs

Jane S. Norbeck, D.N.Sc., RN, FAAN
Dean and Professor
School of Nursing
University of California, San Francisco

The transformation of the health-care system is taking place as you read this, and it can be seen even today in the most common areas.

- A mother brings her child into a clinic for treatment of an earache. Instead of a physician, a nurse practitioner provides the care.
- A patient is readied for surgery. A variety of specialists move about the surgery room, but it's not a specially trained physician administering the anesthetic—it's a certified nurse anesthetist.
- During the recovery from an acute illness, it's decided that the patient no longer needs to stay in the hospital but isn't well enough to return home. It's decided that the best place to continue the recovery is an intermediate care facility. Who makes that decision? A clinical nurse specialist. Who oversees the physical and emotional rehabilitation programs at this facility? Another clinical nurse specialist.

These health-care professionals are all advanced practice nurses (APNs). All have graduate-level degrees, and they serve as proof why, by the year 2000, the demand for nurses with master's and doctoral degrees for advanced practice, clinical specialties, teaching, and research is expected to be double the supply. The federal Health Resources and Services Administration predicted in 1992 that by the turn of the millennium, an estimated 185,000 full-time registered nurses (RNs) with master's and doctoral degrees will be in the workforce, less than half the anticipated demand of 392,000.

The shift to a primary care system will force the health-care industry to maintain quality in a cost-efficient manner. A congressional study done by the Office of Technology Assessment in December 1986 estimated that nurse practitioners can deliver as much as 80 percent of the health services and up to 90 percent of the pediatric care that is provided by primary-care physicians.

Another study estimated the U.S. could save as much as $8.75 billion annually if APNs were used appropriately in the place of physicians. As more and more of the restrictions on APNs succumb to legislative or economic forces, the demand for graduate-level nurses is expected to remain high.

Educational Core for APN

A master's degree in nursing is the educational core that allows advanced practice nurses to work as nurse practitioners, certified nurse midwives, certified clinical nurse specialists, and certified nurse anesthetists.

Nurse practitioners conduct physical exams, diagnose and treat common acute illnesses and injuries, administer immunizations, manage chronic problems such as high blood pressure and diabetes, and order lab services and X rays.

Nurse midwives provide prenatal and gynecological care, deliver babies in hospitals and private settings such as homes, and follow up with postpartum care.

Clinical nurse specialists provide a range of care in specialty areas, such as oncology, pediatrics, and cardiac, neonatal, obstetric/gynecological, neurological, and psychiatric nursing.

Nurse anesthetists administer anesthesia for all types of surgery in operating rooms, dental offices, and outpatient surgical centers.

Master's degrees in nursing administration or nursing education are also available.

There are more than 330 master's degree programs accredited by the National League for Nursing (NLN). The wide spectrum of programs includes the Master of Science in Nursing (M.S.N.) degree, Master of Nursing (M.N.) degree, Master of Science degree with a major in nursing (M.S.), or Master of Arts degree with a nursing major (M.A.). The specific degrees depend on the requirements set by the college or university or by the faculty of the nursing program. There are accelerated programs for RNs, which allow the nurse with a hospital diploma or associate degree to earn both a baccalaureate and master's degree in a condensed program. Some schools offer accelerated master's degree programs for nurses with non-nursing degrees and for non-nursing college graduates. There are joint-degree programs, such as a master's in nursing combined with a Master of Business Administration, Master of Public Health, or Master of Hospital Administration.

Master's Curriculum

The master's degree builds on the baccalaureate degree to enable the student to develop expertise in one area. That specialty can range from running a hospital to providing care for prematurely born babies, from researching the effectiveness of alternative therapies to tackling social and economic causes of health problems. It is an opportunity for the student who has assessed personal career goals and matched them to individual, community, and industry needs. What students can do with their APN degrees is limited only by their imagination.

Full-time master's programs consist of eighteen to twenty-four months of uninterrupted study. Many graduate school students, however, fit their master's-level studies around their work schedule, which can extend the time it takes to graduate.

Master's-level study incorporates theories and concepts of nursing science and their applications, along with the management of health care. Research is used to provide a foundation for the improvement of health-care techniques. Students also have the opportunity to develop the knowledge, leadership skills, and interpersonal skills that will enable them to improve the health-care system.

Classroom and clinical work are involved throughout the master's program. In class, students spend less time listening to lectures and taking notes and more time participating in student- and faculty-led seminars and roundtable discussions. Extended clinical work is generally required.

Graduate-level education in many programs includes courses in statistics, research management, health economics, health policy, health-care ethics, health promotion, nutrition, family planning, mental health, and the prevention of family and social violence. When students begin to concentrate their study in their clinical areas, any number of courses that support their chosen speciality may be included. For example, a nurse wanting to specialize in pediatrics may take courses in child development.

A clinical nurse specialist can focus on acute care, geriatrics, adult health, community health, critical care, gerontology, rehabilitation, and cardiovascular, surgical, oncological, maternity/newborn, pediatric, mental/psychiatric, and women's health nursing. Areas of specialization in nurse practitioner programs include acute care, adult health, child care, community health, emergency care, neonatal health, and primary care.

Admission Requirements

The admission requirements for master's programs in nursing vary a great deal. Generally, a bachelor's degree from a school accredited by the National League for Nursing and a state RN license are required. Scores from the Graduate Record Examinations (GRE) or the Miller Analogies Test (MAT), college transcripts, letters of reference, and an essay are typically required. Non-nurses and nurses with non-nursing degrees have special requirements. The profiles and the two-page descriptions of colleges and universities in this publication will give you an idea of each school's specific requirements.

Proof of some clinical work is typically required for admission into a master's program. However, with the average age of master's program students at 33, many college and university deans are considering waiving this requirement.

It is important to remember that admission officers look at a student's transcripts, clinical work, and letters of reference together. A low grade point average is not an automatic knockout—admissions officers are after a composite package. Also, some specialties require specific courses. Students in the nurse anesthetist program, for instance, must have an upper-level college course in biochemistry. Contact the schools for their specific requirements.

A Master's That's Best for You

Most nurses who think of entering a master's program already have been practicing nursing. They have a good idea what they want to specialize in before they apply for admission. It is crucial to know what you want to study before you enter a master's program.

The best way to ensure success in a master's program is for you to understand your individual strengths and career desires and then find the faculty and college setting that are best suited to help you develop those strengths. Students must make an effort to educate themselves as to the strength of the faculty in each college's master's program. That's the best thing to look for: a strong faculty in one specialty.

This can be tricky. One university's master's program may be rated reasonably high in all fields. Another program might not be rated as high overall, but its cardiovascular program, for example, may be one of the best due to its access to facilities or the fact that its faculty is in the process of developing an innovative new treatment.

This type of information is not hard for the master's candidate to discover; it just takes time. Such information is available from each school's admissions office, which should be more than happy to promote its nursing faculty and support its opinion with proof, such as the research papers that faculty members have published in journals or the number of degrees each faculty member carries.

This type of research is the best way to find a program that meets your needs. The profiles of master's nursing programs in this book should help. If you can, narrow the list to three or four graduate schools and then write each school's admissions department for catalogs and other information. Visit the schools if you can and take time to talk to a guidance counselor from the nursing program.

Other key questions to consider when applying for a master's program are: Does the school offer financial aid, such as loans, scholarships, fellowships, or teaching posts? How much clinical work is needed? Does the clinical work meet your needs, and does the type of clinical work involved match what you understand the health-care system will be using when you graduate?

Is the course work flexible? Can you work part-time and still progress toward a master's degree? This is important to know. A majority of master's program students continue to work while they pursue the degree.

Therefore, master's degree programs may present a flexible offering of short courses to meet the student's schedule demands.

Some programs require a thesis, whereas others provide another type of culminating experience.

The Master's Trends

Today's master's programs have increased the amount of clinical practice that students engage in so that graduates enter the job market ready for certification. There is also a greater emphasis on applying new research findings to methods of patient care. This might involve students' reading literature about new treatments and then incorporating the appropriate changes.

All master's program candidates should consider courses in cost-benefit analysis. As managed-care systems become predominant in the industry, health-care workers will be asked to justify the expense of their treatment as well as its effectiveness. This leads to the crucial issue of quality. There will always be a strong effort to minimize costs in every health-care procedure, but that cannot compromise the quality of care. It's safe to say that discharging a newborn too soon from a hospital due to shortsightedness can be quite costly.

Depending on the specialty, master's candidates entering the job market may be expected to oversee auxiliary care providers, such as nurses aides or other unlicensed employees. They may work in a team structure, and, in this capacity, the nurse specialist may be expected to manage, motivate, and steer the group. This requires team-building as well as other management techniques.

While everyone in the health-care facility will have a part in ensuring patient satisfaction, nurses, particularly advanced practice nurses, will shoulder a great deal of this load. Developing interpersonal and communication skills, as well as having an understanding of human behavior, will make it easier for the advanced practice nurse to help patients to understand modern health-care procedures, which no doubt will improve their feelings of satisfaction.

Finally, nurses at all levels should be aware of the need for flexibility. Many health-care organizations are reducing the number of beds in hospitals, transferring the care of a growing number of patients to other facilities. In light of this trend, it's best for the master's program student to gain experience in a variety of places, such as homes, clinics, and community-based settings.

The demand for quality care will continue to grow. Medical innovations and technological advances will continue. The quality and effectiveness of health care will continue to improve, and nurses with graduate degrees will play an active role in this trend.

The Hot Employment Spots

The health-care industry has undergone such radical transformation in the last five years that administrators feel they cannot predict whether any one geographic region will have more hirings than another. Generally, nurses with master's degrees will be in demand in all regions of the country, in both the U.S. and Canada.

Industry trends indicate that more and more nurses will work outside the hospital in outpatient clinics, community settings, and even businesses. As patients spend less and less time in hospitals, there is a need for nurse specialists to oversee home-care settings and ensure that the quality of care there is high. In this vein, some nurses are taking the initiative and running their own businesses as health-care providers, offering services as they see fit in whatever locations are appropriate.

Immediate Rewards

Advanced practice nurses right out of school can expect annual salaries ranging from $45,000 to $75,000, depending on geographic location and previous experience. However, some rural county health clinics start their nurse practitioners at salaries as low as $32,000 per year.

Certified nurse anesthetists and certified nurse midwives, however, draw larger salaries. Nurse midwives, for example, can draw first-year salaries as high as $80,000 per year. Areas such as the Northeast and the West Coast tend to have nurses in these fields at the higher end of the salary scale. After five years of practice, the salary range for APNs stretches from $50,000 to $100,000 a year. Again, it depends on location. After five years, nurse midwives earn salaries ranging from $65,000 to $120,000 annually.

Salaries for APNs in the year 2005 are not expected to be noticeably higher than they are now. The sizable annual increases, as much as 7 percent per year during the 1980s, have diminished. Projections for first-year salaries in the year 2005 will carry increases tied to normal cost-of-living increases.

Nurse Practitioners: The In-Demand Primary Care Providers

Ted Johnson

Many health-care administrators see a troubling gap developing between the type of care the public will need in the future and who is going to be able to provide that care. The demand will be for primary care that focuses on internal medicine and general or family practice, and it is going to far outweigh the number of physicians who will be providing it.

These administrators realize that relying solely on physicians to deliver this primary care only delays the availability of high-quality care for the public. That is why there is a growing demand for the nurse practitioner (NP) to provide more primary and preventive care.

Front-Line Providers

Nurse practitioners, trained in master's-level advanced practice nursing programs, provide basic health care for infants, children, and adults in community health centers, health maintenance organizations (HMOs), schools, businesses, and homes as well as hospitals. Many practitioners work in clinical specialties, such as pediatrics, family health, women's health, occupational health, and gerontological care.

Nurse practitioners perform physical exams, diagnose and treat common acute illnesses and injuries, immunize, manage chronic problems such as high blood pressure and diabetes, and order and interpret X rays and other lab tests. They also educate patients on healthy lifestyles and health-care options.

The Growing Demand

The demand for nurse practitioners will be great at least until the year 2020. In 1992, there were approximately 30,000 nurses certified as nurse practitioners by national and state certifying organizations. The federal Health Resources and Services Administration predicts that by the year 2000 the demand for nurses trained at the master's and doctoral levels will be just under 400,000, more than twice the projected number of 185,000 anticipated in the workforce. Of those 400,000 jobs, many will be in the nurse practitioner role. Certified nurse midwives, clinical nurse specialists, and certified nurse anesthetists will also be in great demand.

Part of the demand stems from the desire of many physicians to enter specialized practice. Well over 60 percent of the nation's 545,000 active physicians now specialize. The U.S. Bureau of Health Professions last reported to Congress in September 1992 that by the year 2000 the nation will have a surplus of nearly 50,000 physicians, and about 70 percent of all active physicians are expected to be specialists. Some areas report a greater demand for advanced practice nurses than others.

The number of medical school graduates entering residencies in primary care fields from 1986 to 1992 fell by 19 percent. About two thirds of the recent residents in internal medicine entered subspecialties. About 85 percent of medical students said they planned on going into subspecialties. However, studies have shown that when it comes to primary care, the nurse practitioner can be just as effective as a physician.

Better Care, Cheaper

A 1992 American Nursing Association study reported that NPs provided more health promotion activities, such as patient education and exercise prescriptions, scored higher on diagnostic accuracy, and ordered less expensive laboratory tests than physicians. Patients of NPs were more satisfied and demonstrated greater compliance with treatment regimens than patients of physicians. Yet, the education of a nurse practitioner costs at least four to five times less than that of a physician and can be completed at least four years sooner.

This cost-effective method of providing health care is expected to gain popularity in the coming years. Nurse practitioners across the U.S., however, do not assume the same level of responsibility from state to state, with some states being more restrictive than others. Of the forty-eight states that grant nurse practitioners the authority to prescribe medications, only eleven allow them to do it independently of physician supervision. Ten additional states are considering legislation to allow this practice. In twenty states, APNs can practice independently of physician supervision or collaboration.

There is an effort within the nursing profession to create a national standardized certification process for APNs. The American Association of Colleges of Nursing has called for uniform certification to be established by the year 2000 to assure the public of the skill and competency of the advanced practice nurse. Standardized certification, states AACN, must include completion of a graduate degree in nursing as its central requirement.

Ted Johnson is a freelance writer based in Danville, California.

The Nurse Ph.D.: A Vital Profession Needs Leaders

Carole A. Anderson Ph.D., RN, FAAN
Dean and Professor
College of Nursing
Ohio State University

There is no doubt that education is the path for a nurse to achieve clinical expertise and experience. The nursing profession, however, needs more nurses educated at the doctoral level.

It's an undereducated academic work force on two fronts: only about half of the staff on university and college nursing faculties have doctorates. At the same time, there isn't enough research done by doctorally trained nurses.

The lack of nurses prepared at the doctoral level is something the nursing profession needs to address. Compared to other professionals, nurses have more interruptions in their careers. Most members of the profession are females who both work as nurses and fulfill responsibilities as working wives and mothers. Many pursue their education on a part-time basis, juggling the requirements of working, raising a family, and going to school.

The average age of the nursing population is 44.3, with only 11 percent of practicing nurses under the age of 30. Moreover, it's predicted that in the next ten years, much of the nursing population will be retiring.

The greatest job demand for nurses in the next ten years will be for those educated at the master's and doctoral levels, with projections listing the demand as twice as great as the supply. But a majority of nurses are in their 40s by the time they earn their graduate degrees, which leaves less time for them to use their advanced knowledge and experience in their work.

To reverse this trend, nursing faculty are considering waiving the desired clinical experience between the baccalaureate and master's levels. Furthermore, faculties are encouraging more students to carry their education through to the doctoral level, where the options for employment are even greater.

Health-Care Research

When nurses do research for their doctorates, many people tend to think that it focuses primarily on nurses and nursing care. In reality, nurses carry out clinical research in a variety of areas, such as diabetes care, cancer care, and eating disorders.

In the last twenty years advances in medicine have involved advancing treatment, not cures, for the most part. In other words, no cure for the illness has been discovered, but treatment for that illness has improved. However, sometimes the treatment itself causes problems for patients, such as the unwelcome side effects of chemotherapy. Nurses have opportunities to devise solutions to problems like these through research, such as studies on how to manage the illness and its treatment.

The Curricula

Doctoral programs in nursing are aimed at preparing students for careers in health administration, education, clinical research, and advanced clinical practice. Geared around research and creative scholarship, doctoral programs prepare nurses to be leaders and experts within the profession. Through course work, research, and dissertation preparation, students are trained as researchers and scholars to tackle complex health-care questions. Program emphasis may vary, from a focus on health education to a concentration on policy research. The majority of doctoral programs confer the Ph.D. (Doctor of Philosophy) degree, but some award the D.N.Sc. (Doctor of Nursing Science), the D.S.N. (Doctor of Science in Nursing), the N.D. (Doctor of Nursing), the Ed.D. (Doctor of Education), and the D.N.S. (Doctor of Nursing Science).

Doctoral nursing programs traditionally offer courses on the history and philosophy of nursing and the development and testing of nursing and other health-care techniques, as well as the social, economic, political, and ethical issues important to the field. Data management and research methodology are also areas of instruction. Students are expected to work individually on research projects and complete a dissertation.

Doctoral programs allow study on a full- and part-time basis. For graduate students who are employed and therefore seek flexibility in their schedules, many courses are offered on weekends and in the evenings.

Admission Requirements

Admission requirements for doctoral programs vary. Generally a master's degree is necessary, but in some schools a master's degree is completed in conjunction with fulfillment of the doctoral requirements. Standard requirements include an RN license and some clinical experience (usually a year). Graduate Record Examinations (GRE) scores, college transcripts, letters of recommendation, and an essay are frequently required. Students applying for doctoral-level study should have a solid foundation in nursing practice and an interest in research. Programs are usually the equivalent of three years of full-time study.

Selecting a Doctoral Program

Aside from consideration of the type of research and programs available, selecting a doctoral program comes down to personal choice. You'll work closely with professors, and thus the support and mentoring you receive while pursuing your research is as vital as the quality of the facilities. The most important question is whether there is a "match" between your research interest and faculty research. Many of the same questions you'd ask about baccalaureate and master's degree programs apply to doctoral programs. However, in a doctoral program, the contact with professors, the use of research equipment and facilities, and the department's flexibility in allowing you to choose your course of study are critical.

Other questions to consider include: Does the university consider research a priority and have proper funding for it? Is student research assisted through the availability of teaching posts? Are there opportunities to present findings in publications and journals? Is scholarship of faculty, alumni, and students presented at regional and national nursing meetings and subsequently published? Has the body of research done at a university enhanced the knowledge of nursing and health care?

Career Options

Many nurses with doctoral degrees make the natural transition into teaching, but there are many other career options available at this level. Nurses prepared at the doctoral level are often hired by private and public firms as consultants to assess care situations and offer solutions. They are hired by large hospital chains to manage various divisions, and nurses with doctoral degrees manage complex health-care systems. On another front, they research and formulate national and international health-care policy. In short, because of the high level of education, there are more options.

Nurses with higher degrees traditionally have gone into teaching or administration. Professors' salaries vary, ranging from $45,000 to $70,000, depending on location, educational background, and experience. In private industry, nurse executives, many of whom hold doctoral degrees, earn an average of $91,800 annually, according to the American Organization of Nurse Executives. Toward the higher end of the pay scale, the successful for-profit providers of health care often reward their top executives lucratively in base salary and bonuses. The more efficient the care, the more profitable the firm and the higher the pay for executives. A salary of $150,000 plus bonuses is not out of the question for top-level executives.

American Association of Colleges of Nursing's

Indicators of Quality in Doctoral Programs in Nursing

The following indicators apply to the Doctor of Philosophy degree in nursing (Ph.D.), the Doctor of Nursing Science (D.N.S.), and the Doctor of Education in nursing (Ed.D.).

Faculty

1. A diversity of intellectual perspectives is valued and represented by the faculty.
2. Faculty meet the requirements of the parent institution for graduate education, and a substantial proportion of faculty hold earned doctorates in nursing.
3. Faculty conceptualize and implement productive programs of research and scholarship that attract and engage students.
4. Faculty create an environment in which mentoring, socialization of students, and the existence of a community of scholars is evident.
5. Faculty assist students to understand the value of programs of research and scholarship that continue over time and build upon previous work.
6. Faculty identify, generate, and utilize resources within the university and broader community to support program goals.

Programs of Study

1. The emphasis of the program of study is determined by the faculty's areas of expertise and scholarship. Common elements of the program of study include:
   A. History and philosophy of science and their relation to the development of nursing knowledge.
   B. Existing and evolving substantive nursing knowledge.
   C. Methods and processes of theory/knowledge development.
   D. Analytical and leadership strategies for dealing with social, ethical, cultural, economic, and political issues related to nursing, health care, and research.
   E. Research methods and techniques of data analysis.
   F. Progressive, guided, and independent student research experiences.
2. The distribution between nursing and cognate content is consistent with the mission and goals of the program and the student's area of focus.
3. Core content is identifiable. It can be provided through a variety of formal and informal teaching/learning and research activities.
4. Opportunities are provided for role development that complement students' previous experiences and career goals.
5. Requirements and their sequence for progression in the program are clear and available to students in writing.

Resources

1. Sufficient human, financial, and institutional resources are available to accomplish the goals of the unit for research, teaching, and service.
2. Technical and support services are available and accessible to faculty, students, and staff for state of the science information acquisition, communication, and management. This includes computer technology, telecommunication technology, support personnel, and resources for maintenance.
3. Library and data base resources are sufficient to support the scholarly endeavors of faculty and students.
4. Space and equipment are sufficient, including appropriate computer and laboratory facilities, offices, seminar rooms, and study and social areas for doctoral students.
5. Adequate university and clinical resources are available and accessible to faculty and students to support program goals.
6. The interests of the program are represented by faculty and students at the institutional level, and resources for research and student support are equitably allocated within the institution.

Students

1. Students are selected from a pool of highly qualified and motivated applicants who represent diverse populations.
2. Admission criteria are based on standards consistent with those of the institution and provide an

opportunity to consider exceptional students. These criteria should be sufficiently rigorous to admit students who will excel.

3. Students' goals and objectives are congruent with faculty expertise and institutional resources.
4. Students are successful in obtaining financial support through intramural and extramural academic and research awards.
5. Students actively prepare to assume leadership roles after they graduate.
6. Students commit a significant portion of their time to the program and complete the program in a timely fashion.
7. Students establish a pattern of productive scholarship, collaborating with faculty and peers in scientific endeavors that result in the presentation and publication of scholarly work that continues after graduation.

Research

1. Research is an explicit component of the mission of the parent institution and the nursing unit.
2. The university and the nursing unit value, support, and reward faculty and student research and scholarship.
3. Programs of research that are developed over time and build upon previous work exist and are congruent with research priorities within nursing and its constituent communities.
4. A variety of mechanisms, e.g., peer review, mentoring, and consultation, exist that foster high-quality research.
5. Sufficient research exists to support the goals of the program.

Evaluation

The evaluation plan:

1. Is systematic, ongoing, comprehensive, and focuses on the university's and program's specific mission and goals.
2. Includes both process and outcome data related to the indicators of quality in doctoral programs.
3. Adheres to established ethical and process standards for formal program evaluation, e.g., confidentiality and rigorous quantitative and qualitative analyses.
4. Includes data from a variety of internal and external constituencies, e.g., students, graduates, program faculty, employers of graduates, peer groups within nursing, and external funding bodies.
5. Provides for comparison of program processes and outcomes to the standards of its parent graduate school/university and selected peer groups within nursing.
6. Includes ongoing feedback to program faculty and administrators to promote program improvement.
7. Provides comprehensive data in order to determine patterns and trends and recommend future directions at regular intervals.
8. Is supported with adequate human, financial, and institutional resources.

Approved by AACN Membership October 25, 1993

RNs Returning to School: Choosing a Nursing Program

Marilyn Oermann, Ph.D., RN, FAAN
Professor
College of Nursing
Wayne State University

If you are thinking of returning to school to complete your baccalaureate degree or to pursue a graduate degree in nursing, you are not alone. Registered nurses (RNs) are returning to school in record numbers, many seeking advancement or transition to new roles in nursing. There are expanded opportunities for nurses with baccalaureate degrees in nursing. Over the last two decades, the number of RNs prepared initially in diploma and A.D. nursing programs who have graduated from baccalaureate nursing degree programs has more than doubled, according to the American Association of Colleges of Nursing. Although the decision to return to school means considerable investment of time, financial resources, and effort, the benefits can be overwhelmingly positive.

Higher education in nursing opens doors to many opportunities for career growth not otherwise available. By continuing your education, you can:

- update your knowledge and skills, critical today in light of rapid advances in health care and the movement of care toward the community
- move more easily into a new role within your organization or in other health-care settings
- pursue a different career path within nursing

Moreover, returning to school brings personal fulfillment and satisfaction gained through learning more about nursing and the changing health-care system and using that knowledge in the delivery and management of patient care.

More Skills and Flexibility Needed

If you are contemplating returning to school, here are some facts to consider. The health-care system is undergoing dramatic changes. These changes include the movement of care toward the community; a greater role for nurses in primary care, health promotion, and health education; and the need for nurses to care for patients and families in multiple settings, such as schools, workplaces, homes, clinics, and outpatient facilities, as well as hospitals. More and more nurses will be needed to deliver care to patients and families in their homes and within community settings. Moreover, as hospitals continue to become centers for acute and critical care, the nurse's role in patient care and management of other health-care providers has become more complex, requiring advanced knowledge and skills.

Because of the complexity of today's health-care environment, the American Association of Colleges of Nursing and other leading nursing organizations have called for the baccalaureate degree as the minimum educational requirement for professional nursing practice. In fact, nurse executives in hospitals have indicated their desire for the majority of nurses on staff to be prepared at least at the baccalaureate level to handle the increasingly complex demands of patient care and management of health-care delivery. The baccalaureate nursing degree is essential for nurses who must function in different management roles, move across employment settings, and have the flexibility to change positions within nursing. It is also the best way to advance one's career. Baccalaureate nursing degree programs prepare the nurse for a broader role within the health-care system and for practice in community settings, home health care, neighborhood clinics, and other outpatient settings. Continuing education provides the means for nurses to prepare themselves for a future role in nursing.

Despite increased numbers of graduates of baccalaureate and graduate nursing programs, the demand for nurses with baccalaureate and more advanced degrees will continue to grow. The U.S. Department of Health and Human Services predicts that by the year 2000 there will be an excess of nurses prepared at the associate-degree level, a mounting shortage of baccalaureate-prepared nurses, and only half as many nurses prepared at master's and doctoral levels as needed. Nurses with baccalaureate nursing degrees will be needed in all areas of health care, and the demand for nurses with master's and doctoral preparation for advanced practice, management, teaching, and research will continue.

Identifying Strategies

The decision to return to school marks the beginning of a new phase in your career development. It is essential for you to plan this future carefully. Why are you thinking about going to school, and what do you want to accomplish by doing so? Understanding why you want to go back will help you select the best program for you. Knowing what you want to accomplish will help you to focus on your goals and overcome the obstacles that could prevent you from achieving your full potential.

Even if you decide that additional education will help you reach your professional goals, you may also have a list of reasons why you think you cannot return to school—no time, limited financial resources, fear of failure, and concerns about meeting family responsibilities, among others. If you are concerned about the demands of school combined with existing responsibilities, begin by identifying strategies for incorporating classes and study time into your present schedule. Remember, you can start your program with one course and reevaluate your time at the end of the term.

Many programs meet the needs of RNs by offering options such as accelerated course work, advanced placement, and evening and weekend classes.

Research and anecdotal evidence from adults returning to college indicate that despite their need to balance school work with a career and, often, family responsibilities, these adult learners experience less stress and manage their lives better than they had thought possible. Many of these adult learners report that the satisfaction gained from their education more than compensates for any added stress. Furthermore, studies of nurses who have returned to school suggest that while their education may create stress for them, most nurses cope effectively with the demands of advanced education.

If costs are of concern, it is best to investigate tuition-reimbursement opportunities where you are employed, scholarships from the nursing program and other nursing organizations, and loans. This guide contains informative articles about financial aid on pages 43–47 that will give you an overview. The financial aid officer at the program you are considering is probably the best available resource to answer your questions.

If you are unsure of what to expect when returning to school, remember that such feelings are natural for anyone facing a new situation. If you are motivated and committed to pursuing your degree, you will succeed. Most nursing programs offer resources, such as test-taking, study skills, and time-management workshops, as well as assistance with academic problems. You can combine school, work, family, and other responsibilities. Even with these greater demands, the benefits of education outweigh the difficulties.

Clarifying Career Goals

Nursing, unlike many other professions, has a variety of educational paths for nurses returning for advanced education. You should decide if baccalaureate- or graduate-level work is congruent with your career goals. The next step in this process is to reexamine your specific career goals, both immediate and long-term, to determine the level and type of nursing education you will need to meet them. Ask yourself what you want to be doing in the next five to ten years. Discuss your ideas with a counselor in a nursing education program, nurses who are practicing in roles you are considering, and others who are enrolled in a nursing program or who have recently completed a nursing degree.

Graduates of baccalaureate programs are prepared as generalists for practice in all health-care settings. Graduate nursing education occurs at two levels—master's and doctoral. Master's programs vary in length, typically between one and two years. Preparation for roles in advanced practice as nurse practitioners, certified nurse midwives, clinical nurse specialists, registered nurse anesthetists, nursing administrators, or nursing educators requires a master's degree in nursing. Many programs meet the needs of RNs by offering options such as accelerated course work, advanced placement, and evening and weekend classes.

A trend in education for RNs is accelerated programs that combine the baccalaureate and master's nursing programs. These combined programs are designed for RNs without degrees whose career goals involve advanced nursing practice and other roles requiring a master's degree. Nurses who complete these combined programs may be awarded both a baccalaureate and master's degree in nursing or a master's degree only.

At the doctoral level, nurses are prepared for a variety of roles, including research and teaching. Doctoral programs generally consist of three years of full-time study beyond the master's degree, although some programs admit baccalaureate graduates and include master's-level requirements and degrees within the doctoral program.

Matching the Program to Your Needs

Once you have defined your career goals and the level of nursing education they will require, the next step is matching your needs with the offerings and characteristics of specific nursing programs. Some of the criteria you may want to consider in evaluating potential schools of nursing include the types of programs offered, the school's approach to nursing education, length of the program and its specific requirements, availability of full- and part-time study and number of credits required for part-time study, flexibility of the program, and the days, times, and sites at which classes and clinical experiences are offered as they relate to your work schedule. Take into consideration the program's accreditation status; faculty qualifications in terms of research, teaching, and practice; and the resources of the school of nursing and of the college/university, such as library holdings, computer services, and statistical consultants. Also consider the clinical settings used in the curriculum and their relationship to your career goals, as well as the availability of financial aid.

Carefully review the admission criteria, including minimum grade point average; scores required on any admission tests, such as the Graduate Record Examinations for master's and doctoral programs; and any requirements in terms of work experience. For students returning for a baccalaureate degree, prior nursing knowledge may be validated through testing, transfer of courses, and other mechanisms. Review these options prior to applying to a program.

While the intrinsic quality and characteristics of the program are important, your own personal needs have to be included in your decision. Consider commuting distance, costs in relation to your financial resources, program design, and flexibility of the curriculum in relation to your work, family, and personal responsibilities. While the majority of nursing programs offer part-time study, many programs also schedule classes to accommodate work situations.

Ensure Your Success

Once you have made the decision to return to school and have chosen the program that best meets your needs, identify the support you will need, both academic and personal, to ensure your success in the nursing program. Academic support is provided by the institution and may include tutoring services, learning resource centers, computer facilities, and other resources to support your learning. You should take advantage of available support services and seek out resources for areas in which you are weak or need review. Academic support services, however, need to be complemented by personal support through family, friends, and peers. With a firm commitment to pursuing advanced education, a clear choice of a nursing program to meet your goals, and support from others, you are certain to find success in returning to school.

The International Nursing Student—What You Need to Know About Applying to and Attending U.S. or Canadian Schools

Nursing Education in the U.S. and Canada

For many international students completing baccalaureate, master's, or doctoral nursing programs, their choice of learning institutions was obvious: U.S. and Canadian colleges and universities are considered to offer the finest programs of nursing education available anywhere in the world. U.S. and Canadian nursing programs are renowned for their breadth and flexibility, for the excellence of their basic curriculum structure, and for their commitment to extensive on-site clinical training. Nursing study in the U.S. and Canada also affords students the opportunity for "hands-on" learning and practice in the world's most technologically advanced health-care systems. For many international nursing students, and especially for students hailing from countries that are medically underserved, these features make U.S. and Canadian nursing programs unsurpassed.

Applying to Nursing School

The application process for international students often involves the completion of two separate written applications. Many colleges screen international candidates with a brief preliminary application requesting basic biographical and educational information. This document helps the admission officer determine whether you have the minimum credentials for admission before requiring you to commence the lengthy process of completing and submitting final application forms.

Final applications to U.S. and Canadian colleges and universities vary widely in length and complexity, just as specific admission requirements vary from institution to institution. However, international nursing students must typically meet these basic requirements: a satisfactory scholastic record and demonstrated proficiency in English. To be admitted to any postsecondary institutions in the United States or Canada, you must have satisfactorily completed a minimum of twelve years of elementary and secondary education. The customary cycle for this education includes a six-year elementary program, a three-year intermediate program, and a three-year postsecondary program, generally referred to as high school in the U.S. In addition, nursing school programs generally require successful completion of several years of high school–level mathematics and science.

The documentation of satisfactory completion of secondary schooling (and university education, in the case of graduate-level applicants) is achieved through submission of school reports, transcripts, and teacher recommendations. Because academic records and systems of evaluation differ widely from one educational system to the next, request that your school include a guide to grading standards. If you have received your secondary education at a school in which English is not the language of instruction, be certain to include official translations of all documents.

International students who have completed some university-level course work in their native country may be eligible to receive credit for equivalent courses at the U.S. or Canadian institution in which they enroll. Under special circumstances, practical nursing experience may also qualify for university credit. Policies regarding the transfer of or qualification for credits based on education or nursing experience outside of the U.S. (or Canada for Canadian schools) vary widely, so be certain to inquire about these policies at the universities or colleges that interest you.

Language skills are a key to scholastic success. "The ability to speak, write, and understand English is an important determinant of success," says Joann Weiss, Professor and Director of the Nursing and Latin American Studies dual degree programs at the University of New Mexico in Albuquerque. Her advice for potential international applicants is simple: "Develop a true command of written and spoken English." English proficiency for students who have not received formal education in English-speaking schools is usually demonstrated via the Test of English as a Foreign Language (TOEFL); minimum test scores of 550 to 580 are commonly required. This policy, as well as the level of proficiency required, varies from school to school, so be sure to investigate each college's policies.

In addition, most universities offer some form of English language instruction for international students, often under the rubric ESL (English as a second language). Students who require additional language study to meet admission requirements, or students who wish to deepen their skills in written or verbal English, should inquire about ESL program availability.

Many colleges and universities also require that all undergraduate applicants take a standardized test—either the Scholastic Assessment Test (SAT I) and the three subject-oriented SAT II Subject Tests or the ACT Assessment. Like their U.S. and Canadian counterparts, international applicants to graduate-level nursing programs are required by most institutions to take the standardized Graduate Record Examinations (GRE).

Applicants should also be aware that financial assistance for international students is usually quite limited. To spare international students economic hardship during their schooling in the U.S. or Canada, many colleges and universities require them to demonstrate the availability of sufficient financial resources for tuition and minimum living expenses and supplies. As with so many admission requirements, policies regarding financial aid vary considerably; find out early what the policies are at the colleges that interest you.

Attending School in the U.S. or Canada

Once you are accepted by the college or university of your choice, take full advantage of the academic and personal advising systems offered to international students. Most institutions of higher education in the U.S. and Canada maintain an international student advisory office staffed with trained counselors. In addition to general academic counseling and planning, an international adviser can assist in a broad range of matters ranging from immigration and visa concerns to employment opportunities and health-care issues.

With few exceptions, all university students also obtain specialized academic counseling from an assigned faculty adviser. Faculty advisers monitor academic performance and progress and try to ensure that students meet the institutional requirements for their degree. Faculty advisers are excellent sources of information regarding course selection, and some advisers offer tutorials or special language or educational support to international students.

Although all university students face academic challenges, international students often find life outside the classroom equally demanding. Suddenly introduced into a new culture where the way of life may be dramatically different from that of their native country, international students often face a variety of social, domestic, medical, religious, or emotional concerns. Questions about social conventions, meal preparation, or other personal concerns can often be addressed by your international or faculty adviser.

Lorraine Rudowski, Assistant Professor and International Faculty Adviser at the School of Nursing, George Mason University, in Fairfax, Virginia, emphasizes the benefits of a strong relationship with your advisers: "My job as an adviser is to provide comprehensive support to my students—from academic counseling and opportunities for language development to emotional support and guidance to attending parties or other informal social events to ease the sense of social and personal isolation often experienced by foreign students."

Dr. Rudowski says international students would do well to find a sponsor or confidant within the university, someone who understands the conventions of the student's native country. "A culturally sensitive sponsor is better equipped to understand the unique needs of each international student and is much more likely to help students obtain the assistance they need, whether we're talking about religious issues, help with study methods or social skills, or simply knowing how to deal with such everyday chores as cooking and cleaning. All of these matters can be sources of deep concern to international students."

Yet for all the academic, social, and personal challenges facing international nursing students, there is good news. Deans of nursing, professors, and advisers typically praise the motivation and determination of their international students, and international nursing students often boast matriculation rates that match or exceed those of their U.S. and Canadian counterparts.

For more information about the rules and regulations governing international students' entrance to U.S. schools, request the free publication entitled *Predeparture Orientation Handbook for Foreign Students and Scholars Planning Study in the United States* from a United States Information Service (USIS) counseling center.

Quick Reference to Programs Offered

	Baccalaureate	Master's	Joint Degree	Post-Master's	Doctoral	Post-doctoral	Continuing Education
UNITED STATES							
Alabama							
Auburn University	•						•
Auburn University at Montgomery	•						
Jacksonville State University	•						•
Oakwood College	•						
Samford University	•	•					
Troy State University	•	•					
Tuskegee University	•						•
University of Alabama	•						•
University of Alabama at Birmingham	•	•	•		•	•	•
University of Alabama in Huntsville	•	•		•			•
University of Mobile	•	•					
University of North Alabama	•						
University of South Alabama	•	•					
Alaska							
University of Alaska Anchorage	•	•					
Arizona							
Arizona State University	•	•					•
Grand Canyon University	•						
Northern Arizona University	•	•					
University of Arizona	•	•	•	•	•	•	•
University of Phoenix	•	•					
Arkansas							
Arkansas State University	•	•					
Arkansas Tech University	•						
Harding University	•						•
Henderson State University	•						
University of Arkansas	•	•					
University of Arkansas at Pine Bluff	•						
University of Arkansas for Medical Sciences	•	•		•	•		•
University of Central Arkansas	•	•					
California							
Azusa Pacific University	•	•					•
Biola University	•						•
California State University, Bakersfield	•	•					•
California State University, Chico	•	•					•
California State University, Dominguez Hills	•	•					•
California State University, Fresno	•	•		•			•
California State University, Fullerton	•						
California State University, Hayward	•						
California State University, Long Beach	•	•					
California State University, Los Angeles	•	•					

	Baccalaureate	Master's	Joint Degree	Post-Master's	Doctoral	Post-doctoral	Continuing Education
California State University, Sacramento	•	•					
California State University, San Bernardino	•						
California State University, Stanislaus	•						
Dominican College of San Rafael	•						•
Holy Names College	•	•					
Humboldt State University	•						
Loma Linda University	•	•		•			
Mount St. Mary's College	•						
Pacific Union College	•						
Point Loma Nazarene College	•						
Samuel Merritt College	•	•					•
San Diego State University	•	•					
San Francisco State University	•	•					
San Jose State University	•	•		•			•
Sonoma State University	•	•		•			
University of California, Los Angeles	•	•	•		•	•	•
University of California, San Francisco		•			•	•	
University of San Diego	•	•	•	•	•		
University of San Francisco	•	•	•				
University of Southern California	•	•	•	•			•
Colorado							
Beth-El College of Nursing and Health Sciences	•	•					
Mesa State College	•						
Metropolitan State College of Denver	•						
Regis University	•	•					
University of Colorado Health Sciences Center	•	•	•		•		•
University of Northern Colorado	•	•					
University of Southern Colorado	•						
Connecticut							
Central Connecticut State University	•						
Fairfield University	•	•					•
Quinnipiac College	•						•
Sacred Heart University	•	•	•				
Saint Joseph College	•	•					
Southern Connecticut State University	•	•		•			
University of Connecticut	•	•	•		•		•
University of Hartford	•	•	•				•
Western Connecticut State University	•	•					
Yale University		•	•	•	•		
Delaware							
Delaware State University	•						
University of Delaware	•	•		•			•
Wilmington College	•	•					
District of Columbia							
Catholic University of America	•	•	•	•	•		
Georgetown University	•	•					•
Howard University	•	•		•			
University of the District of Columbia	•						
Florida							
Barry University	•	•	•	•	•		

	Baccalaureate	Master's	Joint Degree	Post-Master's	Doctoral	Post-doctoral	Continuing Education
Florida Agricultural and Mechanical University	•						
Florida Atlantic University	•	•					
Florida International University	•	•					
Florida State University	•	•		•			•
Jacksonville University	•						
University of Central Florida	•	•					
University of Florida	•	•		•	•		
University of Miami	•	•			•		
University of North Florida	•						
University of South Florida	•	•					
University of Tampa	•	•					
University of West Florida	•						
Georgia							
Albany State College	•	•					
Armstrong Atlantic State University	•	•					
Brenau University	•	•					
Clayton State College	•						•
Columbus College	•						
Emory University	•	•	•	•			
Georgia Baptist College of Nursing	•						
Georgia College	•	•	•				
Georgia Southern University	•	•					
Georgia Southwestern State University	•						•
Georgia State University	•	•			•		
Kennesaw State University	•	•					
Medical College of Georgia	•	•			•		•
North Georgia College and State University	•						
Valdosta State University	•	•					
West Georgia College	•						
Hawaii							
Hawaii Pacific University	•						
University of Hawaii at Manoa	•	•		•			
Idaho							
Boise State University	•						
Idaho State University	•	•					
Lewis-Clark State College	•						•
Illinois							
Aurora University	•						
Barat College	•						•
Blessing-Rieman College of Nursing	•						
Bradley University	•	•					
Chicago State University	•						
Concordia University	•						
DePaul University	•	•	•				•
Elmhurst College	•						
Governors State University	•	•					•
Illinois Benedictine University	•						
Illinois Wesleyan University	•						
Lewis University	•	•					
Loyola University Chicago	•	•	•		•		
MacMurray College	•						

	Baccalaureate	Master's	Joint Degree	Post-Master's	Doctoral	Post-doctoral	Continuing Education
McKendree College	•						
Mennonite College of Nursing	•	•					
Millikin University	•						
Northern Illinois University	•	•		•			
North Park College	•	•	•	•			
Olivet Nazarene University	•						
Rockford College	•						
Rush University	•	•	•		•	•	•
Saint Francis Medical Center College of Nursing	•						
Saint Joseph College of Nursing	•						
Saint Xavier University	•	•	•				•
Southern Illinois University at Edwardsville	•	•					•
Trinity Christian College	•						
University of Illinois at Chicago	•	•	•	•	•		
University of Illinois at Springfield	•						
West Suburban College of Nursing	•						
Indiana							
Anderson University	•						
Ball State University	•	•					•
Bethel College	•						
Goshen College	•						
Indiana State University	•	•					•
Indiana University East	•						
Indiana University Kokomo	•						•
Indiana University Northwest	•						•
Indiana University–Purdue University Fort Wayne	•	•					
Indiana University–Purdue University Indianapolis	•	•	•		•	•	•
Indiana University South Bend	•						
Indiana University Southeast	•						
Indiana Wesleyan University	•	•		•			
Marian College	•						
Purdue University	•						
Purdue University Calumet	•	•					
Saint Francis College	•	•					•
Saint Mary's College	•						
University of Evansville	•	•					
University of Indianapolis	•	•					
University of Southern Indiana	•	•					•
Valparaiso University	•	•					
Iowa							
Briar Cliff College	•						
Clarke College	•						
Coe College	•						
Drake University	•	•		•			
Graceland College	•	•		•			
Grand View College	•						•
Iowa Wesleyan College	•						•
Luther College	•						•
Morningside College	•						•
Mount Mercy College	•						•

	Baccalaureate	Master's	Joint Degree	Post-Master's	Doctoral	Post-doctoral	Continuing Education
Teikyo Marycrest University	•						
University of Iowa	•	•	•		•	•	•
Kansas							
Baker University	•						•
Bethel College	•						
Fort Hays State University	•	•		•			
Kansas Newman College	•						
Kansas Wesleyan University	•						
MidAmerica Nazarene College	•						•
Pittsburg State University	•	•					
Southwestern College	•						
University of Kansas	•	•	•		•		•
Washburn University of Topeka	•						•
Wichita State University	•	•					•
Kentucky							
Bellarmine College	•	•					•
Berea College	•						•
Eastern Kentucky University	•	•					
Midway College	•						
Morehead State University	•						•
Murray State University	•	•		•			
Northern Kentucky University	•	•		•			
Spalding University	•	•					
Thomas More College	•						
University of Kentucky	•	•		•	•		•
University of Louisville	•	•					
Western Kentucky University	•	•					•
Louisiana							
Dillard University	•						
Grambling State University	•						
Louisiana College	•						
Louisiana State University Medical Center	•	•			•		•
Loyola University, New Orleans	•	•					
McNeese State University	•	•					
Nicholls State University	•						
Northeast Louisiana University	•						
Northwestern State University of Louisiana	•	•					
Our Lady of Holy Cross College	•						
Southeastern Louisiana University	•	•					
Southern University and Agricultural and Mechanical College	•	•					
University of Southwestern Louisiana	•						
Maine							
Husson College	•						
Saint Joseph's College	•	•					
University of Maine	•	•		•			
University of Maine at Fort Kent	•						•
University of New England–University Campus	•	•					
University of New England–Westbrook College Campus	•	•					
University of Southern Maine	•	•		•			•

	Baccalaureate	Master's	Joint Degree	Post-Master's	Doctoral	Post-doctoral	Continuing Education
Maryland							
Bowie State University	•	•					•
College of Notre Dame of Maryland	•						
Columbia Union College	•						•
Coppin State College	•						
Johns Hopkins University	•	•	•	•	•	•	
Salisbury State University	•	•		•			
Towson State University	•						
University of Maryland at Baltimore	•	•	•	•	•		•
Villa Julie College	•						
Massachusetts							
American International College	•						
Anna Maria College	•						
Atlantic Union College	•						
Boston College	•	•	•		•		•
College of Our Lady of the Elms	•						
Curry College	•						•
Emmanuel College	•						
Fitchburg State College	•	•					
Framingham State College	•						
Massachusetts College of Pharmacy and Allied Health Sciences	•						
MGH Institute of Health Professions		•		•			
Northeastern University	•	•	•	•			
Regis College	•	•		•			•
Salem State College	•	•					
Simmons College	•	•		•			
University of Massachusetts Amherst	•	•			•		•
University of Massachusetts Boston	•	•	•		•		
University of Massachusetts Dartmouth	•	•					•
University of Massachusetts Lowell	•	•			•		
University of Massachusetts Worcester		•		•	•		•
Worcester State College	•						
Michigan							
Andrews University	•	•					
Calvin College	•						
Eastern Michigan University	•	•					
Ferris State University	•						
Grand Valley State University	•	•					•
Hope College	•						
Lake Superior State University	•						•
Madonna University	•	•	•				•
Michigan State University	•	•					•
Northern Michigan University	•	•					•
Oakland University	•	•		•			
Saginaw Valley State University	•	•					•
University of Detroit Mercy	•						
University of Michigan	•	•	•		•	•	
University of Michigan–Flint	•						
Wayne State University	•	•			•	•	
Minnesota							
Augsburg College	•						
Bemidji State University	•						

	Baccalaureate	Master's	Joint Degree	Post-Master's	Doctoral	Post-doctoral	Continuing Education
Bethel College	•						
College of Saint Benedict	•						
College of St. Catherine	•	•		•			
College of St. Scholastica	•	•					•
Concordia College	•						
Gustavus Adolphus College	•						
Mankato State University	•	•					•
Metropolitan State University	•	•					
Moorhead State University	•						
St. Olaf College	•						•
University of Minnesota, Twin Cities Campus	•	•			•		•
Winona State University	•	•		•			
Mississippi							
Alcorn State University	•						
Delta State University	•	•		•			
Mississippi College	•						
Mississippi University for Women	•	•					
University of Mississippi Medical Center	•	•		•	•		•
University of Southern Mississippi	•	•					
William Carey College	•						
Missouri							
Avila College	•						•
Central Missouri State University	•						
Culver-Stockton College	•						
Deaconess College of Nursing	•						
Maryville University of Saint Louis	•						
Missouri Southern State College	•						
Missouri Western State College	•						•
Research College of Nursing–Rockhurst College	•	•					
Saint Louis University	•	•	•	•	•		•
Saint Luke's College	•						
Southeast Missouri State University	•	•					
Southwest Baptist University	•						
Southwest Missouri State University	•	•					
Truman State University	•						
University of Missouri–Columbia	•	•			•		•
University of Missouri–Kansas City	•	•			•		
University of Missouri–St. Louis	•	•		•	•		
Webster University	•	•					
William Jewell College	•						
Montana							
Carroll College	•						
Montana State University–Bozeman	•	•					
Montana State University–Northern	•						
Nebraska							
Clarkson College	•	•		•			•
College of Saint Mary	•						
Creighton University	•	•					
Midland Lutheran College	•						•
Nebraska Methodist College of Nursing and Allied Health	•						

	Baccalaureate	Master's	Joint Degree	Post-Master's	Doctoral	Post-doctoral	Continuing Education
Nebraska Wesleyan University	•						
Union College	•						
University of Nebraska Medical Center	•	•			•		•
Nevada							
University of Nevada, Las Vegas	•	•					•
University of Nevada, Reno	•	•		•			
New Hampshire							
Colby-Sawyer College	•						
Rivier College	•	•					
Saint Anselm College	•						•
University of New Hampshire	•	•					
New Jersey							
Bloomfield College	•						
College of New Jersey	•	•					
College of Saint Elizabeth	•						•
Fairleigh Dickinson University, Teaneck-Hackensack Campus	•	•					
Jersey City State College	•						•
Kean College of New Jersey	•	•					
Monmouth University	•	•					
Richard Stockton College of New Jersey	•						
Rutgers, The State University of New Jersey, Camden College of Arts and Sciences	•	•					
Rutgers, The State University of New Jersey, College of Nursing	•	•			•		•
Saint Peter's College	•						•
Seton Hall University	•	•		•			
Thomas Edison State College	•						
University of Medicine and Dentistry of New Jersey		•		•			•
William Paterson College of New Jersey	•	•					
New Mexico							
New Mexico State University	•	•					
University of New Mexico	•	•	•	•			•
New York							
Adelphi University	•	•					
College of Mount Saint Vincent	•	•					•
College of New Rochelle	•	•		•			•
College of Staten Island of the City University of New York	•						•
Columbia University	•	•	•		•		•
Daemen College	•						
Dominican College of Blauvelt	•						
D'Youville College	•	•					•
Elmira College	•						•
Hartwick College	•						
Hunter College of the City University of New York	•	•	•				
Keuka College	•						
Lehman College of the City University of New York	•	•					•

	Baccalaureate	Master's	Joint Degree	Post-Master's	Doctoral	Post-doctoral	Continuing Education
Long Island University, Brooklyn Campus	•	•					
Long Island University, C.W. Post Campus	•	•					
Medgar Evers College of the City University of New York	•						
Mercy College	•	•					
Molloy College	•	•		•			•
Mount Saint Mary College	•	•					
Nazareth College of Rochester	•	•					
New York University	•	•	•		•		•
Niagara University	•	•					
Pace University	•	•		•			•
Roberts Wesleyan College	•						•
Russell Sage College	•	•	•	•			
St. John Fisher College	•	•					•
St. Joseph's College, New York	•						
State University of New York at Binghamton	•	•		•			•
State University of New York at Buffalo	•	•			•		•
State University of New York at New Paltz	•	•					
State University of New York at Stony Brook	•	•		•			•
State University of New York College at Brockport	•						
State University of New York College at Plattsburgh	•						
State University of New York Health Science Center at Brooklyn	•	•					
State University of New York Health Science Center at Syracuse	•	•		•			
State University of New York Institute of Technology at Utica/Rome	•	•					
Syracuse University	•	•	•	•			
Teachers College, Columbia University		•			•		
University of Rochester	•	•			•	•	
University of the State of New York, Regents College	•						•
Utica College of Syracuse University	•						
Wagner College	•	•		•			•
York College of the City University of New York	•						
North Carolina							
Barton College	•						
Duke University		•		•			
East Carolina University	•	•					
Gardner-Webb University	•						
Lenoir-Rhyne College	•						
North Carolina Agricultural and Technical State University	•						
North Carolina Central University	•						
Queens College	•						
University of North Carolina at Chapel Hill	•	•		•	•	•	•
University of North Carolina at Charlotte	•	•	•				•

	Baccalaureate	Master's	Joint Degree	Post-Master's	Doctoral	Post-doctoral	Continuing Education
University of North Carolina at Greensboro	•	•					
University of North Carolina at Wilmington	•						
Western Carolina University	•						
Winston-Salem State University	•						
North Dakota							
Dickinson State University	•						
Jamestown College	•						
Medcenter One College of Nursing	•						
Minot State University	•						•
North Dakota State University	•						
University of Mary	•	•					
University of North Dakota	•	•					
Ohio							
Ashland University	•						
Bowling Green State University	•						
Capital University	•	•	•				
Case Western Reserve University	•	•	•	•	•		•
Cedarville College	•						
Cleveland State University	•						•
College of Mount St. Joseph	•						
Franciscan University of Steubenville	•						
Franklin University	•						
Kent State University	•	•	•	•			
Lourdes College	•						•
Malone College	•						
Medical College of Ohio		•		•			•
Miami University	•						
Ohio State University	•	•	•		•		
Ohio University	•						
Otterbein College	•	•					•
University of Akron	•	•					•
University of Cincinnati	•	•	•		•		•
University of Toledo	•						
Ursuline College	•						•
Walsh University	•						
Wright State University	•	•	•				
Xavier University	•	•					
Youngstown State University	•						
Oklahoma							
East Central University	•						
Langston University	•						
Northeastern State University	•						
Northwestern Oklahoma State University	•						
Oklahoma Baptist University	•						
Oklahoma City University	•						
Oral Roberts University	•						
Southern Nazarene University	•						
Southwestern Oklahoma State University	•						
University of Central Oklahoma	•						

	Baccalaureate	Master's	Joint Degree	Post-Master's	Doctoral	Post-doctoral	Continuing Education
University of Oklahoma Health Sciences Center	•	•					•
University of Tulsa	•						
Oregon							
Linfield College	•						•
Oregon Health Sciences University	•	•	•	•	•	•	
University of Portland	•	•					
Pennsylvania							
Allegheny University of the Health Sciences	•	•					•
Allentown College of St. Francis de Sales	•	•					
Bloomsburg University of Pennsylvania	•	•					
California University of Pennsylvania	•						
Carlow College	•	•					
Cedar Crest College	•	•					
Clarion University of Pennsylvania	•	•					•
College Misericordia	•	•	•				
Duquesne University	•	•	•	•	•		•
Eastern College	•						
East Stroudsburg University of Pennsylvania	•						
Edinboro University of Pennsylvania	•	•					
Gannon University	•	•	•				
Gwynedd-Mercy College	•	•					•
Holy Family College	•	•					
Immaculata College	•						
Indiana University of Pennsylvania	•	•					
Kutztown University of Pennsylvania	•						
La Roche College	•	•					•
La Salle University	•	•					
Lycoming College	•						
Mansfield University of Pennsylvania	•						
Marywood College	•						•
Messiah College	•						
Millersville University of Pennsylvania	•	•					
Neumann College	•	•					
Pennsylvania State University, University Park Campus	•	•		•			•
Saint Francis College	•						
Slippery Rock University of Pennsylvania	•	•		•			
Temple University	•	•					
Thiel College	•						
Thomas Jefferson University	•	•					
University of Pennsylvania	•	•	•	•	•	•	•
University of Pittsburgh	•	•			•	•	•
University of Scranton	•	•					
Villanova University	•	•					•
Waynesburg College	•						•
West Chester University of Pennsylvania	•	•					
Widener University	•	•		•	•		
Wilkes University	•	•					
York College of Pennsylvania	•						

	Baccalaureate	Master's	Joint Degree	Post-Master's	Doctoral	Post-doctoral	Continuing Education
Puerto Rico							
Inter American University of Puerto Rico, Metropolitan Campus	•						•
Pontifical Catholic University of Puerto Rico	•	•					
Universidad Metropolitana	•						
University of Puerto Rico, Humacao University College	•						
University of Puerto Rico, Mayagüez Campus	•						•
University of Puerto Rico, Medical Sciences Campus	•	•					•
University of the Sacred Heart	•						•
Rhode Island							
Rhode Island College	•						
Salve Regina University	•						
University of Rhode Island	•	•			•		
South Carolina							
Clemson University	•	•					•
Lander University	•						
Medical University of South Carolina	•	•		•	•		•
South Carolina State University	•						
University of South Carolina	•	•	•	•	•		
University of South Carolina–Aiken	•						
University of South Carolina–Spartanburg	•						
South Dakota							
Augustana College	•	•					
Mount Marty College	•						
Presentation College	•						
South Dakota State University	•	•					•
Tennessee							
Austin Peay State University	•						
Belmont University	•						
Carson-Newman College	•						
East Tennessee State University	•	•		•			
Middle Tennessee State University	•						•
Southern Adventist University	•						
Tennessee State University	•	•					
Tennessee Technological University	•						•
Union University	•						
University of Memphis	•						•
University of Tennessee at Chattanooga	•	•					•
University of Tennessee at Martin	•						
University of Tennessee, Knoxville	•	•			•		•
University of Tennessee, Memphis		•		•	•		•
Vanderbilt University		•	•	•	•		
Texas							
Abilene Christian University	•	•					
Angelo State University	•	•					
Baylor University	•	•					
Hardin-Simmons University	•	•					

	Baccalaureate	Master's	Joint Degree	Post-Master's	Doctoral	Post-doctoral	Continuing Education
Houston Baptist University	•	•					
Incarnate Word College	•	•	•				•
Lamar University–Beaumont	•						
McMurry University	•						
Midwestern State University	•	•					•
Prairie View A&M University	•						
Southwestern Adventist College	•						
Stephen F. Austin State University	•						
Texas A&M University–Corpus Christi	•	•					
Texas Christian University	•						•
Texas Tech University Health Sciences Center	•	•	•	•			•
Texas Woman's University	•	•			•		
University of Mary Hardin-Baylor	•						
University of Texas at Arlington	•	•					•
University of Texas at Austin	•	•	•		•		
University of Texas at El Paso	•	•		•			•
University of Texas at Tyler	•	•	•	•			
University of Texas Health Science Center at San Antonio	•	•			•		•
University of Texas–Houston Health Science Center	•	•	•	•	•		•
University of Texas Medical Branch at Galveston	•	•		•			•
University of Texas–Pan American	•	•					
West Texas A&M University	•	•					
Utah							
Brigham Young University	•	•	•				
University of Utah	•	•		•	•	•	•
Weber State University	•						
Westminster College of Salt Lake City	•	•					
Vermont							
Norwich University	•						
University of Vermont	•	•		•			
Virginia							
Christopher Newport University	•	•					
Eastern Mennonite University	•						
George Mason University	•	•	•		•		
Hampton University	•	•					
James Madison University	•						
Liberty University	•						
Lynchburg College	•						
Marymount University	•	•					
Norfolk State University	•						
Old Dominion University	•	•					•
Radford University	•	•					•
University of Virginia	•	•	•		•		•
Virginia Commonwealth University	•	•			•		
Virgin Islands							
University of the Virgin Islands	•						
Washington							
Eastern Washington University	•	•					•
Gonzaga University	•	•		•			

	Baccalaureate	Master's	Joint Degree	Post-Master's	Doctoral	Post-doctoral	Continuing Education
Pacific Lutheran University	•	•					•
Saint Martin's College	•	•					•
Seattle Pacific University	•	•		•			
Seattle University	•	•					
University of Washington	•	•	•		•	•	•
Walla Walla College	•						
Washington State University	•	•					•
Whitworth College	•	•					•
West Virginia							
Alderson-Broaddus College	•						
Marshall University	•	•					
Shepherd College	•						
University of Charleston	•						
West Liberty State College	•						
West Virginia University	•	•		•			
West Virginia Wesleyan College	•						
Wheeling Jesuit College	•	•					
Wisconsin							
Alverno College	•						•
Bellin College of Nursing	•						•
Cardinal Stritch College	•	•					
Columbia College of Nursing	•						
Concordia University Wisconsin	•	•					•
Edgewood College	•	•					
Marian College of Fond du Lac	•						
Marquette University	•	•		•			•
University of Wisconsin–Eau Claire	•	•					•
University of Wisconsin–Green Bay	•						•
University of Wisconsin–Madison	•	•		•	•		•
University of Wisconsin–Milwaukee	•	•			•		•
University of Wisconsin–Oshkosh	•	•					•
Viterbo College	•						
Wyoming							
University of Wyoming	•	•		•			•
CANADA							
Alberta							
Athabasca University	•						
University of Alberta	•	•			•	•	
University of Calgary	•	•			•		
University of Lethbridge	•						
British Columbia							
University of British Columbia	•	•			•		
University of Victoria	•	•			•		•
Manitoba							
Brandon University	•						
University of Manitoba	•	•					•
New Brunswick							
Université de Moncton							
University of New Brunswick	•	•					

	Baccalaureate	Master's	Joint Degree	Post-Master's	Doctoral	Post-doctoral	Continuing Education
Newfoundland							
Memorial University of Newfoundland	•	•					
Nova Scotia							
Dalhousie University	•	•	•				
St. Francis Xavier University	•						•
Ontario							
Lakehead University	•						
Laurentian University	•						
McMaster University	•						
Queen's University at Kingston	•	•					
Ryerson Polytechnic University	•						
University of Ottawa	•	•					
University of Toronto	•	•			•		
University of Western Ontario	•	•					
University of Windsor	•	•					
York University	•						•
Prince Edward Island							
University of Prince Edward Island	•						
Quebec							
McGill University	•	•			•		
Université de Montréal	•	•			•		•
Université de Sherbrooke	•						
Université du Québec à Hull	•						
Université du Québec à Rimouski	•						
Université Laval	•	•					
Saskatchewan							
University of Saskatchewan	•	•					•

SPECIALTY NURSING ORGANIZATIONS

Academy of Medical-Surgical Nurses
East Holly Avenue, Box 56
Pitman, NJ 08071-0056
609-256-2323
http://www.inurse.com/~amsn/

American Academy of Ambulatory Care Nursing
East Holly Avenue, Box 56
Pitman, NJ 08071-0056
609-256-2350
http://www.inurse.com/~aaacn/

American Association of Critical-Care Nurses
101 Columbia
Aliso Viejo, CA 92656-1491
714-362-2000
http://www.aacn.org/

American Association of Diabetes Educators
444 North Michigan Avenue, Suite 1240
Chicago, IL 60611-3901
312-644-AADE or 800-338-DMED (toll-free)

American Association of Neuroscience Nurses
224 North Des Plaines, #601
Chicago, IL 60661
312-993-0043
http://www.aann.org/

American Association of Nurse Anesthetists
222 South Prospect Avenue
Park Ridge, IL 60068-4001
847-692-7050

American Association of Occupational Health Nurses
50 Lenox Pointe
Atlanta, GA 30324-3176
404-262-1162
http://www.aaohn.org/

American Association of Spinal Cord Injury Nurses
75-20 Astoria Boulevard
Jackson Heights, NY 11370-1177
718-803-3782

American College of Nurse-Midwives
818 Connecticut Avenue, NW, Suite 900
Washington, DC 20006
202-728-9860

American Holistic Nurses' Association
4101 Lake Boone Trail, Suite 201
Raleigh, NC 27607
800-278-2462 (toll-free)
http://www.ahna.org/

American Nephrology Nurses' Association
East Holly Avenue, Box 56
Pitman, NJ 08071-0056
609-256-2320
http://www.inurse.com/~anna/

American Psychiatric Nurses' Association
1200 Nineteenth Street, NW, Suite 300
Washington, DC 20036
202-857-1133

American Public Health Association/
Public Health Nursing Section
1015 Fifteenth Street, NW, Suite 300
Washington, DC 20005
202-789-5600
http://www.apha.org/apha/Sections/aphaphn.htm

American Radiological Nurses Association
2021 Spring Road, Suite 600
Oak Brook, IL 60521
630-571-9072
http://www.rsna.org/about/orgs/arna.html

American Society of Ophthalmic Registered Nurses
P.O. Box 193030
San Francisco, CA 94119
415-561-8513

American Society of PeriAnesthesia Nurses
6900 Grove Road
Thorofare, NJ 08086
609-845-5557
http://www.aspan.org/

American Society of Plastic and
Reconstructive Surgical Nurses
East Holly Avenue, Box 56
Pitman, NJ 08071-0056
609-256-2340

Association for Professionals in Infection Control and
Epidemiology, Inc.
1016 Sixteenth Street, NW, Sixth Floor
Washington, DC 20036
202-296-2742

Association of Nurses in AIDS Care
11250 Roger Bacon Drive, Suite 8
Reston, VA 20190-5202
703-437-4377
http://www.anacnet.org/aids/

Association of Operating Room Nurses
2170 South Parker Road, #300
Denver, CO 80231-5711
303-755-6300

Association of Pediatric Oncology Nurses
4700 West Lake Avenue
Glenview, IL 60025-1485
847-375-4724
http://www.apon.org/

Association of Rehabilitation Nurses
4700 West Lake Avenue
Glenview, IL 60025
800-229-7530 (toll-free)
http://www.rehabnurse.org/

Association of Women's Health, Obstetric, and
Neonatal Nurses
700 Fourteenth Street, NW, Suite 600
Washington, DC 20005-2019
800-673-8499 (toll-free)
http://www.awhonn.org/

Dermatology Nurses' Association
East Holly Avenue, Box 56
Pitman, NJ 08071-0056
609-256-2330
http://www.inurse.com/~dna/

Emergency Nurses Association
216 Higgins Road
Park Ridge, IL 60068-5736
847-698-9400
http://www.ena.org/

Hospice Nurses Association
Medical Center East, Suite 375
211 North Whitfield Street
Pittsburgh, PA 15206-3031
412-361-2470
http://www.roxane.com/Roxane/rpi/Hospice/HealthcarePro/hna/

Intravenous Nurses Society
Fresh Pond Square
10 Fawcett Street
Cambridge, MA 02138
617-441-3008

National Alliance of Nurse Practitioners
325 Pennsylvania Avenue, SE
Washington, DC 20003-1100
202-675-6350

National Association of Directors of Nursing Administration in Long Term Care
10999 Reed Hartman Highway, Suite 229
Cincinnati, OH 45242
800-222-0539 (toll-free)

National Association of Home Care
228 Seventh Street, SE
Washington, DC 20003
202-547-7424
http://www.nahc.org/home.html

National Association of Neonatal Nurses
1304 South Point Boulevard, Suite 280
Petaluma, CA 94954-6861
800-451-3795 (toll-free)
http://www.ajn.org/ajnnet/nrsorgs/nann/

National Association of Nurse Practitioners in Reproductive Health
2401 Pennsylvania Avenue, NW, Suite 350
Washington, DC 20037-1718
202-408-7050

National Association of Orthopaedic Nurses
East Holly Avenue, Box 56
Pitman, NJ 08071-0056
609-256-2310
http://www.inurse.com/~naon/

National Association of Pediatric Nurse Associates and Practitioners
1101 Kings Highway North, Suite 206
Cherry Hill, NJ 08034
609-667-1773

National Association of School Nurses
P.O. Box 1300
Scarborough, ME 04070-1300
207-883-2117

National Flight Nurses Association
216 Higgins Road
Park Ridge, IL 60068-5736
847-698-1733

National Gerontological Nursing Association
7250 Parkway Drive, Suite 510
Hanover, MD 21076
800-723-0560 (toll-free)
http://www.ajn.org/ajnnet/nrsorgs/ngna/

Oncology Nursing Society
501 Holiday Drive
Pittsburgh, PA 15220-2749
412-921-7373
http://www.ons.org/

Respiratory Nursing Society
4700 West Lake Avenue
Glenview, IL 60025
847-375-4700

Society for Vascular Nursing
309 Winter Street
Norwood, MA 02062
617-762-3630

Society of Gastroenterology Nurses and Associates
401 North Michigan Avenue
Chicago, IL 60611-4267
800-245-7462 (toll-free)

Society of Otorhinolaryngology and Head-Neck Nurses
116 Canal Street, Suite A
New Smyrna Beach, FL 32168-7004
904-428-1695

Society of Urological Nurses and Associates
East Holly Avenue, Box 56
Pitman, NJ 08071-0056
609-256-2335
http://www.inurse.com/~suna/

Paying for Your Nursing Education

Whether you're considering a baccalaureate degree in nursing or have completed your undergraduate education and are planning to attend graduate school, finding a way to pay for that education is an essential part of your planning.

The expense of attending college is considerable and is increasing each year at a rate faster than most other products and services. In fact, the cost of a nursing education at a public four-year college can be over $13,000 per year, including tuition, fees, books, room and board, transportation, and miscellaneous expenses. The cost at a private college or university, at either the graduate or undergraduate level, can be over $30,000 per year.

This is where financial aid comes in. Financial aid is money made available by the government and other sources to help students who otherwise would be unable to attend college. Almost $50 billion in aid is given or lent to students each year. Most college students in this country receive some sort of aid, and all prospective students should investigate what may be available. Most of this aid is given to students because neither they nor their families have sufficient personal resources to pay for college. This kind of aid is referred to as need-based aid. Recipients of need-based aid include traditional students just out of high school or college, as well as older, nontraditional students who are returning to college or graduate school.

There is also merit-based aid, which is awarded to students who display a particular talent, show extraordinary promise, or are members of groups that are underrepresented in college. Many colleges and graduate schools offer merit-based aid to their students in addition to need-based aid.

Types and Sources of Financial Aid

There are three types of aid—*scholarships* (also known as grants or gift aid), *loans,* and *student employment* (including fellowships and assistantships). Scholarships and grants are outright gifts and do not have to be repaid. Loans are borrowed money that must be repaid with interest, usually after graduation. Student employment provides jobs during the academic year for which students are paid. For graduate students, student employment also includes fellowships in which students work, receive free or reduced tuition, and are paid a stipend for living expenses.

Most of the aid available to students is need-based and comes from the federal government through six large financial aid programs (see Table 1). Two of these programs are grant-based—the Federal Pell Grant and the Federal Supplemental Educational Opportunity Grant—and are only available to undergraduate students. Three are loan programs—the Federal Perkins Loan, the Federal Family of Education Loans, and the William Ford Federal Direct Loan—that are provided to both undergraduate and graduate students. The sixth program is a student employment program called Federal Work-Study, also awarded to undergraduate and graduate students.

Table 1: Federal Financial Aid Programs

Program	**Maximum/year**
Federal Pell Grant	$2,700 (undergraduate only)
Federal Supplemental Educational Opportunity Grant	$4,000 (undergraduate only)
Federal Perkins Loan	$3,000 (undergraduate) $5,000 (graduate)
Federal Stafford/ Direct Loan (subsidized)	$2,625 (freshman) $3,500 (sophomore) $5,500 (junior/senior)
Federal Stafford/ Direct Loan (unsubsidized)	$2,625 (freshman) $3,500 (sophomore) $5,500 (junior/senior) $6,625 (independent 1st & 2nd year students) $10,500 (independent 3rd & 4th year students) $18,500 (graduate)
Federal PLUS loan	Up to cost of education (for parents only)

The second-largest source of aid is the colleges and universities themselves. Almost all colleges make funds available, most of which are grants, scholarships, and fellowships. These can either be need- or merit-based.

A third source of aid is state governments. Nearly every state provides aid for students attending college in their home state, although most only have programs for undergraduates. Almost all state aid programs are scholarships and grants, but a few states have loan and work-study programs.

A fourth source of aid is private sources such as corporations, civic associations, unions, fraternal organizations, foundations, and religious groups that bestow scholarships, grants, and fellowships to students. Most of these are not based on need, although the amount of the scholarship may vary depending upon one's financial need. The competition for these scholarships can be formidable, but the rewards are well worth the process. Many companies also offer tuition reimbursement to employees and their dependents. Check with the personnel or human resources department at your or your parents' place of employment for benefit and eligibility information. A partial list of the largest private sources of aid specifically for nursing students immediately follows on page 48.

Eligibility for Financial Aid

Since most of the financial aid that college students receive is based on need, colleges employ a process called "need analysis" to determine student awards. For most applicants, there is one form that the student and parents (if the student is a dependent) fill out on which family income, assets, size, etc., are reported. This form is the Free Application for Federal Student Aid (FAFSA). A formula has been devised that takes into account these and a few other criteria. The end result of this need analysis is the student's expected "family contribution" or FC, representing the amount a family is able to contribute toward educational expenses.

Who's in Your Family: Dependent or Independent

The basic principle of government financial aid is that the primary responsibility for paying college expenses resides with the family. In determining your family contribution, you will first need to know who makes up your "family." That will tell you whose income is counted when the need analysis is done.

Graduate Students: By definition, all graduate nursing students are considered independent. Therefore, only your income (and your spouse's if you are married) counts in determining your expected family contribution.

Undergraduate Students: If you are financially dependent upon your parents, then their income and assets, as well as yours, are counted toward the family contribution. But if you are considered independent of your parents, only your income (and your spouse's if you are married) counts in the calculation.

In order to be considered independent for financial aid, you must meet any ONE of the following:

- You must be at least 24 years old, or
- You must be a veteran of the U.S. Armed Forces, or
- You must be a graduate student, or
- You must be married, or
- You must be an orphan or a ward of the court (or were a ward of the court until you were 18 years old), or
- You have legal dependents other than a spouse

If you meet any one of these conditions, you are considered independent and only your income (and your spouse's if you are married) counts toward your family contribution. Remember, if you are attending school as a graduate student, you are automatically independent.

If there are extraordinary circumstances, the financial aid administrator at the college you will be attending has the authority to make exceptions to the rules. Extensive documentation of the extraordinary situation will have to be provided by you.

If you are a dependent student, you can use the table that appears on page 47 to help you estimate your expected "Family Contribution." If you are considered an independent student, take your total family income for the previous year, subtract all state and federal taxes paid (including FICA), subtract another $3,000 ($6,000 if you are married), and divide the result in half. If your family income is less than $50,000, this is your estimated expected family contribution (EFC). If your income is greater than $50,000, add 35 percent (12 percent if you have children) of your total assets (bank accounts, stocks, etc.). This result is your estimated EFC.

Determining Your Cost and Need

Now that you know approximately how much you and your family will be expected to contribute toward your college expenses, you can subtract the family contribution from the total cost of attending a college or graduate school to determine the amount of need-based financial aid for which you will be eligible. The average costs we have listed as a guide assume that you will be attending nursing school full-time. If you will be attending part-time, you should adjust costs accordingly.

Applying for Financial Aid

After you have subtracted your family contribution from the cost of your education and found that you have financial need, you will want to apply for financial aid to meet that need. The process for applying for aid sometimes is a bit complicated. We suggest you contact the colleges directly for immediate help and precisely relevant information.

Undergraduate and graduate students applying for aid must fill out the Free Application for Federal Student Aid (FAFSA). This form is a four-page application available in high school guidance offices, college financial aid offices, state education department offices, many local libraries, and even the local office of your congressional representative. The FAFSA first becomes available in November or December, almost a year before the fall term in which you will enroll, but you cannot complete it until after January 1.

After you and your parents (if appropriate) have signed your completed FAFSA, you send it to a processing center in the envelope provided. Do not send any additional materials, but do make a copy of what you filled out. Users of the Internet can apply electronically through the Department of Education's on-line *FAFSA Express.*

The processing center enters the data into a computer that runs the federal methodology of need analysis to calculate your family contribution. This center then distributes the information to the schools and agencies you listed on the FAFSA. The actual determination of need and the awarding of aid is handled by each college financial aid office.

It is generally recommended that you complete the FAFSA as soon after January 1 as possible. If it is much later, even while you are actually enrolled in college, it is not too late to qualify for financial aid. If, for example, you decided not to go to college or graduate school until just before classes began, you can still complete the FAFSA and be eligible for many federal and state financial aid programs.

What Happens After You Submit the FAFSA

Two to four weeks after you send in your completed FAFSA, you will receive a Student Aid Report (SAR) that shows the information you reported and your calculated expected Family Contribution. This is an opportunity for you to make corrections or to have the information sent to another school you are considering. The SAR contains instructions on how to make corrections or to designate additional schools.

At the same time that you receive the SAR, the college(s) you specified also receive the information. The financial aid office at the school may request additional information from you or may ask you to provide documentation verifying the information you reported on the FAFSA. For example, they may ask you for a copy of your (and your parent's) income tax return or official forms verifying any untaxed income you or your parents received (e.g., Social Security, disability, or welfare benefits).

Once the financial aid office is satisfied that the information is correct and has determined that you have need, a financial aid offer will be made. Many colleges like to make this offer in the spring prior to the fall enrollment so that students have ample opportunity to make their plans; however, some colleges will wait until summer to notify you.

Some Schools Use a Separate Application

The FAFSA is the only form you use to apply for financial aid. However, many colleges and graduate schools do not utilize the FAFSA to initiate the financial aid application process. Nearly 500 colleges and universities, plus over two hundred private scholarship programs, employ a form called the Financial Aid PROFILE from the College Scholarship Service (CSS). While the form is similar to the FAFSA, several additional questions must be answered for colleges awarding their own funds. You begin the process in October or November by completing a PROFILE Registration form on which you designate the schools to which you are applying. A few weeks later, you will receive a customized, individualized application that you complete and send back to CSS. They, in turn, forward your application information to the schools you selected.

Your Financial Aid Offer

If you are determined to have need, a college will typically offer a combination of the three types of assistance: scholarship/grant, loan, and work-study, to meet this need. You may accept all or part of the financial aid offer; an offer is usually made with the stipulation that you will be attending full-time. If you plan on attending less than full-time, you should contact the financial aid office. It is quite possible your award will be less, partially because colleges recognize that as a part-time student you will have the opportunity to earn more money. In addition, your total costs will likely decrease.

If you are awarded Federal Work-Study, the amount you are awarded—plus the total of any unmet need and your family contribution—is the total you are allowed to earn for the year. If you are already employed, chances are that your job will pay more than a Federal Work-Study job or a job on campus, so you will probably want to talk with your employer about working part-time to attend school.

If you are applying to a school that requests the Financial Aid PROFILE, you will have to start the financial aid application process earlier—in October or November, one year before you plan on enrolling.

If you earn more on your job than the amount you are awarded in Federal Work-Study and receive other need-based aid, there is a possibility you will receive more than the total cost of attending college for the year. In this case, you might want to turn down some of the loan portion of your financial aid offer to avoid "overawarding" and to reduce the amount you will owe when your schooling is complete.

One thing to keep in mind is that the student budget used to establish eligibility for financial aid is based on averages. It may not reflect your actual expenses. Student budgets usually reflect most expenses for categories of students (for example, single students living in their parents' home, single parents living in an apartment or house near campus, etc.). But if you have expenses that are not included, you should talk with someone in the financial aid office about making a budget adjustment. Often, students are permitted to earn or borrow more in order to meet expenses not normally counted in the student budget. On occasion, more grant money is awarded. More often than not, however, if a budget adjustment is made, students are awarded more loan money or work-study or are allowed to earn more in their own jobs.

If Your Family or Job Situation Changes

Because a family contribution is based on the previous year's income, many nursing students find they do not qualify for need-based aid (or not enough to pay their full expenses). This is particularly true of older students who were working full-time last year but are no longer doing so, or who will not work during the academic year. If this

Employer-Paid Financial Aid

Bob Atwater is a certified personnel consultant and vice president for HRA Health Care Services in Atlanta, a consulting firm for the employment and recruitment of physician assistants, nurse practitioners, and certified nurse midwives.

Health-care administrators, Atwater says, have coined a phrase to characterize their efforts to meet the growing demand for nurses with better skills and training: "Grow your own."

"Constant training through the course of a nursing career is the only way to keep pace with the technological and medical advances, but it can be a financial burden on the nurse," Atwater says.

That is why many employers now give qualified employees a benefits package that includes a "continuing education allowance."

For the employer, this type of benefits package can help to recruit candidates willing to further their careers through education. Administrators feel it is the best way to build a staff of nurses with up-to-date certifications in all areas.

In a constantly expanding field, nurses should be required to continue and update their education. The nurses get a paid education, can keep their job, and work flexible hours while they are going to school. Inquiries about these allowances should be made during an interview with the company's human resources department.

---

is your situation, you should speak to a counselor in the financial aid office about making an adjustment in your family contribution need analysis. Financial aid administrators may make changes to any of the elements that go into a need analysis or to the calculated family contribution, if there are conditions that merit a change.

If You Still Don't Qualify for Need-Based Aid

If you still don't qualify for need-based aid but feel you do not have the resources necessary to pay for college or graduate school, you still have several options available.

First, there are two loan programs for students for which need is not a consideration. These two programs are the Unsubsidized Federal Stafford Loan and the Unsubsidized Direct Loan. There is also a non-need-based loan program for parents of dependent children called the Federal PLUS loan. If you or your parents are interested in borrowing through one of these programs, you should check with the financial aid office for more information. For many students, borrowing to pay for a nursing education can be an excellent investment in one's future. At the same time, be sure that you do not overburden yourself when it comes to paying back the loans. Before you accept a student loan, the financial aid office will schedule a counseling session to make certain that you know the terms of the loan and that you understand the ramifications of borrowing. If you can do without, it is often suggested that you postpone student loans until they are absolutely necessary.

A second option, if you do not qualify for aid, is to search for scholarships that are not based on need. Be wary of scholarship search agencies that promise to find you scholarships but ask you to pay a fee. There are many resources providing lists of scholarships, including the annually published *Peterson's Scholarships, Grants & Prizes*, that are available in libraries, counselors' offices, and bookstores. Non-need scholarships require application forms and are extremely competitive; only a handful of students from thousands of applicants receive awards.

Another practical option is to work more hours at an existing job or to find a paying position if you do not already have one. You will probably be on your own when it comes to finding summer work, but the student employment office at your college should be able to help you with a school-year job, either on or off campus. Many colleges have vacancies remaining after they have placed aid students in their work-study jobs.

You should always contact the financial aid office at the school you plan to attend for advice concerning sources of college-based and private aid that may be familiar to them.

Table 2: Approximate Expected Family Contribution for 1997–98

		INCOME BEFORE TAXES								
ASSETS▼		$ 20,000	30,000	40,000	50,000	60,000	70,000	80,000	90,000	100,000
$ 20,000										
FAMILY SIZE	3	$ 800	2,700	4,400	6,800	9,500	12,600	15,600	18,500	21,400
	4	0	2,000	2,600	4,700	8,200	11,400	14,300	17,200	20,200
	5	0	900	1,900	3,700	7,000	10,200	13,100	16,000	19,000
	6	0	0	1,200	2,800	5,800	8,800	11,800	14,700	17,600
$ 30,000										
FAMILY SIZE	3	$ 800	2,700	3,400	5,800	9,500	12,600	15,600	18,500	21,400
	4	0	2,000	2,600	4,700	8,200	11,400	14,300	17,200	20,200
	5	0	900	1,900	3,700	7,000	10,200	13,100	16,000	19,000
	6	0	0	1,200	2,800	5,800	8,800	11,800	14,700	17,600
$ 40,000										
FAMILY SIZE	3	$ 800	2,700	3,400	5,800	9,500	12,600	15,600	18,500	21,400
	4	0	2,000	2,600	4,700	8,200	11,400	14,300	17,200	20,200
	5	0	900	1,900	3,700	7,000	10,200	13,100	16,000	19,000
	6	0	0	1,200	2,800	5,800	8,800	11,800	14,700	17,600
$ 50,000										
FAMILY SIZE	3	$ 1,000	2,900	4,300	7,300	10,100	13,600	16,100	19,100	22,000
	4	400	2,300	3,500	6,200	8,800	11,900	14,900	17,800	20,700
	5	0	1,700	2,800	5,000	7,600	10,700	13,700	16,600	19,500
	6	0	200	2,100	4,000	6,300	9,400	12,300	15,300	18,200
$ 60,000										
FAMILY SIZE	3	$ 1,300	3,200	4,100	7,900	10,600	14,100	16,700	19,600	22,700
	4	700	2,500	3,200	6,700	9,400	12,900	15,400	18,300	21,400
	5	300	1,900	2,500	5,500	8,200	11,700	14,200	17,200	20,200
	6	0	1,200	1,700	4,500	6,800	10,400	12,900	15,800	18,800
$ 80,000										
FAMILY SIZE	3	$ 1,800	3,800	5,800	9,000	11,800	14,900	17,800	20,700	23,700
	4	900	3,000	4,700	7,700	10,500	13,600	16,500	19,400	22,400
	5	400	2,400	3,900	6,400	9,300	12,400	15,400	18,200	21,200
	6	0	1,700	3,100	5,200	7,900	11,100	14,000	16,800	19,900
$100,000										
FAMILY SIZE	3	$ 2,800	4,000	6,900	10,200	12,900	16,000	19,000	21,800	24,800
	4	1,500	3,200	5,700	8,900	11,600	14,800	17,700	20,500	23,500
	5	900	2,500	4,700	7,500	10,400	13,600	16,500	19,300	22,300
	6	400	1,800	3,800	6,100	9,100	12,200	15,100	18,000	21,000
$120,000										
FAMILY SIZE	3	$ 3,900	4,900	8,000	11,300	14,000	17,100	21,000	23,200	25,800
	4	2,600	4,000	6,500	10,100	12,700	15,900	18,800	21,700	24,600
	5	1,900	3,200	5,400	8,800	11,500	14,700	17,600	20,500	23,400
	6	1,200	2,500	4,300	7,200	10,200	13,300	16,300	19,200	22,400
$140,000										
FAMILY SIZE	3	$ 4,600	5,900	9,200	12,400	15,400	18,200	21,200	23,800	28,200
	4	3,200	4,800	7,800	11,100	13,900	17,000	19,900	21,900	26,900
	5	2,500	3,900	6,400	9,800	12,700	15,800	18,800	21,700	25,700
	6	1,700	3,200	5,200	8,300	11,300	14,500	17,400	20,300	23,300

Sources of Financial Aid for Nursing Students

The largest proportion of financial aid for college expenses comes from the federal government and is given on the basis of financial need. Beyond this federal need-based aid, which should always be the primary source of financial aid that a prospective student investigates and which is given regardless of one's field of study, a sizable amount of scholarship help is also available from government agencies, associations, civic or fraternal organizations, and corporations, specifically meant to help students in nursing programs. These sources of aid can be particularly attractive for students who may be disqualified for need-based aid. The following presents some of the major sources of financial aid specifically for nursing students. Not in this list are scholarships that are specific to individual colleges and universities, or are limited to residents of a particular place, or to individuals who have relatively unusual qualifications. Students seeking financial aid should investigate all appropriate possibilities including those sources not listed here. A student can find in libraries, bookstores, and guidance offices guides designed to provide this information, including two Peterson's annually updated publications: *Peterson's College Money Handbook*, for information about undergraduate awards given by the federal government, state governments, and specific colleges, and *Peterson's Scholarships, Grants & Prizes*, for information about awards from private sources.

American Association of Critical Care Nurses
Award Name: AACN Educational Advancement Scholarships
Program Description: Nonrenewable scholarships for AACN members currently enrolled in undergraduate or graduate NLN-accredited programs. The undergraduate award is for use in the junior or senior year. Minimum 3.0 GPA.
Application Contact: American Association of Critical Care Nurses
Educational Advancement Scholarship
101 Columbia
Aliso Viejo, CA 92656

American Cancer Society
Award Name: Scholarships in Cancer Nursing
Program Description: Renewable awards for graduate students in nursing pursuing advanced preparation in cancer nursing: research, education, administration, or clinical practice. Must be U.S. citizen.
Application Contact: American Cancer Society
Department of Detection and Treatment
1599 Clifton Road, NE
Atlanta, GA 30329-4251

American Legion Eight and Forty
Award Name: Eight and Forty Lung/Respiratory Nursing Scholarships
Program Description: Available to RNs with work experience who are taking courses leading to full-time employment in lung or respiratory disease nursing and/or teaching. In most states, the American Legion or American Legion Auxiliary provides scholarships to nurses who are residents of that specific state. Qualifications vary, but usually require that the student be a child or grandchild of a veteran. Contact your local American Legion Post or state headquarters for further information about these awards.
Application Contact: American Legion
Eight and Forty
1599 Clifton Road, NE
Atlanta, GA 30329-4251

Association of Operating Room Nurses
Award Name: AORN Foundation Scholarships
Program Description: Applicant must be an active RN and member of AORN for twelve consecutive months prior to application. Reapplication for each period is required. For baccalaureate, master's of nursing, or doctoral degree at an accredited institution. Minimum 3.0 GPA required.
Application Contact: AORN Scholarship Board
2170 South Parker Road, Suite 300
Denver, CO 80231

Business and Professional Women's Foundation
Award Name: New York Life Foundation Scholarships for Women in Health
Program Description: For women in the last two years of undergraduate study pursuing a health-care career. Must be at least 25 and graduate within two years. Submit proof of enrollment. Must send a double self-addressed stamped envelope for information on this nonrenewable award.
Application Contact: Scholarships/Loans
Business and Professional Women's Foundation
2012 Massachusetts Avenue, NW
Washington, DC 20036

Foundation of National Student Nurses Association
Award Names: FNSNA Scholarships, FNSNA Career Mobility Scholarships, FNSNA Specialty Scholarships, Breakthrough to Nursing Scholarships
Program Description: One-time awards available to nursing students in various educational situations: enrolled in programs leading to an RN license; RNs enrolled in programs leading to a B.A. in nursing; enrolled in a state-approved school in a specialty area of nursing; minority students enrolled in nursing or prenursing programs. Based on financial need, academic ability, and health-related nursing and community activities. Application fee of $10. Send self-addressed stamped envelope with two stamps along with application request.
Application Contact: Scholarship Administrator
Foundation of the National Student Nurses Association
555 West 57th Street, Room 1327
New York, NY 10019

International Order of the King's Daughters and Sons
Award Name: International Order of King's Daughters/Sons Health Scholarships
Program Description: For study in the health fields. No biology, premedical, or veterinary applicants accepted.

B.A./B.S. students are eligible in junior year. Medical/dental students must have finished first year of school. Send #10 self-addressed stamped envelope for application and information.
Application Contact: Mrs. Merle Raber, Director
Health Careers Department
6024 East Chicago Road
Jonesville, MI 49250-9752

Maternity Center Association
Award Name: Hazel Corbin Assistance Fund
Program Description: Applicant must be an RN and accepted into a nurse-midwifery program accredited by the American College of Nurse-Midwives.
Application Contact: Maternity Center Association
48 East 92nd Street
New York, NY 10128-1397

National Association of Hispanic Nurses
Award Name: NAHN National Scholarship Awards
Program Description: One-time award to an outstanding Hispanic nursing student. Must have at least a 3.0 GPA and be a member of NAHN. Based on academic merit, potential contribution to nursing, and financial need.
Application Contact: National Association of Hispanic Nurses
National Scholarship Award Chairperson
1501 16th Street, NW
Washington, DC 20036

National Association of Pediatric Nurse Associates and Practitioners
Award Name: NAPNAP McNeil Scholarships
Program Description: For students enrolled in a pediatric nurse practitioner program. Must be an RN with work experience in pediatrics.
Application Contact: National Association of Pediatric Nurse Associates and Practitioners
1101 Kings Highway North, Suite 206
Cherry Hill, NJ 08034-1912

National Black Nurses' Association
Award Names: NBNA Scholarships; Dr. Lauranne Sams Scholarships
Program Description: Scholarships available to nursing students who are members of NBNA and are enrolled in an accredited school of nursing. Must demonstrate involvement in African-American community and present letter of recommendation from local chapter of NBNA. Send self-addressed stamped envelope with 78 cents postage.
Application Contact: Millicent Gorham, Executive Director
National Black Nurses' Association
1511 K Street, NW, Suite 415
Washington, DC 20005

National Foundation for Long-Term Health Care
Award Name: James D. Durante Nurse Scholarships
Program Description: For students accepted or enrolled in an accredited LPN/RN program and currently employed by an American Health Care Association nursing facility. Winners volunteer 25 hours of service to an AHCA facility. Send legal-size self-addressed stamped envelope for application.
Application Contact: National Foundation for Long-Term Health Care
Durante Nurse Scholarship Program
1201 L Street, NW
Washington, DC 20005-4014

National Institutes of Health
Award Name: NIH Undergraduate Scholarships
Program Description: Awards for students from disadvantaged backgrounds to pursue undergraduate degrees in the life sciences that support professions needed by the NIH. Students must demonstrate a sincere interest in pursuing a career in biomedical research. Must be a U.S. citizen, national, or permanent resident. Must have a GPA of 3.5 or better. Must work for NIH for ten consecutive weeks during the sponsored year and, upon graduation, twelve months for each year's award. Initial award for one year, but renewable for up to four years.
Application Contact: NIH Undergraduate Scholarship Program
National Institutes of Health
Federal Building, Room 604
7550 Wisconsin Avenue
Bethesda, MD 20892-9121

National Society of the Colonial Dames of America
Award Name: Colonial Dames Indian Nurse Scholarships
Program Description: Renewable awards for Native American nursing students of good academic standing within two years of completing courses in a prenursing program. Must be a full-time student recommended by the college, with financial need, but not receiving Indian Health Service Scholarship.
Application Contact: Mrs. Leslie N. Boney Jr.
Colonial Dames Indian Nurse Scholarship
2305 Gillette Avenue
Wilmington, NC 28403

Nurses' Educational Funds, Inc.
Award Names: Nurses' Educational Fund Scholarships, NEF Carnegie and Osborne Scholarships
Program Description: Full-time student at master's level, full-time or part-time at doctoral level. For RNs who are U.S. citizens and members of a national professional nursing association. The Carnegie and Osborne Scholarships are specifically for African Americans. Five-dollar fee for application.
Application Contact: Nurses' Educational Funds, Inc.
555 West 57th Street, 13th Floor
New York, NY 10019

Oncology Nursing Foundation
Award Name: Scholarships
Program Description: ONF offers nearly a dozen one-time scholarships and awards at all levels of study, with various requirements and purposes, to nursing students who are interested in pursuing oncology nursing. Contact the Foundation for details about appropriate awards. Application fee: $5.
Application Contact: Oncology Nursing Foundation
Development Coordinator
501 Holiday Drive
Pittsburgh, PA 15220-2749

United States Air Force Reserve Officer Training Corps
Award Name: Air Force ROTC Nursing Scholarships
Program Description: One to four-year programs available to students of nursing and high school seniors. Nursing graduates agree to accept a commission in the Air Force Nurse Corps and serve four years on active duty after successfully completing their licensing examination. Must have a 2.5 GPA for one- and four-year scholarships, or a 2.65 GPA for two- and three-year scholarships. Two exam failures result in a four-year assignment as an Air Force line officer.
Application Contact: Air Force ROTC
Recruiting Branch
551 East Maxwell Boulevard
Maxwell AFB, AL 36112-6106

United States Army Reserve Officer Training Corps
Award Name: Army ROTC Nursing Scholarships
Program Description: Two- to four-year programs available to students of nursing and high school seniors. Nursing graduates agree to accept a commission in the Army Nurse Corps and serve in the military for a period of eight years. This may be fulfilled by serving on active duty two to four years, followed by service in the Army National Guard or the United States Army Reserve, or in the Inactive Ready Reserve for the remainder of the eight-year obligation.
Application Contact: College Army ROTC
P.O. Box 3279
Warminster, PA 18974-9872

United States Department of Health and Human Services
Award Name: DHHS Scholarships for Disadvantaged Students
Program Description: For U.S. citizens who are full-time disadvantaged students pursuing a degree in nursing or other health-care professions. Schools determine deadlines and awards.
Application Contact: Division of Student Assistance
Bureau of Health Professions
5600 Fishers Lane, Suite 8-34
Rockville, MD 20857

United States Department of Health and Human Services
Award Name: National Health Service Corps Scholarships
Program Description: For U.S. citizens enrolled or accepted into an accredited U.S. institution to become family nurse practitioner, physician's assistant, certified nurse-midwife, or other primary care provider. National Health Service Corps scholarship entails one-year service as an NHSC member providing health care in underserved areas for each year of assistance, with a two-year minimum.
Application Contact: National Health Service Corps Scholarships
United States Public Health Service Recruitment
1010 Wayne Avenue, Suite 120
Silver Spring, MD 20910

Abbreviations Used in This Guide

AACN	American Association of Colleges of Nursing
AACSB	American Assembly of Collegiate Schools of Business
AAHC	Association of Academic Health Centers
AAS	Associate in Applied Science
ACT	American College Testing
ACT ASSET	American College Testing Assessment of Skills for Successful Entry and Transfer
ACT COMP	American College Testing College Outcomes Measures Program
ACT PEP	American College Testing Proficiency Examination Program
AD	Associate Degree
ADN	Associate Degree in Nursing
AHNP	Adult Health Nurse Practitioner
ALE	American Language Exam
AMEDD	Army Medical Department
ANA	American Nurses Association
ANP	Adult Nurse Practitioner
APN	Advanced Practice Nurse
ARNP	Advanced Registered Nurse Practitioner
AS	Associate of Science
ASN	Associate of Science in Nursing
BA	Bachelor of Arts
BAA	Bachelor of Applied Arts
BN	Bachelor of Nursing
BNSc	Bachelor of Nursing Science
BRN	Baccalaureate for the Registered Nurse
BS	Bachelor of Science
BScMH	Bachelor of Science in Mental Health
BScN	Bachelor of Science in Nursing
BSN	Bachelor of Science in Nursing
CAI	computer-assisted instruction
CAUSN	Canadian Association of University Schools of Nursing
CCRN	Critical Care Registered Nurse
CGFNS	Commission on Graduates of Foreign Nursing Schools
C!NAHL	Cumulative Index to Nursing and Allied Health Literature
CLAST	College-Level Academic Skills Test
CLEP	College-Level Examination Program
CNA	Certified Nurse Assistant, Certified Nursing Assistant, Certified Nurse's Aide
CNAT	Canadian Nurses Association Testing
CNM	Certified Nurse-Midwife
CNS	Clinical Nurse Specialist
CODEC	coder/decoder
CPR	cardiopulmonary resuscitation
CRNA	Certified Registered Nurse Anesthetist
CS	Certified Specialist
DNS	Doctor of Nursing Science
DNSc	Doctor of Nursing Science
DrPH	Doctor of Public Health
DSN	Doctor of Science in Nursing
EdD	Doctor of Education
ERIC	Educational Resources Information Center
ESL	English as a second language
ETN	Enterostomal Nurse
FAAN	Fellow in the American Academy of Nursing
FAF	Financial Aid Form
FAFSA	Free Application for Federal Student Aid
FNP	Family Nurse Practitioner
FSEOG	Federal Supplemental Educational Opportunity Grant
GED	General Educational Development
GMAT	Graduate Management Admission Test
GPA	grade point average
GPO	Government Printing Office
GRE	Graduate Record Examinations
gyn	gynecology
HIV	human immunodeficiency virus
HMO	health maintenance organization
ICEOP	Illinois Consortium for Educational Opportunities Program
ICU	intensive care unit
ITV	Interactive television
LD	Licensed Dietician
LPN	Licensed Practical Nurse
LVN	Licensed Vocational Nurse
MA	Master of Arts
MAT	Miller Analogies Test
MBA	Master of Business Administration
MCSc	Master of Clinical Science
MDiv	Master of Divinity
MEd	Master of Education
MELAB	Michigan English Language Assessment Battery
MHA	Master of Hospital Administration Master of Health Administration
MHSA	Master of Health Service Administration
MN	Master of Nursing
MNSc	Master of Nursing Science
MOM	Master of Organizational Management
MPA	Master of Public Administration
MPH	Master of Public Health
MPS	Master of Public Service
MS	Master of Science
MSA	Master of Science in Administration
MSc	Master of Science
MSc(A)	Master of Science (Applied)
MScN	Master of Science in Nursing
MSN	Master of Science in Nursing
MSOB	Master of Science in Organizational Behavior

NCLEX-RN	National Council Licensure Examination for Registered Nurses
ND	Doctor of Nursing
NLN	National League for Nursing
NNP	Neonatal Nurse Practitioner
NP	Nurse Practitioner
NSNA	National Student Nurses Association
OB	Organizational Behavior
ob/gyn	obstetrics/gynecology
OCLC	Online Computer Library Center
OM	Organizational Management
PEP	Proficiency Examination Program
PhD	Doctor of Philosophy
PHEAA	Pennsylvania Higher Education Assistance Agency
PHS	Public Health Service
PLUS	Parents' Loan for Undergraduate Students
PNNP	Perinatal Nurse Practitioner
PNP	Pediatric Nurse Practitioner
PSAT	Preliminary Scholastic Assessment Test
RD	Registered Dietician
RN	Registered Nurse
RN,C	Registered Nurse, Certified
RN,CNA	Registered Nurse, Certified in Nursing Administration
RN,CNAA	Registered Nurse, Certified in Nursing Administration, Advanced
RN,CS	Registered Nurse, Certified Specialist
ROTC	Reserve Officers' Training Corps
RPN	Registered Psychiatric Nurse
SAT	Scholastic Assessment Test
SLS	Supplemental Loans to Students
SNA	Student Nurses Association
SNAP	Student Nurses Acting for Progress
SNO	Student Nurses Organization
TB	tuberculosis
TOEFL	Test of English as a Foreign Language
TSE	Test of Spoken English
TWE	Test of Written English
WHNP	Women's Health Nurse Practitioner

PROFILES OF NURSING PROGRAMS

This section contains factual profiles of colleges, with a focus on their nursing programs. It covers such items as enrollment figures, faculty size, admission and degree requirements, costs, financial aid, areas of study, and whom to contact for more information. In addition, presented here are "Noteworthy" items from nursing school or department administrators about unique features of nursing programs, new programs, or interesting aspects of the school or its facilities.

The information in each of these profiles, collected during winter 1996–97, comes from Peterson's Survey of Nursing Programs, which was sent to the Dean or Director of Nursing at each institution.

UNITED STATES

ALABAMA

AUBURN UNIVERSITY
School of Nursing
Auburn University, Alabama

Programs • Generic Baccalaureate • Accelerated RN Baccalaureate • Baccalaureate for Second Degree • Continuing Education

The University State-supported coed university. Founded: 1856. *Primary accreditation:* regional. *Setting:* 1,875-acre small-town campus. *Total enrollment:* 22,122.

The School of Nursing Founded in 1979. *Nursing program faculty:* 14 (57% with doctorates).

Academic Facilities *Campus library:* 1.7 million volumes (6,856 in health, 4,645 in nursing); 21,100 periodical subscriptions (272 health-care related). *Nursing school resources:* CAI, computer lab, nursing audiovisuals, interactive nursing skills videos, learning resource lab.

Student Life *Student services:* health clinic, personal counseling, career counseling, institutionally sponsored work-study program, job placement, campus safety program, special assistance for disabled students. *International student services:* counseling/support. *Nursing student activities:* Sigma Theta Tau, student nurses association, Chi Eta Phi.

Calendar Quarters.

NURSING STUDENT PROFILE

Undergraduate **Enrollment:** 138
Women: 83%; **Men:** 17%; **Minority:** 7%; **International:** 0%; **Part-time:** 7%

BACCALAUREATE PROGRAMS

Contact Ms. Stephanie Parker, Senior Academic Adviser, 101 Miller Hall, School of Nursing, Auburn University, AL 36849-5055, 334-844-5665. *Fax:* 334-844-4177.

Expenses *State resident tuition:* $3000 full-time, $62 part-time. *Nonresident tuition:* $9000 full-time, $186 part-time. *Full-time mandatory fees:* $15. *Room only:* $1410–$2025.

Financial Aid Institutionally sponsored need-based grants/scholarships, institutionally sponsored non-need grants/scholarships, Federal Nursing Student Loans, Federal Work-Study. *Application deadline:* 8/1.

Generic Baccalaureate Program (BSN)

Applying *Required:* SAT I or ACT, TOEFL for nonnative speakers of English, minimum high school GPA of 2.5, minimum college GPA of 2.5, 3 years of high school math, 2 years of high school science, high school biology, high school transcript, 2 letters of recommendation, transcript of college record. 100 prerequisite credits must be completed before admission to the nursing program. *Options:* May apply for transfer of up to 100 total credits. *Application deadline:* 3/1.

Degree Requirements 210 total credit hours, 110 in nursing.

Accelerated RN Baccalaureate Program (BSN)

Applying *Required:* SAT I or ACT, TOEFL for nonnative speakers of English, minimum high school GPA of 2.5, minimum college GPA of 2.5, 3 years of high school math, 2 years of high school science, high school biology, RN license, diploma or AD in nursing, high school transcript, 2 letters of recommendation, transcript of college record. 102 prerequisite credits must be completed before admission to the nursing program. *Options:* May apply for transfer of up to 100 total credits. *Application deadline:* 3/1.

Degree Requirements 210 total credit hours, 110 in nursing.

Baccalaureate for Second Degree Program (BSN)

Applying *Required:* SAT I or ACT, TOEFL for nonnative speakers of English, minimum college GPA of 2.5, interview, 2 letters of recommendation, transcript of college record. 102 prerequisite credits must be completed before admission to the nursing program. *Options:* May apply for transfer of up to 100 total credits. *Application deadline:* 3/1.

Degree Requirements 210 total credit hours, 110 in nursing.

CONTINUING EDUCATION PROGRAM

Contact Dr. Barbara Wilder, Special Projects, Miller Hall, School of Nursing, Auburn University, AL 36849-5055, 334-844-5665. *Fax:* 334-844-4177. *E-mail:* wildebf@mail.auburn.edu

AUBURN UNIVERSITY AT MONTGOMERY
School of Nursing
Montgomery, Alabama

Programs • Generic Baccalaureate • Accelerated RN Baccalaureate

The University State-supported comprehensive coed institution. Part of Auburn University. Founded: 1967. *Primary accreditation:* regional. *Setting:* 500-acre suburban campus. *Total enrollment:* 5,882.

The School of Nursing Founded in 1979. *Nursing program faculty:* 10 (30% with doctorates).

Academic Facilities *Campus library:* 243,788 volumes (10,889 in health, 9,199 in nursing); 1,507 periodical subscriptions (60 health-care related). *Nursing school resources:* CAI, computer lab, nursing audiovisuals, interactive nursing skills videos, learning resource lab.

Student Life *Student services:* health clinic, personal counseling, career counseling, institutionally sponsored work-study program, job placement, special assistance for disabled students. *International student services:* counseling/support, special assistance for nonnative speakers of English, ESL courses. *Nursing student activities:* Sigma Theta Tau, student nurses association.

Calendar Quarters.

NURSING STUDENT PROFILE

Undergraduate **Enrollment:** 156
Women: 83%; **Men:** 17%; **Minority:** 19%; **International:** 1%; **Part-time:** 8%

BACCALAUREATE PROGRAMS

Contact Ms. Lori Stutheit, Adviser, School of Nursing, Auburn University at Montgomery, 7300 University Drive, Montgomery, AL 36117-3596, 205-244-3658. *Fax:* 205-244-3243.

Expenses *State resident tuition:* $2130 full-time, $56 per credit hours part-time. *Nonresident tuition:* $6390 full-time, $168 per credit hours part-time. *Full-time mandatory fees:* $125–$150. *Room only:* $1770–$2000. *Books and supplies per academic year:* ranges from $500 to $650.

Financial Aid Institutionally sponsored non-need grants/scholarships, Federal Pell Grants, Federal Perkins Loans, Federal Supplemental Educational Opportunity Grants, Federal Work-Study. *Application deadline:* 7/1.

Generic Baccalaureate Program (BSN)

Applying *Required:* SAT I, TOEFL for nonnative speakers of English, minimum college GPA of 2.5, transcript of college record. 100 prerequisite credits must be completed before admission to the nursing program. *Options:* May apply for transfer of up to 100 total credits. *Application deadline:* 2/3. *Application fee:* $25.

Degree Requirements 202 total credit hours, 102 in nursing.

Accelerated RN Baccalaureate Program (BSN)

Applying *Required:* SAT I, TOEFL for nonnative speakers of English, minimum college GPA of 2.5, RN license, diploma or AD in nursing, interview, transcript of college record. *Options:* May apply for transfer of up to 100 total credits. *Application deadline:* 2/3 (summer). *Application fee:* $25.

Degree Requirements 202 total credit hours, 102 in nursing.

JACKSONVILLE STATE UNIVERSITY
Lurleen B. Wallace College of Nursing
Jacksonville, Alabama

Programs • Generic Baccalaureate • Accelerated RN Baccalaureate • Continuing Education

The University State-supported comprehensive coed institution. Founded: 1883. *Primary accreditation:* regional. *Setting:* 345-acre small-town campus. *Total enrollment:* 7,697.

The Lurleen B. Wallace College of Nursing Founded in 1967. *Nursing program faculty:* 14 (86% with doctorates).

Academic Facilities *Campus library:* 620,000 volumes (80,000 in health, 22,000 in nursing); 1,558 periodical subscriptions (200 health-care related). *Nursing school resources:* CAI, computer lab, nursing audiovisuals, learning resource lab.

Student Life *Student services:* health clinic, child-care facilities, personal counseling, career counseling, institutionally sponsored work-study program, job placement, campus safety program, special assistance for disabled students, center for individual instruction. *Nursing student activities:* Sigma Theta Tau, recruiter club, student nurses association, Nurses Christian Fellowship.

Calendar Semesters.

NURSING STUDENT PROFILE

Undergraduate **Enrollment:** 647
Women: 84%; **Men:** 16%; **Minority:** 23%; **International:** 1%; **Part-time:** 0%

BACCALAUREATE PROGRAMS

Contact Dr. Beth Hembree, Student Services Coordinator, Lurleen B. Wallace College of Nursing, Jacksonville State University, 700 Pelham Road, North, Jacksonville, AL 36265-9982, 205-782-5276. *Fax:* 205-782-5406.

Expenses *State resident tuition:* $1940 full-time, $81 per hour part-time. *Nonresident tuition:* $2910 full-time, $122 per hour part-time. *Full-time mandatory fees:* $10–$180. *Room only:* $1080–$1330. *Books and supplies per academic year:* ranges from $250 to $750.

Financial Aid Institutionally sponsored need-based grants/scholarships, institutionally sponsored non-need grants/scholarships, Federal Supplemental Educational Opportunity Grants, Federal Work-Study. *Application deadline:* 3/15.

Generic Baccalaureate Program (BS)

Applying *Required:* SAT I or ACT, 3 years of high school math, 2 years of high school science, high school transcript, written essay, transcript of college record. 45 prerequisite credits must be completed before admission to the nursing program. *Options:* May apply for transfer of up to 56 total credits. *Application deadlines:* 6/1 (fall), 10/1 (spring). *Application fee:* $20.

Degree Requirements 129 total credit hours, 70 in nursing. English competency exam.

Distance learning Courses provided through video.

Accelerated RN Baccalaureate Program (BS)

Applying *Required:* SAT I or ACT, RN license, diploma or AD in nursing, high school transcript, transcript of college record. 45 prerequisite credits must be completed before admission to the nursing program. *Options:* Advanced standing available through advanced placement exams. May apply for transfer of up to 64 total credits. *Application deadlines:* 6/1 (fall), 10/1 (spring). *Application fee:* $20.

Degree Requirements 129 total credit hours, 70 in nursing. English competency exam.

Distance learning Courses provided through video.

CONTINUING EDUCATION PROGRAM

Contact Dr. Beth Hembree, Student Services Coordinator, Lurleen B. Wallace College of Nursing, Jacksonville State University, 700 Pelham Road, North, Jacksonville, AL 36265-9882, 205-782-5276. *Fax:* 205-782-5406.

OAKWOOD COLLEGE
Department of Nursing
Huntsville, Alabama

Program • RN Baccalaureate

The College Independent Seventh-day Adventist 4-year coed college. Founded: 1896. *Primary accreditation:* regional. *Setting:* 1,200-acre campus. *Total enrollment:* 1,626.

The Department of Nursing Founded in 1973.

BACCALAUREATE PROGRAM

Contact Dr. Caryll Dormer, BSN Coordinator, Department of Nursing, Oakwood College, Oakwood Road, NW, Huntsville, AL 35896, 205-726-7000. *Fax:* 205-726-7409.

Expenses *Tuition:* $7440 full-time, $310 per credit hour part-time.

RN Baccalaureate Program (BSN)

Applying *Required:* SAT I or ACT, TOEFL for nonnative speakers of English, minimum high school GPA of 2.0, RN license, diploma or AD in nursing, high school transcript, 2 letters of recommendation. *Application fee:* $45.

SAMFORD UNIVERSITY
Ida V. Moffett School of Nursing
Birmingham, Alabama

Programs • Generic Baccalaureate • RN Baccalaureate • RN to Master's

The University Independent Baptist coed university. Founded: 1841. *Primary accreditation:* regional. *Setting:* 280-acre suburban campus. *Total enrollment:* 4,630.

The Ida V. Moffett School of Nursing Founded in 1973. *Nursing program faculty:* 26 (33% with doctorates).

Academic Facilities *Campus library:* 762,867 volumes (2,000 in health, 12,000 in nursing); 175 periodical subscriptions (175 health-care related). *Nursing school resources:* CAI, computer lab, nursing audiovisuals, learning resource lab.

Student Life *Student services:* health clinic, personal counseling, career counseling, institutionally sponsored work-study program, job placement, campus safety program, special assistance for disabled students, Elder Care (day time) facilities. *International student services:* counseling/support. *Nursing student activities:* Sigma Theta Tau, student nurses association, Nurses Christian Fellowship.

Calendar Semesters, January term (3 weeks).

NURSING STUDENT PROFILE

Undergraduate **Enrollment:** 241
Women: 91%; **Men:** 9%; **Minority:** 8%; **International:** 4%; **Part-time:** 29%
Graduate **Enrollment:** 15
Women: 73%; **Men:** 27%; **Minority:** 20%; **International:** 0%; **Part-time:** 60%

BACCALAUREATE PROGRAMS

Contact Jan Paine, Assistant to the Dean for Enrollment Management, Ida V. Moffett School of Nursing, Samford University, 800 Lakeshore Drive, Birmingham, AL 35229, 205-870-2872. *Fax:* 205-870-2219. *E-mail:* jgpaine@samford.edu

Expenses *Tuition:* $9070 full-time, $300 per hour part-time. *Full-time mandatory fees:* $430. *Room and board:* $4030. *Room only:* $1970. *Books and supplies per academic year:* $550.

Financial Aid Institutionally sponsored need-based grants/scholarships, institutionally sponsored non-need grants/scholarships, Federal Nursing Student Loans, Federal Pell Grants, Federal Supplemental Educational Opportunity Grants, Federal Work-Study. 60% of undergraduate students in nursing programs received some form of financial aid in 1995–96. *Application deadline:* 3/1.

Generic Baccalaureate Program (BSN)

Applying *Required:* SAT I or ACT, TOEFL for nonnative speakers of English, Nursing Entrance Test, minimum high school GPA of 3.0, high school chemistry, high school biology, diploma or AD in nursing, high school transcript, 2 letters of recommendation, written essay, transcript of college record. *Options:* Advanced standing available through the following means: advanced placement exams, credit by exam. May apply for transfer of up to 64 total credits. *Application deadlines:* 8/1 (fall), 1/1 (spring). *Application fee:* $25.

Degree Requirements 71 total credit hours in nursing.

RN Baccalaureate Program (BSN)

Applying *Required:* TOEFL for nonnative speakers of English, RN license, diploma or AD in nursing, 2 letters of recommendation, written essay, transcript of college record, minimum 2.5 GPA in nursing. *Options:* Course work may be accelerated. May apply for transfer of up to 64 total credits. *Application deadline:* rolling. *Application fee:* $25.

Degree Requirements 71 total credit hours in nursing.

MASTER'S PROGRAM

Contact Jan Paine, Assistant to the Dean for Enrollment Management, Ida V. Moffett School of Nursing, Samford University, 800 Lakeshore Drive, Birmingham, AL 35229, 205-870-2872. *Fax:* 205-870-2219. *E-mail:* jgpaine@samford.edu

Areas of Study Nursing administration; nursing education; nurse practitioner program in family health.

Expenses *Tuition:* $6120 full-time, $340 per semester hour part-time. *Full-time mandatory fees:* $0. *Part-time mandatory fees:* $0. *Books and supplies per academic year:* ranges from $300 to $500.

Financial Aid Federal Direct Loans, institutionally sponsored loans, employment opportunities. *Application deadline:* 3/1.

RN to Master's Program (MSN)

Applying *Required:* GRE General Test, Miller Analogies Test, TOEFL for nonnative speakers of English, bachelor's degree in nursing, minimum GPA of 3.0, RN license, 1 year of clinical experience, physical assessment course, statistics course, professional liability/malpractice insurance, essay, interview, 3 letters of recommendation, transcript of college record. *Application deadline:* 5/10. *Application fee:* $25.

Degree Requirements 47–54 total credit hours dependent upon track, 31–47 in nursing, 20–42 in business, education, or missions.

TROY STATE UNIVERSITY
School of Nursing
Troy, Alabama

Programs • Generic Baccalaureate • RN Baccalaureate • MSN

The University State-supported comprehensive coed institution. Part of Troy State University System. Founded: 1887. *Primary accreditation:* regional. *Setting:* 500-acre small-town campus. *Total enrollment:* 5,420.

The School of Nursing Founded in 1969. *Nursing program faculty:* 22. *Off-campus program sites:* Montgomery, Phenix City, Dothan.

Academic Facilities *Campus library:* 27,000 volumes in health. *Nursing school resources:* CAI, computer lab, nursing audiovisuals, learning resource lab.

Student Life *Student services:* health clinic, child-care facilities, personal counseling, career counseling, institutionally sponsored work-study program, job placement, campus safety program, special assistance for disabled students. *International student services:* counseling/support. *Nursing student activities:* Sigma Theta Tau, nursing club, student nurses association.

Calendar Quarters.

NURSING STUDENT PROFILE

Undergraduate **Enrollment:** 536
Women: 90%; **Men:** 10%; **International:** 1%; **Part-time:** 26%

Graduate **Enrollment:** 37
Women: 100%; **Minority:** 22%; **Part-time:** 49%

BACCALAUREATE PROGRAMS

Contact Dr. Donna H. Bedsole, Assistant Dean for Baccalaureate Programs, School of Nursing, Troy State University, Troy, AL 36082, 334-670-3428. *Fax:* 334-670-3744.

Expenses *State resident tuition:* $2640 full-time, $53 per credit hour part-time. *Nonresident tuition:* $5280 full-time, $105 per credit hour part-time. *Room only:* $3690. *Books and supplies per academic year:* $350.

Financial Aid Institutionally sponsored non-need grants/scholarships, Federal Direct Loans, Federal Nursing Student Loans.

Generic Baccalaureate Program (BSN)

Applying *Required:* SAT I, ACT, math and English proficiency test, minimum high school GPA of 2.0, high school transcript. 90 prerequisite credits must be completed before admission to the nursing program. *Options:* Advanced standing available through credit by exam. *Application deadlines:* 4/15 (fall), 10/15 (spring).

Degree Requirements 200 total credit hours, 105 in nursing.

RN Baccalaureate Program (BSN)

Applying *Required:* math and English proficiency test, RN license, diploma or AD in nursing, transcript of college record. 90 prerequisite credits must be completed before admission to the nursing program. *Options:* Advanced standing available through credit by exam. *Application deadline:* rolling.

Degree Requirements 200 total credit hours, 105 in nursing.

MASTER'S PROGRAM

Contact Dr. Charlene Schwab, Assistant Dean for MSN Program, School of Nursing, Troy State University, 305 South Ripley Street, Montgomery, AL 36104, 334-834-2320. *Fax:* 334-262-4167.

Areas of Study Clinical nurse specialist programs in adult health nursing, maternity-newborn nursing; nursing administration; nursing education; nurse practitioner program in family health.

Expenses *State resident tuition:* $71 per credit hour. *Nonresident tuition:* $142 per credit hour.

Financial Aid Nurse traineeships, fellowships.

MSN Program

Applying *Required:* GRE General Test, Miller Analogies Test, bachelor's degree in nursing, minimum GPA of 3.0, RN license, physical assessment course, 3 letters of recommendation, transcript of college record. *Application deadline:* rolling.

Degree Requirements 48 total credit hours, 43 in nursing.

Distance learning Courses provided on-line.

TUSKEGEE UNIVERSITY
School of Nursing and Allied Health
Tuskegee, Alabama

Programs • Generic Baccalaureate • RN Baccalaureate • Continuing Education

The University Independent comprehensive coed institution. Founded: 1881. *Primary accreditation:* regional. *Setting:* 5,000-acre small-town campus. *Total enrollment:* 3,100.

The School of Nursing and Allied Health Founded in 1892. *Nursing program faculty:* 12 (36% with doctorates). *Off-campus program site:* Atlanta, GA.

Academic Facilities *Campus library:* 283,000 volumes (167 in health, 1,279 in nursing); 299 periodical subscriptions (125 health-care related). *Nursing school resources:* CAI, computer lab, nursing audiovisuals, learning resource lab.

Student Life *Student services:* health clinic, personal counseling, career counseling, institutionally sponsored work-study program, job placement, campus safety program, special assistance for disabled students, tutoring. *International student services:* counseling/support. *Nursing student activities:* Sigma Theta Tau, nursing club, student nurses association, Chi Eta Phi.

Calendar Semesters.

NURSING STUDENT PROFILE

Undergraduate **Enrollment:** 127
Women: 99%; **Men:** 1%; **Minority:** 99%; **International:** 0%

BACCALAUREATE PROGRAMS

Contact Dr. Mildred Gardner, Associate Dean, School of Nursing and Allied Health, Tuskegee University, Tuskegee, AL 36088, 334-727-8185. *Fax:* 334-727-5461.

Expenses *State resident tuition:* $8020 full-time, $324 per credit part-time. *Full-time mandatory fees:* $225. *Room and board:* $3750. *Books and supplies per academic year:* ranges from $350 to $400.

Financial Aid Institutionally sponsored need-based grants/scholarships, institutionally sponsored non-need grants/scholarships, Federal Direct

Tuskegee University (continued)

Loans, Federal Nursing Student Loans, Federal Perkins Loans, Federal Supplemental Educational Opportunity Grants, Federal Work-Study. *Application deadline:* 3/31.

Generic Baccalaureate Program (BSN)

Applying *Required:* SAT I or ACT, minimum high school GPA of 2.5, minimum college GPA of 2.5, 2 years of high school math, high school chemistry, high school biology, high school transcript, transcript of college record. *Options:* Advanced standing available through the following means: advanced placement exams, credit by exam. May apply for transfer of up to 60 total credits. *Application deadline:* rolling. *Application fee:* $20.

Degree Requirements 130 total credit hours, 69 in nursing.

RN Baccalaureate Program (BSN)

Applying *Required:* SAT I or ACT, RN license, diploma or AD in nursing, transcript of college record. *Options:* Advanced standing available through the following means: advanced placement exams, credit by exam. May apply for transfer of up to 60 total credits. *Application deadline:* rolling. *Application fee:* $20.

Degree Requirements 130 total credit hours, 69 in nursing.

CONTINUING EDUCATION PROGRAM

Contact Mr. Michael Johnson, Director of Gerontology Program, School of Nursing and Allied Health, Tuskegee University, Tuskegee, AL 36088, 334-727-8187. *Fax:* 334-727-5461.

UNIVERSITY OF ALABAMA

Capstone College of Nursing
Tuscaloosa, Alabama

Programs • Generic Baccalaureate • RN Baccalaureate • Continuing Education

The University State-supported coed university. Part of University of Alabama System. Founded: 1831. *Primary accreditation:* regional. *Setting:* 1,000-acre suburban campus. *Total enrollment:* 18,513.

The Capstone College of Nursing Founded in 1976. *Nursing program faculty:* 28 (53% with doctorates).

Academic Facilities *Campus library:* 1.9 million volumes (25,000 in health, 3,500 in nursing); 16,878 periodical subscriptions (1,500 health-care related). *Nursing school resources:* CAI, computer lab, nursing audiovisuals, interactive nursing skills videos, learning resource lab.

Student Life *Student services:* health clinic, child-care facilities, personal counseling, career counseling, institutionally sponsored work-study program, job placement, campus safety program, special assistance for disabled students. *International student services:* counseling/support, special assistance for nonnative speakers of English. *Nursing student activities:* Sigma Theta Tau, student nurses association, student government.

Calendar Semesters.

NURSING STUDENT PROFILE

Undergraduate **Enrollment:** 571
Women: 86%; **Men:** 14%; **Minority:** 23%; **International:** 1%

BACCALAUREATE PROGRAMS

Contact Dr. Tom Buttram, Director, Office of Student Services, Capstone College of Nursing, University of Alabama, Box 870358, Tuscaloosa, AL 35487-0358, 205-348-6640. *Fax:* 205-348-5559. *E-mail:* tbuttram@uaivm.ua.edu

Expenses *State resident tuition:* $2470 per academic year. *Nonresident tuition:* $6268 per academic year. *Room and board:* $1840. *Room only:* $1030. *Books and supplies per academic year:* ranges from $850 to $900.

Financial Aid Institutionally sponsored need-based grants/scholarships, institutionally sponsored non-need grants/scholarships, Federal Direct Loans, Federal Pell Grants, Federal Perkins Loans, Federal Supplemental Educational Opportunity Grants, Federal Work-Study. 49% of undergraduate students in nursing programs received some form of financial aid in 1995–96. *Application deadline:* 3/1.

Generic Baccalaureate Program (BSN)

Applying *Required:* SAT I, ACT, TOEFL for nonnative speakers of English, minimum college GPA of 2.5, high school transcript, transcript of college record. 64 prerequisite credits must be completed before admission to the nursing program. *Options:* Advanced standing available through the following means: advanced placement exams, credit by exam. Course work may be accelerated. May apply for transfer of up to 64 total credits. *Application deadlines:* 7/14 (fall), 12/9 (spring). *Application fee:* $20.

Degree Requirements 128 total credit hours, 64 in nursing.

RN Baccalaureate Program (BSN)

Applying *Required:* minimum college GPA of 2.5, RN license, diploma or AD in nursing, transcript of college record. *Options:* May apply for transfer of up to 64 total credits. *Application deadlines:* 7/14 (fall), 12/9 (spring).

Degree Requirements 130 total credit hours, 64 in nursing.

CONTINUING EDUCATION PROGRAM

Contact Ms. Geri L. Stone, Director, Professional and Management Programs, College of Continuing Studies, University of Alabama, Box 870388, Tuscaloosa, AL 35487-0388, 205-348-6225.

UNIVERSITY OF ALABAMA AT BIRMINGHAM

School of Nursing
Birmingham, Alabama

Programs • Generic Baccalaureate • Accelerated RN Baccalaureate • MSN • RN to Master's • MSN/MPH • DSN • Postdoctoral • Continuing Education

The University State-supported coed university. Part of University of Alabama System. Founded: 1969. *Primary accreditation:* regional. *Setting:* 265-acre urban campus. *Total enrollment:* 16,452.

The School of Nursing Founded in 1950. *Nursing program faculty:* 81 (73% with doctorates). *Off-campus program site:* Tuscaloosa.

Academic Facilities *Campus library:* 1.1 million volumes (266,988 in health); 5,254 periodical subscriptions (2,532 health-care related). *Nursing school resources:* CAI, computer lab, nursing audiovisuals, interactive nursing skills videos, center for nursing research.

Student Life *Student services:* health clinic, child-care facilities, personal counseling, career counseling, institutionally sponsored work-study program, job placement, campus safety program, special assistance for disabled students. *International student services:* counseling/support, special assistance for nonnative speakers of English. *Nursing student activities:* Sigma Theta Tau, student nurses association.

Calendar Quarters.

NURSING STUDENT PROFILE

Undergraduate **Enrollment:** 382
Women: 78%; **Men:** 22%; **Minority:** 18%; **International:** 1%; **Part-time:** 14%
Graduate **Enrollment:** 309
Women: 94%; **Men:** 6%; **Minority:** 19%; **International:** 4%; **Part-time:** 50%

BACCALAUREATE PROGRAMS

Contact Dr. Jerry Beavers, Director of Student Affairs, School of Nursing, University of Alabama at Birmingham, 1701 University Boulevard, Birmingham, AL 35294-1210, 205-934-5490.

Expenses *State resident tuition:* $2700 full-time, $90 per semester credit hour part-time. *Nonresident tuition:* $5100 full-time, $170 per semester credit hour part-time. *Full-time mandatory fees:* $394–$403. *Part-time mandatory fees:* $191–$194. *Room and board:* $4788. *Room only:* $1467. *Books and supplies per academic year:* $750.

Financial Aid Institutionally sponsored need-based grants/scholarships, institutionally sponsored non-need grants/scholarships, Federal Supplemental Educational Opportunity Grants, Federal Work-Study. 71% of undergraduate students in nursing programs received some form of financial aid in 1995–96. *Application deadline:* 8/1.

Generic Baccalaureate Program (BSN)

Applying *Required:* ACT, TOEFL for nonnative speakers of English, minimum high school GPA of 2.0, minimum college GPA of 2.5, high school transcript, written essay, transcript of college record. 61 prerequisite credits must be completed before admission to the nursing program. *Options:* Advanced standing available through the following means: advanced placement exams, credit by exam. May apply for transfer of up to 64 total credits. *Application deadlines:* 6/14 (fall), 1/12 (spring), 10/11 (winter). *Application fee:* $25.

Degree Requirements 132 total credit hours, 68 in nursing.

Accelerated RN Baccalaureate Program (BSN)

Applying *Required:* ACT, TOEFL for nonnative speakers of English, minimum high school GPA of 2.0, minimum college GPA of 2.5, RN license, diploma or AD in nursing, high school transcript, written essay, transcript of college record, current experience as an RN in a clinical setting. 53 prerequisite credits must be completed before admission to the nursing program. *Options:* Advanced standing available through the following means: advanced placement exams, advanced placement without credit, credit by exam. May apply for transfer of up to 64 total credits. *Application deadlines:* 6/13 (fall), 1/10 (spring), 10/10 (winter). *Application fee:* $25.

Degree Requirements 132 total credit hours, 68 in nursing.

MASTER'S PROGRAMS

Contact Dr. Linda Miers, Chair, Graduate Studies, School of Nursing, University of Alabama at Birmingham, 1701 University Boulevard, Birmingham, AL 35294-1210, 205-934-6102. *E-mail:* miersl@admin.son.uab.edu

Areas of Study Nurse practitioner programs in acute care, adult health, child care/pediatrics, family health, gerontology, neonatal health, occupational health, primary care, women's health.

Expenses *State resident tuition:* $3330 full-time, $111 per semester credit hour part-time. *Nonresident tuition:* $6060 full-time, $202 per semester credit hour part-time. *Full-time mandatory fees:* $321–$330. *Part-time mandatory fees:* $167–$170. *Room and board:* $4788. *Room only:* $1467. *Books and supplies per academic year:* $750.

Financial Aid Graduate assistantships, nurse traineeships, Federal Direct Loans, Federal Nursing Student Loans, employment opportunities, scholarships. 15% of master's level students in nursing programs received some form of financial aid in 1995-96. *Application deadline:* 8/1.

MSN Program

Applying *Required:* GRE General Test (minimum combined score of 1200 on three tests), TOEFL for nonnative speakers of English, bachelor's degree in nursing, minimum GPA of 3.0, RN license, physical assessment course, statistics course, professional liability/malpractice insurance, essay, interview, 2 letters of recommendation, transcript of college record. *Application deadlines:* 5/30 (fall), 12/6 (spring). *Application fee:* $25.

Degree Requirements 44–52 total credit hours dependent upon track, 24–26 in nursing, 20–26 in pharmacology, pathophysiology, health promotion research. Thesis or research project.

Distance learning Courses provided through video. Specific degree requirements include presence at one of two outreach sites: Auburn University School of Nursing or Capstone College of Nursing at the University of Alabama in Tuscaloosa.

RN to Master's Program (MSN)

Applying *Required:* GRE General Test (minimum combined score of 1200 on three tests), minimum GPA of 3.0, RN license, physical assessment course, professional liability/malpractice insurance, essay, interview, 3 letters of recommendation, transcript of college record. *Application deadlines:* 5/30 (fall), 12/6 (spring). *Application fee:* $25.

Degree Requirements 43 total credit hours, 41 in nursing. Thesis or research project.

MSN/MPH Program

Applying *Required:* GRE General Test (minimum combined score of 1200 on three tests), TOEFL for nonnative speakers of English, bachelor's degree in nursing, minimum GPA of 3.0, RN license, physical assessment course, statistics course, professional liability/malpractice insurance, essay, interview, letter of recommendation, transcript of college record. *Application deadlines:* 5/30 (fall), 12/6 (spring). *Application fee:* $25.

Degree Requirements 68 total credit hours, 35 in nursing, 33 in public health and maternal-child health. Thesis or research project.

DOCTORAL PROGRAM

Contact Dr. Carol Dashiff, Associate Dean, Graduate Studies, School of Nursing, University of Alabama at Birmingham, 1701 University Boulevard, Birmingham, AL 35294-1210, 205-934-3485. *E-mail:* dashiffc@admin.son.uab.edu

Areas of Study Nursing administration, nursing education, clinical practice, nursing policy.

Expenses *State resident tuition:* $3330 full-time, $111 per semester credit hour part-time. *Nonresident tuition:* $6060 full-time, $202 per semester credit hour part-time. *Full-time mandatory fees:* $321–$330. *Part-time mandatory fees:* $167–$170. *Room and board:* $4788. *Room only:* $1467. *Books and supplies per academic year:* $750.

Financial Aid Graduate assistantships, nurse traineeships, fellowships, grants, opportunities for employment, institutionally sponsored non-need-based grants/scholarships. *Application deadline:* 8/1.

DSN Program

Applying *Required:* GRE General Test, TOEFL for nonnative speakers of English, master's degree in nursing, statistics course, interview, letter of recommendation, writing sample. *Application deadlines:* 6/2 (fall), 12/1 (spring), 2/16 (summer). *Application fee:* $30.

Degree Requirements 63–70 total credit hours dependent upon track; dissertation; oral exam; written exam; defense of dissertation; residency.

POSTDOCTORAL PROGRAM

Contact Dr. Carol Dashiff, Associate Dean, Graduate Studies, School of Nursing, University of Alabama at Birmingham, 1701 University Boulevard, Birmingham, AL 35294-1210, 205-934-3485. *E-mail:* dashiffc@admin.son.uab.edu

Areas of Study Nursing theory, practice, research, and role development.

CONTINUING EDUCATION PROGRAM

Contact Dr. Mable Lamb, Coordinator of Development and Education, 1917 Building, Room 220, Organizational Development and Education, University of Alabama at Birmingham, Birmingham, AL 35294-6901, 205-934-5041. *E-mail:* lamb-m@nursing.his.uab.edu

THE UNIVERSITY OF ALABAMA IN HUNTSVILLE

College of Nursing
Huntsville, Alabama

Programs • Generic Baccalaureate • Accelerated RN Baccalaureate • Post-Master's • Continuing Education

The University State-supported coed university. Part of University of Alabama System. Founded: 1950. *Primary accreditation:* regional. *Setting:* 337-acre urban campus. *Total enrollment:* 7,264.

The College of Nursing Founded in 1972. *Nursing program faculty:* 33 (34% with doctorates). *Off-campus program sites:* Decatur, Rainsville.

Academic Facilities *Campus library:* 394,334 volumes (9,000 in health, 11,562 in nursing); 3,250 periodical subscriptions (650 health-care related). *Nursing school resources:* CAI, computer lab, nursing audiovisuals, interactive nursing skills videos, learning resource lab.

Student Life *Student services:* health clinic, child-care facilities, personal counseling, career counseling, institutionally sponsored work-study program, job placement, campus safety program, special assistance for disabled students. *International student services:* counseling/support, special assistance for nonnative speakers of English, ESL courses. *Nursing student activities:* Sigma Theta Tau, student nurses association.

Calendar Semesters.

NURSING STUDENT PROFILE

Undergraduate **Enrollment:** 482
Women: 85%; **Men:** 15%; **Minority:** 7%; **International:** 0%; **Part-time:** 6%
Graduate **Enrollment:** 147
Women: 90%; **Men:** 10%; **Minority:** 10%; **International:** 0%; **Part-time:** 22%

BACCALAUREATE PROGRAMS

Contact Ms. Mary Beth Magathan, Director, Nursing Student Affairs, College of Nursing, University of Alabama in Huntsville, Huntsville, AL 35899, 205-890-6742. *Fax:* 205-890-6026. *E-mail:* magathm@email.uah.edu

Expenses *State resident tuition:* $2978 full-time, $1594 per academic year part-time. *Nonresident tuition:* $6246 full-time, $3340 per academic year

The University of Alabama in Huntsville (continued)

part-time. *Full-time mandatory fees:* $690–$840. *Part-time mandatory fees:* $350–$400. *Room and board:* $2390–$3570. *Room only:* $1390–$2570. *Books and supplies per academic year:* ranges from $500 to $700.

Financial Aid Institutionally sponsored need-based grants/scholarships, institutionally sponsored non-need grants/scholarships, Federal Supplemental Educational Opportunity Grants, Federal Work-Study. 41% of undergraduate students in nursing programs received some form of financial aid in 1995–96. *Application deadline:* 3/15.

Generic Baccalaureate Program (BSN)

Applying *Required:* SAT I, ACT, TOEFL for nonnative speakers of English, minimum high school GPA of 2.0, minimum college GPA of 2.0, high school transcript, transcript of college record. 60 prerequisite credits must be completed before admission to the nursing program. *Options:* Advanced standing available through the following means: advanced placement exams, credit by exam. Course work may be accelerated. May apply for transfer of up to 96 total credits. *Application deadline:* 3/1. *Application fee:* $20.

Degree Requirements 128 total credit hours, 66 in nursing.

Accelerated RN Baccalaureate Program (BSN)

Applying *Required:* TOEFL for nonnative speakers of English, minimum high school GPA of 2.0, minimum college GPA of 2.0, RN license, diploma or AD in nursing, high school transcript, transcript of college record. 59 prerequisite credits must be completed before admission to the nursing program. *Options:* Course work may be accelerated. May apply for transfer of up to 96 total credits. *Application deadline:* 4/1 (summer). *Application fee:* $20.

Degree Requirements 128 total credit hours, 60 in nursing.

MASTER'S PROGRAM

Contact Ms. Mary Beth Magathan, Director, Nursing Student Affairs, College of Nursing, University of Alabama in Huntsville, Huntsville, AL 35899, 205-890-6742. *Fax:* 205-890-6026. *E-mail:* magathm@email.uah.edu

Areas of Study Nursing administration; nurse practitioner programs in acute care, family health.

Expenses *State resident tuition:* $3386 full-time, $1922 per academic year part-time. *Nonresident tuition:* $6918 full-time, $3306 per academic year part-time. *Full-time mandatory fees:* $225–$565. *Part-time mandatory fees:* $110–$280. *Books and supplies per academic year:* ranges from $500 to $700.

Financial Aid Graduate assistantships, nurse traineeships, employment opportunities, institutionally sponsored non-need-based grants/scholarships. 34% of master's level students in nursing programs received some form of financial aid in 1995-96. *Application deadline:* 5/2.

Post-Master's Program

Applying *Required:* RN license, physical assessment course, professional liability/malpractice insurance, essay, 2 letters of recommendation, transcript of college record, pathophysiology course; MSN. *Application deadline:* 11/1. *Application fee:* $20.

Degree Requirements 18 total credit hours, 18 in nursing.

CONTINUING EDUCATION PROGRAM

Contact Dr. Fay Raines, Dean, College of Nursing, University of Alabama in Huntsville, Huntsville, AL 35899, 205-890-6345. *Fax:* 205-890-6026. *E-mail:* rainesc@email.uah.edu

See full description on page 518.

UNIVERSITY OF MOBILE

School of Nursing
Mobile, Alabama

Programs • Generic Baccalaureate • RN Baccalaureate • MSN

The University Independent Southern Baptist comprehensive coed institution. Founded: 1961. *Primary accreditation:* regional. *Setting:* 830-acre suburban campus. *Total enrollment:* 2,156.

The School of Nursing Founded in 1973. *Nursing program faculty:* 24 (38% with doctorates).

Academic Facilities *Campus library:* 113,698 volumes (7,846 in health, 6,500 in nursing); 571 periodical subscriptions (109 health-care related). *Nursing school resources:* CAI, computer lab, nursing audiovisuals, interactive nursing skills videos, learning resource lab.

Student Life *Student services:* child-care facilities, personal counseling, career counseling, institutionally sponsored work-study program, job placement. *International student services:* counseling/support, ESL courses. *Nursing student activities:* nursing club, student nurses association.

Calendar Semesters.

NURSING STUDENT PROFILE

Undergraduate **Enrollment:** 180
Women: 80%; **Men:** 20%; **Minority:** 25%; **International:** 5%; **Part-time:** 5%
Graduate **Enrollment:** 56
Women: 90%; **Men:** 10%; **Minority:** 30%; **International:** 0%; **Part-time:** 75%

BACCALAUREATE PROGRAMS

Contact Dr. Rosemary Adams, Dean, School of Nursing, University of Mobile, PO Box 13220, Mobile, AL 36663-0220, 205-675-5990. *Fax:* 205-679-0875.

Expenses *Tuition:* $6840 full-time, $228 per hour part-time. *Full-time mandatory fees:* $200–$300. *Part-time mandatory fees:* $50–$100. *Room and board:* $1940–$2040. *Books and supplies per academic year:* ranges from $250 to $300.

Financial Aid Federal Pell Grants, Federal Supplemental Educational Opportunity Grants, Federal Work-Study. 89% of undergraduate students in nursing programs received some form of financial aid in 1995–96. *Application deadline:* 8/1.

Generic Baccalaureate Program (BSN)

Applying *Required:* ACT, TOEFL for nonnative speakers of English, minimum college GPA of 2.5, high school transcript, transcript of college record. 54 prerequisite credits must be completed before admission to the nursing program. *Options:* Course work may be accelerated. May apply for transfer of up to 96 total credits. *Application deadline:* rolling. *Application fee:* $30.

Degree Requirements 128 total credit hours, 58 in nursing.

RN Baccalaureate Program (BSN)

Applying *Required:* TOEFL for nonnative speakers of English, minimum college GPA of 2.5, RN license, diploma or AD in nursing, transcript of college record. *Options:* Course work may be accelerated. May apply for transfer of up to 96 total credits. *Application deadline:* rolling. *Application fee:* $30.

Degree Requirements 128 total credit hours, 54 in nursing.

MASTER'S PROGRAM

Contact Dr. Rosemary Adams, Dean, School of Nursing, University of Mobile, PO Box 13220, Mobile, AL 36663-0220, 205-675-5990. *Fax:* 205-679-0875.

Areas of Study Clinical nurse specialist program in adult health nursing; nursing administration; nurse practitioner program in family health.

Expenses *Tuition:* $2700 full-time, $150 per semester hour part-time. *Full-time mandatory fees:* $150. *Room and board:* $1940–$2040. *Books and supplies per academic year:* ranges from $200 to $300.

MSN Program

Applying *Required:* GRE General Test, Miller Analogies Test, bachelor's degree in nursing, minimum GPA of 3.0, RN license, physical assessment course, statistics course, transcript of college record. *Application deadline:* rolling.

Degree Requirements 36 total credit hours, 33 in nursing.

UNIVERSITY OF NORTH ALABAMA
College of Nursing
Florence, Alabama

Programs • Generic Baccalaureate • RN Baccalaureate

The University State-supported comprehensive coed institution. Part of Alabama Commission on Higher Education. Founded: 1872. *Primary accreditation:* regional. *Setting:* 100-acre urban campus. *Total enrollment:* 5,437.

The College of Nursing Founded in 1973. *Nursing program faculty:* 14 (36% with doctorates).

Academic Facilities *Campus library:* 294,359 volumes; 2,128 periodical subscriptions. *Nursing school resources:* CAI, computer lab, nursing audiovisuals, interactive nursing skills videos.

Student Life *Student services:* health clinic, child-care facilities, career counseling, institutionally sponsored work-study program, campus safety program, special assistance for disabled students. *International student services:* special assistance for nonnative speakers of English, ESL courses. *Nursing student activities:* student nurses association.

Calendar Semesters.

NURSING STUDENT PROFILE

Undergraduate **Enrollment:** 225
Women: 90%; **Men:** 10%; **Minority:** 10%; **International:** 1%

BACCALAUREATE PROGRAMS

Contact Dr. Frenesi P. Wilson, Dean, Stevens Hall, College of Nursing, University of North Alabama, Florence, AL 35632-0001, 205-760-4311. *Fax:* 205-760-4664.

Expenses *State resident tuition:* $2082 full-time, $79 per semester hour part-time. *Nonresident tuition:* $3804 full-time, $159 per semester hour part-time. *Full-time mandatory fees:* $240–$300. *Room and board:* $1926–$4120. *Room only:* $1470–$2270. *Books and supplies per academic year:* ranges from $300 to $450.

Financial Aid Federal Pell Grants, Federal Perkins Loans, Federal Supplemental Educational Opportunity Grants, Federal Work-Study. *Application deadline:* 4/1.

Generic Baccalaureate Program (BSN)

Applying *Required:* SAT I or ACT, TOEFL for nonnative speakers of English, minimum college GPA of 2.1, high school transcript. 60 prerequisite credits must be completed before admission to the nursing program. *Options:* May apply for transfer of up to 64 total credits. *Application deadlines:* 3/1 (fall), 10/1 (spring). *Application fee:* $20.

Degree Requirements 128 total credit hours, 60 in nursing.

RN Baccalaureate Program (BSN)

Applying *Required:* ACT, TOEFL for nonnative speakers of English, minimum college GPA of 2.1, RN license, diploma or AD in nursing. 60 prerequisite credits must be completed before admission to the nursing program. *Options:* Advanced standing available through credit by exam. May apply for transfer of up to 60–64 total credits. *Application deadlines:* 3/1 (fall), 11/1 (spring).

Degree Requirements 128 total credit hours, 60 in nursing.

UNIVERSITY OF SOUTH ALABAMA
College of Nursing
Mobile, Alabama

Programs • Generic Baccalaureate • Accelerated RN Baccalaureate • RN to Master's • Master's for Nurses with Non-Nursing Degrees

The University State-supported coed university. Founded: 1963. *Primary accreditation:* regional. *Setting:* 1,215-acre suburban campus. *Total enrollment:* 12,254.

The College of Nursing Founded in 1974. *Nursing program faculty:* 45 (38% with doctorates).

Academic Facilities *Campus library:* 74,000 volumes (12,500 in health, 3,200 in nursing); 1,322 periodical subscriptions (1,322 health-care related). *Nursing school resources:* CAI, computer lab, nursing audiovisuals, interactive nursing skills videos, learning resource lab.

Student Life *Student services:* health clinic, personal counseling, career counseling, institutionally sponsored work-study program, job placement, campus safety program, special assistance for disabled students. *International student services:* counseling/support, special assistance for nonnative speakers of English, ESL courses. *Nursing student activities:* Sigma Theta Tau, student nurses association, Phi Kappa Phi, Golden Key.

Calendar Quarters.

NURSING STUDENT PROFILE

Undergraduate **Enrollment:** 919
Women: 79%; **Men:** 21%; **Minority:** 20%; **International:** 1%; **Part-time:** 34%
Graduate **Enrollment:** 274
Women: 74%; **Men:** 26%; **Minority:** 17%; **International:** 1%; **Part-time:** 51%

BACCALAUREATE PROGRAMS

Contact Ms. Bettye B. Odom, Director of Admissions and Advisement, College of Nursing, University of South Alabama, Mobile, AL 36688-0002, 334-434-3410. *Fax:* 334-434-3413.

Expenses *State resident tuition:* $3500 full-time, $58 per credit part-time. *Nonresident tuition:* $4000 full-time, $58 per credit part-time. *Full-time mandatory fees:* $289. *Part-time mandatory fees:* $233. *Room only:* $1980–$2660. *Books and supplies per academic year:* $1000.

Financial Aid Institutionally sponsored need-based grants/scholarships, institutionally sponsored non-need grants/scholarships, Federal Supplemental Educational Opportunity Grants, Federal Work-Study. 64% of undergraduate students in nursing programs received some form of financial aid in 1995–96. *Application deadline:* 8/1.

Generic Baccalaureate Program (BSN)

Applying *Required:* ACT, TOEFL for nonnative speakers of English, minimum college GPA of 2.5, letter of recommendation, transcript of college record. *Options:* May apply for transfer of up to 96 total credits. *Application deadlines:* 9/10 (fall), 3/10 (spring), 12/10 (winter). *Application fee:* $25.

Degree Requirements 200 total credit hours, 111 in nursing.

Accelerated RN Baccalaureate Program (BSN)

Applying *Required:* TOEFL for nonnative speakers of English, minimum college GPA of 2.5, RN license, diploma or AD in nursing, letter of recommendation, transcript of college record. *Options:* Advanced standing available through the following means: advanced placement exams, credit by exam. May apply for transfer of up to 96 total credits. *Application deadlines:* 9/10 (fall), 3/10 (spring), 12/10 (winter). *Application fee:* $25.

Degree Requirements 200 total credit hours, 111 in nursing.

MASTER'S PROGRAMS

Contact Dr. Debra C. Davis, Associate Dean and Director of Graduate Studies, College of Nursing, University of South Alabama, Mobile, AL 36688-0002, 334-434-3410. *Fax:* 334-434-3413.

Areas of Study Clinical nurse specialist programs in adult health nursing, community health nursing, maternity-newborn nursing, pediatric nursing, psychiatric–mental health nursing, women's health nursing; nursing administration; nursing education; nurse practitioner programs in family health, neonatal health, adult acute care.

Expenses *State resident tuition:* $3500 full-time, $68 per credit part-time. *Nonresident tuition:* $4000 full-time, $68 per credit part-time. *Full-time mandatory fees:* $289. *Part-time mandatory fees:* $233. *Room only:* $1980–$2660. *Books and supplies per academic year:* $1500.

Financial Aid Graduate assistantships, nurse traineeships. *Application deadline:* 8/1.

RN to Master's Program (MSN)

Applying *Required:* Miller Analogies Test, bachelor's degree in nursing, minimum GPA of 2.5, RN license, physical assessment course, 2 letters of recommendation, transcript of college record, 3 years of administration experience, 2 years of level II or III nursery care for neonatal nurse practitioners, 2 years for family nurse practitioners, 2 years for adult acute care practitioners. *Application deadlines:* 9/10 (fall), 3/10 (spring), 12/10 (winter). *Application fee:* $25.

Degree Requirements 52–60 total credit hours dependent upon track, 48–60 in nursing, 4 in administration only. Thesis or research project.

University of South Alabama (continued)

Master's for Nurses with Non-Nursing Degrees Program (MSN)

Applying *Required:* Miller Analogies Test, bachelor's degree, minimum GPA of 2.5, RN license, 2 letters of recommendation, transcript of college record. *Application deadlines:* 9/10 (fall), 3/10 (spring), 12/10 (winter). *Application fee:* $25.

Degree Requirements 75–83 total credit hours dependent upon track, 71–83 in nursing, 4 in ex administration only. Thesis or research project.

See full description on page 556.

ALASKA

UNIVERSITY OF ALASKA ANCHORAGE
School of Nursing and Health Sciences
Anchorage, Alaska

Programs • Generic Baccalaureate • Accelerated RN Baccalaureate • MS

The University State-supported comprehensive coed institution. Part of University of Alaska System. Founded: 1954. *Primary accreditation:* regional. *Setting:* 428-acre urban campus. *Total enrollment:* 13,002.

The School of Nursing and Health Sciences Founded in 1970. *Nursing program faculty:* 22 (50% with doctorates).

Academic Facilities *Campus library:* 420,071 volumes (23,000 in health); 3,547 periodical subscriptions (780 health-care related). *Nursing school resources:* CAI, computer lab, nursing audiovisuals, interactive nursing skills videos, learning resource lab, clinical simulation lab.

Student Life *Student services:* health clinic, child-care facilities, personal counseling, career counseling, institutionally sponsored work-study program, campus safety program, special assistance for disabled students. *International student services:* counseling/support, ESL courses. *Nursing student activities:* Sigma Theta Tau, student nurses association.

Calendar Semesters.

NURSING STUDENT PROFILE

Undergraduate **Enrollment:** 255
Women: 89%; **Men:** 11%; **Minority:** 15%; **International:** 0%; **Part-time:** 44%

Graduate **Enrollment:** 56
Women: 96%; **Men:** 4%; **Minority:** 4%; **International:** 0%; **Part-time:** 77%

BACCALAUREATE PROGRAMS

Contact Ms. Marie Samson, Coordinator of Student Affairs, School of Nursing, University of Alaska Anchorage, 3211 Providence Drive, Anchorage, AK 99508, 907-786-4550. *Fax:* 907-786-4550.

Expenses *State resident tuition:* $1078 full-time, $77 per credit part-time. *Nonresident tuition:* $2156 full-time, $154 per credit part-time. *Full-time mandatory fees:* $194–$250. *Part-time mandatory fees:* $100–$150. *Books and supplies per academic year:* ranges from $250 to $500.

Financial Aid Institutionally sponsored need-based grants/scholarships, Federal Pell Grants, Federal Perkins Loans, Federal Work-Study, Alaska student loans. *Application deadline:* 2/1.

Generic Baccalaureate Program (BS)

Applying *Required:* SAT I, ACT, TOEFL for nonnative speakers of English, minimum high school GPA of 2.5, minimum college GPA of 2.7, high school chemistry, high school biology, high school transcript, 3 letters of recommendation, written essay, transcript of college record. 17 prerequisite credits must be completed before admission to the nursing program. *Options:* Advanced standing available through the following means: advanced placement exams, credit by exam. *Application deadlines:* 2/15 (fall), 10/15 (spring). *Application fee:* $35.

Degree Requirements 126 total credit hours, 63 in nursing.

Accelerated RN Baccalaureate Program (BS)

Applying *Required:* minimum college GPA of 2.0, 3 letters of recommendation, transcript of college record, RN license in Alaska. *Options:* Advanced standing available through the following means: advanced placement exams, credit by exam. *Application deadlines:* 2/15 (fall), 10/15 (spring). *Application fee:* $35.

Degree Requirements 126 total credit hours, 63 in nursing.

MASTER'S PROGRAM

Contact Ms. Marie Samson, Coordinator of Student Affairs, School of Nursing and Health Sciences, University of Alaska Anchorage, 3211 Providence Drive, Anchorage, AK 99508, 907-786-4550. *Fax:* 907-786-4550.

Areas of Study Clinical nurse specialist programs in community health nursing, psychiatric–mental health nursing; nursing administration; nurse practitioner program in family health.

Expenses *State resident tuition:* $1530 full-time, $153 per credit part-time. *Nonresident tuition:* $3060 full-time, $306 per credit part-time. *Full-time mandatory fees:* $200–$300. *Part-time mandatory fees:* $100–$200. *Books and supplies per academic year:* ranges from $300 to $700.

Financial Aid Graduate assistantships, nurse traineeships. *Application deadline:* 2/1.

MS Program

Applying *Required:* GRE General Test or Miller Analogies Test, bachelor's degree in nursing, minimum GPA of 3.0, RN license, 1 year of clinical experience, statistics course, professional liability/malpractice insurance, essay, 3 letters of recommendation, transcript of college record, physical assessment course, immunizations for family nurse practitioner track. *Application deadline:* 3/1. *Application fee:* $45.

Degree Requirements 40–43 total credit hours dependent upon track, 34–40 in nursing. Thesis required.

ARIZONA

ARIZONA STATE UNIVERSITY
College of Nursing
Tempe, Arizona

Programs • Generic Baccalaureate • RN Baccalaureate • MS • Continuing Education

The University State-supported coed university. Founded: 1885. *Primary accreditation:* regional. *Setting:* 814-acre suburban campus. *Total enrollment:* 42,040.

The College of Nursing Founded in 1957. *Nursing program faculty:* 48 (60% with doctorates). *Off-campus program sites:* Phoenix, Glendale.

Academic Facilities *Campus library:* 3.4 million volumes (51,000 in health, 8,200 in nursing); 29,645 periodical subscriptions (600 health-care related). *Nursing school resources:* CAI, computer lab, nursing audiovisuals, interactive nursing skills videos, learning resource lab.

Student Life *Student services:* health clinic, child-care facilities, personal counseling, career counseling, institutionally sponsored work-study program, job placement, campus safety program, special assistance for disabled students, community services program. *International student services:* counseling/support, ESL courses. *Nursing student activities:* Sigma Theta Tau, nursing club, student nurses association, College Council of Nursing Students (CCNS).

Calendar Semesters, Winter interim and summer school available.

NURSING STUDENT PROFILE

Undergraduate **Enrollment:** 879
Women: 81%; **Men:** 19%; **Minority:** 16%; **International:** 1%; **Part-time:** 32%

Graduate **Enrollment:** 268
Women: 96%; **Men:** 4%; **Minority:** 7%; **International:** 1%; **Part-time:** 49%

BACCALAUREATE PROGRAMS

Contact Ms. Maurine Lee, Office of Student Services, College of Nursing, Arizona State University, Tempe, AZ 85287-2602, 602-965-2987. *Fax:* 602-965-8468. *E-mail:* icmol@asuvm.inre.asu.edu

Expenses *State resident tuition:* $1884 full-time, $99 per credit hour part-time. *Nonresident tuition:* $7912 full-time, $330 per credit hour part-time.

Full-time mandatory fees: $356. *Room and board:* $4301–$5526. *Room only:* $2130–$3355. *Books and supplies per academic year:* ranges from $800 to $1000.

Financial Aid Institutionally sponsored need-based grants/scholarships, institutionally sponsored non-need grants/scholarships, Federal Direct Loans, Federal Nursing Student Loans, Federal Pell Grants, Federal Perkins Loans, Federal Supplemental Educational Opportunity Grants, Federal Work-Study, PHS Indian Health Service Scholarship, Scholarship for Disadvantaged Students Program. 84% of undergraduate students in nursing programs received some form of financial aid in 1995–96. *Application deadline:* 3/15.

Generic Baccalaureate Program (BSN)

Applying *Required:* SAT I, ACT, TOEFL for nonnative speakers of English, minimum high school GPA of 3.0, 3 years of high school math, 2 years of high school science, high school transcript, transcript of college record, high school class rank: top 25%. 1year each of high school social science and American history; 4 years of high school English. 47 prerequisite credits must be completed before admission to the nursing program. *Options:* Advanced standing available through the following means: advanced placement exams, credit by exam. May apply for transfer of up to 90 total credits. *Application deadlines:* 12/1 (fall), 7/1 (spring). *Application fee:* $35.

Degree Requirements 120 total credit hours, 64 in nursing. University's general education requirements, 50 hours of upper division course work.

Distance learning Courses provided through correspondence.

RN Baccalaureate Program (BSN)

Applying *Required:* TOEFL for nonnative speakers of English, minimum college GPA of 2.75, 3 years of high school math, 2 years of high school science, high school chemistry, RN license, high school transcript, transcript of college record. 82 prerequisite credits must be completed before admission to the nursing program. *Options:* Advanced standing available through the following means: advanced placement exams, credit by exam. May apply for transfer of up to 90 total credits. *Application deadlines:* 12/1 (fall), 7/1 (spring). *Application fee:* $35.

Degree Requirements 120 total credit hours, 61–64 in nursing. University's general education requirements, 50 hours of upper division course work.

Distance learning Courses provided through correspondence.

MASTER'S PROGRAM

Contact Ms. Maurine Lee, Office of Student Services, College of Nursing, Arizona State University, Tempe, AZ 85287-2602, 602-965-2987. *Fax:* 602-965-8468. *E-mail:* icmol@asuvm.inre.asu.edu

Areas of Study Clinical nurse specialist programs in adult health nursing, community health nursing, pediatric nursing, psychiatric–mental health nursing, women's health nursing; nurse midwifery; nursing administration; nursing education; nurse practitioner programs in adult health, child care/pediatrics, family health, psychiatric–mental health, women's health.

Expenses *State resident tuition:* $1884 full-time, $99 per credit hour part-time. *Nonresident tuition:* $7912 full-time, $330 per credit hour part-time. *Full-time mandatory fees:* $66–$96. *Room and board:* $4301–$5526. *Room only:* $2130–$3355. *Books and supplies per academic year:* ranges from $800 to $1000.

Financial Aid Graduate assistantships, nurse traineeships, Federal Nursing Student Loans, institutionally sponsored loans, employment opportunities, institutionally sponsored need-based grants/scholarships, institutionally sponsored non-need-based grants/scholarships. 15% of master's level students in nursing programs received some form of financial aid in 1995-96. *Application deadline:* 3/1.

MS Program

Applying *Required:* GRE General Test (minimum combined score of 1500 on three tests), TOEFL for nonnative speakers of English, bachelor's degree in nursing, minimum GPA of 3.0, RN license, 1 year of clinical experience, physical assessment course, statistics course, essay, interview, 3 letters of recommendation, transcript of college record. *Application deadline:* 2/1. *Application fee:* $35.

Degree Requirements 40–52 total credit hours dependent upon track, 37+ in nursing. Thesis or applied project.

CONTINUING EDUCATION PROGRAM

Contact Mr. David Hrabe, Director of Continuing and Extended Education, Continuing Education Department, College of Nursing, Arizona State University, Box 872602, Tempe, AZ 85287-2602, 602-965-7431. *Fax:* 602-965-0212. *E-mail:* icdph@asuvm.inre.asu.edu

GRAND CANYON UNIVERSITY
Samaritan College of Nursing
Phoenix, Arizona

Program • Generic Baccalaureate

The University Independent Southern Baptist comprehensive coed institution. Founded: 1949. *Primary accreditation:* regional. *Setting:* 70-acre suburban campus. *Total enrollment:* 2,119.

The Samaritan College of Nursing Founded in 1981. *Nursing program faculty:* 23 (4% with doctorates).

Academic Facilities *Campus library:* 76,000 volumes (1,837 in health); 642 periodical subscriptions (139 health-care related). *Nursing school resources:* CAI, computer lab, nursing audiovisuals, learning resource lab.

Student Life *Student services:* health clinic, career counseling, institutionally sponsored work-study program. *International student services:* special assistance for nonnative speakers of English. *Nursing student activities:* Sigma Theta Tau, student nurses association.

Calendar Semesters.

NURSING STUDENT PROFILE

Undergraduate **Enrollment:** 139

Women: 90%; **Men:** 10%; **Minority:** 6%; **International:** 1%; **Part-time:** 0%

BACCALAUREATE PROGRAM

Contact Dr. Jennifer A. Wilson, Dean, Samaritan College of Nursing, Grand Canyon University, 3300 West Camelback Road, Phoenix, AZ 85017, 602-589-2431. *Fax:* 602-589-2895.

Expenses *Tuition:* $4824 full-time, $268 per semester credit hour part-time. *Full-time mandatory fees:* $370. *Room and board:* $3160–$3260. *Books and supplies per academic year:* $400.

Financial Aid Institutionally sponsored need-based grants/scholarships, institutionally sponsored non-need grants/scholarships, Federal Nursing Student Loans, Federal Perkins Loans, Federal Supplemental Educational Opportunity Grants, Federal Work-Study. *Application deadline:* 3/15.

Generic Baccalaureate Program (BSN)

Applying *Required:* minimum college GPA of 2.5, interview, 3 letters of recommendation, written essay, transcript of college record. 37 prerequisite credits must be completed before admission to the nursing program. *Options:* May apply for transfer of up to 64 total credits. *Application deadlines:* 1/31 (fall), 9/24 (spring).

Degree Requirements 128 total credit hours, 63 in nursing.

NORTHERN ARIZONA UNIVERSITY
Department of Nursing
Flagstaff, Arizona

Programs • Generic Baccalaureate • RN Baccalaureate • BSN to Master's • Master's for Second Degree

The University State-supported coed university. Founded: 1899. *Primary accreditation:* regional. *Setting:* 730-acre small-town campus. *Total enrollment:* 20,131.

The Department of Nursing Founded in 1962. *Nursing program faculty:* 19 (47% with doctorates). *Off-campus program sites:* Yuma, Prescott, Kingman.

Academic Facilities *Campus library:* 523,568 volumes (18,500 in health, 1,530 in nursing); 6,148 periodical subscriptions (158 health-care related). *Nursing school resources:* CAI, computer lab, nursing audiovisuals, learning resource lab.

Student Life *Student services:* health clinic, child-care facilities, personal counseling, career counseling, institutionally sponsored work-study program, job placement, campus safety program, special assistance for

Northern Arizona University (continued)

disabled students. *International student services:* counseling/support, special assistance for nonnative speakers of English, ESL courses. *Nursing student activities:* Sigma Theta Tau, student nurses association.

Calendar Semesters.

NURSING STUDENT PROFILE

Undergraduate **Enrollment:** 178
Women: 84%; **Men:** 16%; **Minority:** 19%; **International:** 1%; **Part-time:** 38%
Graduate **Enrollment:** 20
Women: 90%; **Men:** 10%; **Minority:** 5%; **International:** 0%; **Part-time:** 20%

BACCALAUREATE PROGRAMS

Contact Ms. Ruth Nicolls, Assistant Chair, Box 15035, Department of Nursing, Northern Arizona University, Flagstaff, AZ 86011, 520-523-6711/2671. *Fax:* 520-523-7171. *E-mail:* nicolls@nauvax.ucc.nau.edu

Expenses *State resident tuition:* $1940 full-time, $102 per hour part-time. *Nonresident tuition:* $7456 full-time, $311 per hour part-time. *Full-time mandatory fees:* $816–$916. *Room and board:* $2076–$3334. *Room only:* $1576–$1704. *Books and supplies per academic year:* ranges from $250 to $300.

Financial Aid Institutionally sponsored need-based grants/scholarships, Federal Direct Loans, Federal Perkins Loans, Federal Supplemental Educational Opportunity Grants, Federal Work-Study. *Application deadline:* 4/15.

Generic Baccalaureate Program (BS)

Applying *Required:* SAT I or ACT, TOEFL for nonnative speakers of English, minimum college GPA of 2.5, 2 letters of recommendation, written essay, transcript of college record. *Options:* May apply for transfer of up to 70 total credits. *Application deadline:* 2/15. *Application fee:* $30.

Degree Requirements 129 total credit hours, 71 in nursing.

RN Baccalaureate Program (BS)

Applying *Required:* TOEFL for nonnative speakers of English, ACT PEP, minimum college GPA of 2.5, RN license, 2 letters of recommendation, written essay, transcript of college record. 69 prerequisite credits must be completed before admission to the nursing program. *Options:* May apply for transfer of up to 70 total credits. *Application deadline:* 2/15. *Application fee:* $15.

Degree Requirements 129 total credit hours, 71 in nursing.

Distance learning Courses provided through computer-based media, on-line, interactive instructional television.

MASTER'S PROGRAMS

Contact Dr. Carol Craig, Co-coordinator Graduate Program, Department of Nursing, Northern Arizona University, Box 15035, Flagstaff, AZ 86011, 520-523-6707. *Fax:* 520-523-7171. *E-mail:* carol.craig@nau.edu

Areas of Study Clinical nurse specialist program in rural health; nurse practitioner program in family health.

Expenses *State resident tuition:* $1940 full-time, $102 per hour part-time. *Nonresident tuition:* $7456 full-time, $311 per hour part-time. *Full-time mandatory fees:* $816–$916.

Financial Aid Graduate assistantships, nurse traineeships, Federal Direct Loans, Federal Nursing Student Loans, employment opportunities, institutionally sponsored need-based grants/scholarships, institutionally sponsored non-need-based grants/scholarships.

BSN to Master's Program (MS)

Applying *Required:* GRE General Test, bachelor's degree in nursing, RN license, 1 year of clinical experience, physical assessment course, statistics course, essay, 3 letters of recommendation, transcript of college record, minimum 3.0 GPA in last two years of baccalaureate program, must be accepted by the Graduate College and Department of Nursing.. *Application deadline:* 2/15. *Application fee:* $35.

Degree Requirements 36 total credit hours, 30 in nursing. 45 hours in nursing and 3 elective hours for family nurse practitioner track. Thesis required.

Master's for Second Degree Program (MS)

Applying *Required:* GRE General Test, bachelor's degree in nursing, RN license, 1 year of clinical experience, physical assessment course, statistics course, essay, 3 letters of recommendation, transcript of college record, MSN, 3.0 GPA in last two years of baccalaureate program. *Application deadline:* 2/15. *Application fee:* $35.

Degree Requirements 36 total credit hours, 36 in nursing.

UNIVERSITY OF ARIZONA
College of Nursing
Tucson, Arizona

Programs • Generic Baccalaureate • RN Baccalaureate • Baccalaureate for Second Degree • MS/MBA • Post-Master's • PhD • Postdoctoral • Continuing Education

The University State-supported coed university. Founded: 1885. *Primary accreditation:* regional. *Setting:* 347-acre urban campus. *Total enrollment:* 34,777.

The College of Nursing Founded in 1957. *Nursing program faculty:* 58 (50% with doctorates).

Academic Facilities *Campus library:* 3.0 million volumes (195,000 in health); 30,000 periodical subscriptions (2,500 health-care related). *Nursing school resources:* CAI, computer lab, nursing audiovisuals, interactive nursing skills videos, learning resource lab.

Student Life *Student services:* health clinic, personal counseling, career counseling, institutionally sponsored work-study program, job placement, campus safety program, special assistance for disabled students. *International student services:* counseling/support, special assistance for nonnative speakers of English, ESL courses, orientation for registration. *Nursing student activities:* Sigma Theta Tau, student nurses association.

Calendar Semesters.

NURSING STUDENT PROFILE

Undergraduate **Enrollment:** 249
Women: 89%; **Men:** 11%; **Minority:** 22%; **Part-time:** 16%
Graduate **Enrollment:** 159
Women: 89%; **Men:** 11%; **Minority:** 14%; **International:** 5%; **Part-time:** 77%

BACCALAUREATE PROGRAMS

Contact Ms. Mary E. Henkel, Coordinator of Undergraduate Student Affairs, College of Nursing, University of Arizona, PO Box 210203, Tucson, AZ 85721-0203, 520-626-6161. *Fax:* 520-626-2211.

Expenses *State resident tuition:* $1940 full-time, $102 per credit hour part-time. *Nonresident tuition:* $8308 full-time, $346 per credit hour part-time. *Full-time mandatory fees:* $10–$50. *Room only:* $1745–$4026. *Books and supplies per academic year:* ranges from $400 to $600.

Financial Aid Institutionally sponsored need-based grants/scholarships, institutionally sponsored non need grants/scholarships, Federal Nursing Student Loans, Federal Pell Grants, Federal Supplemental Educational Opportunity Grants, Federal Work-Study. *Application deadline:* 3/1.

Generic Baccalaureate Program (BSN)

Applying *Required:* SAT I or ACT, TOEFL for nonnative speakers of English, minimum high school GPA of 2.5, minimum college GPA of 2.75, 3 years of high school math, 2 years of high school science, high school transcript, 3 letters of recommendation, written essay, transcript of college record. 51 prerequisite credits must be completed before admission to the nursing program. *Options:* Advanced standing available through the following means: advanced placement exams, credit by exam. Course work may be accelerated. May apply for transfer of up to 102 total credits. *Application deadlines:* 12/1 (fall), 7/1 (spring).

Degree Requirements 129 total credit hours, 62 in nursing. Computer literacy, writing proficiency exam.

RN Baccalaureate Program (BSN)

Applying *Required:* minimum college GPA of 2.75, RN license, diploma or AD in nursing, high school transcript, 3 letters of recommendation, written essay, transcript of college record. 52 prerequisite credits must be completed before admission to the nursing program. *Options:* Advanced standing available through the following means: advanced placement exams, credit by exam. Course work may be accelerated. May apply for transfer of up to 93 total credits. *Application deadlines:* 12/1 (fall), 7/1 (spring).

Degree Requirements 123 total credit hours, 56 in nursing. Computer literacy, writing proficiency exam.

Baccalaureate for Second Degree Program (BSN)

Applying *Required:* minimum college GPA of 3.0, 3 letters of recommendation, written essay, transcript of college record. 36 prerequisite credits must be completed before admission to the nursing program. *Options:*

Advanced standing available through credit by exam. Course work may be accelerated. May apply for transfer of up to 39 total credits. *Application deadline:* 7/1.

Degree Requirements 86 total credit hours, 47 in nursing.

MASTER'S PROGRAMS

Contact Ms. Gloria Thompson, Administrative Secretary, College of Nursing, University of Arizona, PO Box 210203, Tucson, AZ 85721-0203, 520-626-6154. *Fax:* 520-626-2669.

Areas of Study Clinical nurse specialist program in nurse case management with a clinical nursing focus; nurse practitioner programs in adult health, family health, gerontology, psychiatric–mental health.

Expenses *State resident tuition:* $1940 full-time, $102 per credit hour part-time. *Nonresident tuition:* ranges from $6228 to $8308 full-time, $346 per credit hour part-time. *Room and board:* $2245–$4526. *Room only:* $1745–$4026. *Books and supplies per academic year:* ranges from $620 to $650.

Financial Aid Graduate assistantships, nurse traineeships, fellowships, Federal Nursing Student Loans. 16% of master's level students in nursing programs received some form of financial aid in 1995-96. *Application deadline:* 3/1.

MS/MBA Program

Applying *Required:* GRE General Test, TOEFL for nonnative speakers of English, bachelor's degree in nursing, bachelor's degree, minimum GPA of 3.0, RN license, physical assessment course, statistics course, professional liability/malpractice insurance, essay, 3 letters of recommendation, transcript of college record. *Application deadlines:* 3/15 (fall), 10/1 (spring). *Application fee:* $35.

Degree Requirements 36–47 total credit hours dependent upon track, 33 in nursing, 3 in elective. Thesis required.

Post-Master's Program

Applying *Required:* RN license, professional liability/malpractice insurance, essay, 3 letters of recommendation, transcript of college record. *Application deadline:* 5/1. *Application fee:* $10.

Degree Requirements 28 total credit hours, 21 in nursing.

DOCTORAL PROGRAM

Contact Ms. Gloria Thompson, Administrative Secretary, College of Nursing, University of Arizona, PO Box 210203, Tucson, AZ 85721-0203, 520-626-6154. *Fax:* 520-626-2211.

Areas of Study Nursing research.

Expenses *State resident tuition:* $1940 full-time, $102 per credit hour part-time. *Nonresident tuition:* ranges from $6228 to $8308 full-time, $346 per credit hour part-time. *Room and board:* $2245–$4526. *Room only:* $1745–$4026. *Books and supplies per academic year:* ranges from $500 to $750.

Financial Aid Graduate assistantships, fellowships. *Application deadline:* 3/1.

PhD Program

Applying *Required:* GRE General Test, TOEFL for nonnative speakers of English, 3 scholarly papers, statistics course, interview, 3 letters of recommendation, vitae, writing sample, competitive review by faculty committee. *Application deadlines:* 4/1 (fall), 10/1 (spring). *Application fee:* $35.

Degree Requirements 75–111 total credit hours dependent upon track; dissertation; oral exam; written exam; defense of dissertation; residency.

POSTDOCTORAL PROGRAM

Contact Dr. Pamela Reed, Associate Dean for Academic Affairs, College of Nursing, University of Arizona, PO Box 210203, Tucson, AZ 85721-0203, 520-626-6151. *Fax:* 520-626-2669.

CONTINUING EDUCATION PROGRAM

Contact Dr. Dona Pardo, Coordinator of Continuing Education, College of Nursing, University of Arizona, PO Box 210203, Tucson, AZ 85721-0203, 520-626-6767. *Fax:* 520-626-2211.

See full description on page 522.

UNIVERSITY OF PHOENIX

Department of Health Care Professions
Phoenix, Arizona

Programs • Accelerated RN Baccalaureate • MN • Master's for Nurses with Non-Nursing Degrees

The University Proprietary comprehensive coed institution. Founded: 1976. *Primary accreditation:* regional. *Total enrollment:* 27,139.

The Department of Health Care Professions Founded in 1982. *Nursing program faculty:* 400. *Off-campus program sites:* Tucson, AZ; Sacramento, CA; Colorado Springs, CO.

Calendar Semesters.

NURSING STUDENT PROFILE

Undergraduate **Enrollment:** 1800
Women: 87%; **Men:** 13%
Graduate **Enrollment:** 350
Women: 85%; **Men:** 15%

BACCALAUREATE PROGRAM

Contact local branch campus.

Financial Aid Federal Pell Grants, Federal PLUS Loans, Federal Stafford Loans.

Accelerated RN Baccalaureate Program (BSN)

Applying *Required:* TOEFL for nonnative speakers of English, minimum college GPA of 2.0, RN license, diploma or AD in nursing, transcript of college record, 1 year of experience as an RN, medical documentation, professional liability/malpractice insurance. 56 prerequisite credits must be completed before admission to the nursing program. *Application deadline:* rolling. *Application fee:* $55.

Degree Requirements 126 total credit hours, 36 in nursing.

MASTER'S PROGRAMS

Contact local branch campus.

Areas of Study Nursing administration; nursing education; nurse practitioner program in women's health.

MN Program

Applying *Required:* TOEFL for nonnative speakers of English, bachelor's degree in nursing, minimum GPA of 2.5, RN license, 3 years of clinical experience, 2 letters of recommendation, transcript of college record. *Application deadline:* rolling. *Application fee:* $55.

Degree Requirements 39 total credit hours.

Master's for Nurses with Non-Nursing Degrees Program (MN)

Applying *Required:* bachelor's degree, minimum GPA of 2.5, RN license, 3 years of clinical experience, transcript of college record, 3 bridge courses. *Application deadline:* rolling. *Application fee:* $55.

Degree Requirements 39 total credit hours.

ARKANSAS

ARKANSAS STATE UNIVERSITY

Department of Nursing
State University, Arkansas

Programs • Generic Baccalaureate • RN Baccalaureate • LPN to Baccalaureate • MSN

Arkansas State University (continued)

The University State-supported comprehensive coed institution. Founded: 1909. *Primary accreditation:* regional. *Setting:* 800-acre small-town campus. *Total enrollment:* 9,807.

The Department of Nursing Founded in 1969. *Nursing program faculty:* 24 (16% with doctorates). *Off-campus program sites:* Melbourne, Mountain Home, Beebe.

Academic Facilities *Campus library:* 465,883 volumes (13,951 in nursing); 2,600 periodical subscriptions. *Nursing school resources:* CAI, computer lab, nursing audiovisuals, interactive nursing skills videos, learning resource lab.

Student Life *Student services:* health clinic, personal counseling, career counseling, institutionally sponsored work-study program, job placement, campus safety program, special assistance for disabled students. *International student services:* counseling/support, special assistance for nonnative speakers of English, ESL courses. *Nursing student activities:* Sigma Theta Tau, student nurses association, Eta Theta Honor Society for Allied Health and Nursing.

Calendar Semesters.

NURSING STUDENT PROFILE

Undergraduate **Enrollment:** 367
Women: 84%; **Men:** 16%; **Minority:** 6%; **International:** 1%; **Part-time:** 5%

Graduate **Enrollment:** 86
Women: 89%; **Men:** 11%; **Minority:** 17%; **International:** 0%; **Part-time:** 90%

BACCALAUREATE PROGRAMS

Contact Mrs. Shirley Basinger, Nursing Adviser, Department of Nursing, Arkansas State University, PO Box 69, State University, AR 72467, 501-972-3074. *Fax:* 501-972-2954. *E-mail:* sbasinge@crow.astate.edu

Expenses *State resident tuition:* $1950 full-time, $82 per credit hour part-time. *Nonresident tuition:* $5040 full-time, $211 per credit hour part-time. *Full-time mandatory fees:* $15. *Room and board:* $1250–$1505. *Books and supplies per academic year:* ranges from $100 to $500.

Financial Aid Institutionally sponsored need-based grants/scholarships, institutionally sponsored non-need grants/scholarships, Federal Direct Loans, Federal Perkins Loans, Federal Supplemental Educational Opportunity Grants, Federal Work-Study. *Application deadline:* 7/1.

Generic Baccalaureate Program (BSN)

Applying *Required:* ACT, TOEFL for nonnative speakers of English, minimum college GPA of 2.0, transcript of college record, minimum 2.0 GPA in 8 hours of science course work. 30 prerequisite credits must be completed before admission to the nursing program. *Options:* May apply for transfer of up to 103 total credits. *Application deadlines:* 6/15 (fall), 11/15 (spring), 11/15 (early admissions).

Degree Requirements 135 total credit hours, 69 in nursing.

RN Baccalaureate Program (BSN)

Applying *Required:* ACT, TOEFL for nonnative speakers of English, minimum college GPA of 2.0, RN license, diploma or AD in nursing, transcript of college record. *Options:* Advanced standing available through the following means: advanced placement exams, credit by exam. May apply for transfer of up to 99 total credits. *Application deadlines:* 6/15 (fall), 11/15 (spring).

Degree Requirements 131 total credit hours, 65 in nursing.

LPN to Baccalaureate Program (BSN)

Applying *Required:* ACT, TOEFL for nonnative speakers of English, minimum college GPA of 2.0, transcript of college record, LPN license. *Options:* Advanced standing available through advanced placement exams. *Application deadlines:* 6/15 (fall), 11/15 (spring).

Degree Requirements 135 total credit hours, 69 in nursing.

MASTER'S PROGRAM

Contact Dr. Elizabeth Stokes, Director, MSN Programs, Department of Nursing, Arkansas State University, PO Box 69, State University, AR 72467, 501-972-3074. *Fax:* 501-972-2954. *E-mail:* estokes@crow.astate.edu

Areas of Study Clinical nurse specialist program in adult health nursing.

Expenses *State resident tuition:* $2340 full-time, $98 per credit hour part-time. *Nonresident tuition:* $9120 full-time, $256 per credit hour part-time. *Full-time mandatory fees:* $80. *Room and board:* $1250–$1505. *Books and supplies per academic year:* ranges from $300 to $500.

Financial Aid Graduate assistantships, nurse traineeships. *Application deadline:* 7/1.

MSN Program

Applying *Required:* GRE General Test, Miller Analogies Test, bachelor's degree in nursing, minimum GPA of 2.75, RN license, physical assessment course, statistics course, professional liability/malpractice insurance, transcript of college record. *Application deadline:* rolling.

Degree Requirements 36 total credit hours, 30 in nursing.

ARKANSAS TECH UNIVERSITY
Department of Nursing
Russellville, Arkansas

Programs • Generic Baccalaureate • RN Baccalaureate • Baccalaureate for Second Degree

The University State-supported comprehensive coed institution. Founded: 1909. *Primary accreditation:* regional. *Setting:* 517-acre small-town campus. *Total enrollment:* 4,593.

The Department of Nursing Founded in 1974. *Nursing program faculty:* 12 (12% with doctorates). *Off-campus program site:* Fort Smith.

Academic Facilities *Campus library:* 136,000 volumes (10,050 in health, 8,525 in nursing); 1,298 periodical subscriptions (70 health-care related). *Nursing school resources:* CAI, computer lab, nursing audiovisuals, learning resource lab.

Student Life *Student services:* health clinic, child-care facilities, personal counseling, career counseling, institutionally sponsored work-study program, job placement, campus safety program, special assistance for disabled students. *International student services:* counseling/support, special assistance for nonnative speakers of English. *Nursing student activities:* Sigma Theta Tau, student nurses association.

Calendar Semesters.

NURSING STUDENT PROFILE

Undergraduate **Enrollment:** 64
Women: 94%; **Men:** 6%; **Minority:** 2%; **International:** 2%; **Part-time:** 16%

BACCALAUREATE PROGRAMS

Contact Dr. Audrey R. Owens, Head, Dean Hall, Department of Nursing, Arkansas Tech University, Russellville, AR 72801-2222, 501-968-0383. *Fax:* 501-968-0219.

Expenses *State resident tuition:* $1820 full-time, $84 per credit hour part-time. *Nonresident tuition:* $3740 full-time, $168 per credit hour part-time. *Full-time mandatory fees:* $40–$85. *Part-time mandatory fees:* $40–$85. *Room and board:* $1290–$1330. *Books and supplies per academic year:* ranges from $100 to $250.

Financial Aid Institutionally sponsored need-based grants/scholarships, institutionally sponsored non-need grants/scholarships, Federal Supplemental Educational Opportunity Grants. 95% of undergraduate students in nursing programs received some form of financial aid in 1995–96. *Application deadline:* 1/1.

Generic Baccalaureate Program (BSN)

Applying *Required:* articulation model, minimum college GPA of 2.75, CPR certification, professional liability/malpractice insurance, health certification, Hepatitis B vaccine series. 62 prerequisite credits must be completed before admission to the nursing program. *Options:* Advanced standing available through the following means: advanced placement exams, credit by exam. Course work may be accelerated. May apply for transfer of up to 68 total credits. *Application deadlines:* 3/1 (fall), 10/1 (spring).

Degree Requirements 124 total credit hours, 62 in nursing.

Distance learning Courses provided through correspondence, video.

RN Baccalaureate Program (BSN)

Applying *Required:* minimum college GPA of 2.75, RN license, diploma or AD in nursing, transcript of college record, CPR certification, professional liability/malpractice insurance, health certification, Hepatitis B vaccine series. 62 prerequisite credits must be completed before admission to the nursing program. *Options:* Advanced standing available through the following means: advanced placement exams, credit by exam. Course work may be accelerated. May apply for transfer of up to 68 total credits. *Application deadlines:* 3/1 (fall), 10/1 (spring).

Degree Requirements 124 total credit hours, 62 in nursing.

Distance learning Courses provided through correspondence, video.

Baccalaureate for Second Degree Program (BSN)

Applying *Required:* minimum college GPA of 2.75, transcript of college record, CPR certification, professional liability/malpractice insurance, health certification, Hepatitis B vaccine series. *Options:* Course work may be accelerated. May apply for transfer of up to 68 total credits. *Application deadlines:* 3/1 (fall), 10/1 (spring).

Degree Requirements 124 total credit hours, 62 in nursing.

Distance learning Courses provided through correspondence, video.

HARDING UNIVERSITY
School of Nursing
Searcy, Arkansas

Programs • Generic Baccalaureate • Accelerated RN Baccalaureate • Baccalaureate for Second Degree • Continuing Education

The University Independent comprehensive coed institution, affiliated with Church of Christ. Founded: 1924. *Primary accreditation:* regional. *Setting:* 200-acre small-town campus. *Total enrollment:* 4,071.

The School of Nursing Founded in 1975. *Nursing program faculty:* 15 (20% with doctorates).

Academic Facilities *Campus library:* 396,411 volumes (5,000 in health, 1,729 in nursing); 1,152 periodical subscriptions (145 health-care related). *Nursing school resources:* CAI, computer lab, nursing audiovisuals, interactive nursing skills videos, learning resource lab.

Student Life *Student services:* health clinic, personal counseling, career counseling, institutionally sponsored work-study program, job placement, special assistance for disabled students. *International student services:* counseling/support, special assistance for nonnative speakers of English. *Nursing student activities:* Sigma Theta Tau, student nurses association.

Calendar Semesters.

NURSING STUDENT PROFILE

Undergraduate **Enrollment:** 105

Women: 84%; **Men:** 16%; **Minority:** 10%; **International:** 1%; **Part-time:** 1%

BACCALAUREATE PROGRAMS

Contact Mr. Tod J. Martin, Assistant to the Dean, School of Nursing, Harding University, PO Box 2265, Searcy, AR 72149-0001, 501-279-4682. *Fax:* 501-279-4669. *E-mail:* tmartin@harding.edu

Expenses *Tuition:* $6825 full-time, $228 per hour part-time. *Full-time mandatory fees:* $930–$1100. *Room and board:* $3800–$4000. *Room only:* $1650–$2000. *Books and supplies per academic year:* ranges from $500 to $1000.

Financial Aid Institutionally sponsored need-based grants/scholarships, institutionally sponsored non-need grants/scholarships, Federal Nursing Student Loans, Federal Supplemental Educational Opportunity Grants, Federal Work-Study. *Application deadline:* 5/1.

Generic Baccalaureate Program (BSN)

Applying *Required:* SAT I, ACT, TOEFL for nonnative speakers of English, minimum college GPA of 2.0, high school transcript, 2 letters of recommendation, transcript of college record, minimum 2.5 GPA in nursing prerequisite courses. 40 prerequisite credits must be completed before admission to the nursing program. *Options:* May apply for transfer of up to 96 total credits. *Application deadlines:* 10/1 (fall), 10/1 (spring).

Degree Requirements 129 total credit hours, 60 in nursing.

Accelerated RN Baccalaureate Program (BSN)

Applying *Required:* RN license, diploma or AD in nursing, 2 letters of recommendation, transcript of college record. 40 prerequisite credits must be completed before admission to the nursing program. *Options:* May apply for transfer of up to 96 total credits. *Application deadlines:* 10/1 (fall), 10/1 (spring).

Degree Requirements 129 total credit hours, 60 in nursing.

Baccalaureate for Second Degree Program (BSN)

Applying *Required:* minimum college GPA of 2.0, 2 letters of recommendation, transcript of college record, minimum 2.5 GPA in nursing. 40 prerequisite credits must be completed before admission to the nursing program. *Options:* May apply for transfer of up to 96 total credits. *Application deadlines:* 10/1 (fall), 10/1 (spring).

Degree Requirements 129 total credit hours, 60 in nursing.

CONTINUING EDUCATION PROGRAM

Contact Dr. Cathleen M. Shultz, Dean and Professor, School of Nursing, Harding University, PO Box 2265, Searcy, AR 72149-0001, 501-279-4476. *Fax:* 501-279-4669.

HENDERSON STATE UNIVERSITY
Nursing Department
Arkadelphia, Arkansas

Programs • Generic Baccalaureate • RN Baccalaureate • LPN to Baccalaureate

The University State-supported comprehensive coed institution. Founded: 1890. *Primary accreditation:* regional. *Setting:* 132-acre small-town campus. *Total enrollment:* 3,614.

The Nursing Department Founded in 1975. *Nursing program faculty:* 11 (36% with doctorates). *Off-campus program site:* Hot Springs.

Academic Facilities *Campus library:* 244,000 volumes (8,100 in health, 6,000 in nursing); 1,501 periodical subscriptions (57 health-care related). *Nursing school resources:* CAI, computer lab, nursing audiovisuals, learning resource lab.

Student Life *Student services:* health clinic, personal counseling, career counseling, institutionally sponsored work-study program, job placement, campus safety program, special assistance for disabled students, tutoring. *International student services:* counseling/support, special assistance for nonnative speakers of English, tutoring. *Nursing student activities:* nursing club, student nurses association.

Calendar Semesters.

NURSING STUDENT PROFILE

Undergraduate **Enrollment:** 243

Women: 80%; **Men:** 20%; **Minority:** 22%; **International:** 0%; **Part-time:** 25%

BACCALAUREATE PROGRAMS

Contact Dr. Rita Monsen, Chairperson, Nursing Department, Henderson State University, 1100 Henderson Street, Box 7803, Arkadelphia, AR 71999-0001, 501-230-5015. *Fax:* 501-230-5144. *E-mail:* monsenr@holly.hsu.edu

Expenses *State resident tuition:* $864 full-time, $80 per semester hour part-time. *Nonresident tuition:* $1728 full-time, $160 per semester hour part-time. *Full-time mandatory fees:* $70. *Part-time mandatory fees:* $70. *Books and supplies per academic year:* ranges from $100 to $500.

Financial Aid Institutionally sponsored need-based grants/scholarships, institutionally sponsored non-need grants/scholarships, Federal Nursing Student Loans, Federal Pell Grants, Federal Perkins Loans, Federal Supplemental Educational Opportunity Grants, Federal Work-Study. 80% of undergraduate students in nursing programs received some form of financial aid in 1995–96. *Application deadline:* 8/15.

Generic Baccalaureate Program (BSN)

Applying *Required:* ACT, ASSET (for students age 21 or more without previous college credit), minimum college GPA of 2.5, high school transcript. 34 prerequisite credits must be completed before admission to the nursing program. *Options:* Advanced standing available through credit by exam. May apply for transfer of up to 94 total credits. *Application deadline:* 6/1. *Application fee:* $35.

Degree Requirements 126 total credit hours, 58 in nursing. English proficiency exam.

RN Baccalaureate Program (BSN)

Applying *Required:* minimum college GPA of 2.5, RN license, diploma or AD in nursing, high school transcript. 34 prerequisite credits must be completed before admission to the nursing program. *Options:* Advanced standing available through credit by exam. May apply for transfer of up to 94 total credits. *Application deadline:* 11/1. *Application fee:* $35.

Degree Requirements 126 total credit hours, 58 in nursing. English proficiency exam.

Henderson State University (continued)

LPN to Baccalaureate Program (BSN)

Applying *Required:* ACT, minimum college GPA of 2.5, high school transcript, LPN license. 34 prerequisite credits must be completed before admission to the nursing program. *Options:* May apply for transfer of up to 94 total credits. *Application fee:* $35.

Degree Requirements 126 total credit hours, 58 in nursing. English proficiency exam.

UNIVERSITY OF ARKANSAS

Department of Nursing
Fayetteville, Arkansas

Programs • Generic Baccalaureate • RN Baccalaureate • MNSc

The University State-supported coed university. Part of University of Arkansas System. Founded: 1871. *Primary accreditation:* regional. *Setting:* 420-acre small-town campus. *Total enrollment:* 14,692.

The Department of Nursing *Nursing program faculty:* 11.

Academic Facilities *Campus library:* 1.0 million volumes; 16,000 periodical subscriptions.

Calendar Semesters.

BACCALAUREATE PROGRAMS

Contact Head, Ozark Hall 217, Department of Nursing, University of Arkansas, Fayetteville, AR 72701, 501-575-3904.

Expenses *State resident tuition:* $0 per academic year. *Nonresident tuition:* $3562 full-time, $221 per credit hour part-time. *Full-time mandatory fees:* $2568. *Part-time mandatory fees:* $84+. *Room and board:* $3656–$3981. *Books and supplies per academic year:* ranges from $500 to $1000.

Financial Aid Institutionally sponsored need-based grants/scholarships, institutionally sponsored non-need grants/scholarships, Federal Work-Study, Federal PLUS Loans, Federal Stafford Loans. *Application deadline:* 4/1.

Generic Baccalaureate Program (BSN)

Applying *Required:* SAT I or ACT, TOEFL for nonnative speakers of English, minimum college GPA of 2.75, high school math, high school science, high school chemistry, high school biology, high school transcript, CPR certification, immunization. 64 prerequisite credits must be completed before admission to the nursing program. *Application deadline:* rolling. *Application fee:* $15.

Degree Requirements 132 total credit hours, 67 in nursing.

RN Baccalaureate Program (BSN)

Applying *Required:* minimum college GPA of 2.75, RN license, diploma or AD in nursing, transcript of college record, immunizations. *Application deadline:* rolling. *Application fee:* $15.

Degree Requirements 132 total credit hours, 67 in nursing.

MASTER'S PROGRAM

Contact Beth C. Vaughn-Wrobel, Associate Dean for Academic Programs, University of Arkansas, 4301 West Markham, Little Rock, AR 72205, 501-686-5374.

Areas of Study Nursing administration; nursing education.

Expenses *State resident tuition:* $0 per academic year. *Nonresident tuition:* $4368 full-time, $323 per credit hour part-time. *Full-time mandatory fees:* $3716. *Room and board:* $3656–$3966. *Books and supplies per academic year:* ranges from $500 to $1000.

MNSc Program

Applying *Required:* GRE General Test (minimum combined score of 1000 on three tests) or Miller Analogies Test, TOEFL for nonnative speakers of English, bachelor's degree in nursing, minimum GPA of 2.85, RN license, physical assessment course, statistics course, transcript of college record. *Application fee:* $25.

Degree Requirements 39–46 total credit hours dependent upon track, 39–46 in nursing. Thesis, research practicum, or research project.

UNIVERSITY OF ARKANSAS AT PINE BLUFF

Department of Nursing
Pine Bluff, Arkansas

Programs • Generic Baccalaureate • RN Baccalaureate

The University State-supported comprehensive coed institution. Part of University of Arkansas System. Founded: 1873. *Primary accreditation:* regional. *Setting:* 327-acre urban campus. *Total enrollment:* 3,242.

The Department of Nursing Founded in 1978. *Nursing program faculty:* 8 (12% with doctorates).

Academic Facilities *Campus library:* 357,950 volumes; 46 health-care related periodical subscriptions. *Nursing school resources:* CAI, computer lab, nursing audiovisuals, interactive nursing skills videos, learning resource lab.

Student Life *Student services:* health clinic, child-care facilities, personal counseling, career counseling, institutionally sponsored work-study program, job placement, campus safety program, special assistance for disabled students. *International student services:* counseling/support. *Nursing student activities:* student nurses association.

Calendar Semesters.

NURSING STUDENT PROFILE

Undergraduate **Enrollment:** 45

Women: 75%; **Men:** 25%; **Minority:** 90%; **International:** 2%; **Part-time:** 0%

BACCALAUREATE PROGRAMS

Contact Irene T. Henderson, Department Chairperson, 1200 North University Drive, PO Box 4973, Pine Bluff, AR 71611, 501-543-8220. *Fax:* 501-543-8229.

Expenses *State resident tuition:* $1680 full-time, $70 per hour part-time. *Nonresident tuition:* $3888 full-time, $162 per hour part-time. *Full-time mandatory fees:* $123. *Room and board:* $1508–$1740. *Books and supplies per academic year:* $410.

Financial Aid Institutionally sponsored need-based grants/scholarships, institutionally sponsored non-need grants/scholarships, Federal Pell Grants, Federal Perkins Loans, Federal Supplemental Educational Opportunity Grants, Federal Work-Study, Federal SDS. 89% of undergraduate students in nursing programs received some form of financial aid in 1995–96. *Application deadline:* 4/15.

Generic Baccalaureate Program (BSN)

Applying *Required:* SAT I or ACT, NLN Preadmission Examination-RN, minimum high school GPA of 2.5, minimum college GPA of 2.5, 3 years of high school math, 2 years of high school science, high school foreign language, high school transcript, interview, 3 letters of recommendation. 41 prerequisite credits must be completed before admission to the nursing program. *Options:* Advanced standing available through advanced placement exams. *Application deadline:* rolling.

Degree Requirements 129–131 total credit hours dependent upon track, 69 in nursing.

RN Baccalaureate Program (BSN)

Applying *Required:* minimum high school GPA of 2.5, minimum college GPA of 2.5, RN license, diploma or AD in nursing, high school transcript, interview, 3 letters of recommendation, written essay, transcript of college record. *Options:* Advanced standing available through advanced placement exams. *Application deadline:* rolling.

Degree Requirements 129–131 total credit hours dependent upon track, 69 in nursing.

UNIVERSITY OF ARKANSAS FOR MEDICAL SCIENCES
College of Nursing
Little Rock, Arkansas

Programs • Generic Baccalaureate • RN Baccalaureate • MNSc • Master's for Nurses with Non-Nursing Degrees • Post-Master's • PhD • Continuing Education

The University State-supported coed university. Part of University of Arkansas System. Founded: 1879. *Primary accreditation:* regional. *Setting:* 5-acre urban campus. *Total enrollment:* 1,791.

The College of Nursing Founded in 1953. *Nursing program faculty:* 59 (49% with doctorates). *Off-campus program sites:* El Dorado, Helena, Texarkana.

Academic Facilities *Campus library:* 170,000 volumes; 1,719 periodical subscriptions (1,719 health-care related). *Nursing school resources:* CAI, computer lab, nursing audiovisuals, interactive nursing skills videos, learning resource lab.

Student Life *Student services:* health clinic, personal counseling, institutionally sponsored work-study program, campus safety program. *Nursing student activities:* Sigma Theta Tau, student nurses association.

Calendar Semesters.

NURSING STUDENT PROFILE

Undergraduate **Enrollment:** 186
Women: 87%; **Men:** 13%; **Minority:** 9%; **International:** 0%; **Part-time:** 20%

Graduate **Enrollment:** 188
Women: 91%; **Men:** 9%; **Minority:** 3%; **International:** 0%; **Part-time:** 88%

BACCALAUREATE PROGRAMS

Contact Ms. Mary G. Robertson, Director of Admissions and Registrar, College of Nursing, University of Arkansas for Medical Sciences, 4301 West Markham, Slot 529, Little Rock, AR 72205-7199, 501-686-5224. *Fax:* 501-686-8350. *E-mail:* mgrobertson@con.uams.edu

Expenses *State resident tuition:* $2100 full-time, $88 per credit hour part-time. *Nonresident tuition:* $5250 full-time, $219 per credit hour part-time. *Full-time mandatory fees:* $13–$78. *Room only:* $1530–$4320. *Books and supplies per academic year:* ranges from $600 to $700.

Financial Aid Federal Nursing Student Loans, Federal Pell Grants, Federal Perkins Loans, Federal Supplemental Educational Opportunity Grants.

GENERIC BACCALAUREATE PROGRAM (BSN)

Applying *Required:* TOEFL for nonnative speakers of English, NLN Preadmission Examination, minimum college GPA of 2.5, transcript of college record. 64 prerequisite credits must be completed before admission to the nursing program. *Options:* May apply for transfer of up to 64 total credits. *Application deadline:* 2/1 (summer).

Degree Requirements 124 total credit hours, 60 in nursing.

RN BACCALAUREATE PROGRAM (BSN)

Applying *Required:* minimum college GPA of 2.5, RN license, diploma or AD in nursing, transcript of college record, clinical experience or advanced placement exam. 64 prerequisite credits must be completed before admission to the nursing program. *Options:* Advanced standing available through advanced placement exams. Course work may be accelerated. May apply for transfer of up to 64 total credits. *Application deadlines:* 2/1 (fall), 2/1 (summer).

Degree Requirements 125 total credit hours, 60 in nursing.

Distance learning Courses provided through video.

MASTER'S PROGRAMS

Contact Dr. Beth C. Vaughan-Wrobel, Associate Dean for Academic Programs, College of Nursing, University of Arkansas for Medical Sciences, 4301 West Markham, Slot 529, Little Rock, AR 72205-7199, 501-686-5453. *Fax:* 501-686-8350. *E-mail:* bcwrobel@con.uams.edu

Areas of Study Clinical nurse specialist programs in adult health nursing, pediatric nursing; nursing administration; nurse practitioner programs in acute care, child care/pediatrics, family health, gerontology, women's health.

Expenses *State resident tuition:* $2770 full-time, $139 per credit hour part-time. *Nonresident tuition:* $5940 full-time, $297 per credit hour part-time. *Full-time mandatory fees:* $60–$150. *Room only:* $1530–$4320. *Books and supplies per academic year:* ranges from $600 to $700.

Financial Aid Nurse traineeships, Federal Nursing Student Loans.

MNSc PROGRAM

Applying *Required:* GRE General Test, Miller Analogies Test, TOEFL for nonnative speakers of English, bachelor's degree in nursing, minimum GPA of 2.85, RN license, physical assessment course, statistics course, professional liability/malpractice insurance, transcript of college record. *Application deadlines:* 4/1 (fall), 9/1 (spring).

Degree Requirements 39–46 total credit hours dependent upon track, 39–46 in nursing.

MASTER'S FOR NURSES WITH NON-NURSING DEGREES PROGRAM (MNSc)

Applying *Required:* GRE General Test, Miller Analogies Test, TOEFL for nonnative speakers of English, bachelor's degree, minimum GPA of 2.85, RN license, physical assessment course, statistics course, professional liability/malpractice insurance, transcript of college record, portfolio or completion of undergraduate deficiencies. *Application deadlines:* 4/1 (fall), 9/1 (spring). *Application fee:* $50.

Degree Requirements 39–46 total credit hours dependent upon track, 39–46 in nursing.

POST-MASTER'S PROGRAM

Applying *Required:* TOEFL for nonnative speakers of English, RN license, professional liability/malpractice insurance, interview, 3 letters of recommendation, transcript of college record, master's degree. *Application deadlines:* 4/1 (fall), 9/1 (spring).

Degree Requirements 20–32 total credit hours dependent upon track, 20–32 in nursing.

DOCTORAL PROGRAM

Contact Dr. Beth C. Vaughan-Wrobel, Associate Dean for Academic Programs, College of Nursing, University of Arkansas for Medical Sciences, 4301 West Markham, Slot 529, Little Rock, AR 72205-7199, 501-686-5453. *Fax:* 501-686-8350. *E-mail:* bcwrobel@con.uams.edu

Areas of Study Nursing research.

Expenses *State resident tuition:* $2770 full-time, $139 per credit hour part-time. *Nonresident tuition:* $5940 full-time, $297 per credit hour part-time.

Financial Aid Graduate assistantships, nurse traineeships.

PhD PROGRAM

Applying *Required:* TOEFL for nonnative speakers of English, GRE General Test (minimum combined score of 1100 on two sections), master's degree in nursing, 1 scholarly paper, statistics course, interview, 3 letters of recommendation, writing sample, competitive review by faculty committee. *Application deadline:* 1/15. *Application fee:* $50.

Degree Requirements 60 total credit hours; dissertation; written exam; defense of dissertation; residency.

CONTINUING EDUCATION PROGRAM

Contact Ms. Benni Odgen, Director of Continuing Education, College of Nursing, University of Arkansas for Medical Sciences, 4301 West Markham, Slot 529, Little Rock, AR 72205-7199, 501-686-5374. *Fax:* 501-686-8350.

UNIVERSITY OF CENTRAL ARKANSAS
Department of Nursing
Conway, Arkansas

Programs • Generic Baccalaureate • RN Baccalaureate • LPN to Baccalaureate • MSN • RN to Master's

University of Central Arkansas (continued)

The University State-supported comprehensive coed institution. Founded: 1907. *Primary accreditation:* regional. *Setting:* 256-acre small-town campus. *Total enrollment:* 8,882.

The Department of Nursing Founded in 1967. *Nursing program faculty:* 16 (44% with doctorates). *Off-campus program sites:* Fort Smith, Harrison.

Academic Facilities *Campus library:* 1.2 million volumes (10,000 in health, 4,500 in nursing); 2,652 periodical subscriptions (347 health-care related). *Nursing school resources:* CAI, computer lab, nursing audiovisuals, interactive nursing skills videos, learning resource lab.

Student Life *Student services:* health clinic, personal counseling, career counseling, institutionally sponsored work-study program, job placement, campus safety program, special assistance for disabled students. *International student services:* counseling/support, special assistance for nonnative speakers of English, ESL courses. *Nursing student activities:* Sigma Theta Tau, student nurses association.

Calendar Semesters.

NURSING STUDENT PROFILE

Undergraduate **Enrollment:** 155
Women: 79%; **Men:** 21%; **Minority:** 10%; **International:** 90%; **Part-time:** 20%
Graduate **Enrollment:** 46
Part-time: 80%

BACCALAUREATE PROGRAMS

Contact Ms. Ann Mattison, Program Coordinator, Department of Nursing, University of Central Arkansas, 201 Donaghey Avenue, Conway, AR 72035, 501-450-3120. *Fax:* 501-450-5560. *E-mail:* annm@ccl.uca.edu

Expenses *State resident tuition:* $909 full-time, $76 per credit hour part-time. *Nonresident tuition:* $1895 full-time, $158 per credit hour part-time. *Full-time mandatory fees:* $150. *Part-time mandatory fees:* $75. *Books and supplies per academic year:* $100.

Financial Aid Institutionally sponsored need-based grants/scholarships, institutionally sponsored non-need grants/scholarships, Federal Supplemental Educational Opportunity Grants, Federal Work-Study. *Application deadline:* 4/15.

GENERIC BACCALAUREATE PROGRAM (BSN)

Applying *Required:* ACT, minimum college GPA of 2.5, written essay, transcript of college record. 34 prerequisite credits must be completed before admission to the nursing program. *Options:* May apply for transfer of up to 74 total credits. *Application deadline:* 3/1.

Degree Requirements 131 total credit hours, 57 in nursing.

RN BACCALAUREATE PROGRAM (BSN)

Applying *Required:* TOEFL for nonnative speakers of English, minimum college GPA of 2.5, RN license, diploma or AD in nursing, written essay, transcript of college record. 30 prerequisite credits must be completed before admission to the nursing program. *Options:* Advanced standing available through the following means: advanced placement exams, advanced placement without credit. May apply for transfer of up to 106 total credits. *Application deadlines:* 3/1 (fall), 10/1 (spring).

Degree Requirements 133 total credit hours, 61 in nursing.

Distance learning Courses provided through compressed video.

LPN TO BACCALAUREATE PROGRAM (BSN)

Applying *Required:* minimum college GPA of 2.5, transcript of college record, LPN license. 34 prerequisite credits must be completed before admission to the nursing program. *Options:* Advanced standing available through the following means: advanced placement exams, advanced placement without credit. May apply for transfer of up to 81 total credits. *Application deadline:* 3/1.

Degree Requirements 133 total credit hours, 61 in nursing.

MASTER'S PROGRAMS

Contact Dr. Rebecca Lancaster, Director of Graduate Program, Department of Nursing, University of Central Arkansas, 201 Donaghey Avenue, Conway, AR 72035, 501-450-3119. *Fax:* 501-450-5503. *E-mail:* beckyl@ccl.uca.edu

Areas of Study Clinical nurse specialist programs in adult health nursing, community health nursing, psychiatric–mental health nursing; nursing education; nurse practitioner programs in adult health, primary care.

Expenses *State resident tuition:* $1000 full-time, $100 per credit hour part-time. *Nonresident tuition:* $2088 full-time, $209 per credit hour part-time. *Full-time mandatory fees:* $150. *Part-time mandatory fees:* $75. *Books and supplies per academic year:* $150.

Financial Aid Graduate assistantships, nurse traineeships. *Application deadline:* 4/15.

MSN PROGRAM

Applying *Required:* bachelor's degree in nursing, minimum GPA of 2.7, RN license, 1 year of clinical experience, statistics course, professional liability/malpractice insurance, essay, interview, 2 letters of recommendation, transcript of college record, professional resume. *Application deadlines:* 7/1 (fall), 12/1 (spring).

Degree Requirements 42–45 total credit hours dependent upon track, 42–45 in nursing.

Distance learning Courses provided through compressed video.

RN TO MASTER'S PROGRAM (MSN)

Applying *Required:* minimum GPA of 3.0, RN license, 2 years of clinical experience, statistics course, professional liability/malpractice insurance, transcript of college record, challenge of sophomore and junior nursing courses. *Application deadline:* 3/1.

Degree Requirements 165 total credit hours, 55 in nursing.

Distance learning Courses provided through compressed video.

CALIFORNIA

AZUSA PACIFIC UNIVERSITY
School of Nursing
Azusa, California

Programs • Generic Baccalaureate • Accelerated RN Baccalaureate • Baccalaureate for Second Degree • MSN • Master's for Nurses with Non-Nursing Degrees • Continuing Education

The University Independent nondenominational comprehensive coed institution. Founded: 1899. *Primary accreditation:* regional. *Setting:* 60-acre small-town campus. *Total enrollment:* 4,360.

The School of Nursing Founded in 1975. *Nursing program faculty:* 42 (19% with doctorates).

► ***NOTEWORTHY***

Azusa Pacific University, located 26 miles northeast of Los Angeles in Azusa, California, provides baccalaureate and master's clinical nurse specialization and family nurse practitioner programs, with an emphasis on academic excellence in a caring Christian university environment. The attractive, well-landscaped campus includes many contemporary facilities. APU offers numerous extracurricular activities and is close to mountains, beaches, and desert. The School of Nursing seeks to provide students with the opportunity to grow intellectually, physically, emotionally, and spiritually. Clinical courses, offered each semester, provide a wide range of clinical experiences with a student-faculty ratio of no more than 11:1.

Academic Facilities *Campus library:* 115,000 volumes (14,005 in health, 4,692 in nursing); 1,200 periodical subscriptions (394 health-care related). *Nursing school resources:* computer lab, nursing audiovisuals, learning resource lab.

Student Life *Student services:* health clinic, personal counseling, career counseling, institutionally sponsored work-study program, job placement, campus safety program, special assistance for disabled students, tutoring. *International student services:* counseling/support, special assistance for nonnative speakers of English, ESL courses. *Nursing student activities:* Sigma Theta Tau, nursing club, student nurses association.

Calendar Semesters.

NURSING STUDENT PROFILE

Undergraduate **Enrollment:** 208
Women: 93%; **Men:** 7%; **Minority:** 37%; **International:** 0%; **Part-time:** 14%
Graduate **Enrollment:** 116
Women: 98%; **Men:** 2%; **Minority:** 27%; **International:** 0%; **Part-time:** 14%

BACCALAUREATE PROGRAMS

Contact Admissions Office, School of Nursing, Azusa Pacific University, 901 East Alosta Avenue, Azusa, CA 91702, 818-812-3016. *Fax:* 818-815-3865.

Expenses *Tuition:* $13,020 full-time, $545 per unit part-time. *Full-time mandatory fees:* $317. *Room and board:* $4190–$5170. *Room only:* $1880–$2860. *Books and supplies per academic year:* ranges from $825 to $975.

Financial Aid Institutionally sponsored need-based grants/scholarships, institutionally sponsored non-need grants/scholarships, Federal Nursing Student Loans, Federal Supplemental Educational Opportunity Grants. *Application deadline:* 7/1.

Generic Baccalaureate Program (BSN)

Applying *Required:* SAT I, ACT, TOEFL for nonnative speakers of English, minimum high school GPA of 2.7, minimum college GPA of 2.0, 2 years of high school math, high school chemistry, high school biology, high school transcript, interview, 3 letters of recommendation, written essay, transcript of college record. *Options:* Advanced standing available through credit by exam. Course work may be accelerated. May apply for transfer of up to 61 total credits. *Application deadline:* 4/1. *Application fee:* $45.

Degree Requirements 136 total credit hours, 64 in nursing. Participation in 3 community service/ministry experiences.

Accelerated RN Baccalaureate Program (BSN)

Applying *Required:* SAT I, ACT, TOEFL for nonnative speakers of English, minimum high school GPA of 2.7, minimum college GPA of 3.0, RN license, diploma or AD in nursing, high school transcript, interview, 3 letters of recommendation, written essay, transcript of college record. *Options:* May apply for transfer of up to 61 total credits. *Application deadline:* rolling. *Application fee:* $45.

Degree Requirements 126 total credit hours, 24 in nursing. Participation in community service/ministry experiences.

Baccalaureate for Second Degree Program (BSN)

Applying *Required:* SAT I, ACT, TOEFL for nonnative speakers of English, minimum college GPA of 3.0, interview, 3 letters of recommendation, written essay, transcript of college record. *Options:* Course work may be accelerated. May apply for transfer of up to 61 total credits. *Application deadline:* rolling. *Application fee:* $45.

Degree Requirements 126 total credit hours, 67 in nursing.

MASTER'S PROGRAMS

Contact Ms. Barb Barthelmess, Secretary, Graduate Program, School of Nursing, Azusa Pacific University, 901 East Alosta Avenue, Azusa, CA 91702, 818-815-5391. *Fax:* 818-815-5414.

Areas of Study Clinical nurse specialist programs in adult health nursing, community health nursing, home health nursing; nursing administration; nursing education; nurse practitioner program in family health.

Expenses *Tuition:* ranges from $325 to $350 per unit. *Full-time mandatory fees:* $152. *Books and supplies per academic year:* $700+.

Financial Aid Nurse traineeships. 75% of master's level students in nursing programs received some form of financial aid in 1995-96. *Application deadline:* 7/15.

MSN Program

Applying *Required:* bachelor's degree in nursing, minimum GPA of 3.0, RN license, professional liability/malpractice insurance, essay, interview, 3 letters of recommendation, transcript of college record. *Application deadline:* rolling. *Application fee:* $40–60.

Degree Requirements 42 total credit hours, 38–39 in nursing. Thesis or comprehensive exam.

Master's for Nurses with Non-Nursing Degrees Program (MSN)

Applying *Required:* bachelor's degree, minimum GPA of 3.0, RN license, 3 letters of recommendation, transcript of college record. *Application deadline:* rolling. *Application fee:* $40–60.

Degree Requirements 42 total credit hours, 42 in nursing. Thesis or comprehensive exam.

CONTINUING EDUCATION PROGRAM

Contact Mrs. Kathie Speck, Undergraduate and Continuing Education Secretary, School of Nursing, Azusa Pacific University, 901 East Alosta Avenue, Azusa, CA 91702, 818-815-5385. *Fax:* 818-815-5414.

BIOLA UNIVERSITY
Department of Baccalaureate Nursing
La Mirada, California

Programs • Generic Baccalaureate • Accelerated RN Baccalaureate • Baccalaureate for Second Degree • Continuing Education

The University Independent nondenominational coed university. Founded: 1908. *Primary accreditation:* regional. *Setting:* 95-acre suburban campus. *Total enrollment:* 3,039.

The Department of Baccalaureate Nursing Founded in 1964. *Nursing program faculty:* 12 (25% with doctorates).

Academic Facilities *Campus library:* 208,614 volumes (4,372 in health, 3,877 in nursing); 1,174 periodical subscriptions (70 health-care related). *Nursing school resources:* CAI, computer lab, nursing audiovisuals, learning resource lab.

Student Life *Student services:* health clinic, personal counseling, career counseling, institutionally sponsored work-study program, job placement, campus safety program, special assistance for disabled students. *International student services:* counseling/support, special assistance for nonnative speakers of English, ESL courses. *Nursing student activities:* nursing club, student nurses association, Nurses Christian Fellowship.

Calendar Semesters.

NURSING STUDENT PROFILE

Undergraduate **Enrollment:** 144
Women: 90%; **Men:** 10%; **Minority:** 42%; **International:** 15%; **Part-time:** 10%

BACCALAUREATE PROGRAMS

Contact Ms. Cynthia Westcott, Associate Chair, Department of Baccalaureate Nursing, Biola University, 13800 Biola Avenue, La Mirada, CA 90639, 310-903-4850. *Fax:* 310-903-4851. *E-mail:* cheryll_cole@peter.biola.edu

Expenses *Tuition:* $13,408 full-time, $599 per unit part-time. *Full-time mandatory fees:* $150. *Room and board:* $4300–$5012. *Room only:* $2296–$2798. *Books and supplies per academic year:* ranges from $150 to $500.

Financial Aid Institutionally sponsored need-based grants/scholarships, institutionally sponsored non-need grants/scholarships, Federal Direct Loans, Federal Nursing Student Loans, Federal Perkins Loans, Federal Supplemental Educational Opportunity Grants, Federal Work-Study. 80% of undergraduate students in nursing programs received some form of financial aid in 1995–96. *Application deadline:* 3/1.

Generic Baccalaureate Program (BS)

Applying *Required:* SAT I or ACT, TOEFL for nonnative speakers of English, NLN Preadmission Examination-RN, minimum college GPA of 2.8, 2 years of high school math, 2 years of high school science, high school chemistry, high school biology, high school foreign language, high school transcript, interview, 2 letters of recommendation, written essay, transcript of college record. 30 prerequisite credits must be completed before admission to the nursing program. *Options:* Advanced standing available through the following means: advanced placement exams, credit by exam. May apply for transfer of up to 70 total credits. *Application deadlines:* 6/1 (fall), 1/1 (spring). *Application fee:* $55.

Degree Requirements 142 total credit hours, 61 in nursing. 30 units of biblical studies.

Biola University (continued)

Accelerated RN Baccalaureate Program (BS)

Applying *Required:* SAT I, TOEFL for nonnative speakers of English, minimum college GPA of 2.8, 2 years of high school math, 2 years of high school science, high school chemistry, high school biology, RN license, diploma or AD in nursing, high school foreign language, high school transcript, interview, 2 letters of recommendation, written essay, transcript of college record. 30 prerequisite credits must be completed before admission to the nursing program. *Options:* Advanced standing available through the following means: advanced placement exams, credit by exam. May apply for transfer of up to 70 total credits. *Application deadlines:* 6/1 (fall), 1/1 (spring). *Application fee:* $55.

Degree Requirements 142 total credit hours, 61 in nursing. 30 units of biblical studies.

Baccalaureate for Second Degree Program (BS)

Applying *Required:* SAT I, TOEFL for nonnative speakers of English, minimum college GPA of 2.8, 2 years of high school math, 2 years of high school science, high school chemistry, high school biology, high school foreign language, high school transcript, interview, 2 letters of recommendation, written essay, transcript of college record. 30 prerequisite credits must be completed before admission to the nursing program. *Options:* Advanced standing available through the following means: advanced placement exams, credit by exam. May apply for transfer of up to 70 total credits. *Application deadlines:* 6/1 (fall), 1/1 (spring). *Application fee:* $55.

Degree Requirements 142 total credit hours, 61 in nursing. 30 units of biblical studies.

CONTINUING EDUCATION PROGRAM

Contact Ms. Anne Gewe, Associate Professor, Biola University, 13800 Biola Avenue, La Mirada, CA 90639, 310-903-4850. *Fax:* 310-903-4748. *E-mail:* anne_gewe@peter.biola.edu

CALIFORNIA STATE UNIVERSITY, BAKERSFIELD

Department of Nursing
Bakersfield, California

Programs • Generic Baccalaureate • RN Baccalaureate • Accelerated RN Baccalaureate • MSN • Continuing Education

The University State-supported comprehensive coed institution. Part of California State University System. Founded: 1970. *Primary accreditation:* regional. *Setting:* 575-acre urban campus. *Total enrollment:* 5,319.

The Department of Nursing Founded in 1972. *Nursing program faculty:* 15 (33% with doctorates).

Academic Facilities *Campus library:* 46,752 volumes; 2,331 periodical subscriptions (96 health-care related). *Nursing school resources:* CAI, computer lab, nursing audiovisuals, interactive nursing skills videos.

Student Life *Student services:* health clinic, child-care facilities, personal counseling, career counseling, institutionally sponsored work-study program, job placement, campus safety program, special assistance for disabled students. *International student services:* counseling/support, special assistance for nonnative speakers of English. *Nursing student activities:* Sigma Theta Tau, nursing club, student nurses association.

Calendar Quarters.

NURSING STUDENT PROFILE

Undergraduate **Enrollment:** 210
Women: 97%; **Men:** 3%; **Minority:** 40%
Graduate **Enrollment:** 40
Women: 99%; **Men:** 1%; **Minority:** 20%; **Part-time:** 50%

BACCALAUREATE PROGRAMS

Contact Ms. Nancy Haley, Secretary, Department of Nursing, California State University, Bakersfield, 9001 Stockdale Highway, Bakersfield, CA 93311-1099, 805-664-3103. *Fax:* 805-665-6903. *E-mail:* nhaley@csubak.edu

Expenses *Nonresident tuition:* $2952 full-time, $164 per unit part-time. *Full-time mandatory fees:* $1953. *Part-time mandatory fees:* $1287. *Room and board:* $4070.

Financial Aid Institutionally sponsored need-based grants/scholarships, institutionally sponsored non-need grants/scholarships, Federal Direct Loans, Federal Nursing Student Loans, Federal Perkins Loans, Federal Supplemental Educational Opportunity Grants. 50% of undergraduate students in nursing programs received some form of financial aid in 1995–96. *Application deadline:* 3/2.

Generic Baccalaureate Program (BSN)

Applying *Required:* SAT I or ACT, TOEFL for nonnative speakers of English, minimum high school GPA of 2.0, minimum college GPA of 2.5, 3 years of high school math, 3 years of high school science, high school foreign language, high school transcript, transcript of college record. 45 prerequisite credits must be completed before admission to the nursing program. *Options:* May apply for transfer of up to 105 total credits. *Application deadline:* 1/31. *Application fee:* $55.

Degree Requirements 192 total credit hours, 84 in nursing.

RN Baccalaureate Program (BSN)

Applying *Required:* TOEFL for nonnative speakers of English, minimum high school GPA of 2.0, minimum college GPA of 2.0, RN license, diploma or AD in nursing, 3 letters of recommendation, transcript of college record. 90 prerequisite credits must be completed before admission to the nursing program. *Options:* Advanced standing available through credit by exam. May apply for transfer of up to 105 total credits. *Application deadline:* 5/30. *Application fee:* $55.

Degree Requirements 186 total credit hours, 82 in nursing.

Accelerated RN Baccalaureate Program (BSN)

Applying *Required:* TOEFL for nonnative speakers of English, minimum high school GPA of 2.0, minimum college GPA of 3.0, RN license, 3 letters of recommendation, transcript of college record. 90 prerequisite credits must be completed before admission to the nursing program. *Options:* Advanced standing available through advanced placement exams. Course work may be accelerated. May apply for transfer of up to 105 total credits. *Application deadline:* 5/30. *Application fee:* $55.

Degree Requirements 186 total credit hours, 82 in nursing.

MASTER'S PROGRAM

Contact Dr. Colette York, Graduate Coordinator and Professor, Department of Nursing, California State University, Bakersfield, 9001 Stockdale Highway, Bakersfield, CA 93311-1099, 805-664-3115. *Fax:* 805-665-6903. *E-mail:* cyork@csubak.edu

Areas of Study Nursing administration; nursing education; nurse practitioner program in family health.

Expenses *Nonresident tuition:* $2952 full-time, $164 per unit part-time. *Full-time mandatory fees:* $1953. *Part-time mandatory fees:* $1287.

Financial Aid Nurse traineeships, institutionally sponsored need-based grants/scholarships, institutionally sponsored non-need-based grants/scholarships. 40% of master's level students in nursing programs received some form of financial aid in 1995-96. *Application deadline:* 5/15.

MSN Program

Applying *Required:* TOEFL for nonnative speakers of English, GRE General Test (minimum combined score of 900 on quantitative and verbal sections) required only if GPA is below 3.0 on last 60 quarter units, bachelor's degree in nursing, bachelor's degree, RN license, 1 year of clinical experience, physical assessment course, statistics course, professional liability/malpractice insurance, 3 letters of recommendation, transcript of college record. *Application deadlines:* 5/15 (family nurse practitioner track), rolling. *Application fee:* $55.

Degree Requirements 54–59 total credit hours dependent upon track, 39–59 in nursing, 15 in administration, education. Thesis or special project.

CONTINUING EDUCATION PROGRAM

Contact Dr. David H. Ost, Dean, Extended University, California State University, Bakersfield, 9001 Stockdale Highway, Bakersfield, CA 93311-1099, 805-664-2441. *Fax:* 805-664-2447. *E-mail:* dost@csubak.edu

CALIFORNIA STATE UNIVERSITY, CHICO

School of Nursing
Chico, California

Programs • Generic Baccalaureate • Accelerated RN Baccalaureate • Baccalaureate for Second Degree • BSN to Master's • Continuing Education

The University State-supported comprehensive coed institution. Part of California State University System. Founded: 1887. *Primary accreditation:* regional. *Setting:* 119-acre small-town campus. *Total enrollment:* 13,798.

The School of Nursing Founded in 1952. *Nursing program faculty:* 20 (21% with doctorates).

Academic Facilities *Campus library:* 1.3 million volumes (17,727 in health, 1,467 in nursing); 4,124 periodical subscriptions (133 health-care related). *Nursing school resources:* CAI, computer lab, nursing audiovisuals, interactive nursing skills videos, learning resource lab.

Student Life *Student services:* health clinic, child-care facilities, personal counseling, career counseling, institutionally sponsored work-study program, job placement, campus safety program, special assistance for disabled students. *International student services:* counseling/support, special assistance for nonnative speakers of English, ESL courses. *Nursing student activities:* Sigma Theta Tau, nursing club, student nurses association.

Calendar Semesters.

NURSING STUDENT PROFILE

Undergraduate **Enrollment:** 150
Women: 78%; **Men:** 22%; **Minority:** 13%; **International:** 0%; **Part-time:** 6%
Graduate **Enrollment:** 15
Women: 94%; **Men:** 6%; **Minority:** 0%; **International:** 0%; **Part-time:** 100%

BACCALAUREATE PROGRAMS

Contact Dr. Sherry D. Fox, Director, School of Nursing, California State University, Chico, Chico, CA 95929-0200, 916-898-5891. *Fax:* 916-898-4363.

Expenses *Nonresident tuition:* $5688 full-time, $237 per unit part-time. *Full-time mandatory fees:* $2037. *Part-time mandatory fees:* $1370. *Room and board:* $4632.

Financial Aid Institutionally sponsored need-based grants/scholarships, institutionally sponsored non-need grants/scholarships, Federal Pell Grants, Federal Supplemental Educational Opportunity Grants, Federal Work-Study.

Generic Baccalaureate Program (BSN)

Applying *Required:* minimum college GPA of 2.5, transcript of college record. 28 prerequisite credits must be completed before admission to the nursing program. *Options:* Course work may be accelerated. May apply for transfer of up to 70 total credits. *Application deadlines:* 11/30 (fall), 8/30 (spring). *Application fee:* $55.

Degree Requirements 128 total credit hours, 58 in nursing.

Accelerated RN Baccalaureate Program (BSN)

Applying *Required:* minimum college GPA of 2.3, RN license, diploma or AD in nursing, transcript of college record. 25 prerequisite credits must be completed before admission to the nursing program. *Options:* Advanced standing available through credit by exam. Course work may be accelerated. May apply for transfer of up to 70 total credits. *Application deadlines:* 11/30 (fall), 8/30 (spring). *Application fee:* $55.

Degree Requirements 128 total credit hours, 58 in nursing.

Baccalaureate for Second Degree Program (BSN)

Applying *Required:* minimum college GPA of 2.5, transcript of college record. 25 prerequisite credits must be completed before admission to the nursing program. *Options:* Course work may be accelerated. May apply for transfer of up to 70 total credits. *Application deadlines:* 11/30 (fall), 8/30 (spring). *Application fee:* $55.

Degree Requirements 128 total credit hours, 58 in nursing.

MASTER'S PROGRAM

Contact Shelley Young, Graduate Coordinator, School of Nursing, California State University, Chico, Chico, CA 95929-0200, 916-898-6207. *Fax:* 916-898-4363.

Areas of Study Clinical nurse specialist program in adult health nursing; nursing education.

Expenses *Nonresident tuition:* $5688 full-time, $237 per unit part-time. *Full-time mandatory fees:* $2032. *Part-time mandatory fees:* $1370. *Room and board:* $4632.

Financial Aid Institutionally sponsored loans, institutionally sponsored need-based grants/scholarships, institutionally sponsored non-need-based grants/scholarships.

BSN to Master's Program (MSN)

Applying *Required:* Miller Analogies Test, bachelor's degree in nursing, minimum GPA of 3.0, RN license, physical assessment course, statistics course, professional liability/malpractice insurance, transcript of college record. *Application deadline:* rolling. *Application fee:* $55.

Degree Requirements 30 total credit hours, 24 in nursing, 6 in electives. Thesis required.

CONTINUING EDUCATION PROGRAM

Contact Ms. Deborah Barger, Continuing Education, School of Nursing, California State University, Chico, Chico, CA 95929-0020, 916-898-6105. *Fax:* 916-898-4363.

CALIFORNIA STATE UNIVERSITY, DOMINGUEZ HILLS

Division of Nursing
Carson, California

Programs • RN Baccalaureate • MSN • Master's for Nurses with Non-Nursing Degrees • Continuing Education

The University State-supported comprehensive coed institution. Part of California State University System. Founded: 1960. *Primary accreditation:* regional. *Setting:* 350-acre urban campus. *Total enrollment:* 9,977.

The Division of Nursing Founded in 1981. *Nursing program faculty:* 21 (95% with doctorates).

Academic Facilities *Campus library:* 423,939 volumes (10,065 in health, 6,200 in nursing); 3,350 periodical subscriptions. *Nursing school resources:* CAI, computer lab, learning resource lab, CINAHL, ERIC, Medline, Psychlit, Sociofile, Business, General Science, GPO, Humanities, Social Sciences indices.

Student Life *Student services:* health clinic, child-care facilities, personal counseling, career counseling, institutionally sponsored work-study program, job placement, campus safety program, special assistance for disabled students, nationwide computer support. *International student services:* special assistance for nonnative speakers of English, ESL courses. *Nursing student activities:* Sigma Theta Tau, student nurses association.

Calendar Trimesters for national delivery, semesters for California delivery.

NURSING STUDENT PROFILE

Undergraduate **Enrollment:** 1700
Women: 95%; **Men:** 5%; **Minority:** 32%; **Part-time:** 92%
Graduate **Enrollment:** 550
Women: 95%; **Men:** 5%; **Minority:** 22%; **Part-time:** 90%

BACCALAUREATE PROGRAM

Contact Dr. Angela Albright, Chair, Undergraduate Program in Nursing Science, Division of Nursing, California State University, Dominguez Hills, Carson, CA 90747, 310-516-4040. *Fax:* 310-516-3542. *E-mail:* aalbright@dhvx20.csudh.edu

Expenses *State resident tuition:* $0 full-time, $0 part-time. *Nonresident tuition:* $5904 full-time, $246 per unit part-time. *Full-time mandatory fees:* $1741. *Part-time mandatory fees:* $1074.

Financial Aid Institutionally sponsored need-based grants/scholarships, Federal Direct Loans, Federal Nursing Student Loans, Federal Supplemental Educational Opportunity Grants, Federal Work-Study.

California State University, Dominguez Hills (continued)

RN Baccalaureate Program (BSN)

Applying *Required:* TOEFL for nonnative speakers of English, RN license, diploma or AD in nursing, transcript of college record. 56 prerequisite credits must be completed before admission to the nursing program. *Options:* Advanced standing available through the following means: advanced placement exams, credit by exam. Course work may be accelerated. May apply for transfer of up to 96 total credits. *Application deadlines:* 11/30 (fall), 4/30 (spring). *Application fee:* $55.

Degree Requirements 126 total credit hours, 53 in nursing. Graduate writing requirement.

Distance learning Courses provided through video, computer-based media, on-line. Specific degree requirements include live seminar classes at 170 sites in California.

MASTER'S PROGRAMS

Contact Dr. Margaret Wallace, Chair, Graduate Program in Nursing Science, Division of Nursing, California State University, Dominguez Hills, Carson, CA 90747, 310-243-2050. *Fax:* 310-516-3542. *E-mail:* mwallace@dhvx20.csudh.edu

Areas of Study Clinical nurse specialist programs in gerontological nursing, maternity-newborn nursing; nursing administration; nursing education; nurse practitioner program in family health.

Expenses *State resident tuition:* $0 full-time, $0 part-time. *Nonresident tuition:* $246 per unit. *Full-time mandatory fees:* $1074–$1740.

Financial Aid Nurse traineeships, Federal Nursing Student Loans.

MSN Program

Applying *Required:* bachelor's degree in nursing, bachelor's degree, minimum GPA of 3.0, RN license, physical assessment course, statistics course, professional liability/malpractice insurance, transcript of college record. *Application deadlines:* 11/30 (fall), 4/30 (spring). *Application fee:* $55.

Degree Requirements 36 total credit hours, 36 in nursing. Project or comprehensive exam, 52 total credit hours for nurse practitioner program.

Distance learning Courses provided through video, computer-based media, on-line.

Master's for Nurses with Non-Nursing Degrees Program (MSN)

Applying *Required:* bachelor's degree, minimum GPA of 3.0, RN license, physical assessment course, statistics course, professional liability/malpractice insurance, transcript of college record. *Application deadlines:* 11/30 (fall), 4/30 (spring). *Application fee:* $55.

Degree Requirements 36 total credit hours, 36 in nursing. Project or comprehensive exam, 52 total credit hours for nurse practitioner program.

Distance learning Courses provided through video, computer-based media, on-line.

CONTINUING EDUCATION PROGRAM

Contact Ms. M. Kathleen Johnston, Coordinator of Development, Division of Nursing, California State University, Dominguez Hills, Carson, CA 90747, 310-243-2021. *Fax:* 310-516-3542. *E-mail:* kjohnston@dhvx20.csudh.edu

CALIFORNIA STATE UNIVERSITY, FRESNO

Department of Nursing
Fresno, California

Programs • Generic Baccalaureate • RN Baccalaureate • MSN • Post-Master's • Continuing Education

The University State-supported comprehensive coed institution. Part of California State University System. Founded: 1911. *Primary accreditation:* regional. *Setting:* 1,410-acre urban campus. *Total enrollment:* 17,460.

The Department of Nursing Founded in 1957. *Nursing program faculty:* 36 (44% with doctorates). *Off-campus program site:* Visalia.

Academic Facilities *Campus library:* 866,211 volumes (28,855 in health, 2,111 in nursing); 2,845 periodical subscriptions (135 health-care related). *Nursing school resources:* CAI, computer lab, nursing audiovisuals, interactive nursing skills videos, learning resource lab.

Student Life *Student services:* health clinic, child-care facilities, personal counseling, career counseling, institutionally sponsored work-study program, job placement, campus safety program, special assistance for disabled students, educational opportunity program, migrant services, reentry programs. *International student services:* counseling/support, special assistance for nonnative speakers of English, ESL courses. *Nursing student activities:* Sigma Theta Tau, student nurses association, mentoring program.

Calendar Semesters.

NURSING STUDENT PROFILE

Undergraduate **Enrollment:** 256
Women: 71%; **Men:** 29%; **Minority:** 56%; **International:** 1%; **Part-time:** 17%
Graduate **Enrollment:** 81
Women: 84%; **Men:** 16%; **Minority:** 39%; **International:** 1%; **Part-time:** 72%

BACCALAUREATE PROGRAMS

Contact Georgia Porcella, Admissions Coordinator, Department of Nursing, California State University, Fresno, 2345 East San Ramon Avenue, Fresno, CA 93740-8031, 209-278-6579. *Fax:* 209-278-6360. *E-mail:* georgia_porcella@csufresno.edu

Expenses *State resident tuition:* $0 per academic year. *Nonresident tuition:* $5904 full-time, $246 per unit part-time. *Full-time mandatory fees:* $1008–$1740. *Part-time mandatory fees:* $1140. *Room and board:* $5140. *Books and supplies per academic year:* $1300.

Financial Aid Institutionally sponsored need-based grants/scholarships, institutionally sponsored non-need grants/scholarships, Federal Nursing Student Loans, Federal Pell Grants, Federal Perkins Loans, Federal Supplemental Educational Opportunity Grants, Federal Work-Study, scholarships for disadvantaged students. 85% of undergraduate students in nursing programs received some form of financial aid in 1995–96. *Application deadline:* 3/1.

Generic Baccalaureate Program (BSN)

Applying *Required:* SAT I or ACT, TOEFL for nonnative speakers of English, English placement test, entry-level math test, minimum high school GPA of 2.0, minimum college GPA of 2.5, 3 years of high school math, 1 year of high school science, high school foreign language, high school transcript, transcript of college record. 32 prerequisite credits must be completed before admission to the nursing program. *Application deadline:* 2/15. *Application fee:* $55.

Degree Requirements 130 total credit hours, 65 in nursing.

RN Baccalaureate Program (BSN)

Applying *Required:* TOEFL for nonnative speakers of English, English placement test, entry-level math test, minimum high school GPA of 2.0, minimum college GPA of 2.5, 3 years of high school math, 1 year of high school science, RN license, diploma or AD in nursing, high school transcript, transcript of college record. 32 prerequisite credits must be completed before admission to the nursing program. *Options:* Advanced standing available through credit by exam. May apply for transfer of up to 33 total credits. *Application deadline:* rolling. *Application fee:* $55.

Degree Requirements 130 total credit hours, 65 in nursing.

MASTER'S PROGRAMS

Contact Dr. Michael Russler, Graduate Coordinator, Department of Nursing, California State University, Fresno, 2345 East San Ramon Avenue, Fresno, CA 93740-8031, 209-278-2041. *Fax:* 209-278-6360. *E-mail:* michael_russler@csufresno.edu

Areas of Study Nurse practitioner programs in child care/pediatrics, family health, gerontology, primary care, school health.

Expenses *State resident tuition:* $0 per academic year. *Nonresident tuition:* $4428 full-time, $246 per unit part-time. *Full-time mandatory fees:* $1008–$1740. *Part-time mandatory fees:* $1140. *Room and board:* $5610. *Books and supplies per academic year:* $750.

Financial Aid Graduate assistantships, nurse traineeships, Federal Nursing Student Loans. 51% of master's level students in nursing programs received some form of financial aid in 1995-96. *Application deadline:* 3/1.

MSN Program

Applying *Required:* GRE General Test, bachelor's degree in nursing, bachelor's degree, minimum GPA of 3.0, RN license, 1 year of clinical experience, physical assessment course, statistics course, professional liability/malpractice insurance, essay, 3 letters of recommendation, transcript of college record. *Application deadline:* 3/1. *Application fee:* $55.

Degree Requirements 36–47 total credit hours dependent upon track, 36 in nursing. Thesis, project, or comprehensive exam.

Post-Master's Program

Applying *Required:* bachelor's degree in nursing, bachelor's degree, minimum GPA of 3.0, RN license, 1 year of clinical experience, physical assessment course, professional liability/malpractice insurance, essay, 3 letters of recommendation, transcript of college record, MSN. *Application deadline:* 3/1. *Application fee:* $55.

Degree Requirements 24 total credit hours, 24 in nursing.

CONTINUING EDUCATION PROGRAM

Contact Dr. Audrey Anderson, Dean, Extended Education, California State University, Fresno, 5005 North Maple Avenue, Fresno, CA 93740-0076, 209-278-0333.

CALIFORNIA STATE UNIVERSITY, FULLERTON
Department of Nursing
Fullerton, California

Programs • RN Baccalaureate • RN Baccalaureate

The University State-supported comprehensive coed institution. Part of California State University System. Founded: 1957. *Primary accreditation:* regional. *Setting:* 225-acre suburban campus. *Total enrollment:* 22,097.

The Department of Nursing Founded in 1974. *Nursing program faculty:* 9 (22% with doctorates). *Off-campus program site:* Mission Viejo.

Academic Facilities *Nursing school resources:* computer lab, nursing audiovisuals.

Student Life *Student services:* health clinic, child-care facilities, personal counseling, career counseling, institutionally sponsored work-study program, job placement, campus safety program, special assistance for disabled students. *International student services:* counseling/support, special assistance for nonnative speakers of English, ESL courses. *Nursing student activities:* student nurses association, Nursing Honor Society.

Calendar Semesters.

NURSING STUDENT PROFILE

Undergraduate **Enrollment:** 153
Women: 96%; **Men:** 4%; **Minority:** 45%; **International:** 2%

BACCALAUREATE PROGRAMS

Contact Dr. Julia B. George, Head, Department of Nursing, California State University, Fullerton, PO Box 34080, Fullerton, CA 92634-9480, 714-773-3145. *Fax:* 714-773-3314. *E-mail:* jgeorge@fullerton.edu

Expenses *State resident tuition:* $0 per academic year. *Nonresident tuition:* $7830 full-time, $246 per unit part-time. *Full-time mandatory fees:* $1261–$1927. *Books and supplies per academic year:* $600.

Financial Aid Institutionally sponsored need-based grants/scholarships, institutionally sponsored non-need grants/scholarships, Federal Direct Loans. *Application deadline:* 3/1.

RN Baccalaureate Program (BScN)

Applying *Required:* RN license, diploma or AD in nursing, letter of recommendation, transcript of college record. *Options:* May apply for transfer of up to 70 total credits.

Degree Requirements 128 total credit hours, 42 in nursing. Statistics.

Distance learning Courses provided through satellite.

RN Baccalaureate Program (BS)

Applying *Required:* minimum college GPA of 2.0, RN license, diploma or AD in nursing, 2 letters of recommendation, transcript of college record. 56 prerequisite credits must be completed before admission to the nursing program. *Options:* May apply for transfer of up to 70 total credits. *Application deadlines:* 8/1 (fall), 1/1 (spring). *Application fee:* $55.

Degree Requirements 128 total credit hours, 43 in nursing. Upper division statistics course.

Distance learning Courses provided through satellite.

CALIFORNIA STATE UNIVERSITY, HAYWARD
Department of Nursing
Hayward, California

Programs • Generic Baccalaureate • RN Baccalaureate

The University State-supported comprehensive coed institution. Part of California State University System. Founded: 1957. *Primary accreditation:* regional. *Setting:* 343-acre suburban campus. *Total enrollment:* 12,650.

The Department of Nursing Founded in 1971.

Academic Facilities *Campus library:* 800,000 volumes; 2,200 periodical subscriptions.

Calendar Quarters.

BACCALAUREATE PROGRAMS

Contact Chair, Department of Nursing, California State University, Hayward, Hayward, CA 94542-3012, 510-885-3481. *Fax:* 510-885-2156.

Expenses *State resident tuition:* $0 per academic year. *Nonresident tuition:* $7380 full-time, $164 per unit part-time. *Full-time mandatory fees:* $1108–$1774.

Generic Baccalaureate Program (BS)

Applying *Required:* SAT I or ACT, TOEFL for nonnative speakers of English, minimum high school GPA of 2.0, 3 years of high school math, high school transcript. *Application deadlines:* 11/2 (fall), 8/2 (spring), 2/1 (winter; 6/1 summer). *Application fee:* $55.

Degree Requirements 186 total credit hours, 137–139 in nursing.

RN Baccalaureate Program (BS)

Applying *Application fee:* $55.

Degree Requirements 186 total credit hours, 101–103 in nursing.

CALIFORNIA STATE UNIVERSITY, LONG BEACH
Department of Nursing
Long Beach, California

Programs • Generic Baccalaureate • RN Baccalaureate • BSN to Master's • Accelerated RN to Master's

The University State-supported comprehensive coed institution. Part of California State University System. Founded: 1949. *Primary accreditation:* regional. *Setting:* 320-acre suburban campus. *Total enrollment:* 26,403.

The Department of Nursing Founded in 1965.

Calendar Semesters.

BACCALAUREATE PROGRAMS

Contact Assistant Director of Undergraduate Program, Department of Nursing, California State University, Long Beach, 1250 Bellflower Boulevard, Long Beach, CA 90840-0119, 310-985-4582. *Fax:* 310-985-2382.

Generic Baccalaureate Program (BSN)

Applying *Required:* SAT I or ACT, TOEFL for nonnative speakers of English, writing proficiency exam, critical thinking test, minimum college GPA of 2.5, interview, transcript of college record. *Application deadlines:* 11/1 (fall), 8/2 (spring). *Application fee:* $55.

Degree Requirements 132 total credit hours.

RN Baccalaureate Program (BSN)

Applying *Required:* TOEFL for nonnative speakers of English, writing proficiency exam, critical thinking test, minimum college GPA of 2.5, RN license, interview, transcript of college record. 56 prerequisite credits must be completed before admission to the nursing program. *Application deadlines:* 11/1 (fall), 8/2 (spring). *Application fee:* $55.

Degree Requirements 132 total credit hours.

MASTER'S PROGRAMS

Contact Graduate Adviser, Department of Nursing, California State University, Long Beach, 1250 Bellflower Boulevard, Long Beach, CA 90840-0119, 310-985-4469. *Fax:* 310-985-2382.

California State University, Long Beach (continued)

BSN to Master's Program (MS)

Applying *Required:* TOEFL for nonnative speakers of English, bachelor's degree in nursing, RN license, physical assessment course, statistics course, pathophysiology course, community health nursing course. *Application deadlines:* 3/15 (fall), 10/15 (spring). *Application fee:* $55.

Degree Requirements 27 total credit hours in nursing. Thesis or comprehensive exam and an overall 3.0 GPA.

Accelerated RN to Master's Program (MS)

Applying *Required:* RN license. *Application fee:* $55.

Degree Requirements 36 total credit hours. Thesis or comprehensive exam and an overall 3.0 GPA.

CALIFORNIA STATE UNIVERSITY, LOS ANGELES

Department of Nursing
Los Angeles, California

Programs • Generic Baccalaureate • RN Baccalaureate • MSN • Accelerated RN to Master's • Accelerated Master's for Nurses with Non-Nursing Degrees

The University State-supported comprehensive coed institution. Part of California State University System. Founded: 1947. *Primary accreditation:* regional. *Setting:* 173-acre urban campus. *Total enrollment:* 18,224.

The Department of Nursing Founded in 1956.

Academic Facilities *Campus library:* 1.0 million volumes; 2,500 periodical subscriptions.

Calendar Quarters.

BACCALAUREATE PROGRAMS

Contact Professor and Primary Undergraduate Adviser, Department of Nursing, California State University, Los Angeles, 5151 State University Drive, Los Angeles, CA 90032, 213-343-4700. *Fax:* 213-343-6454.

Expenses *State resident tuition:* $0 per academic year. *Nonresident tuition:* $7380 full-time, $164 per unit part-time. *Full-time mandatory fees:* $1044–$1710.

Generic Baccalaureate Program (BS)

Applying *Required:* SAT I or ACT, TOEFL for nonnative speakers of English. *Application deadlines:* 11/1 (fall), 8/1 (spring), 2/1 (winter; 6/1 summer). *Application fee:* $55.

Degree Requirements 198 total credit hours, 120–121 in nursing.

RN Baccalaureate Program (BS)

Applying *Required:* TOEFL for nonnative speakers of English. *Application deadline:* 2/1 (winter; 6/1 summer). *Application fee:* $55.

Degree Requirements 198 total credit hours, 120–121 in nursing.

MASTER'S PROGRAMS

Contact Chair, Department of Nursing, California State University, Los Angeles, 5151 State University Drive, Los Angeles, CA 90032, 213-343-4700. *Fax:* 213-343-6454.

Areas of Study Clinical nurse specialist programs in adult health nursing, parent-child nursing; nursing administration; nursing education; nurse practitioner programs in child care/pediatrics, women's health.

MSN Program

Applying *Required:* bachelor's degree in nursing, minimum GPA of 3.0.

Accelerated RN to Master's Program (MSN)

Applying *Required:* minimum GPA of 2.75, RN license, 1 year of clinical experience, associate's degree in nursing.

Accelerated Master's for Nurses with Non-Nursing Degrees Program (MSN)

Applying *Required:* bachelor's degree, minimum GPA of 2.75, RN license, associate's degree in nursing.

CALIFORNIA STATE UNIVERSITY, SACRAMENTO

Division of Nursing
Sacramento, California

Programs • Generic Baccalaureate • RN Baccalaureate • Baccalaureate for Second Degree • MSN

The University State-supported comprehensive coed institution. Part of California State University System. Founded: 1947. *Primary accreditation:* regional. *Setting:* 288-acre urban campus. *Total enrollment:* 22,796.

The Division of Nursing Founded in 1958.

Academic Facilities *Campus library:* 912,000 volumes (33,000 in health); 5,425 periodical subscriptions (327 health-care related).

Calendar Semesters.

BACCALAUREATE PROGRAMS

Contact Chairperson, Division of Nursing, California State University, Sacramento, 6000 J Street, Sacramento, CA 95819-6096, 916-278-6525. *Fax:* 916-278-6311.

Expenses *State resident tuition:* $0 per academic year. *Nonresident tuition:* $8118 full-time, $246 per unit part-time. *Full-time mandatory fees:* $1260–$1926.

Financial Aid Institutionally sponsored need-based grants/scholarships, institutionally sponsored non-need grants/scholarships, Federal Pell Grants, Federal Supplemental Educational Opportunity Grants, Federal Work-Study, Federal PLUS Loans, state university grant. *Application deadline:* 3/2.

Generic Baccalaureate Program (BS)

Degree Requirements 132 total credit hours, 88–91 in nursing.

RN Baccalaureate Program (BS)

Applying *Required:* SAT I or ACT. 45 prerequisite credits must be completed before admission to the nursing program.

Degree Requirements 132 total credit hours, 88–91 in nursing.

Baccalaureate for Second Degree Program (BS)

Degree Requirements 132 total credit hours, 88–91 in nursing.

MASTER'S PROGRAM

Contact Graduate Coordinator, Division of Nursing, California State University, Sacramento, 6000 J Street, Sacramento, CA 95819-6096, 916-278-6525. *Fax:* 916-278-6311.

Areas of Study Clinical nurse specialist programs in adult health nursing, community health nursing, family health nursing, school nursing; nursing administration; nursing education; nurse practitioner program in primary care.

Expenses *State resident tuition:* $0 per academic year. *Nonresident tuition:* $6354 full-time, $246 per unit part-time. *Full-time mandatory fees:* $150–$1926.

MSN Program

Applying *Required:* essay, 3 letters of recommendation, transcript of college record, physical examination, immunization, CPR certification. *Application deadline:* 1/30.

Degree Requirements 36 total credit hours, 30 in nursing, 6 in electives. Thesis or project.

CALIFORNIA STATE UNIVERSITY, SAN BERNARDINO

Nursing Department
San Bernardino, California

Program • Generic Baccalaureate

The University State-supported comprehensive coed institution. Part of California State University System. Founded: 1965. *Primary accreditation:* regional. *Setting:* 430-acre suburban campus. *Total enrollment:* 11,864.

The Nursing Department Founded in 1977.

Academic Facilities *Campus library:* 580,000 volumes (32,000 in health, 1,760 in nursing); 1,600 periodical subscriptions (345 health-care related).

Calendar Quarters.

BACCALAUREATE PROGRAM

Contact Ms. Mary Martin, Secretary, Nursing Department, California State University, San Bernardino, 5500 University Parkway, San Bernardino, CA 92407, 909-880-5380.

CALIFORNIA STATE UNIVERSITY, STANISLAUS
Department of Nursing
Turlock, California

Programs • RN Baccalaureate • Baccalaureate for Second Degree

The University State-supported comprehensive coed institution. Part of California State University System. Founded: 1957. *Primary accreditation:* regional. *Setting:* 220-acre small-town campus. *Total enrollment:* 5,972.

The Department of Nursing Founded in 1978. *Nursing program faculty:* 5 (40% with doctorates). *Off-campus program site:* Stockton.

Academic Facilities *Campus library:* 257,000 volumes (9,525 in health, 1,200 in nursing); 2,326 periodical subscriptions (116 health-care related). *Nursing school resources:* CAI, computer lab, nursing audiovisuals.

Student Life *Student services:* health clinic, child-care facilities, personal counseling, career counseling, institutionally sponsored work-study program, job placement, campus safety program, special assistance for disabled students. *International student services:* counseling/support, special assistance for nonnative speakers of English, ESL courses. *Nursing student activities:* Sigma Theta Tau.

Calendar 4-1-4.

NURSING STUDENT PROFILE

Undergraduate **Enrollment:** 106

Women: 87%; **Men:** 13%; **Minority:** 38%; **International:** 6%; **Part-time:** 75%

BACCALAUREATE PROGRAMS

Contact Dr. June L. Boffman, Chair, Department of Nursing, California State University, Stanislaus, 801 Monte Vista Avenue, Turlock, CA 95382, 209-667-3141. *Fax:* 209-664-7067. *E-mail:* june@toto.csustan.edu

Expenses *State resident tuition:* $0 full-time, $0 part-time. *Nonresident tuition:* $7626 full-time, $246 per credit hour part-time. *Full-time mandatory fees:* $553–$1910. *Part-time mandatory fees:* $537. *Room and board:* $5000. *Room only:* $3150. *Books and supplies per academic year:* ranges from $300 to $400.

Financial Aid Institutionally sponsored need-based grants/scholarships, institutionally sponsored non-need grants/scholarships, Federal Supplemental Educational Opportunity Grants, Federal Work-Study.

RN Baccalaureate Program (BSN)

Applying *Required:* SAT I, TOEFL for nonnative speakers of English, minimum college GPA of 2.0, 3 years of high school math, 3 years of high school science, high school chemistry, RN license, diploma or AD in nursing, high school transcript, letter of recommendation, transcript of college record, minimum 2.0 GPA in 3 semester-unit college-level English composition and chemistry courses. 60 prerequisite credits must be completed before admission to the nursing program. *Options:* May apply for transfer of up to 70 total credits. *Application deadline:* rolling. *Application fee:* $55.

Degree Requirements 124 total credit hours, 37 in nursing.

Baccalaureate for Second Degree Program (BSN)

Applying *Required:* minimum college GPA of 2.0, 3 years of high school math, 3 years of high school science, high school chemistry, high school biology, RN license, diploma or AD in nursing, letter of recommendation, transcript of college record, minimum 2.0 GPA in 3 semester-unit college-level English composition, and chemistry courses. 60 prerequisite credits must be completed before admission to the nursing program. *Options:* Course work may be accelerated. *Application deadline:* rolling. *Application fee:* $55.

Degree Requirements 124 total credit hours, 37 in nursing.

DOMINICAN COLLEGE OF SAN RAFAEL
School of Nursing and Allied Health Professions
San Rafael, California

Programs • Generic Baccalaureate • Continuing Education

The College Independent Roman Catholic comprehensive coed institution. Founded: 1890. *Primary accreditation:* regional. *Setting:* 80-acre suburban campus. *Total enrollment:* 1,364.

The School of Nursing and Allied Health Professions Founded in 1983. *Nursing program faculty:* 23 (23% with doctorates).

Academic Facilities *Campus library:* 94,584 volumes (600 in health, 535 in nursing); 469 periodical subscriptions (48 health-care related). *Nursing school resources:* CAI, computer lab, nursing audiovisuals, interactive nursing skills videos, learning resource lab.

Student Life *Student services:* health clinic, personal counseling, career counseling, institutionally sponsored work-study program. *International student services:* ESL courses. *Nursing student activities:* student nurses association, Nursing Honor Society.

Calendar Semesters.

NURSING STUDENT PROFILE

Undergraduate **Enrollment:** 271

Women: 89%; **Men:** 11%; **Minority:** 43%; **International:** 1%; **Part-time:** 36%

BACCALAUREATE PROGRAM

Contact Dr. Martha A. Nelson, Director and Dean, School of Nursing, Dominican College of San Rafael, 50 Acacia Avenue, San Rafael, CA 94901-8008, 415-485-3295. *Fax:* 415-485-3205.

Expenses *Tuition:* $14,380 full-time, $600 per unit part-time. *Full-time mandatory fees:* $670. *Room and board:* $6240–$6700. *Books and supplies per academic year:* ranges from $350 to $500.

Financial Aid Institutionally sponsored need-based grants/scholarships, institutionally sponsored non-need grants/scholarships, Federal Nursing Student Loans, Federal Perkins Loans, Federal Supplemental Educational Opportunity Grants, Federal Work-Study, Federal Stafford Loans. *Application deadline:* 3/2.

Generic Baccalaureate Program (BS)

Applying *Required:* SAT I or ACT, TOEFL for nonnative speakers of English, minimum high school GPA of 2.5, minimum college GPA of 2.5, 2 letters of recommendation, written essay, transcript of college record. *Options:* Advanced standing available through the following means: advanced placement exams, credit by exam. May apply for transfer of up to 70 total credits. *Application deadline:* rolling. *Application fee:* $35.

Degree Requirements 126 total credit hours, 60 in nursing.

CONTINUING EDUCATION PROGRAM

Contact Bonnie Sullivan, Director, Academy For Professional Development, Dominican College of San Rafael, 50 Acacia Avenue, San Rafael, CA 94901-2298, 415-485-3255.

See full description on page 440.

HOLY NAMES COLLEGE
Department of Nursing
Oakland, California

Programs • RN Baccalaureate • Accelerated RN Baccalaureate • RN to Master's

Holy Names College (continued)

The College Independent Roman Catholic comprehensive coed institution. Founded: 1868. *Primary accreditation:* regional. *Setting:* 60-acre urban campus. *Total enrollment:* 975.

The Department of Nursing Founded in 1975. *Nursing program faculty:* 20 (60% with doctorates).

Academic Facilities *Campus library:* 180,000 volumes (15,000 in health, 4,800 in nursing); 670 periodical subscriptions (150 health-care related). *Nursing school resources:* CAI, computer lab, nursing audiovisuals, interactive nursing skills videos, learning resource lab.

Student Life *Student services:* health clinic, child-care facilities, personal counseling, career counseling, institutionally sponsored work-study program, job placement, campus safety program, special assistance for disabled students. *International student services:* counseling/support, special assistance for nonnative speakers of English, ESL courses. *Nursing student activities:* Sigma Theta Tau, nursing club.

Calendar Semesters, Trimesters.

NURSING STUDENT PROFILE

Undergraduate **Enrollment:** 204
Women: 90%; **Men:** 10%; **Minority:** 45%; **International:** 20%; **Part-time:** 88%

BACCALAUREATE PROGRAMS

Contact Dr. Arlene Sargent, Chairperson and Professor, Department of Nursing, Holy Names College, 3500 Mountain Boulevard, Oakland, CA 94619-1699, 510-436-1127. *Fax:* 510-436-1376. *E-mail:* sargent@academmail.hnc.edu

Expenses *Tuition:* $375 per unit. *Full-time mandatory fees:* $15–$75. *Books and supplies per academic year:* ranges from $30 to $200.

Financial Aid Institutionally sponsored need-based grants/scholarships, Federal Direct Loans, Federal Nursing Student Loans, Federal Pell Grants, Federal Perkins Loans, Federal Supplemental Educational Opportunity Grants, Federal Work-Study. 70% of undergraduate students in nursing programs received some form of financial aid in 1995–96. *Application deadline:* 7/15.

RN Baccalaureate Program (BSN)

Applying *Required:* TOEFL for nonnative speakers of English, minimum high school GPA of 2.5, 3 years of high school math, RN license, diploma or AD in nursing, high school transcript, interview, 2 letters of recommendation, written essay, transcript of college record. 60 prerequisite credits must be completed before admission to the nursing program. *Options:* Advanced standing available through the following means: advanced placement exams, credit by exam. May apply for transfer of up to 75 total credits. *Application deadlines:* 7/1 (fall), 12/1 (spring). *Application fee:* $35.

Degree Requirements 120 total credit hours, 33 in nursing. Statistics, epidemiology, senior colloquium.

Distance learning Courses provided through interactive teleconference.

Accelerated RN Baccalaureate Program (BSN)

Applying *Required:* TOEFL for nonnative speakers of English, minimum high school GPA of 2.5, 3 years of high school math, RN license, diploma or AD in nursing, high school transcript, interview, letter of recommendation, written essay, transcript of college record. 60 prerequisite credits must be completed before admission to the nursing program. *Options:* Advanced standing available through credit by exam. *Application deadline:* 3/2. *Application fee:* $35.

Degree Requirements 120 total credit hours, 33 in nursing.

Distance learning Courses provided through interactive teleconferencing.

MASTER'S PROGRAM

Contact Dr. Aida Sahud, Director of Graduate Program, Department of Nursing, Holy Names College, 3500 Mountain Boulevard, Oakland, CA 94619, 510-436-1239. *Fax:* 510-436-1376. *E-mail:* sahud@academmail.hnc.edu

Areas of Study Nurse practitioner programs in community health, family health.

Expenses *Tuition:* $450 per unit. *Part-time mandatory fees:* $75–$150. *Books and supplies per academic year:* ranges from $150 to $300.

Financial Aid Federal Direct Loans, employment opportunities.

RN to Master's Program (MSN)

Applying *Required:* TOEFL for nonnative speakers of English, bachelor's degree, minimum GPA of 3.0, RN license, statistics course, professional liability/malpractice insurance, essay, 2 letters of recommendation, transcript of college record. *Application deadline:* 3/31. *Application fee:* $35.

Degree Requirements 30–40 total credit hours dependent upon track, 30–40 in nursing. Intensive clinical project or other final project.

Distance learning Courses provided on-line. Specific degree requirements include 4 consecutive days per month on campus.

HUMBOLDT STATE UNIVERSITY

Department of Nursing
Arcata, California

Programs • Generic Baccalaureate • Accelerated RN Baccalaureate

The University State-supported comprehensive coed institution. Part of California State University System. Founded: 1913. *Primary accreditation:* regional. *Setting:* 161-acre rural campus. *Total enrollment:* 7,427.

The Department of Nursing Founded in 1958. *Nursing program faculty:* 12 (8% with doctorates).

Academic Facilities *Campus library:* 439,868 volumes (16,000 in health, 750 in nursing); 2,203 periodical subscriptions (152 health-care related). *Nursing school resources:* CAI, computer lab, nursing audiovisuals, interactive nursing skills videos, learning resource lab.

Student Life *Student services:* health clinic, personal counseling, career counseling, institutionally sponsored work-study program, job placement. *International student services:* ESL courses. *Nursing student activities:* nursing club.

Calendar Semesters.

NURSING STUDENT PROFILE

Undergraduate **Enrollment:** 136
Women: 82%; **Men:** 18%; **Minority:** 7%; **Part-time:** 14%

BACCALAUREATE PROGRAMS

Contact Dr. Noreen Frisch, Chair and Professor, Department of Nursing, Humboldt State University, Arcata, CA 95521-8299, 707-826-3215. *Fax:* 707-826-5141.

Expenses *State resident tuition:* $0 per academic year. *Nonresident tuition:* ranges from $7872 to $8364 full-time, $246 per unit part-time. *Full-time mandatory fees:* $1900. *Part-time mandatory fees:* $459. *Room and board:* $7050–$9500. *Room only:* $4000. *Books and supplies per academic year:* ranges from $650 to $1000.

Financial Aid Institutionally sponsored need-based grants/scholarships, institutionally sponsored non-need grants/scholarships, Federal Supplemental Educational Opportunity Grants, Federal Work-Study. *Application deadline:* 2/28.

Generic Baccalaureate Program (BS)

Applying *Required:* SAT I or ACT, minimum college GPA of 2.0, high school transcript, written essay, transcript of college record, residence in California. 5 prerequisite credits must be completed before admission to the nursing program. *Options:* May apply for transfer of up to 70 total credits. *Application deadlines:* 11/30 (fall), 8/30 (spring). *Application fee:* $45.

Degree Requirements 124 total credit hours, 52 in nursing.

Accelerated RN Baccalaureate Program (BS)

Applying *Required:* minimum college GPA of 2.0, RN license, diploma or AD in nursing, transcript of college record, residence in California. *Options:* Advanced standing available through advanced placement exams. May apply for transfer of up to 70 total credits. *Application deadlines:* 11/30 (fall), 8/30 (spring). *Application fee:* $45.

Degree Requirements 124 total credit hours, 52 in nursing.

LOMA LINDA UNIVERSITY
School of Nursing
Loma Linda, California

Programs • Generic Baccalaureate • RN Baccalaureate • Accelerated Baccalaureate for Second Degree • LPN to Baccalaureate • MS • Post-Master's

The University Seventh-day Adventist.

The School of Nursing Founded in 1905. *Nursing program faculty:* 39 (49% with doctorates).

Academic Facilities *Campus library:* 182,587 volumes (30,431 in health, 3,916 in nursing); 2,703 periodical subscriptions (253 health-care related). *Nursing school resources:* computer lab, nursing audiovisuals, interactive nursing skills videos, learning resource lab.

Student Life *Student services:* health clinic, child-care facilities, personal counseling, institutionally sponsored work-study program, campus safety program. *International student services:* counseling/support, special assistance for nonnative speakers of English, ESL courses. *Nursing student activities:* Sigma Theta Tau, student nurses association.

Calendar Quarters.

NURSING STUDENT PROFILE

Undergraduate **Enrollment:** 305

Women: 80%; **Men:** 20%; **Minority:** 53%; **International:** 21%; **Part-time:** 10%

Graduate **Enrollment:** 72

Women: 96%; **Men:** 4%; **Minority:** 33%; **International:** 17%; **Part-time:** 45%

BACCALAUREATE PROGRAMS

Contact Ms. Judy Peters, Director of Admissions, School of Nursing, Loma Linda University, Loma Linda, CA 92350, 909-824-4923. *Fax:* 909-824-4134.

Expenses *Tuition:* $13,650 full-time, ranges from $175 to $350 part-time. *Full-time mandatory fees:* $0–$250.

Financial Aid Institutionally sponsored need-based grants/scholarships, institutionally sponsored non-need grants/scholarships, Federal Nursing Student Loans, Federal Supplemental Educational Opportunity Grants, Federal Work-Study. *Application deadline:* 4/15.

Generic Baccalaureate Program (BS)

Applying *Required:* TOEFL for nonnative speakers of English, NLN Preadmission Examination-RN, minimum college GPA of 3.0, 2 years of high school math, high school transcript, interview, written essay, transcript of college record, 2 reference forms. 48 prerequisite credits must be completed before admission to the nursing program. *Options:* Course work may be accelerated. May apply for transfer of up to 105 total credits. *Application deadlines:* 3/31 (fall), 12/31 (spring), 9/30 (winter). *Application fee:* $75.

Degree Requirements 191 total credit hours, 93 in nursing.

RN Baccalaureate Program (BS)

Applying *Required:* minimum college GPA of 2.5, 2 years of high school math, RN license, diploma or AD in nursing, high school transcript, interview, written essay, transcript of college record, 2 reference forms. *Options:* Course work may be accelerated. *Application deadlines:* 3/31 (fall), 12/31 (spring), 9/30 (winter). *Application fee:* $75.

Degree Requirements 190 total credit hours, 93 in nursing.

Accelerated Baccalaureate for Second Degree Program (BS)

Applying *Required:* TOEFL for nonnative speakers of English, minimum college GPA of 3.0, 2 years of high school math, high school transcript, interview, 2 letters of recommendation, written essay, transcript of college record. *Options:* Course work may be accelerated. *Application deadlines:* 3/31 (fall), 12/15 (spring), 9/30 (winter). *Application fee:* $75.

LPN to Baccalaureate Program (BS)

Applying *Required:* TOEFL for nonnative speakers of English, minimum college GPA of 3.0, 2 years of high school math, high school transcript, interview, 2 letters of recommendation, written essay, transcript of college record, LVN license. *Options:* Course work may be accelerated. *Application deadlines:* 3/31 (fall), 12/15 (spring), 9/30 (winter). *Application fee:* $75.

MASTER'S PROGRAMS

Contact Ms. Joyce Bates, Administrative Assistant, School of Nursing, Loma Linda University, Loma Linda, CA 92350, 909-478-8061. *Fax:* 909-824-4134.

Areas of Study Clinical nurse specialist programs in adult health nursing, critical care nursing, pediatric nursing, school health nursing; nursing administration; nurse practitioner programs in adult health, child care/pediatrics, family health, neonatal health, pediatric critical care.

Expenses *Tuition:* $8400 full-time, $350 per unit part-time. *Full-time mandatory fees:* $0.

Financial Aid Nurse traineeships, Federal Direct Loans, institutionally sponsored loans, institutionally sponsored non-need-based grants/scholarships. *Application deadline:* 9/15.

MS Program

Applying *Required:* TOEFL for nonnative speakers of English, bachelor's degree in nursing, minimum GPA of 3.0, RN license, 1 year of clinical experience, statistics course, essay, interview, 3 letters of recommendation, transcript of college record. *Application deadline:* rolling. *Application fee:* $50.

Degree Requirements 53–67 total credit hours dependent upon track.

Post-Master's Program

Applying *Required:* minimum GPA of 3.0, RN license, 1 year of clinical experience, physical assessment course, 3 letters of recommendation, transcript of college record, MSN with clinical major. *Application deadline:* rolling. *Application fee:* $50.

Degree Requirements 31–35 total credit hours dependent upon track, 31 in nursing.

MOUNT ST. MARY'S COLLEGE
Department of Nursing
Los Angeles, California

Programs • Generic Baccalaureate • RN Baccalaureate • Accelerated Baccalaureate for Second Degree

The College Independent Roman Catholic comprehensive primarily women's institution. Founded: 1925. *Primary accreditation:* regional. *Setting:* 71-acre suburban campus. *Total enrollment:* 1,974.

The Department of Nursing Founded in 1952. *Nursing program faculty:* 29 (8% with doctorates).

Academic Facilities *Campus library:* 140,000 volumes (4,000 in health, 1,000 in nursing); 800 periodical subscriptions (150 health-care related). *Nursing school resources:* CAI, computer lab, nursing audiovisuals, interactive nursing skills videos, learning resource lab.

Student Life *Student services:* health clinic, personal counseling, career counseling, institutionally sponsored work-study program, campus safety program, special assistance for disabled students, learning assistance center. *International student services:* counseling/support, special assistance for nonnative speakers of English. *Nursing student activities:* student nurses association, Alpha Tau Delta.

Calendar Semesters.

NURSING STUDENT PROFILE

Undergraduate **Enrollment:** 224

Women: 95%; **Men:** 5%; **Minority:** 62%; **International:** 1%; **Part-time:** 0%

BACCALAUREATE PROGRAMS

Contact Ms. Jeanette Stone, Admissions Counselor, Admissions Office, Mount St. Mary's College, 12001 Chalon Road, Los Angeles, CA 90049, 310-476-2237. *Fax:* 310-440-3258.

Expenses *Tuition:* $14,014 full-time, $533 per unit part-time. *Full-time mandatory fees:* $110–$350. *Room and board:* $5084–$7116. *Books and supplies per academic year:* ranges from $400 to $700.

Financial Aid Institutionally sponsored need-based grants/scholarships, institutionally sponsored non-need grants/scholarships, Federal Nursing Student Loans, Federal Pell Grants, Federal Perkins Loans, Federal Supplemental Educational Opportunity Grants, Federal Work-Study, Federal Stafford Loans. 93% of undergraduate students in nursing programs received some form of financial aid in 1995–96. *Application deadline:* 3/1.

Mount St. Mary's College (continued)

GENERIC BACCALAUREATE PROGRAM (BSN)

Applying *Required:* SAT I, ACT, TOEFL for nonnative speakers of English, minimum college GPA of 2.7, high school chemistry, high school biology, high school foreign language, high school transcript, letter of recommendation, written essay, transcript of college record, minimum 2.5 GPA in science courses. 31 prerequisite credits must be completed before admission to the nursing program. *Options:* May apply for transfer of up to 66 total credits. *Application deadline:* 2/1. *Application fee:* $30.

Degree Requirements 127 total credit hours, 64 in nursing. 15 units of philosophy/religion, 9 of units psychology.

RN BACCALAUREATE PROGRAM (BSN)

Applying *Required:* advanced placement exam, minimum college GPA of 2.7, RN license, diploma or AD in nursing, interview, written essay, transcript of college record. *Options:* Advanced standing available through credit by exam. May apply for transfer of up to 66 total credits. *Application deadline:* rolling. *Application fee:* $30.

Degree Requirements 124 total credit hours, 22 in nursing.

ACCELERATED BACCALAUREATE FOR SECOND DEGREE PROGRAM (BSN)

Applying *Required:* minimum college GPA of 2.8, interview, 2 letters of recommendation, written essay, transcript of college record. 57 prerequisite credits must be completed before admission to the nursing program. *Application deadlines:* 2/1 (fall), 11/1 (summer). *Application fee:* $30.

Degree Requirements 124 total credit hours, 56 in nursing.

PACIFIC UNION COLLEGE
Department of Nursing
Angwin, California

Program • RN Baccalaureate

The College Independent Seventh-day Adventist comprehensive coed institution. Founded: 1882. *Primary accreditation:* regional. *Setting:* 200-acre rural campus. *Total enrollment:* 1,640.

The Department of Nursing Founded in 1981. *Nursing program faculty:* 20.

Academic Facilities *Campus library:* 237,438 volumes; 1,044 periodical subscriptions.

Calendar Quarters.

BACCALAUREATE PROGRAM

Contact Julia Pearce, Chair, 116 Davidian Hall, Department of Nursing, Pacific Union College, Angwin, CA 94508, 707-965-7262.

Expenses *Tuition:* $12,960 full-time, $375 per quarter hour part-time.

Financial Aid Institutionally sponsored need-based grants/scholarships, institutionally sponsored non-need grants/scholarships, Federal Pell Grants, Federal Perkins Loans, Federal Supplemental Educational Opportunity Grants, Federal Work-Study, Federal PLUS Loans, Federal Stafford Loans, Bureau of Indian Affairs grants, state aid. *Application deadline:* 3/2.

RN BACCALAUREATE PROGRAM (BSN)

Applying *Required:* SAT I, RN license, diploma or AD in nursing, high school transcript, interview, 2 letters of recommendation, transcript of college record. *Options:* Advanced standing available through credit by exam. May apply for transfer of up to 57 total credits. *Application fee:* $30.

Degree Requirements 192 total credit hours.

POINT LOMA NAZARENE COLLEGE
Department of Nursing
San Diego, California

Programs • Generic Baccalaureate • LPN to Baccalaureate

The College Independent Nazarene comprehensive coed institution. Founded: 1902. *Primary accreditation:* regional. *Setting:* 88-acre suburban campus. *Total enrollment:* 2,459.

The Department of Nursing Founded in 1971. *Nursing program faculty:* 16 (19% with doctorates).

Academic Facilities *Campus library:* 143,577 volumes; 613 periodical subscriptions. *Nursing school resources:* CAI, computer lab, nursing audiovisuals, interactive nursing skills videos, learning resource lab, Internet.

Student Life *Student services:* health clinic, personal counseling, career counseling, institutionally sponsored work-study program, job placement, campus safety program. *International student services:* ESL courses. *Nursing student activities:* Sigma Theta Tau, student nurses association, Nurses Christian Fellowship.

Calendar Semesters.

NURSING STUDENT PROFILE

Undergraduate **Enrollment:** 120

Women: 95%; **Men:** 5%; **Minority:** 16%; **International:** 2%

BACCALAUREATE PROGRAMS

Contact Mr. Bill Young, Executive Director for Enrollment Services, Department of Nursing, Point Loma Nazarene College, 3900 Lomaland Drive, San Diego, CA 92106, 619-849-2225. *Fax:* 619-849-2579.

Expenses *Tuition:* $11,584 full-time, ranges from $362 to $398 per semester unit part-time. *Full-time mandatory fees:* $258. *Room and board:* $4730. *Books and supplies per academic year:* ranges from $200 to $500.

Financial Aid Institutionally sponsored need-based grants/scholarships, institutionally sponsored non-need grants/scholarships, Federal Direct Loans, Federal Nursing Student Loans, Federal Pell Grants, Federal Perkins Loans, Federal Supplemental Educational Opportunity Grants, Federal Work-Study. *Application deadline:* 6/15.

GENERIC BACCALAUREATE PROGRAM (BSN)

Applying *Required:* SAT I, ACT, minimum high school GPA of 2.5, minimum college GPA of 2.7, high school transcript, 3 letters of recommendation, written essay, transcript of college record. 20 prerequisite credits must be completed before admission to the nursing program. *Options:* Advanced standing available through the following means: advanced placement exams, advanced placement without credit, credit by exam. *Application deadlines:* 3/1 (fall), 4/1 (nursing program). *Application fee:* $20.

Degree Requirements 128 total credit hours, 52 in nursing.

LPN TO BACCALAUREATE PROGRAM (BSN)

Applying *Required:* minimum high school GPA of 2.5, minimum college GPA of 2.7, California LVN or LPN. *Options:* Advanced standing available through credit by exam. Course work may be accelerated. *Application deadlines:* 3/1 (fall), 4/1 (Department of Nursing). *Application fee:* $20.

Degree Requirements 128 total credit hours, 52 in nursing.

SAMUEL MERRITT COLLEGE
Intercollegiate Nursing Program
Oakland, California

Programs • Generic Baccalaureate • RN Baccalaureate • BSN to Master's • Master's for Non-Nursing College Graduates • Continuing Education

The College Independent comprehensive specialized primarily women's institution. Founded: 1909. *Primary accreditation:* regional. *Setting:* 1-acre urban campus. *Total enrollment:* 576.

The Intercollegiate Nursing Program Founded in 1909. *Nursing program faculty:* 57 (24% with doctorates). *Off-campus program site:* Moraga.

Academic Facilities *Campus library:* 7,000 volumes (14,437 in health); 430 periodical subscriptions (430 health-care related). *Nursing school resources:* CAI, computer lab, nursing audiovisuals, interactive nursing skills videos, learning resource lab, TV production studio.

Student Life *Student services:* health clinic, career counseling, institutionally sponsored work-study program, campus safety program, special assistance for disabled students. *International student services:* counseling/

support, special assistance for nonnative speakers of English, ESL courses. *Nursing student activities:* Sigma Theta Tau, student nurses association.

Calendar 4-1-4.

NURSING STUDENT PROFILE

Undergraduate **Enrollment:** 309
Women: 90%; **Men:** 10%; **Minority:** 31%; **International:** 1%; **Part-time:** 9%
Graduate **Enrollment:** 128
Women: 83%; **Men:** 17%; **Minority:** 27%; **International:** 10%; **Part-time:** 16%

BACCALAUREATE PROGRAMS

Contact Mr. John Garten-Shuman, Director of Admissions, Samuel Merritt College, 370 Hawthorne Avenue, Oakland, CA 94609, 510-869-6576. *Fax:* 510-869-6525. *E-mail:* jgartenshuman@compuserve.com

Expenses *Tuition:* $13,865 full-time, $580 per unit part-time. *Full-time mandatory fees:* $65. *Room only:* $3300–$4400.

Financial Aid Institutionally sponsored need-based grants/scholarships, institutionally sponsored non-need grants/scholarships, Federal Direct Loans, Federal Nursing Student Loans, Federal Pell Grants, Federal Perkins Loans, Federal Supplemental Educational Opportunity Grants, Federal Work-Study. 85% of undergraduate students in nursing programs received some form of financial aid in 1995–96. *Application deadline:* 3/2.

Generic Baccalaureate Program (BSN)

Applying *Required:* SAT I, ACT, TOEFL for nonnative speakers of English, minimum high school GPA of 2.5, minimum college GPA of 2.5, 2 years of high school math, 2 years of high school science, high school chemistry, high school biology, high school transcript, interview, letter of recommendation, written essay, transcript of college record. *Options:* Advanced standing available through credit by exam. Course work may be accelerated. *Application deadlines:* 3/1 (fall), 9/1 (spring). *Application fee:* $35.

Degree Requirements 128 total credit hours. 615 clinical hours.

RN Baccalaureate Program (BSN)

Applying *Required:* TOEFL for nonnative speakers of English, minimum college GPA of 2.5, RN license, diploma or AD in nursing, letter of recommendation, written essay, transcript of college record. *Options:* Advanced standing available through credit by exam. Course work may be accelerated. *Application deadlines:* 10/1 (fall), 5/1 (spring). *Application fee:* $35.

Degree Requirements 128 total credit hours.

MASTER'S PROGRAMS

Contact John Garten-Shuman, Director of Admission, Samuel Merritt College, 370 Hawthorne Avenue, Oakland, CA 94609, 510-869-6576. *Fax:* 510-869-6525. *E-mail:* jgartenshuman@compuserve.com

Areas of Study Clinical nurse specialist program in case management; nurse anesthesia; nurse practitioner program in family health.

Expenses *Tuition:* ranges from $8880 to $15,540 full-time, $555 per unit part-time. *Full-time mandatory fees:* $25.

BSN to Master's Program (MSN)

Applying *Required:* TOEFL for nonnative speakers of English, GRE for certified registered nurse anesthetist track, bachelor's degree, minimum GPA of 3., RN license, 1 year of clinical experience, essay, interview, 2 letters of recommendation, transcript of college record, statistics course for certified registered nurse anesthetist track. *Application deadline:* 2/1. *Application fee:* $50.

Degree Requirements 49–63 total credit hours dependent upon track, 49–63 in nursing. 675 clinical hours for family nurse practitioner track.

Master's for Non-Nursing College Graduates Program (MSN)

Applying *Required:* TOEFL for nonnative speakers of English, bachelor's degree, minimum GPA of 3.0, statistics course, essay, interview, 2 letters of recommendation, transcript of college record. *Application deadline:* 2/1. *Application fee:* $50.

Degree Requirements 90 total credit hours, 90 in nursing.

CONTINUING EDUCATION PROGRAM

Contact Sarah Keating, Dean, Intercollegiate Nursing Program, Samuel Merritt College, 370 Hawthorne Avenue, Oakland, CA 94609, 510-869-6129. *Fax:* 510-869-6525.

See full description on page 500.

SAN DIEGO STATE UNIVERSITY
School of Nursing
San Diego, California

Programs • Generic Baccalaureate • RN Baccalaureate • MSN

The University State-supported coed university. Part of California State University System. Founded: 1897. *Primary accreditation:* regional. *Setting:* 300-acre urban campus. *Total enrollment:* 28,724.

The School of Nursing Founded in 1953. *Nursing program faculty:* 39 (71% with doctorates).

Academic Facilities *Campus library:* 1.1 million volumes (35,000 in health, 13,000 in nursing); 6,230 periodical subscriptions (335 health-care related). *Nursing school resources:* CAI, computer lab, nursing audiovisuals, interactive nursing skills videos, learning resource lab.

Student Life *Student services:* health clinic, personal counseling, career counseling, institutionally sponsored work-study program, special assistance for disabled students. *International student services:* counseling/support, special assistance for nonnative speakers of English, ESL courses. *Nursing student activities:* Sigma Theta Tau, student nurses association.

Calendar Semesters.

NURSING STUDENT PROFILE

Undergraduate **Enrollment:** 307
Women: 90%; **Men:** 10%; **Minority:** 53%; **International:** 1%; **Part-time:** 2%
Graduate **Enrollment:** 98
Women: 96%; **Men:** 4%; **Minority:** 12%; **International:** 0%; **Part-time:** 90%

BACCALAUREATE PROGRAMS

Contact Dr. Myrna Moffett, Assistant Professor, Hardy Tower 58, School of Nursing, San Diego State University, 5500 Campanile Drive, San Diego, CA 92182-4158, 619-594-6384. *Fax:* 619-594-2765. *E-mail:* mmoffett@mail.sdsu.edu

Expenses *State resident tuition:* $0 per academic year. *Nonresident tuition:* $7872 full-time, $246 per unit part-time. *Full-time mandatory fees:* $1236–$1902. *Part-time mandatory fees:* $618. *Room and board:* $5624. *Books and supplies per academic year:* ranges from $650 to $850.

Financial Aid Institutionally sponsored need-based grants/scholarships, institutionally sponsored non-need grants/scholarships, Federal Direct Loans, Federal Nursing Student Loans. 24% of undergraduate students in nursing programs received some form of financial aid in 1995–96. *Application deadline:* 1/1.

Generic Baccalaureate Program (BS)

Applying *Required:* SAT I or ACT, TOEFL for nonnative speakers of English, minimum high school GPA of 2.0, minimum college GPA of 2.5, 3 years of high school math, 1 year of high school science, high school foreign language, high school transcript, written essay, transcript of college record. 18 prerequisite credits must be completed before admission to the nursing program. *Options:* May apply for transfer of up to 56 total credits. *Application deadlines:* 11/1 (fall), 8/1 (spring). *Application fee:* $55.

Degree Requirements 128 total credit hours, 58 in nursing.

RN Baccalaureate Program (BS)

Applying *Required:* TOEFL for nonnative speakers of English, RN license, diploma or AD in nursing, transcript of college record. 21 prerequisite credits must be completed before admission to the nursing program. *Options:* Advanced standing available through credit by exam. May apply for transfer of up to 27 total credits. *Application deadlines:* 11/1 (fall), 8/1 (spring). *Application fee:* $55.

Degree Requirements 128 total credit hours, 66 in nursing.

MASTER'S PROGRAM

Contact Dr. Carolyn Walker, Professor and Graduate Adviser, Hardy Tower 58, School of Nursing, San Diego State University, 5500 Campanile Drive, San Diego, CA 92182-4158, 619-594-6386. *Fax:* 619-594-2765. *E-mail:* cwalker@mail.sdsu.edu

Areas of Study Clinical nurse specialist programs in community health nursing, critical care nursing, school health nursing, pediatric critical

San Diego State University (continued)
care nursing; nurse midwifery; nursing administration; nurse practitioner programs in adult health, family health, gerontology.

Expenses *State resident tuition:* $0 per academic year. *Nonresident tuition:* $4428 full-time, $246 per unit part-time. *Full-time mandatory fees:* $1236–$1902. *Part-time mandatory fees:* $618. *Books and supplies per academic year:* ranges from $700 to $1000.

Financial Aid Graduate assistantships, nurse traineeships, Federal Direct Loans, Federal Nursing Student Loans, employment opportunities, institutionally sponsored need-based grants/scholarships, institutionally sponsored non-need-based grants/scholarships. 26% of master's level students in nursing programs received some form of financial aid in 1995-96. *Application deadline:* 1/1.

MSN Program

Applying *Required:* GRE General Test, bachelor's degree in nursing, minimum GPA of 3.0, RN license, 1 year of clinical experience, physical assessment course, statistics course, professional liability/malpractice insurance, essay, interview, 3 letters of recommendation, transcript of college record, 1 year obstetrics experience for midwives. *Application deadlines:* 1/15 (nurse practitioner program), rolling. *Application fee:* $55.

Degree Requirements 39–54 total credit hours dependent upon track, 33–39 in nursing. Thesis, project, or comprehensive exam.

See full description on page 502.

SAN FRANCISCO STATE UNIVERSITY
School of Nursing
San Francisco, California

Programs • Generic Baccalaureate • RN Baccalaureate • Accelerated RN Baccalaureate • Baccalaureate for Second Degree • LPN to Baccalaureate • MSN • Master's for Nurses with Non-Nursing Degrees • Master's for Non-Nursing College Graduates

The University State-supported comprehensive coed institution. Part of California State University System. Founded: 1899. *Primary accreditation:* regional. *Setting:* 90-acre urban campus. *Total enrollment:* 26,791.

The School of Nursing Founded in 1954. *Nursing program faculty:* 40 (60% with doctorates). *Off-campus program sites:* Oakland, San Jose, San Mateo.

▶ ***NOTEWORTHY***

The School of Nursing graduate program offers advanced preparation in case management/long-term care, case management in primary care (family nurse practitioner), community/public health, and a new emphasis in entrepreneurial leadership. These programs develop nurse leaders able to collaborate with interdisciplinary health-care teams and consumers within multicultural environments. The entrepreneurial leadership program integrates traditional management skills within a community-based framework. Graduates of all tracks are able to develop, implement, provide, and evaluate culturally appropriate services.

Academic Facilities *Campus library:* 2.5 million volumes (11,000 in health, 1,500 in nursing); 6,700 periodical subscriptions (200 health-care related). *Nursing school resources:* CAI, computer lab, nursing audiovisuals, interactive nursing skills videos, learning resource lab.

Student Life *Student services:* health clinic, child-care facilities, personal counseling, career counseling, institutionally sponsored work-study program, job placement, campus safety program, special assistance for disabled students. *International student services:* counseling/support, special assistance for nonnative speakers of English, ESL courses. *Nursing student activities:* Sigma Theta Tau, nursing club, student nurses association.

Calendar Semesters.

NURSING STUDENT PROFILE

Undergraduate **Enrollment:** 250
Women: 88%; **Men:** 12%; **Minority:** 53%; **International:** 1%; **Part-time:** 5%
Graduate **Enrollment:** 180
Women: 80%; **Men:** 20%; **Minority:** 40%; **International:** 1%; **Part-time:** 40%

BACCALAUREATE PROGRAMS

Contact Dr. Karen Johnson-Brennan, Associate Director, BSN Program, School of Nursing, San Francisco State University, San Francisco, CA 94132, 415-338-2315. *Fax:* 415-338-0555.

Expenses *State resident tuition:* $0 per academic year. *Full-time mandatory fees:* $1316–$1982. *Room and board:* $5100–$5400. *Room only:* $4100. *Books and supplies per academic year:* ranges from $300 to $400.

Financial Aid Institutionally sponsored need-based grants/scholarships, institutionally sponsored non-need grants/scholarships, Federal Nursing Student Loans, Federal Pell Grants, Federal Supplemental Educational Opportunity Grants. 52% of undergraduate students in nursing programs received some form of financial aid in 1995–96. *Application deadline:* 5/1.

Generic Baccalaureate Program (BSN)

Applying *Required:* SAT I or ACT, TOEFL for nonnative speakers of English, minimum high school GPA of 2.0, minimum college GPA of 2.5, 3 years of high school math, high school foreign language, high school transcript, letter of recommendation, transcript of college record. 38 prerequisite credits must be completed before admission to the nursing program. *Options:* Advanced standing available through the following means: advanced placement exams, credit by exam. Course work may be accelerated. May apply for transfer of up to 70 total credits. *Application deadlines:* 11/30 (fall), 11/30 (spring). *Application fee:* $55.

Degree Requirements 124 total credit hours, 50 in nursing.

RN Baccalaureate Program (BSN)

Applying *Required:* TOEFL for nonnative speakers of English, minimum college GPA of 2.0, RN license, diploma or AD in nursing, transcript of college record, minimum 2.5 GPA in nursing courses. 38 prerequisite credits must be completed before admission to the nursing program. *Options:* Advanced standing available through the following means: advanced placement exams, credit by exam. Course work may be accelerated. May apply for transfer of up to 70 total credits. *Application deadlines:* 11/30 (fall), 11/30 (spring). *Application fee:* $55.

Degree Requirements 124 total credit hours, 50 in nursing.

Accelerated RN Baccalaureate Program (BSN)

Applying *Required:* TOEFL for nonnative speakers of English, minimum college GPA of 2.0, RN license, diploma or AD in nursing, transcript of college record. 38 prerequisite credits must be completed before admission to the nursing program. *Options:* Advanced standing available through the following means: advanced placement exams, credit by exam. Course work may be accelerated. May apply for transfer of up to 70 total credits. *Application deadlines:* 11/30 (fall), 11/30 (spring). *Application fee:* $55.

Degree Requirements 124 total credit hours, 50 in nursing.

Baccalaureate for Second Degree Program (BSN)

Applying *Required:* SAT I or ACT, TOEFL for nonnative speakers of English, minimum college GPA of 2.5, transcript of college record, BA or BS. 38 prerequisite credits must be completed before admission to the nursing program. *Options:* Advanced standing available through the following means: advanced placement exams, credit by exam. Course work may be accelerated. May apply for transfer of up to 70 total credits. *Application deadlines:* 11/30 (fall), 11/30 (spring). *Application fee:* $55.

Degree Requirements 124 total credit hours, 50 in nursing.

LPN to Baccalaureate Program (BSN)

Applying *Required:* SAT I, TOEFL for nonnative speakers of English, minimum college GPA of 2.5, letter of recommendation, written essay, transcript of college record, high school class rank: top 33%. *Options:* Advanced standing available through advanced placement exams. Course work may be accelerated. May apply for transfer of up to 70 total credits. *Application deadlines:* 11/30 (fall), 11/30 (spring). *Application fee:* $55.

Degree Requirements 124 total credit hours, 50 in nursing.

MASTER'S PROGRAMS

Contact Frank McLaughlin, Graduate Coordinator, School of Nursing, San Francisco State University, San Francisco, CA 94132, 415-338-1802. *Fax:* 415-338-0555.

Areas of Study Nursing administration; nursing education; nurse practitioner programs in family health, primary care.

Expenses *State resident tuition:* $0 per academic year. *Full-time mandatory fees:* $1316. *Room and board:* $5100–$5400. *Room only:* $4100. *Books and supplies per academic year:* ranges from $500 to $600.

Financial Aid Nurse traineeships, Federal Nursing Student Loans, work-study. 24% of master's level students in nursing programs received some form of financial aid in 1995-96. *Application deadline:* 8/15.

MSN Program

Applying *Required:* TOEFL for nonnative speakers of English, bachelor's degree in nursing, minimum GPA of 3.0, RN license, statistics course, professional liability/malpractice insurance, essay, 3 letters of recommendation, transcript of college record, resume; 2 years clinical experience, physical assessment course for family nurse practitioner track. *Application deadlines:* 5/15 (fall), 11/30 (spring), 3/1 (family nurse practitioner track). *Application fee:* $55.

Degree Requirements 36–45 total credit hours dependent upon track, 30–34 in nursing, 6 in other specified areas. Culminating experience for family nurse practitioner track.

Master's for Nurses with Non-Nursing Degrees Program (MSN)

Applying *Required:* TOEFL for nonnative speakers of English, bachelor's degree, minimum GPA of 3.0, RN license, statistics course, professional liability/malpractice insurance, essay, 3 letters of recommendation, transcript of college record, resume. *Application deadlines:* 5/15 (fall), 11/30 (spring). *Application fee:* $55.

Degree Requirements 36 total credit hours, 30 in nursing, 6 in other specified areas. Culminating experience.

Master's for Non-Nursing College Graduates Program (MSN)

Applying *Required:* TOEFL for nonnative speakers of English, bachelor's degree, minimum GPA of 3.0, statistics course, professional liability/malpractice insurance, essay, 3 letters of recommendation, transcript of college record, resume. *Application deadline:* 11/30. *Application fee:* $55.

Degree Requirements 36 total credit hours, 30 in nursing, 6 in research and other specified areas. Culminating experience.

SAN JOSE STATE UNIVERSITY
School of Nursing
San Jose, California

Programs • Generic Baccalaureate • RN Baccalaureate • Accelerated RN Baccalaureate • MS • Master's for Nurses with Non-Nursing Degrees • Post-Master's • Continuing Education

The University State-supported comprehensive coed institution. Part of California State University System. Founded: 1857. *Primary accreditation:* regional. *Setting:* 104-acre urban campus. *Total enrollment:* 26,299.

The School of Nursing Founded in 1955. *Nursing program faculty:* 46 (56% with doctorates). *Off-campus program site:* Salinas.

Academic Facilities *Campus library:* 887,609 volumes (2,060 in nursing); 3,137 periodical subscriptions (234 health-care related). *Nursing school resources:* CAI, computer lab, nursing audiovisuals, interactive nursing skills videos, learning resource lab.

Student Life *Student services:* health clinic, personal counseling, career counseling, institutionally sponsored work-study program, job placement, campus safety program, special assistance for disabled students. *International student services:* counseling/support, special assistance for nonnative speakers of English, ESL courses. *Nursing student activities:* Sigma Theta Tau, student nurses association.

Calendar Semesters.

NURSING STUDENT PROFILE

Undergraduate **Enrollment:** 515
Women: 90%; **Men:** 10%; **Minority:** 68%; **International:** 0%; **Part-time:** 16%
Graduate **Enrollment:** 106
Women: 98%; **Men:** 2%; **Minority:** 25%; **International:** 0%; **Part-time:** 75%

BACCALAUREATE PROGRAMS

Contact Dr. Kathy Abriam-Yago, Student Retention Coordinator, School of Nursing, San Jose State University, 1 Washington Square, San Jose, CA 95192, 408-924-3159. *Fax:* 408-924-3135.

Expenses *State resident tuition:* $0 per academic year. *Full-time mandatory fees:* $1304–$1970. *Books and supplies per academic year:* ranges from $200 to $400.

Financial Aid Institutionally sponsored need-based grants/scholarships, institutionally sponsored non-need grants/scholarships. *Application deadline:* 3/1.

Generic Baccalaureate Program (BS)

Applying *Required:* TOEFL for nonnative speakers of English, entry-level math test, NLN Preadmission Examination, minimum high school GPA of 2.0, minimum college GPA of 2.3, 3 years of high school math, high school transcript, residence in California. 33 prerequisite credits must be completed before admission to the nursing program. *Options:* Advanced standing available through credit by exam. May apply for transfer of up to 65 total credits. *Application deadlines:* 11/30 (fall), 8/31 (spring). *Application fee:* $55.

Degree Requirements 129 total credit hours, 62 in nursing.

RN Baccalaureate Program (BS)

Applying *Required:* TOEFL for nonnative speakers of English, minimum high school GPA of 2.0, minimum college GPA of 2.3, RN license, diploma or AD in nursing, residence in California. *Options:* Advanced standing available through credit by exam. May apply for transfer of up to 70 total credits. *Application deadlines:* 11/30 (fall), 8/31 (spring). *Application fee:* $55.

Degree Requirements 129 total credit hours, 56 in nursing.

Accelerated RN Baccalaureate Program (BS)

Applying *Required:* entry-level math test, minimum high school GPA of 2.0, minimum college GPA of 2.3, 3 years of high school math, RN license, diploma or AD in nursing, interview, residence in California. *Options:* Advanced standing available through credit by exam. *Application deadlines:* 11/30 (fall), 8/31 (spring). *Application fee:* $55.

Degree Requirements 129 total credit hours, 56 in nursing.

MASTER'S PROGRAMS

Contact Dr. Coleen Saylor, Graduate Coordinator, School of Nursing, San Jose State University, 1 Washington Square, San Jose, CA 95192, 408-924-1321. *Fax:* 408-924-3135.

Areas of Study Clinical nurse specialist programs in gerontological nursing, school health nursing; nursing administration; nursing education.

Expenses *Full-time mandatory fees:* $1304–$1970. *Room and board:* $3500.

Financial Aid Nurse traineeships. *Application deadline:* 3/1.

MS Program

Applying *Required:* TOEFL for nonnative speakers of English, bachelor's degree in nursing, minimum GPA of 3.0, RN license, physical assessment course, statistics course, professional liability/malpractice insurance, essay, 2 letters of recommendation, transcript of college record. *Application deadlines:* 11/1 (fall), 11/1 (spring). *Application fee:* $55.

Degree Requirements 36 total credit hours, 30 in nursing. Thesis required.

Master's for Nurses with Non-Nursing Degrees Program (MS)

Applying *Required:* minimum GPA of 3.0, RN license, physical assessment course, statistics course, essay, 2 letters of recommendation, transcript of college record. *Application deadlines:* 11/1 (fall), 1/1 (spring). *Application fee:* $55.

Degree Requirements 36 total credit hours, 30 in nursing.

San Jose State University (continued)

POST-MASTER'S PROGRAM

Applying *Required:* minimum GPA of 3.0, RN license, physical assessment course, professional liability/malpractice insurance, 3 letters of recommendation, transcript of college record. *Application deadline:* 3/15. *Application fee:* $55.

Degree Requirements 30 total credit hours, 30 in nursing.

CONTINUING EDUCATION PROGRAM

Contact Dr. Sharon Hogan, Continuing Education Director, School of Nursing, San Jose State University, 1 Washington Square, San Jose, CA 95192, 408-924-3120. *Fax:* 408-924-3135.

SONOMA STATE UNIVERSITY

Department of Nursing
Rohnert Park, California

Programs • Generic Baccalaureate • RN Baccalaureate • BSN to Master's • Post-Master's

The University State-supported comprehensive coed institution. Part of California State University System. Founded: 1960. *Primary accreditation:* regional. *Setting:* 220-acre small-town campus. *Total enrollment:* 6,778.

The Department of Nursing Founded in 1972. *Nursing program faculty:* 19 (42% with doctorates). *Off-campus program sites:* Oakland, Santa Rosa, Arcata.

Academic Facilities *Campus library:* 453,462 volumes (23,478 in health, 14,345 in nursing); 111 health-care related periodical subscriptions. *Nursing school resources:* CAI, computer lab, nursing audiovisuals, interactive nursing skills videos, learning resource lab, Internet.

Student Life *Student services:* health clinic, child-care facilities, personal counseling, career counseling, institutionally sponsored work-study program, job placement, campus safety program, special assistance for disabled students. *International student services:* counseling/support, special assistance for nonnative speakers of English, ESL courses. *Nursing student activities:* Sigma Theta Tau, student nurses association.

Calendar Semesters.

NURSING STUDENT PROFILE

Undergraduate **Enrollment:** 135
Women: 93%; **Men:** 7%; **Minority:** 41%; **Part-time:** 42%
Graduate **Enrollment:** 96
Women: 96%; **Men:** 4%; **Minority:** 13%; **International:** 0%; **Part-time:** 30%

BACCALAUREATE PROGRAMS

Contact Dr. Janice Hitchcock, Acting Chairperson, Department of Nursing, Sonoma State University, 1801 East Cotati Avenue, Rohnert Park, CA 94928, 707-664-2465. *Fax:* 707-664-2653. *E-mail:* janice.hitchcock@sonoma.edu

Expenses *Nonresident tuition:* $7810 full-time, $246 per unit part-time. *Full-time mandatory fees:* $2130. *Part-time mandatory fees:* $1464. *Room and board:* $4343–$5495. *Room only:* $2768–$4073. *Books and supplies per academic year:* $1000.

Financial Aid Institutionally sponsored need-based grants/scholarships, institutionally sponsored non-need grants/scholarships, Federal Direct Loans, Federal Nursing Student Loans, Federal Pell Grants, Federal Perkins Loans, Federal Supplemental Educational Opportunity Grants, Federal Work-Study. *Application deadline:* 5/31.

GENERIC BACCALAUREATE PROGRAM (BSN)

Applying *Required:* SAT I, ACT, minimum high school GPA of 2.0, minimum college GPA of 2.5, 3 years of high school math, high school chemistry, high school biology, high school foreign language, high school transcript, 2 letters of recommendation, written essay, transcript of college record. *Options:* Advanced standing available through the following means: advanced placement exams, credit by exam. May apply for transfer of up to 70 total credits. *Application deadline:* 1/31. *Application fee:* $55.

Degree Requirements 127 total credit hours, 56 in nursing.

RN BACCALAUREATE PROGRAM (BSN)

Applying *Required:* minimum college GPA of 2.0, RN license, diploma or AD in nursing, transcript of college record. 60 prerequisite credits must be completed before admission to the nursing program. *Options:* May apply for transfer of up to 70 total credits. *Application deadline:* 1/31. *Application fee:* $55.

Degree Requirements 127 total credit hours, 33 in nursing.

MASTER'S PROGRAMS

Contact Becky Cohen, Secretary, Department of Nursing, Sonoma State University, 1801 East Cotati Avenue, Rohnert Park, CA 94928, 707-664-2465. *Fax:* 707-664-2653. *E-mail:* becky.cohen@sonoma.edu

Areas of Study Nursing administration; nurse practitioner program in family health.

Expenses *Nonresident tuition:* ranges from $2952 to $5904 full-time, $246 per unit part-time. *Full-time mandatory fees:* $2130. *Part-time mandatory fees:* $1464. *Books and supplies per academic year:* $1000.

Financial Aid Nurse traineeships, Federal Nursing Student Loans.

BSN TO MASTER'S PROGRAM (MSN)

Applying *Required:* GRE General Test, bachelor's degree in nursing, minimum GPA of 3.0, RN license, 2 years of clinical experience, physical assessment course, statistics course, professional liability/malpractice insurance, essay, interview, 3 letters of recommendation, transcript of college record, demonstrated computer literacy for leadership and management/case management track. *Application deadline:* 1/31. *Application fee:* $55.

Degree Requirements 39–40 total credit hours dependent upon track, 39–40 in nursing. Thesis or comprehensive exam.

Distance learning Courses provided through live teleconference.

POST-MASTER'S PROGRAM

Applying *Required:* minimum GPA of 3.0, RN license, 2 years of clinical experience, physical assessment course, professional liability/malpractice insurance, essay, interview, 3 letters of recommendation, transcript of college record, MSN. *Application deadline:* 1/31.

Degree Requirements 30 total credit hours, 30 in nursing.

UNIVERSITY OF CALIFORNIA, LOS ANGELES

School of Nursing
Los Angeles, California

Programs • Generic Baccalaureate • RN Baccalaureate • MSN • MSN/MBA • PhD • Postdoctoral • Continuing Education

The University State-supported coed university. Part of University of California System. Founded: 1919. *Primary accreditation:* regional. *Setting:* 419-acre urban campus. *Total enrollment:* 34,713.

The School of Nursing Founded in 1949. *Nursing program faculty:* 58 (53% with doctorates).

Academic Facilities *Campus library:* 6.0 million volumes (500,000 in health); 95,000 periodical subscriptions (6,000 health-care related). *Nursing school resources:* CAI, computer lab, nursing audiovisuals, interactive nursing skills videos, learning resource lab.

Student Life *Student services:* health clinic, child-care facilities, personal counseling, career counseling, institutionally sponsored work-study program, campus safety program, special assistance for disabled students.

International student services: counseling/support, ESL courses. *Nursing student activities:* Sigma Theta Tau, student nurses association.

Calendar Quarters.

NURSING STUDENT PROFILE

Undergraduate **Enrollment:** 33
Women: 91%; **Men:** 9%; **Minority:** 66%; **International:** 0%; **Part-time:** 1%
Graduate **Enrollment:** 230
Women: 96%; **Men:** 4%; **Minority:** 39%; **International:** 2%; **Part-time:** 3%

BACCALAUREATE PROGRAMS

Contact Student Affairs Office, School of Nursing, University of California, Los Angeles, 700 Tiverton Avenue, Box 951702, Los Angeles, CA 90095-1702, 310-825-7181. *Fax:* 310-206-7433.

Expenses *State resident tuition:* $0 per academic year. *Nonresident tuition:* $7699 per academic year. *Full-time mandatory fees:* $4001. *Room and board:* $3163–$6828. *Books and supplies per academic year:* ranges from $904 to $2519.

Financial Aid Institutionally sponsored need-based grants/scholarships, institutionally sponsored non-need grants/scholarships, Federal Direct Loans, Federal Nursing Student Loans, Federal Pell Grants, Federal Perkins Loans, Federal Supplemental Educational Opportunity Grants, Federal Work-Study. 58% of undergraduate students in nursing programs received some form of financial aid in 1995–96. *Application deadline:* 3/2.

Generic Baccalaureate Program (BS)

Applying *Required:* SAT I, ACT, College Board Achievements, minimum college GPA of 2.8, 3 years of high school math, 2 years of high school science, 3 letters of recommendation, written essay, transcript of college record. 84 prerequisite credits must be completed before admission to the nursing program. *Application fee:* $40.

Degree Requirements 180 total credit hours, 105 in nursing.

RN Baccalaureate Program (BS)

Applying *Required:* minimum college GPA of 2.8, high school math, high school science, RN license, letter of recommendation, written essay, transcript of college record. 84 prerequisite credits must be completed before admission to the nursing program. *Application fee:* $40.

Degree Requirements 180 total credit hours, 105 in nursing.

MASTER'S PROGRAMS

Contact Student Affairs Office, School of Nursing, University of California, Los Angeles, 700 Tiverton Avenue, Box 951702, Los Angeles, CA 90095-1702, 310-825-7181. *Fax:* 310-206-7433. *E-mail:* sonsaff@ucla.edu

Areas of Study Clinical nurse specialist programs in gerontological nursing, oncology nursing, acute care; nurse midwifery; nursing administration; nurse practitioner programs in acute care, child care/pediatrics, family health, gerontology, occupational health, oncology.

Expenses *State resident tuition:* $0. *Nonresident tuition:* $7699 per academic year. *Full-time mandatory fees:* $5943. *Room and board:* $8463. *Books and supplies per academic year:* $3771.

Financial Aid Graduate assistantships, nurse traineeships, fellowships, Federal Direct Loans, Federal Nursing Student Loans, institutionally sponsored loans, employment opportunities, institutionally sponsored need-based grants/scholarships, institutionally sponsored non-need-based grants/scholarships. 50% of master's level students in nursing programs received some form of financial aid in 1995-96. *Application deadline:* 7/1.

MSN Program

Applying *Required:* TOEFL for nonnative speakers of English, Commission on Graduates of Foreign Nursing Schools exam for international students, bachelor's degree in nursing, minimum GPA of 3.0, RN license, physical assessment course, statistics course, essay, 3 letters of recommendation, transcript of college record, human physiology, research. *Application deadline:* 2/1. *Application fee:* $40.

Degree Requirements 49–69 total credit hours dependent upon track. Comprehensive exam.

MSN/MBA Program

Applying *Required:* GMAT, bachelor's degree in nursing, RN license, statistics course, essay, 3 letters of recommendation, transcript of college record, nursing research course. *Application deadline:* 2/1. *Application fee:* $40.

Degree Requirements 125 total credit hours, 37 in nursing. Comprehensive exam.

DOCTORAL PROGRAM

Contact Student Affairs Office, School of Nursing, University of California, Los Angeles, 700 Tiverton Avenue, Box 951702, Los Angeles, CA 90095-1702, 310-825-7181. *Fax:* 310-206-7433. *E-mail:* sonsaff@ucla.edu

Areas of Study Bio-behavioral research or health systems research.

Expenses *State resident tuition:* $0 per academic year. *Nonresident tuition:* $7699 per academic year. *Full-time mandatory fees:* $4443. *Room and board:* $8463. *Books and supplies per academic year:* $3771.

Financial Aid Graduate assistantships, fellowships, dissertation grants, grants, Federal Direct Loans, Federal Nursing Student Loans, institutionally sponsored loans, opportunities for employment, institutionally sponsored need-based grants/scholarships, institutionally sponsored non-need-based grants/scholarships. *Application deadline:* 9/1.

PhD Program

Applying *Required:* GRE General Test (minimum combined score of 1500 on three tests), TOEFL for nonnative speakers of English, Commission on Graduates of Foreign Nursing Schools (CGFNS), master's degree in nursing, master's degree, 2 scholarly papers, statistics course, 4 letters of recommendation, vitae, writing sample, competitive review by faculty committee, scholarly papers or creative work, minimum 3.5 GPA, research and theory. *Application deadline:* 2/1. *Application fee:* $40.

Degree Requirements dissertation; oral exam; written exam; defense of dissertation.

POSTDOCTORAL PROGRAM

Contact Dr. Geraldine Padilla, Associate Dean for Research, School of Nursing, University of California, Los Angeles, 700 Tiverton Avenue, Box 951702, Los Angeles, CA 90095-1702, 310-206-2032. *Fax:* 310-206-7433.

Areas of Study Nursing research in health quality of life outcomes, intervention for minority partners of persons with AIDS, vulnerable population.

CONTINUING EDUCATION PROGRAM

Contact Extension Division, Nursing Education, University of California, Los Angeles, 614 UNEX, PO Box 24901, Los Angeles, CA 90024-0901, 310-825-8423.

UNIVERSITY OF CALIFORNIA, SAN FRANCISCO

School of Nursing
San Francisco, California

Programs • MSN • Master's for Non-Nursing College Graduates • PhD • Postdoctoral

The University State-supported graduate specialized coed institution. Part of University of California System. Founded: 1864. *Primary accreditation:* regional. *Total enrollment:* 3,695.

The School of Nursing Founded in 1907. *Nursing program faculty:* 122 (63% with doctorates). *Off-campus program site:* Fresno.

Academic Facilities *Campus library:* 873,642 volumes (856,169 in health, 131,046 in nursing); 3,337 periodical subscriptions (3,270 health-care related). *Nursing school resources:* computer lab, nursing audiovisuals, interactive nursing skills videos, learning resource lab.

Student Life *Student services:* health clinic, child-care facilities, personal counseling, career counseling, institutionally sponsored work-study program, job placement, campus safety program, special assistance for

University of California, San Francisco (continued)
disabled students. *International student services:* counseling/support, ESL courses. *Nursing student activities:* Sigma Theta Tau, student nurses association.

Calendar Quarters.

NURSING STUDENT PROFILE

Graduate **Enrollment:** 467
Women: 93%; **Men:** 7%; **Minority:** 25%; **International:** 5%; **Part-time:** 2%

MASTER'S PROGRAMS

Contact Mr. Jeff Kilmer, Director, Office of Student and Curricular Affairs, School of Nursing, University of California, San Francisco, N319X, San Francisco, CA 94143-0602, 415-476-1435. *Fax:* 415-476-9707. *E-mail:* jeff_kilmer_at_nursing@ccmail.ucsf.edu

Areas of Study Clinical nurse specialist programs in cardiovascular nursing, community health nursing, critical care nursing, gerontological nursing, occupational health nursing, oncology nursing, perinatal nursing, psychiatric–mental health nursing; nurse anesthesia; nurse midwifery; nursing administration; nurse practitioner programs in acute care, adult health, child care/pediatrics, family health, gerontology, neonatal health, occupational health, psychiatric–mental health, school health, women's health.

Expenses *State resident tuition:* $0 full-time, $0 part-time. *Nonresident tuition:* $8394 per academic year. *Full-time mandatory fees:* $5804. *Room only:* $605–$915. *Books and supplies per academic year:* ranges from $920 to $1100.

Financial Aid Graduate assistantships, nurse traineeships, Federal Direct Loans, Federal Nursing Student Loans, institutionally sponsored loans, employment opportunities, institutionally sponsored need-based grants/scholarships. 48% of master's level students in nursing programs received some form of financial aid in 1995-96.

MSN Program

Applying *Required:* GRE General Test, TOEFL for nonnative speakers of English, bachelor's degree in nursing, minimum GPA of 3.0, RN license, 1 year of clinical experience, statistics course, essay, 4 letters of recommendation, transcript of college record. *Application deadline:* 2/1. *Application fee:* $40.

Degree Requirements 30–110 total credit hours dependent upon track, 18 in nursing. Thesis or comprehensive exam, 8 units clinical work.

Master's for Non-Nursing College Graduates Program (MSN)

Applying *Required:* GRE General Test, bachelor's degree, minimum GPA of 3.0, statistics course, essay, 4 letters of recommendation, transcript of college record. *Application deadline:* 10/1 (summer). *Application fee:* $40.

Degree Requirements 30–110 total credit hours dependent upon track, 18 in nursing. Thesis or comprehensive exam, 8 units clinical work.

DOCTORAL PROGRAM

Contact Mr. Jeff Kilmer, Director, Office of Student and Curricular Affairs, School of Nursing, University of California, San Francisco, N319X, San Francisco, CA 94143-0602, 415-476-1435. *Fax:* 415-476-9707.

Areas of Study Nursing research, nursing science, theory development.

Expenses *State resident tuition:* $0 per academic year. *Nonresident tuition:* $8394 per academic year. *Full-time mandatory fees:* $5804. *Room only:* $605–$915. *Books and supplies per academic year:* ranges from $920 to $1100.

Financial Aid Graduate assistantships, nurse traineeships, fellowships, dissertation grants, grants, Federal Direct Loans, institutionally sponsored loans, opportunities for employment, institutionally sponsored need-based grants/scholarships, National Research Student Award.

PhD Program

Applying *Required:* GRE General Test, TOEFL for nonnative speakers of English, statistics course, 4 letters of recommendation, writing sample, competitive review by faculty committee, minimum 3.2 undergraduate GPA, minimum 3.5 graduate GPA, RN license, 1 year nursing experience. *Application deadline:* 12/1. *Application fee:* $40.

Degree Requirements dissertation; oral exam; written exam; defense of dissertation; residency.

POSTDOCTORAL PROGRAM

Contact Mr. Jeff Kilmer, Director, Office of Student and Curricular Affairs, School of Nursing, University of California, San Francisco, N319X, San Francisco, CA 94143-0602, 415-476-1435. *Fax:* 415-476-9707.

Areas of Study Individualized study.

See full description on page 524.

UNIVERSITY OF SAN DIEGO
Philip Y. Hahn School of Nursing
San Diego, California

Programs • RN Baccalaureate • RN to Master's • MSN/MBA • Post-Master's • DNSc

The University Independent Roman Catholic coed university. Founded: 1949. *Primary accreditation:* regional. *Setting:* 180-acre urban campus. *Total enrollment:* 6,416.

The Philip Y. Hahn School of Nursing Founded in 1974. *Nursing program faculty:* 33 (100% with doctorates).

Academic Facilities *Campus library:* 620,000 volumes (25,000 in health, 15,000 in nursing); 6,000 periodical subscriptions (200 health-care related). *Nursing school resources:* computer lab, nursing audiovisuals, interactive nursing skills videos, learning resource lab.

Student Life *Student services:* health clinic, child-care facilities, personal counseling, career counseling, institutionally sponsored work-study program, job placement, campus safety program, special assistance for disabled students. *International student services:* counseling/support, special assistance for nonnative speakers of English. *Nursing student activities:* Sigma Theta Tau, student nurses association.

Calendar Semesters.

NURSING STUDENT PROFILE

Undergraduate **Enrollment:** 30
Women: 99%; **Men:** 1%; **Minority:** 13%; **International:** 0%; **Part-time:** 55%
Graduate **Enrollment:** 210
Women: 95%; **Men:** 5%; **Minority:** 14%; **International:** 1%; **Part-time:** 79%

BACCALAUREATE PROGRAM

Contact Ms. Cathleen Mumper, Student Services Director, Philip Y. Hahn School of Nursing, University of San Diego, 5998 Alcala Park, San Diego, CA 92110-2492, 619-260-4548. *Fax:* 619-260-6814. *E-mail:* cmm@teetot.acusd.edu

Expenses *Tuition:* ranges from $1530 to $6100 full-time, $510 per unit part-time. *Full-time mandatory fees:* $100–$200. *Part-time mandatory fees:* $100–$200. *Books and supplies per academic year:* ranges from $100 to $400.

Financial Aid Institutionally sponsored need-based grants/scholarships, institutionally sponsored non-need grants/scholarships, Federal Pell Grants, Federal Perkins Loans, Federal Supplemental Educational Opportunity Grants, Federal Work-Study. 77% of undergraduate students in nursing programs received some form of financial aid in 1995–96. *Application deadline:* 2/20.

RN Baccalaureate Program (BSN)

Applying *Required:* TOEFL for nonnative speakers of English, ACT PEP for diploma RNs, minimum college GPA of 3.0, RN license, diploma or AD in nursing, high school transcript, 3 letters of recommendation, written essay, transcript of college record. 57 prerequisite credits must be completed before admission to the nursing program. *Options:* May apply for transfer of up to 87 total credits. *Application deadline:* rolling. *Application fee:* $45.

Degree Requirements 124 total credit hours, 64 in nursing.

MASTER'S PROGRAMS

Contact Ms. Cathleen Mumper, Student Services Director, Philip Y. Hahn School of Nursing, University of San Diego, 5998 Alcala Park, San Diego, CA 92110-2492, 619-260-4548. *Fax:* 619-260-6814. *E-mail:* cmm@teetot.acusd.edu

Areas of Study Nursing administration; nurse practitioner programs in adult health, child care/pediatrics, family health, gerontology, school health.

Expenses *Tuition:* $525 per unit. *Full-time mandatory fees:* $100–$200. *Part-time mandatory fees:* $100–$200. *Books and supplies per academic year:* ranges from $100 to $600.

Financial Aid Graduate assistantships, nurse traineeships, fellowships, institutionally sponsored loans, institutionally sponsored need-based grants/scholarships, institutionally sponsored non-need-based grants/ scholarships. 70% of master's level students in nursing programs received some form of financial aid in 1995-96. *Application deadline:* 5/1.

RN to Master's Program (MSN)

Applying *Required:* GRE General Test, Miller Analogies Test, TOEFL for nonnative speakers of English, ACT PEP for diploma RNs, minimum GPA of 3.0, RN license, 1 year of clinical experience, statistics course, professional liability/malpractice insurance, essay, interview, 3 letters of recommendation, transcript of college record. *Application deadlines:* 3/1 (fall), 11/1 (spring). *Application fee:* $45.

Degree Requirements 152–164 total credit hours dependent upon track, 95–107 in nursing.

MSN/MBA Program

Applying *Required:* GRE General Test or Miller Analogies Test, TOEFL for nonnative speakers of English, GMAT, bachelor's degree in nursing, minimum GPA of 3.0, RN license, 1 year of clinical experience, statistics course, professional liability/malpractice insurance, essay, 3 letters of recommendation, transcript of college record. *Application deadlines:* 3/1 (fall), 11/1 (spring). *Application fee:* $45.

Degree Requirements 78 total credit hours, 30 in nursing, 48 in business.

Post-Master's Program

Applying *Required:* TOEFL for nonnative speakers of English, minimum GPA of 3.0, RN license, 1 year of clinical experience, professional liability/malpractice insurance, essay, interview, 3 letters of recommendation, transcript of college record, master's degree in nursing. *Application deadlines:* 3/1 (fall), 11/1 (spring). *Application fee:* $45.

Degree Requirements 33–40 total credit hours dependent upon track.

DOCTORAL PROGRAM

Contact Ms. Cathleen Mumper, Student Services Director, Philip Y. Hahn School of Nursing, University of San Diego, 5998 Alcala Park, San Diego, CA 92110-2492, 619-260-4548. *Fax:* 619-260-6814.

Areas of Study Nursing administration, nursing education, clinical practice.

Expenses *Tuition:* ranges from $1620 to $9720 full-time, $540 per unit part-time. *Full-time mandatory fees:* $100–$200. *Part-time mandatory fees:* $100–$200. *Books and supplies per academic year:* ranges from $100 to $400.

Financial Aid Graduate assistantships, nurse traineeships, fellowships, institutionally sponsored loans, institutionally sponsored need-based grants/scholarships, institutionally sponsored non-need-based grants/ scholarships. *Application deadline:* 5/1.

DNSc Program

Applying *Required:* GRE General Test, Miller Analogies Test, TOEFL for nonnative speakers of English, master's degree in nursing, 1 year of clinical experience, 1 scholarly paper, statistics course, interview, 3 letters of recommendation, vitae, writing sample, competitive review by faculty committee. *Application deadlines:* 2/15 (fall), 9/15 (spring), 2/15 (summer). *Application fee:* $45.

Degree Requirements 54 total credit hours; 18 units in core requirements, 15 units in cognates, 9 units in electives, 12 units in dissertation research; dissertation; oral exam; written exam; defense of dissertation; residency.

See full description on page 552.

UNIVERSITY OF SAN FRANCISCO

School of Nursing
San Francisco, California

Programs • Generic Baccalaureate • RN Baccalaureate • MSN • MSN/ MBA

The University Independent Roman Catholic (Jesuit) coed university. Founded: 1855. *Primary accreditation:* regional. *Setting:* 55-acre urban campus. *Total enrollment:* 7,833.

The School of Nursing Founded in 1954.

Academic Facilities *Campus library:* 588,300 volumes (2,444 in nursing); 2,409 periodical subscriptions (92 health-care related).

Calendar Semesters.

BACCALAUREATE PROGRAMS

Contact Assistant to the Dean for Student Services, School of Nursing, University of San Francisco, 2130 Fulton Street, San Francisco, CA 94117-1080, 415-666-6694. *Fax:* 415-666-6877.

Expenses *Tuition:* $14,920 full-time, $545 per unit part-time.

Financial Aid Institutionally sponsored need-based grants/scholarships, institutionally sponsored non-need grants/scholarships, Federal Direct Loans, Federal Nursing Student Loans, Federal Perkins Loans, Federal Supplemental Educational Opportunity Grants, Federal PLUS Loans, Federal Stafford Loans, state aid. *Application deadline:* 2/15.

Generic Baccalaureate Program (BSN)

Applying *Required:* SAT I or ACT, TOEFL for nonnative speakers of English, high school transcript, 2 letters of recommendation, written essay. *Options:* Advanced standing available through the following means: advanced placement exams, credit by exam. *Application fee:* $35.

Degree Requirements 128 total credit hours, 64 in nursing.

RN Baccalaureate Program (BSN)

Applying *Required:* TOEFL for nonnative speakers of English, RN license, diploma or AD in nursing, high school transcript, 2 letters of recommendation, transcript of college record. *Options:* Advanced standing available through credit by exam. *Application fee:* $35.

Degree Requirements 128 total credit hours, 64 in nursing.

MASTER'S PROGRAMS

Contact Assistant to the Dean for Student Services, School of Nursing, University of San Francisco, 2130 Fulton Street, San Francisco, CA 94117-1080, 415-666-6694. *Fax:* 415-666-6877.

Areas of Study Clinical nurse specialist program in advanced practice nursing; nursing administration.

Expenses *Tuition:* $590 per unit.

MSN Program

Applying *Required:* TOEFL for nonnative speakers of English, bachelor's degree in nursing, minimum GPA of 3.0, RN license, 1 year of clinical experience, statistics course, 3 letters of recommendation, transcript of college record. *Application fee:* $40.

Degree Requirements 36–47 total credit hours dependent upon track, 36–47 in nursing. Comprehensive exam.

MSN/MBA Program

Applying *Required:* TOEFL for nonnative speakers of English, GMAT, bachelor's degree in nursing, minimum GPA of 3.0, RN license, 1 year of clinical experience, 3 letters of recommendation, transcript of college record. *Application fee:* $40.

Degree Requirements 36 total credit hours in nursing.

See full description on page 554.

UNIVERSITY OF SOUTHERN CALIFORNIA

Department of Nursing
Los Angeles, California

Programs • Generic Baccalaureate • RN Baccalaureate • Baccalaureate for Second Degree • MSN • MSN/MBA • Post-Master's • Continuing Education

The University Independent coed university. Founded: 1880. *Primary accreditation:* regional. *Setting:* 150-acre urban campus. *Total enrollment:* 27,589.

The Department of Nursing Founded in 1981. *Nursing program faculty:* 36 (41% with doctorates).

Academic Facilities *Campus library:* 2.7 million volumes (156,200 in health); 36,844 periodical subscriptions (2,627 health-care related). *Nursing school resources:* CAI, computer lab, nursing audiovisuals, interactive nursing skills videos, learning resource lab.

Student Life *Student services:* health clinic, child-care facilities, personal counseling, career counseling, institutionally sponsored work-study program, job placement, campus safety program, special assistance for

University of Southern California (continued)
disabled students. *International student services:* counseling/support, special assistance for nonnative speakers of English, ESL courses. *Nursing student activities:* Sigma Theta Tau, nursing club, student nurses association, Chi Eta Phi.

Calendar Semesters.

NURSING STUDENT PROFILE

Undergraduate **Enrollment:** 343
Women: 82%; **Men:** 18%; **Minority:** 65%
Graduate **Enrollment:** 68
Women: 85%; **Men:** 15%; **Minority:** 31%; **Part-time:** 26%

BACCALAUREATE PROGRAMS

Contact Ms. Lynette Merriman, Director, Admissions and Student Affairs, CHP 222, Department of Nursing, University of Southern California, 1540 East Alcazar Street, Los Angeles, CA 90033, 213-342-2020. *Fax:* 213-342-2091.

Expenses *Tuition:* $19,140 full-time, $644 per unit part-time. *Full-time mandatory fees:* $740. *Books and supplies per academic year:* ranges from $700 to $1000.

Financial Aid Institutionally sponsored need-based grants/scholarships, institutionally sponsored non-need grants/scholarships, Federal Direct Loans, Federal Nursing Student Loans, Federal Pell Grants, Federal Perkins Loans, Federal Supplemental Educational Opportunity Grants, Federal Work-Study, California grants. 90% of undergraduate students in nursing programs received some form of financial aid in 1995–96. *Application deadline:* 2/15.

Generic Baccalaureate Program (BSN)

Applying *Required:* SAT I or ACT, minimum high school GPA of 3.0, minimum college GPA of 3.0, high school chemistry, high school biology, high school transcript, 2 letters of recommendation, written essay, transcript of college record, resume. 60 prerequisite credits must be completed before admission to the nursing program. *Options:* May apply for transfer of up to 70 total credits. *Application deadlines:* 1/31 (fall), 11/1 (spring). *Application fee:* $50.

Degree Requirements 130 total credit hours, 70 in nursing.

RN Baccalaureate Program (BSN)

Applying *Required:* TOEFL for nonnative speakers of English, minimum college GPA of 3.0, high school chemistry, RN license, diploma or AD in nursing, 2 letters of recommendation, written essay, transcript of college record. 62 prerequisite credits must be completed before admission to the nursing program. *Options:* Advanced standing available through credit by exam. Course work may be accelerated. May apply for transfer of up to 70 total credits. *Application deadlines:* 1/31 (fall), 11/1 (spring). *Application fee:* $50.

Degree Requirements 130 total credit hours, 70 in nursing.

Baccalaureate for Second Degree Program (BSN)

Applying *Required:* SAT I or ACT, minimum high school GPA of 3.0, minimum college GPA of 3.0, high school chemistry, high school biology, high school transcript, letter of recommendation, written essay, transcript of college record, resume. 60 prerequisite credits must be completed before admission to the nursing program. *Options:* May apply for transfer of up to 80 total credits. *Application deadlines:* 1/31 (fall), 11/1 (spring). *Application fee:* $50.

Degree Requirements 130 total credit hours, 70 in nursing.

MASTER'S PROGRAMS

Contact Ms. Allison Frierson, Recruitment Coordinator, CHP 222, Department of Nursing, University of Southern California, 1540 East Alcazar Street, Los Angeles, CA 90033, 213-342-2020. *Fax:* 213-342-2091. *E-mail:* frierson@hsc.usc.edu

Areas of Study Clinical nurse specialist program in enterostomal therapy nursing; nurse anesthesia; nurse midwifery; nursing administration; nurse practitioner programs in family health, gerontology.

Expenses *Tuition:* $19,140 full-time, $644 per unit part-time. *Full-time mandatory fees:* $700. *Part-time mandatory fees:* $400–$700.

Financial Aid Graduate assistantships, nurse traineeships, Federal Nursing Student Loans, institutionally sponsored loans. *Application deadline:* 2/15.

MSN Program

Applying *Required:* GRE General Test, bachelor's degree in nursing, minimum GPA of 3.0, RN license, 1 year of clinical experience, physical assessment course, statistics course, professional liability/malpractice insurance, essay, interview, 3 letters of recommendation, transcript of college record. *Application deadlines:* 8/1 (fall), 11/1 (spring). *Application fee:* $50.

Degree Requirements 40–41 total credit hours dependent upon track, 37–38 in nursing, 3 in business and other specified areas. Project.

MSN/MBA Program

Applying *Required:* GRE General Test, GMAT, bachelor's degree in nursing, minimum GPA of 3.0, RN license, statistics course, professional liability/malpractice insurance, essay, 3 letters of recommendation, transcript of college record. *Application deadlines:* 8/1 (fall), 11/1 (spring). *Application fee:* $50.

Degree Requirements 70 total credit hours, 27 in nursing, 43 in business.

Post-Master's Program

Applying *Required:* minimum GPA of 3.0, RN license, 1 year of clinical experience, physical assessment course, professional liability/malpractice insurance, essay, 3 letters of recommendation, transcript of college record. *Application deadlines:* 8/1 (fall), 11/1 (spring). *Application fee:* $50.

Degree Requirements 30 total credit hours, 27 in nursing, 3 in other specified areas.

CONTINUING EDUCATION PROGRAM

Contact Ms. Peggy Kalowes, Director, Continuing Education, CHP 222, Department of Nursing, University of Southern California, 1540 East Alcazar Street, Los Angeles, CA 90033, 213-342-2001. *Fax:* 213-342-2091. *E-mail:* kalowes@hsc.usc.edu

See full description on page 558.

COLORADO

BETH-EL COLLEGE OF NURSING AND HEALTH SCIENCES

Beth-El College of Nursing
Colorado Springs, Colorado

Programs • Accelerated RN Baccalaureate • Master's

The College City-supported comprehensive specialized primarily women's institution. Founded: 1904. *Primary accreditation:* regional. *Setting:* 1-acre urban campus. *Total enrollment:* 460.

The Beth-El College of Nursing Founded in 1904. *Nursing program faculty:* 40 (25% with doctorates).

Academic Facilities *Nursing school resources:* computer lab, nursing audiovisuals, interactive nursing skills videos.

Student Life *Student services:* personal counseling, career counseling, institutionally sponsored work-study program, campus safety program. *Nursing student activities:* Sigma Theta Tau, student nurses association.

Calendar Semesters.

NURSING STUDENT PROFILE

Undergraduate **Enrollment:** 335
Women: 90%; **Men:** 10%; **Minority:** 10%; **International:** 0%; **Part-time:** 60%
Graduate **Enrollment:** 104
Women: 95%; **Men:** 5%; **Minority:** 3%; **International:** 0%; **Part-time:** 60%

BACCALAUREATE PROGRAM

Contact Ms. Marilyn J. Atwood, Director of Student Affairs, Beth-El College of Nursing, Beth-El College of Nursing and Health Sciences, 2790 North Academy Boulevard, Suite 200, Colorado Springs, CO 80917, 719-475-5170. *Fax:* 719-475-5198.

Expenses *State resident tuition:* $4300 full-time, $179 per credit part-time. *Nonresident tuition:* $4300 full-time, $179 per credit part-time. *Full-time*

mandatory fees: $105. *Part-time mandatory fees:* $105. *Books and supplies per academic year:* ranges from $250 to $500.

Financial Aid Institutionally sponsored need-based grants/scholarships, Federal Perkins Loans, Federal Supplemental Educational Opportunity Grants, Federal Work-Study. 46% of undergraduate students in nursing programs received some form of financial aid in 1995–96. *Application deadline:* 6/1.

ACCELERATED RN BACCALAUREATE PROGRAM (BSN)

Applying *Required:* ACT, minimum high school GPA of 2.8, minimum college GPA of 2.8, 3 years of high school math, 3 years of high school science, high school chemistry, high school biology, RN license, diploma or AD in nursing, high school foreign language, high school transcript, 2 letters of recommendation, written essay, transcript of college record, high school class rank: top 40%. *Options:* Advanced standing available through credit by exam. Course work may be accelerated. May apply for transfer of up to 105 total credits. *Application deadlines:* 2/1 (fall), 10/15 (spring). *Application fee:* $30.

Degree Requirements 129 total credit hours, 75 in nursing.

MASTER'S PROGRAM

Contact Barbara Joyce Nagata, Chair, Department of Graduate Studies, Beth-El College of Nursing, 2790 North Academy, Suite 200, Colorado Springs, CO 80917, 719-475-5170.

MESA STATE COLLEGE
Department of Nursing and Radiologic Science
Grand Junction, Colorado

Program • Generic Baccalaureate

The College State-supported 4-year coed college. Part of State Colleges in Colorado. Founded: 1925. *Primary accreditation:* regional. *Setting:* 42-acre small-town campus. *Total enrollment:* 4,721.

The Department of Nursing and Radiologic Science Founded in 1979. *Nursing program faculty:* 11 (22% with doctorates).

Academic Facilities *Campus library:* 150,902 volumes (9,500 in health, 6,485 in nursing); 976 periodical subscriptions (121 health-care related). *Nursing school resources:* computer lab, nursing audiovisuals, learning resource lab.

Student Life *Student services:* health clinic, child-care facilities, personal counseling, career counseling, institutionally sponsored work-study program, job placement, campus safety program, special assistance for disabled students. *Nursing student activities:* Sigma Theta Tau, student nurses association.

Calendar Semesters.

NURSING STUDENT PROFILE

Undergraduate **Enrollment:** 83

Women: 80%; **Men:** 20%; **Minority:** 7%; **International:** 0%; **Part-time:** 14%

BACCALAUREATE PROGRAM

Contact Dr. Sandy Forrest, Chair, Department of Nursing and Radiologic Science, Mesa State College, 1175 Texas Avenue, PO Box 2647, Grand Junction, CO 81502, 970-248-1522. *Fax:* 970-248-1923.

Expenses *State resident tuition:* $2250 full-time, $75 per credit hour part-time. *Nonresident tuition:* $8190 full-time, $273 per credit part-time. *Room and board:* $3870–$4830. *Room only:* $2106–$2670. *Books and supplies per academic year:* $300.

Financial Aid Institutionally sponsored need-based grants/scholarships, institutionally sponsored non-need grants/scholarships, Federal Supplemental Educational Opportunity Grants, Federal Work-Study. *Application deadline:* 3/1.

GENERIC BACCALAUREATE PROGRAM (BSN)

Applying *Required:* SAT I, ACT, minimum college GPA of 2.75, written essay, transcript of college record. 45 prerequisite credits must be completed before admission to the nursing program. *Application deadline:* 10/1.

Degree Requirements 120 total credit hours, 54 in nursing.

METROPOLITAN STATE COLLEGE OF DENVER
Department of Nursing and Health Care Management
Denver, Colorado

Program • RN Baccalaureate

The College State-supported 4-year coed college. Part of State Colleges in Colorado. Founded: 1963. *Primary accreditation:* regional. *Setting:* 171-acre urban campus. *Total enrollment:* 16,815.

The Department of Nursing and Health Care Management Founded in 1974.

Academic Facilities *Campus library:* 731,000 volumes (16,770 in health); 3,581 periodical subscriptions (259 health-care related).

Student Life *Student services:* health clinic, campus safety program. *Nursing student activities:* nursing club.

Calendar Semesters.

BACCALAUREATE PROGRAM

Contact Dr. Kathleen McGuire-Mahony, Chair, Department of Nursing and Health Care Management, Metropolitan State College of Denver, PO Box 173362, Denver, CO 80217-3362, 303-556-3130. *Fax:* 303-556-3439.

Expenses *State resident tuition:* $1632 full-time, $68 per credit hour part-time. *Nonresident tuition:* $6432 full-time, $268 per credit hour part-time. *Full-time mandatory fees:* $155.

Financial Aid Federal Pell Grants, Federal Supplemental Educational Opportunity Grants, Federal Work-Study, Federal PLUS Loans, Federal Stafford Loans, state aid. *Application deadline:* 3/1.

RN BACCALAUREATE PROGRAM (BS)

Applying *Required:* SAT I, ACT, RN license, diploma or AD in nursing, high school transcript, transcript of college record, basic life support certificate, professional liability/malpractice insurance, immunizations, Colorado RN license, recent clinical experience, qualify for Colorado Articulation Model/Agreement. 30 prerequisite credits must be completed before admission to the nursing program. *Application fee:* $25.

Degree Requirements 30 total credit hours in nursing.

REGIS UNIVERSITY
Department of Nursing
Denver, Colorado

Programs • Generic Baccalaureate • RN Baccalaureate • Accelerated Baccalaureate for Second Degree • MSN

The University Independent Roman Catholic (Jesuit) comprehensive coed institution. Founded: 1877. *Primary accreditation:* regional. *Setting:* 90-acre suburban campus. *Total enrollment:* 6,806.

The Department of Nursing Founded in 1948. *Nursing program faculty:* 18 (22% with doctorates). *Off-campus program site:* Colorado Springs.

Academic Facilities *Campus library:* 260,891 volumes (682 in health, 815 in nursing); 1,993 periodical subscriptions (165 health-care related). *Nursing school resources:* computer lab, learning resource lab, health-specific databases.

Regis University (continued)

Student Life *Student services:* health clinic, personal counseling, career counseling, institutionally sponsored work-study program, job placement, campus safety program. *International student services:* ESL courses. *Nursing student activities:* Sigma Theta Tau, student nurses association.

Calendar Semesters, 8-week evening sessions, 10-week alternating weekend sessions.

NURSING STUDENT PROFILE

Undergraduate **Enrollment:** 325
Women: 88%; **Men:** 12%; **Minority:** 8%; **International:** 1%; **Part-time:** 42%
Graduate **Enrollment:** 58
Women: 97%; **Men:** 3%; **Minority:** 7%; **International:** 0%; **Part-time:** 21%

BACCALAUREATE PROGRAMS

Contact Admissions Counselor, Department of Nursing, Regis University, 3333 Regis Boulevard, Denver, CO 80221-1099, 800-388-2366. *Fax:* 303-964-5533. *E-mail:* rooney@regis.edu

Expenses *Tuition:* $7050 full-time, ranges from $199 to $440 per semester hour part-time. *Full-time mandatory fees:* $65. *Room and board:* $5280–$7760. *Room only:* $2980–$4760. *Books and supplies per academic year:* $550.

Financial Aid Institutionally sponsored need-based grants/scholarships, institutionally sponsored non-need grants/scholarships, Federal Nursing Student Loans, Federal Perkins Loans, Federal Supplemental Educational Opportunity Grants, Federal Work-Study. 61% of undergraduate students in nursing programs received some form of financial aid in 1995–96. *Application deadline:* 3/15.

Generic Baccalaureate Program (BSN)

Applying *Required:* SAT I, ACT, TOEFL for nonnative speakers of English, minimum high school GPA of 2.2, minimum college GPA of 2.5, 2 letters of recommendation, written essay, transcript of college record. 60 prerequisite credits must be completed before admission to the nursing program. *Options:* Advanced standing available through the following means: advanced placement exams, credit by exam. May apply for transfer of up to 71 total credits. *Application deadline:* 2/15. *Application fee:* $40.

Degree Requirements 128 total credit hours, 60 in nursing.

RN Baccalaureate Program (BSN)

Applying *Required:* TOEFL for nonnative speakers of English, RN license, diploma or AD in nursing. 69 prerequisite credits must be completed before admission to the nursing program. *Options:* Advanced standing available through credit by exam. May apply for transfer of up to 98 total credits. *Application deadline:* rolling. *Application fee:* $40.

Degree Requirements 128 total credit hours, 30 in nursing.

Accelerated Baccalaureate for Second Degree Program (BSN)

Applying *Required:* TOEFL for nonnative speakers of English, minimum college GPA of 2.5, 2 letters of recommendation, written essay, transcript of college record. 43 prerequisite credits must be completed before admission to the nursing program. *Options:* Course work may be accelerated. *Application deadline:* 7/15. *Application fee:* $40.

Degree Requirements 128 total credit hours, 57 in nursing.

MASTER'S PROGRAM

Contact Admissions Counselor, MSN Program, Department of Nursing, Regis University, 3333 Regis Boulevard, Denver, CO 80221-1099, 800-388-2366. *Fax:* 303-364-5533.

Areas of Study Nursing administration; nurse practitioner programs in family health, perinatal nursing.

Expenses *Tuition:* $238 per semester hour. *Full-time mandatory fees:* $25–$115. *Books and supplies per academic year:* ranges from $350 to $450.

Financial Aid Nurse traineeships. 60% of master's level students in nursing programs received some form of financial aid in 1995-96. *Application deadline:* 3/15.

MSN Program

Applying *Required:* Miller Analogies Test, TOEFL for nonnative speakers of English, bachelor's degree in nursing, minimum GPA of 2.75, RN license, 2 years of clinical experience, statistics course, essay, 3 letters of recommendation, transcript of college record, perinatal nurse practitioner emphasis requires 2 years of high-risk labor/delivery. *Application fee:* $40–50.

Degree Requirements 36–48 total credit hours dependent upon track. Thesis or project.

Distance learning Courses provided through video, computer-based media. Specific degree requirements include emphasis in perinatal nurse practitioner only.

UNIVERSITY OF COLORADO HEALTH SCIENCES CENTER
School of Nursing
Denver, Colorado

Programs • Generic Baccalaureate • MS • RN to Master's • MS/MBA • PhD • ND • Continuing Education

The University State-supported upper-level coed institution. Part of University of Colorado System. Founded: 1883. *Primary accreditation:* regional. *Setting:* 40-acre urban campus. *Total enrollment:* 2,260.

The School of Nursing Founded in 1898. *Nursing program faculty:* 84 (70% with doctorates). *Off-campus program sites:* Grand Junction, Durango, La Junta.

Academic Facilities *Campus library:* 225,452 volumes (225,452 in health); 1,943 periodical subscriptions (1,943 health-care related). *Nursing school resources:* CAI, computer lab, nursing audiovisuals, interactive nursing skills videos, learning resource lab.

Student Life *Student services:* health clinic, personal counseling, institutionally sponsored work-study program, special assistance for disabled students. *International student services:* counseling/support. *Nursing student activities:* Sigma Theta Tau, student nurses association.

Calendar Semesters.

NURSING STUDENT PROFILE

Undergraduate **Enrollment:** 166
Women: 95%; **Men:** 5%; **Minority:** 17%; **International:** 0%; **Part-time:** 5%
Graduate **Enrollment:** 393
Women: 95%; **Men:** 5%; **Minority:** 6%; **International:** 1%; **Part-time:** 18%

BACCALAUREATE PROGRAM

Contact Gwendolyn Hill, Director, Office of Admissions and Student Support, School of Nursing, University of Colorado Health Sciences Center, 4200 East 9th Avenue, Box C288, Denver, CO 80262, 303-315-5592. *Fax:* 303-315-8660. *E-mail:* gwendolyn.hill@uchsc.edu

Expenses *State resident tuition:* $4290 full-time, $143 per credit hour part-time. *Nonresident tuition:* $14,100 full-time, $470 per credit hour part-time. *Full-time mandatory fees:* $1580. *Books and supplies per academic year:* ranges from $1314 to $1524.

Financial Aid Institutionally sponsored need-based grants/scholarships, institutionally sponsored non-need grants/scholarships, Federal Direct Loans, Federal Nursing Student Loans, Federal Perkins Loans, Federal Supplemental Educational Opportunity Grants, Federal Work-Study. *Application deadline:* 3/1.

Generic Baccalaureate Program (BS)

Applying *Required:* TOEFL for nonnative speakers of English, minimum college GPA of 2.75, written essay, transcript of college record. 60 prerequisite credits must be completed before admission to the nursing program. *Options:* Advanced standing available through the following means: advanced placement exams, credit by exam. May apply for transfer of up to 60 total credits. *Application deadline:* 10/1. *Application fee:* $35.

Degree Requirements 127 total credit hours, 67 in nursing.

MASTER'S PROGRAMS

Contact Gwendolyn Hill, Director, Office of Admissions and Student Support, School of Nursing, University of Colorado Health Sciences Center, 4200 East 9th Avenue, Box C288, Denver, CO 80262, 303-315-5592. *Fax:* 303-315-8660. *E-mail:* gwendolyn.hill@uchsc.edu

Areas of Study Clinical nurse specialist programs in adult health nursing, community health nursing, critical care nursing, oncology nursing, psychiatric–mental health nursing, school nursing; nurse midwifery; nursing administration; nurse practitioner programs in adult health, child care/pediatrics, family health, gerontology, women's health.

Expenses *State resident tuition:* $2256 full-time, $188 per credit hour part-time. *Nonresident tuition:* $7332 full-time, $611 per credit hour part-time. *Full-time mandatory fees:* $1490. *Books and supplies per academic year:* ranges from $1204 to $1424.

Financial Aid Graduate assistantships, nurse traineeships, Federal Direct Loans, Federal Nursing Student Loans, employment opportunities, institutionally sponsored non-need-based grants/scholarships. *Application deadline:* 3/1.

MS Program

Applying *Required:* GRE General Test, TOEFL for nonnative speakers of English, bachelor's degree in nursing, minimum GPA of 2.75, RN license, statistics course, essay, interview, 4 letters of recommendation, transcript of college record. *Application deadlines:* 2/1 (fall), 9/1 (spring). *Application fee:* $35.

Degree Requirements 30–63 total credit hours dependent upon track, 30–63 in nursing.

Distance learning Courses provided through video.

RN to Master's Program (MS)

Applying *Required:* GRE General Test, TOEFL for nonnative speakers of English, bachelor's degree in nursing, minimum GPA of 2.75, RN license, essay, interview, 4 letters of recommendation, transcript of college record, portfolio. *Application deadline:* 9/1. *Application fee:* $45.

Degree Requirements 45–78 total credit hours dependent upon track, 45–78 in nursing.

MS/MBA Program

Applying *Required:* GRE General Test, TOEFL for nonnative speakers of English, bachelor's degree in nursing, minimum GPA of 2.75, RN license, statistics course, essay, interview, 4 letters of recommendation, transcript of college record. *Application deadlines:* 9/1 (fall), 3/1 (spring). *Application fee:* $85.

Degree Requirements 64 total credit hours, 31 in nursing, 39 in business, health administration, and other specified areas.

DOCTORAL PROGRAMS

Contact Gwendolyn Hill, Director, Office of Admissions and Student Support, School of Nursing, University of Colorado Health Sciences Center, 4200 East 9th Avenue, Box C288, Denver, CO 80262, 303-315-5592. *Fax:* 303-315-8660. *E-mail:* gwendolyn.hill@uchsc.edu

Areas of Study Nursing research.

Expenses *State resident tuition:* $1980 full-time, $165 per credit hour part-time. *Nonresident tuition:* $6480 full-time, $540 per credit hour part-time. *Full-time mandatory fees:* $1490–$1730. *Books and supplies per academic year:* ranges from $1418 to $1628.

Financial Aid Graduate assistantships, nurse traineeships, fellowships, dissertation grants, grants, Federal Direct Loans, Federal Nursing Student Loans, opportunities for employment. *Application deadline:* 3/1.

PhD Program

Applying *Required:* GRE General Test, TOEFL for nonnative speakers of English, master's degree, statistics course, interview, 4 letters of recommendation, vitae, competitive review by faculty committee, nursing portfolio, minimum 2.75 undergraduate GPA. *Application deadline:* 9/1. *Application fee:* $35.

Degree Requirements 75 total credit hours; 30 hours dissertation research; dissertation; oral exam; written exam; defense of dissertation.

ND Program

Applying *Required:* TOEFL for nonnative speakers of English, master's degree in nursing, statistics course, interview, 3 letters of recommendation, competitive review by faculty committee, baccalaureate degree, minimum 120 hours of completed college course work in a non-nursing field. *Application deadline:* 12/1. *Application fee:* $40.

Degree Requirements 114 total credit hours; 95 hours in nursing, 19 hours in clinical science and electives; 3 years of course work, 1 year of clinical residency in hospital or health-care agency.

CONTINUING EDUCATION PROGRAM

Contact Dr. Ann Smith, Director, Extended Studies and Continuing Education and Assistant Professor, School of Nursing, University of Colorado Health Sciences Center, 4200 East 9th Avenue, Box C288, Denver, CO 80262, 303-315-8691. *Fax:* 303-315-8660. *E-mail:* ann.smith@uchsc.edu

UNIVERSITY OF NORTHERN COLORADO
School of Nursing
Greeley, Colorado

Programs • Generic Baccalaureate • RN Baccalaureate • MS

The University State-supported coed university. Founded: 1890. *Primary accreditation:* regional. *Setting:* 240-acre suburban campus. *Total enrollment:* 10,352.

The School of Nursing Founded in 1963. *Nursing program faculty:* 23 (44% with doctorates).

Academic Facilities *Campus library:* 390,802 volumes (17,525 in health, 4,160 in nursing); 4,091 periodical subscriptions (353 health-care related). *Nursing school resources:* CAI, computer lab, nursing audiovisuals, interactive nursing skills videos, learning resource lab.

Student Life *Student services:* health clinic, child-care facilities, personal counseling, career counseling, institutionally sponsored work-study program, job placement, campus safety program, special assistance for disabled students. *International student services:* counseling/support, special assistance for nonnative speakers of English, ESL courses. *Nursing student activities:* Sigma Theta Tau, student nurses association.

Calendar Semesters.

NURSING STUDENT PROFILE

Undergraduate **Enrollment:** 180
Women: 90%; **Men:** 10%; **Minority:** 20%; **International:** 0%; **Part-time:** 10%

Graduate **Enrollment:** 55
Women: 95%; **Men:** 5%; **Minority:** 3%; **International:** 0%; **Part-time:** 80%

BACCALAUREATE PROGRAMS

Contact Ms. Diane Peters, Assistant Director, School of Nursing, University of Northern Colorado, Greeley, CO 80639, 303-351-1691. *Fax:* 303-351-1707. *E-mail:* dpeters@bentley.univnorthco.edu

Expenses *State resident tuition:* $1914 full-time, $106 per hour part-time. *Nonresident tuition:* $8416 full-time, $468 per hour part-time. *Full-time mandatory fees:* $1080. *Part-time mandatory fees:* $324. *Room and board:* $4270. *Books and supplies per academic year:* ranges from $180 to $250.

Financial Aid Institutionally sponsored need-based grants/scholarships, institutionally sponsored non-need grants/scholarships, Federal Supplemental Educational Opportunity Grants, Federal Work-Study. *Application deadline:* 3/1.

Generic Baccalaureate Program (BS)

Applying *Required:* SAT I or ACT, TOEFL for nonnative speakers of English, minimum high school GPA of 2.8, minimum college GPA of 2.5, 2 years of high school math, 2 years of high school science, high school chemistry, high school biology, high school transcript, letter of recommendation, written essay, transcript of college record. 41 prerequisite credits must be completed before admission to the nursing program. *Options:* Advanced standing available through the following means: advanced placement exams, credit by exam. May apply for transfer of up to 90 total credits. *Application deadlines:* 1/15 (fall), 1/15 (summer). *Application fee:* $30.

Degree Requirements 127 total credit hours, 66 in nursing. Summer semester in junior year.

RN Baccalaureate Program (BS)

Applying *Required:* minimum college GPA of 3.0, RN license, diploma or AD in nursing, high school transcript, letter of recommendation, transcript of college record, 1,000 hours of work experience. 41 prerequisite credits must be completed before admission to the nursing program. *Options:* Advanced standing available through credit by exam. May apply for transfer of up to 90 total credits. *Application deadline:* rolling. *Application fee:* $30.

Degree Requirements 120 total credit hours, 67 in nursing.

University of Northern Colorado (continued)

MASTER'S PROGRAM

Contact Dr. Judy Richter, MS Program Coordinator and Professor, School of Nursing, University of Northern Colorado, Greeley, CO 80639, 303-351-2663. *Fax:* 303-351-1707.

Areas of Study Clinical nurse specialist program in chronic illness nursing; nursing education; nurse practitioner program in family health.

Expenses *State resident tuition:* $2264 full-time, $126 per hour part-time. *Nonresident tuition:* $8958 full-time, $498 per hour part-time. *Full-time mandatory fees:* $1080. *Part-time mandatory fees:* $324+. *Room and board:* $4270.

Financial Aid Graduate assistantships, nurse traineeships, fellowships. *Application deadline:* 8/1.

MS PROGRAM

Applying *Required:* GRE General Test or Miller Analogies Test, bachelor's degree in nursing, minimum GPA of 3.0, RN license, 1 year of clinical experience, statistics course, essay, interview, 2 letters of recommendation, transcript of college record, physical assessment course for family nurse practitioner program only, undergraduate level research course. *Application deadlines:* 1/1 (family nurse practitioner program), rolling. *Application fee:* $30.

Degree Requirements 38–43 total credit hours dependent upon track, 32–43 in nursing, 6 in education.

UNIVERSITY OF SOUTHERN COLORADO

Department of Nursing
Pueblo, Colorado

Programs • Generic Baccalaureate • RN Baccalaureate

The University State-supported comprehensive coed institution. Part of Colorado State University System. Founded: 1933. *Primary accreditation:* regional. *Setting:* 275-acre suburban campus. *Total enrollment:* 4,331.

The Department of Nursing Founded in 1985. *Nursing program faculty:* 8 (25% with doctorates).

Academic Facilities *Campus library:* 185,604 volumes; 1,300 periodical subscriptions. *Nursing school resources:* computer lab, nursing audiovisuals, learning resource lab.

Student Life *Student services:* health clinic, child-care facilities, personal counseling, career counseling, institutionally sponsored work-study program, job placement, campus safety program, special assistance for disabled students. *International student services:* counseling/support. *Nursing student activities:* Sigma Theta Tau, student nurses association.

Calendar Semesters.

NURSING STUDENT PROFILE

Undergraduate **Enrollment:** 99
Women: 88%; **Men:** 12%; **Minority:** 14%; **International:** 2%; **Part-time:** 0%

BACCALAUREATE PROGRAMS

Contact Melva J. Steen, Director and Chair, Department of Nursing, University of Southern Colorado, 2200 Bonforte Boulevard, Pueblo, CO 81001, 719-549-2401. *Fax:* 719-549-2732.

Expenses *State resident tuition:* $1720 per academic year. *Nonresident tuition:* $7720 per academic year. *Full-time mandatory fees:* $434. *Room and board:* $4176–$5308. *Room only:* $1912–$2860.

Financial Aid Institutionally sponsored need-based grants/scholarships, institutionally sponsored non-need grants/scholarships, Federal Work-Study.

GENERIC BACCALAUREATE PROGRAM (BSN)

Applying *Required:* SAT I or ACT, minimum college GPA of 2.75, transcript of college record, CPR certification, immunizations. 40 prerequisite credits must be completed before admission to the nursing program. *Options:* May apply for transfer of up to 64 total credits. *Application deadline:* 5/1.

Degree Requirements 128 total credit hours, 68 in nursing.

RN BACCALAUREATE PROGRAM (BSN)

Applying *Required:* RN license, diploma or AD in nursing, transcript of college record, CPR certification, immunizations. 77 prerequisite credits must be completed before admission to the nursing program. *Options:* May apply for transfer of up to 64 total credits. *Application deadline:* rolling.

Degree Requirements 128 total credit hours, 68 in nursing.

CONNECTICUT

CENTRAL CONNECTICUT STATE UNIVERSITY

Department of Health and Human Service Professions
New Britain, Connecticut

Program • RN Baccalaureate

The University State-supported comprehensive coed institution. Part of Connecticut State University System. Founded: 1849. *Primary accreditation:* regional. *Setting:* 176-acre suburban campus. *Total enrollment:* 9,525.

The Department of Health and Human Service Professions Founded in 1981. *Nursing program faculty:* 4 (100% with doctorates).

Academic Facilities *Campus library:* 560,765 volumes (10,525 in health, 1,741 in nursing); 77,000 periodical subscriptions (5,000 health-care related). *Nursing school resources:* computer lab, nursing audiovisuals.

Student Life *Student services:* health clinic, child-care facilities, personal counseling, career counseling, institutionally sponsored work-study program, job placement, campus safety program, special assistance for disabled students. *International student services:* counseling/support, special assistance for nonnative speakers of English, ESL courses. *Nursing student activities:* nursing club, student nurses association.

Calendar Semesters.

NURSING STUDENT PROFILE

Undergraduate **Enrollment:** 360
Women: 95%; **Men:** 5%; **Minority:** 3%; **Part-time:** 99%

BACCALAUREATE PROGRAM

Contact Dr. Judith Hriceniak, Chairperson, Department of Health and Human Service Professions, Central Connecticut University, 1615 Stanley Street, New Britain, CT 06050-4010, 203-832-2145. *Fax:* 203-832-2109. *E-mail:* hriceniak@ccsuctstateu.edu

Expenses *State resident tuition:* $2012 full-time, $150 per credit part-time. *Nonresident tuition:* $6510 full-time, $150 per credit part-time. *Full-time mandatory fees:* $1530. *Part-time mandatory fees:* $82. *Room and board:* $4952. *Room only:* $2912. *Books and supplies per academic year:* ranges from $250 to $500.

Financial Aid Institutionally sponsored need-based grants/scholarships, institutionally sponsored non-need grants/scholarships, Federal Direct Loans, Federal Supplemental Educational Opportunity Grants, Federal Work-Study. 1% of undergraduate students in nursing programs received some form of financial aid in 1995–96. *Application deadline:* 4/22.

RN BACCALAUREATE PROGRAM (BSN)

Applying *Required:* TOEFL for nonnative speakers of English, RN license, diploma or AD in nursing, transcript of college record, transfer students must have taken 45 credits at CCSU. 45 prerequisite credits must be completed before admission to the nursing program. *Options:* Advanced standing available through the following means: advanced placement exams, credit by exam. Course work may be accelerated. *Application deadlines:* 5/1 (fall), 11/1 (spring). *Application fee:* $40.

Degree Requirements 130 total credit hours, 31 in nursing.

FAIRFIELD UNIVERSITY
School of Nursing
Fairfield, Connecticut

Programs • Generic Baccalaureate • RN Baccalaureate • Accelerated Baccalaureate for Second Degree • BSN to Master's • Continuing Education

The University Independent Roman Catholic (Jesuit) comprehensive coed institution. Founded: 1942. *Primary accreditation:* regional. *Setting:* 200-acre suburban campus. *Total enrollment:* 4,980.

The School of Nursing Founded in 1970. *Nursing program faculty:* 13 (70% with doctorates).

▶ *NOTEWORTHY*

Founded by the Jesuits in 1942, Fairfield University is a comprehensive university and close-knit community located in southern Connecticut. Generic students enroll in their first nursing course as freshmen, begin clinical courses as sophomores, and conclude with a transition course. RN-BSN students earn credit through transfer or challenge exams and complete required courses on a full-time or part-time, day or evening basis. Individuals with a degree in another field complete the nursing curriculum in an intensive 18-month program. The master's program focuses on advanced practice in family (family nurse practitioner) and mental health (psychiatric nurse practitioner). The well-rounded Fairfield education takes place in an environment characterized by a genuine sense of caring and community.

Academic Facilities *Campus library:* 265,000 volumes (21,267 in health, 9,500 in nursing); 1,900 periodical subscriptions (134 health-care related). *Nursing school resources:* CAI, computer lab, nursing audiovisuals, interactive nursing skills videos, learning resource lab.

Student Life *Student services:* health clinic, personal counseling, career counseling, institutionally sponsored work-study program, job placement, campus safety program, special assistance for disabled students. *International student services:* counseling/support. *Nursing student activities:* Sigma Theta Tau, nursing club, student nurses association.

Calendar Semesters.

NURSING STUDENT PROFILE

Undergraduate **Enrollment:** 284
Women: 95%; **Men:** 5%; **Minority:** 6%; **International:** 0%; **Part-time:** 18%

Graduate **Enrollment:** 47
Women: 96%; **Men:** 4%; **Minority:** 11%; **International:** 0%; **Part-time:** 40%

BACCALAUREATE PROGRAMS

Contact Dr. Suzanne MacAvoy, Director, Undergraduate Program, School of Nursing, Fairfield University, North Benson Road, Fairfield, CT 06430-5195, 203-254-4000 Ext. 2709. *Fax:* 203-254-4126. *E-mail:* smacavoy@fair1.fairfield.edu

Expenses *Tuition:* $17,360 full-time, $295 per credit part-time. *Full-time mandatory fees:* $505. *Part-time mandatory fees:* $505. *Room and board:* $6800. *Books and supplies per academic year:* ranges from $500 to $600.

Financial Aid Institutionally sponsored need-based grants/scholarships, institutionally sponsored non-need grants/scholarships, Federal Nursing Student Loans, Federal Supplemental Educational Opportunity Grants, Federal Work-Study. 80% of undergraduate students in nursing programs received some form of financial aid in 1995–96. *Application deadline:* 2/15.

Generic Baccalaureate Program (BS)

Applying *Required:* SAT I, ACT, 3 years of high school math, 3 years of high school science, high school chemistry, high school biology, high school foreign language, high school transcript, interview recommended. *Options:* Advanced standing available through advanced placement exams. May apply for transfer of up to 60 total credits. *Application deadlines:* 3/1 (fall), 12/1 (spring). *Application fee:* $40.

Degree Requirements 131 total credit hours, 51 in nursing.

RN Baccalaureate Program (BS)

Applying *Required:* RN license, diploma or AD in nursing, high school transcript, transcript of college record. *Options:* Advanced standing available through the following means: advanced placement exams, credit by exam. Course work may be accelerated. May apply for transfer of up to 66 total credits. *Application deadline:* rolling. *Application fee:* $40.

Degree Requirements 131 total credit hours, 51 in nursing.

Accelerated Baccalaureate for Second Degree Program (BS)

Applying *Required:* SAT I, ACT, minimum college GPA of 2.5, high school transcript, transcript of college record, BS or BA in discipline other than nursing. 16 prerequisite credits must be completed before admission to the nursing program. *Options:* Advanced standing available through advanced placement exams. Course work may be accelerated. May apply for transfer of up to 66 total credits. *Application deadline:* 12/1 (summer). *Application fee:* $40.

Degree Requirements 131 total credit hours, 51 in nursing.

MASTER'S PROGRAM

Contact Dr. Kathleen Wheeler, Director, Graduate Program, School of Nursing, Fairfield University, North Benson Road, Fairfield, CT 06430-5195, 203-254-4000 Ext. 2708. *Fax:* 203-254-4126. *E-mail:* kwheeler@fair1.fairfield.edu

Areas of Study Nurse practitioner programs in family health, psychiatric–mental health.

Expenses *Tuition:* $8910 full-time, $4950 per year part-time. *Full-time mandatory fees:* $500. *Part-time mandatory fees:* $500. *Books and supplies per academic year:* $1000.

Financial Aid Nurse traineeships. 32% of master's level students in nursing programs received some form of financial aid in 1995-96. *Application deadline:* 8/1.

BSN to Master's Program (MSN)

Applying *Required:* GRE General Test (minimum combined score of 1500 on three tests) or Miller Analogies Test, bachelor's degree in nursing, minimum GPA of 3.0, RN license, 1 year of clinical experience, physical assessment course, statistics course, professional liability/malpractice insurance, interview, 2 letters of recommendation, transcript of college record. *Application deadline:* rolling. *Application fee:* $50.

Degree Requirements 45 total credit hours, 42 in nursing, 3 in marriage and family therapy. Thesis required.

CONTINUING EDUCATION PROGRAM

Contact Terry Quell, RN, Assistant to the Dean, School of Nursing, Fairfield University, North Benson Road, Fairfield, CT 06430-5195, 203-254-4000 Ext. 2704. *Fax:* 203-254-4126. *E-mail:* tquell@fair1.fairfield.edu

QUINNIPIAC COLLEGE
Department of Nursing
Hamden, Connecticut

Programs • Generic Baccalaureate • RN Baccalaureate • Continuing Education

The College Independent comprehensive coed institution. Founded: 1929. *Primary accreditation:* regional. *Setting:* 185-acre suburban campus. *Total enrollment:* 5,117.

The Department of Nursing Founded in 1968. *Nursing program faculty:* 20 (15% with doctorates).

Academic Facilities *Campus library:* 304,857 volumes; 4,291 periodical subscriptions. *Nursing school resources:* CAI, computer lab, nursing audiovisuals, interactive nursing skills videos, learning resource lab.

Quinnipiac College (continued)

Student Life *Student services:* health clinic, personal counseling, career counseling, institutionally sponsored work-study program, job placement, campus safety program, special assistance for disabled students. *International student services:* counseling/support. *Nursing student activities:* student nurses association.

Calendar Semesters.

NURSING STUDENT PROFILE

Undergraduate **Enrollment:** 265
Women: 80%; **Men:** 20%; **Minority:** 5%; **International:** 1%; **Part-time:** 1%

BACCALAUREATE PROGRAMS

Contact Ms. Joan Isaac Mohr, Vice President and Dean of Admissions, Admissions Office, Quinnipiac College, Mount Carmel Avenue, Hamden, CT 06518, 203-281-8600. *Fax:* 203-281-8906. *E-mail:* admissions@quinnipiac.edu

Expenses *Tuition:* $14,120 full-time, $450 per credit hour part-time. *Full-time mandatory fees:* $35. *Room and board:* $6770–$7690. *Books and supplies per academic year:* ranges from $500 to $1200.

Financial Aid Institutionally sponsored need-based grants/scholarships, institutionally sponsored non-need grants/scholarships, Federal Nursing Student Loans, Federal Perkins Loans, Federal Supplemental Educational Opportunity Grants, Federal Work-Study. 60% of undergraduate students in nursing programs received some form of financial aid in 1995–96. *Application deadline:* 3/1.

Generic Baccalaureate Program (BS)

Applying *Required:* SAT I, ACT, minimum high school GPA of 2.5, minimum college GPA of 2.0, 3 years of high school math, 3 years of high school science, high school chemistry, high school biology, high school transcript, written essay, transcript of college record, high school class rank: top 50%. *Options:* Advanced standing available through advanced placement exams. *Application deadline:* rolling. *Application fee:* $45.

Degree Requirements 134 total credit hours, 50 in nursing. Clinical experience.

RN Baccalaureate Program (BS)

Applying *Required:* minimum college GPA of 2.5, RN license, diploma or AD in nursing, written essay, transcript of college record. *Options:* Advanced standing available through advanced placement exams. *Application deadline:* rolling. *Application fee:* $45.

Degree Requirements 140 total credit hours, 61 in nursing. Clinical experience.

CONTINUING EDUCATION PROGRAM

Contact Ms. Rosemarie DeVivo, Assistant Dean, Graduate and Continuing Education, Quinnipiac College, Mount Carmel Avenue, Hamden, CT 06518, 203-281-8612. *Fax:* 203-281-8749.

See full description on page 492.

SACRED HEART UNIVERSITY
Nursing Programs
Fairfield, Connecticut

Programs • Generic Baccalaureate • RN Baccalaureate • RN to Master's • MSN/MBA

The University Independent Roman Catholic comprehensive coed institution. Founded: 1963. *Primary accreditation:* regional. *Setting:* 56-acre suburban campus. *Total enrollment:* 5,545.

The Nursing Programs Founded in 1980. *Nursing program faculty:* 8 (50% with doctorates). *Off-campus program site:* New Haven.

Academic Facilities *Campus library:* 153,000 volumes (4,500 in health, 3,900 in nursing); 1,090 periodical subscriptions (75 health-care related). *Nursing school resources:* CAI, computer lab, nursing audiovisuals, interactive nursing skills videos, learning resource lab.

Student Life *Student services:* health clinic, personal counseling, career counseling, institutionally sponsored work-study program. *International student services:* counseling/support, special assistance for nonnative speakers of English, ESL courses. *Nursing student activities:* Sigma Theta Tau, student nurses association.

Calendar Semesters.

NURSING STUDENT PROFILE

Undergraduate **Enrollment:** 200
Women: 98%; **Men:** 2%; **Minority:** 5%; **International:** 0%; **Part-time:** 80%
Graduate **Enrollment:** 76
Women: 99%; **Men:** 1%; **Minority:** 7%; **International:** 0%; **Part-time:** 95%

BACCALAUREATE PROGRAMS

Contact Dr. Constance Young, Associate Director, Undergraduate Programs, Nursing Programs, Sacred Heart University, 5151 Park Avenue, Fairfield, CT 06432, 203-371-7844. *Fax:* 203-365-7662.

Expenses *Tuition:* $12,212 full-time, ranges from $265 to $400 per credit part-time. *Full-time mandatory fees:* $502. *Part-time mandatory fees:* $220. *Room and board:* $5960–$6380. *Room only:* $4490. *Books and supplies per academic year:* ranges from $400 to $800.

Financial Aid Institutionally sponsored need-based grants/scholarships, institutionally sponsored non-need grants/scholarships, Federal Supplemental Educational Opportunity Grants, Federal Work-Study. *Application deadline:* 3/1.

Generic Baccalaureate Program (BS)

Applying *Required:* SAT I or ACT, TOEFL for nonnative speakers of English, minimum high school GPA of 3.0, minimum college GPA of 2.5, 3 years of high school math, 3 years of high school science, high school chemistry, high school biology, high school transcript, 2 letters of recommendation, written essay, transcript of college record, high school class rank: top 50%. 34 prerequisite credits must be completed before admission to the nursing program. *Options:* Advanced standing available through the following means: advanced placement exams, credit by exam. May apply for transfer of up to 60–90 total credits. *Application deadline:* rolling. *Application fee:* $30.

Degree Requirements 126 total credit hours, 57 in nursing.

RN Baccalaureate Program (BS)

Applying *Required:* minimum college GPA of 2.5, RN license, diploma or AD in nursing, 2 letters of recommendation, transcript of college record. 41 prerequisite credits must be completed before admission to the nursing program. *Options:* Advanced standing available through credit by exam. May apply for transfer of up to 60–90 total credits. *Application deadline:* rolling. *Application fee:* $30.

Degree Requirements 125 total credit hours, 57 in nursing. Portfolio evaluation of lower division nursing work.

MASTER'S PROGRAMS

Contact Dr. Anne M. Barker, Director, Nursing Programs, Sacred Heart University, 5151 Park Avenue, Fairfield, CT 06432, 203-371-7715. *Fax:* 203-365-7662.

Areas of Study Nursing administration; nurse practitioner program in family health.

Expenses *Tuition:* ranges from $340 to $440 per credit. *Full-time mandatory fees:* $71.

Financial Aid Graduate assistantships, nurse traineeships, Federal Nursing Student Loans, institutionally sponsored loans, employment opportunities. *Application deadline:* 3/1.

RN to Master's Program (MSN)

Applying *Required:* Miller Analogies Test, minimum GPA of 3.2, RN license, 2 years of clinical experience, statistics course, professional liability/malpractice insurance, essay, interview, 2 letters of recommendation, transcript of college record. *Application deadline:* rolling. *Application fee:* $40.

Degree Requirements 154 total credit hours, 45 in nursing, 107 in business, humanities, liberal arts, science. Portfolio evaluation of lower division nursing work. Thesis required.

MSN/MBA Program

Applying *Required:* Miller Analogies Test, bachelor's degree, minimum GPA of 3.0, RN license, statistics course, professional liability/malpractice insurance, essay, interview, 2 letters of recommendation, transcript of college record, physical assessment course of at least 30 hours and nursing research required for nurse practitioner track. *Application deadlines:* 5/1 (fall), 12/1 (spring), 5/1 (nurse practitioner). *Application fee:* $35.

Degree Requirements 45–72 total credit hours dependent upon track, 15 in nursing, 30 in business. 30 hours in nursing and 15 hours in family health for nurse practitioner track. Thesis required.

SAINT JOSEPH COLLEGE
Division of Nursing
West Hartford, Connecticut

Programs • Generic Baccalaureate • RN Baccalaureate • Baccalaureate for Second Degree • BSN to Master's • Master's for Nurses with Non-Nursing Degrees

The College Independent Roman Catholic comprehensive women's institution. Founded: 1932. *Primary accreditation:* regional. *Setting:* 84-acre suburban campus. *Total enrollment:* 1,916.

The Division of Nursing Founded in 1975. *Nursing program faculty:* 25 (50% with doctorates).

Academic Facilities *Campus library:* 133,000 volumes (4,940 in nursing); 641 periodical subscriptions (90 health-care related). *Nursing school resources:* CAI, computer lab, nursing audiovisuals, interactive nursing skills videos, learning resource lab.

Student Life *Student services:* health clinic, child-care facilities, personal counseling, career counseling, institutionally sponsored work-study program, job placement, campus safety program, special assistance for disabled students. *International student services:* counseling/support, special assistance for nonnative speakers of English. *Nursing student activities:* Sigma Theta Tau, nursing club, student nurses association.

Calendar Semesters.

NURSING STUDENT PROFILE

Undergraduate **Enrollment:** 355
Women: 99%; **Men:** 1%; **Minority:** 12%; **International:** 1%; **Part-time:** 53%
Graduate **Enrollment:** 78
Women: 94%; **Men:** 6%; **Minority:** 4%; **International:** 0%; **Part-time:** 99%

BACCALAUREATE PROGRAMS

Contact Ms. Tina Demo, Director of Admissions, Division of Nursing, Saint Joseph College, West Hartford, CT 06117, 203-232-4571. *Fax:* 203-233-5695.

Expenses *Tuition:* $13,800 full-time, $345 per credit part-time. *Full-time mandatory fees:* $0. *Room and board:* $2800. *Room only:* $2500. *Books and supplies per academic year:* ranges from $250 to $400.

Financial Aid Institutionally sponsored need-based grants/scholarships, institutionally sponsored non-need grants/scholarships, Federal Pell Grants, Federal Perkins Loans, Federal Supplemental Educational Opportunity Grants, Federal Work-Study, Federal Stafford Loans. 34% of undergraduate students in nursing programs received some form of financial aid in 1995–96. *Application deadline:* 2/15.

Generic Baccalaureate Program (BS)

Applying *Required:* SAT I, TOEFL for nonnative speakers of English, minimum college GPA of 2.8, 3 years of high school math, 3 years of high school science, high school transcript, interview, letter of recommendation. 45 prerequisite credits must be completed before admission to the nursing program. *Options:* Advanced standing available through credit by exam. Course work may be accelerated. May apply for transfer of up to 60 total credits. *Application deadline:* rolling. *Application fee:* $25.

Degree Requirements 128 total credit hours, 51 in nursing. Biology, chemistry, math, psychology, sociology, nutrition, general education, theme courses.

RN Baccalaureate Program (BS)

Applying *Required:* TOEFL for nonnative speakers of English, minimum college GPA of 2.8, RN license, diploma or AD in nursing, interview, letter of recommendation, transcript of college record. *Options:* Advanced standing available through credit by exam. Course work may be accelerated. May apply for transfer of up to 60 total credits. *Application deadline:* rolling. *Application fee:* $25.

Degree Requirements 128 total credit hours.

Baccalaureate for Second Degree Program (BSN)

Applying *Required:* TOEFL for nonnative speakers of English, minimum college GPA of 2.8. *Options:* Advanced standing available through credit by exam. Course work may be accelerated. *Application deadline:* rolling. *Application fee:* $25.

MASTER'S PROGRAMS

Contact Ms. Virginia Knowlden, Director, Master's Programs in Advanced Practice Nursing, Division of Nursing, Saint Joseph College, West Hartford, CT 06117, 203-232-4571. *Fax:* 203-233-5695. *E-mail:* vknowlden@mercy.sjc.edu

Areas of Study Clinical nurse specialist programs in family health nursing, psychiatric–mental health nursing; nurse practitioner program in family health.

Expenses *Tuition:* $360 per credit. *Full-time mandatory fees:* $0. *Room and board:* $2500–$2800. *Books and supplies per academic year:* ranges from $250 to $400.

Financial Aid Graduate assistantships, nurse traineeships, employment opportunities, Federal Stafford Loans. 13% of master's level students in nursing programs received some form of financial aid in 1995-96. *Application deadline:* 2/15.

BSN to Master's Program (MS)

Applying *Required:* Miller Analogies Test, GRE General Test (minimum combined score of 1000 on two sections), bachelor's degree in nursing, bachelor's degree, minimum GPA of 3.0, RN license, physical assessment course, statistics course, professional liability/malpractice insurance, essay, interview, 2 letters of recommendation, transcript of college record, research. *Application deadline:* rolling. *Application fee:* $25.

Degree Requirements 50 total credit hours, 38 in nursing, 6 in other specified areas. Thesis required.

Master's for Nurses with Non-Nursing Degrees Program (MS)

Applying *Required:* GRE General Test, Miller Analogies Test, NLN Comprehensive Exam, bachelor's degree, minimum GPA of 3.0, RN license, physical assessment course, statistics course, professional liability/malpractice insurance, essay, interview, letter of recommendation, transcript of college record, research. *Application deadline:* rolling. *Application fee:* $25.

Degree Requirements 50 total credit hours, 38 in nursing, 6 in other specified areas. Thesis required.

SOUTHERN CONNECTICUT STATE UNIVERSITY
Department of Nursing
New Haven, Connecticut

Programs • Generic Baccalaureate • Accelerated RN Baccalaureate • MSN • Post-Master's

The University State-supported comprehensive coed institution. Part of Connecticut State University System. Founded: 1893. *Primary accreditation:* regional. *Setting:* 168-acre urban campus. *Total enrollment:* 11,591.

The Department of Nursing Founded in 1973. *Nursing program faculty:* 24 (33% with doctorates).

Academic Facilities *Campus library:* 384,987 volumes; 3,291 periodical subscriptions (200 health-care related). *Nursing school resources:* CAI, computer lab, nursing audiovisuals, interactive nursing skills videos, learning resource lab.

Student Life *Student services:* health clinic, child-care facilities, personal counseling, career counseling, institutionally sponsored work-study program, campus safety program, special assistance for disabled students.

Southern Connecticut State University (continued)

International student services: counseling/support, ESL courses. *Nursing student activities:* Sigma Theta Tau, nursing club, student nurses association.

Calendar Semesters.

NURSING STUDENT PROFILE

Undergraduate **Enrollment:** 139
Women: 85%; **Men:** 15%; **Minority:** 10%; **International:** 0%; **Part-time:** 6%
Graduate **Enrollment:** 51
Women: 98%; **Men:** 2%; **Minority:** 10%; **International:** 0%; **Part-time:** 90%

BACCALAUREATE PROGRAMS

Contact Dr. Cesarina Thompson, Chairperson, Department of Nursing, Southern Connecticut State University, 501 Crescent Street, New Haven, CT 06515, 203-392-6487. *Fax:* 203-392-6493.

Expenses *State resident tuition:* $2012 full-time, $186 per credit part-time. *Nonresident tuition:* $6510 per academic year. *Full-time mandatory fees:* $378. *Room and board:* $4846. *Room only:* $2616.

Financial Aid Institutionally sponsored need-based grants/scholarships, institutionally sponsored non-need grants/scholarships, department scholarship fund.

Generic Baccalaureate Program (BSN)

Applying *Required:* SAT I, pre-nursing exam, minimum college GPA of 2.4, 3 years of high school math, high school transcript, written essay, transcript of college record. 62 prerequisite credits must be completed before admission to the nursing program. *Options:* May apply for transfer of up to 90 total credits. *Application deadline:* 2/1. *Application fee:* $20.

Degree Requirements 124 total credit hours, 49 in nursing.

Accelerated RN Baccalaureate Program (BSN)

Applying *Required:* minimum college GPA of 2.4, RN license, diploma or AD in nursing, written essay, transcript of college record. *Options:* Advanced standing available through credit by exam. May apply for transfer of up to 90 total credits. *Application deadline:* rolling.

Degree Requirements 124 total credit hours, 17 in nursing.

MASTER'S PROGRAMS

Contact Dr. Ellen Russell Beatty, Coordinator, MSN Program, Department of Nursing, Southern Connecticut State University, 501 Crescent Street, New Haven, CT 06515, 203-392-6477. *Fax:* 203-392-6493.

Areas of Study Nursing administration; nursing education; nurse practitioner program in family health.

Expenses *State resident tuition:* $1944 full-time, $200 per credit part-time. *Nonresident tuition:* $4600 per academic year. *Full-time mandatory fees:* $400.

Financial Aid Graduate assistantships, nurse traineeships.

MSN Program

Applying *Required:* GRE General Test or Miller Analogies Test, pre-admission exam for nurse practitioner track, bachelor's degree in nursing, minimum GPA of 2.8, RN license, 1 year of clinical experience, statistics course, professional liability/malpractice insurance, interview, 2 letters of recommendation, transcript of college record. *Application deadline:* rolling. *Application fee:* $20.

Degree Requirements 36 total credit hours, 27–33 in nursing, 3–9 in education or administration. Thesis required.

Post-Master's Program

Applying *Required:* pre-admission exam for nurse practitioner track, bachelor's degree in nursing, minimum GPA of 2.8, RN license, 1 year of clinical experience, physical assessment course, statistics course, professional liability/malpractice insurance, interview, 2 letters of recommendation, transcript of college record, master's degree in nursing. *Application deadline:* rolling. *Application fee:* $20.

Degree Requirements 24 total credit hours, 24 in nursing. Thesis required.

UNIVERSITY OF CONNECTICUT

School of Nursing
Storrs, Connecticut

Programs • Generic Baccalaureate • RN Baccalaureate • MS • Master's for Nurses with Non-Nursing Degrees • MS/MBA • MS/MPH • PhD • Continuing Education

The University State-supported coed university. Founded: 1881. *Primary accreditation:* regional. *Setting:* 4,000-acre rural campus. *Total enrollment:* 15,735.

The School of Nursing Founded in 1942. *Nursing program faculty:* 37 (81% with doctorates). *Off-campus program site:* Farmington.

Academic Facilities *Campus library:* 2.4 million volumes; 18,200 periodical subscriptions. *Nursing school resources:* CAI, computer lab, nursing audiovisuals, interactive nursing skills videos, learning resource lab.

Student Life *Student services:* health clinic, child-care facilities, personal counseling, career counseling, institutionally sponsored work-study program, job placement, campus safety program, special assistance for disabled students. *International student services:* counseling/support, special assistance for nonnative speakers of English, ESL courses. *Nursing student activities:* Sigma Theta Tau, nursing club, student nurses association.

Calendar Semesters.

NURSING STUDENT PROFILE

Undergraduate **Enrollment:** 400
Women: 80%; **Men:** 20%; **Minority:** 10%; **International:** 0%; **Part-time:** 7%
Graduate **Enrollment:** 197
Women: 97%; **Men:** 3%; **Minority:** 5%; **International:** 0%; **Part-time:** 75%

BACCALAUREATE PROGRAMS

Contact Ms. Eva Gorbants, Director, Academic Advisory Center, School of Nursing, University of Connecticut, 231 Glenbrook Road, Storrs, CT 06269-2026, 860-486-4730. *Fax:* 860-486-0001. *E-mail:* nuradm04@uconnvm.uconn.edu

Expenses *State resident tuition:* $4360 per academic year. *Nonresident tuition:* $12,306 per academic year. *Full-time mandatory fees:* $1000–$1200. *Room and board:* $6304. *Books and supplies per academic year:* ranges from $600 to $800.

Financial Aid Institutionally sponsored need-based grants/scholarships, institutionally sponsored non-need grants/scholarships, Federal Direct Loans, Federal Nursing Student Loans, Federal Pell Grants, Federal Perkins Loans, Federal Supplemental Educational Opportunity Grants, Federal Work-Study. *Application deadline:* 3/1.

Generic Baccalaureate Program (BS)

Applying *Required:* SAT I, TOEFL for nonnative speakers of English, minimum high school GPA of 3.0, minimum college GPA of 2.5, 3 years of high school math, high school chemistry, high school biology, high school foreign language, high school transcript, transcript of college record. *Options:* Advanced standing available through the following means: advanced placement exams, credit by exam. May apply for transfer of up to 90 total credits. *Application deadlines:* 4/1 (fall), 10/15 (spring). *Application fee:* $40.

Degree Requirements 130 total credit hours, 65 in nursing.

RN Baccalaureate Program (BS)

Applying *Required:* minimum college GPA of 2.8, RN license, diploma or AD in nursing, high school transcript, transcript of college record. *Options:* Advanced standing available through the following means: advanced placement exams, credit by exam. Course work may be accelerated. May apply for transfer of up to 90 total credits. *Application deadlines:* 4/1 (fall), 10/15 (spring). *Application fee:* $40.

Degree Requirements 130 total credit hours, 65 in nursing.

MASTER'S PROGRAMS

Contact Ms. Eva Gorbants, Director, Academic Advisory Center, School of Nursing, University of Connecticut, 231 Glenbrook Road, Storrs, CT 06269-2026, 860-486-4730. *Fax:* 860-486-0001. *E-mail:* nuradm08@uconnvm.uconn.edu

Areas of Study Clinical nurse specialist programs in community health nursing, perinatal nursing, psychiatric–mental health nursing, perioperative nursing; nursing administration; nurse practitioner programs in acute care, adult health, gerontology, neonatal health, primary care.

Expenses *State resident tuition:* $4968 full-time, $276 per credit part-time. *Nonresident tuition:* $12,910 full-time, $717 per credit part-time. *Full-time mandatory fees:* $369. *Part-time mandatory fees:* $369.

Financial Aid Graduate assistantships, nurse traineeships, Federal Direct Loans, Federal Nursing Student Loans, employment opportunities. *Application deadline:* 3/1.

MS Program

Applying *Required:* GRE General Test for ACNP track, bachelor's degree in nursing, minimum GPA of 3.0, RN license, 1 year of clinical experience, physical assessment course, professional liability/malpractice insurance, essay, 3 letters of recommendation, transcript of college record. *Application deadline:* 3/1. *Application fee:* $40.

Degree Requirements 39 total credit hours, 39 in nursing.

Master's for Nurses with Non-Nursing Degrees Program (MS)

Applying *Required:* TOEFL for nonnative speakers of English, GRE General Test for ACNP track, bachelor's degree, minimum GPA of 3.0, RN license, 1 year of clinical experience, physical assessment course, professional liability/malpractice insurance, essay, 3 letters of recommendation, transcript of college record. *Application deadline:* 3/1. *Application fee:* $40.

Degree Requirements 59 total credit hours, 39 in nursing.

MS/MBA Program

Applying *Required:* GMAT, bachelor's degree in nursing, minimum GPA of 3.0, RN license, statistics course, professional liability/malpractice insurance, essay, interview, 3 letters of recommendation, transcript of college record, college-level calculus. *Application deadline:* 3/1. *Application fee:* $40.

Degree Requirements 69 total credit hours, 27 in nursing, 42 in business.

MS/MPH Program

Applying *Required:* bachelor's degree in nursing, minimum GPA of 3.0, RN license, physical assessment course, statistics course, professional liability/malpractice insurance, essay, interview, 3 letters of recommendation, transcript of college record. *Application deadline:* 3/1. *Application fee:* $40.

Degree Requirements 63 total credit hours, 27 in nursing, 36 in public health.

DOCTORAL PROGRAM

Contact Ms. Eva Gorbants, Director, Academic Advisory Center, School of Nursing, University of Connecticut, 231 Glenbrook Road, Storrs, CT 06269-2026, 860-486-4730. *Fax:* 860-486-0001. *E-mail:* nuradm08@uconnvm.uconn.edu

Areas of Study Nursing research.

Expenses *State resident tuition:* $4968 full-time, $276 per credit part-time. *Nonresident tuition:* $12,910 full-time, $717 per credit part-time. *Full-time mandatory fees:* $369.

Financial Aid Graduate assistantships, nurse traineeships, fellowships, dissertation grants, Federal Direct Loans, Federal Nursing Student Loans, opportunities for employment, institutionally sponsored non-need-based grants/scholarships. *Application deadline:* 3/1.

PhD Program

Applying *Required:* GRE General Test, TOEFL for nonnative speakers of English, master's degree in nursing, 3 scholarly papers, interview, letter of recommendation, vitae, competitive review by faculty committee. *Application deadline:* 3/1. *Application fee:* $40.

Degree Requirements 36 total credit hours; dissertation; written exam; defense of dissertation; residency.

CONTINUING EDUCATION PROGRAM

Contact Dr. Kay Bruttomerso, Associate Dean, School of Nursing, University of Connecticut, 231 Glenbrook Road, Storrs, CT 06269-2026, 860-486-3716. *Fax:* 860-486-0001. *E-mail:* bruttome@uconnvm.uconn.edu

See full description on page 528.

UNIVERSITY OF HARTFORD
Division of Nursing
West Hartford, Connecticut

Programs • RN Baccalaureate • MSN • MSN/MSOB • Continuing Education

The University Independent comprehensive coed institution. Founded: 1877. *Primary accreditation:* regional. *Total enrollment:* 7,022.

The Division of Nursing Founded in 1977. *Nursing program faculty:* 7 (70% with doctorates).

Academic Facilities *Nursing school resources:* CAI, nursing audiovisuals.

Student Life *Student services:* health clinic, personal counseling, career counseling, job placement, campus safety program, special assistance for disabled students. *International student services:* counseling/support, special assistance for nonnative speakers of English, ESL courses. *Nursing student activities:* Sigma Theta Tau.

Calendar Semesters.

NURSING STUDENT PROFILE

Undergraduate **Enrollment:** 78
Women: 95%; **Men:** 5%; **Minority:** 14%; **International:** 0%; **Part-time:** 100%
Graduate **Enrollment:** 113
Women: 98%; **Men:** 2%; **Minority:** 4%; **International:** 0%; **Part-time:** 100%

BACCALAUREATE PROGRAM

Contact Ms. Marlene J. Hall, Counselor and Recruiter, Division of Nursing, University of Hartford, 200 Bloomfield Avenue, West Hartford, CT 06117, 860-768-4213. *Fax:* 860-768-5346. *E-mail:* mhall@uhavax.hartford.edu

Expenses *Tuition:* $7714 full-time, $255 per credit part-time. *Books and supplies per academic year:* ranges from $400 to $500.

RN Baccalaureate Program (BSN)

Applying *Required:* TOEFL for nonnative speakers of English, NLN Achievement Tests, minimum college GPA of 2.0, RN license, diploma or AD in nursing, transcript of college record. *Options:* May apply for transfer of up to 90 total credits. *Application deadline:* rolling. *Application fee:* $35.

Degree Requirements 121 total credit hours, 31 in nursing.

MASTER'S PROGRAMS

Contact Ms. Marlene J. Hall, Counselor/Recruiter, Division of Nursing, University of Hartford, 200 Bloomfield Avenue, West Hartford, CT 06117, 860-768-4213. *Fax:* 860-768-5346. *E-mail:* mhall@uhavax.hartford.edu

Areas of Study Nursing administration; nursing education.

Expenses *Tuition:* $275 per credit. *Part-time mandatory fees:* $110+. *Books and supplies per academic year:* ranges from $400 to $500.

Financial Aid Federal Stafford Loans.

MSN Program

Applying *Required:* bachelor's degree in nursing, minimum GPA of 3.0, RN license, 1 year of clinical experience, professional liability/malpractice insurance, essay, 2 letters of recommendation, transcript of college record. *Application deadline:* 4/30. *Application fee:* $35.

Degree Requirements 33 total credit hours, 24 in nursing, 9 in management or education. Research project.

MSN/MSOB Program

Applying *Required:* bachelor's degree, minimum GPA of 3.0, RN license, 1 year of clinical experience, professional liability/malpractice insurance, essay, letter of recommendation, transcript of college record, statistics, physical assessment for non-BSN students. *Application deadline:* 4/30. *Application fee:* $35.

Degree Requirements 46 total credit hours, 25–28 in nursing, 18–21 in organizational behavior. Research project.

University of Hartford (continued)

CONTINUING EDUCATION PROGRAM

Contact Ms. Shelly Hartnett, Professional and Continuing Education, University of Hartford, 99 Pratt Street, Hartford, CT 06103, 860-524-7739. *Fax:* 860-524-7744.

WESTERN CONNECTICUT STATE UNIVERSITY

Department of Nursing
Danbury, Connecticut

Programs • Generic Baccalaureate • RN Baccalaureate • RN to Master's • Master's for Nurses with Non-Nursing Degrees

The University State-supported comprehensive coed institution. Part of Connecticut State University System. Founded: 1903. *Primary accreditation:* regional. *Setting:* 340-acre urban campus. *Total enrollment:* 5,607.

The Department of Nursing Founded in 1965. *Nursing program faculty:* 16 (63% with doctorates).

Academic Facilities *Campus library:* 200,000 volumes; 1,584 periodical subscriptions. *Nursing school resources:* CAI, computer lab, nursing audiovisuals, learning resource lab, advanced technology classroom.

Student Life *Student services:* health clinic, personal counseling, career counseling, institutionally sponsored work-study program, job placement, campus safety program, special assistance for disabled students. *International student services:* counseling/support, ESL courses. *Nursing student activities:* Sigma Theta Tau, nursing club.

Calendar Semesters.

NURSING STUDENT PROFILE

Undergraduate **Enrollment:** 150
Women: 90%; **Men:** 10%; **Part-time:** 33%
Graduate **Enrollment:** 50
Women: 100%; **Minority:** 3%; **Part-time:** 100%

BACCALAUREATE PROGRAMS

Contact Dr. Barbara Piscopo, Chair, Department of Nursing, Western Connecticut State University, 181 White Street, Danbury, CT 06810, 203-837-8556. *Fax:* 203-837-8526. *E-mail:* piscopo@wcsub.ctstateu.edu

Expenses *State resident tuition:* $2012 full-time, $147 per semester hour part-time. *Nonresident tuition:* $6510 full-time, $147 per semester hour part-time. *Full-time mandatory fees:* $1462–$2297. *Room and board:* $4476. *Room only:* $2478. *Books and supplies per academic year:* $1050.

Financial Aid Institutionally sponsored need-based grants/scholarships, institutionally sponsored non-need grants/scholarships, Federal Direct Loans, Federal Pell Grants, Federal Perkins Loans, Federal Supplemental Educational Opportunity Grants, Federal Work-Study, Federal Family Education Loan Program (FFELP), Connecticut Aid for Public University. *Application deadline:* 4/1.

Generic Baccalaureate Program (BS)

Applying *Required:* SAT I, ACT, TOEFL for nonnative speakers of English, minimum high school GPA of 2.5, minimum college GPA of 2.25, 3 years of high school math, high school chemistry, high school biology, high school foreign language, high school transcript, transcript of college record. 28 prerequisite credits must be completed before admission to the nursing program. *Options:* Advanced standing available through credit by exam. May apply for transfer of up to 90 total credits. *Application deadline:* rolling. *Application fee:* $40.

Degree Requirements 125 total credit hours, 51 in nursing.

RN Baccalaureate Program (BS)

Applying *Required:* minimum college GPA of 2.25, RN license, diploma or AD in nursing, high school transcript, transcript of college record. 28 prerequisite credits must be completed before admission to the nursing program. *Options:* Advanced standing available through credit by exam. May apply for transfer of up to 90 total credits. *Application deadline:* rolling. *Application fee:* $40.

Degree Requirements 125 total credit hours, 51 in nursing.

MASTER'S PROGRAMS

Contact Dr. Andrea O'Connor, MSN Coordinator, Department of Nursing, Western Connecticut State University, 181 White Street, Danbury, CT 06810, 203-837-8564. *Fax:* 203-837-8526. *E-mail:* occonora@wcsub.ctstateu.edu

Areas of Study Clinical nurse specialist programs in adult health nursing, medical-surgical nursing; nursing administration; nurse practitioner program in adult health.

Expenses *State resident tuition:* $145. *Nonresident tuition:* $145. *Part-time mandatory fees:* $10.

Financial Aid Graduate assistantships.

RN to Master's Program (MSN)

Applying *Required:* Miller Analogies Test, bachelor's degree in nursing, minimum GPA of 3.0, RN license, 1 year of clinical experience, statistics course, interview, 2 letters of recommendation. *Application deadline:* rolling. *Application fee:* $40.

Degree Requirements 36 total credit hours, 20–36 in nursing. Thesis or project.

Master's for Nurses with Non-Nursing Degrees Program (MSN)

Applying *Required:* Miller Analogies Test, minimum GPA of 3.0, RN license, 1 year of clinical experience, physical assessment course, statistics course, interview, 2 letters of recommendation. *Application deadline:* rolling. *Application fee:* $20.

Degree Requirements 36 total credit hours, 20–36 in nursing. Thesis or project.

YALE UNIVERSITY

School of Nursing
New Haven, Connecticut

Programs • MSN • Master's for Nurses with Non-Nursing Degrees • Master's for Non-Nursing College Graduates • MSN/MPH • MSN/MPPM • Post-Master's • DNSc

The University Independent coed university. Founded: 1701. *Primary accreditation:* regional. *Setting:* 170-acre urban campus. *Total enrollment:* 10,986.

The School of Nursing Founded in 1923. *Nursing program faculty:* 85 (25% with doctorates).

Academic Facilities *Campus library:* 10,986 volumes (381,000 in health); 3,800 periodical subscriptions (2,500 health-care related). *Nursing school resources:* computer lab, nursing audiovisuals.

Student Life *Student services:* health clinic, child-care facilities, personal counseling, career counseling, institutionally sponsored work-study program, campus safety program, special assistance for disabled students. *International student services:* counseling/support. *Nursing student activities:* Sigma Theta Tau.

Calendar Semesters.

NURSING STUDENT PROFILE

Graduate **Enrollment:** 268
Women: 92%; **Men:** 8%; **Minority:** 12%; **International:** 1%; **Part-time:** 29%

MASTER'S PROGRAMS

Contact Ms. Cassy D. Pollack, Associate Dean for Students, School of Nursing, Yale University, 100 Church Street South, PO Box 9740, New Haven, CT 06536-0740, 203-785-2393. *Fax:* 203-785-3554. *E-mail:* cassy.pollack@yale.edu

Areas of Study Clinical nurse specialist programs in cardiovascular nursing, oncology nursing, psychiatric–mental health nursing; nurse midwifery; nurse practitioner programs in adult health, child care/pediatrics, family health, gerontology, school health.

Expenses *Tuition:* $17,600 full-time, ranges from $8800 to $11,734 per year part-time. *Full-time mandatory fees:* $700. *Room and board:* $8470–$11,400. *Books and supplies per academic year:* ranges from $1800 to $2100.

Financial Aid Graduate assistantships, nurse traineeships, Federal Nursing Student Loans, institutionally sponsored loans, employment opportunities, institutionally sponsored need-based grants/scholarships. 63% of master's level students in nursing programs received some form of financial aid in 1995-96. *Application deadline:* 4/30.

MSN Program

Master's for Nurses with Non-Nursing Degrees Program

Applying *Required:* GRE General Test, TOEFL for nonnative speakers of English, bachelor's degree, RN license, statistics course, essay, interview, 3 letters of recommendation, transcript of college record. *Application deadline:* 1/15. *Application fee:* $35.

Degree Requirements 40 total credit hours, 40 in nursing. Thesis required.

Master's for Non-Nursing College Graduates Program (MSN)

Applying *Required:* GRE General Test, TOEFL for nonnative speakers of English, bachelor's degree, statistics course, essay, interview, 3 letters of recommendation, transcript of college record. *Application deadline:* 11/30. *Application fee:* $35.

Degree Requirements 81 total credit hours, 81 in nursing. Thesis required.

MSN/MPH Program

Applying *Required:* GRE General Test, TOEFL for nonnative speakers of English, bachelor's degree, RN license, statistics course, essay, interview, 3 letters of recommendation, transcript of college record. *Application deadline:* 1/15. *Application fee:* $35.

Degree Requirements 40 total credit hours in nursing. Thesis required.

MSN/MPPM Program

Applying *Required:* GRE General Test, TOEFL for nonnative speakers of English, bachelor's degree, RN license, statistics course, essay, interview, 3 letters of recommendation, transcript of college record. *Application deadline:* 1/15. *Application fee:* $35.

Degree Requirements 40 total credit hours in nursing. Thesis required.

Post-Master's Program

Applying *Required:* bachelor's degree, RN license, essay, interview, letter of recommendation, transcript of college record, master's degree in nursing. *Application deadline:* 1/15. *Application fee:* $35.

Degree Requirements 21–31 total credit hours dependent upon track, 21–31 in nursing.

DOCTORAL PROGRAM

Contact Dr. Margaret Grey, Associate Dean for Research and Doctoral Studies, School of Nursing, Yale University, 25 Park Street, PO Box 9740, New Haven, CT 06536-0740, 203-785-2393. *Fax:* 203-785-3554. *E-mail:* margaret.grey@yale.edu

Areas of Study Nursing research, clinical practice, nursing policy.

Expenses *Tuition:* $17,600 full-time, $8800 per year part-time. *Full-time mandatory fees:* $750. *Part-time mandatory fees:* $750. *Room and board:* $8470. *Books and supplies per academic year:* $640.

Financial Aid Nurse traineeships, fellowships, dissertation grants, grants, opportunities for employment. *Application deadline:* 4/15.

DNSc Program

Applying *Required:* GRE General Test, TOEFL for nonnative speakers of English, master's degree in nursing, 2 years of clinical experience, 1 year in proposed area of specialization, statistics course, interview, 3 letters of recommendation, vitae, writing sample, competitive review by faculty committee. *Application deadline:* 3/15. *Application fee:* $35.

Degree Requirements 62 total credit hours; dissertation; oral exam; written exam; defense of dissertation.

See full description on page 576.

DELAWARE

DELAWARE STATE UNIVERSITY

Department of Nursing
Dover, Delaware

Programs • Generic Baccalaureate • RN Baccalaureate

The University State-supported comprehensive coed institution. Part of Delaware Higher Education Commission. Founded: 1891. *Primary accreditation:* regional. *Setting:* 400-acre small-town campus. *Total enrollment:* 3,175.

The Department of Nursing Founded in 1974. *Nursing program faculty:* 12 (33% with doctorates). *Off-campus program sites:* Georgetown, Wilmington.

Academic Facilities *Campus library:* 2,850 volumes (500 in health, 350 in nursing); 1,251 periodical subscriptions (70 health-care related). *Nursing school resources:* CAI, computer lab, nursing audiovisuals, interactive nursing skills videos, learning resource lab.

Student Life *Student services:* health clinic, child-care facilities, personal counseling, career counseling, institutionally sponsored work-study program, job placement, campus safety program, special assistance for disabled students. *International student services:* counseling/support, special assistance for nonnative speakers of English, ESL courses. *Nursing student activities:* nursing club, student nurses association, Nursing Honor Society.

Calendar Semesters.

NURSING STUDENT PROFILE

Undergraduate **Enrollment:** 294

Women: 96%; **Men:** 4%; **Minority:** 57%; **International:** 4%; **Part-time:** 10%

BACCALAUREATE PROGRAMS

Contact Dr. Mary P. Watkins, Chairperson, Department of Nursing, Delaware State University, 1200 North DuPont Highway, Dover, DE 19901-2275, 302-739-4933. *Fax:* 302-739-2952.

Expenses *State resident tuition:* $2496 full-time, $104 per credit part-time. *Nonresident tuition:* $6096 full-time, $254 per credit part-time. *Full-time mandatory fees:* $50–$75. *Room and board:* $4364–$4704. *Room only:* $2500–$2840.

Financial Aid Institutionally sponsored need-based grants/scholarships, Federal Direct Loans, Federal Perkins Loans, Federal Supplemental Educational Opportunity Grants, Federal Work-Study. 97% of undergraduate students in nursing programs received some form of financial aid in 1995–96. *Application deadline:* 4/1.

Generic Baccalaureate Program (BSN)

Applying *Required:* SAT I, ACT, Nursing Entrance Test, minimum high school GPA of 2.0, minimum college GPA of 2.5, high school chemistry, high school biology, high school transcript, 3 letters of recommendation, transcript of college record. *Options:* Advanced standing available through the following means: advanced placement exams, credit by exam. Course work may be accelerated. May apply for transfer of up to 70 total credits. *Application deadlines:* 6/1 (fall), 11/1 (spring). *Application fee:* $10.

Degree Requirements 131 total credit hours, 62 in nursing.

RN Baccalaureate Program (BSN)

Applying *Required:* SAT I, ACT, minimum high school GPA of 2.5, minimum college GPA of 2.5, RN license, diploma or AD in nursing, high school transcript, transcript of college record. *Options:* Course work may be accelerated. May apply for transfer of up to 70 total credits. *Application deadlines:* 6/1 (fall), 11/1 (spring). *Application fee:* $10.

Degree Requirements 121 total credit hours, 60 in nursing.

UNIVERSITY OF DELAWARE

College of Health and Nursing Sciences
Newark, Delaware

Programs • Generic Baccalaureate • RN Baccalaureate • Accelerated Baccalaureate for Second Degree • MSN • Post-Master's • Continuing Education

The University State-related coed university. Founded: 1743. *Primary accreditation:* regional. *Setting:* 1,000-acre small-town campus. *Total enrollment:* 17,892.

The College of Health and Nursing Sciences Founded in 1966. *Nursing program faculty:* 41 (49% with doctorates).

▶ *NOTEWORTHY*

The Baccalaureate for the Registered Nurse (BRN) is an innovative program—both nursing and support courses are offered in a distance learning format. All RN students must enroll in three 1-credit weekend courses held on the Newark campus. The College also offers an accelerated degree option for adults who have earned a baccalaureate degree in another discipline. All prerequisites must be completed before students begin the intense accelerated sequence. A GPI of 3.0 or higher is required for admission.

University of Delaware (continued)

Academic Facilities *Campus library:* 2.1 million volumes; 20,000 periodical subscriptions. *Nursing school resources:* CAI, computer lab, nursing audiovisuals, interactive nursing skills videos, learning resource lab.

Student Life *Student services:* health clinic, child-care facilities, personal counseling, career counseling, institutionally sponsored work-study program, job placement, campus safety program, special assistance for disabled students. *International student services:* counseling/support, special assistance for nonnative speakers of English, ESL courses. *Nursing student activities:* Sigma Theta Tau, nursing club, student nurses association.

Calendar Semesters.

NURSING STUDENT PROFILE

Undergraduate **Enrollment:** 619

Women: 92%; **Men:** 8%; **Minority:** 9%; **International:** 1%; **Part-time:** 32%

Graduate **Enrollment:** 152

Women: 95%; **Men:** 5%; **Minority:** 7%; **International:** 0%; **Part-time:** 89%

BACCALAUREATE PROGRAMS

Contact Dr. Pamela Beeman, Associate Dean, College of Health and Nursing Sciences, University of Delaware, Newark, DE 19716, 302-831-2381. *Fax:* 302-831-2382.

Expenses *State resident tuition:* $3990 full-time, $166 per credit part-time. *Nonresident tuition:* $11,250 full-time, $469 per credit part-time. *Full-time mandatory fees:* $440. *Part-time mandatory fees:* $15. *Room and board:* $4420–$5070. *Room only:* $2480–$3150. *Books and supplies per academic year:* $530.

Financial Aid Institutionally sponsored need-based grants/scholarships, institutionally sponsored non-need grants/scholarships, Federal Nursing Student Loans, Federal Work-Study. *Application deadline:* 3/1.

Generic Baccalaureate Program (BSN)

Applying *Required:* SAT I, minimum high school GPA of 3.0, minimum college GPA of 3.0, 3 years of high school math, 3 years of high school science, high school chemistry, high school biology, high school transcript, transcript of college record. *Options:* Advanced standing available through advanced placement exams. Course work may be accelerated. May apply for transfer of up to 96 total credits. *Application deadlines:* 3/1 (fall), 11/15 (spring). *Application fee:* $40.

Degree Requirements 126 total credit hours, 58 in nursing.

RN Baccalaureate Program (BSN)

Applying *Required:* minimum college GPA of 2.5, RN license, diploma or AD in nursing, high school transcript, transcript of college record. 30 prerequisite credits must be completed before admission to the nursing program. *Options:* Course work may be accelerated. May apply for transfer of up to 96 total credits. *Application deadline:* rolling. *Application fee:* $40.

Degree Requirements 125 total credit hours, 59 in nursing.

Distance learning Courses provided through video, computer-based media. Specific degree requirements include 3 one-credit weekend courses at the Newark campus.

Accelerated Baccalaureate for Second Degree Program (BSN)

Applying *Required:* SAT I, minimum college GPA of 3.0, interview, transcript of college record. *Options:* May apply for transfer of up to 96 total credits. *Application deadline:* rolling. *Application fee:* $40.

Degree Requirements 126 total credit hours, 58 in nursing.

MASTER'S PROGRAMS

Contact Dr. Janice Selekman, Chairperson, College of Health and Nursing Sciences, University of Delaware, Newark, DE 19716, 302-831-2193. *Fax:* 302-831-2382.

Areas of Study Clinical nurse specialist programs in cardiovascular nursing, gerontological nursing, maternity-newborn nursing, medical-surgical nursing, oncology nursing, pediatric nursing; nursing administration; nurse practitioner programs in adult health, child care/pediatrics, family health, gerontology, women's health.

Expenses *State resident tuition:* $3990 full-time, $222 per credit part-time. *Nonresident tuition:* $11,250 full-time, $625 per credit part-time. *Full-time mandatory fees:* $178.

Financial Aid Graduate assistantships, nurse traineeships. 11% of master's level students in nursing programs received some form of financial aid in 1995-96. *Application deadline:* 7/1.

MSN Program

Applying *Required:* GRE General Test, bachelor's degree in nursing, minimum GPA, RN license, 1 year of clinical experience, physical assessment course, statistics course, professional liability/malpractice insurance, interview, 3 letters of recommendation, transcript of college record, written essay for family nurse practitioner track. *Application deadlines:* 7/1 (fall), 12/1 (spring). *Application fee:* $50.

Degree Requirements 34–46 total credit hours dependent upon track, 34–46 in nursing. Thesis, scholarly project, or research utilization course.

Post-Master's Program

Applying *Required:* RN license, physical assessment course, professional liability/malpractice insurance, essay, interview, 3 letters of recommendation, transcript of college record. *Application deadlines:* 7/1 (fall), 12/1 (spring). *Application fee:* $40.

Degree Requirements 16–28 total credit hours dependent upon track, 16–28 in nursing.

CONTINUING EDUCATION PROGRAM

Contact Dr. Madeline E. Lambrecht, Director, Division of Special Programs, McDowell Hall, College of Health and Nursing Sciences, University of Delaware, Newark, DE 19716, 800-400-6877. *Fax:* 302-831-4550. *E-mail:* dsp@mvs.udel.edu

See full description on page 530.

WILMINGTON COLLEGE
Division of Nursing
New Castle, Delaware

Programs • RN Baccalaureate • RN to Master's

The College Independent comprehensive coed institution. Founded: 1967. *Primary accreditation:* regional. *Setting:* 13-acre suburban campus. *Total enrollment:* 3,800.

The Division of Nursing Founded in 1985. *Nursing program faculty:* 30 (13% with doctorates). *Off-campus program sites:* Dover, Georgetown, Wilmington.

▶ *NOTEWORTHY*

Wilmington College offers 2 levels of nursing education: a BSN program for registered nurses and an MSN program with a family nurse practitioner concentration. Each student's academic and professional growth is fostered by the small college environment in which individual attention is emphasized. The expertise and commitment of the faculty contribute to the strength of both programs. A unique feature is the availability of both programs at several locations throughout Delaware. The 8-week sessions provide an accelerated yet manageable format for adult learners.

Academic Facilities *Campus library:* 110,000 volumes (2,300 in nursing); 345 periodical subscriptions (46 health-care related). *Nursing school resources:* CAI, computer lab, nursing audiovisuals, learning resource lab.

Student Life *Student services:* career counseling, institutionally sponsored work-study program, job placement, campus safety program. *Nursing student activities:* Nursing Honor Society.

Calendar Six 8-week sessions.

NURSING STUDENT PROFILE

Undergraduate

Women: 95%; **Men:** 5%; **Minority:** 6%; **International:** 0%; **Part-time:** 92%

Graduate **Enrollment:** 100

Women: 95%; **Men:** 5%; **Minority:** 6%; **International:** 0%; **Part-time:** 92%

BACCALAUREATE PROGRAM

Contact Dr. Betty Caffo, Chair, Division of Nursing, Wilmington College, 320 DuPont Highway, New Castle, DE 19720, 302-328-9401. *Fax:* 302-328-5902.

Expenses *Tuition:* $5700 full-time, $190 per credit part-time. *Full-time mandatory fees:* $50. *Books and supplies per academic year:* $500.

Financial Aid Institutionally sponsored need-based grants/scholarships, Federal Work-Study. *Application deadline:* 8/1.

RN Baccalaureate Program (BSN)

Applying *Required:* RN license, diploma or AD in nursing, transcript of college record. *Options:* Course work may be accelerated. May apply for transfer of up to 75 total credits. *Application deadline:* rolling. *Application fee:* $25.

Degree Requirements 120 total credit hours, 61 in nursing.

MASTER'S PROGRAM

Contact Dianna Nefosky, Admissions Assistant, 320 Dupont Highway, New Castle, DE 19720, 302-328-9407. *Fax:* 302-328-5902.

Areas of Study Nurse practitioner program in family health.

Expenses *Tuition:* $702 per credits. *Full-time mandatory fees:* $50.

Financial Aid 20% of master's level students in nursing programs received some form of financial aid in 1995-96. *Application deadline:* 8/1.

RN to Master's Program (MSN)

Applying *Required:* bachelor's degree in nursing, bachelor's degree, RN license, interview, transcript of college record. *Application deadline:* 12/20. *Application fee:* $25.

Degree Requirements 42 total credit hours.

DISTRICT OF COLUMBIA

THE CATHOLIC UNIVERSITY OF AMERICA
School of Nursing
Washington, District of Columbia

Programs • Generic Baccalaureate • RN Baccalaureate • Accelerated Baccalaureate for Second Degree • BSN to Master's • RN to Master's • MSN/Master's in Health Service Management • Post-Master's • DNSc

The University Independent coed university, affiliated with Roman Catholic Church. Founded: 1887. *Primary accreditation:* regional. *Setting:* 155-acre urban campus. *Total enrollment:* 6,108.

The School of Nursing Founded in 1932. *Nursing program faculty:* 26 (66% with doctorates).

Academic Facilities *Campus library:* 1.3 million volumes (38,876 in nursing); 8,929 periodical subscriptions (316 health-care related). *Nursing school resources:* CAI, computer lab, nursing audiovisuals, interactive nursing skills videos, learning resource lab, study and writing skills center, Donley Technology Center.

Student Life *Student services:* health clinic, child-care facilities, personal counseling, career counseling, institutionally sponsored work-study program, campus safety program, special assistance for disabled students, campus ministry. *International student services:* counseling/support, special assistance for nonnative speakers of English, ESL courses. *Nursing student activities:* Sigma Theta Tau, nursing club, student nurses association.

Calendar Semesters.

NURSING STUDENT PROFILE

Undergraduate **Enrollment:** 267

Women: 90%; **Men:** 10%; **Minority:** 25%; **International:** 7%; **Part-time:** 7%

Graduate **Enrollment:** 132

Women: 97%; **Men:** 3%; **Minority:** 10%; **International:** 12%; **Part-time:** 75%

BACCALAUREATE PROGRAMS

Contact Ms. Carolyn S. d'Avis, Director, Baccalaureate Program, School of Nursing, Catholic University of America, Washington, DC 20064, 202-319-6457. *Fax:* 202-319-6485. *E-mail:* davis@cua.edu

Expenses *Tuition:* $15,562 full-time, $600 per hour part-time. *Full-time mandatory fees:* $1200–$1340. *Room and board:* $6148–$7338. *Room only:* $3376–$4454. *Books and supplies per academic year:* ranges from $500 to $1000.

Financial Aid Institutionally sponsored need-based grants/scholarships, institutionally sponsored non-need grants/scholarships, Federal Nursing Student Loans, Federal Pell Grants, Federal Perkins Loans, Federal Supplemental Educational Opportunity Grants, Federal Work-Study. *Application deadline:* 4/1.

Generic Baccalaureate Program (BSN)

Applying *Required:* SAT I or ACT, TOEFL for nonnative speakers of English, minimum high school GPA of 3.0, 3 years of high school math, 3 years of high school science, high school chemistry, high school biology, high school transcript, 2 letters of recommendation, written essay. *Options:* Advanced standing available through the following means: advanced placement exams, advanced placement without credit. Course work may be accelerated. May apply for transfer of up to 99 total credits. *Application deadlines:* 6/1 (fall), 12/1 (spring). *Application fee:* $50.

Degree Requirements 129 total credit hours, 64 in nursing. Philosophy, religion courses.

RN Baccalaureate Program (BSN)

Applying *Required:* TOEFL for nonnative speakers of English, ACT PEP for diploma RNs, minimum high school GPA of 3.0, minimum college GPA of 2.5, RN license, diploma or AD in nursing, high school transcript, 2 letters of recommendation, written essay, transcript of college record, transcript evaluation for international students. 94 prerequisite credits must be completed before admission to the nursing program. *Options:* Advanced standing available through credit by exam. May apply for transfer of up to 94 total credits. *Application deadlines:* 6/1 (fall), 12/1 (spring). *Application fee:* $50.

Degree Requirements 126 total credit hours, 32 in nursing.

Accelerated Baccalaureate for Second Degree Program (BSN)

Applying *Required:* minimum college GPA of 3.0, 2 letters of recommendation, written essay, transcript of college record. 68 prerequisite credits must be completed before admission to the nursing program. *Options:* May apply for transfer of up to 68 total credits. *Application deadline:* 6/1. *Application fee:* $50.

Degree Requirements 129 total credit hours, 61 in nursing.

MASTER'S PROGRAMS

Contact Sr. Mary Jean Flaherty, Dean, School of Nursing, Catholic University of America, Washington, DC 20064, 202-319-5403. *Fax:* 202-319-6485.

Areas of Study Clinical nurse specialist program in cardiovascular nursing; nursing administration; nursing education; nurse practitioner programs in adult health, child care/pediatrics, family health, gerontology, psychiatric–mental health, school health, advanced practice psychiatric-mental health nursing.

Expenses *Tuition:* $15,562 full-time, $600 per hour part-time. *Full-time mandatory fees:* $1200–$1340. *Room and board:* $6364–$7600. *Room only:* $3474–$4610. *Books and supplies per academic year:* ranges from $750 to $1000.

Financial Aid Nurse traineeships, Federal Nursing Student Loans, institutionally sponsored need-based grants/scholarships, institutionally sponsored non-need-based grants/scholarships. *Application deadline:* 4/1.

BSN to Master's Program (MSN)

Applying *Required:* GRE General Test, TOEFL for nonnative speakers of English, bachelor's degree in nursing, minimum GPA of 3.0, RN license, 2 years of clinical experience, statistics course, professional liability/malpractice insurance, 3 letters of recommendation, transcript of college record. *Application deadlines:* 7/1 (fall), 12/1 (spring). *Application fee:* $50.

Degree Requirements 41–46 total credit hours dependent upon track, 29–34 in nursing, 12 in philosophy, natural and/or behavioral science, and other specified areas. Capstone research project.

RN to Master's Program (MSN)

Applying *Required:* GRE General Test, minimum GPA of 3.0, RN license, 2 years of clinical experience, statistics course, professional liability/malpractice insurance, interview, 3 letters of recommendation, transcript of college record. *Application deadlines:* 7/1 (fall), 12/1 (spring). *Application fee:* $50.

Degree Requirements 63–68 total credit hours dependent upon track, 48–53 in nursing, 15 in philosophy, natural and/or behavioral science, and other specified areas. Capstone research project.

MSN/Master's in Health Service Management Program

Applying *Required:* GRE General Test, TOEFL for nonnative speakers of English, bachelor's degree in nursing, minimum GPA of 3.0, RN license,

The Catholic University of America (continued)

2 years of clinical experience, statistics course, professional liability/malpractice insurance, interview, 3 letters of recommendation, transcript of college record. *Application deadlines:* 7/1 (fall), 12/1 (spring). *Application fee:* $50.

Degree Requirements 61 total credit hours, 31 in nursing, 30 in health services management. Capstone research project.

Post-Master's Program

Applying *Required:* minimum GPA of 3.0, RN license, 2 years of clinical experience, professional liability/malpractice insurance, interview, 3 letters of recommendation, transcript of college record. *Application deadlines:* 7/1 (fall), 12/1 (spring). *Application fee:* $50.

Degree Requirements 19–22 total credit hours dependent upon track, 13–16 in nursing, 6 in pathophysiology, pharmacology.

DOCTORAL PROGRAM

Contact Sr. Mary Jean Flaherty, Dean, School of Nursing, Catholic University of America, Washington, DC 20064, 202-319-5109. *Fax:* 202-319-6485.

Areas of Study Nursing administration, nursing education, nursing research, clinical practice.

Expenses *Tuition:* $15,562 full-time, $600 per hour part-time. *Full-time mandatory fees:* $1200–$1340. *Room and board:* $6148–$7338. *Room only:* $3376–$4454.

Financial Aid Graduate assistantships, dissertation grants, opportunities for employment. *Application deadline:* 2/1.

DNSc Program

Applying *Required:* GRE General Test, TOEFL for nonnative speakers of English, master's degree in nursing, 2 years of clinical experience, 1 scholarly paper, statistics course, interview, 3 letters of recommendation, writing sample. *Application deadline:* 3/1. *Application fee:* $50.

Degree Requirements 66 total credit hours; dissertation; oral exam; written exam; defense of dissertation; residency.

GEORGETOWN UNIVERSITY

School of Nursing
Washington, District of Columbia

Programs • Generic Baccalaureate • RN Baccalaureate • Baccalaureate for Second Degree • MSN • Continuing Education

The University Independent Roman Catholic (Jesuit) coed university. Founded: 1789. *Primary accreditation:* regional. *Setting:* 110-acre urban campus. *Total enrollment:* 12,618.

The School of Nursing Founded in 1903. *Nursing program faculty:* 51 (75% with doctorates).

Academic Facilities *Campus library:* 171,000 volumes (36,000 in health, 20,000 in nursing); 1,841 periodical subscriptions (92 health-care related). *Nursing school resources:* CAI, computer lab, nursing audiovisuals, interactive nursing skills videos, learning resource lab.

Student Life *Student services:* health clinic, personal counseling, career counseling, institutionally sponsored work-study program, job placement, campus safety program, special assistance for disabled students. *International student services:* counseling/support, special assistance for nonnative speakers of English. *Nursing student activities:* Sigma Theta Tau, student nurses association, student academic council.

Calendar Semesters.

NURSING STUDENT PROFILE

Undergraduate **Enrollment:** 298

Women: 95%; **Men:** 5%; **Minority:** 21%; **International:** 1%; **Part-time:** 6%

Graduate **Enrollment:** 172

Women: 80%; **Men:** 20%; **Minority:** 8%; **International:** 0%; **Part-time:** 57%

BACCALAUREATE PROGRAMS

Contact Sharon Murray, Coordinator of Admissions and Recruitment, School of Nursing, Georgetown University, 3700 Reservoir Road, NW, Washington, DC 20007, 202-687-2781. *Fax:* 202-687-5553.

Expenses *Tuition:* $19,696 per academic year. *Full-time mandatory fees:* $337. *Room and board:* $4100–$7462. *Books and supplies per academic year:* ranges from $600 to $1000.

Financial Aid Institutionally sponsored need-based grants/scholarships, Federal Direct Loans, Federal Nursing Student Loans, Federal Perkins Loans, Federal Supplemental Educational Opportunity Grants, Federal Work-Study. *Application deadline:* 2/1.

Generic Baccalaureate Program (BSN)

Applying *Required:* SAT I or ACT, 3 College Board Achievements, TOEFL for nonnative speakers of English, minimum high school GPA of 3.0, minimum college GPA of 3.0, 3 years of high school math, 3 years of high school science, high school chemistry, high school biology, high school foreign language, high school transcript, interview, 3 letters of recommendation, written essay. *Options:* Advanced standing available through advanced placement exams. Course work may be accelerated. May apply for transfer of up to 60 total credits. *Application deadlines:* 1/10 (fall), 11/15 (early decision). *Application fee:* $50.

Degree Requirements 130 total credit hours, 65 in nursing.

RN Baccalaureate Program (BSN)

Applying *Required:* SAT I or ACT, TOEFL for nonnative speakers of English, minimum college GPA of 3.0, RN license, diploma or AD in nursing, interview, 2 letters of recommendation, transcript of college record. *Options:* Advanced standing available through credit by exam. Course work may be accelerated. May apply for transfer of up to 60 total credits. *Application deadline:* 3/1. *Application fee:* $50.

Degree Requirements 121 total credit hours, 56 in nursing.

Baccalaureate for Second Degree Program (BSN)

Applying *Required:* TOEFL for nonnative speakers of English, minimum college GPA of 3.0, high school chemistry, high school biology, high school transcript, 2 letters of recommendation, written essay, transcript of college record. 59 prerequisite credits must be completed before admission to the nursing program. *Options:* Course work may be accelerated. May apply for transfer of up to 59 total credits. *Application deadline:* 3/1. *Application fee:* $50.

Degree Requirements 120 total credit hours, 61 in nursing.

MASTER'S PROGRAM

Contact Sharon Murray, Coordinator of Admissions and Recruitment, School of Nursing, Georgetown University, 3700 Reservoir Road, NW, Washington, DC 20007, 202-687-2781. *Fax:* 202-687-5553.

Areas of Study Nurse anesthesia; nurse midwifery; nurse practitioner programs in acute care, family health.

Expenses *Tuition:* $16,670 per academic year. *Full-time mandatory fees:* $180. *Room and board:* $8034. *Books and supplies per academic year:* ranges from $600 to $1000.

Financial Aid Graduate assistantships, nurse traineeships, Federal Direct Loans, Federal Nursing Student Loans, employment opportunities. *Application deadline:* 4/1.

MSN Program

Applying *Required:* GRE General Test, Miller Analogies Test, TOEFL for nonnative speakers of English, GRE General Test for nurse anesthesia track, bachelor's degree in nursing, minimum GPA of 3.0, RN license, 1 year of clinical experience, statistics course, professional liability/malpractice insurance, essay, 3 letters of recommendation, transcript of college record, interview for nurse-midwifery and nurse anesthesia tracks. *Application deadlines:* 2/1 (fall), 11/1 (spring), 6/15 (acute care nurse practitioner). *Application fee:* $50.

Degree Requirements 36–45 total credit hours dependent upon track, 36–45 in nursing.

CONTINUING EDUCATION PROGRAM

Contact Sharon Murray, Coordinator of Admissions and Recruitment, School of Nursing, Georgetown University, 3700 Resevoir Road, NW, Washington, DC 20007, 202-687-2781. *Fax:* 202-687-5553.

See full description on page 450.

HOWARD UNIVERSITY
College of Nursing
Washington, District of Columbia

Programs • Generic Baccalaureate • RN Baccalaureate • Baccalaureate for Second Degree • MSN • Post-Master's

The University Independent coed university. Founded: 1867. *Primary accreditation:* regional. *Setting:* 242-acre urban campus. *Total enrollment:* 10,332.

The College of Nursing Founded in 1968. *Nursing program faculty:* 32 (43% with doctorates).

Academic Facilities *Campus library:* 1.9 million volumes (219,448 in health, 4,300 in nursing); 26,038 periodical subscriptions (5,247 health-care related). *Nursing school resources:* CAI, computer lab, nursing audiovisuals, interactive nursing skills videos, learning resource lab.

Student Life *Student services:* health clinic, personal counseling, career counseling, institutionally sponsored work-study program, job placement. *International student services:* counseling/support. *Nursing student activities:* Sigma Theta Tau, student nurses association.

Calendar Semesters.

NURSING STUDENT PROFILE

Undergraduate **Enrollment:** 416
Women: 90%; **Men:** 10%; **Minority:** 98%; **International:** 8%; **Part-time:** 44%
Graduate **Enrollment:** 58
Women: 92%; **Men:** 8%; **Minority:** 98%; **International:** 12%; **Part-time:** 75%

BACCALAUREATE PROGRAMS

Contact Ms. Carolyn J. Harris, Assistant Dean, Student Affairs, College of Nursing, Howard University, 501 Bryant Street, NW, Washington, DC 20059, 202-806-7483. *Fax:* 202-806-5958.

Expenses *Tuition:* $8320 full-time, $346 per credit hour part-time. *Full-time mandatory fees:* $202–$350. *Room and board:* $2000–$7200. *Books and supplies per academic year:* ranges from $900 to $1050.

Financial Aid Institutionally sponsored need-based grants/scholarships, institutionally sponsored non-need grants/scholarships, Federal Direct Loans, Federal Nursing Student Loans, Federal Work-Study. *Application deadline:* 2/1.

Generic Baccalaureate Program (BSN)

Applying *Required:* SAT I, ACT, TOEFL for nonnative speakers of English, minimum high school GPA of 2.5, high school chemistry, high school biology, high school transcript, transcript of college record. *Options:* Course work may be accelerated. *Application deadlines:* 2/1 (fall), 11/1 (spring). *Application fee:* $45.

Degree Requirements 127 total credit hours, 57 in nursing.

RN Baccalaureate Program (BSN)

Applying *Required:* TOEFL for nonnative speakers of English, minimum college GPA of 2.5, RN license, diploma or AD in nursing, transcript of college record. 63 prerequisite credits must be completed before admission to the nursing program. *Options:* Advanced standing available through advanced placement exams. Course work may be accelerated. May apply for transfer of up to 67 total credits. *Application deadlines:* 2/1 (fall), 11/1 (spring). *Application fee:* $45.

Degree Requirements 124 total credit hours, 30 in nursing.

Baccalaureate for Second Degree Program (BSN)

Applying *Required:* TOEFL for nonnative speakers of English, minimum college GPA of 2.5, transcript of college record. 55 prerequisite credits must be completed before admission to the nursing program. *Options:* Advanced standing available through advanced placement exams. Course work may be accelerated. *Application deadlines:* 2/1 (fall), 11/1 (spring). *Application fee:* $45.

Degree Requirements 126 total credit hours, 56 in nursing.

MASTER'S PROGRAMS

Contact Dr. Coralease Ruff, Assistant Dean, Graduate Studies, College of Nursing, Howard University, 501 Bryant Street, NW, Washington, DC 20059, 202-806-7460. *Fax:* 202-806-5958.

Areas of Study Nurse practitioner program in family health.

Expenses *Tuition:* $9000 full-time, $533 per credit hour part-time. *Full-time mandatory fees:* $185–$335. *Books and supplies per academic year:* ranges from $425 to $825.

Financial Aid Graduate assistantships, nurse traineeships, institutionally sponsored loans. *Application deadline:* 2/1.

MSN Program

Applying *Required:* GRE General Test, TOEFL for nonnative speakers of English, bachelor's degree in nursing, minimum GPA of 3.0, RN license, physical assessment course, statistics course, professional liability/malpractice insurance, essay, interview, 3 letters of recommendation, transcript of college record. *Application deadlines:* 2/1 (fall), 11/1 (spring). *Application fee:* $45.

Degree Requirements 42 total credit hours, 36 in nursing, 3 in educational research.

Post-Master's Program

Applying *Required:* minimum GPA of 3.0, RN license, professional liability/malpractice insurance, essay, interview, 3 letters of recommendation, transcript of college record, MSN. *Application deadlines:* 2/1 (fall), 11/1 (spring). *Application fee:* $45.

Degree Requirements 23 total credit hours, 23 in nursing. Basic health assessment course.

UNIVERSITY OF THE DISTRICT OF COLUMBIA
Nursing Education Program
Washington, District of Columbia

Programs • Generic Baccalaureate • RN Baccalaureate

The University District-supported comprehensive coed institution. Founded: 1976. *Primary accreditation:* regional. *Setting:* 28-acre urban campus. *Total enrollment:* 9,660.

The Nursing Education Program Founded in 1968. *Nursing program faculty:* 10 (20% with doctorates).

Calendar Semesters.

NURSING STUDENT PROFILE

Undergraduate **Enrollment:** 45
Women: 80%; **Men:** 20%; **Minority:** 99%; **International:** 50%

BACCALAUREATE PROGRAMS

Contact Dr. Hazel Marshall, Interim Director, Nursing Education Program, University of the District of Columbia, 4200 Connecticut Avenue, NW, Washington, DC 20008.

Expenses *State resident tuition:* $1392 full-time, $58 per credit hour part-time. *Nonresident tuition:* $4224 full-time, $176 per credit hour part-time. *Full-time mandatory fees:* $110.

Financial Aid Federal Work-Study, Federal and state grants and loans.

Generic Baccalaureate Program (BSN)

Applying *Options:* Advanced standing available through credit by exam. *Application deadline:* 3/1. *Application fee:* $20.

Degree Requirements 120 total credit hours, 68 in nursing.

RN Baccalaureate Program (BSN)

Applying *Required:* RN license, diploma or AD in nursing. *Application deadline:* 3/1. *Application fee:* $20.

Degree Requirements 120 total credit hours, 68 in nursing.

FLORIDA

BARRY UNIVERSITY
School of Nursing
Miami Shores, Florida

Programs • Generic Baccalaureate • Accelerated Baccalaureate • RN Baccalaureate • Accelerated Baccalaureate for Second Degree • LPN to Baccalaureate • MSN • RN to Master's • MSN/MBA • Post-Master's • PhD

The University Independent Roman Catholic comprehensive coed institution. Founded: 1940. *Primary accreditation:* regional. *Setting:* 90-acre suburban campus. *Total enrollment:* 7,098.

The School of Nursing Founded in 1953. *Nursing program faculty:* 34 (39% with doctorates). *Off-campus program sites:* Fort Lauderdale, Palm Beach, Port St. Lucie.

Academic Facilities *Campus library:* 550,000 volumes (14,000 in health, 8,000 in nursing); 2,000 periodical subscriptions (300 health-care related). *Nursing school resources:* CAI, computer lab, nursing audiovisuals, interactive nursing skills videos, learning resource lab.

Student Life *Student services:* health clinic, personal counseling, career counseling, institutionally sponsored work-study program, job placement, campus safety program, special assistance for disabled students. *International student services:* counseling/support, special assistance for nonnative speakers of English, ESL courses. *Nursing student activities:* Sigma Theta Tau, student nurses association.

Calendar Semesters.

NURSING STUDENT PROFILE

Undergraduate **Enrollment:** 329
Women: 90%; **Men:** 10%; **Minority:** 54%; **International:** 2%; **Part-time:** 53%
Graduate **Enrollment:** 205
Women: 94%; **Men:** 6%; **Minority:** 40%; **International:** 1%; **Part-time:** 88%

BACCALAUREATE PROGRAMS

Contact Dr. Victoria Schoolcraft, Associate Dean, School of Nursing, Barry University, 11300 Northeast 2nd Avenue, Miami Shores, FL 33161-6695, 305-899-3800. *Fax:* 305-899-3831. *E-mail:* schoolcraft@diana.barry.edu

Expenses *Tuition:* $12,790 full-time, $365 per credit part-time. *Full-time mandatory fees:* $200–$400. *Part-time mandatory fees:* $60–$120. *Room and board:* $5200–$6160. *Books and supplies per academic year:* ranges from $200 to $300.

Financial Aid Institutionally sponsored need-based grants/scholarships, institutionally sponsored non-need grants/scholarships, Federal Direct Loans, Federal Nursing Student Loans, Federal Pell Grants, Federal Perkins Loans, Federal Supplemental Educational Opportunity Grants. 75% of undergraduate students in nursing programs received some form of financial aid in 1995–96. *Application deadline:* 2/15.

Generic Baccalaureate Program (BSN)

Applying *Required:* ACT, SAT II Writing Test, SAT II Subject Test, TOEFL for nonnative speakers of English, minimum high school GPA of 2.7, minimum college GPA of 2.7, 3 years of high school math, 3 years of high school science, high school chemistry, high school transcript, 2 letters of recommendation, written essay, transcript of college record. 30 prerequisite credits must be completed before admission to the nursing program. *Options:* Advanced standing available through credit by exam. Course work may be accelerated. May apply for transfer of up to 90 total credits. *Application deadline:* rolling. *Application fee:* $30.

Degree Requirements 126 total credit hours, 55 in nursing.

Accelerated Baccalaureate Program (BSN)

Applying *Required:* ACT, SAT II Writing Test, SAT II Subject Test, TOEFL for nonnative speakers of English, minimum high school GPA of 3.0, high school math, high school science, high school chemistry, high school transcript, 2 letters of recommendation, written essay, transcript of college record. 30 prerequisite credits must be completed before admission to the nursing program. *Options:* Advanced standing available through credit by exam. Course work may be accelerated. May apply for transfer of up to 90 total credits. *Application deadline:* rolling. *Application fee:* $30.

Degree Requirements 126 total credit hours, 55 in nursing.

RN Baccalaureate Program (BSN)

Applying *Required:* TOEFL for nonnative speakers of English, minimum college GPA of 2.7, RN license, diploma or AD in nursing, letter of recommendation, written essay, transcript of college record. 30 prerequisite credits must be completed before admission to the nursing program. *Options:* Advanced standing available through credit by exam. Course work may be accelerated. May apply for transfer of up to 90 total credits. *Application deadline:* rolling. *Application fee:* $30.

Degree Requirements 120 total credit hours, 59 in nursing.

Accelerated Baccalaureate for Second Degree Program (BSN)

Applying *Required:* TOEFL for nonnative speakers of English, minimum college GPA of 2.7, letter of recommendation, written essay, transcript of college record, letter of intent. 43 prerequisite credits must be completed before admission to the nursing program. *Options:* Advanced standing available through credit by exam. Course work may be accelerated. May apply for transfer of up to 43 total credits. *Application deadline:* rolling. *Application fee:* $30.

Degree Requirements 96 total credit hours, 55 in nursing.

LPN to Baccalaureate Program (BSN)

Applying *Required:* ACT, SAT II Writing Test, SAT II Subject Test, minimum college GPA of 2.7, high school chemistry, high school biology, letter of recommendation, written essay, transcript of college record, LPN license or proof of eligibility to sit for the NCLEX-Practical Nurse exam. 30 prerequisite credits must be completed before admission to the nursing program. *Options:* Advanced standing available through credit by exam. Course work may be accelerated. May apply for transfer of up to 90 total credits. *Application deadline:* rolling. *Application fee:* $30.

Degree Requirements 125 total credit hours, 55 in nursing.

MASTER'S PROGRAMS

Contact Dr. Patricia Munhall, Associate Dean, School of Nursing, Barry University, 11300 Northeast 2nd Avenue, Miami Shores, FL 33161-6695, 305-899-3800. *Fax:* 305-899-3831. *E-mail:* munhall@diana.barry.edu

Areas of Study Nursing administration; nursing education; nurse practitioner programs in acute care, adult health, community health, family health.

Expenses *Tuition:* $7290 full-time, $405 per credit part-time. *Full-time mandatory fees:* $200–$250. *Room and board:* $5200–$6160. *Books and supplies per academic year:* ranges from $150 to $200.

Financial Aid Graduate assistantships, nurse traineeships, institutionally sponsored loans, employment opportunities. 50% of master's level students in nursing programs received some form of financial aid in 1995-96. *Application deadline:* 2/15.

MSN Program

Applying *Required:* GRE General Test (minimum combined score of 900 on three tests), Miller Analogies Test, bachelor's degree in nursing, minimum GPA of 3.0, RN license, 1 year of clinical experience, statistics course, professional liability/malpractice insurance, essay, 2 letters of recommendation, transcript of college record. *Application deadline:* rolling. *Application fee:* $30.

Degree Requirements 45 total credit hours, 39 in nursing, 6 in other specified areas. Thesis or research project.

RN to Master's Program (MSN)

Applying *Required:* GRE General Test (minimum combined score of 900 on three tests), Miller Analogies Test, minimum GPA of 3.0, RN license, professional liability/malpractice insurance, essay, 3 letters of recommendation, transcript of college record, diploma or AD in nursing. *Application deadline:* rolling.

Degree Requirements 167 total credit hours, 106 in nursing, 61 in other specified areas. Thesis or research project.

MSN/MBA Program

Applying *Required:* GRE General Test (minimum combined score of 900 on three tests), Miller Analogies Test, bachelor's degree in nursing, minimum GPA of 3.0, RN license, 1 year of clinical experience, statistics course, professional liability/malpractice insurance, essay, 2 letters of recommendation, transcript of college record. *Application deadline:* rolling. *Application fee:* $30.

Degree Requirements 63 total credit hours, 36 in nursing, 27 in business. Thesis or research project.

Post-Master's Program

Applying *Required:* GRE General Test (minimum combined score of 900 on three tests), Miller Analogies Test, minimum GPA of 3.0, RN license, 1 year of clinical experience, physical assessment course, statistics course, professional liability/malpractice insurance, essay, 2 letters of recommendation, transcript of college record. *Application deadline:* rolling. *Application fee:* $30.

Degree Requirements 25 total credit hours, 25 in nursing.

DOCTORAL PROGRAM

Contact Dr. Patricia Munhall, Associate Dean, School of Nursing, Barry University, 11300 North East 2nd Avenue, Miami Shores, FL 33161, 305-899-3800. *Fax:* 305-899-3831. *E-mail:* munhall@diana.barry.edu

Areas of Study Nursing administration, nursing education, nursing research.

Expenses *Tuition:* $9180 full-time, $510 per credit part-time. *Full-time mandatory fees:* $200–$250. *Books and supplies per academic year:* ranges from $200 to $300.

Financial Aid Graduate assistantships, opportunities for employment. *Application deadline:* 2/15.

PhD Program

Applying *Required:* GRE General Test (minimum combined score of 1000 on three tests), Miller Analogies Test, master's degree in nursing, master's degree, statistics course, interview, 2 letters of recommendation, writing sample, competitive review by faculty committee, graduate-level research courses. *Application deadline:* rolling. *Application fee:* $30.

Degree Requirements 45 total credit hours; dissertation; oral exam; defense of dissertation.

FLORIDA AGRICULTURAL AND MECHANICAL UNIVERSITY
School of Nursing
Tallahassee, Florida

Programs • Generic Baccalaureate • RN Baccalaureate

The University State-supported coed university. Part of State University System of Florida. Founded: 1887. *Primary accreditation:* regional. *Setting:* 419-acre suburban campus. *Total enrollment:* 10,324.

The School of Nursing Founded in 1904. *Nursing program faculty:* 20.

Academic Facilities *Campus library:* 500,000 volumes; 3,500 periodical subscriptions.

Calendar Semesters.

BACCALAUREATE PROGRAMS

Contact Dean, School of Nursing, Florida Agricultural and Mechanical University, Tallahassee, FL 32307, 904-599-3017. *Fax:* 904-599-3847.

Expenses *State resident tuition:* $2480 full-time, $62 per credit hour part-time. *Nonresident tuition:* $4720 full-time, $118 per credit hour part-time. *Full-time mandatory fees:* $34–$130. *Room and board:* $3176–$3280. *Room only:* $1980.

Generic Baccalaureate Program (BS)

Applying *Required:* SAT I or ACT, TOEFL for nonnative speakers of English, minimum high school GPA of 3.0, minimum college GPA of 2.5, 3 years of high school math, 3 years of high school science, high school foreign language, interview, 3 letters of recommendation, health exam. *Application deadlines:* 5/1 (fall), 9/15 (spring).

Degree Requirements 120 total credit hours, 61 in nursing.

RN Baccalaureate Program (BS)

Applying *Required:* minimum college GPA of 2.5, interview, 3 letters of recommendation. *Application deadlines:* 5/1 (fall), 9/15 (spring).

Degree Requirements 120 total credit hours, 61 in nursing.

FLORIDA ATLANTIC UNIVERSITY
College of Nursing
Boca Raton, Florida

Programs • Generic Baccalaureate • RN Baccalaureate • MSN • Master's for Nurses with Non-Nursing Degrees

The University State-supported coed university. Part of State University System of Florida. Founded: 1961. *Primary accreditation:* regional. *Setting:* 850-acre suburban campus. *Total enrollment:* 17,843.

The College of Nursing Founded in 1979. *Nursing program faculty:* 19 (89% with doctorates). *Off-campus program sites:* Port St. Lucie, Palm Beach, Davie.

Academic Facilities *Campus library:* 592,131 volumes (14,025 in health, 1,800 in nursing); 4,079 periodical subscriptions (237 health-care related). *Nursing school resources:* CAI, computer lab, nursing audiovisuals, interactive nursing skills videos, learning resource lab.

Student Life *Student services:* health clinic, child-care facilities, personal counseling, career counseling, institutionally sponsored work-study program, job placement, campus safety program, special assistance for disabled students. *International student services:* counseling/support, special assistance for nonnative speakers of English, ESL courses. *Nursing student activities:* Sigma Theta Tau, student nurses association.

Calendar Semesters.

NURSING STUDENT PROFILE

Undergraduate **Enrollment:** 210
Women: 88%; **Men:** 12%; **Minority:** 18%; **Part-time:** 12%
Graduate **Enrollment:** 117
Women: 99%; **Men:** 1%; **Minority:** 1%; **Part-time:** 99%

BACCALAUREATE PROGRAMS

Contact Dr. Rozzano Locsin, Undergraduate Program Coordinator and Associate Professor, College of Nursing, Florida Atlantic University, 777 Glades Road, Boca Raton, FL 33431, 561-367-2875. *Fax:* 561-367-3652. *E-mail:* locsin@acc.fau.edu

Expenses *State resident tuition:* $845 full-time, $423 per academic year part-time. *Nonresident tuition:* $4428 full-time, $2214 per academic year part-time. *Full-time mandatory fees:* $20. *Books and supplies per academic year:* ranges from $400 to $500.

Financial Aid Institutionally sponsored need-based grants/scholarships, institutionally sponsored non-need grants/scholarships. 45% of undergraduate students in nursing programs received some form of financial aid in 1995–96. *Application deadline:* 4/1.

Generic Baccalaureate Program (BSN)

Applying *Required:* SAT I, ACT, TOEFL for nonnative speakers of English, minimum high school GPA of 3.0, minimum college GPA of 2.75, 3 years of high school math, 3 years of high school science, high school biology, high school foreign language, high school transcript, transcript of college record. 60 prerequisite credits must be completed before admission to the nursing program. *Options:* May apply for transfer of up to 60 total credits. *Application deadlines:* 3/15 (fall), 11/1 (spring). *Application fee:* $25.

Degree Requirements 120 total credit hours, 48 in nursing.

Distance learning Courses provided through video, audio.

RN Baccalaureate Program (BSN)

Applying *Required:* TOEFL for nonnative speakers of English, minimum college GPA of 2.5, RN license, diploma or AD in nursing, transcript of college record, CPR certification, physical exam. 60 prerequisite credits must be completed before admission to the nursing program. *Options:* May apply for transfer of up to 60 total credits. *Application deadlines:* 3/15 (fall), 11/1 (spring). *Application fee:* $25.

Degree Requirements 120 total credit hours, 30 in nursing.

Distance learning Courses provided through video, audio.

Florida Atlantic University (continued)

MASTER'S PROGRAMS

Contact Dr. Edward Freeman, Associate Professor and Graduate Program Coordinator, College of Nursing, Florida Atlantic University, 777 Glades Road, Boca Raton, FL 33431, 561-367-3384. *Fax:* 561-367-3687. *E-mail:* efreeman@acc.fau.edu

Areas of Study Nursing administration; nurse practitioner programs in adult health, family health.

Expenses *State resident tuition:* $2846 full-time, $2135 per year part-time. *Nonresident tuition:* $9336 full-time, $7002 per year part-time. *Full-time mandatory fees:* $150–$200. *Part-time mandatory fees:* $150–$200. *Books and supplies per academic year:* ranges from $400 to $500.

Financial Aid Graduate assistantships, nurse traineeships. *Application deadline:* 4/1.

MSN Program

Applying *Required:* GRE General Test, bachelor's degree in nursing, minimum GPA of 3.0, RN license, physical assessment course, statistics course, professional liability/malpractice insurance, essay, 2 letters of recommendation, transcript of college record. *Application deadlines:* 6/1 (fall), 11/1 (spring), 3/15 (summer). *Application fee:* $20.

Degree Requirements 35–49 total credit hours dependent upon track, 32–43 in nursing, 3–6 in other specified areas. Thesis or project for nurse practitioner track.

Master's for Nurses with Non-Nursing Degrees Program (MSN)

Applying *Required:* GRE General Test, bachelor's degree, minimum GPA of 3.0, RN license, physical assessment course, statistics course, professional liability/malpractice insurance, 2 letters of recommendation, transcript of college record. *Application deadlines:* 6/1 (fall), 11/1 (spring), 3/15 (summer). *Application fee:* $20.

Degree Requirements 35–49 total credit hours dependent upon track, 32–43 in nursing, 3–6 in other specified areas. Thesis or project.

FLORIDA INTERNATIONAL UNIVERSITY

School of Nursing
North Miami, Florida

Programs • Generic Baccalaureate • RN Baccalaureate • MSN

The University State-supported coed university. Part of State University System of Florida. Founded: 1965. *Primary accreditation:* regional. *Setting:* 544-acre urban campus. *Total enrollment:* 23,303.

The School of Nursing Founded in 1982. *Nursing program faculty:* 42 (70% with doctorates).

Academic Facilities *Nursing school resources:* CAI, computer lab, nursing audiovisuals, learning resource lab.

Student Life *Student services:* health clinic, child-care facilities, personal counseling, career counseling, institutionally sponsored work-study program, job placement, special assistance for disabled students. *International student services:* counseling/support. *Nursing student activities:* National Student Nurses Association, Nursing Honor Society.

Calendar Semesters.

NURSING STUDENT PROFILE

Undergraduate **Enrollment:** 348

Graduate **Enrollment:** 70

BACCALAUREATE PROGRAMS

Contact Mrs. Rosa Thornton, Academic Adviser, School of Nursing, Florida International University, North Campus, 151st Street at Biscayne Boulevard, North Miami, FL 33181, 305-940-5915. *Fax:* 305-919-5395.

Expenses *State resident tuition:* $1814 full-time, $59 per credit hour part-time. *Nonresident tuition:* $7196 full-time, $234 per credit hour part-time. *Full-time mandatory fees:* $46. *Part-time mandatory fees:* $46.

Financial Aid Federal Pell Grants, Federal Work-Study. 75% of undergraduate students in nursing programs received some form of financial aid in 1995–96.

Generic Baccalaureate Program (BSN)

Applying *Required:* SAT I or ACT, minimum college GPA of 3.0, high school foreign language, high school transcript, written essay, transcript of college record. 60 prerequisite credits must be completed before admission to the nursing program. *Options:* Advanced standing available through advanced placement exams. May apply for transfer of up to 60 total credits. *Application deadline:* rolling.

Degree Requirements 123 total credit hours, 63 in nursing.

RN Baccalaureate Program (BSN)

Applying *Required:* minimum college GPA of 2.5, RN license, diploma or AD in nursing, high school transcript, written essay, transcript of college record. *Options:* Advanced standing available through credit by exam. *Application deadline:* rolling.

Degree Requirements 123 total credit hours.

MASTER'S PROGRAM

Contact Dr. Divina Grossman, Department Chair, School of Nursing, Florida International University, North Campus, 151st Street at Biscayne Boulevard, North Miami, FL 33181, 305-940-5915. *Fax:* 305-956-5395.

Areas of Study Nursing administration; nursing education; nurse practitioner programs in adult health, child care/pediatrics, psychiatric–mental health.

Expenses *State resident tuition:* $2415 full-time, $115 per credit part-time. *Nonresident tuition:* $8064 full-time, $384 per credit part-time. *Full-time mandatory fees:* $46. *Part-time mandatory fees:* $46.

Financial Aid Nurse traineeships.

MSN Program

Applying *Required:* GRE General Test, TOEFL for nonnative speakers of English, bachelor's degree in nursing, minimum GPA of 3.0, RN license, 1 year of clinical experience, physical assessment course, statistics course, essay, interview, 3 letters of recommendation, transcript of college record, computer literacy. *Application deadline:* rolling.

Degree Requirements 42 total credit hours, 39 in nursing. Paper or thesis.

FLORIDA STATE UNIVERSITY

School of Nursing
Tallahassee, Florida

Programs • Generic Baccalaureate • RN Baccalaureate • MSN • RN to Master's • Post-Master's • Continuing Education

The University State-supported coed university. Part of State University System of Florida. Founded: 1857. *Primary accreditation:* regional. *Setting:* 451-acre suburban campus. *Total enrollment:* 30,268.

The School of Nursing Founded in 1950. *Nursing program faculty:* 45 (36% with doctorates). *Off-campus program site:* Panama City.

Academic Facilities *Campus library:* 1.9 million volumes (220,248 in nursing). *Nursing school resources:* CAI, computer lab, nursing audiovisuals, interactive nursing skills videos, learning resource lab, satellite television.

Student Life *Student services:* health clinic, child-care facilities, personal counseling, career counseling, institutionally sponsored work-study program, job placement, campus safety program, special assistance for disabled students. *International student services:* counseling/support, special assistance for nonnative speakers of English, ESL courses. *Nursing student activities:* Sigma Theta Tau, student nurses association.

Calendar Semesters, One summer semester required.

NURSING STUDENT PROFILE

Undergraduate **Enrollment:** 258

Women: 83%; **Men:** 17%; **Minority:** 14%; **International:** 0%; **Part-time:** 2%

Graduate **Enrollment:** 89

Women: 90%; **Men:** 10%; **Minority:** 16%; **International:** 0%; **Part-time:** 80%

BACCALAUREATE PROGRAMS

Contact Ms. Mary Lee Kight, Academic Adviser, School of Nursing, Florida State University, Tallahassee, FL 32306-3051, 904-644-5107. *Fax:* 904-644-7660. *E-mail:* mlkight@mailer.fsu.edu

Expenses *State resident tuition:* $1800 full-time, $60 per semester hour part-time. *Nonresident tuition:* $6700 full-time, $223 per semester hour part-time. *Full-time mandatory fees:* $128–$141. *Room and board:* $4720. *Room only:* $2080. *Books and supplies per academic year:* $700.

Financial Aid *Application deadline:* 3/10.

Generic Baccalaureate Program (BSN)

Applying *Required:* minimum college GPA of 2.7, high school foreign language, high school transcript, transcript of college record, minimum 2.5 GPA in science courses, questionnaire accompanying application. 62 prerequisite credits must be completed before admission to the nursing program. *Application deadlines:* 5/20 (fall), 11/1 (spring). *Application fee:* $20.

Degree Requirements 124 total credit hours, 64 in nursing.

RN Baccalaureate Program (BSN)

Applying *Required:* NLN Mobility Profile II, minimum college GPA of 2.7, RN license, high school foreign language, high school transcript, transcript of college record, minimum 2.5 GPA in science courses, questionnaire accompanying nursing application. 88 prerequisite credits must be completed before admission to the nursing program. *Options:* Course work may be accelerated. May apply for transfer of up to 90 total credits. *Application deadlines:* 5/20 (fall), 11/1 (spring). *Application fee:* $20.

Degree Requirements 120 total credit hours, 60 in nursing.

MASTER'S PROGRAMS

Contact Dr. Deborah Frank, Graduate Program Director, School of Nursing, Florida State University, Tallahassee, FL 32306-3051, 904-644-5974. *Fax:* 904-644-7660.

Areas of Study Nurse practitioner programs in acute care, adult health, child care/pediatrics, family health, gerontology, primary care, women's health.

Expenses *State resident tuition:* $2957 full-time, $118 per semester hour part-time. *Nonresident tuition:* $9726 full-time, $389 per semester hour part-time. *Full-time mandatory fees:* $128–$141. *Books and supplies per academic year:* ranges from $300 to $500.

Financial Aid Graduate assistantships, nurse traineeships, Federal Nursing Student Loans, institutionally sponsored loans, employment opportunities. *Application deadline:* 4/15.

MSN Program

Applying *Required:* TOEFL for nonnative speakers of English, GRE General Test (minimum combined score of 1000 on verbal and quantitative sections), bachelor's degree in nursing, minimum GPA of 3.0, RN license, 2 years of clinical experience, statistics course, 3 letters of recommendation, transcript of college record. *Application deadlines:* 7/13 (fall), 11/15 (spring). *Application fee:* $20.

Degree Requirements 45 total credit hours, 38 in nursing. Thesis required.

RN to Master's Program (MSN)

Applying *Required:* GRE General Test (minimum combined score of 1000 on three tests), minimum GPA of 3.0, RN license, 2 years of clinical experience, transcript of college record. *Application deadlines:* 5/20 (fall), 10/1 (spring). *Application fee:* $20.

Degree Requirements 158 total credit hours, 100 in nursing. Thesis required.

Post-Master's Program

Applying *Required:* GRE General Test (minimum combined score of 1000 on verbal and quantitative sections), minimum GPA of 3.0, RN license, 2 years of clinical experience, statistics course, professional liability/malpractice insurance, 3 letters of recommendation, transcript of college record. *Application deadlines:* 7/13 (fall), 11/15 (spring). *Application fee:* $20.

Degree Requirements 25 total credit hours, 25 in nursing.

CONTINUING EDUCATION PROGRAM

Contact Dr. Evelyn T. Singer, Dean, School of Nursing, Florida State University, Tallahassee, FL 32306-3051, 904-644-3299. *Fax:* 904-644-7660.

JACKSONVILLE UNIVERSITY
School of Nursing
Jacksonville, Florida

Programs • Generic Baccalaureate • RN Baccalaureate

The University Independent comprehensive coed institution. Founded: 1934. *Primary accreditation:* regional. *Setting:* 260-acre suburban campus. *Total enrollment:* 2,416.

The School of Nursing Founded in 1982. *Nursing program faculty:* 15 (27% with doctorates).

Academic Facilities *Campus library:* 176,849 volumes (3,000 in health, 300 in nursing); 750 periodical subscriptions (46 health-care related). *Nursing school resources:* CAI, computer lab, nursing audiovisuals, interactive nursing skills videos, learning resource lab.

Student Life *Student services:* health clinic, personal counseling, career counseling, institutionally sponsored work-study program, job placement, campus safety program, special assistance for disabled students. *International student services:* counseling/support, special assistance for nonnative speakers of English, ESL courses. *Nursing student activities:* Sigma Theta Tau, student nurses association.

Calendar Semesters.

NURSING STUDENT PROFILE	
Undergraduate	Enrollment: 140
Women: 73%; Men: 27%; Minority: 14%; International: 2%; Part-time: 20%	

BACCALAUREATE PROGRAMS

Contact Dr. Linda Miller, Director, School of Nursing, Jacksonville University, 2800 University Boulevard North, Jacksonville, FL 32211, 904-745-7280. *Fax:* 904-745-7287. *E-mail:* lmiller@junix.ju.edu

Expenses *Tuition:* $12,000 full-time, $165 per credit hour part-time. *Full-time mandatory fees:* $200. *Room and board:* $4230–$4598. *Room only:* $2190. *Books and supplies per academic year:* ranges from $450 to $500.

Financial Aid Institutionally sponsored need-based grants/scholarships, institutionally sponsored non-need grants/scholarships, Federal Pell Grants, Federal Supplemental Educational Opportunity Grants, Federal Work-Study. 93% of undergraduate students in nursing programs received some form of financial aid in 1995–96.

Generic Baccalaureate Program (BSN)

Applying *Required:* SAT I, ACT, minimum college GPA of 2.5, interview, 3 letters of recommendation, written essay, transcript of college record. 28 prerequisite credits must be completed before admission to the nursing program. *Options:* May apply for transfer of up to 64 total credits. *Application deadline:* 4/30. *Application fee:* $25.

Degree Requirements 133 total credit hours, 70 in nursing.

RN Baccalaureate Program (BSN)

Applying *Required:* minimum college GPA of 2.5, RN license, interview, 3 letters of recommendation, written essay, transcript of college record. *Options:* May apply for transfer of up to 64 total credits. *Application deadline:* rolling. *Application fee:* $25.

Degree Requirements 128 total credit hours, 64 in nursing.

UNIVERSITY OF CENTRAL FLORIDA
School of Nursing
Orlando, Florida

Programs • Generic Baccalaureate • RN Baccalaureate • Baccalaureate for Second Degree • BSN to Master's

The University State-supported coed university. Part of State University System of Florida. Founded: 1963. *Primary accreditation:* regional. *Setting:* 1,445-acre suburban campus. *Total enrollment:* 26,174.

The School of Nursing Founded in 1980. *Nursing program faculty:* 35 (52% with doctorates). *Off-campus program sites:* Cocoa Beach, Daytona Beach.

Academic Facilities *Campus library:* 897,500 volumes (5,000 in health, 3,780 in nursing); 5,000 periodical subscriptions (300 health-care related). *Nursing school resources:* CAI, computer lab, nursing audiovisuals, interactive nursing skills videos, learning resource lab, clinical skills lab.

Student Life *Student services:* health clinic, child-care facilities, personal counseling, career counseling, institutionally sponsored work-study program, job placement, campus safety program, special assistance for disabled students, wellness center. *International student services:* counseling/

University of Central Florida (continued)
support, special assistance for nonnative speakers of English, ESL courses, student center. *Nursing student activities:* Sigma Theta Tau, nursing club, student nurses association.

Calendar Semesters.

NURSING STUDENT PROFILE

Undergraduate **Enrollment:** 178
Women: 89%; **Men:** 11%; **Minority:** 11%; **International:** 0%; **Part-time:** 34%
Graduate **Enrollment:** 50
Women: 95%; **Men:** 5%; **Minority:** 6%; **International:** 0%; **Part-time:** 25%

BACCALAUREATE PROGRAMS

Contact Dr. Elizabeth Stullenbarger, Director, School of Nursing, University of Central Florida, PO Box 162210, Orlando, FL 32816-2210, 407-823-2744. *Fax:* 407-823-5675.

Expenses *State resident tuition:* $915 full-time, $61 per credit hour part-time. *Nonresident tuition:* $3537 full-time, $236 per credit hour part-time. *Full-time mandatory fees:* $94. *Books and supplies per academic year:* $500.

Financial Aid Institutionally sponsored need-based grants/scholarships, institutionally sponsored non-need grants/scholarships, Federal Nursing Student Loans, Federal Supplemental Educational Opportunity Grants, Federal Work-Study. 34% of undergraduate students in nursing programs received some form of financial aid in 1995–96. *Application deadline:* 3/16.

Generic Baccalaureate Program (BSN)

Applying *Required:* SAT I, CLAST, minimum high school GPA of 2.5, minimum college GPA of 2.5, 3 years of high school math, high school foreign language, high school transcript, written essay, transcript of college record. 27 prerequisite credits must be completed before admission to the nursing program. *Options:* May apply for transfer of up to 60 total credits. *Application deadline:* 2/1. *Application fee:* $15.

Degree Requirements 124 total credit hours, 67 in nursing. CLAST.

Distance learning Courses provided through video, computer-based media, on-line.

RN Baccalaureate Program (BSN)

Applying *Required:* minimum high school GPA of 2.5, minimum college GPA of 2.5, 3 years of high school math, 3 years of high school science, RN license, diploma or AD in nursing, high school foreign language, high school transcript, written essay, transcript of college record. 8 prerequisite credits must be completed before admission to the nursing program. *Application deadline:* rolling. *Application fee:* $15.

Degree Requirements 120 total credit hours, 36 in nursing.

Distance learning Courses provided through video, computer-based media, on-line.

Baccalaureate for Second Degree Program (BSN)

Applying *Required:* SAT I, minimum high school GPA of 2.5, minimum college GPA of 2.5, 3 years of high school math, high school foreign language, high school transcript, written essay, transcript of college record. 27 prerequisite credits must be completed before admission to the nursing program. *Options:* May apply for transfer of up to 60 total credits. *Application deadline:* 2/1. *Application fee:* $15.

Degree Requirements 124 total credit hours, 67 in nursing. CLAST.

Distance learning Courses provided through video, computer-based media, on-line.

MASTER'S PROGRAM

Contact Mary Lou Sole, Associate Professor, School of Nursing, University of Central Florida, PO Box 162210, Orlando, FL 32816-2210, 407-823-2744. *E-mail:* msole@pegasus.cc.ucf.edu

Areas of Study Nursing administration; nurse practitioner program in family health.

Expenses *State resident tuition:* $1399 full-time, $117 per credit hour part-time. *Nonresident tuition:* $4647 full-time, $387 per credit hour part-time.

Financial Aid Graduate assistantships, nurse traineeships, fellowships, Federal Nursing Student Loans, employment opportunities. 30% of master's level students in nursing programs received some form of financial aid in 1995-96. *Application deadline:* 3/16.

BSN to Master's Program (MSN)

Applying *Required:* GRE General Test, TOEFL for nonnative speakers of English, bachelor's degree in nursing, minimum GPA of 3.0, RN license, 1 year of clinical experience, statistics course, 2 letters of recommendation, transcript of college record. *Application deadline:* 2/1. *Application fee:* $25.

Degree Requirements 36–43 total credit hours dependent upon track, 30–43 in nursing, 6 in health services administration course for nursing administration track. Thesis or culminating project.

UNIVERSITY OF FLORIDA
College of Nursing
Gainesville, Florida

Programs • Generic Baccalaureate • RN Baccalaureate • MN • MSN • Master's for Nurses with Non-Nursing Degrees • Post-Master's • Doctorate in Nursing Sciences

The University State-supported coed university. Part of State University System of Florida. Founded: 1853. *Primary accreditation:* regional. *Setting:* 2,000-acre suburban campus. *Total enrollment:* 39,439.

The College of Nursing Founded in 1956. *Nursing program faculty:* 68 (54% with doctorates). *Off-campus program sites:* Jacksonville, Orlando.

Academic Facilities *Campus library:* 3.1 million volumes (259,318 in health, 2,916 in nursing); 3,510 periodical subscriptions (51 health-care related). *Nursing school resources:* CAI, computer lab, nursing audiovisuals, interactive nursing skills videos, learning resource lab.

Student Life *Student services:* health clinic, personal counseling, career counseling, institutionally sponsored work-study program, job placement, campus safety program, special assistance for disabled students. *International student services:* counseling/support, special assistance for nonnative speakers of English, ESL courses. *Nursing student activities:* Sigma Theta Tau, student nurses association.

Calendar Semesters.

NURSING STUDENT PROFILE

Undergraduate **Enrollment:** 293
Women: 86%; **Men:** 14%; **Minority:** 12%; **International:** 0%; **Part-time:** 9%
Graduate **Enrollment:** 318
Women: 96%; **Men:** 4%; **Minority:** 10%; **International:** 1%; **Part-time:** 84%

BACCALAUREATE PROGRAMS

Contact Ms. Patricia M. Bivens, Admissions Officer and Registrar, J.H. Miller Health Center, College of Nursing, University of Florida, PO Box 100197, Gainesville, FL 32610-0197, 352-392-3518. *Fax:* 352-392-8100.

Expenses *State resident tuition:* $1790 per academic year. *Nonresident tuition:* $7040 per academic year. *Full-time mandatory fees:* $57–$213. *Room and board:* $4080–$4710. *Room only:* $1890–$2520. *Books and supplies per academic year:* $600.

Financial Aid Institutionally sponsored need-based grants/scholarships, institutionally sponsored non-need grants/scholarships, Federal Nursing Student Loans. *Application deadline:* 8/1.

Generic Baccalaureate Program (BSN)

Applying *Required:* SAT I, TOEFL for nonnative speakers of English, minimum college GPA of 2.8, high school foreign language, high school transcript, transcript of college record. 64 prerequisite credits must be completed before admission to the nursing program. *Options:* May apply for transfer of up to 64 total credits. *Application deadlines:* 2/1 (fall), 10/1 (spring), 1/31 (summer). *Application fee:* $20.

Degree Requirements 124 total credit hours, 64 in nursing.

RN Baccalaureate Program (BSN)

Applying *Required:* SAT I, CLAST, minimum college GPA of 2.8, RN license, diploma or AD in nursing, high school foreign language, high school transcript, transcript of college record. 64 prerequisite credits must be completed before admission to the nursing program. *Options:* Course work may be accelerated. May apply for transfer of up to 64 total credits. *Application deadlines:* 6/10 (fall), 11/1 (spring), 3/1 (summer). *Application fee:* $20.

Degree Requirements 124 total credit hours, 64 in nursing.

MASTER'S PROGRAMS

Contact Ms. Patricia M. Bivens, Admissions Officer and Registrar, J.H. Miller Health Center, College of Nursing, University of Florida, PO Box 100197, Gainesville, FL 32610-0197, 352-392-3518. *Fax:* 352-392-8100.

Areas of Study Clinical nurse specialist programs in adult health nursing, community health nursing, critical care nursing, family health nursing, gerontological nursing, maternity-newborn nursing, oncology nursing, pediatric nursing, psychiatric–mental health nursing, women's health nursing; nurse midwifery; nursing administration; nurse practitioner programs in child care/pediatrics, family health, gerontology.

Expenses *State resident tuition:* $2770 per academic year. *Nonresident tuition:* $9270 per academic year. *Full-time mandatory fees:* $109–$350. *Room and board:* $4080–$4710. *Room only:* $1890–$2520. *Books and supplies per academic year:* $600.

Financial Aid Graduate assistantships, nurse traineeships, Federal Nursing Student Loans, institutionally sponsored loans, employment opportunities. *Application deadline:* 8/1.

MN Program

Applying *Required:* GRE General Test, bachelor's degree in nursing, minimum GPA of 3.0, RN license, 1 year of clinical experience, physical assessment course, statistics course, professional liability/malpractice insurance, 2 letters of recommendation, transcript of college record. *Application deadlines:* 6/10 (fall), 11/1 (spring), 3/1 (summer). *Application fee:* $20.

Degree Requirements 48 total credit hours, 40 in nursing, 8 in support courses. Project.

MSN Program

Applying *Required:* GRE General Test, bachelor's degree in nursing, minimum GPA of 3.0, RN license, 1 year of clinical experience, physical assessment course, statistics course, professional liability/malpractice insurance, 2 letters of recommendation, transcript of college record. *Application deadlines:* 6/10 (fall), 11/1 (spring), 3/1 (summer). *Application fee:* $20.

Degree Requirements 48 total credit hours, 40 in nursing, 8 in support courses. Thesis required.

Master's for Nurses with Non-Nursing Degrees Program (MSN)

Applying *Required:* GRE General Test, minimum GPA of 3.0, RN license, 1 year of clinical experience, physical assessment course, statistics course, professional liability/malpractice insurance, 2 letters of recommendation, transcript of college record. *Application deadlines:* 6/10 (fall), 11/1 (spring), 3/1 (summer). *Application fee:* $20.

Degree Requirements 48 total credit hours, 40 in nursing, 8 in support courses. Thesis required.

Post-Master's Program

Applying *Required:* GRE General Test (minimum combined score of 1000 on three tests), minimum GPA of 3.0, RN license, 1 year of clinical experience, professional liability/malpractice insurance, interview, 2 letters of recommendation, transcript of college record. *Application deadlines:* 6/1 (fall), 11/1 (spring), 3/1 (summer). *Application fee:* $20.

Degree Requirements 20 total credit hours, 20 in nursing.

DOCTORAL PROGRAM

Contact Ms. Patricia M. Bivens, Admissions Officer and Registrar, J.H. Miller Health Center, College of Nursing, University of Florida, PO Box 100197, Gainesville, FL 32610-0197, 352-392-3518. *Fax:* 352-392-8100.

Areas of Study Nursing research.

Expenses *State resident tuition:* $2770 per academic year. *Nonresident tuition:* $9270 per academic year. *Full-time mandatory fees:* $109–$350. *Room and board:* $4080–$4710. *Room only:* $1890–$2520.

Financial Aid Graduate assistantships, nurse traineeships, fellowships, dissertation grants, grants. *Application deadline:* 8/1.

Doctorate in Nursing Sciences Program (PhD)

Applying *Required:* GRE General Test, master's degree in nursing, 1 year of clinical experience, 1 year in proposed area of specialization, 3 letters of recommendation, vitae, completed course work in research from an NLN-accredited school, statement of professional goals. *Application deadlines:* 6/10 (fall), 11/1 (spring), 3/1 (summer). *Application fee:* $20.

Degree Requirements 90 total credit hours; 9 credit hours of theory, 12 credit hours in research, 3 credit hours of professional practice, 12 credit hours in electives, 12 credit hours in minor, 12 credit hours in dissertation research; dissertation; oral exam; written exam; defense of dissertation; residency.

See full description on page 532.

UNIVERSITY OF MIAMI

School of Nursing
Coral Gables, Florida

Programs • Generic Baccalaureate • Accelerated RN Baccalaureate • Baccalaureate for Second Degree • Master's • Doctoral

The University Independent coed university. Founded: 1925. *Primary accreditation:* regional. *Setting:* 260-acre suburban campus. *Total enrollment:* 13,541.

The School of Nursing Founded in 1948.

Academic Facilities *Campus library:* 1.7 million volumes; 15,849 periodical subscriptions.

Calendar Semesters.

BACCALAUREATE PROGRAMS

Contact Administrative Assistant to the Dean of Student Services, School of Nursing, University of Miami, 5801 Red Road, Coral Gables, FL 33143, 305-284-4096. *Fax:* 305-284-5686.

Expenses *Tuition:* $18,220 full-time, $742 per credit part-time. *Full-time mandatory fees:* $372.

Generic Baccalaureate Program (BSN)

Applying *Required:* SAT I or ACT, written essay. *Options:* Advanced standing available through advanced placement exams.

Degree Requirements 120 total credit hours, 64 in nursing.

Accelerated RN Baccalaureate Program (BSN)

Applying *Required:* minimum college GPA of 2.5.

Degree Requirements 120 total credit hours, 30 in nursing.

Baccalaureate for Second Degree Program (BSN)

Degree Requirements 120 total credit hours, 64 in nursing.

MASTER'S PROGRAMS

Contact Administrative Assistant for Student Admission and Records, School of Nursing, University of Miami, 5801 Red Road, Coral Gables, FL 33143, 305-284-4325. *Fax:* 305-284-5686.

DOCTORAL PROGRAM

Contact Associate Dean, School of Nursing, University of Miami, 5801 Red Road, Coral Gables, FL 33143, 305-284-2904. *Fax:* 305-284-5686.

UNIVERSITY OF NORTH FLORIDA

College of Health, Department of Nursing
Jacksonville, Florida

Programs • Generic Baccalaureate • RN Baccalaureate

The University State-supported comprehensive coed institution. Part of State University System of Florida. Founded: 1965. *Primary accreditation:* regional. *Setting:* 1,000-acre urban campus. *Total enrollment:* 10,463.

The College of Health, Department of Nursing Founded in 1975. *Nursing program faculty:* 14 (50% with doctorates). *Off-campus program site:* Orange Park.

Academic Facilities *Campus library:* 600,000 volumes (60,000 in health, 18,000 in nursing); 3,000 periodical subscriptions (360 health-care related). *Nursing school resources:* CAI, computer lab, nursing audiovisuals, interactive nursing skills videos, learning resource lab.

Student Life *Student services:* health clinic, child-care facilities, personal counseling, career counseling, institutionally sponsored work-study program, job placement, campus safety program, special assistance for

University of North Florida (continued)

disabled students. *International student services:* counseling/support. *Nursing student activities:* Sigma Theta Tau, student nurses association.

Calendar Semesters.

NURSING STUDENT PROFILE

Undergraduate **Enrollment:** 269

Women: 88%; **Men:** 12%; **Minority:** 17%; **International:** 0%; **Part-time:** 44%

BACCALAUREATE PROGRAMS

Contact Ms. Ludella Wilson, Assistant Professor and Academic Adviser, College of Health, Department of Nursing, University of North Florida, 4567 St. Johns Bluff Road South, Jacksonville, FL 32224-2645, 904-646-2812. *Fax:* 904-646-2848. *E-mail:* lwilson@unf.edu

Expenses *State resident tuition:* $1806 full-time, $58 per credit hour part-time. *Nonresident tuition:* $6873 full-time, $222 per credit hour part-time. *Full-time mandatory fees:* $125.

Financial Aid Institutionally sponsored need-based grants/scholarships, institutionally sponsored non-need grants/scholarships, Federal Pell Grants, Federal Perkins Loans, Federal Supplemental Educational Opportunity Grants, Federal Work-Study. *Application deadline:* 4/1.

Generic Baccalaureate Program (BSN)

Applying *Required:* minimum college GPA of 2.5, high school foreign language, interview, transcript of college record, professional liability/malpractice insurance, CPR certification, immunizations. 60 prerequisite credits must be completed before admission to the nursing program. *Options:* May apply for transfer of up to 60 total credits. *Application deadlines:* 4/1 (spring), 1/15 (summer). *Application fee:* $20.

Degree Requirements 124 total credit hours, 64 in nursing.

RN Baccalaureate Program (BSN)

Applying *Required:* minimum college GPA of 2.5, RN license, diploma or AD in nursing, transcript of college record, professional liability/malpractice insurance, CPR certification, immunizations. 60 prerequisite credits must be completed before admission to the nursing program. *Application deadlines:* 7/5 (fall), 11/1 (spring), 3/12 (summer). *Application fee:* $20.

Degree Requirements 124 total credit hours, 64 in nursing.

UNIVERSITY OF SOUTH FLORIDA
College of Nursing
Tampa, Florida

Programs • Generic Baccalaureate • RN Baccalaureate • MS

The University State-supported coed university. Part of State University System of Florida. Founded: 1956. *Primary accreditation:* regional. *Setting:* 1,695-acre suburban campus. *Total enrollment:* 36,146.

The College of Nursing Founded in 1973. *Nursing program faculty:* 37 (78% with doctorates). *Off-campus program sites:* Ft. Myers, Sarasota, St. Petersberg.

▶ *NOTEWORTHY*

The College of Nursing at the University of South Florida is an active participant in the Health Sciences Center, the academic campus, and the Tampa Bay community. Established in 1973, the College of Nursing offers NLN-accredited programs for basic and RN students at the baccalaureate level and 6 concentration areas at the master's level. Approximately 80% of the nursing faculty members hold doctoral degrees. Students in the College of Nursing benefit from the resources of a research university that serves more than 36,000 students as well as from the culturally diverse opportunities in the Tampa Bay area.

Academic Facilities *Campus library:* 859,472 volumes (106,028 in health, 3,898 in nursing); 1,581 periodical subscriptions (1,581 health-care related). *Nursing school resources:* CAI, computer lab, nursing audiovisuals, interactive nursing skills videos, learning resource lab.

Student Life *Student services:* health clinic, child-care facilities, personal counseling, career counseling, job placement, campus safety program, special assistance for disabled students. *International student services:* counseling/support. *Nursing student activities:* Sigma Theta Tau, student nurses association.

Calendar Semesters.

NURSING STUDENT PROFILE

Undergraduate **Enrollment:** 304

Women: 87%; **Men:** 13%; **Minority:** 30%; **Part-time:** 40%

Graduate **Enrollment:** 239

Women: 95%; **Men:** 5%; **Minority:** 10%; **International:** 1%; **Part-time:** 63%

BACCALAUREATE PROGRAMS

Contact Dr. Lois Lowry, Associate Dean for Undergraduate Studies, College of Nursing, University of South Florida, 12901 Bruce B. Downs Boulevard, MDC Box 22, Tampa, FL 33612-4799, 813-974-2191. *Fax:* 813-974-5418.

Expenses *State resident tuition:* $3644 full-time, $65 per credit hour part-time. *Nonresident tuition:* $5764 full-time, $240 per credit hour part-time. *Room only:* $1003. *Books and supplies per academic year:* ranges from $300 to $500.

Financial Aid Institutionally sponsored need-based grants/scholarships, institutionally sponsored non-need grants/scholarships, Federal Direct Loans, Federal Pell Grants, Federal Perkins Loans.

Generic Baccalaureate Program (BS)

Applying *Required:* SAT I, ACT, TOEFL for nonnative speakers of English, minimum high school GPA of 3.0, minimum college GPA of 2.5, 3 years of high school math, 3 years of high school science, high school foreign language, transcript of college record, computer literacy. 60 prerequisite credits must be completed before admission to the nursing program. *Options:* Course work may be accelerated. May apply for transfer of up to 90 total credits. *Application deadline:* 1/1.

Degree Requirements 124 total credit hours, 61 in nursing.

RN Baccalaureate Program (BS)

Applying *Required:* SAT I, ACT, TOEFL for nonnative speakers of English, minimum high school GPA of 3.0, minimum college GPA of 2.5, 3 years of high school math, 3 years of high school science, RN license, diploma or AD in nursing, high school foreign language, transcript of college record, computer literacy. 60 prerequisite credits must be completed before admission to the nursing program. *Options:* Advanced standing available through credit by exam. Course work may be accelerated. May apply for transfer of up to 90 total credits. *Application deadlines:* 1/1 (fall), 9/1 (spring).

Degree Requirements 124 total credit hours, 61 in nursing.

MASTER'S PROGRAM

Contact Dr. Linda Moody, Associate Dean for Graduate Studies, College of Nursing, University of South Florida, 12901 Bruce B. Downs Boulevard, MDC Box 22, Tampa, FL 33612-4799, 813-974-2191. *Fax:* 813-974-5418.

Areas of Study Clinical nurse specialist programs in adult health nursing, community health nursing, critical care nursing, family health nursing, gerontological nursing, oncology nursing, pediatric nursing, psychiatric–mental health nursing; nurse practitioner programs in acute care, adult health, child care/pediatrics, family health, gerontology.

Expenses *State resident tuition:* $2176 full-time, $121 per credit hour part-time. *Nonresident tuition:* $7050 full-time, $392 per credit hour part-time. *Books and supplies per academic year:* $300.

Financial Aid Graduate assistantships, nurse traineeships, institutionally sponsored need-based grants/scholarships, institutionally sponsored non-need-based grants/scholarships. *Application deadline:* 8/25.

MS Program

Applying *Required:* GRE General Test, TOEFL for nonnative speakers of English, bachelor's degree in nursing, minimum GPA of 3.0, RN license, physical assessment course, statistics course, essay, interview, 3 letters of recommendation, transcript of college record. *Application deadlines:* 4/1 (fall), 9/1 (spring). *Application fee:* $20.

Degree Requirements 44 total credit hours, 38 in nursing, 3–6 in other specified areas.

THE UNIVERSITY OF TAMPA
Nursing Department
Tampa, Florida

Programs • RN Baccalaureate • BSN to Master's • Master's for Nurses with Non-Nursing Degrees

The University Independent comprehensive coed institution. Founded: 1931. *Primary accreditation:* regional. *Setting:* 69-acre urban campus. *Total enrollment:* 2,529.

The Nursing Department Founded in 1982.

Academic Facilities *Campus library:* 222,425 volumes (8,000 in health, 5,000 in nursing); 1,883 periodical subscriptions (100 health-care related).

Calendar Semesters.

BACCALAUREATE PROGRAM

Contact Director and Chair, Nursing Department, University of Tampa, 401 West Kennedy Boulevard, Tampa, FL 33606-1490, 813-253-6223. *Fax:* 813-258-7426.

Expenses *Tuition:* $6710 full-time, $285 per credit hour part-time. *Full-time mandatory fees:* $356. *Room and board:* $2205–$2925. *Room only:* $990–$1595.

RN Baccalaureate Program (BSN)

Applying *Required:* minimum college GPA of 2.0, RN license. *Options:* May apply for transfer of up to 64 total credits.

Degree Requirements 124 total credit hours.

MASTER'S PROGRAMS

Expenses *Tuition:* $295 per credit hour.

BSN to Master's Program (MSN)

Applying *Required:* GRE General Test, score of 1000 or higher on both verbal and quantitative sections, minimum GPA of 3.0, RN license, interview, 2 letters of recommendation, evidence of computer literacy. *Application fee:* $35.

Degree Requirements 37+ total credit hours dependent upon track.

Master's for Nurses with Non-Nursing Degrees Program (MSN)

Applying *Required:* GRE General Test, score of 1000 or higher on both verbal and quantitative sections, minimum GPA of 3.0, RN license, interview, 2 letters of recommendation, evidence of computer literacy. *Application fee:* $35.

Degree Requirements 37+ total credit hours dependent upon track.

UNIVERSITY OF WEST FLORIDA
Department of Nursing
Pensacola, Florida

Program • RN Baccalaureate

The University State-supported comprehensive coed institution. Part of State University System of Florida. Founded: 1963. *Primary accreditation:* regional. *Setting:* 1,000-acre suburban campus. *Total enrollment:* 8,000.

The Department of Nursing Founded in 1975. *Nursing program faculty:* 5 (20% with doctorates). *Off-campus program site:* Fort Walton Beach.

Academic Facilities *Campus library:* 559,000 volumes (20,000 in health, 4,500 in nursing); 3,470 periodical subscriptions (200 health-care related). *Nursing school resources:* CAI, computer lab, nursing audiovisuals, learning resource lab.

Student Life *Student services:* health clinic, child-care facilities, personal counseling, career counseling, institutionally sponsored work-study program, job placement, campus safety program, special assistance for disabled students. *International student services:* counseling/support, special assistance for nonnative speakers of English, ESL courses. *Nursing student activities:* student nurses association.

Calendar Semesters.

NURSING STUDENT PROFILE	
Undergraduate	Enrollment: 90
Women: 95%; Men: 5%; Minority: 10%; International: 2%; Part-time: 98%	

BACCALAUREATE PROGRAM

Contact Dr. Marilyn L. Lamborn, RN, Chairperson, Department of Nursing, University of West Florida, 11000 University Parkway, Pensacola, FL 32514-5751, 904-474-2884. *Fax:* 904-474-3128. *E-mail:* mlamborn@uwf.cc.uwf.edu

Expenses *State resident tuition:* $1455 full-time, $61 per semester part-time. *Nonresident tuition:* $5652 full-time, $235 per semester part-time. *Full-time mandatory fees:* $100–$300. *Part-time mandatory fees:* $50–$100. *Books and supplies per academic year:* ranges from $250 to $500.

Financial Aid Institutionally sponsored non-need grants/scholarships, Federal Perkins Loans, Federal Supplemental Educational Opportunity Grants, Federal Work-Study. 56% of undergraduate students in nursing programs received some form of financial aid in 1995–96. *Application deadline:* 4/1.

RN Baccalaureate Program (BSN)

Applying *Required:* SAT I, TOEFL for nonnative speakers of English, minimum high school GPA of 2.0, minimum college GPA of 2.0, RN license, diploma or AD in nursing, high school transcript, transcript of college record, new graduates with diploma or ADN must take boards at first offering. 65 prerequisite credits must be completed before admission to the nursing program. *Options:* May apply for transfer of up to 20 total credits. *Application deadlines:* 6/30 (fall), 12/1 (spring), 3/11 (summer). *Application fee:* $20.

Degree Requirements 120 total credit hours, 36 in nursing.

GEORGIA

ALBANY STATE COLLEGE
School of Nursing and Allied Health
Albany, Georgia

Programs • Generic Baccalaureate • RN Baccalaureate • MS

The College State-supported comprehensive coed institution. Part of University System of Georgia. Founded: 1903. *Primary accreditation:* regional. *Setting:* 131-acre urban campus. *Total enrollment:* 3,151.

The School of Nursing and Allied Health Founded in 1961.

Academic Facilities *Campus library:* 170,000 volumes; 600 periodical subscriptions.

Calendar Quarters.

BACCALAUREATE PROGRAMS

Contact Dean, School of Nursing and Allied Health, Albany State College, Albany, GA 31705, 912-430-4624.

Expenses *State resident tuition:* $1494 full-time, $42 per quarter hour part-time. *Nonresident tuition:* $4704 full-time, $132 per quarter hour part-time. *Full-time mandatory fees:* $405. *Part-time mandatory fees:* $405. *Room and board:* $2610. *Room only:* $1320.

Financial Aid Federal Nursing Student Loans, Federal Pell Grants, Federal Perkins Loans, Federal Supplemental Educational Opportunity Grants, Federal Work-Study, Federal PLUS Loans, Federal Stafford Loans, Federal Supplemental Loans for Students, Georgia Student Incentive Grant. *Application deadline:* 4/15.

Generic Baccalaureate Program (BSN)

Applying *Required:* SAT I or ACT, TOEFL for nonnative speakers of English, Regents exam, minimum college GPA of 3.0, 3 years of high school math, high school transcript, interview, health exam, GED certificate or high school transcript. *Application fee:* $10.

Degree Requirements 194 total credit hours, 31 in nursing. 2.0 overall GPA, 20 credit hours in humanities, 20 in mathematics and natural science, and 20 in social sciences.

Albany State College (continued)

RN Baccalaureate Program (BSN)

Applying *Required:* SAT I or ACT, TOEFL for nonnative speakers of English. *Application fee:* $10.

Degree Requirements 194 total credit hours, 31 in nursing. 2.0 overall GPA, 20 credit hours in humanities, 20 in mathematics and natural science, and 20 in social sciences.

MASTER'S PROGRAM

Contact Coordinator, Graduate Nursing Program, School of Nursing and Allied Health, Albany State College, Albany, GA 31705, 912-430-4727.

Areas of Study Clinical nurse specialist programs in community health nursing, maternity-newborn nursing.

MS Program

Applying *Required:* GRE General Test or Miller Analogies Test, bachelor's degree in nursing, minimum GPA of 2.5.

ARMSTRONG ATLANTIC STATE UNIVERSITY
Division of Nursing
Savannah, Georgia

Programs • Generic Baccalaureate • RN Baccalaureate • MSN

The University State-supported comprehensive coed institution. Part of University System of Georgia. Founded: 1935. *Primary accreditation:* regional. *Setting:* 250-acre suburban campus. *Total enrollment:* 5,348.

The Division of Nursing Founded in 1978. *Nursing program faculty:* 16 (44% with doctorates). *Off-campus program site:* Brunswick.

Academic Facilities *Campus library:* 172,000 volumes (5,649 in health, 1,250 in nursing); 1,188 periodical subscriptions (200 health-care related). *Nursing school resources:* computer lab, nursing audiovisuals.

Student Life *Student services:* career counseling, institutionally sponsored work-study program, job placement, campus safety program, special assistance for disabled students. *Nursing student activities:* Sigma Theta Tau, student nurses association.

Calendar Quarters.

NURSING STUDENT PROFILE

Undergraduate **Enrollment:** 103
Women: 95%; **Men:** 5%; **Minority:** 12%; **International:** 0%; **Part-time:** 0%
Graduate **Enrollment:** 25
Women: 100%; **Minority:** 20%; **International:** 0%; **Part-time:** 100%

BACCALAUREATE PROGRAMS

Contact Dr. Carole M. Massey, Program Coordinator, Baccalaureate Nursing Program, Division of Nursing, Armstrong State College, 11935 Abercorn Street, Savannah, GA 31419-1997, 912-927-5302. *Fax:* 912-921-5585.

Expenses *State resident tuition:* $1719 full-time, $42 per quarter hour part-time. *Nonresident tuition:* $4929 full-time, $132 per quarter hour part-time. *Full-time mandatory fees:* $75. *Room and board:* $3726–$4278. *Books and supplies per academic year:* ranges from $300 to $2000.

Financial Aid Institutionally sponsored need-based grants/scholarships, institutionally sponsored non-need grants/scholarships, Federal Supplemental Educational Opportunity Grants, Federal Work-Study.

Generic Baccalaureate Program (BS)

Applying *Required:* SAT I or ACT, minimum high school GPA of 2.0, minimum college GPA of 2.5, 3 years of high school math, 3 years of high school science, high school foreign language, high school transcript, transcript of college record. 45 prerequisite credits must be completed before admission to the nursing program. *Application deadline:* 12/1. *Application fee:* $10.

Degree Requirements 91 total credit hours, 82 in nursing. Exit exam.

RN Baccalaureate Program (BS)

Applying *Required:* SAT I or ACT, minimum high school GPA of 2.0, minimum college GPA of 2.5, 3 years of high school math, 3 years of high school science, RN license, diploma or AD in nursing, high school foreign language, high school transcript, transcript of college record. 45 prerequisite credits must be completed before admission to the nursing program. *Application deadline:* 12/1. *Application fee:* $10.

Degree Requirements 91 total credit hours, 82 in nursing. Exit exam.

MASTER'S PROGRAM

Contact Dr. Camille P. Stern, Program Coordinator, Graduate Nursing Program, Division of Nursing, Armstrong State College, 11935 Abercorn Street, Savannah, GA 31419-1997, 912-921-5721. *Fax:* 912-921-5585.

Areas of Study Clinical nurse specialist program in adult health nursing; nursing administration.

Expenses *State resident tuition:* $2292 full-time, $53 per quarter hour part-time. *Nonresident tuition:* $6572 full-time, $90 per quarter hour part-time. *Full-time mandatory fees:* $75.

MSN Program

Applying *Required:* GRE General Test, Miller Analogies Test, bachelor's degree in nursing, minimum GPA of 2.5, RN license, 1 year of clinical experience, physical assessment course, statistics course, professional liability/malpractice insurance, 3 letters of recommendation, transcript of college record.

BRENAU UNIVERSITY
Department of Nursing
Gainesville, Georgia

Programs • Generic Baccalaureate • RN Baccalaureate • BSN to Master's

The University Independent comprehensive primarily women's institution. Founded: 1878. *Primary accreditation:* regional. *Setting:* 50-acre small-town campus. *Total enrollment:* 2,225.

The Department of Nursing Founded in 1978. *Nursing program faculty:* 14 (36% with doctorates). *Off-campus program sites:* Atlanta, Athens.

Academic Facilities *Campus library:* 80,000 volumes (6,000 in health, 5,000 in nursing); 1,000 periodical subscriptions (75 health-care related). *Nursing school resources:* CAI, computer lab, nursing audiovisuals, interactive nursing skills videos, learning resource lab.

Student Life *Student services:* health clinic, child-care facilities, personal counseling, career counseling, institutionally sponsored work-study program, job placement, campus safety program, special assistance for disabled students. *International student services:* counseling/support, ESL courses. *Nursing student activities:* Sigma Theta Tau, student nurses association.

Calendar Semesters.

NURSING STUDENT PROFILE

Undergraduate **Enrollment:** 150
Women: 95%; **Men:** 5%; **Minority:** 5%; **International:** 0%; **Part-time:** 10%
Graduate **Enrollment:** 29
Women: 100%; **Minority:** 5%; **International:** 0%; **Part-time:** 100%

BACCALAUREATE PROGRAMS

Contact Dr. John Upchurch, Director of Admissions, Brenau University, One Centennial Circle, Gainesville, GA 30501, 770-534-6100. *Fax:* 770-534-6114.

Expenses *Tuition:* $16,680 full-time, $345 per hour part-time. *Full-time mandatory fees:* $140. *Books and supplies per academic year:* ranges from $200 to $500.

Financial Aid Institutionally sponsored need-based grants/scholarships, institutionally sponsored non-need grants/scholarships, Federal Direct Loans, Federal Nursing Student Loans, Federal Pell Grants, Federal Perkins Loans, Federal Supplemental Educational Opportunity Grants, Federal Work-Study. 100% of undergraduate students in nursing programs received some form of financial aid in 1995–96. *Application deadline:* 4/15.

Generic Baccalaureate Program (BSN)

Applying *Required:* SAT I, ACT, TOEFL for nonnative speakers of English, minimum college GPA of 2.5, high school transcript, transcript of college record. 60 prerequisite credits must be completed before admission to the nursing program. *Application deadline:* rolling. *Application fee:* $30.

Degree Requirements 120 total credit hours, 60 in nursing.

RN Baccalaureate Program (BSN)

Applying *Required:* TOEFL for nonnative speakers of English, minimum college GPA of 2.5, RN license, diploma or AD in nursing, transcript of college record. 60 prerequisite credits must be completed before admission to the nursing program. *Options:* Advanced standing available through credit by exam. *Application deadline:* rolling. *Application fee:* $30.

Degree Requirements 120 total credit hours, 60 in nursing.

MASTER'S PROGRAM

Contact Ms. Cathy Cobb, Graduate Admissions Coordinator, Brenau University, 1 Centennial Circle, Gainesville, GA 30501, 770-534-6162.

Areas of Study Nurse practitioner program in family health.

Expenses *Tuition:* $411 per hour. *Part-time mandatory fees:* $80.

BSN to Master's Program (MS)

Applying *Required:* GRE General Test or Miller Analogies Test, TOEFL for nonnative speakers of English, bachelor's degree in nursing, minimum GPA of 3.0, RN license, 1 year of clinical experience, physical assessment course, statistics course, professional liability/malpractice insurance, essay, 3 letters of recommendation, transcript of college record. *Application deadline:* rolling. *Application fee:* $30.

Degree Requirements 49 total credit hours, 46 in nursing, 3 in pathophysiology.

CLAYTON STATE COLLEGE
School of Health Sciences, Department of Baccalaureate Degree Nursing
Morrow, Georgia

Programs • Generic Baccalaureate • RN Baccalaureate • Accelerated RN Baccalaureate • Continuing Education

The College State-supported 4-year coed college. Part of University System of Georgia. Founded: 1969. *Primary accreditation:* regional. *Setting:* 163-acre suburban campus. *Total enrollment:* 5,020.

The School of Health Sciences, Department of Baccalaureate Degree Nursing Founded in 1987. *Nursing program faculty:* 17 (33% with doctorates). *Off-campus program sites:* Rockdale, Fayette, De Kalb.

Academic Facilities *Campus library:* 75,000 volumes (3,450 in health, 1,800 in nursing); 780 periodical subscriptions (151 health-care related). *Nursing school resources:* CAI, computer lab, nursing audiovisuals, learning resource lab.

Student Life *Student services:* health clinic, personal counseling, career counseling, institutionally sponsored work-study program, job placement, campus safety program, special assistance for disabled students. *International student services:* counseling/support, special assistance for nonnative speakers of English. *Nursing student activities:* Sigma Theta Tau, student nurses association.

Calendar Quarters.

NURSING STUDENT PROFILE

Undergraduate **Enrollment:** 320

Women: 80%; **Men:** 20%; **Minority:** 35%; **International:** 15%; **Part-time:** 80%

BACCALAUREATE PROGRAMS

Contact Dr. Linda F. Samson, Dean, School of Health Sciences, Department of Baccalaureate Nursing, Clayton State College, 5900 North Lee Street, Morrow, GA 30260, 770-961-3484. *Fax:* 770-961-3700. *E-mail:* samson@cc.csc.peachnet.edu

Expenses *State resident tuition:* ranges from $2002 to $2024 full-time, $44 per credit hour part-time. *Nonresident tuition:* ranges from $6916 to $6992 full-time, $152 per credit hour part-time. *Full-time mandatory fees:* $66–$86. *Books and supplies per academic year:* ranges from $100 to $150.

Financial Aid Institutionally sponsored need-based grants/scholarships, institutionally sponsored non-need grants/scholarships, Federal Nursing Student Loans, Federal Work-Study, HOPE Scholarships. *Application deadline:* 2/15.

Generic Baccalaureate Program (BSN)

Applying *Required:* SAT I, TOEFL for nonnative speakers of English, COMPASS test, minimum high school GPA of 2.5, minimum college GPA of 2.5, written essay, transcript of college record, college-prep curriculum. 90 prerequisite credits must be completed before admission to the nursing program. *Options:* Advanced standing available through the following means: advanced placement exams, credit by exam. *Application deadlines:* 2/15 (fall), 10/15 (spring).

Degree Requirements 182 total credit hours, 102 in nursing.

RN Baccalaureate Program (BSN)

Applying *Required:* RN license, diploma or AD in nursing, transcript of college record. *Options:* Course work may be accelerated. May apply for transfer of up to 145 total credits. *Application deadlines:* 8/15 (fall), 2/15 (spring), 6/1 (summer).

Degree Requirements 184 total credit hours, 95 in nursing.

Accelerated RN Baccalaureate Program (BSN)

Applying *Required:* RN license, diploma or AD in nursing, transcript of college record. *Options:* May apply for transfer of up to 145 total credits. *Application deadlines:* 8/15 (fall), 2/15 (spring), 6/1 (summer).

Degree Requirements 184 total credit hours, 111 in nursing.

CONTINUING EDUCATION PROGRAM

Contact Dr. Bryan Edwards, Director, Continuing Education, Clayton State College, PO Box 285, Morrow, GA 30260, 770-961-3550.

See full description on page 426.

COLUMBUS COLLEGE
Department of Nursing
Columbus, Georgia

Programs • Generic Baccalaureate • RN Baccalaureate

The College State-supported comprehensive coed institution. Part of University System of Georgia. Founded: 1958. *Primary accreditation:* regional. *Setting:* 132-acre suburban campus. *Total enrollment:* 5,738.

The Department of Nursing Founded in 1984.

Academic Facilities *Campus library:* 242,294 volumes (34,509 in health, 11,409 in nursing); 1,389 periodical subscriptions (150 health-care related).

Calendar Quarters.

NURSING STUDENT PROFILE

Undergraduate **Enrollment:** 72

Women: 87%; **Men:** 13%; **Minority:** 22%; **International:** 1%; **Part-time:** 1%

BACCALAUREATE PROGRAMS

Contact Admissions Office, Department of Nursing, Columbus College, Columbus, GA 31907-2079, 706-568-2035. *Fax:* 706-569-3101.

Expenses *State resident tuition:* $2460 full-time, $82 per quarter hour part-time. *Nonresident tuition:* $7632 full-time, $190 per quarter hour part-time. *Full-time mandatory fees:* $300–$350.

Financial Aid Institutionally sponsored non-need grants/scholarships, Federal Direct Loans, Federal Perkins Loans, Federal Supplemental Educational Opportunity Grants, Federal Work-Study, state-sponsored loans and scholarships.

Generic Baccalaureate Program (BSN)

Applying *Required:* SAT I or ACT, TOEFL for nonnative speakers of English, minimum college GPA of 2.5, 3 years of high school math, 3 years of high school science, high school foreign language, high school transcript, 3 letters of recommendation, written essay, transcript of college record. *Options:* Advanced standing available through credit by exam. *Application fee:* $20.

Degree Requirements 183 total credit hours.

RN Baccalaureate Program (BSN)

Applying *Required:* SAT I or ACT, TOEFL for nonnative speakers of English, minimum college GPA of 2.5, 3 years of high school math, 3 years of high school science, RN license, diploma or AD in nursing, high school

Columbus College (continued)
foreign language, high school transcript, 3 letters of recommendation, written essay, transcript of college record. *Options:* Advanced standing available through credit by exam. *Application fee:* $20.

Degree Requirements 183 total credit hours.

EMORY UNIVERSITY
Nell Hodgson Woodruff School of Nursing
Atlanta, Georgia

Programs • Generic Baccalaureate • MSN • RN to Master's • MSN/MPH • Post-Master's

The University Independent Methodist coed university. Founded: 1836. *Primary accreditation:* regional. *Setting:* 631-acre suburban campus. *Total enrollment:* 11,308.

The Nell Hodgson Woodruff School of Nursing Founded in 1905. *Nursing program faculty:* 100 (45% with doctorates).

Academic Facilities *Campus library:* 1.5 million volumes (210,813 in health); 15,458 periodical subscriptions. *Nursing school resources:* CAI, computer lab, nursing audiovisuals, interactive nursing skills videos, learning resource lab.

Student Life *Student services:* health clinic, child-care facilities, personal counseling, career counseling, institutionally sponsored work-study program, job placement, campus safety program, special assistance for disabled students. *International student services:* counseling/support, ESL courses. *Nursing student activities:* Sigma Theta Tau, student nurses association.

Calendar Semesters.

NURSING STUDENT PROFILE

Undergraduate **Enrollment:** 239
Women: 92%; **Men:** 8%; **Minority:** 15%; **International:** 13%; **Part-time:** 4%
Graduate **Enrollment:** 220
Women: 94%; **Men:** 6%; **Minority:** 15%; **International:** 2%; **Part-time:** 51%

BACCALAUREATE PROGRAM

Contact Mrs. B. J. Amini, Acting Co-Director, Office of Student Affairs, Nell Hodgson Woodruff School of Nursing, Emory University, 531 Asbury Circle, Atlanta, GA 30322, 404-727-7980. *Fax:* 404-727-0536. *E-mail:* nurswi@nurse.emory.edu

Expenses *Tuition:* $15,970 full-time, $665 per hour part-time. *Full-time mandatory fees:* $230. *Room and board:* $3724–$4024. *Books and supplies per academic year:* $1580.

Financial Aid Institutionally sponsored need-based grants/scholarships, institutionally sponsored non-need grants/scholarships, Federal Nursing Student Loans, Federal Pell Grants, Federal Perkins Loans, Federal Work-Study. *Application deadline:* 2/15.

GENERIC BACCALAUREATE PROGRAM (BSN)

Applying *Required:* TOEFL for nonnative speakers of English, minimum college GPA of 2.5, 3 letters of recommendation, written essay, transcript of college record. 60 prerequisite credits must be completed before admission to the nursing program. *Options:* May apply for transfer of up to 15 total credits. *Application fee:* $35.

Degree Requirements 120 total credit hours, 61 in nursing.

MASTER'S PROGRAMS

Contact Mr. Edward J. Weaver, Co-Director, Office of Student Affairs, Nell Hodgson Woodruff School of Nursing, Emory University, 531 Asbury Circle, Atlanta, GA 30322, 404-727-7980. *Fax:* 404-727-0536. *E-mail:* nurew@nurse.emory.edu

Areas of Study Clinical nurse specialist programs in adult health nursing, critical care nursing, maternity-newborn nursing, medical-surgical nursing, oncology nursing, pediatric nursing, perinatal nursing, psychiatric–mental health nursing; nurse midwifery; nurse practitioner programs in acute care, adult health, child care/pediatrics, family health, gerontology, neonatal health, psychiatric–mental health, oncology.

Expenses *Tuition:* $16,270 full-time, $677 per hour part-time. *Full-time mandatory fees:* $180. *Room and board:* $4658. *Books and supplies per academic year:* $2100.

Financial Aid Graduate assistantships, nurse traineeships, fellowships, Federal Nursing Student Loans, institutionally sponsored loans, employment opportunities, institutionally sponsored need-based grants/scholarships, institutionally sponsored non-need-based grants/scholarships. *Application deadline:* 2/15.

MSN PROGRAM

Applying *Required:* GRE General Test (minimum combined score of 1500 on three tests), Miller Analogies Test, TOEFL for nonnative speakers of English, bachelor's degree in nursing, minimum GPA of 3.0, RN license, 1 year of clinical experience, physical assessment course, statistics course, essay, interview, 3 letters of recommendation, transcript of college record, CPR certification. *Application deadlines:* 4/1 (fall), 2/1 (nurse midwifery and community-based nurse practitioner tracks). *Application fee:* $35.

Degree Requirements 48 total credit hours, 48 in nursing.

RN TO MASTER'S PROGRAM (MSN)

Applying *Required:* GRE General Test or Miller Analogies Test, TOEFL for nonnative speakers of English, minimum GPA of 3.0, RN license, 1 year of clinical experience, physical assessment course, statistics course, professional liability/malpractice insurance, essay, interview, 3 letters of recommendation, transcript of college record, CPR certification. *Application deadlines:* 4/1 (fall), 2/1 (nurse midwifery and community-based nurse practitioner tracks). *Application fee:* $35.

Degree Requirements 71 total credit hours, 71 in nursing.

MSN/MPH PROGRAM

Applying *Required:* GRE General Test, TOEFL for nonnative speakers of English, bachelor's degree in nursing, minimum GPA of 3.0, RN license, 1 year of clinical experience, physical assessment course, statistics course, professional liability/malpractice insurance, essay, interview, 3 letters of recommendation, transcript of college record, CPR certification. *Application deadlines:* 4/1 (fall), 2/1 (nurse midwifery and community-based nurse practitioner tracks). *Application fee:* $35.

Degree Requirements 72 total credit hours, 40 in nursing.

POST-MASTER'S PROGRAM

Applying *Required:* GRE General Test or Miller Analogies Test, TOEFL for nonnative speakers of English, minimum GPA of 3.0, RN license, 1 year of clinical experience, physical assessment course, statistics course, professional liability/malpractice insurance, essay, interview, 3 letters of recommendation, transcript of college record, pathophysiology or advanced physiology course and master's in nursing. *Application deadline:* 11/1. *Application fee:* $35.

Degree Requirements 19–34 total credit hours dependent upon track, 19–34 in nursing.

GEORGIA BAPTIST COLLEGE OF NURSING
Department of Nursing
Atlanta, Georgia

Programs • Generic Baccalaureate • RN Baccalaureate

The College Independent Baptist 4-year specialized women's college. Founded: 1988. *Primary accreditation:* regional. *Setting:* 20-acre urban campus. *Total enrollment:* 374.

The Department of Nursing Founded in 1989. *Nursing program faculty:* 41 (29% with doctorates).

Academic Facilities *Campus library:* 11,000 volumes (3,000 in health, 4,500 in nursing); 160 periodical subscriptions (140 health-care related). *Nursing school resources:* CAI, computer lab, nursing audiovisuals, interactive nursing skills videos, learning resource lab, Internet, Galileo, various CD-ROM resources.

Student Life *Student services:* health clinic, child-care facilities, personal counseling, career counseling, campus safety program, special assistance for disabled students. *International student services:* counseling/support, special assistance for nonnative speakers of English. *Nursing student activities:* recruiter club, nursing club, student nurses association, Nursing Honor Society.

Calendar Quarters.

NURSING STUDENT PROFILE

Undergraduate **Enrollment:** 334
Women: 100%; **Minority:** 15%; **International:** 3%; **Part-time:** 9%

BACCALAUREATE PROGRAMS

Contact Ms. Judy Craven, Director of Admissions, Georgia Baptist College of Nursing, 274 Boulevard, Atlanta, GA 30312, 404-265-4800. *Fax:* 404-265-3811. *E-mail:* gbenadm@mindspring.com

Expenses *Tuition:* $4861 full-time, $125 per quarter hour part-time. *Full-time mandatory fees:* $75–$250. *Room only:* $1134–$1638. *Books and supplies per academic year:* ranges from $400 to $1200.

Financial Aid Institutionally sponsored need-based grants/scholarships, institutionally sponsored non-need grants/scholarships, Federal Pell Grants, Federal Supplemental Educational Opportunity Grants, Federal PLUS Loans, Federal Stafford Loans.

Generic Baccalaureate Program (BSN)

Applying *Required:* SAT I, ACT, TOEFL for nonnative speakers of English, 3 years of high school math, 3 years of high school science, high school chemistry, high school biology, high school foreign language, high school transcript, letter of recommendation, written essay, transcript of college record. *Options:* Advanced standing available through the following means: advanced placement exams, credit by exam. May apply for transfer of up to 141 total credits. *Application deadlines:* 4/15 (fall), 1/7 (spring). *Application fee:* $20.

Degree Requirements 188 total credit hours, 103 in nursing. Computer literacy.

RN Baccalaureate Program (BSN)

Applying *Required:* TOEFL for nonnative speakers of English, RN license, diploma or AD in nursing, 2 letters of recommendation, written essay, transcript of college record. *Options:* Advanced standing available through the following means: advanced placement exams, credit by exam. *Application deadline:* rolling. *Application fee:* $20.

Degree Requirements 188 total credit hours, 48 in nursing. Computer literacy.

GEORGIA COLLEGE
School of Nursing
Milledgeville, Georgia

Programs • Generic Baccalaureate • RN Baccalaureate • MSN • MSN/MBA

The College State-supported comprehensive coed institution. Part of University System of Georgia. Founded: 1889. *Primary accreditation:* regional. *Setting:* 696-acre small-town campus. *Total enrollment:* 5,710.

The School of Nursing Founded in 1982. *Nursing program faculty:* 19 (32% with doctorates). *Off-campus program sites:* Macon, Dublin.

Student Life *Student services:* health clinic, child-care facilities, personal counseling, career counseling, institutionally sponsored work-study program, job placement, campus safety program, special assistance for disabled students. *International student services:* counseling/support. *Nursing student activities:* Sigma Theta Tau, nursing club, student nurses association.

Calendar Quarters.

NURSING STUDENT PROFILE

Undergraduate **Enrollment:** 260
Women: 90%; **Men:** 10%; **Minority:** 2%; **International:** 1%
Graduate **Enrollment:** 60
Part-time: 100%

BACCALAUREATE PROGRAMS

Contact School of Nursing, Georgia College, Milledgeville, GA 31061, 912-453-4004.

Expenses *State resident tuition:* $1922 full-time, $44 per quarter hour part-time. *Nonresident tuition:* $5801 full-time, $152 per quarter hour part-time. *Full-time mandatory fees:* $200–$250. *Room and board:* $1755–$2850. *Books and supplies per academic year:* ranges from $400 to $600.

Financial Aid Institutionally sponsored need based grants/scholarships, institutionally sponsored non-need grants/scholarships, Federal Direct Loans, Federal Nursing Student Loans, Federal Pell Grants, Federal Perkins Loans, Federal Supplemental Educational Opportunity Grants, Federal Work-Study, HOPE Scholarships. 90% of undergraduate students in nursing programs received some form of financial aid in 1995–96. *Application deadline:* 7/1.

Generic Baccalaureate Program (BSN)

Applying *Required:* SAT I, 3 years of high school math, 3 years of high school science, high school chemistry, high school biology, high school foreign language, high school transcript, immunizations, CPR certification, health exam, professional liability/malpractice insurance. *Application deadline:* 4/1. *Application fee:* $10.

RN Baccalaureate Program (BSN)

Applying *Required:* minimum college GPA of 2.5, RN license, diploma or AD in nursing, transcript of college record, immunizations, CPR certification, health exam, professional liability/malpractice insurance. *Application deadline:* 4/1. *Application fee:* $10.

MASTER'S PROGRAMS

Contact Dr. Cheryl Kish, Graduate Coordinator, School of Nursing, Georgia College, Milledgeville, GA 31061, 912-453-4004.

Areas of Study Clinical nurse specialist programs in adult health nursing, family health nursing; nursing administration; nurse practitioner program in family health.

Expenses *State resident tuition:* $2028 full-time, $47 per hour part-time. *Nonresident tuition:* $6134 full-time, $161 per hour part-time. *Part-time mandatory fees:* $0–$300.

MSN Program

Applying *Required:* GRE General Test or Miller Analogies Test, bachelor's degree in nursing, minimum GPA of 3.0, RN license, 1 year of clinical experience, statistics course, professional liability/malpractice insurance, transcript of college record. *Application deadline:* 7/1.

Degree Requirements 60–85 total credit hours dependent upon track.

MSN/MBA Program

Applying *Required:* GMAT, bachelor's degree in nursing, minimum GPA of 3.0, RN license, 1 year of clinical experience, statistics course, professional liability/malpractice insurance, transcript of college record. *Application deadline:* 7/1.

GEORGIA SOUTHERN UNIVERSITY
Department of Nursing
Statesboro, Georgia

Programs • Generic Baccalaureate • RN Baccalaureate • MSN

The University State-supported comprehensive coed institution. Part of University System of Georgia. Founded: 1906. *Primary accreditation:* regional. *Setting:* 601-acre small-town campus. *Total enrollment:* 14,157.

The Department of Nursing Founded in 1980. *Nursing program faculty:* 26 (52% with doctorates).

Academic Facilities *Campus library:* 451,292 volumes (11,850 in nursing); 3,362 periodical subscriptions (750 health-care related). *Nursing school resources:* CAI, computer lab, nursing audiovisuals, interactive nursing skills videos, learning resource lab.

Student Life *Student services:* health clinic, child-care facilities, personal counseling, career counseling, institutionally sponsored work-study program, job placement, campus safety program, special assistance for

Georgia Southern University (continued)
disabled students. *International student services:* counseling/support, special assistance for nonnative speakers of English, ESL courses. *Nursing student activities:* Sigma Theta Tau, student nurses association.

Calendar Quarters.

NURSING STUDENT PROFILE

Undergraduate **Enrollment:** 273
Women: 88%; **Men:** 12%; **Minority:** 26%; **Part-time:** 5%
Graduate **Enrollment:** 99
Women: 95%; **Men:** 5%; **Minority:** 16%; **Part-time:** 48%

BACCALAUREATE PROGRAMS

Contact Dr. Kathy Koon, Director, BSN Program, LB 8158, Department of Nursing, Georgia Southern University, Statesboro, GA 30460-8158, 912-681-5454. *Fax:* 912-681-0536. *E-mail:* kkoon@gsvus2.cc.gasou.edu

Expenses *State resident tuition:* $1584 full-time, $44 per credit hour part-time. *Nonresident tuition:* $3879 full-time, $108 per credit hour part-time. *Full-time mandatory fees:* up to $471. *Part-time mandatory fees:* up to $471. *Room and board:* $2490–$3750. *Room only:* $330–$700. *Books and supplies per academic year:* ranges from $300 to $750.

Financial Aid Institutionally sponsored need-based grants/scholarships, institutionally sponsored non-need grants/scholarships, Federal Nursing Student Loans, Federal Work-Study, HOPE Scholarships. 96% of undergraduate students in nursing programs received some form of financial aid in 1995–96. *Application deadline:* 8/1.

Generic Baccalaureate Program (BSN)

Applying *Required:* SAT I, minimum college GPA of 2.7, 3 years of high school math, 3 years of high school science, high school foreign language, high school transcript, 3 letters of recommendation, written essay, transcript of college record, desire to work and live in rural or underserved areas. 45 prerequisite credits must be completed before admission to the nursing program. *Options:* May apply for transfer of up to 45 total credits. *Application deadline:* rolling.

Degree Requirements 200 total credit hours, 99 in nursing.

RN Baccalaureate Program (BSN)

Applying *Required:* minimum college GPA of 2.7, RN license, diploma or AD in nursing, 3 letters of recommendation. 87 prerequisite credits must be completed before admission to the nursing program. *Options:* Advanced standing available through advanced placement without credit. May apply for transfer of up to 49 total credits. *Application deadline:* rolling.

Degree Requirements 200 total credit hours, 99 in nursing.

Distance learning Courses provided through on-line.

MASTER'S PROGRAM

Contact Dr. Donna Hodnicki, Director, MSN Program, LB 8158, Department of Nursing, Georgia Southern University, Statesboro, GA 30460-8158, 912-681-5056. *Fax:* 912-681-0536. *E-mail:* dhodnicki@gsums2.cc.gasou.edu

Areas of Study Clinical nurse specialist program in community health nursing; nurse practitioner program in family health.

Expenses *State resident tuition:* $1584 full-time, $44 per credit hour part-time. *Nonresident tuition:* $3879 full-time, $108 per credit hour part-time. *Full-time mandatory fees:* $471. *Part-time mandatory fees:* $471. *Books and supplies per academic year:* ranges from $360 to $750.

Financial Aid Graduate assistantships, nurse traineeships, Federal Nursing Student Loans, institutionally sponsored loans. 88% of master's level students in nursing programs received some form of financial aid in 1995-96. *Application deadline:* 8/1.

MSN Program

Applying *Required:* GRE General Test, Miller Analogies Test, bachelor's degree in nursing, minimum GPA of 3.0, RN license, 1 year of clinical experience, physical assessment course, statistics course, professional liability/malpractice insurance, interview, 3 letters of recommendation, transcript of college record, desire to work and live in rural or underserved areas. *Application deadlines:* 8/16 (fall), 2/25 (spring), 11/18 (winter).

Degree Requirements 60–75 total credit hours dependent upon track, 55 in nursing. Thesis or project.

Distance learning Courses provided on-line.

GEORGIA SOUTHWESTERN STATE UNIVERSITY

School of Nursing
Americus, Georgia

Programs • RN Baccalaureate • Continuing Education

The University State-supported comprehensive coed institution. Part of University System of Georgia. Founded: 1906. *Primary accreditation:* regional. *Setting:* 187-acre small-town campus. *Total enrollment:* 2,607.

The School of Nursing Founded in 1974. *Nursing program faculty:* 5 (60% with doctorates).

Academic Facilities *Campus library:* 156,457 volumes (7,100 in health); 845 periodical subscriptions (31 health-care related). *Nursing school resources:* CAI, computer lab, nursing audiovisuals, learning resource lab.

Student Life *Student services:* health clinic, personal counseling, career counseling, institutionally sponsored work-study program, job placement, campus safety program, special assistance for disabled students. *International student services:* counseling/support, ESL courses. *Nursing student activities:* Sigma Theta Tau, student nurses association.

Calendar Quarters.

NURSING STUDENT PROFILE

Undergraduate **Enrollment:** 65
Women: 92%; **Men:** 8%; **Minority:** 18%; **International:** 0%; **Part-time:** 50%

BACCALAUREATE PROGRAM

Contact Dr. Martha Buhler, Chair, BSN Department, School of Nursing, Georgia Southwestern State University, 800 Wheatley Street, Americus, GA 31709, 912-931-2662. *Fax:* 912-931-2288.

Expenses *State resident tuition:* $1584 full-time, $44 per quarter hour part-time. *Nonresident tuition:* $5463 full-time, $152 per quarter hour part-time. *Full-time mandatory fees:* $480. *Part-time mandatory fees:* $0–$480. *Room and board:* $2925–$3555. *Room only:* $1425–$2055.

RN Baccalaureate Program (BSN)

Applying *Required:* RN license, diploma or AD in nursing, high school transcript, interview, 3 letters of recommendation, transcript of college record, Georgia RN license. *Options:* May apply for transfer of up to 100 total credits. *Application deadlines:* 8/27 (fall), 3/9 (spring), 12/15 (winter). *Application fee:* $10.

Degree Requirements 91 total credit hours, 56 in nursing. 35 quarter credits of upper division non-nursing courses.

CONTINUING EDUCATION PROGRAM

Contact Dr. Martha S. Buhler, Acting Dean, School of Nursing, Georgia Southwestern State University, 800 Wheatley Street, Americus, GA 31709, 912-931-2275. *Fax:* 912-931-2288.

GEORGIA STATE UNIVERSITY

School of Nursing
Atlanta, Georgia

Programs • Generic Baccalaureate • Accelerated RN Baccalaureate • MS • RN to Master's • PhD

The University State-supported coed university. Part of University System of Georgia. Founded: 1913. *Primary accreditation:* regional. *Setting:* 24-acre urban campus. *Total enrollment:* 24,316.

The School of Nursing Founded in 1969. *Nursing program faculty:* 37 (75% with doctorates).

Academic Facilities *Campus library:* 1.5 million volumes (52,835 in health, 2,641 in nursing); 11,129 periodical subscriptions (460 health-care related). *Nursing school resources:* CAI, computer lab, nursing audiovisuals, learning resource lab.

Student Life *Student services:* health clinic, child-care facilities, personal counseling, institutionally sponsored work-study program, job placement.

International student services: special assistance for nonnative speakers of English, ESL courses. *Nursing student activities:* Sigma Theta Tau, student nurses association.

Calendar Quarters.

NURSING STUDENT PROFILE

Undergraduate **Enrollment:** 190
Women: 85%; **Men:** 15%; **Minority:** 26%; **International:** 2%; **Part-time:** 63%
Graduate **Enrollment:** 310
Women: 96%; **Men:** 4%; **Minority:** 19%; **International:** 0%; **Part-time:** 56%

BACCALAUREATE PROGRAMS

Contact Dr. Judith Wold, Director, Undergraduate Nursing Programs, School of Nursing, Georgia State University, PO Box 4019, Atlanta, GA 30302-4019, 404-651-4275. *Fax:* 404-651-4969. *E-mail:* nurjlw@panther.gsu.edu

Expenses *State resident tuition:* $2124 full-time, $472 per quarter part-time. *Nonresident tuition:* $8379 full-time, $1862 per quarter part-time. *Full-time mandatory fees:* $250–$300. *Books and supplies per academic year:* ranges from $400 to $600.

Financial Aid Institutionally sponsored need-based grants/scholarships, Federal Work-Study. *Application deadline:* 5/1.

Generic Baccalaureate Program (BS)

Applying *Required:* SAT I, ACT, TOEFL for nonnative speakers of English, minimum high school GPA of 2.0, minimum college GPA of 2.5, high school chemistry, high school biology, high school transcript, transcript of college record. 55 prerequisite credits must be completed before admission to the nursing program. *Options:* May apply for transfer of up to 140 total credits. *Application deadline:* 4/15. *Application fee:* $10.

Degree Requirements 192 total credit hours, 84 in nursing.

Accelerated RN Baccalaureate Program (BS)

Applying *Required:* minimum college GPA of 2.5, RN license, diploma or AD in nursing, interview, 2 letters of recommendation, transcript of college record, recent practice as RN. 55 prerequisite credits must be completed before admission to the nursing program. *Options:* May apply for transfer of up to 140 total credits. *Application deadlines:* 4/15 (fall), 4/15 (summer). *Application fee:* $10.

Degree Requirements 192 total credit hours, 41 in nursing.

MASTER'S PROGRAMS

Contact Dr. Dee Baldwin, Director, Graduate Nursing Programs, School of Nursing, Georgia State University, PO Box 4019, Atlanta, GA 30302-4019, 404-651-4028. *Fax:* 404-651-4969. *E-mail:* nurdmb@panther.gsu.edu

Areas of Study Clinical nurse specialist programs in adult health nursing, psychiatric–mental health nursing; nurse practitioner programs in child care/pediatrics, community health, women's health.

Expenses *State resident tuition:* $2124 full-time, $472 per quarter part-time. *Nonresident tuition:* $8379 full-time, $1862 per quarter part-time. *Full-time mandatory fees:* $58–$75. *Books and supplies per academic year:* ranges from $400 to $600.

Financial Aid Graduate assistantships, nurse traineeships. *Application deadline:* 5/1.

MS Program

Applying *Required:* bachelor's degree in nursing, minimum GPA of 2.75, RN license, 1 year of clinical experience, statistics course, professional liability/malpractice insurance, interview, 2 letters of recommendation, transcript of college record. *Application deadlines:* 7/15 (fall), 4/15 (summer). *Application fee:* $10.

Degree Requirements 65–75 total credit hours dependent upon track, 45 in nursing, 20 in biology, statistics, and other specified areas. Thesis required.

RN to Master's Program (MS)

Applying *Required:* minimum GPA of 2.75, RN license, 1 year of clinical experience, statistics course, professional liability/malpractice insurance, interview, 2 letters of recommendation, transcript of college record. *Application deadlines:* 7/15 (fall), 4/15 (summer). *Application fee:* $10.

Degree Requirements 65–75 total credit hours dependent upon track, 45 in nursing, 20 in biology, statistics, and other specified areas. Thesis required.

DOCTORAL PROGRAM

Contact Dr. Dee Baldwin, Director, Graduate Nursing Programs, School of Nursing, Georgia State University, PO Box 4019, Atlanta, GA 30302-4019, 404-651-4028. *Fax:* 404-651-4969. *E-mail:* nurdmb@panther.gsu.edu

Areas of Study Nursing education, family nursing, community nursing.

Expenses *State resident tuition:* $2124 full-time, $472 per quarter part-time. *Nonresident tuition:* $8379 full-time, $1862 per quarter part-time. *Full-time mandatory fees:* $250–$300. *Books and supplies per academic year:* ranges from $400 to $600.

Financial Aid Graduate assistantships, nurse traineeships. *Application deadline:* 5/1.

PhD Program

Applying *Required:* GRE General Test, master's degree in nursing, 1 scholarly paper, interview, 3 letters of recommendation, vitae, writing sample, competitive review by faculty committee. *Application fee:* $10.

Degree Requirements 105 total credit hours; written exam; residency.

KENNESAW STATE UNIVERSITY
School of Nursing
Kennesaw, Georgia

Programs • Generic Baccalaureate • RN Baccalaureate • BSN to Master's

The University State-supported comprehensive coed institution. Part of University System of Georgia. Founded: 1963. *Primary accreditation:* regional. *Setting:* 186-acre suburban campus. *Total enrollment:* 12,100.

The School of Nursing Founded in 1985. *Nursing program faculty:* 13 (54% with doctorates).

Academic Facilities *Nursing school resources:* CAI, computer lab, interactive nursing skills videos, learning resource lab.

Student Life *Student services:* personal counseling, career counseling, institutionally sponsored work-study program, job placement, campus safety program, special assistance for disabled students. *International student services:* counseling/support, ESL courses. *Nursing student activities:* Sigma Theta Tau, student nurses association.

Calendar Quarters.

NURSING STUDENT PROFILE

Undergraduate **Enrollment:** 160
Women: 85%; **Men:** 15%; **Minority:** 8%; **International:** 2%; **Part-time:** 50%
Graduate **Enrollment:** 44
Women: 93%; **Men:** 7%; **Minority:** 9%; **International:** 7%; **Part-time:** 0%

BACCALAUREATE PROGRAMS

Contact Dr. David Bennett, Department Chair, Department of Baccalaureate Degree Nursing, Kennesaw State University, 1000 Chastain Road, Kennesaw, GA 30144, 770-423-6061. *Fax:* 770-423-6627. *E-mail:* dbennett@ksc.mail.kennesaw.edu

Expenses *State resident tuition:* $1974 full-time, $44 per credit hour part-time. *Nonresident tuition:* $5853 full-time, $152 per credit hour part-time. *Full-time mandatory fees:* $295. *Part-time mandatory fees:* $295. *Books and supplies per academic year:* ranges from $480 to $680.

Financial Aid Institutionally sponsored need-based grants/scholarships, institutionally sponsored non-need grants/scholarships, Federal Pell Grants, Federal Perkins Loans, Federal Supplemental Educational Opportunity Grants, Federal Work-Study, Federal Stafford Loans, service-cancelable loans. *Application deadline:* 4/1.

Generic Baccalaureate Program (BSN)

Applying *Required:* SAT I, ACT, TOEFL for nonnative speakers of English, minimum high school GPA of 2.0, minimum college GPA of 2.5, 3 years of high school math, 3 years of high school science, letter of recommendation, transcript of college record. 35 prerequisite credits must be completed before admission to the nursing program. *Application deadlines:* 6/1 (fall), 9/1 (spring).

Degree Requirements 193 total credit hours, 77 in nursing. Foreign language for students without a baccalaureate degree.

Kennesaw State University (continued)

RN Baccalaureate Program (BSN)

Applying *Required:* SAT I, ACT, minimum high school GPA of 2.0, minimum college GPA of 2.5, 3 years of high school math, 3 years of high school science, RN license, diploma or AD in nursing, letter of recommendation, transcript of college record. 68 prerequisite credits must be completed before admission to the nursing program. *Application deadlines:* 6/1 (fall), 9/1 (spring).

Degree Requirements 193 total credit hours, 77 in nursing.

MASTER'S PROGRAM

Contact Dr. Regina Dorman, Director, School of Nursing, Kennesaw State University, 1000 Chastain Road, Kennesaw, GA 30144, 770-423-6061. *Fax:* 770-423-6627. *E-mail:* gdorman@ksumail.kennesaw.edu

Areas of Study Nurse practitioner program in family health.

Expenses *State resident tuition:* $3000 per academic year. *Nonresident tuition:* $6500 per academic year. *Full-time mandatory fees:* $295. *Room and board:* $150–$350.

Financial Aid Federal Nursing Student Loans, institutionally sponsored loans, employment opportunities. *Application deadline:* 7/31.

BSN to Master's Program (MSN)

Applying *Required:* GRE General Test (minimum combined score of 1300 on three tests), TOEFL for nonnative speakers of English, bachelor's degree in nursing, bachelor's degree, minimum GPA of 2.5, RN license, physical assessment course, professional liability/malpractice insurance, essay, transcript of college record, 3 years of direct patient care experience, resume. *Application deadline:* 7/31. *Application fee:* $20.

Degree Requirements 60 total credit hours, 60 in nursing. 600 clinical hours.

See full description on page 466.

MEDICAL COLLEGE OF GEORGIA

School of Nursing
Augusta, Georgia

Programs • Generic Baccalaureate • RN Baccalaureate • MN • MSN • PhD • Continuing Education

The College State-supported coed university. Part of University System of Georgia. Founded: 1828. *Primary accreditation:* regional. *Setting:* 100-acre urban campus. *Total enrollment:* 2,015.

The School of Nursing Founded in 1943. *Nursing program faculty:* 65 (46% with doctorates). *Off-campus program sites:* Athens, Barnesville.

Academic Facilities *Campus library:* 159,834 volumes (147,846 in health, 11,988 in nursing); 1,410 periodical subscriptions (1,410 health-care related). *Nursing school resources:* computer lab, nursing audiovisuals, interactive nursing skills videos, learning resource lab.

Student Life *Student services:* health clinic, child-care facilities, personal counseling, career counseling, institutionally sponsored work-study program, job placement, campus safety program, special assistance for disabled students. *International student services:* counseling/support. *Nursing student activities:* Sigma Theta Tau, student nurses association.

Calendar Quarters.

NURSING STUDENT PROFILE

Undergraduate **Enrollment:** 321

Women: 85%; **Men:** 15%; **Minority:** 14%; **International:** 1%; **Part-time:** 2%

Graduate **Enrollment:** 95

Women: 90%; **Men:** 10%; **Minority:** 12%; **International:** 1%; **Part-time:** 66%

BACCALAUREATE PROGRAMS

Contact Ms. Elizabeth Griffin, Director, Academic Admissions, AA-170-Kelly Building, School of Nursing, Medical College of Georgia, Augusta, GA 30912, 706-721-2725. *Fax:* 706-721-0186. *E-mail:* lgriffin@mail.mcg.edu

Expenses *State resident tuition:* $3064 full-time, $59 per credit hour part-time. *Nonresident tuition:* $7545 full-time, $203 per credit hour part-time. *Full-time mandatory fees:* $264. *Part-time mandatory fees:* $15–$83. *Room and board:* $3870–$4734. *Room only:* $1305–$2169. *Books and supplies per academic year:* $700.

Financial Aid Institutionally sponsored need-based grants/scholarships, Federal Nursing Student Loans, Federal Supplemental Educational Opportunity Grants, Federal Work-Study. 73% of undergraduate students in nursing programs received some form of financial aid in 1995–96. *Application deadline:* 3/1.

Generic Baccalaureate Program (BSN)

Applying *Required:* SAT I, ACT, TOEFL for nonnative speakers of English, minimum college GPA of 2.0, 3 years of high school math, 3 years of high school science, high school chemistry, high school biology, high school foreign language, 3 letters of recommendation, written essay, transcript of college record. 90 prerequisite credits must be completed before admission to the nursing program. *Options:* May apply for transfer of up to 90 total credits. *Application deadline:* 3/1.

Degree Requirements 180 total credit hours, 90 in nursing.

Distance learning Courses provided through video.

RN Baccalaureate Program (BSN)

Applying *Required:* SAT I, ACT, TOEFL for nonnative speakers of English, minimum college GPA of 2.0, 3 years of high school math, 3 years of high school science, high school chemistry, high school biology, RN license, diploma or AD in nursing, high school foreign language, 3 letters of recommendation, written essay, transcript of college record. 90 prerequisite credits must be completed before admission to the nursing program. *Options:* May apply for transfer of up to 90 total credits. *Application deadline:* 3/1.

Degree Requirements 180 total credit hours, 90 in nursing.

Distance learning Courses provided through video.

MASTER'S PROGRAMS

Contact Ms. Elizabeth Griffin, Director, Academic Admissions, AA-170, Medical College of Georgia, Augusta, GA 30912, 706-721-2725. *Fax:* 706-721-0186. *E-mail:* lgriffin@mail.mcg.edu

Areas of Study Clinical nurse specialist programs in adult health nursing, community health nursing, parent-child nursing, psychiatric–mental health nursing; nurse anesthesia; nurse practitioner programs in child care/pediatrics, family health, neonatal health.

Expenses *State resident tuition:* $3307 full-time, $62 per credit hour part-time. *Nonresident tuition:* $10,559 full-time, $214 per credit hour part-time. *Full-time mandatory fees:* $347. *Part-time mandatory fees:* $15–$83. *Room and board:* $3870–$4734. *Room only:* $1305–$2169. *Books and supplies per academic year:* $700.

Financial Aid Nurse traineeships, Federal Nursing Student Loans, employment opportunities. 28% of master's level students in nursing programs received some form of financial aid in 1995-96. *Application deadline:* 6/1.

MN Program

Applying *Required:* GRE General Test (minimum combined score of 900 on three tests), TOEFL for nonnative speakers of English, bachelor's degree in nursing, minimum GPA of 3.0, RN license, 1 year of clinical experience, physical assessment course, statistics course, professional liability/malpractice insurance, essay, interview, 3 letters of recommendation, transcript of college record. *Application deadline:* 6/30.

Degree Requirements 60–121 total credit hours dependent upon track, 55–75 in nursing.

MSN Program

Applying *Required:* GRE General Test (minimum combined score of 900 on three tests), TOEFL for nonnative speakers of English, bachelor's degree in nursing, minimum GPA of 3.0, RN license, 1 year of clinical experience, physical assessment course, statistics course, professional liability/malpractice insurance, essay, interview, 3 letters of recommendation, transcript of college record. *Application deadline:* 6/30.

Degree Requirements 60–85 total credit hours dependent upon track, 55–75 in nursing. Thesis, investigative project, or supervised research.

DOCTORAL PROGRAMS

Contact Ms. Elizabeth Griffin, Director, Academic Admissions, AA-170, Medical College of Georgia, Augusta, GA 30912, 706-721-2725. *Fax:* 706-721-0186. *E-mail:* lgriffin@mail.mcg.edu

Areas of Study Nursing administration, health care across the life span.

Expenses *State resident tuition:* $2812 full-time, $62 per credit hour part-time. *Nonresident tuition:* $8892 full-time, $214 per credit hour part-time. *Full-time mandatory fees:* $347. *Room and board:* $3870–$4734. *Room only:* $1305–$2169. *Books and supplies per academic year:* $700.

Financial Aid Nurse traineeships, dissertation grants, opportunities for employment. *Application deadline:* 6/1.

PhD Program

Applying *Required:* GRE General Test (minimum combined score of 1000 on three tests), TOEFL for nonnative speakers of English, master's degree in nursing, 2 years of clinical experience, 1 scholarly paper, statistics course, interview, 3 letters of recommendation, vitae, writing sample, competitive review by faculty committee. *Application deadline:* 3/1.

Degree Requirements 98 total credit hours; 10 hours in statistics; dissertation; oral exam; written exam; defense of dissertation.

Postbaccalaureate Doctorate (PhD)

Applying *Required:* GRE General Test (minimum combined score of 1000 on three tests), TOEFL for nonnative speakers of English, 2 years of clinical experience, 1 scholarly paper, statistics course, interview, 3 letters of recommendation, vitae, writing sample, competitive review by faculty committee. *Application deadline:* 3/1.

Degree Requirements 143 total credit hours; 10 hours in statistics; dissertation; oral exam; written exam; defense of dissertation.

CONTINUING EDUCATION PROGRAM

Contact Ms. Patricia Pennington, Conference Coordinator, Division of Continuing Education, Medical College of Georgia, Augusta, GA 30912, 706-721-3967. *Fax:* 706-721-4642.

See full description on page 478.

NORTH GEORGIA COLLEGE AND STATE UNIVERSITY
Department of Nursing
Dahlonega, Georgia

Programs • RN Baccalaureate • ADN to Baccalaureate

The University State-supported comprehensive coed institution. Part of University System of Georgia. Founded: 1873. *Primary accreditation:* regional. *Setting:* 140-acre small-town campus. *Total enrollment:* 2,973.

The Department of Nursing Founded in 1974. *Nursing program faculty:* 21 (20% with doctorates). *Off-campus program sites:* Atlanta, Gainesville.

Academic Facilities *Campus library:* 106,800 volumes (8,616 in health, 2,500 in nursing); 1,465 periodical subscriptions (69 health-care related). *Nursing school resources:* CAI, computer lab, nursing audiovisuals.

Student Life *Student services:* health clinic, personal counseling, career counseling, institutionally sponsored work-study program, job placement, campus safety program, special assistance for disabled students. *International student services:* counseling/support, special assistance for nonnative speakers of English, ESL courses. *Nursing student activities:* student nurses association.

Calendar Quarters.

NURSING STUDENT PROFILE

Undergraduate **Enrollment:** 181
Women: 90%; **Men:** 10%; **Minority:** 1%; **International:** 1%; **Part-time:** 65%

BACCALAUREATE PROGRAMS

Contact Dr. Linda Roberts-Betsch, Head and Professor, Department of Nursing, North Georgia College, Route 60, Dahlonega, GA 30597, 706-864-1930. *Fax:* 706-864-1668. *E-mail:* lroberts@nugget.ngc.peachnet.edu

Expenses *State resident tuition:* $1584 full-time, $44 per credit hour part-time. *Nonresident tuition:* $3879 full-time, $152 per credit hour part-time. *Full-time mandatory fees:* $125–$300. *Room and board:* $2853. *Room only:* $1365. *Books and supplies per academic year:* ranges from $500 to $700.

Financial Aid Institutionally sponsored need-based grants/scholarships, institutionally sponsored non-need grants/scholarships, Federal Nursing Student Loans, Federal Supplemental Educational Opportunity Grants, Federal Work-Study, HOPE Scholarships.

RN Baccalaureate Program (BSN)

Applying *Required:* SAT I, minimum college GPA of 2.5, 3 years of high school math, 3 years of high school science, high school chemistry, high school biology, RN license, diploma or AD in nursing, high school foreign language, transcript of college record. 95 prerequisite credits must be completed before admission to the nursing program. *Options:* Advanced standing available through the following means: advanced placement exams, credit by exam. Course work may be accelerated. May apply for transfer of up to 130 total credits. *Application deadlines:* 2/1 (fall), 2/1 (summer). *Application fee:* $10.

Degree Requirements 193 total credit hours, 105 in nursing.

ADN to Baccalaureate Program (BSN)

Applying *Required:* SAT I, minimum college GPA of 2.5, 3 years of high school math, 3 years of high school science, high school chemistry, high school biology, diploma or AD in nursing, high school foreign language, transcript of college record. *Options:* Course work may be accelerated. May apply for transfer of up to 45 total credits. *Application deadlines:* 2/1 (fall), 2/1 (summer). *Application fee:* $10.

Degree Requirements 193 total credit hours, 105 in nursing.

VALDOSTA STATE UNIVERSITY
School of Nursing
Valdosta, Georgia

Programs • Generic Baccalaureate • MSN

The University State-supported coed university. Part of University System of Georgia. Founded: 1906. *Primary accreditation:* regional. *Setting:* 168-acre small-town campus. *Total enrollment:* 9,594.

The School of Nursing Founded in 1967.

Calendar Quarters.

BACCALAUREATE PROGRAM

Contact Acting Assistant Dean and Head, Department of Undergraduate Studies, College of Nursing, Valdosta State University, 1300 North Patterson Street, Valdosta, GA 31698, 912-333-5959. *Fax:* 912-333-7300.

Financial Aid Federal Nursing Student Loans.

MASTER'S PROGRAM

Contact Assistant Dean and Head, Graduate Department, College of Nursing, Valdosta State University, 1300 North Patterson Street, Valdosta, GA 31698, 912-333-5959. *Fax:* 912-333-7300.

Expenses *State resident tuition:* $2121 full-time, $235 per 5 hours part-time. *Nonresident tuition:* $6195 full-time, $805 per 5 hours part-time.

MSN Program

Applying *Required:* GRE General Test or Miller Analogies Test, GRE General Test (minimum score of 800 on verbal and analytical sections), minimum GPA of 2.8, transcript of college record, Georgia RN license, minimum of 1 year of experience as a registered nurse.

Degree Requirements 60 total credit hours, 10 in other specified areas. Thesis required.

WEST GEORGIA COLLEGE
Department of Nursing
Carrollton, Georgia

Program • RN Baccalaureate

The College State-supported comprehensive coed institution. Part of University System of Georgia. Founded: 1933. *Primary accreditation:* regional. *Setting:* 400-acre small-town campus. *Total enrollment:* 8,650.

The Department of Nursing Founded in 1976.

West Georgia College (continued)

BACCALAUREATE PROGRAM

Contact Chair, Department of Nursing, West Georgia College, Carrollton, GA 30118, 404-836-6552.

Expenses *State resident tuition:* $1584 full-time, $44 per quarter hour part-time. *Nonresident tuition:* $3879 full-time, $108 per quarter hour part-time. *Room and board:* $2235–$3345. *Room only:* $1635–$1755.

RN Baccalaureate Program (BSN)

Applying *Application fee:* $15.

Degree Requirements 196 total credit hours. Attain a grade of "C" or higher in all nursing courses.

HAWAII

HAWAII PACIFIC UNIVERSITY
Nursing Program, Windward Campus
Honolulu, Hawaii

Programs • Generic Baccalaureate • RN Baccalaureate • Accelerated Baccalaureate for Second Degree • LPN to Baccalaureate

The University Independent comprehensive coed institution. Founded: 1965. *Primary accreditation:* regional. *Setting:* 135-acre urban campus. *Total enrollment:* 8,036.

The Nursing Program, Windward Campus Founded in 1983. *Nursing program faculty:* 51 (75% with doctorates).

▶ *NOTEWORTHY*

Hawaii Pacific University's Nursing Program offers hands-on experiences in both classroom and clinical settings in which transcultural nursing is an everyday opportunity. Students are accepted directly into the Nursing Program when they apply to the University and do not have to wait until they have completed all prerequisites. In the sophomore year, HPU students begin their clinical experiences. Small clinical laboratories (8–10 students) are located throughout the island of Oahu. Hawaii Pacific's Nursing Program is accredited by the National League for Nursing and approved by the State of Hawaii Board of Nursing.

Academic Facilities *Campus library:* 156,000 volumes (4,200 in health, 1,600 in nursing); 3,700 periodical subscriptions (85 health-care related). *Nursing school resources:* CAI, computer lab, nursing audiovisuals, learning resource lab, nursing arts lab.

Student Life *Student services:* health clinic, personal counseling, career counseling, institutionally sponsored work-study program, job placement, campus safety program, special assistance for disabled students. *International student services:* counseling/support, special assistance for nonnative speakers of English, ESL courses, international student organization. *Nursing student activities:* Sigma Theta Tau, nursing club, student nurses association.

Calendar 4-1-4.

NURSING STUDENT PROFILE

Undergraduate **Enrollment:** 561

Women: 88%; **Men:** 12%; **Minority:** 65%; **International:** 2%; **Part-time:** 59%

BACCALAUREATE PROGRAMS

Contact Nancy L. Ellis, Admissions Office, Nursing Program, Hawaii Pacific University, 1164 Bishop Street, Honolulu, HI 96813, 808-544-0238. *Fax:* 808-544-1136.

Expenses *Tuition:* $11,000 full-time, $460 per credit part-time. *Full-time mandatory fees:* $600. *Room and board:* $6500. *Books and supplies per academic year:* ranges from $600 to $800.

Financial Aid Institutionally sponsored need-based grants/scholarships, institutionally sponsored non-need grants/scholarships, Federal Nursing Student Loans, Federal Pell Grants, Federal Perkins Loans, Federal Supplemental Educational Opportunity Grants, Federal Work-Study. 53% of undergraduate students in nursing programs received some form of financial aid in 1995–96. *Application deadline:* 3/1.

Generic Baccalaureate Program (BSN)

Applying *Required:* SAT (recommended), minimum high school GPA of 2.5, minimum college GPA of 2.5, high school transcript, transcript of college record. *Options:* Advanced standing available through the following means: advanced placement exams, advanced placement without credit, credit by exam. Course work may be accelerated. May apply for transfer of up to 64 total credits. *Application deadlines:* 5/16 (summer), rolling. *Application fee:* $50.

Degree Requirements 130 total credit hours, 69 in nursing.

RN Baccalaureate Program (BSN)

Applying *Required:* SAT (recommended), minimum high school GPA of 2.5, minimum college GPA of 2.5, RN license, diploma or AD in nursing, transcript of college record. *Options:* Advanced standing available through the following means: advanced placement exams, advanced placement without credit, credit by exam. Course work may be accelerated. May apply for transfer of up to 64 total credits. *Application deadlines:* 5/16 (summer), rolling. *Application fee:* $50.

Degree Requirements 130 total credit hours, 34 in nursing. NLN Mobility Profile I and II exams for graduates of non-NLN accredited programs.

Accelerated Baccalaureate for Second Degree Program (BSN)

Applying *Required:* SAT (recommended), minimum college GPA of 2.5, transcript of college record. 59 prerequisite credits must be completed before admission to the nursing program. *Options:* Advanced standing available through the following means: advanced placement exams, advanced placement without credit, credit by exam. *Application deadline:* rolling. *Application fee:* $50.

Degree Requirements 130 total credit hours, 69 in nursing.

LPN to Baccalaureate Program (BSN)

Applying *Required:* SAT (recommended), minimum high school GPA of 2.5, minimum college GPA of 2.0, transcript of college record, LPN license. *Options:* Advanced standing available through the following means: advanced placement exams, advanced placement without credit, credit by exam. Course work may be accelerated. May apply for transfer of up to 64 total credits. *Application deadlines:* 5/6 (summer), rolling. *Application fee:* $50.

Degree Requirements 130 total credit hours, 57 in nursing.

See full description on page 454.

UNIVERSITY OF HAWAII AT MANOA
School of Nursing
Honolulu, Hawaii

Programs • Generic Baccalaureate • RN Baccalaureate • MS • Post-Master's

The University State-supported coed university. Part of University of Hawaii System. Founded: 1907. *Primary accreditation:* regional. *Setting:* 300-acre urban campus. *Total enrollment:* 18,300.

The School of Nursing Founded in 1932. *Nursing program faculty:* 55 (49% with doctorates). *Off-campus program sites:* Maui, Kauai, Molokai.

▶ *NOTEWORTHY*

The UH School of Nursing offers programs for nursing careers in a unique multicultural population, which gives students opportunities to interact with people from many cultural backgrounds. The School offers programs leading to the Bachelor of Science and Master of Science degrees and a post-master's certificate in nursing. The undergraduate nursing program provides 2 options: the generic BS degree program admitting students as sophomores and the UH system's articulated AS/BS program in which students enter with an ADN. The MS degree program prepares nurses to function at an advanced level, in a specialty, as a clinical nurse specialist and/or nurse practitioner, or as a nurse executive.

Academic Facilities *Campus library:* 2.0 million volumes; 25,000 periodical subscriptions (80 health-care related). *Nursing school resources:* CAI, computer lab, nursing audiovisuals, interactive nursing skills videos, learning resource lab.

Student Life *Student services:* health clinic, child-care facilities, personal counseling, career counseling, institutionally sponsored work-study program, job placement, special assistance for disabled students. *International*

student services: counseling/support, special assistance for nonnative speakers of English, ESL courses. *Nursing student activities:* Sigma Theta Tau, nursing club, student nurses association.

Calendar Semesters.

NURSING STUDENT PROFILE

Undergraduate **Enrollment:** 248

Women: 81%; **Men:** 19%; **Minority:** 77%; **International:** 3%; **Part-time:** 6%

Graduate **Enrollment:** 117

Women: 88%; **Men:** 12%; **Minority:** 37%; **International:** 4%; **Part-time:** 56%

BACCALAUREATE PROGRAMS

Contact Dr. Lois Magnussen, Director of Student Services, Webster 201, School of Nursing, Student Services, University of Hawaii at Manoa, 2528 The Mall, Honolulu, HI 96822, 808-956-8939. *Fax:* 808-956-5977.

Expenses *State resident tuition:* $2304 full-time, $96 per credit hour part-time. *Nonresident tuition:* $7752 full-time, $323 per credit hour part-time. *Full-time mandatory fees:* $676–$840. *Part-time mandatory fees:* $650–$835. *Room only:* $1800–$3000. *Books and supplies per academic year:* ranges from $1200 to $1600.

Financial Aid Institutionally sponsored need-based grants/scholarships, institutionally sponsored non-need grants/scholarships, Federal Nursing Student Loans. *Application deadline:* 3/1.

Generic Baccalaureate Program (BS)

Applying *Required:* SAT I, ACT, TOEFL for nonnative speakers of English, NLN Preadmission Examination-RN, minimum college GPA of 2.5, 2 years of high school math, 2 years of high school science, high school transcript, transcript of college record, high school class rank: top 40%. 39 prerequisite credits must be completed before admission to the nursing program. *Application deadlines:* 2/1 (fall), 10/1 (spring). *Application fee:* $10.

Degree Requirements 134 total credit hours, 65 in nursing.

RN Baccalaureate Program (BS)

Applying *Required:* TOEFL for nonnative speakers of English, NLN Mobility Profile II for graduates of diploma and non-NLN accredited schools, minimum college GPA of 2.5, RN license, diploma or AD in nursing, transcript of college record. 34 prerequisite credits must be completed before admission to the nursing program. *Options:* May apply for transfer of up to 35 total credits. *Application deadlines:* 2/1 (fall), 10/1 (spring). *Application fee:* $10.

Degree Requirements 134 total credit hours, 34 in nursing.

MASTER'S PROGRAMS

Contact Dr. Lois Magnussen, Director of Student Services, Webster 201, School of Nursing, University of Hawaii at Manoa, 2528 The Mall, Honolulu, HI 96822, 808-956-8939. *Fax:* 808-956-5977.

Areas of Study Clinical nurse specialist programs in adult health nursing, gerontological nursing, psychiatric–mental health nursing, advanced practice nursing; nursing administration; nurse practitioner programs in adult health, child care/pediatrics, family health, gerontology, psychiatric–mental health, women's health, advanced practice nursing.

Expenses *State resident tuition:* $3144 full-time, $131 per credit hour part-time. *Nonresident tuition:* $8088 full-time, $337 per credit hour part-time. *Full-time mandatory fees:* $716–$816. *Room only:* $1800–$3000. *Books and supplies per academic year:* ranges from $600 to $800.

Financial Aid Graduate assistantships, nurse traineeships, Federal Nursing Student Loans, employment opportunities. *Application deadline:* 3/1.

MS Program

Applying *Required:* GRE General Test, TOEFL for nonnative speakers of English, bachelor's degree in nursing, minimum GPA of 3.0, RN license, physical assessment course, statistics course, professional liability/malpractice insurance, essay, interview, 2 letters of recommendation, transcript of college record, CPR certification, research course. *Application deadline:* 3/1. *Application fee:* $10.

Degree Requirements 36–53 total credit hours dependent upon track, 36–53 in nursing. Thesis or scholarly paper.

Post-Master's Program

Applying *Required:* TOEFL for nonnative speakers of English, minimum GPA of 3.0, RN license, physical assessment course, statistics course, professional liability/malpractice insurance, essay, interview, 2 letters of recommendation, transcript of college record. *Application deadline:* 3/1.

Degree Requirements 21–24 total credit hours dependent upon track, 21–24 in nursing.

IDAHO

BOISE STATE UNIVERSITY
Department of Nursing
Boise, Idaho

Programs • Generic Baccalaureate • RN Baccalaureate

The University State-supported comprehensive coed institution. Part of Idaho System of Higher Education. Founded: 1932. *Primary accreditation:* regional. *Setting:* 130-acre urban campus. *Total enrollment:* 14,205.

The Department of Nursing Founded in 1957.

Academic Facilities *Campus library:* 385,000 volumes; 4,700 periodical subscriptions.

BACCALAUREATE PROGRAMS

Contact Advising Office, Department of Nursing, Boise State University, 1910 University Drive, Boise, ID 83725, 208-385-3790.

Financial Aid Federal Direct Loans, Federal Pell Grants, Federal Perkins Loans, Federal Work-Study.

Generic Baccalaureate Program (BS)

Applying *Required:* SAT I or ACT, TOEFL for nonnative speakers of English, high school transcript. *Application deadlines:* 7/31 (fall), 11/27 (spring). *Application fee:* $20.

Degree Requirements 128–129 total credit hours dependent upon track, 55 in nursing.

RN Baccalaureate Program (BS)

Applying *Required:* NLN mobility tests, RN license, diploma or AD in nursing. *Application deadlines:* 7/31 (fall), 11/27 (spring). *Application fee:* $20.

Degree Requirements 128–129 total credit hours dependent upon track, 60 in nursing.

IDAHO STATE UNIVERSITY
Department of Nursing
Pocatello, Idaho

Programs • Generic Baccalaureate • Accelerated RN Baccalaureate • MSN

The University State-supported coed university. Founded: 1901. *Primary accreditation:* regional. *Setting:* 274-acre small-town campus. *Total enrollment:* 12,041.

The Department of Nursing Founded in 1952. *Nursing program faculty:* 16 (66% with doctorates). *Off-campus program sites:* Twin Falls, Boise, Lewiston.

Academic Facilities *Nursing school resources:* computer lab, nursing audio-visuals, learning resource lab.

Student Life *Student services:* health clinic, child-care facilities, personal counseling, career counseling, institutionally sponsored work-study program, job placement, campus safety program, special assistance for

Idaho State University (continued)
disabled students. *International student services:* counseling/support, ESL courses. *Nursing student activities:* Sigma Theta Tau, student nurses association.

Calendar Semesters.

NURSING STUDENT PROFILE

Undergraduate **Enrollment:** 110
Women: 89%; **Men:** 11%; **Minority:** 5%; **International:** 1%; **Part-time:** 10%
Graduate **Enrollment:** 72
Women: 83%; **Men:** 17%; **Minority:** 1%; **International:** 0%; **Part-time:** 82%

BACCALAUREATE PROGRAMS

Contact Dr. Pamela Clarke, Chairperson, Nursing Department, Idaho State University, Box 8101, Pocatello, ID 83209-8101, 208-236-2185. *Fax:* 208-236-4645. *E-mail:* clarpame@isu.edu

Expenses *State resident tuition:* $2326 full-time, $86 per credit part-time. *Nonresident tuition:* $7800 full-time, $168 per credit part-time. *Full-time mandatory fees:* $157–$1570. *Books and supplies per academic year:* $300.

Financial Aid Institutionally sponsored need-based grants/scholarships, institutionally sponsored non-need grants/scholarships, Federal Nursing Student Loans, Federal Supplemental Educational Opportunity Grants, Federal Work-Study. *Application deadline:* 2/15.

Generic Baccalaureate Program (BS)

Applying *Required:* SAT I, ACT, minimum high school GPA of 2.0, minimum college GPA of 2.5, high school transcript, transcript of college record. 44 prerequisite credits must be completed before admission to the nursing program. *Options:* Advanced standing available through credit by exam. Course work may be accelerated. *Application deadline:* 1/15. *Application fee:* $25.

Degree Requirements 128 total credit hours, 49 in nursing.

Accelerated RN Baccalaureate Program (BS)

Applying *Required:* minimum college GPA of 2.5, RN license, diploma or AD in nursing, transcript of college record. 44 prerequisite credits must be completed before admission to the nursing program. *Options:* Advanced standing available through credit by exam. *Application deadline:* 1/15. *Application fee:* $25.

Degree Requirements 128 total credit hours, 49 in nursing.

MASTER'S PROGRAM

Contact Dr. Pamela Clarke, Chairperson, Department of Nursing, Idaho State University, Box 8101, Pocatello, ID 83209-8101, 208-236-2185. *Fax:* 208-236-4645. *E-mail:* clarpame@isu.edu

Areas of Study Nursing administration; nursing education; nurse practitioner program in family health.

Expenses *State resident tuition:* $2636 full-time, $110 per credit part-time. *Nonresident tuition:* $8290 full-time, $192 per credit part-time. *Full-time mandatory fees:* $203–$2039. *Books and supplies per academic year:* ranges from $100 to $550.

Financial Aid Graduate assistantships, nurse traineeships. *Application deadline:* 3/15.

MSN Program

Applying *Required:* GRE General Test, bachelor's degree in nursing, minimum GPA of 3.0, RN license, 2 years of clinical experience, physical assessment course, statistics course, professional liability/malpractice insurance, essay, interview, 3 letters of recommendation, transcript of college record, nursing research course. *Application deadlines:* 5/15 (fall), 10/15 (spring). *Application fee:* $25.

Degree Requirements 36–48 total credit hours dependent upon track, 30–48 in nursing. Thesis, project, or oral and written examinations.

Distance learning Courses provided through video.

LEWIS-CLARK STATE COLLEGE
Division of Nursing
Lewiston, Idaho

Programs • Generic Baccalaureate • RN Baccalaureate • Continuing Education

The College State-supported 4-year coed college. Founded: 1893. *Primary accreditation:* regional. *Setting:* 44-acre rural campus. *Total enrollment:* 3,138.

The Division of Nursing Founded in 1979. *Nursing program faculty:* 13 (31% with doctorates). *Off-campus program site:* Coeur d'Alene.

Academic Facilities *Campus library:* 194,399 volumes (13,199 in health, 2,001 in nursing); 1,763 periodical subscriptions (166 health-care related). *Nursing school resources:* CAI, computer lab, nursing audiovisuals, interactive nursing skills videos, learning resource lab.

Student Life *Student services:* health clinic, child-care facilities, personal counseling, career counseling, institutionally sponsored work-study program, job placement, campus safety program, special assistance for disabled students. *International student services:* counseling/support, special assistance for nonnative speakers of English, ESL courses. *Nursing student activities:* student nurses association.

Calendar Semesters.

NURSING STUDENT PROFILE

Undergraduate **Enrollment:** 162
Women: 82%; **Men:** 18%; **Minority:** 1%; **International:** 2%; **Part-time:** 46%

BACCALAUREATE PROGRAMS

Contact Dr. Mary McFarland, Chair and Professor, Division of Nursing, Lewis-Clark State College, 500 8th Avenue, Lewiston, ID 83501-2698, 208-799-2250. *Fax:* 208-799-2062. *E-mail:* mmcfarla@lcsc.edu

Expenses *State resident tuition:* $1626 full-time, $81 per credit part-time. *Nonresident tuition:* $6352 per academic year. *Full-time mandatory fees:* $100–$200. *Part-time mandatory fees:* $100–$200. *Room and board:* $3220–$3550. *Room only:* $1090–$1580. *Books and supplies per academic year:* ranges from $950 to $1550.

Financial Aid Institutionally sponsored need-based grants/scholarships, institutionally sponsored non-need grants/scholarships, Federal Nursing Student Loans, Federal Pell Grants, Federal Perkins Loans, Federal Supplemental Educational Opportunity Grants, Federal Work-Study. *Application deadline:* 2/1.

Generic Baccalaureate Program (BSN)

Applying *Required:* TOEFL for nonnative speakers of English, PSB Nursing School Aptitude Exam, minimum college GPA of 2.75, high school chemistry, written essay, transcript of college record, curriculum vitae. 21 prerequisite credits must be completed before admission to the nursing program. *Options:* Course work may be accelerated. May apply for transfer of up to 70 total credits. *Application deadline:* 2/14. *Application fee:* $50.

Degree Requirements 128 total credit hours, 61 in nursing. Lower and upper division core courses.

Distance learning Courses provided through video, audio.

RN Baccalaureate Program (BSN)

Applying *Required:* minimum college GPA of 2.75, RN license, diploma or AD in nursing, transcript of college record. 21 prerequisite credits must be completed before admission to the nursing program. *Options:* Advanced standing available through advanced placement exams. Course work may be accelerated. May apply for transfer of up to 70 total credits. *Application deadlines:* 3/3 (fall), 10/1 (spring). *Application fee:* $35.

Degree Requirements 128 total credit hours, 27 in nursing. 34 hours of support and lower and upper division core courses.

Distance learning Courses provided through video, audio.

CONTINUING EDUCATION PROGRAM

Contact Dr. Mary McFarland, Chair and Professor, Division of Nursing, Lewis-Clark State College, 500 8th Avenue, Lewiston, ID 83601-2698, 208-799-2250. *Fax:* 208-799-2062. *E-mail:* mmcfarla@lcsc.edu

ILLINOIS

AURORA UNIVERSITY
School of Nursing
Aurora, Illinois

Programs • Generic Baccalaureate • RN Baccalaureate

The University Independent comprehensive coed institution. Founded: 1893. *Primary accreditation:* regional. *Setting:* 26-acre suburban campus. *Total enrollment:* 2,025.

The School of Nursing Founded in 1979. *Nursing program faculty:* 13 (46% with doctorates). *Off-campus program site:* Chicago.

Academic Facilities *Campus library:* 14,004 volumes; 718 periodical subscriptions (94 health-care related). *Nursing school resources:* CAI, computer lab, nursing audiovisuals, learning resource lab.

Student Life *Student services:* health clinic, personal counseling, career counseling, institutionally sponsored work-study program, job placement, special assistance for disabled students. *Nursing student activities:* Sigma Theta Tau, student nurses association.

Calendar Trimesters.

NURSING STUDENT PROFILE

Undergraduate **Enrollment:** 253
Women: 89%; **Men:** 11%; **Minority:** 49%; **International:** 0%; **Part-time:** 45%

BACCALAUREATE PROGRAMS

Contact Dr. Mary Glenn, Coordinator, Undergraduate Program, School of Nursing, Aurora University, 347 South Gladstone Avenue, Aurora, IL 60506, 630-844-5140. *Fax:* 630-844-7822.

Expenses *Tuition:* $10,800 full-time, $376 per term part-time. *Full-time mandatory fees:* $125. *Part-time mandatory fees:* $30. *Books and supplies per academic year:* ranges from $200 to $300.

Financial Aid Institutionally sponsored need-based grants/scholarships, institutionally sponsored non-need grants/scholarships, Federal Work-Study. *Application deadline:* 5/1.

Generic Baccalaureate Program (BSN)

Applying *Required:* SAT I or ACT, Nursing Entrance Test, minimum college GPA of 2.5, 3 years of high school science, high school transcript, transcript of college record, high school class rank: top 50%. *Options:* Advanced standing available through the following means: advanced placement exams, credit by exam. May apply for transfer of up to 60 total credits. *Application deadline:* rolling. *Application fee:* $25.

Degree Requirements 129 total credit hours, 60 in nursing.

RN Baccalaureate Program (BSN)

Applying *Required:* TOEFL for nonnative speakers of English, ACT PEP or NLN Mobility Profile for clinical placement, minimum college GPA of 2.5, RN license, diploma or AD in nursing, transcript of college record. *Options:* Advanced standing available through credit by exam. May apply for transfer of up to 21 total credits. *Application deadline:* rolling. *Application fee:* $25.

Degree Requirements 129 total credit hours, 60 in nursing.

BARAT COLLEGE
Department of Nursing, Barat College and Finch University of Health Sciences/The Chicago Medical School
North Chicago, Illinois

Programs • RN Baccalaureate • Continuing Education

The College Independent Roman Catholic 4-year coed college. Founded: 1858. *Primary accreditation:* regional. *Setting:* 30-acre suburban campus. *Total enrollment:* 735.

The Department of Nursing, Barat College and Finch University of Health Sciences/The Chicago Medical School Founded in 1986. *Nursing program faculty:* 4 (25% with doctorates).

Academic Facilities *Campus library:* 100,000 volumes (100,000 in health, 1,000 in nursing); 1,100 periodical subscriptions (1,100 health-care related). *Nursing school resources:* CAI, computer lab, nursing audiovisuals, interactive nursing skills videos, learning resource lab.

Calendar Semesters.

NURSING STUDENT PROFILE

Undergraduate **Enrollment:** 48
Women: 96%; **Men:** 4%; **Minority:** 4%; **Part-time:** 85%

BACCALAUREATE PROGRAM

Contact Ms. Patti Mathis, Administrative Assistant, Department of Nursing, Barat College and Finch University of Health Sciences/The Chicago Medical School, 3333 Green Bay Road, North Chicago, IL 60064, 847-578-3324. *Fax:* 847-578-8627.

Expenses *Tuition:* $12,060 full-time, $402 per hour part-time. *Full-time mandatory fees:* $10–$150. *Room and board:* $4680. *Books and supplies per academic year:* $900.

Financial Aid Institutionally sponsored need-based grants/scholarships, institutionally sponsored non-need grants/scholarships, Federal Direct Loans, Federal Pell Grants, Federal Perkins Loans, Federal Supplemental Educational Opportunity Grants, Federal Work-Study. *Application deadline:* 4/15.

RN Baccalaureate Program (BSN)

Applying *Required:* minimum college GPA of 2.0, RN license, diploma or AD in nursing, 2 letters of recommendation, transcript of college record, Illinois RN license. 45 prerequisite credits must be completed before admission to the nursing program. *Options:* Advanced standing available through credit by exam. May apply for transfer of up to 90 total credits. *Application deadline:* rolling. *Application fee:* $20.

Degree Requirements 120 total credit hours, 33 in nursing.

CONTINUING EDUCATION PROGRAM

Contact Dr. Sandra Salloway, Director, Department of Nursing, Barat College and Finch University of Health Sciences/The Chicago Medical School, 3333 Green Bay Road, North Chicago, IL 60064, 847-578-3324. *Fax:* 847-578-8627.

BLESSING-RIEMAN COLLEGE OF NURSING
Quincy, Illinois

Programs • Generic Baccalaureate • RN Baccalaureate

The College Independent 4-year specialized primarily women's college. Founded: 1985. *Primary accreditation:* regional. *Setting:* 1-acre small-town campus. *Total enrollment:* 226. Founded in 1891. *Nursing program faculty:* 13 (8% with doctorates).

▶ ***NOTEWORTHY***

Blessing-Rieman offers a unique joint program with Culver-Stockton College, combining the excellence of a 100+ year-old nursing program with the excellence of a 150+ year-old liberal arts program. Freshman students are accepted as nursing majors. Clinical experiences begin first semester for sophomores and continue for about 1,000 hours through specialty areas and community and critical care. These experiences are held in a regional medical center and more than a dozen community agencies. State-of-the-art clinical and computer laboratories are available for simulated practice. The library holds an extensive nursing collection of bound volumes and periodicals in addition to other learning resources.

Academic Facilities *Campus library:* 3,355 volumes (200 in health, 3,000 in nursing); 88 periodical subscriptions (86 health-care related). *Nursing school resources:* CAI, computer lab, nursing audiovisuals, interactive nursing skills videos, learning resource lab.

Blessing-Rieman College of Nursing (continued)

Student Life *Student services:* health clinic, child-care facilities, personal counseling, career counseling, institutionally sponsored work-study program, job placement, campus safety program. *Nursing student activities:* student nurses association, honor society.

Calendar Semesters.

NURSING STUDENT PROFILE

Undergraduate **Enrollment:** 183
Women: 90%; **Men:** 10%; **Minority:** 4%; **International:** 0%; **Part-time:** 16%

BACCALAUREATE PROGRAMS

Contact Ms. Sharon Wharton, Director of Admissions, Blessing-Rieman College of Nursing, Broadway at 11th Street, Quincy, IL 62305-7005, 217-223-5520 Ext. 6961. *Fax:* 217-223-6400. *E-mail:* swharton@culver.edu

Expenses *Tuition:* $8800 full-time, $370 per credit hour part-time. *Full-time mandatory fees:* $100–$200. *Room and board:* $3800. *Room only:* $1800.

Financial Aid Institutionally sponsored need-based grants/scholarships, institutionally sponsored non-need grants/scholarships, Federal Nursing Student Loans, Federal Pell Grants, Federal Family Education Loan Program (FFELP). 56% of undergraduate students in nursing programs received some form of financial aid in 1995–96. *Application deadline:* 6/1.

Generic Baccalaureate Program (BSN)

Applying *Required:* ACT, TOEFL for nonnative speakers of English, minimum high school GPA of 3.0, minimum college GPA of 2.0, high school chemistry, high school biology, high school transcript, transcript of college record, high school class rank: top 50%. *Application deadline:* rolling.

Degree Requirements 128 total credit hours, 32 in nursing.

RN Baccalaureate Program (BSN)

Applying *Required:* TOEFL for nonnative speakers of English, RN license, diploma or AD in nursing, 40 , transcript of college record. *Options:* Advanced standing available through advanced placement exams. *Application deadline:* rolling.

Degree Requirements 128 total credit hours, 32 in nursing.

See full description on page 434.

BRADLEY UNIVERSITY
Department of Nursing
Peoria, Illinois

Programs • Generic Baccalaureate • Accelerated RN Baccalaureate • LPN to Baccalaureate • Master's

The University Independent comprehensive coed institution. Founded: 1897. *Primary accreditation:* regional. *Setting:* 50-acre urban campus. *Total enrollment:* 5,973.

The Department of Nursing Founded in 1967. *Off-campus program site:* Decatur.

Academic Facilities *Campus library:* 531,744 volumes (120 in health, 37,034 in nursing); 2,100 periodical subscriptions (115 health-care related).

Calendar Semesters.

BACCALAUREATE PROGRAMS

Contact Chairperson, Department of Nursing, Bradley University, Peoria, IL 61625, 309-677-2541. *Fax:* 309-677-2527.

Generic Baccalaureate Program (BSN)

Applying *Required:* SAT I or ACT, TOEFL for nonnative speakers of English, high school math, high school transcript, interview, letter of recommendation, 3 units of high school English, 1 of laboratory science, 2 of social sciences, immunizations, CPR certification. *Application deadline:* rolling.

Degree Requirements 51 total credit hours in nursing.

Accelerated RN Baccalaureate Program (BSN)

Applying *Required:* high school math, interview, letter of recommendation, immunizations, CPR certification. *Application deadline:* rolling.

LPN to Baccalaureate Program (BSN)

Applying *Required:* TOEFL for nonnative speakers of English, NLN Mobility Profile I and II, high school math, interview, letter of recommendation, LPN license, immunizations, CPR certification. *Application deadline:* rolling.

MASTER'S PROGRAMS

Areas of Study Nurse anesthesia; nursing administration.

CHICAGO STATE UNIVERSITY
College of Nursing and Allied Health Professions
Chicago, Illinois

Programs • Generic Baccalaureate • RN Baccalaureate

The University State-supported comprehensive coed institution. Founded: 1867. *Primary accreditation:* regional. *Setting:* 161-acre urban campus. *Total enrollment:* 9,103.

The College of Nursing and Allied Health Professions Founded in 1972. *Nursing program faculty:* 28.

Academic Facilities *Campus library:* 320,000 volumes.

Calendar Semesters.

BACCALAUREATE PROGRAMS

Contact Dr. Linda Hureston, Chair, Business and Health Sciences Building, College of Nursing and Allied Health Professions, Chicago State University, 95th Street at King Drive, Chicago, IL 60628, 312-995-3992.

Expenses *State resident tuition:* $2022 full-time, $84 per credit hour part-time. *Nonresident tuition:* $6066 full-time, $253 per credit hour part-time. *Full-time mandatory fees:* $0–$398. *Part-time mandatory fees:* $0–$131. *Room and board:* $5140.

Financial Aid Institutionally sponsored need-based grants/scholarships, Federal Direct Loans, Federal Pell Grants, Federal Perkins Loans, Federal Supplemental Educational Opportunity Grants, Federal Work-Study, Federal Family Education Loan Program (FFELP), Federal PLUS Loans, Federal Stafford Loans. *Application deadline:* 4/15.

Generic Baccalaureate Program (BSN)

Applying *Required:* ACT, minimum college GPA of 2.5, high school math, high school science, high school transcript, interview, 3 letters of recommendation, immunizations. *Options:* May apply for transfer of up to 0 total credits. *Application deadlines:* 7/15 (fall), 11/15 (spring).

Degree Requirements 120 total credit hours, 60 in nursing. Comprehensive exams.

RN Baccalaureate Program (BSN)

Applying *Required:* ACT, minimum college GPA of 2.5, high school math, high school science, RN license, high school transcript, interview, 3 letters of recommendation, immunizations. *Application deadlines:* 7/15 (fall), 11/15 (spring).

Degree Requirements 120 total credit hours, 60 in nursing. Comprehensive exams.

CONCORDIA UNIVERSITY
Concordia University and West Suburban College of Nursing
Oak Park, Illinois

Programs • Generic Baccalaureate • RN Baccalaureate

The University Independent comprehensive coed institution, Part of Concordia University system. affiliated with Lutheran Church–Missouri Synod. Founded: 1864. *Primary accreditation:* regional. *Setting:* 40-acre suburban campus. *Total enrollment:* 2,418.

The Concordia University and West Suburban College of Nursing Founded in 1982.

Academic Facilities *Campus library:* 153,000 volumes (3,000 in health, 1,000 in nursing); 360 periodical subscriptions (350 health-care related). *Nursing school resources:* CAI, computer lab, nursing audiovisuals, learning resource lab.

Calendar Quarters.

BACCALAUREATE PROGRAMS

Contact Director of Admission, Concordia University and West Suburban College of Nursing, Concordia University, Erie at Austin Boulevard, Oak Park, IL 60302, 708-383-6200 Ext. 6530.

Expenses *Tuition:* ranges from $10,752 to $11,952 full-time, ranges from $224 to $249 per quarter hour part-time. *Full-time mandatory fees:* $83. *Room and board:* $4623. *Room only:* $1635.

Financial Aid Institutionally sponsored need-based grants/scholarships, institutionally sponsored non-need grants/scholarships, Federal Pell Grants, Federal Perkins Loans, Federal Supplemental Educational Opportunity Grants, Federal PLUS Loans, Federal Stafford Loans, SLS program. *Application deadline:* 6/1.

Generic Baccalaureate Program (BS)

Applying *Required:* SAT I or ACT, TOEFL for nonnative speakers of English, high school chemistry, high school biology, high school transcript, letter of recommendation, written essay, high school class rank: top 33%. *Application deadline:* rolling. *Application fee:* $25.

Degree Requirements 192 total credit hours, 84 in nursing.

RN Baccalaureate Program (BS)

Applying *Required:* minimum college GPA of 2.33, RN license, diploma or AD in nursing, letter of recommendation, written essay, transcript of college record. *Options:* Advanced standing available through credit by exam. *Application deadline:* rolling. *Application fee:* $25.

Degree Requirements 192 total credit hours, 84 in nursing.

DEPAUL UNIVERSITY
Department of Nursing
Chicago, Illinois

Programs • RN Baccalaureate • MS • RN to Master's • MS/MPS • Continuing Education

The University Independent Roman Catholic coed university. Founded: 1898. *Primary accreditation:* regional. *Setting:* 36-acre urban campus. *Total enrollment:* 17,133.

The Department of Nursing Founded in 1947. *Nursing program faculty:* 8 (63% with doctorates). *Off-campus program sites:* Arlington Heights, Greyslake, Naperville.

▶ ***NOTEWORTHY***

Located in beautiful Lincoln Park along the north shore of Lake Michigan, DePaul offers the facilities of a major university and the personal attention of a small liberal arts and sciences college. Programs of study meet the needs of today's managed-care environment, using cutting-edge technology. The baccalaureate completion program for registered nurses focuses on case management across the continuum of care. Students with a bachelor's degree can pursue a Certificate of Advanced Study in Managed Care and Case Management. The state-of-the-art master's degree in advanced practice nursing prepares nurses for clinical specialty, nurse practitioner, and case management positions.

Academic Facilities *Campus library:* 700,000 volumes (16,000 in health); 8,500 periodical subscriptions (300 health-care related). *Nursing school resources:* CAI, computer lab, nursing audiovisuals, interactive nursing skills videos, learning resource lab, interactive video classrooms.

Student Life *Student services:* personal counseling, career counseling, institutionally sponsored work-study program, job placement, campus safety program, special assistance for disabled students. *International student services:* counseling/support, ESL courses. *Nursing student activities:* Sigma Theta Tau, membership on department committees.

Calendar Quarters.

NURSING STUDENT PROFILE

Undergraduate **Enrollment:** 32
Women: 75%; **Men:** 25%; **Minority:** 44%; **International:** 10%; **Part-time:** 88%
Graduate **Enrollment:** 79
Women: 97%; **Men:** 3%; **Minority:** 25%; **International:** 5%; **Part-time:** 82%

BACCALAUREATE PROGRAM

Contact Dr. Susan Poslusny, Chairperson and Assistant Professor, Department of Nursing, DePaul University, 802 West Belden Avenue, Chicago, IL 60614, 312-325-7280. *Fax:* 312-325-7282. *E-mail:* sposlusny@condor.depaul.edu

Expenses *Tuition:* $12,750 full-time, $263 per credit part-time. *Full-time mandatory fees:* $10. *Part-time mandatory fees:* $10. *Books and supplies per academic year:* $150.

Financial Aid Institutionally sponsored need-based grants/scholarships, institutionally sponsored non-need grants/scholarships, Federal Nursing Student Loans, Federal Supplemental Educational Opportunity Grants, Federal Work-Study, Federal Scholarship for Disadvantaged Students. 41% of undergraduate students in nursing programs received some form of financial aid in 1995–96. *Application deadline:* 4/1.

RN Baccalaureate Program (BS)

Applying *Required:* TOEFL for nonnative speakers of English, minimum college GPA of 2.5, RN license, diploma or AD in nursing, transcript of college record. *Options:* Advanced standing available through credit by exam. Course work may be accelerated. May apply for transfer of up to 132 total credits. *Application deadline:* rolling. *Application fee:* $25.

Degree Requirements 188 total credit hours, 40 in nursing.

Distance learning Courses provided through video, audio, computer-based media, on-line.

MASTER'S PROGRAMS

Contact Dr. Susan Poslusny, Chairperson and Associate Professor, Department of Nursing, DePaul University, 802 West Belden Avenue, Chicago, IL 60614, 312-325-7280. *Fax:* 312-325-7282. *E-mail:* sposlusn@condor.depaul.edu

Areas of Study Clinical nurse specialist programs in community health nursing, home health care, acute and chronic illness; nurse anesthesia; nursing administration; nursing education; nurse practitioner programs in primary care, psychiatric–mental health.

Expenses *Tuition:* $290 per credit. *Books and supplies per academic year:* $200.

Financial Aid Graduate assistantships, nurse traineeships, Federal Direct Loans, Federal Scholarships for Disadvantaged students. 25% of master's level students in nursing programs received some form of financial aid in 1995-96. *Application deadline:* 4/1.

MS Program

Applying *Required:* GRE General Test, TOEFL for nonnative speakers of English, bachelor's degree in nursing, minimum GPA of 2.8, RN license, 1 year of clinical experience, physical assessment course, statistics course, professional liability/malpractice insurance, 3 letters of recommendation, transcript of college record, 1 year chemistry, critical care experience for nurse anesthesia. *Application deadline:* rolling. *Application fee:* $20.

Degree Requirements 48–64 total credit hours dependent upon track, 48–64 in nursing. Comprehensive exam or research project.

Distance learning Courses provided through interactive video.

RN to Master's Program (MS)

Applying *Required:* GRE General Test, TOEFL for nonnative speakers of English, bachelor's degree, minimum GPA of 3.0, RN license, 1 year of clinical experience, physical assessment course, statistics course, professional liability/malpractice insurance, transcript of college record. *Application deadline:* rolling. *Application fee:* $25.

Degree Requirements 76–92 total credit hours dependent upon track, 64–92 in nursing, up to 12 in other specified areas. Comprehensive exam or research project.

Distance learning Courses provided through interactive video.

DePaul University (continued)

MS/MPS PROGRAM

Applying *Required:* GRE General Test, TOEFL for nonnative speakers of English, bachelor's degree in nursing, minimum GPA of 2.8, RN license, physical assessment course, statistics course, professional liability/ malpractice insurance, 3 letters of recommendation, transcript of college record. *Application deadline:* rolling. *Application fee:* $25.

Degree Requirements 60 total credit hours, 48 in nursing, 12 in public service, nursing. Comprehensive exam or research project.

CONTINUING EDUCATION PROGRAM

Contact Susan Poslusny, Chairperson and Assistant Professor, Department of Nursing, DePaul University, 802 West Belden Avenue, Chicago, IL 60614, 312-325-7280. *Fax:* 312-325-7282. *E-mail:* sposlusny@wppost.depaul.edu

ELMHURST COLLEGE
Deicke Center for Nursing Education
Elmhurst, Illinois

Programs • Generic Baccalaureate • Generic Baccalaureate • RN Baccalaureate • RN Baccalaureate • Baccalaureate for Second Degree • Baccalaureate for Second Degree

The College Independent 4-year coed college, affiliated with United Church of Christ. Founded: 1871. *Primary accreditation:* regional. *Setting:* 38-acre suburban campus. *Total enrollment:* 2,785.

The Deicke Center for Nursing Education Founded in 1971. *Nursing program faculty:* 10 (50% with doctorates). *Off-campus program sites:* Park Ridge, Chicago, Oak Lawn.

Academic Facilities *Campus library:* 240,000 volumes; 1,300 periodical subscriptions. *Nursing school resources:* computer lab, nursing audiovisuals, interactive nursing skills videos, learning resource lab.

Student Life *Student services:* health clinic, personal counseling, career counseling, institutionally sponsored work-study program, job placement, campus safety program. *International student services:* counseling/ support. *Nursing student activities:* Sigma Theta Tau.

Calendar 4-1-4.

NURSING STUDENT PROFILE

Undergraduate **Enrollment:** 145
Women: 96%; **Men:** 4%; **Minority:** 12%; **Part-time:** 30%

BACCALAUREATE PROGRAMS

Contact Dr. Jean Lytle, Director, Deicke Center for Nursing Education, Elmhurst College, 190 Prospect Avenue, Elmhurst, IL 60126, 708-617-3344. *Fax:* 708-617-3237.

Expenses *Tuition:* $10,976 full-time, $320 per semester hour part-time. *Full-time mandatory fees:* $50–$100. *Room and board:* $4660. *Room only:* $2500. *Books and supplies per academic year:* ranges from $500 to $1500.

Financial Aid Institutionally sponsored need-based grants/scholarships, institutionally sponsored non-need grants/scholarships, Federal Direct Loans, Federal Pell Grants, Federal Perkins Loans, Federal Supplemental Educational Opportunity Grants, Federal Work-Study. *Application deadline:* 4/15.

GENERIC BACCALAUREATE PROGRAM (BA)

Applying *Required:* SAT I, ACT, 100% on PC SOLVE CAI, minimum high school GPA of 2.5, minimum college GPA of 2.75, high school chemistry, high school biology, high school foreign language, high school transcript, letter of recommendation, written essay, transcript of college record, high school class rank: top 50%, Student Clinical Nursing Sequence Requirements (available at Deicke Center), minimum 2.0 in all college science courses. 64 prerequisite credits must be completed before admission to the nursing program. *Options:* Advanced standing available through the following means: advanced placement exams, credit by exam. May apply for transfer of up to 64 total credits. *Application deadlines:* 8/1 (fall), 12/15 (spring), 11/1 (nursing program). *Application fee:* $15.

Degree Requirements 128 total credit hours, 40 in nursing.

GENERIC BACCALAUREATE PROGRAM (BS)

Applying *Required:* SAT I, ACT, 100% on PC SOLVE CAI, minimum high school GPA of 2.5, minimum college GPA of 2.75, high school chemistry, high school biology, high school transcript, letter of recommendation, transcript of college record, high school class rank: top 50%, Student Clinical Nursing Sequence Requirements (available at Deicke Center), minimum 2.0 in all college science courses. 64 prerequisite credits must be completed before admission to the nursing program. *Options:* Advanced standing available through the following means: advanced placement exams, credit by exam. May apply for transfer of up to 64 total credits. *Application deadlines:* 8/1 (fall), 12/15 (spring), 11/15 (nursing program). *Application fee:* $15.

Degree Requirements 128 total credit hours, 40 in nursing.

RN BACCALAUREATE PROGRAM (BA)

Applying *Required:* ACT PEP, minimum college GPA of 2.75, RN license, diploma or AD in nursing, letter of recommendation, written essay, transcript of college record, Student Clinical Nursing Sequence Requirements (available at Deicke Center), minimum 2.0 in all college natural science courses. 64 prerequisite credits must be completed before admission to the nursing program. *Options:* Advanced standing available through the following means: advanced placement exams, credit by exam. May apply for transfer of up to 64 total credits. *Application deadlines:* 8/1 (fall), 12/15 (spring). *Application fee:* $15.

Degree Requirements 128 total credit hours, 40 in nursing.

RN BACCALAUREATE PROGRAM (BS)

Applying *Required:* ACT PEP, 100% on PC SOLVE, minimum college GPA of 2.75, RN license, diploma or AD in nursing, letter of recommendation, written essay, transcript of college record, Student Clinical Nursing Sequence Requirements (available at Deicke Center), minimum 2.0 in all college natural science courses. 64 prerequisite credits must be completed before admission to the nursing program. *Options:* Advanced standing available through the following means: advanced placement exams, credit by exam. May apply for transfer of up to 64 total credits. *Application deadlines:* 9/1 (fall), 12/15 (spring). *Application fee:* $15.

Degree Requirements 128 total credit hours, 40 in nursing.

BACCALAUREATE FOR SECOND DEGREE PROGRAM (BA)

Applying *Required:* 100% on PC SOLVE CAI, minimum college GPA of 2.75, high school foreign language, high school transcript, letter of recommendation, written essay, transcript of college record, Student Clinical Nursing Sequence Requirements (available at Deicke Center), minimum 2.0 in all college natural science courses. 64 prerequisite credits must be completed before admission to the nursing program. *Options:* Advanced standing available through the following means: advanced placement exams, credit by exam. *Application deadlines:* 8/1 (fall), 12/15 (spring), 11/1 (nursing program). *Application fee:* $15.

Degree Requirements 40 total credit hours, 40 in nursing.

BACCALAUREATE FOR SECOND DEGREE PROGRAM (BS)

Applying *Required:* 100% on PC SOLVE CAI, minimum college GPA of 2.75, high school foreign language, high school transcript, letter of recommendation, written essay, transcript of college record, Student Clinical Nursing Sequence Requirements (available at Deicke Center), minimum 2.0 in all college natural science courses. 64 prerequisite credits must be completed before admission to the nursing program. *Options:* Advanced standing available through the following means: advanced placement exams, credit by exam. *Application deadlines:* 8/1 (fall), 12/15 (spring), 11/1 (nursing program). *Application fee:* $15.

Degree Requirements 40 total credit hours in nursing.

GOVERNORS STATE UNIVERSITY
Division of Nursing
University Park, Illinois

Programs • RN Baccalaureate • MS • Continuing Education

The University State-supported upper-level coed institution. Founded: 1969. *Primary accreditation:* regional. *Setting:* 750-acre suburban campus. *Total enrollment:* 6,073.

The Division of Nursing Founded in 1971. *Nursing program faculty:* 8 (88% with doctorates). *Off-campus program sites:* Chicago, Kankakee.

Academic Facilities *Campus library:* 179,408 volumes (13,891 in health, 1,499 in nursing); 2,188 periodical subscriptions (420 health-care related).

Nursing school resources: CAI, computer lab, nursing audiovisuals, interactive nursing skills videos, learning resource lab.

Student Life *Student services:* child-care facilities, personal counseling, career counseling, institutionally sponsored work-study program, job placement, special assistance for disabled students, academic support services. *International student services:* counseling/support, mentorship program. *Nursing student activities:* Sigma Theta Tau, nursing club, all-campus student senate.

Calendar Trimesters.

NURSING STUDENT PROFILE

Undergraduate **Enrollment:** 63
Women: 98%; **Men:** 2%; **Minority:** 48%; **International:** 2%; **Part-time:** 100%
Graduate **Enrollment:** 52
Women: 94%; **Men:** 6%; **Minority:** 48%; **International:** 0%; **Part-time:** 100%

BACCALAUREATE PROGRAM

Contact Dr. Annie Lawrence, Chairperson, Division of Nursing, College of Health Professions, Governors State University, University Park, IL 60466, 708-534-4042. *Fax:* 708-534-8958.

Expenses *State resident tuition:* $1014 full-time, $85 per credit hour part-time. *Nonresident tuition:* $3042 full-time, $253 per credit hour part-time. *Full-time mandatory fees:* $85. *Books and supplies per academic year:* $300.

Financial Aid Institutionally sponsored need-based grants/scholarships, institutionally sponsored non-need grants/scholarships, Federal Nursing Student Loans, Federal Supplemental Educational Opportunity Grants, Federal Work-Study. *Application deadline:* 10/1.

RN Baccalaureate Program (BS)

Applying *Required:* ACT, TOEFL for nonnative speakers of English, NLN Mobility Profile II for non-NLN ABN programs, RN license, diploma or AD in nursing, transcript of college record, minimum 2.0 GPA in nursing. 60 prerequisite credits must be completed before admission to the nursing program. *Options:* Course work may be accelerated. May apply for transfer of up to 75 total credits. *Application deadlines:* 7/16 (fall), 11/19 (spring), 4/15 (summer).

Degree Requirements 120 total credit hours, 67 in nursing.

MASTER'S PROGRAM

Contact Dr. Annie Lawrence, Chairperson, Division of Nursing, College of Health Professions, Governors State University, University Park, IL 60466, 708-534-4042.

Areas of Study Clinical nurse specialist programs in critical care nursing, restorative nursing; nursing administration; nursing education.

Expenses *State resident tuition:* $1068 full-time, $89 per credit hour part-time. *Nonresident tuition:* $3204 full-time, $267 per credit hour part-time. *Full-time mandatory fees:* $195. *Books and supplies per academic year:* ranges from $200 to $275.

Financial Aid Graduate assistantships, nurse traineeships, Federal Nursing Student Loans, tuition waivers. 12% of master's level students in nursing programs received some form of financial aid in 1995-96. *Application deadline:* 10/1.

MS Program

Applying *Required:* GRE General Test, bachelor's degree in nursing, minimum GPA of 2.5, RN license, 2 years of clinical experience, physical assessment course, statistics course, professional liability/malpractice insurance, essay, 3 letters of recommendation, transcript of college record, minimum 3.0 GPA in upper-division nursing courses. *Application deadlines:* 7/16 (fall), 11/19 (spring), 4/15 (summer).

Degree Requirements 35–38 total credit hours dependent upon track, 26–27 in nursing, 3–9 in pathophysiology and selective/electives. Comprehensive exam.

CONTINUING EDUCATION PROGRAM

Contact Dr. Annie Lawrence, Chair, Division of Nursing and Health Science, Governors State University, University Park, IL 60460, 708-534-4042. *Fax:* 708-534-8958. *E-mail:* alawrence@csu.edu

ILLINOIS BENEDICTINE UNIVERSITY
Department of Nursing
Lisle, Illinois

Program • Accelerated RN Baccalaureate

The University Independent Roman Catholic comprehensive coed institution. Founded: 1887. *Primary accreditation:* regional. *Setting:* 108-acre suburban campus. *Total enrollment:* 2,485.

The Department of Nursing Founded in 1981. *Nursing program faculty:* 3 (67% with doctorates).

Academic Facilities *Campus library:* 88,900 volumes (1,350 in health, 850 in nursing); 800 periodical subscriptions (169 health-care related). *Nursing school resources:* CAI, computer lab, nursing audiovisuals.

Student Life *Student services:* health clinic, child-care facilities, personal counseling, career counseling, job placement, campus safety program. *International student services:* ESL courses. *Nursing student activities:* Sigma Theta Tau.

Calendar Modular.

NURSING STUDENT PROFILE

Undergraduate **Enrollment:** 54
Women: 100%; **Minority:** 15%; **Part-time:** 94%

BACCALAUREATE PROGRAM

Contact Ms. Barbara Haubec, Nursing Secretary, Department of Nursing, Benedictine University, 5700 College Road, Lisle, IL 60532, 630-829-6580. *Fax:* 630-829-6584.

Expenses *Tuition:* $11,640 full-time, $390 per credit hour part-time. *Full-time mandatory fees:* $200. *Part-time mandatory fees:* $0. *Books and supplies per academic year:* $500.

Financial Aid Institutionally sponsored need-based grants/scholarships. 80% of undergraduate students in nursing programs received some form of financial aid in 1995–96. *Application deadline:* 4/15.

Accelerated RN Baccalaureate Program (BSN)

Applying *Required:* minimum college GPA of 2.0, RN license, diploma or AD in nursing, transcript of college record. *Options:* Advanced standing available through the following means: advanced placement exams, advanced placement without credit, credit by exam. Course work may be accelerated. May apply for transfer of up to 90 total credits. *Application deadline:* rolling. *Application fee:* $30.

Degree Requirements 120 total credit hours, 53 in nursing.

ILLINOIS WESLEYAN UNIVERSITY
School of Nursing
Bloomington, Illinois

Programs • Generic Baccalaureate • RN Baccalaureate • Baccalaureate for Second Degree

The University Independent 4-year coed college. Founded: 1850. *Primary accreditation:* regional. *Setting:* 63-acre suburban campus. *Total enrollment:* 1,875.

The School of Nursing Founded in 1958. *Nursing program faculty:* 13 (64% with doctorates).

Academic Facilities *Campus library:* 194,182 volumes (6,018 in health, 1,009 in nursing); 1,075 periodical subscriptions (120 health-care related). *Nursing school resources:* CAI, computer lab, nursing audiovisuals, interactive nursing skills videos, learning resource lab, Internet and World Wide Web lab.

Student Life *Student services:* health clinic, child-care facilities, personal counseling, career counseling, institutionally sponsored work-study program, job placement, campus safety program. *International student services:*

Illinois Wesleyan University (continued)
counseling/support, special assistance for nonnative speakers of English. *Nursing student activities:* Sigma Theta Tau, student nurses association, Alpha Tau Delta.

Calendar 4-4-1.

NURSING STUDENT PROFILE

Undergraduate **Enrollment:** 100
Women: 95%; **Men:** 5%; **Minority:** 5%; **International:** 2%; **Part-time:** 2%

BACCALAUREATE PROGRAMS

Contact Dr. Donna L. Hartweg, Director, School of Nursing, Illinois Wesleyan University, PO Box 2900, Bloomington, IL 61702-2900, 309-556-3051. *Fax:* 309-556-3043. *E-mail:* dhartweg@titan.iwu.edu

Expenses *Tuition:* $17,380 per academic year. *Full-time mandatory fees:* $110. *Room and board:* $4590. *Room only:* $2640.

Financial Aid Institutionally sponsored need-based grants/scholarships, institutionally sponsored non-need grants/scholarships, Federal Nursing Student Loans, Federal Supplemental Educational Opportunity Grants, Federal Work-Study. *Application deadline:* 3/1.

Generic Baccalaureate Program (BSN)

Applying *Required:* SAT I, ACT, TOEFL for nonnative speakers of English, high school chemistry, high school biology, high school transcript, written essay, high school class rank: top 30%. *Options:* Advanced standing available through the following means: advanced placement exams, advanced placement without credit, credit by exam. May apply for transfer of up to 72 total credits. *Application deadlines:* 5/1 (fall), 12/1 (spring).

Degree Requirements 128 total credit hours, 60 in nursing.

RN Baccalaureate Program (BSN)

Applying *Required:* SAT I, ACT, TOEFL for nonnative speakers of English, minimum college GPA of 3.0, high school chemistry, high school biology, RN license, high school transcript, written essay, transcript of college record. *Options:* Advanced standing available through the following means: advanced placement exams, advanced placement without credit, credit by exam. May apply for transfer of up to 64 total credits. *Application deadlines:* 5/1 (fall), 12/1 (spring).

Degree Requirements 128 total credit hours, 60 in nursing.

Baccalaureate for Second Degree Program (BSN)

Applying *Required:* SAT I, ACT, TOEFL for nonnative speakers of English, minimum college GPA of 3.0, high school chemistry, high school biology, high school transcript, written essay, transcript of college record. *Options:* Advanced standing available through the following means: advanced placement exams, advanced placement without credit, credit by exam. *Application deadlines:* 5/1 (fall), 12/1 (spring).

Degree Requirements 128 total credit hours, 64 in nursing.

See full description on page 460.

LEWIS UNIVERSITY
College of Nursing
Romeoville, Illinois

Programs • Generic Baccalaureate • RN Baccalaureate • Baccalaureate for Second Degree • MSN • RN to Master's • Master's for Nurses with Non-Nursing Degrees

The University Independent comprehensive coed institution, affiliated with Roman Catholic Church. Founded: 1932. *Primary accreditation:* regional. *Setting:* 600-acre small-town campus. *Total enrollment:* 4,348.

The College of Nursing Founded in 1973. *Nursing program faculty:* 50 (20% with doctorates). *Off-campus program sites:* Hickory Hills, Schaumburg.

Academic Facilities *Campus library:* 170,000 volumes (30,000 in health, 20,000 in nursing); 650 periodical subscriptions (200 health-care related). *Nursing school resources:* CAI, computer lab, nursing audiovisuals, interactive nursing skills videos, learning resource lab.

Student Life *Student services:* health clinic, personal counseling, career counseling, institutionally sponsored work-study program, campus safety program. *International student services:* ESL courses. *Nursing student activities:* Sigma Theta Tau, student nurses association.

Calendar Semesters.

NURSING STUDENT PROFILE

Undergraduate **Enrollment:** 600
Women: 94%; **Men:** 6%; **Minority:** 18%; **International:** 0%; **Part-time:** 35%
Graduate **Enrollment:** 80
Women: 95%; **Men:** 5%; **Minority:** 10%; **International:** 0%; **Part-time:** 90%

BACCALAUREATE PROGRAMS

Contact Ms. Nan Yancey, Undergraduate Director, College of Nursing, Lewis University, Route 53, Romeoville, IL 60446-2298, 815-838-0500 Ext. 5359. *Fax:* 815-838-8306.

Expenses *Tuition:* $8880 full-time, $370 per credit part-time. *Full-time mandatory fees:* $0. *Room and board:* $5118. *Books and supplies per academic year:* $300.

Financial Aid Institutionally sponsored need-based grants/scholarships, institutionally sponsored non-need grants/scholarships, Federal Pell Grants, Federal Perkins Loans, Federal Supplemental Educational Opportunity Grants, Federal Work-Study. 50% of undergraduate students in nursing programs received some form of financial aid in 1995–96. *Application deadline:* 4/1.

Generic Baccalaureate Program (BSN)

Applying *Required:* ACT, minimum college GPA of 2.5, 3 years of high school math, 3 years of high school science, high school transcript, transcript of college record. 31 prerequisite credits must be completed before admission to the nursing program. *Options:* May apply for transfer of up to 72–96 total credits. *Application deadline:* rolling. *Application fee:* $50.

Degree Requirements 128 total credit hours, 58 in nursing.

RN Baccalaureate Program (BSN)

Applying *Required:* minimum college GPA of 2.5, RN license, diploma or AD in nursing, transcript of college record. 31 prerequisite credits must be completed before admission to the nursing program. *Options:* Course work may be accelerated. May apply for transfer of up to 96 total credits. *Application deadline:* rolling.

Degree Requirements 128 total credit hours, 19 in nursing. 15 general education credits, last 32 credits must be taken at Lewis University.

Baccalaureate for Second Degree Program (BSN)

Applying *Required:* minimum college GPA of 2.25, transcript of college record. 31 prerequisite credits must be completed before admission to the nursing program. *Options:* May apply for transfer of up to 96 total credits. *Application deadline:* rolling. *Application fee:* $50.

Degree Requirements 58 total credit hours, 58 in nursing. 15 general education credits.

MASTER'S PROGRAMS

Contact Dr. Sue Barrett, Graduate Director, College of Nursing, Lewis University, Route 53, Romeoville, IL 60446-2298, 815-838-0500 Ext. 5363. *Fax:* 815-838-8306.

Areas of Study Clinical nurse specialist program in community health nursing; nursing administration; nursing education.

Expenses *Tuition:* $6660 full-time, $370 per credit part-time. *Full-time mandatory fees:* $0. *Books and supplies per academic year:* $200.

Financial Aid Graduate assistantships, nurse traineeships. 15% of master's level students in nursing programs received some form of financial aid in 1995-96. *Application deadline:* 8/1.

MSN Program

Applying *Required:* GRE or written essay, bachelor's degree in nursing, minimum GPA of 2.5, RN license, 1 year of clinical experience, statistics course, essay, interview, 3 letters of recommendation, transcript of college record. *Application deadline:* rolling.

Degree Requirements 33 total credit hours, 27–33 in nursing, up to 6 in education or business.

RN to Master's Program (MSN)

Applying *Required:* GRE or written essay, minimum GPA of 3.0, RN license, 2 years of clinical experience, statistics course, interview, 3 letters of recommendation, transcript of college record. *Application deadline:* rolling.

Degree Requirements 59–75 total credit hours dependent upon track, 40–46 in nursing, up to 6 in education or business. 13 hours in undergraduate nursing.

Master's for Nurses with Non-Nursing Degrees Program (MSN)

Applying *Required:* GRE or written essay, minimum GPA of 3.0, RN license, 2 years of clinical experience, statistics course, interview, 3 letters of recommendation, transcript of college record. *Application deadline:* rolling.

Degree Requirements 33–44 total credit hours dependent upon track, 27–44 in nursing, up to 6 in education or business.

LOYOLA UNIVERSITY CHICAGO

Marcella Niehoff School of Nursing Chicago, Illinois

Programs • Generic Baccalaureate • Accelerated RN Baccalaureate • Baccalaureate for Second Degree • RN to Master's • MSN/MBA • MSN/MDiv • PhD

The University Independent Roman Catholic (Jesuit) coed university. Founded: 1870. *Primary accreditation:* regional. *Setting:* 105-acre urban campus. *Total enrollment:* 14,001.

The Marcella Niehoff School of Nursing Founded in 1935. *Nursing program faculty:* 46 (83% with doctorates). *Off-campus program site:* Maywood.

Academic Facilities *Campus library:* 1.3 million volumes (51,674 in health, 4,966 in nursing); 11,581 periodical subscriptions (2,630 health-care related). *Nursing school resources:* CAI, computer lab, nursing audiovisuals, interactive nursing skills videos, learning resource lab.

Student Life *Student services:* health clinic, child-care facilities, personal counseling, career counseling, institutionally sponsored work-study program, job placement, campus safety program, special assistance for disabled students. *International student services:* counseling/support, special assistance for nonnative speakers of English, ESL courses. *Nursing student activities:* Sigma Theta Tau, student nurses association.

Calendar Semesters.

NURSING STUDENT PROFILE

Undergraduate **Enrollment:** 420

Women: 94%; **Men:** 6%; **Minority:** 29%; **International:** 1%; **Part-time:** 16%

Graduate **Enrollment:** 230

Women: 97%; **Men:** 3%; **Minority:** 6%; **International:** 1%; **Part-time:** 93%

BACCALAUREATE PROGRAMS

Contact Ms. Sandra LaBlance, Assistant Dean of Students, Marcella Niehoff School of Nursing, Loyola University of Chicago, 6525 North Sheridan Road, Chicago, IL 60626, 773-508-3262. *Fax:* 773-508-3241. *E-mail:* slablan@luc.edu

Expenses *Tuition:* $14,400 full-time, $325 per credit part-time. *Full-time mandatory fees:* $516. *Room and board:* $5776–$6519. *Room only:* $4363–$4548.

Financial Aid Institutionally sponsored need-based grants/scholarships, institutionally sponsored non-need grants/scholarships, Federal Nursing Student Loans, Federal Supplemental Educational Opportunity Grants, Federal Work-Study. *Application deadline:* 2/15.

Generic Baccalaureate Program (BSN)

Applying *Required:* SAT I, ACT, TOEFL for nonnative speakers of English, 3 years of high school math, high school chemistry, high school biology, high school transcript, transcript of college record, health insurance, immunizations, CPR certification. *Options:* May apply for transfer of up to 64 total credits. *Application deadlines:* 3/1 (fall), 12/1 (spring). *Application fee:* $25.

Degree Requirements 130 total credit hours, 51 in nursing.

Accelerated RN Baccalaureate Program (BSN)

Applying *Required:* minimum college GPA of 2.5, RN license, high school transcript, transcript of college record, health insurance, immunizations, CPR certification. 20 prerequisite credits must be completed before admission to the nursing program. *Options:* May apply for transfer of up to 64 total credits. *Application deadline:* rolling. *Application fee:* $25.

Degree Requirements 130 total credit hours, 51 in nursing.

Baccalaureate for Second Degree Program (BSN)

Applying *Required:* minimum college GPA of 3.0, high school transcript, written essay, transcript of college record, health insurance, immunizations, CPR certification. *Options:* May apply for transfer of up to 79 total credits. *Application deadlines:* 2/1 (fall), 2/1 (summer). *Application fee:* $25.

Degree Requirements 130 total credit hours, 51 in nursing.

MASTER'S PROGRAMS

Contact Dr. Marcia C. Maurer, Associate Dean and Director of Graduate Programs, Marcella Niehoff School of Nursing, Loyola University of Chicago, 6525 North Sheridan Road, Chicago, IL 60626, 312-508-3261. *Fax:* 312-508-3241. *E-mail:* mmaurer@luc.edu

Areas of Study Clinical nurse specialist programs in critical care nursing, oncology nursing, cardiac rehabilitation; nursing administration; nurse practitioner programs in adult health, child care/pediatrics, women's health, critical care/trauma.

Expenses *Tuition:* $8568 full-time, $408 per semester hour part-time. *Full-time mandatory fees:* $55. *Part-time mandatory fees:* $40. *Books and supplies per academic year:* ranges from $200 to $500.

Financial Aid Graduate assistantships, nurse traineeships, fellowships, Federal Direct Loans, Federal Nursing Student Loans, institutionally sponsored loans, employment opportunities, ICEOP for Illinois residents. 5% of master's level students in nursing programs received some form of financial aid in 1995-96. *Application deadline:* 5/31.

RN to Master's Program (MSN)

Applying *Required:* GRE General Test, TOEFL for nonnative speakers of English, minimum GPA of 3.0, RN license, 4 years of clinical experience, physical assessment course, statistics course, professional liability/malpractice insurance, essay, interview, 3 letters of recommendation, transcript of college record, ADN or diploma in nursing, professional portfolio. *Application deadlines:* 5/31 (fall), 11/30 (spring). *Application fee:* $30.

Degree Requirements 124 total credit hours, 75 in nursing. Comprehensive exam.

MSN/MBA Program

Applying *Required:* GMAT, bachelor's degree in nursing, minimum GPA of 3.0, RN license, 1 year of clinical experience, statistics course, interview, 3 letters of recommendation, transcript of college record. *Application deadlines:* 5/31 (fall), 11/30 (spring). *Application fee:* $30.

Degree Requirements 75 total credit hours, 36 in nursing, 39 in business administration.

MSN/MDiv Program

Applying *Required:* GRE General Test, TOEFL for nonnative speakers of English, bachelor's degree in nursing, minimum GPA of 3.0, RN license, 1 year of clinical experience, physical assessment course, statistics course, professional liability/malpractice insurance, essay, interview, 3 letters of recommendation, transcript of college record. *Application deadline:* rolling. *Application fee:* $30.

Degree Requirements 75 total credit hours. Thesis or comprehensive exam.

DOCTORAL PROGRAM

Contact Dr. Marcia C. Maurer, Associate Dean and Director of Graduate Programs, Marcella Niehoff School of Nursing, Loyola University of Chicago, 6525 North Sheridan Road, Chicago, IL 60626, 312-508 3261. *Fax:* 312-508-3241.

Areas of Study Nursing research.

Expenses *Tuition:* $408 per semester hour. *Full-time mandatory fees:* $55. *Part-time mandatory fees:* $40. *Books and supplies per academic year:* ranges from $200 to $500.

Financial Aid Graduate assistantships, nurse traineeships, fellowships, dissertation grants, Federal Direct Loans, institutionally sponsored loans. *Application deadline:* 1/1.

Loyola University Chicago (continued)

PhD Program

Applying *Required:* GRE General Test (minimum combined score of 1500 on three tests), TOEFL for nonnative speakers of English, 1 scholarly paper, statistics course, interview, 3 letters of recommendation, vitae, writing sample, BSN, Illinois RN license. *Application deadline:* 1/1. *Application fee:* $30.

Degree Requirements 63 total credit hours; 9 semester hours in philosophy/ethics, 9 semester hours of electives, 15 semester hours in research, 30 semester hours in nursing; dissertation; oral exam; written exam; defense of dissertation; English as a second language course for nonnative English-speaking PhD students.

See full description on page 472.

MACMURRAY COLLEGE
Nursing Department
Jacksonville, Illinois

Programs • Generic Baccalaureate • RN Baccalaureate

The College Independent United Methodist 4-year coed college. Founded: 1846. *Primary accreditation:* regional. *Setting:* 60-acre small-town campus. *Total enrollment:* 693.

The Nursing Department Founded in 1979. *Nursing program faculty:* 5.

▶ ***NOTEWORTHY***

MacMurray College offers a Bachelor of Science in Nursing degree program firmly based on an acclaimed liberal arts core curriculum. Although it is a young program, it has grown rapidly to prominence. It is fully accredited by the National League for Nursing, and its graduates achieve high pass rates on the licensure exam as well as excellent placement in the nursing profession. Passavant Area Hospital in Jacksonville, Memorial Medical Center and St. John's Hospital in nearby Springfield, and area community health agencies provide varied clinical experiences.

Academic Facilities *Campus library:* 145,000 volumes (750 in health, 1,700 in nursing); 450 periodical subscriptions (50 health-care related). *Nursing school resources:* CAI, computer lab, nursing audiovisuals, interactive nursing skills videos, learning resource lab.

Student Life *Student services:* health clinic, personal counseling, career counseling, institutionally sponsored work-study program, job placement, campus safety program, special assistance for disabled students. *Nursing student activities:* student nurses association.

Calendar Semesters.

NURSING STUDENT PROFILE

Undergraduate **Enrollment:** 70

Women: 80%; **Men:** 20%; **Minority:** 4%; **International:** 1%; **Part-time:** 7%

BACCALAUREATE PROGRAMS

Contact Dr. Margaret A. Boudreau, Director of Nursing, Nursing Department, MacMurray College, 447 East College Avenue, Jacksonville, IL 62650, 217-479-7083. *Fax:* 217-479-7086. *E-mail:* macbsn@fgi.net

Expenses *Tuition:* $10,940 full-time, $330 per credit hour part-time. *Full-time mandatory fees:* $200. *Room and board:* $4000. *Room only:* $1800. *Books and supplies per academic year:* ranges from $625 to $800.

Financial Aid Institutionally sponsored need-based grants/scholarships, institutionally sponsored non-need grants/scholarships, Federal Nursing Student Loans, Federal Supplemental Educational Opportunity Grants. 84% of undergraduate students in nursing programs received some form of financial aid in 1995–96. *Application deadline:* 5/1.

Generic Baccalaureate Program (BSN)

Applying *Required:* ACT, minimum high school GPA of 2.5, high school transcript, 2 letters of recommendation, written essay, high school class rank: top 50%. *Options:* May apply for transfer of up to 60 total credits. *Application deadline:* rolling. *Application fee:* $10.

Degree Requirements 126 total credit hours, 51 in nursing.

RN Baccalaureate Program (BSN)

Applying *Required:* RN license, diploma or AD in nursing, interview, transcript of college record. *Options:* May apply for transfer of up to 60 total credits. *Application deadline:* rolling. *Application fee:* $10.

Degree Requirements 126 total credit hours, 51 in nursing.

MCKENDREE COLLEGE
Division of Nursing
Lebanon, Illinois

Program • RN Baccalaureate

The College Independent 4-year coed college, affiliated with United Methodist Church. Founded: 1828. *Primary accreditation:* regional. *Setting:* 50-acre small-town campus. *Total enrollment:* 1,618.

The Division of Nursing Founded in 1978. *Nursing program faculty:* 10 (20% with doctorates). *Off-campus program sites:* Carterville, Ina, Godfrey.

▶ ***NOTEWORTHY***

McKendree College in Lebanon, Illinois, has offered a BSN completion program for registered nurses since 1978. The NLN-accredited, upper-division curriculum is designed exclusively for graduates of diploma and associate degree programs. Combining liberal arts with career-directed studies, the curriculum builds on the registered nurses' previous education and experience while promoting their professional status and career possibilities. The nursing courses consist of 30 hours of upper-level study that can be completed in a format compatible with a working nurse's schedule. Options include 1 day per week, 2 days per week for those interested in full-time study, and evenings at select sites throughout southern Illinois and Kentucky.

Academic Facilities *Campus library:* 75,000 volumes (1,881 in health, 700 in nursing); 514 periodical subscriptions (51 health-care related). *Nursing school resources:* CAI, computer lab, nursing audiovisuals, learning resource lab.

Calendar Semesters.

NURSING STUDENT PROFILE

Undergraduate **Enrollment:** 334

Women: 96%; **Men:** 4%; **Minority:** 5%; **International:** 0%; **Part-time:** 94%

BACCALAUREATE PROGRAM

Contact Ms. Pam Chambers, Admissions Counselor/Nursing Recruiter, Division of Nursing, McKendree College, 701 College Road, Lebanon, IL 62254, 618-537-4481. *Fax:* 618-537-6259.

Expenses *Tuition:* $7200 full-time, $300 per credit hour part-time. *Full-time mandatory fees:* $50. *Room and board:* $3500. *Books and supplies per academic year:* $350.

Financial Aid Institutionally sponsored need-based grants/scholarships, Federal Nursing Student Loans, Federal Supplemental Educational Opportunity Grants, Federal Work-Study. 78% of undergraduate students in nursing programs received some form of financial aid in 1995–96. *Application deadline:* 7/1.

RN Baccalaureate Program (BSN)

Applying *Required:* minimum college GPA of 2.5, high school transcript, transcript of college record. *Options:* Advanced standing available through credit by exam. Course work may be accelerated. May apply for transfer of up to 70–96 total credits. *Application deadlines:* 8/1 (fall), 11/30 (spring).

Degree Requirements 128 total credit hours, 30 in nursing.

MENNONITE COLLEGE OF NURSING
Bloomington, Illinois

Programs • Generic Baccalaureate • RN Baccalaureate • BSN to Master's

The College Independent interdenominational upper-level specialized coed institution. Founded: 1919. *Primary accreditation:* regional. *Setting:* 2-acre urban campus. *Total enrollment:* 198. Founded in 1982. *Nursing program faculty:* 38 (16% with doctorates).

Academic Facilities *Campus library:* 6,822 volumes (5,116 in health, 1,706 in nursing); 550 periodical subscriptions (540 health-care related). *Nursing school resources:* CAI, computer lab, nursing audiovisuals, interactive nursing skills videos, Internet.

Student Life *Student services:* personal counseling, career counseling, institutionally sponsored work-study program, job placement, campus safety program, special assistance for disabled students. *International student services:* Transcultural Nursing Program, Transcultural Nursing Club. *Nursing student activities:* Sigma Theta Tau, nursing club, student nurses association, Nursing Honor Society, Mennonite Student Nursing Organization.

Calendar Semesters.

NURSING STUDENT PROFILE

Undergraduate **Enrollment:** 175
Women: 91%; **Men:** 9%; **Minority:** 6%; **International:** 0%; **Part-time:** 6%
Graduate **Enrollment:** 25
Women: 100%; **Minority:** 4%; **International:** 0%; **Part-time:** 76%

BACCALAUREATE PROGRAMS

Contact Ms. Mary Ann Watkins, Director of Admissions and Financial Aid, Mennonite College of Nursing, 804 North East Street, Bloomington, IL 61701, 309-829-0718. *Fax:* 309-829-0765.

Expenses *Tuition:* $8834 full-time, $368 per credit hour part-time. *Full-time mandatory fees:* $0. *Room and board:* $2556. *Room only:* $2046. *Books and supplies per academic year:* $648.

Financial Aid Institutionally sponsored need-based grants/scholarships, institutionally sponsored non-need grants/scholarships, Federal Nursing Student Loans, Federal Pell Grants, Federal Perkins Loans, Federal Supplemental Educational Opportunity Grants, Federal Work-Study. *Application deadline:* 4/1.

Generic Baccalaureate Program (BSN)

Applying *Required:* SAT I, ACT, minimum college GPA of 2.5, high school transcript, 2 letters of recommendation, transcript of college record, no grade lower than "C" will be accepted. 60 prerequisite credits must be completed before admission to the nursing program. *Options:* May apply for transfer of up to 35 total credits. *Application deadline:* rolling.

Degree Requirements 125 total credit hours, 65 in nursing.

RN Baccalaureate Program (BSN)

Applying *Required:* minimum college GPA of 2.5, RN license, diploma or AD in nursing, 2 letters of recommendation, written essay, transcript of college record, 2.5 GPA for all previous nursing coursework with no grade lower than "C". 60 prerequisite credits must be completed before admission to the nursing program. *Options:* May apply for transfer of up to 9 total credits. *Application deadline:* rolling.

Degree Requirements 125 total credit hours, 65 in nursing.

MASTER'S PROGRAM

Contact Mary Ann Watkins, Director of Admissions and Financial Aid, Mennonite College of Nursing, 804 North East Street, Bloomington, IL 61701, 309-829-0718. *Fax:* 309-829-0765.

Areas of Study Nurse practitioner program in family health.

Expenses *Tuition:* $405 per semester hour. *Full-time mandatory fees:* $0. *Room and board:* $3858. *Books and supplies per academic year:* $384.

Financial Aid Nurse traineeships, Federal Nursing Student Loans, institutionally sponsored loans, institutionally sponsored need-based grants/scholarships. 40% of master's level students in nursing programs received some form of financial aid in 1995-96. *Application deadline:* 4/1.

BSN to Master's Program (MSN)

Applying *Required:* GRE General Test, bachelor's degree in nursing, minimum GPA of 3.0, RN license, 2 years of clinical experience, physical assessment course, statistics course, essay, interview, 3 letters of recommendation, transcript of college record, resume, nursing research course with no grade lower than "C". *Application deadline:* 2/1.

Degree Requirements 43 total credit hours, 43 in nursing. 3.0 overall GPA.

See full description on page 480.

MILLIKIN UNIVERSITY
School of Nursing
Decatur, Illinois

Programs • Generic Baccalaureate • RN Baccalaureate

The University Independent 4-year coed college, affiliated with Presbyterian Church (U.S.A.). Founded: 1901. *Primary accreditation:* regional. *Setting:* 45-acre suburban campus. *Total enrollment:* 1,883.

The School of Nursing Founded in 1979. *Nursing program faculty:* 10 (10% with doctorates).

Academic Facilities *Campus library:* 160,000 volumes (10,000 in health, 6,000 in nursing); 1,000 periodical subscriptions (64 health-care related). *Nursing school resources:* CAI, computer lab, nursing audiovisuals, interactive nursing skills videos, learning resource lab.

Student Life *Student services:* health clinic, personal counseling, career counseling, institutionally sponsored work-study program, job placement, campus safety program. *International student services:* counseling/support. *Nursing student activities:* recruiter club, nursing club, student nurses association, Alpha Tau Delta.

Calendar Semesters.

NURSING STUDENT PROFILE

Undergraduate **Enrollment:** 185
Women: 88%; **Men:** 12%; **Minority:** 5%; **International:** 0%; **Part-time:** 10%

BACCALAUREATE PROGRAMS

Contact Dr. Linda K. Niedringhaus, Dean of Nursing, School of Nursing, Millikin University, 1184 West Main Street, Decatur, IL 62522, 217-424-6348. *Fax:* 217-424-3993. *E-mail:* lniedringhaus@mail.millikin.edu

Expenses *Tuition:* $13,000 full-time, $360 per credit hour part-time. *Full-time mandatory fees:* $90. *Room and board:* $4800. *Room only:* $2500. *Books and supplies per academic year:* ranges from $400 to $500.

Financial Aid Institutionally sponsored need-based grants/scholarships, institutionally sponsored non-need grants/scholarships, Federal Direct Loans, Federal Pell Grants, Federal Perkins Loans, Federal Supplemental Educational Opportunity Grants, Federal Work-Study. 90% of undergraduate students in nursing programs received some form of financial aid in 1995–96. *Application deadline:* 4/30.

Generic Baccalaureate Program (BSN)

Applying *Required:* ACT, TOEFL for nonnative speakers of English, minimum high school GPA of 3.0, minimum college GPA of 2.5, 3 years of high school math, high school chemistry, high school biology, high school transcript, 3 letters of recommendation, transcript of college record, high school class rank: top 25%. 12 prerequisite credits must be completed before admission to the nursing program. *Options:* May apply for transfer of up to 80 total credits. *Application deadlines:* 4/30 (fall), 9/30 (spring).

Degree Requirements 128 total credit hours, 47 in nursing.

RN Baccalaureate Program (BSN)

Applying *Required:* TOEFL for nonnative speakers of English, minimum college GPA of 2.5, RN license, diploma or AD in nursing, high school transcript, 3 letters of recommendation, transcript of college record. 60 prerequisite credits must be completed before admission to the nursing program. *Options:* Advanced standing available through the following means: advanced placement exams, credit by exam. May apply for transfer of up to 80 total credits. *Application deadline:* rolling.

Degree Requirements 128 total credit hours, 47 in nursing.

NORTHERN ILLINOIS UNIVERSITY
School of Nursing
De Kalb, Illinois

Programs • Generic Baccalaureate • RN Baccalaureate • MS • Post-Master's

The University State-supported coed university. Founded: 1895. *Primary accreditation:* regional. *Setting:* 589-acre small-town campus. *Total enrollment:* 22,218.

The School of Nursing Founded in 1959. *Nursing program faculty:* 52 (34% with doctorates). *Off-campus program sites:* Rockford, Hoffman Estates.

Academic Facilities *Campus library:* 1.4 million volumes (40,000 in health); 11,882 periodical subscriptions (388 health-care related). *Nursing school*

Northern Illinois University (continued)
resources: CAI, computer lab, nursing audiovisuals, interactive nursing skills videos, learning resource lab.

Student Life *Student services:* health clinic, child-care facilities, personal counseling, career counseling, institutionally sponsored work-study program, job placement, special assistance for disabled students. *International student services:* counseling/support, special assistance for nonnative speakers of English, ESL courses. *Nursing student activities:* Sigma Theta Tau, student nurses association.

Calendar Semesters.

NURSING STUDENT PROFILE

Undergraduate **Enrollment:** 534
Women: 90%; **Men:** 10%; **Minority:** 11%; **International:** 0%; **Part-time:** 37%
Graduate **Enrollment:** 107
Women: 100%; **Minority:** 7%; **International:** 0%; **Part-time:** 89%

BACCALAUREATE PROGRAMS

Contact Ms. Karen Pickett, Undergraduate Services Coordinator, School of Nursing, Northern Illinois University, 1240 Normal Road, De Kalb, IL 60115-2864, 815-753-1231. *Fax:* 815-753-0814. *E-mail:* kpicket@niu.edu

Expenses *State resident tuition:* $2035 full-time, $95 per hour part-time. *Nonresident tuition:* $7114 full-time, $285 per hour part-time. *Full-time mandatory fees:* $409–$1000. *Part-time mandatory fees:* $34+. *Room and board:* $3600. *Books and supplies per academic year:* ranges from $300 to $500.

Financial Aid Institutionally sponsored need-based grants/scholarships, institutionally sponsored non-need grants/scholarships, Federal Direct Loans, Federal Nursing Student Loans, Federal Pell Grants, Federal Perkins Loans, Federal Supplemental Educational Opportunity Grants, Federal Work-Study. *Application deadline:* 3/1.

Generic Baccalaureate Program (BS)

Applying *Required:* ACT, TOEFL for nonnative speakers of English, minimum college GPA of 2.25, high school transcript, high school class rank: top 30%. 5 prerequisite credits must be completed before admission to the nursing program. *Options:* May apply for transfer of up to 74 total credits. *Application deadline:* 2/15.

Degree Requirements 124 total credit hours, 50 in nursing.

RN Baccalaureate Program (BS)

Applying *Required:* minimum college GPA of 2.25, RN license, diploma or AD in nursing, transcript of college record. 5 prerequisite credits must be completed before admission to the nursing program. *Options:* Advanced standing available through credit by exam. May apply for transfer of up to 74 total credits. *Application deadlines:* 2/15 (fall), 10/15 (spring).

Degree Requirements 124 total credit hours, 50 in nursing.

Distance learning Courses provided through video, audio.

MASTER'S PROGRAMS

Contact Ms. Cindy Luxton, Graduate Student Services Coordinator, School of Nursing, Northern Illinois University, 1240 Normal Road, De Kalb, IL 60115-2864, 815-753-1231. *Fax:* 815-753-0814. *E-mail:* cluxt@niu.edu

Areas of Study Clinical nurse specialist programs in adult health nursing, community health nursing, gerontological nursing, maternity-newborn nursing; nurse practitioner program in family health.

Expenses *State resident tuition:* $1726 full-time, $96 per hour part-time. *Nonresident tuition:* $5178 full-time, $288 per hour part-time. *Full-time mandatory fees:* $450. *Part-time mandatory fees:* $34+. *Room and board:* $3600. *Books and supplies per academic year:* ranges from $550 to $1000.

Financial Aid Graduate assistantships, nurse traineeships, fellowships, Federal Direct Loans, Federal Nursing Student Loans, institutionally sponsored loans, employment opportunities, institutionally sponsored need-based grants/scholarships, institutionally sponsored non-need-based grants/scholarships. *Application deadline:* 3/1.

MS Program

Applying *Required:* GRE General Test, bachelor's degree in nursing, minimum GPA of 2.75, RN license, 1 year of clinical experience, physical assessment course, statistics course, professional liability/malpractice insurance, 2 letters of recommendation, transcript of college record. *Application deadlines:* 6/1 (fall), 11/1 (spring), 4/1 (summer). *Application fee:* $30.

Degree Requirements 36 total credit hours, 30 in nursing.

Distance learning Courses provided through video, audio.

Post-Master's Program

Applying *Required:* bachelor's degree in nursing, RN license, physical assessment course, essay, interview, 2 letters of recommendation, transcript of college record, curriculum vitae, master's degree in nursing. *Application deadline:* 2/1. *Application fee:* $30.

Degree Requirements 26 total credit hours.

NORTH PARK COLLEGE
Division of Nursing
Chicago, Illinois

Programs • Generic Baccalaureate • RN Baccalaureate • Accelerated RN Baccalaureate • MS/MA • BSN to Master's • MS/MBA • Post-Master's

The College Independent comprehensive coed institution, affiliated with Evangelical Covenant Church. Founded: 1891. *Primary accreditation:* regional. *Setting:* 30-acre urban campus. *Total enrollment:* 1,750.

The Division of Nursing Founded in 1964. *Nursing program faculty:* 40 (40% with doctorates).

Academic Facilities *Campus library:* 215,503 volumes (5,200 in nursing); 1,000 periodical subscriptions (140 health-care related). *Nursing school resources:* computer lab, nursing audiovisuals, learning resource lab.

Student Life *Student services:* health clinic, personal counseling, career counseling, institutionally sponsored work-study program, job placement, campus safety program, special assistance for disabled students. *International student services:* counseling/support, special assistance for nonnative speakers of English, ESL courses. *Nursing student activities:* Sigma Theta Tau, student nurses association.

Calendar Semesters.

NURSING STUDENT PROFILE

Undergraduate **Enrollment:** 242
Women: 88%; **Men:** 12%; **Minority:** 40%; **International:** 5%; **Part-time:** 28%
Graduate **Enrollment:** 105
Women: 96%; **Men:** 4%; **Minority:** 43%; **International:** 18%; **Part-time:** 77%

BACCALAUREATE PROGRAMS

Contact Dr. Alma Joel Labunski, Chair and Professor, Division of Nursing, North Park College, 3255 West Foster Avenue, Chicago, IL 60625, 773-244-5691. *Fax:* 773-244-4952.

Expenses *Tuition:* $13,990 full-time, $495 per credit hour part-time. *Full-time mandatory fees:* $90. *Room only:* $2570. *Books and supplies per academic year:* ranges from $200 to $400.

Financial Aid Institutionally sponsored need-based grants/scholarships, institutionally sponsored non-need grants/scholarships, Federal Nursing Student Loans, Federal Supplemental Educational Opportunity Grants, Federal Work-Study. 66% of undergraduate students in nursing programs received some form of financial aid in 1995–96. *Application deadline:* 8/26.

Generic Baccalaureate Program (BS)

Applying *Required:* SAT I or ACT, TOEFL for nonnative speakers of English, minimum high school GPA of 2.5, minimum college GPA of 2.5, 3 years of high school science, high school transcript, 2 letters of recommendation, written essay, transcript of college record. 36 prerequisite credits must be completed before admission to the nursing program. *Options:* Advanced standing available through the following means: advanced placement exams, credit by exam. Course work may be accelerated. May apply for transfer of up to 60 total credits. *Application deadline:* rolling. *Application fee:* $20.

Degree Requirements 120 total credit hours, 51 in nursing.

RN Baccalaureate Program (BS)

Applying *Required:* SAT I or ACT, TOEFL for nonnative speakers of English, ACT PEP, minimum high school GPA of 2.5, minimum college GPA of 2.5, 3 years of high school math, 3 years of high school science, high school chemistry, high school biology, RN license, diploma or AD in nursing, high school transcript, 2 letters of recommendation, transcript of college record. 25 prerequisite credits must be completed before admission to the nursing program. *Options:* Advanced standing available through the following means: advanced placement exams, credit by exam. Course work may be accelerated. May apply for transfer of up to 60 total credits. *Application deadlines:* 8/28 (fall), 1/16 (spring). *Application fee:* $20.

Degree Requirements 120 total credit hours, 23 in nursing.

Accelerated RN Baccalaureate Program (BS)

Applying *Required:* SAT I or ACT, TOEFL for nonnative speakers of English, ACT PEP, minimum high school GPA of 2.5, minimum college GPA of 2.5, 3 years of high school math, 3 years of high school science, high school chemistry, high school biology, RN license, diploma or AD in nursing, high school transcript, 2 letters of recommendation, transcript of college record. 25 prerequisite credits must be completed before admission to the nursing program. *Options:* Advanced standing available through advanced placement exams. May apply for transfer of up to 60 total credits. *Application deadlines:* 8/28 (fall), 1/16 (spring). *Application fee:* $20.

Degree Requirements 120 total credit hours, 23 in nursing.

MASTER'S PROGRAMS

Contact Dr. Alma Joe Labunski, Chair and Professor, Division of Nursing, North Park College, 3225 West Foster Avenue, Chicago, IL 60625, 773-244-5691. *Fax:* 773-244-4952.

Areas of Study Nursing administration; nursing education.

Expenses *Tuition:* $5940 full-time, $330 per semester hour part-time. *Books and supplies per academic year:* ranges from $300 to $400.

Financial Aid Graduate assistantships, Federal Nursing Student Loans, institutionally sponsored loans, employment opportunities, institutionally sponsored need-based grants/scholarships, institutionally sponsored non-need-based grants/scholarships. 80% of master's level students in nursing programs received some form of financial aid in 1995-96. *Application deadline:* 8/26.

MS/MA Program

Applying *Required:* GRE General Test or Miller Analogies Test, TOEFL for nonnative speakers of English, bachelor's degree in nursing, minimum GPA of 3.0, RN license, 1 year of clinical experience, statistics course, professional liability/malpractice insurance, essay, interview, 2 letters of recommendation, transcript of college record. *Application deadline:* rolling. *Application fee:* $20.

Degree Requirements 77 total credit hours, 34 in nursing. Thesis required.

BSN to Master's Program (MS)

Applying *Required:* GRE General Test or Miller Analogies Test, TOEFL for nonnative speakers of English, bachelor's degree in nursing, minimum GPA of 3.0, RN license, 1 year of clinical experience, statistics course, professional liability/malpractice insurance, essay, interview, 2 letters of recommendation, transcript of college record. *Application deadline:* rolling. *Application fee:* $20.

Degree Requirements 37 total credit hours, 37 in nursing. Thesis required.

MS/MBA Program

Applying *Required:* GRE General Test or Miller Analogies Test, TOEFL for nonnative speakers of English, bachelor's degree in nursing, minimum GPA of 3.0, RN license, 1 year of clinical experience, statistics course, professional liability/malpractice insurance, essay, interview, 2 letters of recommendation, transcript of college record. *Application deadline:* rolling. *Application fee:* $20.

Degree Requirements 62 total credit hours, 31 in nursing, 31 in business. Thesis required.

Post-Master's Program

Applying *Required:* GRE General Test or Miller Analogies Test, TOEFL for nonnative speakers of English, bachelor's degree in nursing, minimum GPA of 3.0, RN license, 1 year of clinical experience, statistics course, professional liability/malpractice insurance, essay, interview, 2 letters of recommendation, transcript of college record, master's degree. *Application deadline:* rolling. *Application fee:* $20.

Degree Requirements 25 total credit hours, 25 in nursing. 630 clinical hours.

See full description on page 488.

OLIVET NAZARENE UNIVERSITY
Division of Nursing
Kankakee, Illinois

Programs • Generic Baccalaureate • Accelerated RN Baccalaureate

The University Independent comprehensive coed institution, affiliated with Church of the Nazarene. Founded: 1907. *Primary accreditation:* regional. *Setting:* 168-acre suburban campus. *Total enrollment:* 2,256.

The Division of Nursing Founded in 1968. *Nursing program faculty:* 11 (18% with doctorates).

Academic Facilities *Campus library:* 160,521 volumes (5,920 in health, 4,028 in nursing); 975 periodical subscriptions (78 health-care related). *Nursing school resources:* CAI, computer lab, nursing audiovisuals, learning resource lab, interactive CD-ROM.

Student Life *Student services:* personal counseling, career counseling, institutionally sponsored work-study program, job placement, special assistance for disabled students. *International student services:* counseling/support, special assistance for nonnative speakers of English. *Nursing student activities:* Sigma Theta Tau, student nurses association.

Calendar Semesters.

NURSING STUDENT PROFILE

Undergraduate **Enrollment:** 245

Women: 92%; **Men:** 8%; **Minority:** 26%; **International:** 5%; **Part-time:** 0%

BACCALAUREATE PROGRAMS

Contact John Mongerson, Admissions Office, Olivet Nazarene University, Box 6005, Kankakee, IL 60901, 815-939-5203. *Fax:* 815-939-5069. *E-mail:* admissions@olivet.edu

Expenses *Tuition:* $10,026 per academic year. *Full-time mandatory fees:* $140. *Room and board:* $4460. *Books and supplies per academic year:* $500.

Financial Aid Institutionally sponsored need-based grants/scholarships, institutionally sponsored non-need grants/scholarships, Federal Pell Grants, Federal Perkins Loans, Federal Supplemental Educational Opportunity Grants, Federal Work-Study, Federal Family Education Loan Program (FFELP). 53% of undergraduate students in nursing programs received some form of financial aid in 1995–96. *Application deadline:* 3/1.

Generic Baccalaureate Program (BS)

Applying *Required:* ACT, high school transcript, 2 letters of recommendation, transcript of college record, high school class rank: . *Options:* Advanced standing available through the following means: advanced placement exams, advanced placement without credit, credit by exam. Course work may be accelerated. May apply for transfer of up to 68 total credits. *Application deadline:* rolling.

Degree Requirements 128 total credit hours, 51 in nursing.

Accelerated RN Baccalaureate Program (BS)

Applying *Required:* NLN Mobility Profile II (for graduates of non-NLN accredited programs only), minimum college GPA of 2.2, RN license, diploma or AD in nursing, 2 letters of recommendation, transcript of college record. *Options:* May apply for transfer of up to 82 total credits. *Application deadline:* rolling.

Degree Requirements 128 total credit hours, 51 in nursing.

ROCKFORD COLLEGE
Department of Nursing
Rockford, Illinois

Programs • Generic Baccalaureate • RN Baccalaureate

Rockford College (continued)

The College Independent comprehensive coed institution. Founded: 1847. *Primary accreditation:* regional. *Setting:* 130-acre suburban campus. *Total enrollment:* 1,468.

The Department of Nursing Founded in 1981. *Nursing program faculty:* 6 (33% with doctorates).

Academic Facilities *Campus library:* 175,300 volumes (1,200 in nursing); 850 periodical subscriptions (69 health-care related). *Nursing school resources:* CAI, computer lab, nursing audiovisuals, learning resource lab.

Student Life *Student services:* health clinic, personal counseling, career counseling, institutionally sponsored work-study program, job placement, campus safety program, special assistance for disabled students. *International student services:* counseling/support, ESL courses. *Nursing student activities:* nursing club, student nurses association.

Calendar Semesters.

NURSING STUDENT PROFILE

Undergraduate **Enrollment:** 153
Women: 94%; **Men:** 6%; **Minority:** 16%; **International:** 0%; **Part-time:** 30%

BACCALAUREATE PROGRAMS

Contact Office of Admissions, Department of Nursing, Rockford College, 5050 East State Street, Rockford, IL 61108, 815-226-4050. *E-mail:* admission@rockford.edu

Expenses *Tuition:* $14,100 full-time, $360 per hour part-time. *Room and board:* $4400. *Books and supplies per academic year:* $1000.

Financial Aid Institutionally sponsored need-based grants/scholarships, institutionally sponsored non-need grants/scholarships, Federal Nursing Student Loans, Federal Pell Grants, Federal Supplemental Educational Opportunity Grants, Federal Work-Study. 70% of undergraduate students in nursing programs received some form of financial aid in 1995–96.

Generic Baccalaureate Program (BSN)

Applying *Required:* SAT I, ACT, minimum high school GPA of 2.5, 3 years of high school math, high school chemistry, high school transcript, interview, letter of recommendation, written essay, transcript of college record. 42 prerequisite credits must be completed before admission to the nursing program. *Options:* Advanced standing available through credit by exam. Course work may be accelerated. May apply for transfer of up to 60 total credits. *Application deadline:* rolling. *Application fee:* $35.

Degree Requirements 124 total credit hours, 52 in nursing.

RN Baccalaureate Program (BSN)

Applying *Required:* SAT I or ACT, minimum college GPA of 2.5, RN license, diploma or AD in nursing, high school transcript, interview, letter of recommendation, written essay, transcript of college record. 42 prerequisite credits must be completed before admission to the nursing program. *Options:* Advanced standing available through credit by exam. Course work may be accelerated. May apply for transfer of up to 60 total credits. *Application deadline:* rolling. *Application fee:* $35.

Degree Requirements 124 total credit hours, 52 in nursing.

RUSH UNIVERSITY
College of Nursing
Chicago, Illinois

Programs • Generic Baccalaureate • RN Baccalaureate • RN to Master's • Master's for Nurses with Non-Nursing Degrees • MS/MM • ND • Postdoctoral • Continuing Education

The University Independent upper-level coed institution. Founded: 1969. *Primary accreditation:* regional. *Setting:* 35-acre urban campus. *Total enrollment:* 1,453.

The College of Nursing Founded in 1972. *Nursing program faculty:* 96 (60% with doctorates).

Academic Facilities *Campus library:* 124,120 volumes (12,412 in health, 12,412 in nursing); 2,125 periodical subscriptions (2,083 health-care related). *Nursing school resources:* CAI, computer lab, nursing audiovisuals, learning resource lab.

Student Life *Student services:* health clinic, child-care facilities, personal counseling, career counseling, institutionally sponsored work-study program, job placement, campus safety program, special assistance for disabled students, academic skills counseling. *International student services:* counseling/support. *Nursing student activities:* Sigma Theta Tau, student nurses association, Nurses Christian Fellowship.

Calendar Quarters.

NURSING STUDENT PROFILE

Undergraduate **Enrollment:** 251
Women: 90%; **Men:** 10%; **Minority:** 28%; **International:** 1%; **Part-time:** 8%
Graduate **Enrollment:** 394
Women: 92%; **Men:** 8%; **Minority:** 11%; **International:** 1%; **Part-time:** 95%

BACCALAUREATE PROGRAMS

Contact Armour Academic Center, 1743 West Harrison Street, 600 South Paulina, Chicago, IL 60612, 312-942-7100. *Fax:* 312-942-2219.

Expenses *Tuition:* $3418 full-time, $300 per quarter part-time. *Full-time mandatory fees:* $1260. *Room and board:* $6570. *Books and supplies per academic year:* ranges from $500 to $800.

Financial Aid Institutionally sponsored need-based grants/scholarships, institutionally sponsored non-need grants/scholarships, Federal Nursing Student Loans, Federal Perkins Loans, Federal Supplemental Educational Opportunity Grants, Federal Work-Study. *Application deadline:* 8/15.

Generic Baccalaureate Program (BS)

Applying *Required:* TOEFL for nonnative speakers of English, minimum college GPA of 2.75, 3 letters of recommendation, written essay, transcript of college record. 90 prerequisite credits must be completed before admission to the nursing program. *Options:* Advanced standing available through credit by exam. May apply for transfer of up to 45 total credits. *Application deadlines:* 3/1 (fall), 3/1 (summer). *Application fee:* $25.

Degree Requirements 180 total credit hours, 86 in nursing. 4 required electives.

RN Baccalaureate Program (BS)

Applying *Required:* TOEFL for nonnative speakers of English, minimum college GPA of 2.75, RN license, diploma or AD in nursing, 3 letters of recommendation, written essay, transcript of college record. 90 prerequisite credits must be completed before admission to the nursing program. *Options:* Advanced standing available through credit by exam. May apply for transfer of up to 144 total credits. *Application deadline:* 3/1. *Application fee:* $25.

Degree Requirements 180 total credit hours, 86 in nursing. 4 required electives.

MASTER'S PROGRAMS

Contact Armour Academic Center, 1743 West Harrison Street, 600 South Paulina, Chicago, IL 60612, 312-942-7100. *Fax:* 312-942-2219.

Areas of Study Clinical nurse specialist programs in cardiovascular nursing, community health nursing, critical care nursing, gerontological nursing, maternity-newborn nursing, medical-surgical nursing, oncology nursing, pediatric nursing, psychiatric–mental health nursing, rehabilitation nursing, women's health nursing, transplant nursing, home health nursing; nurse anesthesia; nurse practitioner programs in acute care, adult health, child care/pediatrics, community health, family health, gerontology, neonatal health, primary care, psychiatric–mental health.

Expenses *Tuition:* $3877 full-time, $340 per quarter part-time. *Full-time mandatory fees:* $1680. *Room and board:* $10,080. *Books and supplies per academic year:* ranges from $880 to $1000.

Financial Aid Graduate assistantships, nurse traineeships, Federal Nursing Student Loans, institutionally sponsored loans, employment opportunities, institutionally sponsored need-based grants/scholarships. *Application deadline:* 8/1.

RN to Master's Program (MS)

Applying *Required:* GRE General Test, TOEFL for nonnative speakers of English, ACT PEP, TSE for nonnative speakers of English, bachelor's degree, minimum GPA of 3.0, RN license, essay, interview, 3 letters of recommendation, transcript of college record. *Application deadlines:* 8/1 (fall), 2/15 (spring), 5/1 (summer). *Application fee:* $25.

Degree Requirements 55 total credit hours, 27 in nursing, 12 in clinical practice.

Master's for Nurses with Non-Nursing Degrees Program (MS)

Applying *Required:* GRE General Test, TOEFL for nonnative speakers of English, ACT PEP, TSE for nonnative speakers of English, bachelor's degree, minimum GPA of 3.0, RN license, essay, interview, 3 letters of recommendation, transcript of college record. *Application deadlines:* 8/1 (fall), 2/15 (spring), 5/1 (summer). *Application fee:* $25.

Degree Requirements 55 total credit hours, 27 in nursing, 12 in clinical practice.

MS/MM Program

Applying *Required:* GRE General Test, TOEFL for nonnative speakers of English, TSE for nonnative speakers of English, bachelor's degree in nursing, minimum GPA of 3.0, RN license, essay, interview, 3 letters of recommendation, transcript of college record. *Application deadlines:* 8/1 (fall), 2/15 (spring), 5/1 (summer). *Application fee:* $25.

Degree Requirements 55 total credit hours, 27 in nursing, 12 in clinical practice.

DOCTORAL PROGRAMS

Contact Ms. Phyllis Peterson, Director of Admission Services, Schweppe Sprague Hall, Room 119, College of Nursing, Rush University, 1743 West Harrison Street, Chicago, IL 60612, 312-942-7100. *Fax:* 312-942-2219.

Areas of Study Nursing research, clinical practice, nursing policy.

Expenses *Tuition:* $3877 full-time, $340 per quarter part-time. *Full-time mandatory fees:* $1680. *Room and board:* $10,080. *Books and supplies per academic year:* ranges from $880 to $1000.

Financial Aid Graduate assistantships, nurse traineeships, grants, Federal Nursing Student Loans, institutionally sponsored loans, opportunities for employment, institutionally sponsored need-based grants/scholarships. *Application deadline:* 8/1.

Doctorate in Nursing Sciences Program (DNSc)

Applying *Required:* TOEFL for nonnative speakers of English, GRE for postbaccalaureate entrance, TSE for nonnative speakers of English, statistics course, interview, 3 letters of recommendation, vitae, writing sample, minimum 3.0 GPA in previous degree. Summer option program requires full-time enrollment for 3 consecutive summers, MSN, and graduate-level biostatistics course. *Application deadlines:* 8/1 (fall), 3/31 (summer). *Application fee:* $25.

Degree Requirements 195 total credit hours; 20 hours clinical practica, 12 hours dissertation, 8 hours graduate biostatistics; dissertation; oral exam; written exam; defense of dissertation.

ND Program

Applying *Required:* TOEFL for nonnative speakers of English, GRE for postbaccalaureate entrance, TSE for nonnative speakers of English, interview, 3 letters of recommendation, vitae, writing sample, baccalaureate degree in nursing. *Application deadlines:* 8/1 (fall), 2/15 (spring). *Application fee:* $25.

Degree Requirements 85 total credit hours; 30 quarter hours post-master's minimum, 8 quarter hours clinical practice; written exam; Doctor of Nursing project presentation.

POSTDOCTORAL PROGRAM

Contact Ms. Phyllis Peterson, Director of Admission Services, Schweppe Sprague Hall, Room 119, College of Nursing, Rush University, 1743 West Harrison Street, Chicago, IL 60612, 312-942-7100. *Fax:* 312-942-2219.

CONTINUING EDUCATION PROGRAM

Contact Ms. Mildred Perlia, Director, Nursing Professional Development, Schweppe Sprague Hall, Room 410, College of Nursing, Rush University, 1743 West Harrison Street, Chicago, IL 60612, 312-942-6982. *Fax:* 312-942-3287. *E-mail:* mperlia@cnis.rpslmc.edu

See full description on page 496.

SAINT FRANCIS MEDICAL CENTER COLLEGE OF NURSING
Peoria, Illinois

Program • Generic Baccalaureate

The College Independent Roman Catholic upper-level specialized coed institution. Founded: 1986. *Primary accreditation:* regional. *Total enrollment:* 156. Founded in 1905.

Academic Facilities *Campus library:* 5,150 volumes; 112 periodical subscriptions.

Calendar Semesters.

BACCALAUREATE PROGRAM

Contact Director of Admissions and Registrar, Saint Francis Medical Center College of Nursing, 511 Northeast Greenleaf Street, Peoria, IL 61603-3783, 309-655-2596. *Fax:* 309-655-3648.

SAINT JOSEPH COLLEGE OF NURSING
Joliet, Illinois

Programs • Generic Baccalaureate • Accelerated RN Baccalaureate

The College Independent Roman Catholic upper-level specialized coed institution. Founded: 1989. *Primary accreditation:* regional. *Total enrollment:* 185. Founded in 1920. *Nursing program faculty:* 17 (24% with doctorates).

Academic Facilities *Campus library:* 3,600 volumes (1,100 in health, 2,000 in nursing); 60 periodical subscriptions (60 health-care related). *Nursing school resources:* CAI, computer lab, nursing audiovisuals, interactive nursing skills videos, learning resource lab, video classroom.

Student Life *Student services:* personal counseling, career counseling, job placement, campus safety program, special assistance for disabled students. *Nursing student activities:* student nurses association.

Calendar Semesters.

NURSING STUDENT PROFILE

Undergraduate **Enrollment:** 222

Women: 91%; **Men:** 9%; **Minority:** 16%; **International:** 0%; **Part-time:** 42%

BACCALAUREATE PROGRAMS

Contact Alan Christensen, Director of Admissions, Saint Joseph College of Nursing, 290 North Springfield Avenue, Joliet, IL 60435, 815-741-7382. *Fax:* 815-741-7131.

Expenses *Tuition:* $8512 full-time, $266 per semester hour part-time. *Full-time mandatory fees:* $60. *Part-time mandatory fees:* $30. *Books and supplies per academic year:* ranges from $500 to $1000.

Financial Aid Institutionally sponsored need-based grants/scholarships, institutionally sponsored non-need grants/scholarships, Federal Direct Loans, Federal Pell Grants, Federal Supplemental Educational Opportunity Grants, Federal Work-Study. 76% of undergraduate students in nursing programs received some form of financial aid in 1995–96. *Application deadline:* 6/1.

Generic Baccalaureate Program (BSN)

Applying *Required:* TOEFL for nonnative speakers of English, minimum college GPA of 2.5, high school transcript, 2 letters of recommendation, written essay, transcript of college record. 62 prerequisite credits must be completed before admission to the nursing program. *Options:* Advanced standing available through the following means: advanced placement exams, credit by exam. Course work may be accelerated. May apply for transfer of up to 62 total credits. *Application deadlines:* 4/1 (fall), 8/1 (spring), 12/1 (fall early decision). *Application fee:* $25.

Degree Requirements 128 total credit hours, 66 in nursing.

Accelerated RN Baccalaureate Program (BSN)

Applying *Required:* TOEFL for nonnative speakers of English, minimum college GPA of 2.5, RN license, 2 letters of recommendation, written essay, transcript of college record. 62 prerequisite credits must be completed before admission to the nursing program. *Options:* Advanced standing available through the following means: advanced placement exams, credit by exam. Course work may be accelerated. May apply for transfer of up to 62 total credits. *Application deadlines:* 4/1 (fall), 8/1 (spring), 12/1 (fall early decision). *Application fee:* $25.

Degree Requirements 128 total credit hours, 66 in nursing.

SAINT XAVIER UNIVERSITY
School of Nursing
Chicago, Illinois

Programs • Generic Baccalaureate • RN Baccalaureate • LPN to Baccalaureate • RN to Master's • Master's for Nurses with Non-Nursing Degrees • MS/MBA • Continuing Education

The University Independent Roman Catholic comprehensive coed institution. Founded: 1847. *Primary accreditation:* regional. *Setting:* 55-acre urban campus. *Total enrollment:* 4,442.

The School of Nursing Founded in 1935. *Nursing program faculty:* 56 (34% with doctorates). *Off-campus program sites:* Elk Grove Village, Palos Hills.

Academic Facilities *Campus library:* 161,655 volumes (7,516 in health, 11,250 in nursing); 932 periodical subscriptions (115 health-care related). *Nursing school resources:* CAI, computer lab, nursing audiovisuals, interactive nursing skills videos, learning resource lab, access to on-line databases.

Student Life *Student services:* child-care facilities, personal counseling, career counseling, institutionally sponsored work-study program, job placement, campus safety program, special assistance for disabled students, nursing clinic. *International student services:* counseling/support, special assistance for nonnative speakers of English, ESL courses. *Nursing student activities:* Sigma Theta Tau, student nurses association, nursing center.

Calendar 4-1-4.

NURSING STUDENT PROFILE

Undergraduate **Enrollment:** 518
Women: 94%; **Men:** 6%; **Minority:** 28%; **International:** 1%; **Part-time:** 42%
Graduate **Enrollment:** 125
Women: 99%; **Men:** 1%; **Minority:** 19%; **International:** 0%; **Part-time:** 97%

BACCALAUREATE PROGRAMS

Contact Ms. Darlene O'Callaghan, Assistant Dean, Undergraduate Program, School of Nursing, Saint Xavier University, 3700 West 103rd Street, Chicago, IL 60655, 773-298-3707. *Fax:* 773-779-9061.

Expenses *Tuition:* $11,970 full-time, $399 per semester hour part-time. *Full-time mandatory fees:* $80. *Part-time mandatory fees:* $50. *Room and board:* $4800.

Financial Aid Institutionally sponsored need-based grants/scholarships, institutionally sponsored non-need grants/scholarships, Federal Perkins Loans, Federal Supplemental Educational Opportunity Grants, Federal Work-Study. 80% of undergraduate students in nursing programs received some form of financial aid in 1995–96. *Application deadline:* 3/1.

Generic Baccalaureate Program (BS)

Applying *Required:* ACT, TOEFL for nonnative speakers of English, minimum high school GPA of 2.5, minimum college GPA of 2.5, 3 years of high school math, 3 years of high school science, high school chemistry, high school biology, high school foreign language, high school transcript, 3 letters of recommendation, written essay, transcript of college record. *Options:* May apply for transfer of up to 90 total credits. *Application deadline:* rolling. *Application fee:* $25.

Degree Requirements 124 total credit hours, 49 in nursing.

RN Baccalaureate Program (BS)

Applying *Required:* TOEFL for nonnative speakers of English, minimum high school GPA of 2.5, minimum college GPA of 2.5, 3 years of high school math, 3 years of high school science, high school chemistry, high school biology, RN license, diploma or AD in nursing, high school transcript, written essay, transcript of college record. *Options:* Advanced standing available through credit by exam. Course work may be accelerated. May apply for transfer of up to 90 total credits. *Application deadline:* rolling. *Application fee:* $25.

Degree Requirements 124 total credit hours, 49 in nursing.

LPN to Baccalaureate Program (BS)

Applying *Required:* TOEFL for nonnative speakers of English, minimum high school GPA of 2.5, minimum college GPA of 2.5, 3 years of high school math, 3 years of high school science, high school chemistry, high school biology, high school foreign language, high school transcript, written essay, transcript of college record, LPN license, 1 year of recent work experience as LPN, copy of pharmacology certificate. *Options:* Advanced standing available through credit by exam. May apply for transfer of up to 90 total credits. *Application deadline:* rolling. *Application fee:* $25.

Degree Requirements 124 total credit hours, 49 in nursing.

MASTER'S PROGRAMS

Contact Dr. Joan Hau, Assistant Dean, Graduate Program, School of Nursing, Saint Xavier University, 3700 West 103rd Street, Chicago, IL 60655, 773-298-3708. *Fax:* 773-779-9061. *E-mail:* hau@sxu.edu

Areas of Study Clinical nurse specialist programs in community health nursing, medical-surgical nursing, psychiatric–mental health nursing; nursing administration; nurse practitioner program in family health.

Expenses *Tuition:* $3789 full-time, $421 per semester hour part-time. *Full-time mandatory fees:* $80. *Part-time mandatory fees:* $50.

Financial Aid Graduate assistantships, nurse traineeships, fellowships, employment opportunities, institutionally sponsored need-based grants/scholarships. *Application deadline:* 3/1.

RN to Master's Program (MS)

Applying *Required:* Miller Analogies Test, minimum GPA of 3.0, RN license, professional liability/malpractice insurance, essay, interview, 2 letters of recommendation, transcript of college record. *Application deadline:* rolling. *Application fee:* $35.

Degree Requirements 162 total credit hours, 57 in nursing. Project.

Master's for Nurses with Non-Nursing Degrees Program (MS)

Applying *Required:* Miller Analogies Test, NLN Comprehensive Achievement Test, bachelor's degree, minimum GPA of 3.0, RN license, statistics course, professional liability/malpractice insurance, essay, interview, letter of recommendation, transcript of college record, completion of 3 undergraduate nursing courses with a cumulative GPA of 3.0. *Application deadline:* rolling. *Application fee:* $35.

Degree Requirements 48 total credit hours, 48 in nursing. Project.

MS/MBA Program

Applying *Required:* GMAT, bachelor's degree in nursing, minimum GPA of 3.0, RN license, statistics course, professional liability/malpractice insurance, essay, interview, 2 letters of recommendation, transcript of college record. *Application deadline:* rolling. *Application fee:* $35.

Degree Requirements 55 total credit hours, 38 in nursing, 17 in business. Project.

CONTINUING EDUCATION PROGRAM

Contact Dr. Mary M. Lebold, Dean, School of Nursing, Saint Xavier University, 3700 West 103rd Street, Chicago, IL 60655, 773-298-3700. *Fax:* 773-779-9061. *E-mail:* lebold@sxu.edu

SOUTHERN ILLINOIS UNIVERSITY AT EDWARDSVILLE
School of Nursing
Edwardsville, Illinois

Programs • Generic Baccalaureate • RN Baccalaureate • MS • Continuing Education

The University State-supported comprehensive coed institution. Part of Southern Illinois University. Founded: 1957. *Primary accreditation:* regional. *Setting:* 2,600-acre suburban campus. *Total enrollment:* 11,047.

The School of Nursing Founded in 1965. *Nursing program faculty:* 56 (43% with doctorates). *Off-campus program sites:* Effingham, Olney, Ullin.

Academic Facilities *Campus library:* 800,000 volumes; 6,130 periodical subscriptions. *Nursing school resources:* CAI, computer lab, nursing audiovisuals, interactive nursing skills videos, learning resource lab.

Student Life *Student services:* health clinic, child-care facilities, personal counseling, career counseling, institutionally sponsored work-study program, job placement, campus safety program, special assistance for

disabled students. *International student services:* counseling/support, special assistance for nonnative speakers of English, ESL courses. *Nursing student activities:* Sigma Theta Tau, nursing club, student nurses association.

Calendar Semesters.

NURSING STUDENT PROFILE

Undergraduate **Enrollment:** 345
Women: 80%; **Men:** 20%; **Minority:** 17%; **International:** 0%; **Part-time:** 24%
Graduate **Enrollment:** 141
Women: 91%; **Men:** 9%; **Minority:** 9%; **International:** 0%; **Part-time:** 71%

BACCALAUREATE PROGRAMS

Contact Dr. Mary de Meneses, Associate Dean for Educational Services, School of Nursing, Southern Illinois University at Edwardsville, Box 1066, Edwardsville, IL 62026-1066, 618-692-3972. *Fax:* 618-682-3854. *E-mail:* mdemene@siue.edu

Expenses *State resident tuition:* $2469 full-time, $186 per semester hour part-time. *Nonresident tuition:* $6326 full-time, $346 per semester hour part-time. *Full-time mandatory fees:* $196–$488. *Room and board:* $3960. *Books and supplies per academic year:* $500.

Financial Aid Institutionally sponsored need-based grants/scholarships, institutionally sponsored non-need grants/scholarships, Federal Direct Loans, Federal Nursing Student Loans, Federal Pell Grants, Federal Perkins Loans, Federal Supplemental Educational Opportunity Grants, Federal Work-Study. *Application deadline:* 5/1.

Generic Baccalaureate Program (BS)

Applying *Required:* ACT, TOEFL for nonnative speakers of English, minimum college GPA of 2.7, 3 years of high school math, 3 years of high school science, high school chemistry, high school transcript, transcript of college record. 37 prerequisite credits must be completed before admission to the nursing program. *Options:* Course work may be accelerated. May apply for transfer of up to 58 total credits. *Application deadlines:* 2/28 (fall), 8/31 (spring).

Degree Requirements 124 total credit hours, 66 in nursing.

RN Baccalaureate Program (BS)

Applying *Required:* ACT, minimum college GPA of 2.7, 3 years of high school math, 3 years of high school science, RN license, diploma or AD in nursing, high school transcript, transcript of college record. 48 prerequisite credits must be completed before admission to the nursing program. *Options:* Advanced standing available through the following means: advanced placement exams, advanced placement without credit, credit by exam. Course work may be accelerated.

Degree Requirements 124 total credit hours, 25 in nursing.

Distance learning Courses provided through on-line.

MASTER'S PROGRAM

Contact Ms. Moureen Mattingly, Academic Adviser, School of Nursing, Southern Illinois University at Edwardsville, Box 1066, Edwardsville, IL 62026-1066, 618-692-3930. *Fax:* 618-692-3854. *E-mail:* mmattin@siue.edu

Areas of Study Clinical nurse specialist programs in community health nursing, medical-surgical nursing, psychiatric–mental health nursing; nurse anesthesia; nurse practitioner programs in adult health, family health.

Expenses *State resident tuition:* $2490 full-time, $186 per semester hour part-time. *Nonresident tuition:* $6622 full-time, $358 per semester hour part-time. *Full-time mandatory fees:* $186–$384.

Financial Aid Graduate assistantships, nurse traineeships, Federal Nursing Student Loans, employment opportunities. *Application deadline:* 5/1.

MS Program

Applying *Required:* bachelor's degree in nursing, minimum GPA of 2.5, RN license, physical assessment course, statistics course, professional liability/malpractice insurance, interview, 3 letters of recommendation, transcript of college record, minimum of 1 year of clinical experience for nurse anesthesia track. *Application deadline:* 2/1.

Degree Requirements 34–66 total credit hours dependent upon track, 25–57 in nursing, 3–9 in other specified areas. Thesis or project.

CONTINUING EDUCATION PROGRAM

Contact Ms. Rita Arras, Acting Coordinator of Continuing Education, School of Nursing, Southern Illinois University at Edwardsville, Box 1066, Edwardsville, IL 62026-1066, 618-692-3922. *Fax:* 618-682-3854.

TRINITY CHRISTIAN COLLEGE
Department of Nursing
Palos Heights, Illinois

Programs • Generic Baccalaureate • RN Baccalaureate

The College Independent interdenominational 4-year coed college. Founded: 1959. *Primary accreditation:* regional. *Setting:* 53-acre suburban campus. *Total enrollment:* 636.

The Department of Nursing Founded in 1983. *Nursing program faculty:* 7 (43% with doctorates).

Academic Facilities *Campus library:* 60,500 volumes (200 in health, 400 in nursing); 350 periodical subscriptions (42 health-care related). *Nursing school resources:* CAI, computer lab, nursing audiovisuals, interactive nursing skills videos, learning resource lab.

Student Life *Student services:* personal counseling, career counseling, institutionally sponsored work-study program. *Nursing student activities:* student nurses association, Nursing Honor Society.

Calendar 4-1-4.

NURSING STUDENT PROFILE

Undergraduate **Enrollment:** 64
Women: 94%; **Men:** 6%; **Minority:** 6%; **International:** 0%; **Part-time:** 17%

BACCALAUREATE PROGRAMS

Contact Dr. Cynthia N. Sander, Chairperson, Department of Nursing, Trinity Christian College, 6601 West College Drive, Palos Heights, IL 60463, 708-597-3000 Ext. 335. *Fax:* 708-385-5665. *E-mail:* cynthia.sander@trnty.edu

Expenses *Tuition:* $11,250 full-time, $375 per credit hour part-time. *Full-time mandatory fees:* $85. *Room and board:* $4090–$4435. *Room only:* $2300. *Books and supplies per academic year:* ranges from $200 to $300.

Financial Aid Institutionally sponsored need-based grants/scholarships, institutionally sponsored non-need grants/scholarships, Federal Nursing Student Loans, Federal Supplemental Educational Opportunity Grants, Federal Work-Study. *Application deadline:* 2/15.

Generic Baccalaureate Program (BSN)

Applying *Required:* ACT, TOEFL for nonnative speakers of English, minimum high school GPA of 2.2, minimum college GPA of 2.5, high school transcript, transcript of college record. 60 prerequisite credits must be completed before admission to the nursing program. *Options:* Advanced standing available through the following means: advanced placement exams, credit by exam. *Application deadline:* rolling. *Application fee:* $20.

Degree Requirements 125 total credit hours, 55 in nursing.

RN Baccalaureate Program (BSN)

Applying *Required:* minimum college GPA of 2.5, RN license, diploma or AD in nursing. 35 prerequisite credits must be completed before admission to the nursing program. *Options:* Advanced standing available through the following means: advanced placement exams, credit by exam. May apply for transfer of up to 65 total credits. *Application deadline:* rolling. *Application fee:* $20.

Degree Requirements 125 total credit hours, 55 in nursing.

UNIVERSITY OF ILLINOIS AT CHICAGO
College of Nursing
Chicago, Illinois

Programs • Generic Baccalaureate • RN Baccalaureate • MS • Master's for Nurses with Non-Nursing Degrees • MS/MBA • MS/MPH • Post-Master's • Doctorate in Nursing Sciences

University of Illinois at Chicago (continued)

The University State-supported coed university. Part of University of Illinois System. Founded: 1946. *Primary accreditation:* regional. *Setting:* 200-acre urban campus. *Total enrollment:* 24,589.

The College of Nursing Founded in 1951. *Nursing program faculty:* 123 (60% with doctorates). *Off-campus program sites:* Rockford, Peoria, Urbana-Champaign.

▶ *NOTEWORTHY*

The University of Illinois at Chicago College of Nursing, consistently among the top 10 colleges of nursing in the United States, continues at the forefront of nursing education and research. Graduates, known for producing the nursing knowledge today that will guide the nursing practice of tomorrow, create and maintain high-quality health-care delivery systems and ensure that excellent nursing services are available to the public. An outstanding characteristic is diversity both in the specializations available for study and among the student body, whose background and clinical experiences enrich the broad range of topics that are the focus of study and investigation.

Academic Facilities *Campus library:* 5.7 million volumes (500,000 in health). *Nursing school resources:* computer lab, nursing audiovisuals, interactive nursing skills videos, learning resource lab.

Student Life *Student services:* health clinic, child-care facilities, personal counseling, career counseling, institutionally sponsored work-study program, job placement, campus safety program, special assistance for disabled students. *International student services:* counseling/support, special assistance for nonnative speakers of English, ESL courses. *Nursing student activities:* Sigma Theta Tau, student nurses association.

Calendar Semesters.

NURSING STUDENT PROFILE

Undergraduate **Enrollment:** 630
Women: 82%; **Men:** 18%; **Minority:** 15%; **International:** 1%; **Part-time:** 20%

Graduate **Enrollment:** 590
Women: 95%; **Men:** 5%; **Minority:** 6%; **International:** 20%; **Part-time:** 75%

BACCALAUREATE PROGRAMS

Contact Ms. Leah C. Beckwith, Director of Admissions and Recruitment, College of Nursing, University of Illinois at Chicago, 845 South Damen Avenue, Chicago, IL 60612-7350, 312-996-3566. *Fax:* 312-413-4399. *E-mail:* leahb@uic.edu

Expenses *State resident tuition:* $4200 full-time, ranges from $2124 to $3232 per year part-time. *Nonresident tuition:* $9928 full-time, ranges from $4038 to $7252 per year part-time. *Room and board:* $5000. *Books and supplies per academic year:* ranges from $600 to $700.

Financial Aid Institutionally sponsored need-based grants/scholarships, institutionally sponsored non-need grants/scholarships, Federal Nursing Student Loans, Federal Pell Grants, Federal Supplemental Educational Opportunity Grants, Federal Work-Study. 60% of undergraduate students in nursing programs received some form of financial aid in 1995–96. *Application deadline:* 3/1.

Generic Baccalaureate Program (BSN)

Applying *Required:* SAT I, ACT, TOEFL for nonnative speakers of English, minimum college GPA of 2.5, 3 years of high school math, high school chemistry, high school biology, high school transcript, 2 letters of recommendation, written essay, transcript of college record, high school class rank: top 50%. 49 prerequisite credits must be completed before admission to the nursing program. *Options:* Advanced standing available through advanced placement exams. May apply for transfer of up to 55 total credits. *Application deadline:* 2/28. *Application fee:* $30.

Degree Requirements 133 total credit hours, 78 in nursing.

RN Baccalaureate Program (BSN)

Applying *Required:* TOEFL for nonnative speakers of English, minimum college GPA of 2.5, RN license, diploma or AD in nursing, 2 letters of recommendation, written essay, transcript of college record. 49 prerequisite credits must be completed before admission to the nursing program. *Options:* Advanced standing available through credit by exam. May apply for transfer of up to 55 total credits. *Application deadline:* 2/28. *Application fee:* $30.

Degree Requirements 133 total credit hours, 78 in nursing.

MASTER'S PROGRAMS

Contact Ms. Leah C. Beckwith, Director of Admissions and Recruitment, College of Nursing, University of Illinois at Chicago, 845 South Damen Avenue, Chicago, IL 60612-7350, 312-996-3566. *Fax:* 312-413-4399. *E-mail:* leahb@uic.edu

Areas of Study Clinical nurse specialist programs in cardiovascular nursing, community health nursing, critical care nursing, family health nursing, maternity-newborn nursing, medical-surgical nursing, occupational health nursing, oncology nursing, pediatric nursing, perinatal nursing, psychiatric–mental health nursing, public health nursing, rehabilitation nursing, women's health nursing, cardiopulmonary nursing, home health care administration; nurse midwifery; nursing administration; nurse practitioner programs in acute care, child care/pediatrics, family health, occupational health, school health, women's health, critical care.

Expenses *State resident tuition:* $4748 full-time, ranges from $2312 to $3604 per year part-time. *Nonresident tuition:* $10,534 full-time, ranges from $4396 to $7774 per year part-time. *Room and board:* $5000. *Books and supplies per academic year:* ranges from $750 to $850.

Financial Aid Graduate assistantships, nurse traineeships, fellowships, Federal Nursing Student Loans, institutionally sponsored need-based grants/scholarships, institutionally sponsored non-need-based grants/scholarships. 50% of master's level students in nursing programs received some form of financial aid in 1995-96. *Application deadline:* 3/1.

MS Program

Applying *Required:* GRE General Test, TOEFL for nonnative speakers of English, bachelor's degree in nursing, minimum GPA of 3.0, RN license, statistics course, interview, 3 letters of recommendation, transcript of college record, required clinical experience varies with specialty concentration. *Application deadlines:* 5/30 (fall), 10/27 (spring), 4/15 (summer). *Application fee:* $30–40.

Degree Requirements 36–51 total credit hours dependent upon track, 36–51 in nursing. Thesis or research project.

Master's for Nurses with Non-Nursing Degrees Program (MS)

Applying *Required:* GRE General Test, TOEFL for nonnative speakers of English, bachelor's degree, minimum GPA of 3.0, RN license, statistics course, essay, interview, 3 letters of recommendation, transcript of college record, research course, required clinical experience varies with specialty concentration. *Application deadlines:* 5/30 (fall), 10/30 (spring), 4/15 (summer). *Application fee:* $30–40.

Degree Requirements 36–51 total credit hours dependent upon track, 36–51 in nursing. Thesis or research project.

MS/MBA Program

Applying *Required:* TOEFL for nonnative speakers of English, GMAT, bachelor's degree, minimum GPA of 3.0, RN license, statistics course, essay, interview, 3 letters of recommendation, transcript of college record, research courses, calculus course, computer programming course. *Application deadlines:* 5/30 (fall), 10/30 (spring), 4/15 (summer). *Application fee:* $30–40.

Degree Requirements 67–70 total credit hours dependent upon track, 27 in nursing, 40 in business.

MS/MPH Program

Applying *Required:* GRE General Test, TOEFL for nonnative speakers of English, bachelor's degree, minimum GPA of 3.0, RN license, statistics course, interview, 3 letters of recommendation, transcript of college record. *Application deadlines:* 5/30 (fall), 10/30 (spring). *Application fee:* $30–40.

Degree Requirements 60–62 total credit hours dependent upon track, 28 in nursing, 32–34 in public health. Thesis or project.

Post-Master's Program

Applying *Required:* GRE General Test, bachelor's degree in nursing, minimum GPA of 3.0, RN license, 1 year of clinical experience, physical assessment course, essay, interview, 3 letters of recommendation, transcript of college record, MS in nursing. *Application deadlines:* 5/30 (fall), 10/30 (spring), 4/15 (summer). *Application fee:* $30–40.

Degree Requirements 24–28 total credit hours dependent upon track, 24–28 in nursing.

DOCTORAL PROGRAM

Contact Ms. Leah C. Beckwith, Director of Admissions and Recruitment, College of Nursing, University of Illinois at Chicago, 845 South Damen Avenue, Chicago, IL 60612-7350, 312-996-3566. *Fax:* 312-413-4399. *E-mail:* leahb@uic.edu

Areas of Study Nursing administration, nursing research, clinical practice, nursing policy.

Expenses *State resident tuition:* $4200 full-time, ranges from $2124 to $3232 per year part-time. *Nonresident tuition:* $9928 full-time, ranges from $4038 to $7252 per year part-time. *Room and board:* $5000. *Books and supplies per academic year:* ranges from $600 to $700.

Financial Aid Graduate assistantships, nurse traineeships, fellowships, grants, institutionally sponsored loans, opportunities for employment. *Application deadline:* 3/1.

Doctorate in Nursing Sciences Program (PhD)

Applying *Required:* GRE General Test, TOEFL for nonnative speakers of English, master's degree in nursing, master's degree, statistics course, interview, 3 letters of recommendation, vitae, writing sample, competitive review by faculty committee, research course. *Application deadline:* 5/30. *Application fee:* $30.

Degree Requirements 96 total credit hours; 31 semester hours in research, 33 semester hours of course work, 32 semester hours in master's program; dissertation; defense of dissertation; oral or written preliminary exams.

See full description on page 534.

UNIVERSITY OF ILLINOIS AT SPRINGFIELD

Nursing Program
Springfield, Illinois

Program • RN Baccalaureate

The University State-supported upper-level coed institution. Founded: 1969. *Primary accreditation:* regional. *Setting:* 746-acre suburban campus. *Total enrollment:* 4,702.

The Nursing Program Founded in 1973. *Nursing program faculty:* 9 (44% with doctorates).

Academic Facilities *Campus library:* 528,000 volumes (15,743 in nursing); 2,650 periodical subscriptions (177 health-care related). *Nursing school resources:* computer lab, nursing audiovisuals.

Student Life *Student services:* health clinic, child-care facilities, personal counseling, career counseling, institutionally sponsored work-study program, job placement, campus safety program, special assistance for disabled students, learning center. *International student services:* counseling/support, ESL courses. *Nursing student activities:* Sigma Theta Tau.

Calendar Semesters.

NURSING STUDENT PROFILE

Undergraduate **Enrollment:** 120

Women: 98%; **Men:** 2%; **Minority:** 1%; **International:** 0%; **Part-time:** 73%

BACCALAUREATE PROGRAM

Contact Ms. Margie Williams, Director, Nursing Program, University of Illinois at Springfield, Shepherd Road, Springfield, IL 62794-9243, 217-786-6648. *Fax:* 217-786-7188.

Expenses *State resident tuition:* $5100 full-time, $85 per semester hour part-time. *Nonresident tuition:* $15,300 full-time, $255 per semester hour part-time. *Full-time mandatory fees:* $24–$78. *Room and board:* $549–$2142. *Books and supplies per academic year:* $400.

Financial Aid Institutionally sponsored need-based grants/scholarships.

RN Baccalaureate Program (BSN)

Applying *Required:* NLN Achievement Tests, RN license, diploma or AD in nursing, transfer students only, professional liability/malpractice insurance. 60 prerequisite credits must be completed before admission to the nursing program. *Options:* Advanced standing available through credit by exam. Course work may be accelerated. May apply for transfer of up to 72 total credits. *Application deadline:* rolling.

Degree Requirements 120 total credit hours, 67 in nursing.

WEST SUBURBAN COLLEGE OF NURSING

Concordia University and West Suburban College of Nursing
Oak Park, Illinois

Programs • Generic Baccalaureate • RN Baccalaureate

The College Independent 4-year specialized coed college. Founded: 1982. *Primary accreditation:* regional. *Setting:* 10-acre suburban campus. *Total enrollment:* 258.

The Concordia University and West Suburban College of Nursing Founded in 1982. *Nursing program faculty:* 20 (15% with doctorates). *Off-campus program site:* River Forest.

Academic Facilities *Campus library:* 4,000 volumes (3,000 in health, 1,000 in nursing); 310 periodical subscriptions (300 health-care related). *Nursing school resources:* CAI, computer lab, nursing audiovisuals, learning resource lab.

Student Life *Student services:* personal counseling, career counseling, campus safety program. *Nursing student activities:* nursing club, student nurses association, Nursing Honor Society.

Calendar Semesters.

NURSING STUDENT PROFILE

Undergraduate **Enrollment:** 224

Women: 93%; **Men:** 7%; **Minority:** 32%; **International:** 0%; **Part-time:** 13%

BACCALAUREATE PROGRAMS

Contact Mr. Edward Pryor, Director of Admission, Concordia University and West Suburban College of Nursing, West Suburban College of Nursing, Erie at Austin Boulevard, Oak Park, IL 60302, 708-763-6530. *Fax:* 708-383-8783.

Expenses *Tuition:* $11,200 full-time, ranges from $224 to $249 per credit hour part-time. *Full-time mandatory fees:* $83. *Room and board:* $4623. *Books and supplies per academic year:* $400.

Financial Aid Institutionally sponsored need-based grants/scholarships, institutionally sponsored non-need grants/scholarships, Federal Direct Loans, Federal Pell Grants, Federal Perkins Loans, Federal Supplemental Educational Opportunity Grants, Federal Work-Study, special scholarships administered at West Suburban Hospital Medical Center. 82% of undergraduate students in nursing programs received some form of financial aid in 1995–96. *Application deadline:* 6/1.

Generic Baccalaureate Program (BScN)

Applying *Required:* ACT, TOEFL for nonnative speakers of English, minimum high school GPA of 2.5, minimum college GPA of 2.5, high school chemistry, high school biology, high school transcript, letter of recommendation, written essay, transcript of college record, high school class rank: top 33%. *Options:* May apply for transfer of up to 100 total credits. *Application deadline:* rolling. *Application fee:* $25.

Degree Requirements 131 total credit hours, 66 in nursing.

RN Baccalaureate Program (BScN)

Applying *Required:* TOEFL for nonnative speakers of English, minimum college GPA of 2.5, RN license, diploma or AD in nursing, letter of recommendation, transcript of college record. *Options:* Advanced standing available through credit by exam. May apply for transfer of up to 66 total credits. *Application deadline:* rolling. *Application fee:* $25.

Degree Requirements 131 total credit hours, 66 in nursing.

INDIANA

ANDERSON UNIVERSITY

School of Nursing
Anderson, Indiana

Programs • Generic Baccalaureate • Accelerated RN Baccalaureate

The University Independent comprehensive coed institution, affiliated with Church of God. Founded: 1917. *Primary accreditation:* regional. *Setting:* 100-acre suburban campus. *Total enrollment:* 2,261.

The School of Nursing Founded in 1973. *Nursing program faculty:* 9 (23% with doctorates).

Anderson University (continued)

▶ ***NOTEWORTHY***

Anderson University offers an innovative nursing program that integrates liberal arts with sciences and professional nursing. Students begin the practice of nursing in the sophomore year with individual, family, and community clients. All types of community agencies, including churches, are clinical settings. Intercultural nursing is stressed, including 3 weeks practicing in another culture during the senior year. RN students entering the nursing major receive credit for their previous nursing and general education. Transition courses are offered in the summer, with the senior year of the major offered on weekends. The BSN can usually be earned in 2 calendar years and 1 summer.

Academic Facilities *Campus library:* 240,269 volumes (6,127 in nursing); 940 periodical subscriptions (113 health-care related). *Nursing school resources:* CAI, computer lab, nursing audiovisuals, interactive nursing skills videos, learning resource lab.

Student Life *Student services:* health clinic, personal counseling, career counseling, institutionally sponsored work-study program, job placement, campus safety program, special assistance for disabled students. *International student services:* counseling/support, special assistance for nonnative speakers of English. *Nursing student activities:* Sigma Theta Tau, student nurses association, Nursing Honor Society.

Calendar Semesters.

NURSING STUDENT PROFILE

Undergraduate **Enrollment:** 105

Women: 90%; **Men:** 10%; **Minority:** 4%; **Part-time:** 13%

BACCALAUREATE PROGRAMS

Contact Dr. Patricia Bennett, Director, School of Nursing, Anderson University, 1100 East 5th Street, Anderson, IN 46012, 317-641-4380. *Fax:* 317-641-3851. *E-mail:* pbennett@kirk.anderson.edu

Expenses *Tuition:* $11,840 full-time, $494 per credit hour part-time. *Full-time mandatory fees:* $65. *Room and board:* $3980. *Room only:* $2200. *Books and supplies per academic year:* $400.

Financial Aid Institutionally sponsored need-based grants/scholarships, institutionally sponsored non-need grants/scholarships, Federal Pell Grants, Federal Perkins Loans, Federal Supplemental Educational Opportunity Grants, Federal Work-Study. 90% of undergraduate students in nursing programs received some form of financial aid in 1995–96. *Application deadline:* 3/1.

Generic Baccalaureate Program (BSN)

Applying *Required:* SAT I, ACT, minimum high school GPA of 3.0, minimum college GPA of 2.5, 3 years of high school science, high school chemistry, high school biology, high school transcript, 3 letters of recommendation, written essay, transcript of college record, high school class rank: top 33%, immunizations. 28 prerequisite credits must be completed before admission to the nursing program. *Options:* Advanced standing available through the following means: advanced placement exams, advanced placement without credit, credit by exam. Course work may be accelerated. May apply for transfer of up to 80 total credits. *Application deadline:* 3/1. *Application fee:* $20.

Degree Requirements 124 total credit hours, 52 in nursing. Intercultural project in senior year.

Accelerated RN Baccalaureate Program (BSN)

Applying *Required:* SAT I, ACT, minimum college GPA of 2.5, RN license, diploma or AD in nursing, interview, 3 letters of recommendation, written essay, transcript of college record, immunizations, SPR, 1000 hours work experience. 45 prerequisite credits must be completed before admission to the nursing program. *Options:* Advanced standing available through the following means: advanced placement exams, advanced placement without credit, credit by exam. May apply for transfer of up to 80 total credits. *Application deadline:* 3/1. *Application fee:* $25.

Degree Requirements 124 total credit hours, 52 in nursing. Intercultural project.

BALL STATE UNIVERSITY
School of Nursing
Muncie, Indiana

Programs • Generic Baccalaureate • RN Baccalaureate • MS • Continuing Education

The University State-supported coed university. Founded: 1918. *Primary accreditation:* regional. *Setting:* 955-acre urban campus. *Total enrollment:* 19,115.

The School of Nursing Founded in 1964. *Nursing program faculty:* 31 (45% with doctorates). *Off-campus program sites:* Fort Wayne, Indianapolis.

Academic Facilities *Campus library:* 1.2 million volumes (22,500 in health, 4,200 in nursing); 3,900 periodical subscriptions (180 health-care related). *Nursing school resources:* CAI, computer lab, nursing audiovisuals, interactive nursing skills videos, learning resource lab.

Student Life *Student services:* health clinic, child-care facilities, personal counseling, career counseling, institutionally sponsored work-study program, job placement, campus safety program, special assistance for disabled students. *International student services:* counseling/support, ESL courses. *Nursing student activities:* Sigma Theta Tau, student nurses association.

Calendar Semesters.

NURSING STUDENT PROFILE

Undergraduate **Enrollment:** 184

Women: 92%; **Men:** 8%; **International:** 1%; **Part-time:** 10%

Graduate **Enrollment:** 121

Women: 98%; **Men:** 2%; **Minority:** 2%; **International:** 2%; **Part-time:** 97%

BACCALAUREATE PROGRAMS

Contact Dr. Nancy Dillard, Associate Director, School of Nursing, Ball State University, Muncie, IN 47306, 317-285-5589. *Fax:* 317-285-2169. *E-mail:* nldillard@bsuvc.bsu.edu

Expenses *State resident tuition:* $3188 full-time, $1008 per semester part-time. *Nonresident tuition:* $8448 full-time, $2506 per semester part-time. *Full-time mandatory fees:* $50–$77. *Part-time mandatory fees:* $50–$77. *Room and board:* $3952. *Books and supplies per academic year:* ranges from $250 to $500.

Financial Aid Institutionally sponsored need-based grants/scholarships, institutionally sponsored non-need grants/scholarships, Federal Direct Loans, Federal Pell Grants, Federal Perkins Loans, Federal Supplemental Educational Opportunity Grants, Federal Work-Study. 33% of undergraduate students in nursing programs received some form of financial aid in 1995–96. *Application deadline:* 3/1.

Generic Baccalaureate Program (BS)

Applying *Required:* SAT I, ACT, TOEFL for nonnative speakers of English, minimum college GPA of 2.75, transcript of college record, high school transcript or GED certificate. 30 prerequisite credits must be completed before admission to the nursing program. *Options:* May apply for transfer of up to 90 total credits. *Application deadline:* rolling. *Application fee:* $25.

Degree Requirements 126 total credit hours, 46 in nursing.

RN Baccalaureate Program (BS)

Applying *Required:* SAT I, ACT, TOEFL for nonnative speakers of English, minimum college GPA of 2.75, RN license, diploma or AD in nursing, high school transcript or GED certificate. 30 prerequisite credits must be completed before admission to the nursing program. *Options:* May apply for transfer of up to 90 total credits. *Application deadline:* rolling. *Application fee:* $25.

Degree Requirements 126 total credit hours, 46 in nursing.

Distance learning Courses provided through computer-based media, interactive television.

MASTER'S PROGRAM

Contact Dr. Marilyn Ryan, Associate Director, Graduate Program, School of Nursing, Ball State University, Muncie, IN 47306, 317-285-5764. *E-mail:* meryan@bsuvc.bsu.edu

Areas of Study Clinical nurse specialist program in adult health nursing; nursing administration; nursing education; nurse practitioner programs in adult health, family health.

Expenses *State resident tuition:* $2016 full-time, $478 per hour part-time. *Nonresident tuition:* $5000 full-time, $1108 per hour part-time. *Full-time*

mandatory fees: $234–$288. *Part-time mandatory fees:* $120–$144. *Room and board:* $4064–$4568. *Books and supplies per academic year:* ranges from $200 to $300.

Financial Aid Nurse traineeships, Federal Direct Loans, institutionally sponsored loans, employment opportunities. 8% of master's level students in nursing programs received some form of financial aid in 1995-96. *Application deadline:* 3/1.

MS Program

Applying *Required:* bachelor's degree in nursing, minimum GPA of 2.8, RN license, 2 years of clinical experience, physical assessment course, professional liability/malpractice insurance, transcript of college record, Universal Precautions Verified Training, TB test. *Application deadline:* rolling. *Application fee:* $15.

Degree Requirements 39–48 total credit hours dependent upon track, 36–45 in nursing. Practicum for teachers, administrators, and NP certificate.

CONTINUING EDUCATION PROGRAM

Contact Dr. Carole Brigham, Coordinator, Continuing Education and Faculty Development, School of Nursing, Ball State University, Muncie, IN 47306, 317-285-5575. *Fax:* 317-285-2169. *E-mail:* cjbrigham@bsuvc.bsu.edu

BETHEL COLLEGE
Division of Nursing
Mishawaka, Indiana

Programs • Generic Baccalaureate • RN Baccalaureate

The College Independent comprehensive coed institution, affiliated with Missionary Church. Founded: 1947. *Primary accreditation:* regional. *Setting:* 65-acre suburban campus. *Total enrollment:* 1,352.

The Division of Nursing Founded in 1985. *Nursing program faculty:* 18 (6% with doctorates). *Off-campus program site:* Plymouth.

Academic Facilities *Campus library:* 73,000 volumes (100 in health, 2,000 in nursing); 430 periodical subscriptions (100 health-care related). *Nursing school resources:* CAI, computer lab, nursing audiovisuals, interactive nursing skills videos, learning resource lab.

Student Life *Student services:* health clinic, personal counseling, career counseling, institutionally sponsored work-study program, job placement, campus safety program, special assistance for disabled students. *International student services:* counseling/support, special assistance for nonnative speakers of English. *Nursing student activities:* Sigma Theta Tau, student nurses association.

Calendar Semesters.

NURSING STUDENT PROFILE

Undergraduate **Enrollment:** 175
Women: 90%; **Men:** 10%; **Minority:** 5%; **Part-time:** 40%

BACCALAUREATE PROGRAMS

Contact Ms. Cheryl Martin, Admission Coordinator, Division of Nursing, Bethel College, 1001 West McKinley Street, Mishawaka, IN 46545, 219-257-3368.

Expenses *Tuition:* $10,350 per academic year. *Room and board:* $3300–$3300. *Room only:* $1450. *Books and supplies per academic year:* ranges from $200 to $500.

Financial Aid Institutionally sponsored long-term loans, institutionally sponsored non-need grants/scholarships, Federal Perkins Loans. *Application deadline:* 3/1.

Generic Baccalaureate Program (BSN)

Applying *Required:* SAT I or ACT, minimum high school GPA of 2.25, minimum college GPA of 2.25, high school chemistry, high school biology, interview, 2 letters of recommendation, written essay, transcript of college record, immunizations, physical exam. 30 prerequisite credits must be completed before admission to the nursing program. *Options:* Advanced standing available through credit by exam. Course work may be accelerated. May apply for transfer of up to 96 total credits. *Application deadline:* rolling. *Application fee:* $50.

Degree Requirements 126 total credit hours, 56 in nursing.

RN Baccalaureate Program (BSN)

Applying *Required:* SAT I or ACT, minimum high school GPA of 2.25, minimum college GPA of 2.25, RN license, diploma or AD in nursing, interview, 2 letters of recommendation, written essay, transcript of college record, immunizations, physical exam. 36 prerequisite credits must be completed before admission to the nursing program. *Options:* Course work may be accelerated. May apply for transfer of up to 96 total credits. *Application deadline:* rolling. *Application fee:* $50.

Degree Requirements 126 total credit hours, 56 in nursing. Independent project.

GOSHEN COLLEGE
Department of Nursing
Goshen, Indiana

Programs • Generic Baccalaureate • Accelerated RN Baccalaureate

The College Independent Mennonite 4-year coed college. Founded: 1894. *Primary accreditation:* regional. *Setting:* 135-acre small-town campus. *Total enrollment:* 1,071.

The Department of Nursing Founded in 1950. *Nursing program faculty:* 10 (20% with doctorates).

▶ *NOTEWORTHY*

Goshen College is home to the oldest private baccalaureate nursing program in Indiana. The program has had NLN accreditation since 1962. Goshen College, a 4-year liberal arts Christian college, is known for its focus on intercultural awareness and peace and justice issues. The Study Service Term Abroad, an integral part of the general education program, provides students with an immersion experience in another culture. Clinical assignments in the nursing major include a wide range of hospital and community experiences. Goshen College also offers a BSN completion option for RNs with evening classes and individually arranged clinical experiences.

Academic Facilities *Campus library:* 117,600 volumes (80 in health, 750 in nursing); 830 periodical subscriptions (67 health-care related). *Nursing school resources:* CAI, computer lab, nursing audiovisuals, interactive nursing skills videos, learning resource lab.

Student Life *Student services:* health clinic, child-care facilities, personal counseling, career counseling, institutionally sponsored work-study program, job placement, campus safety program, special assistance for disabled students. *International student services:* counseling/support, special assistance for nonnative speakers of English, ESL courses. *Nursing student activities:* Sigma Theta Tau, student nurses association.

Calendar Semesters plus May term concentration.

NURSING STUDENT PROFILE

Undergraduate **Enrollment:** 76
Women: 96%; **Men:** 4%; **Minority:** 5%; **International:** 4%; **Part-time:** 3%

BACCALAUREATE PROGRAMS

Contact Dr. Miriam Martin, Professor and Director, Department of Nursing, Goshen College, Goshen, IN 46526, 219-535-7369. *Fax:* 219-535-7660. *E-mail:* miriamem@goshen.edu

Expenses *Tuition:* $10,900 full-time, $430 per credit hour part-time. *Full-time mandatory fees:* $770. *Room and board:* $3880. *Room only:* $1920. *Books and supplies per academic year:* $400.

Financial Aid Institutionally sponsored need-based grants/scholarships, institutionally sponsored non-need grants/scholarships, Federal Direct Loans, Federal Nursing Student Loans, Federal Pell Grants, Federal Perkins Loans, Federal Supplemental Educational Opportunity Grants, Federal Work-Study, state scholarships. 99% of undergraduate students in nursing programs received some form of financial aid in 1995–96. *Application deadline:* 3/1.

Generic Baccalaureate Program (BSN)

Applying *Required:* SAT I, TOEFL for nonnative speakers of English, assessment examination, minimum high school GPA of 2.5, minimum college GPA of 2.5, 3 years of high school math, 3 years of high school science, high school chemistry, high school foreign language, high school transcript, 2 letters of recommendation, transcript of college record, security check. 29 prerequisite credits must be completed before

Goshen College (continued)

admission to the nursing program. *Options:* Advanced standing available through the following means: advanced placement exams, advanced placement without credit, credit by exam. Course work may be accelerated. May apply for transfer of up to 30 total credits. *Application deadline:* 5/15. *Application fee:* $15.

Degree Requirements 124 total credit hours, 46 in nursing.

Accelerated RN Baccalaureate Program (BSN)

Applying *Required:* SAT I, TOEFL for nonnative speakers of English, minimum high school GPA of 2.5, minimum college GPA of 2.5, 3 years of high school math, 3 years of high school science, high school chemistry, RN license, diploma or AD in nursing, high school foreign language, high school transcript, 2 letters of recommendation, transcript of college record. 60 prerequisite credits must be completed before admission to the nursing program. *Options:* Advanced standing available through the following means: advanced placement exams, credit by exam. May apply for transfer of up to 31 total credits. *Application deadline:* rolling. *Application fee:* $15.

Degree Requirements 124 total credit hours, 30 in nursing.

INDIANA STATE UNIVERSITY
School of Nursing
Terre Haute, Indiana

Programs • Generic Baccalaureate • RN Baccalaureate • MS • Continuing Education

The University State-supported coed university. Founded: 1865. *Primary accreditation:* regional. *Setting:* 91-acre urban campus. *Total enrollment:* 11,184.

The School of Nursing Founded in 1963. *Nursing program faculty:* 31 (29% with doctorates). *Off-campus program site:* Vincennes.

▶ *NOTEWORTHY*

Indiana State University School of Nursing is committed to high-quality undergraduate and graduate education. The School includes an academic nursing center that provides learning experiences for all levels of students as well as service and research opportunities. There are optional international nursing opportunities for undergraduate and graduate students. In cooperation with the School of Business, graduate students can pursue an MS/MBA dual-degree option. A post-master's family nurse practitioner track is available for registered nurses with an earned graduate degree in nursing. The School collaborates with the Terre Haute Center for Medical Education and the Midwest Center for Rural Health for interdisciplinary education of students in rural health care.

Academic Facilities *Campus library:* 1.2 million volumes (22,860 in health, 4,399 in nursing); 4,267 periodical subscriptions (170 health-care related). *Nursing school resources:* CAI, computer lab, nursing audiovisuals, learning resource lab.

Student Life *Student services:* health clinic, child-care facilities, personal counseling, career counseling, institutionally sponsored work-study program, job placement, campus safety program, special assistance for disabled students. *International student services:* counseling/support, special assistance for nonnative speakers of English, ESL courses. *Nursing student activities:* Sigma Theta Tau, student nurses association.

Calendar Semesters.

NURSING STUDENT PROFILE

Undergraduate **Enrollment:** 420

Women: 88%; **Men:** 12%; **Minority:** 5%; **International:** 1%; **Part-time:** 45%

Graduate **Enrollment:** 40

Women: 100%; **Minority:** 1%; **International:** 0%; **Part-time:** 88%

BACCALAUREATE PROGRAMS

Contact Ms. Linda S. Harbour, Director of Student Affairs, School of Nursing, Indiana State University, Terre Haute, IN 47809, 812-237-2316. *Fax:* 812-237-4300. *E-mail:* nuharbo@befac.indstate.edu

Expenses *State resident tuition:* $1536 full-time, $110 per credit hour part-time. *Nonresident tuition:* $3802 full-time, $266 per credit hour part-time. *Full-time mandatory fees:* $20–$80. *Part-time mandatory fees:* $20–$40. *Room and board:* $3995–$4105. *Books and supplies per academic year:* ranges from $500 to $1000.

Financial Aid Institutionally sponsored need-based grants/scholarships, institutionally sponsored non-need grants/scholarships, Federal Nursing Student Loans, Federal Pell Grants, Federal Perkins Loans, Federal Supplemental Educational Opportunity Grants, Federal Work-Study. 65% of undergraduate students in nursing programs received some form of financial aid in 1995–96. *Application deadline:* 3/1.

Generic Baccalaureate Program (BS)

Applying *Required:* SAT I, minimum high school GPA of 2.0, 2 years of high school math, high school chemistry, high school transcript, high school class rank: top 25%. *Options:* Advanced standing available through the following means: advanced placement exams, advanced placement without credit, credit by exam. Course work may be accelerated. May apply for transfer of up to 85 total credits. *Application deadline:* rolling. *Application fee:* $20.

Degree Requirements 124 total credit hours, 66 in nursing.

RN Baccalaureate Program (BS)

Applying *Required:* RN license, high school transcript, high school or college-level algebra and chemistry. *Options:* Advanced standing available through the following means: advanced placement exams, advanced placement without credit, credit by exam. Course work may be accelerated. May apply for transfer of up to 85 total credits. *Application deadline:* rolling. *Application fee:* $20.

Degree Requirements 124 total credit hours, 66 in nursing.

MASTER'S PROGRAM

Contact Ms. Linda S. Harbour, Director of Student Affairs, School of Nursing, Indiana State University, Terre Haute, IN 47809, 812-237-2316. *Fax:* 812-237-4300. *E-mail:* nuharbo@befac.indstate.edu

Areas of Study Clinical nurse specialist programs in adult health nursing, community health nursing; nursing administration; nursing education; nurse practitioner program in family health.

Expenses *State resident tuition:* $3696 full-time, $132 per credit part-time. *Nonresident tuition:* $8372 full-time, $299 per credit part-time. *Room and board:* $3995–$4105. *Books and supplies per academic year:* ranges from $500 to $1500.

Financial Aid Graduate assistantships, nurse traineeships. 13% of master's level students in nursing programs received some form of financial aid in 1995-96. *Application deadline:* 3/1.

MS Program

Applying *Required:* GRE General Test, bachelor's degree in nursing, RN license, physical assessment course, essay, 3 letters of recommendation, transcript of college record. *Application fee:* $20.

Degree Requirements 34 total credit hours, 28 in nursing.

CONTINUING EDUCATION PROGRAM

Contact Ms. Deborah Barnhart, Director of Continuing Education, School of Nursing, Indiana State University, Terre Haute, IN 47809, 812-237-3696. *Fax:* 812-237-4300. *E-mail:* nubarn@befac.indstate.edu

INDIANA UNIVERSITY EAST
School of Nursing
Richmond, Indiana

Program • Generic Baccalaureate

The University State-supported 4-year coed college. Part of Indiana University System. Founded: 1971. *Primary accreditation:* regional. *Setting:* 194-acre small-town campus. *Total enrollment:* 2,390.

The School of Nursing Founded in 1988. *Nursing program faculty:* 16 (19% with doctorates).

Academic Facilities *Campus library:* 56,677 volumes (1,621 in health, 3,418 in nursing); 600 periodical subscriptions (70 health-care related). *Nursing school resources:* CAI, computer lab, nursing audiovisuals, interactive nursing skills videos, learning resource lab.

Student Life *Student services:* personal counseling, career counseling, institutionally sponsored work-study program, job placement, campus safety program, special assistance for disabled students, wellness center. *Nursing student activities:* Sigma Theta Tau, student nurses association, student government/newspaper.

Calendar Semesters.

NURSING STUDENT PROFILE

Undergraduate **Enrollment:** 46
Women: 88%; **Men:** 12%; **Minority:** 0%; **International:** 0%; **Part-time:** 100%

BACCALAUREATE PROGRAM

Contact Jan Robey Marker, Coordinator of Nursing Student Services, School of Nursing, Indiana University East, Richmond, IN 47374-1289, 317-973-8225. *Fax:* 317-973-8523. *E-mail:* jmarker@indiana.edu

Expenses *State resident tuition:* $2612 full-time, $87 per credit hour part-time. *Nonresident tuition:* $6773 full-time, $226 per credit hour part-time. *Full-time mandatory fees:* $183–$200. *Part-time mandatory fees:* $25+. *Books and supplies per academic year:* ranges from $700 to $1000.

Financial Aid Institutionally sponsored need-based grants/scholarships, institutionally sponsored non-need grants/scholarships, Federal Direct Loans, Federal Pell Grants, Federal Perkins Loans, Federal Work-Study. *Application deadline:* 3/1.

Generic Baccalaureate Program (BSN)

Applying *Required:* SAT I, ACT, minimum college GPA of 2.5, minimum 2.0 GPA in all prerequisites. 67 prerequisite credits must be completed before admission to the nursing program. *Options:* Advanced standing available through credit by exam.

Degree Requirements 122 total credit hours, 55 in nursing. CPR certification.

INDIANA UNIVERSITY KOKOMO
School of Nursing
Kokomo, Indiana

Programs • Generic Baccalaureate • Accelerated RN Baccalaureate • Baccalaureate for Second Degree • Continuing Education

The University State-supported comprehensive coed institution. Part of Indiana University System. Founded: 1945. *Primary accreditation:* regional. *Setting:* 51-acre small-town campus. *Total enrollment:* 3,065.

The School of Nursing Founded in 1967. *Nursing program faculty:* 16 (19% with doctorates).

Academic Facilities *Campus library:* 114,956 volumes (2,043 in health, 1,374 in nursing); 1,505 periodical subscriptions (78 health-care related). *Nursing school resources:* CAI, computer lab, nursing audiovisuals, interactive nursing skills videos, learning resource lab.

Student Life *Student services:* child-care facilities, personal counseling, career counseling, job placement, special assistance for disabled students, tutoring in science and nursing courses. *Nursing student activities:* Sigma Theta Tau, student nurses association.

Calendar Semesters.

NURSING STUDENT PROFILE

Undergraduate **Enrollment:** 479
Women: 91%; **Men:** 9%; **Minority:** 1%; **International:** 1%; **Part-time:** 65%

BACCALAUREATE PROGRAMS

Contact Dr. Nancy Schlapman, Coordinator of BSN Program, School of Nursing, Indiana University Kokomo, 2300 Washington Street, PO Box 9003, Kokomo, IN 46904-9003, 317-455-9334. *Fax:* 317-455-9421. *E-mail:* nschlapm@iukfs1.iuk.indiana.edu

Expenses *State resident tuition:* $3800 full-time, $122 per credit hour part-time. *Nonresident tuition:* $226 per credit hour. *Full-time mandatory fees:* $600–$700. *Books and supplies per academic year:* $600.

Financial Aid Institutionally sponsored need-based grants/scholarships, institutionally sponsored non-need grants/scholarships, Federal Nursing Student Loans, Federal Perkins Loans, Federal Supplemental Educational Opportunity Grants, Federal Work-Study, Federal Stafford Loans, state grants. *Application deadline:* 3/1.

Generic Baccalaureate Program (BSN)

Applying *Required:* SAT I, ACT, minimum high school GPA of 2.0, minimum college GPA of 2.5, 4 years of high school math, 1 year of high school science, high school chemistry, high school biology, high school transcript, transcript of college record, high school class rank: top 50%, math, English, reading placement tests. 67 prerequisite credits must be completed before admission to the nursing program. *Options:* Advanced standing available through the following means: advanced placement exams, credit by exam. *Application deadline:* rolling. *Application fee:* $30.

Degree Requirements 125 total credit hours, 58 in nursing. Fundamental skills course requirements.

Accelerated RN Baccalaureate Program (BSN)

Applying *Required:* SAT I, ACT, minimum high school GPA of 2.0, minimum college GPA of 2.0, 4 years of high school math, 1 year of high school science, high school chemistry, high school biology, RN license, diploma or AD in nursing, high school transcript, transcript of college record, high school class rank: top 50%, math, English, reading placement tests. 67 prerequisite credits must be completed before admission to the nursing program. *Options:* Advanced standing available through the following means: advanced placement exams, credit by exam. Course work may be accelerated. *Application deadline:* rolling. *Application fee:* $30.

Degree Requirements 125 total credit hours, 58 in nursing. Fundamental skills course requirements.

Baccalaureate for Second Degree Program (BSN)

Applying *Required:* SAT I or ACT, minimum high school GPA of 2.0, minimum college GPA of 2.0, 4 years of high school math, 1 year of high school science, high school chemistry, high school biology, high school transcript, transcript of college record, high school class rank: top 50%, math, English, reading placement tests. *Options:* Advanced standing available through the following means: advanced placement exams, credit by exam. Course work may be accelerated. *Application deadline:* rolling. *Application fee:* $30.

Degree Requirements 125 total credit hours, 58 in nursing. Fundamental skills course requirements.

CONTINUING EDUCATION PROGRAM

Contact Mrs. Susan Ardrey, Coordinator, Continuing Education, Indiana University Kokomo, 2300 South Washington Street, PO Box 9003, Kokomo, IN 46904-9003, 317-455-9251. *Fax:* 317-455-9421. *E-mail:* sardrey@iukfs1.indiana.edu

INDIANA UNIVERSITY NORTHWEST
School of Nursing
Gary, Indiana

Programs • Generic Baccalaureate • RN Baccalaureate • Continuing Education

The University State-supported comprehensive coed institution. Part of Indiana University System. Founded: 1959. *Primary accreditation:* regional. *Setting:* 27-acre urban campus. *Total enrollment:* 5,301.

The School of Nursing Founded in 1965. *Nursing program faculty:* 21 (14% with doctorates).

Academic Facilities *Campus library:* 210,000 volumes (42,000 in health, 15,000 in nursing); 11,000 periodical subscriptions (200 health-care related). *Nursing school resources:* CAI, computer lab, nursing audiovisuals, interactive nursing skills videos, learning resource lab.

Student Life *Student services:* child-care facilities, personal counseling, career counseling, institutionally sponsored work-study program, job placement, campus safety program, special assistance for disabled students. *Nursing student activities:* Sigma Theta Tau, student nurses association.

Calendar Semesters.

NURSING STUDENT PROFILE

Undergraduate **Enrollment:** 285
Women: 85%; **Men:** 15%; **Minority:** 24%; **International:** 0%

BACCALAUREATE PROGRAMS

Contact Donna Brown Russell, Coordinator of BSN Program, School of Nursing, Indiana University Northwest, 3400 Broadway, Gary, IN 46408-1197, 219-980-6606. *Fax:* 219-980-6578. *E-mail:* drussell@iunhawl.iun.indiana.edu

Expenses *State resident tuition:* $2900 full-time, $87 per credit hour part-time. *Nonresident tuition:* $7450 full-time, $226 per credit hour part-time.

Indiana University Northwest (continued)

Full-time mandatory fees: $195–$666. *Books and supplies per academic year:* ranges from $600 to $800.

Financial Aid Institutionally sponsored need-based grants/scholarships, institutionally sponsored non-need grants/scholarships, Federal Nursing Student Loans, Federal Perkins Loans, Federal Supplemental Educational Opportunity Grants, Federal Work-Study. *Application deadline:* 3/1.

GENERIC BACCALAUREATE PROGRAM (BSN)

Applying *Required:* SAT I, SAT II Writing Test, TOEFL for nonnative speakers of English, minimum college GPA of 2.3, 3 years of high school math, 3 years of high school science, high school chemistry, high school biology, high school foreign language, high school transcript, transcript of college record, high school class rank: top 50%. 67 prerequisite credits must be completed before admission to the nursing program. *Options:* May apply for transfer of up to 90 total credits. *Application deadline:* 4/15. *Application fee:* $25.

Degree Requirements 124 total credit hours, 69 in nursing.

RN BACCALAUREATE PROGRAM (BSN)

Applying *Required:* SAT I, TOEFL for nonnative speakers of English, minimum college GPA of 2.3, RN license, diploma or AD in nursing, high school transcript, transcript of college record. 67 prerequisite credits must be completed before admission to the nursing program. *Options:* Advanced standing available through the following means: advanced placement exams, advanced placement without credit, credit by exam. Course work may be accelerated. May apply for transfer of up to 90 total credits. *Application deadline:* 4/15. *Application fee:* $25.

Degree Requirements 124 total credit hours, 69 in nursing.

CONTINUING EDUCATION PROGRAM

Contact Doris R. Blaney, Dean, School of Nursing, Indiana University Northwest, 3400 Broadway, Gary, IN 46408-1197, 219-980-6603. *Fax:* 219-980-6578. *E-mail:* dblaney@iunhawl.iun.indiana.edu

INDIANA UNIVERSITY–PURDUE UNIVERSITY FORT WAYNE

Indiana University–Purdue University Fort Wayne/Parkview Nursing Program
Fort Wayne, Indiana

Programs • RN Baccalaureate • MS

The University State-supported comprehensive coed institution. Part of Indiana and Purdue University Systems. Founded: 1917. *Primary accreditation:* regional. *Setting:* 412-acre urban campus. *Total enrollment:* 11,011.

The Indiana University–Purdue University Fort Wayne/Parkview Nursing Program Founded in 1964. *Nursing program faculty:* 14 (29% with doctorates).

Academic Facilities *Campus library:* 299,235 volumes (20,000 in health, 2,000 in nursing); 2,568 periodical subscriptions (129 health-care related). *Nursing school resources:* CAI, computer lab, nursing audiovisuals, interactive nursing skills videos, learning resource lab.

Student Life *Student services:* child-care facilities, personal counseling, career counseling, institutionally sponsored work-study program, job placement, campus safety program, special assistance for disabled students. *International student services:* counseling/support, special assistance for nonnative speakers of English, ESL courses. *Nursing student activities:* student nurses association.

Calendar Semesters.

NURSING STUDENT PROFILE

Undergraduate **Enrollment:** 385
Women: 90%; **Men:** 10%; **Part-time:** 77%

BACCALAUREATE PROGRAM

Contact Dr. Elaine W. Cowen, Chair, Indiana University-Purdue University Fort Wayne/Parkview Nursing Program, 2101 Coliseum Boulevard, East, Fort Wayne, IN 46805, 219-481-6816. *Fax:* 219-481-6083. *E-mail:* cowen@smtplink.ipfw.indiana.edu

Expenses *State resident tuition:* $3003 full-time, $94 per credit hour part-time. *Nonresident tuition:* $7189 full-time, $225 per credit hour part-time. *Full-time mandatory fees:* $21–$148. *Books and supplies per academic year:* ranges from $300 to $500.

Financial Aid Institutionally sponsored need-based grants/scholarships, institutionally sponsored non-need grants/scholarships, Federal Pell Grants, Federal Perkins Loans, Federal Supplemental Educational Opportunity Grants, Federal Work-Study. *Application deadline:* 3/1.

RN BACCALAUREATE PROGRAM (BS)

Applying *Required:* minimum college GPA of 2.3, RN license, diploma or AD in nursing, high school transcript, transcript of college record. 60 prerequisite credits must be completed before admission to the nursing program. *Options:* Advanced standing available through the following means: advanced placement exams, credit by exam. May apply for transfer of up to 96 total credits. *Application deadline:* rolling. *Application fee:* $30.

Degree Requirements 128 total credit hours, 31 in nursing.

MASTER'S PROGRAM

Contact Audré McLoughlin, Director, Neff Hall B50, Parkview Nursing Program, Indiana University-Purdue University Fort Wayne, 2101 Coliseum Boulevard, East, Fort Wayne, IN 46805, 219-481-6816. *Fax:* 219-481-6083.

Areas of Study Nursing administration.

Expenses *State resident tuition:* $121. *Nonresident tuition:* $265. *Full-time mandatory fees:* $18–$81.

MS PROGRAM

Applying *Required:* GRE if GPA is less than 3.0, bachelor's degree in nursing, bachelor's degree, RN license, statistics course, professional liability/malpractice insurance, essay, 3 letters of recommendation, transcript of college record, accounting course, economics course, mathematics course. *Application deadlines:* 8/1 (fall), 12/15 (spring), 5/1 (summer). *Application fee:* $30.

Degree Requirements 39–41 total credit hours dependent upon track, 21–23 in nursing.

Distance learning Courses provided through correspondence, video, audio.

INDIANA UNIVERSITY–PURDUE UNIVERSITY INDIANAPOLIS

School of Nursing
Indianapolis, Indiana

Programs • Generic Baccalaureate • RN Baccalaureate • MSN • RN to Master's • MSN/MPA • PhD • Postdoctoral • Continuing Education

The University State-supported coed university. Part of Indiana and Purdue University Systems. Founded: 1969. *Primary accreditation:* regional. *Setting:* 370-acre urban campus. *Total enrollment:* 26,939.

The School of Nursing Founded in 1914. *Nursing program faculty:* 156 (38% with doctorates).

Academic Facilities *Campus library:* 699,368 volumes (209,344 in health, 3,002 in nursing); 15,198 periodical subscriptions (2,717 health-care related). *Nursing school resources:* CAI, computer lab, nursing audiovisuals, interactive nursing skills videos, learning resource lab.

Student Life *Student services:* health clinic, child-care facilities, personal counseling, career counseling, institutionally sponsored work-study program, job placement, campus safety program, special assistance for

disabled students. *International student services:* counseling/support, ESL courses. *Nursing student activities:* Sigma Theta Tau, nursing club, student nurses association.

Calendar Semesters.

NURSING STUDENT PROFILE

Undergraduate **Enrollment:** 530

Women: 93%; **Men:** 7%; **Minority:** 9%; **International:** 1%; **Part-time:** 14%

Graduate **Enrollment:** 426

Women: 96%; **Men:** 4%; **Minority:** 7%; **International:** 1%; **Part-time:** 88%

BACCALAUREATE PROGRAMS

Contact Dr. Donna Boland, Associate Dean for Undergraduate Programs, School of Nursing, Indiana University-Purdue University Indianapolis, 1111 Middle Drive, NU 140, Indianapolis, IN 46202, 317-274-8038. *Fax:* 317-274-2996. *E-mail:* klynn@wpo.iupui.edu

Expenses *State resident tuition:* $3162 full-time, $102 per credit hour part-time. *Nonresident tuition:* $9765 full-time, $315 per credit hour part-time. *Full-time mandatory fees:* $140–$400. *Books and supplies per academic year:* ranges from $600 to $1000.

Financial Aid Institutionally sponsored need-based grants/scholarships, institutionally sponsored non-need grants/scholarships, Federal Nursing Student Loans, Federal Supplemental Educational Opportunity Grants, Federal Work-Study. *Application deadline:* 3/1.

Generic Baccalaureate Program (BSN)

Applying *Required:* SAT I, ACT, SAT II Writing Test, TOEFL for nonnative speakers of English, minimum college GPA of 2.5, 3 years of high school math, 3 years of high school science, high school chemistry, high school biology, high school transcript, transcript of college record, high school class rank: top 50%. 67 prerequisite credits must be completed before admission to the nursing program. *Options:* May apply for transfer of up to 31 total credits. *Application deadlines:* 4/15 (fall), 9/15 (spring).

Degree Requirements 124 total credit hours, 57 in nursing.

RN Baccalaureate Program (BSN)

Applying *Required:* minimum college GPA of 2.5, RN license, diploma or AD in nursing, transcript of college record. *Application deadlines:* 4/15 (fall), 10/15 (spring).

Degree Requirements 34 total credit hours in nursing.

MASTER'S PROGRAMS

Contact Dr. Linda Finke, Associate Dean for Graduate Programs, School of Nursing, Indiana University-Purdue University at Indianapolis, 1111 Middle Drive, NU 136, Indianapolis, IN 46202, 317-274-3115. *Fax:* 317-274-2996. *E-mail:* lfinke@wpo.iupui.edu

Areas of Study Clinical nurse specialist programs in adult health nursing, cardiovascular nursing, community health nursing, critical care nursing, gerontological nursing, oncology nursing, psychiatric–mental health nursing, rehabilitation nursing, women's health nursing; nursing administration; nurse practitioner programs in adult health, child care/pediatrics, family health, gerontology, women's health.

Expenses *State resident tuition:* ranges from $3330 to $4995 full-time, $139 per credit hour part-time. *Nonresident tuition:* ranges from $9606 to $14,409 full-time, $400 per credit hour part-time. *Full-time mandatory fees:* $766. *Room and board:* $550.

Financial Aid Graduate assistantships, nurse traineeships, fellowships, institutionally sponsored loans, employment opportunities. *Application deadline:* 5/1.

MSN Program

Applying *Required:* GRE General Test, TOEFL for nonnative speakers of English, bachelor's degree in nursing, minimum GPA of 3.0, RN license, 2 years of clinical experience, physical assessment course, statistics course, 3 letters of recommendation, transcript of college record. *Application deadlines:* 4/1 (fall), 10/1 (spring). *Application fee:* $50.

Degree Requirements 42 total credit hours, 36 in nursing. Nursing study.

RN to Master's Program (MSN)

Applying *Required:* GRE General Test, TOEFL for nonnative speakers of English, minimum GPA of 3.0, RN license, 2 years of clinical experience, physical assessment course, statistics course, 3 letters of recommendation, transcript of college record. *Application deadlines:* 4/1 (fall), 10/1 (spring). *Application fee:* $50.

Degree Requirements 42 total credit hours, 36 in nursing. Nursing study or thesis.

MSN/MPA Program

Applying *Required:* GRE General Test, TOEFL for nonnative speakers of English, minimum GPA of 3.0, RN license, 2 years of clinical experience, physical assessment course, statistics course, 3 letters of recommendation, transcript of college record, computer literacy. *Application deadlines:* 4/1 (fall), 10/1 (spring). *Application fee:* $50.

Degree Requirements 42 total credit hours, 36 in nursing. Nursing study or thesis.

DOCTORAL PROGRAM

Contact Dr. Linda Finke, Associate Dean for Graduate Programs, School of Nursing, Indiana University-Purdue University at Indianapolis, 1111 Middle Drive, NU 136, Indianapolis, IN 46202, 317-274-3115. *Fax:* 317-274-2996. *E-mail:* lfinke@wpo.iupui.edu

Areas of Study Nursing administration, nursing education, nursing research, nursing policy, information systems.

Expenses *State resident tuition:* ranges from $3330 to $4995 full-time, $139 per credit hour part-time. *Nonresident tuition:* ranges from $9606 to $14,409 full-time, $400 per credit hour part-time. *Full-time mandatory fees:* $556. *Books and supplies per academic year:* $550.

Financial Aid Graduate assistantships, fellowships, dissertation grants, institutionally sponsored loans, opportunities for employment. *Application deadline:* 5/1.

PhD Program

Applying *Required:* GRE General Test, TOEFL for nonnative speakers of English, 1 scholarly paper, statistics course, interview, 3 letters of recommendation, vitae, writing sample, competitive review by faculty committee. *Application deadline:* 2/1. *Application fee:* $50.

Degree Requirements 90 total credit hours; dissertation; written exam; defense of dissertation; residency.

POSTDOCTORAL PROGRAM

Contact Dr. Linda Finke, Associate Dean for Graduate Programs, School of Nursing, Indiana University-Purdue University at Indianapolis, 1111 Middle Drive, NU 136, Indianapolis, IN 46202, 317-274-3115. *Fax:* 317-274-2996. *E-mail:* lfinke@wpo.iupui.edu

Areas of Study Adolescent health, family adaptation.

CONTINUING EDUCATION PROGRAM

Contact Dr. Charlotte Carlley, Assistant Dean for Continuing Education, School of Nursing, Indiana University-Purdue University at Indianapolis, 1111 Middle Drive, NU 337, Indianapolis, IN 46202, 317-274-7779. *Fax:* 317-274-0012. *E-mail:* ccarlley@wpo.iupui.edu

See full description on page 462.

INDIANA UNIVERSITY SOUTH BEND

School of Nursing
South Bend, Indiana

Programs • Generic Baccalaureate • Accelerated RN Baccalaureate

The University State-supported comprehensive coed institution. Part of Indiana University System. Founded: 1922. *Primary accreditation:* regional. *Setting:* 40-acre suburban campus. *Total enrollment:* 7,544.

The School of Nursing Founded in 1988. *Nursing program faculty:* 20 (20% with doctorates). *Off-campus program site:* Elkhart.

Academic Facilities *Campus library:* 200,000 volumes (2,100 in health, 4,150 in nursing); 2,100 periodical subscriptions (145 health-care related). *Nursing school resources:* CAI, computer lab, nursing audiovisuals, interactive nursing skills videos, learning resource lab.

Student Life *Student services:* child-care facilities, personal counseling, career counseling, institutionally sponsored work-study program, job placement, campus safety program, special assistance for disabled students.

Indiana University South Bend (continued)

International student services: counseling/support, special assistance for nonnative speakers of English, ESL courses. *Nursing student activities:* Sigma Theta Tau, recruiter club, student nurses association.

Calendar Semesters.

NURSING STUDENT PROFILE

Undergraduate **Enrollment:** 485
Women: 80%; **Men:** 20%; **Minority:** 10%; **International:** 0%; **Part-time:** 40%

BACCALAUREATE PROGRAMS

Contact Dr. Marian Martin Pettengill, Dean, School of Nursing, Indiana University South Bend, 1700 Mishawaka, PO Box 7111, South Bend, IN 46634-7111, 219-237-4207. *Fax:* 219-237-4461. *E-mail:* mpettengill@iusb.edu

Expenses *State resident tuition:* $3933 full-time, $100 per credit hour part-time. *Nonresident tuition:* $8391 full-time, $264 per credit hour part-time. *Full-time mandatory fees:* $518–$1032. *Books and supplies per academic year:* ranges from $220 to $600.

Financial Aid Institutionally sponsored need-based grants/scholarships, institutionally sponsored non-need grants/scholarships, Federal Direct Loans, Federal Perkins Loans, Federal Supplemental Educational Opportunity Grants, Federal Work-Study, community work-study, Michiana Transfer Award. *Application deadline:* 3/1.

Generic Baccalaureate Program (BSN)

Applying *Required:* SAT I or ACT, TOEFL for nonnative speakers of English, math, English composition, and remedial reading exams, minimum college GPA of 2.5, high school math, high school chemistry, high school biology, high school transcript, transcript of college record, high school class rank: top 50%. 60 prerequisite credits must be completed before admission to the nursing program. *Options:* Advanced standing available through the following means: advanced placement exams, credit by exam. *Application deadlines:* 9/30 (fall), 4/15 (spring).

Degree Requirements 122 total credit hours, 62 in nursing.

Accelerated RN Baccalaureate Program (BSN)

Applying *Required:* minimum college GPA of 2.5, high school chemistry, RN license, diploma or AD in nursing, transcript of college record. 60 prerequisite credits must be completed before admission to the nursing program. *Options:* Advanced standing available through the following means: advanced placement exams, credit by exam. *Application deadlines:* 9/30 (fall), 4/15 (spring).

Degree Requirements 122 total credit hours, 62 in nursing.

INDIANA UNIVERSITY SOUTHEAST

Division of Nursing
New Albany, Indiana

Programs • Generic Baccalaureate • RN Baccalaureate

The University State-supported comprehensive coed institution. Part of Indiana University System. Founded: 1941. *Primary accreditation:* regional. *Setting:* 177-acre suburban campus. *Total enrollment:* 5,464.

The Division of Nursing Founded in 1941. *Nursing program faculty:* 18 (6% with doctorates).

Academic Facilities *Campus library:* 250,000 volumes.

Student Life *Student services:* personal counseling, career counseling. *Nursing student activities:* Sigma Theta Tau, student nurses association.

Calendar Semesters.

NURSING STUDENT PROFILE

Undergraduate **Enrollment:** 103
Women: 89%; **Men:** 11%; **Minority:** 0%; **International:** 2%; **Part-time:** 0%

BACCALAUREATE PROGRAMS

Contact Pamela White, Counselor, Division of Nursing, Indiana University Southeast, 4201 Grant Line Road, New Albany, IN 47105-6405, 812-941-2341. *Fax:* 812-941-2687.

Expenses *State resident tuition:* $2653 full-time, $87 per credit hour part-time. *Nonresident tuition:* $6893 full-time, $226 per credit hour part-time. *Full-time mandatory fees:* $224.

Generic Baccalaureate Program (BSN)

Applying *Required:* SAT I, 2 years of high school math, 1 year of high school science, high school class rank: top 50%. *Options:* Advanced standing available through the following means: advanced placement exams, credit by exam. *Application deadlines:* 7/15 (fall), 12/1 (spring). *Application fee:* $20.

Degree Requirements 122 total credit hours.

RN Baccalaureate Program (BSN)

Applying *Required:* minimum college GPA of 2.0, RN license, diploma or AD in nursing, transcript of college record. *Options:* Advanced standing available through the following means: advanced placement exams, credit by exam. *Application deadlines:* 7/15 (fall), 12/1 (spring). *Application fee:* $20.

Degree Requirements 122 total credit hours.

INDIANA WESLEYAN UNIVERSITY

Division of Nursing Education
Marion, Indiana

Programs • Generic Baccalaureate • Accelerated RN Baccalaureate • MS • Post-Master's

The University Independent Wesleyan comprehensive coed institution. Founded: 1920. *Primary accreditation:* regional. *Setting:* 132-acre small-town campus. *Total enrollment:* 5,069.

The Division of Nursing Education Founded in 1973. *Nursing program faculty:* 15 (38% with doctorates). *Off-campus program sites:* Anderson, Indianapolis, Kokomo.

▶ ***NOTEWORTHY***

Indiana Wesleyan University has been educating nurses since 1973. The Division of Nursing Education attempts to create a Christ-centered educational climate where students are equipped for lifelong learning and service. The philosophy of the Division of Nursing is based on the faculty's belief that man is created by a direct act of God and has intrinsic worth and value. Faith founded on Judeo-Christian principles is integrated in the learning process. The curricular emphasis on diversity enables undergraduate students to complete a clinical course in intercultural nursing. The graduate program prepares nurses for advanced practice in multicultural settings and provides a foundation for doctoral studies.

Academic Facilities *Campus library:* 93,047 volumes (1,175 in health, 1,050 in nursing); 1,340 periodical subscriptions (152 health-care related). *Nursing school resources:* computer lab, nursing audiovisuals, interactive nursing skills videos, learning resource lab.

Student Life *Student services:* health clinic, child-care facilities, personal counseling, career counseling, institutionally sponsored work-study program, campus safety program, special assistance for disabled students. *International student services:* counseling/support, special assistance for nonnative speakers of English, ESL courses. *Nursing student activities:* Sigma Theta Tau, nursing club, Nurses Christian Fellowship.

Calendar Semesters.

NURSING STUDENT PROFILE

Undergraduate **Enrollment:** 503
Women: 96%; **Men:** 4%; **Minority:** 3%; **International:** 1%; **Part-time:** 6%
Graduate **Enrollment:** 107
Women: 95%; **Men:** 5%; **Minority:** 7%; **International:** 1%; **Part-time:** 64%

BACCALAUREATE PROGRAMS

Contact Ms. Joyce McDonald, Office Manager, Division of Nursing Education, Indiana Wesleyan University, 4201 South Washington Street, Marion, IN 46953, 317-677-2269. *Fax:* 317-677-2284. *E-mail:* jmcdonald@indwes.edu

Expenses *Tuition:* $10,260 full-time, $218 per credit hour part-time. *Full-time mandatory fees:* $75–$150. *Part-time mandatory fees:* $75–$150. *Room and board:* $3596–$4042. *Room only:* $1684. *Books and supplies per academic year:* $600.

Financial Aid Institutionally sponsored need-based grants/scholarships, institutionally sponsored non-need grants/scholarships, Federal Nursing

Student Loans, Federal Pell Grants, Federal Perkins Loans, Federal Supplemental Educational Opportunity Grants, Federal Work-Study. 34% of undergraduate students in nursing programs received some form of financial aid in 1995–96. *Application deadline:* 3/1.

Generic Baccalaureate Program (BS)

Applying *Required:* SAT I or ACT, TOEFL for nonnative speakers of English, NLN Preadmission Examination, minimum high school GPA of 2.0, minimum college GPA of 2.5, high school transcript, letter of recommendation, transcript of college record. 29 prerequisite credits must be completed before admission to the nursing program. *Options:* Advanced standing available through the following means: advanced placement exams, credit by exam. May apply for transfer of up to 62 total credits. *Application deadlines:* 9/1 (fall), 1/1 (spring). *Application fee:* $15.

Degree Requirements 124 total credit hours, 58 in nursing.

Accelerated RN Baccalaureate Program (BS)

Applying *Required:* SAT I, TOEFL for nonnative speakers of English, minimum college GPA of 2.5, RN license, diploma or AD in nursing, 2 letters of recommendation, written essay, transcript of college record. 60 prerequisite credits must be completed before admission to the nursing program. *Application deadline:* rolling. *Application fee:* $15.

Degree Requirements 124 total credit hours, 61 in nursing.

MASTER'S PROGRAMS

Contact Dr. Susan Stranahan, Director, Graduate Studies in Nursing Education, Division of Nursing Education, Indiana Wesleyan University, 4201 South Washington Street, Marion, IN 46953, 317-677-2148. *Fax:* 317-677-2284. *E-mail:* sstranahan@indwes.edu

Areas of Study Clinical nurse specialist program in community health nursing; nurse practitioner programs in adult health, family health, gerontology.

Expenses *Tuition:* $368 per credit hour. *Full-time mandatory fees:* $45–$210. *Room and board:* $750. *Books and supplies per academic year:* ranges from $750 to $1000.

Financial Aid Graduate assistantships, nurse traineeships, employment opportunities, institutionally sponsored need-based grants/scholarships. 19% of master's level students in nursing programs received some form of financial aid in 1995-96. *Application deadline:* 4/1.

MS Program

Applying *Required:* GRE General Test, bachelor's degree in nursing, RN license, 1 year of clinical experience, statistics course, interview, 3 letters of recommendation, transcript of college record, professional liability/malpractice insurance for primary care nursing track. *Application deadlines:* 7/31 (fall), 11/30 (spring), 3/30 (May and summer terms).

Degree Requirements 36 total credit hours. Thesis required.

Post-Master's Program

Applying *Required:* GRE General Test, TOEFL for nonnative speakers of English, bachelor's degree in nursing, minimum GPA of 3.0, RN license, 1 year of clinical experience, professional liability/malpractice insurance, interview, 3 letters of recommendation, transcript of college record, master's degree in nursing. *Application deadlines:* 7/31 (fall), 11/30 (spring), 3/30 (May and summer terms).

Degree Requirements 22–25 total credit hours dependent upon track.

MARIAN COLLEGE
Department of Nursing
Indianapolis, Indiana

Programs • Generic Baccalaureate • RN Baccalaureate • Baccalaureate for Second Degree

The College Independent Roman Catholic 4-year coed college. Founded: 1851. *Primary accreditation:* regional. *Setting:* 114-acre urban campus. *Total enrollment:* 1,352.

The Department of Nursing Founded in 1985. *Nursing program faculty:* 10 (10% with doctorates).

Academic Facilities *Campus library:* 123,467 volumes (1,100 in health, 2,000 in nursing); 300 periodical subscriptions (93 health-care related). *Nursing school resources:* CAI, computer lab, nursing audiovisuals, interactive nursing skills videos, learning resource lab.

Student Life *Student services:* health clinic, personal counseling, career counseling, institutionally sponsored work-study program, job placement, campus safety program. *International student services:* counseling/support, special assistance for nonnative speakers of English, ESL courses. *Nursing student activities:* Sigma Theta Tau, nursing club, student nurses association.

Calendar Semesters.

NURSING STUDENT PROFILE

Undergraduate **Enrollment:** 200
Women: 91%; **Men:** 9%; **Minority:** 17%; **International:** 0%; **Part-time:** 7%

BACCALAUREATE PROGRAMS

Contact Ms. Liane Ammerman, BSN Adviser, Department of Nursing, Marian College, 3200 Cold Spring Road, Indianapolis, IN 46222, 317-929-0603. *Fax:* 317-929-0263.

Expenses *Tuition:* $10,790 full-time, $299 per credit part-time. *Full-time mandatory fees:* $252–$652. *Room and board:* $1866–$2112. *Books and supplies per academic year:* ranges from $200 to $400.

Financial Aid Institutionally sponsored need-based grants/scholarships, institutionally sponsored non-need grants/scholarships, Federal Nursing Student Loans, Federal Pell Grants, Federal Supplemental Educational Opportunity Grants, Federal Work-Study. 41% of undergraduate students in nursing programs received some form of financial aid in 1995–96. *Application deadline:* 3/1.

Generic Baccalaureate Program (BSN)

Applying *Required:* SAT I, minimum high school GPA of 2.5, minimum college GPA of 2.5, high school chemistry, high school biology, high school transcript, transcript of college record. 30 prerequisite credits must be completed before admission to the nursing program. *Options:* Advanced standing available through credit by exam. May apply for transfer of up to 30 total credits. *Application deadlines:* 6/1 (fall), 11/1 (spring). *Application fee:* $20.

Degree Requirements 128 total credit hours, 53 in nursing.

RN Baccalaureate Program (BSN)

Applying *Required:* NLN Mobility Profile II for diploma graduates, minimum college GPA of 2.3, RN license, diploma or AD in nursing, transcript of college record. 15 prerequisite credits must be completed before admission to the nursing program. *Options:* Course work may be accelerated. May apply for transfer of up to 30 total credits. *Application deadline:* rolling. *Application fee:* $20.

Degree Requirements 128 total credit hours, 53 in nursing.

Baccalaureate for Second Degree Program (BSN)

Applying *Required:* minimum college GPA of 2.7, interview, transcript of college record. 39 prerequisite credits must be completed before admission to the nursing program. *Options:* Advanced standing available through credit by exam. Course work may be accelerated. May apply for transfer of up to 30 total credits. *Application deadline:* rolling. *Application fee:* $20.

Degree Requirements 128 total credit hours, 53 in nursing.

PURDUE UNIVERSITY
School of Nursing
West Lafayette, Indiana

Programs • Generic Baccalaureate • RN Baccalaureate

The University State-supported coed university. Part of Purdue University System. Founded: 1869. *Primary accreditation:* regional. *Setting:* 1,579-acre suburban campus. *Total enrollment:* 34,685.

The School of Nursing Founded in 1963. *Nursing program faculty:* 35 (29% with doctorates).

Academic Facilities *Campus library:* 2.1 million volumes (200,000 in health, 10,000 in nursing); 10,000 periodical subscriptions (1,000 health-care related). *Nursing school resources:* computer lab.

Calendar Semesters.

Purdue University (continued)

BACCALAUREATE PROGRAMS

Contact Assistant Head for Student Affairs, 1336 Johnson Hall of Nursing, School of Nursing, Purdue University, West Lafayette, IN 47907-1337, 317-494-4008. *Fax:* 317-496-1800.

Expenses *State resident tuition:* $3208 full-time, $115 per credit hour part-time. *Nonresident tuition:* $10,636 full-time, $351 per credit hour part-time.

Financial Aid Institutionally sponsored need-based grants/scholarships, institutionally sponsored non-need grants/scholarships. *Application deadline:* 3/1.

Generic Baccalaureate Program (BS)

Applying *Required:* SAT I or ACT, TOEFL for nonnative speakers of English, 4 years of high school math, 4 years of high school science, high school transcript, health exam, immunizations, CPR certification. *Options:* Advanced standing available through advanced placement exams. *Application deadline:* 11/15.

Degree Requirements 128 total credit hours, 61 in nursing.

RN Baccalaureate Program (BS)

Applying *Required:* SAT I or ACT, TOEFL for nonnative speakers of English, minimum college GPA of 2.5, RN license, diploma or AD in nursing, interview, transcript of college record, health exam, immunizations, CPR certification. *Application deadline:* 2/1.

Degree Requirements 128 total credit hours, 64 in nursing.

PURDUE UNIVERSITY CALUMET
Department of Nursing
Hammond, Indiana

Programs • RN Baccalaureate • MS

The University State-supported comprehensive coed institution. Part of Purdue University System. Founded: 1951. *Primary accreditation:* regional. *Setting:* 167-acre urban campus. *Total enrollment:* 8,975.

The Department of Nursing Founded in 1965. *Nursing program faculty:* 27 (30% with doctorates).

Academic Facilities *Campus library:* 262,355 volumes (15,000 in health, 9,647 in nursing); 66,579 periodical subscriptions (3,158 health-care related). *Nursing school resources:* CAI, computer lab, nursing audiovisuals, interactive nursing skills videos, learning resource lab.

Student Life *Student services:* child-care facilities, personal counseling, career counseling, institutionally sponsored work-study program, job placement, campus safety program, special assistance for disabled students. *Nursing student activities:* Sigma Theta Tau.

Calendar Semesters.

NURSING STUDENT PROFILE

Undergraduate **Enrollment:** 300
Women: 92%; **Men:** 8%; **Minority:** 20%; **International:** 0%; **Part-time:** 84%
Graduate **Enrollment:** 90
Women: 95%; **Men:** 5%; **Minority:** 24%; **Part-time:** 83%

BACCALAUREATE PROGRAM

Contact Gil Wegner, Associate Professor, Department of Nursing, Purdue University Calumet, Hammond, IN 46323-2094, 219-989-2818. *Fax:* 219-989-2848.

Expenses *State resident tuition:* $4000 full-time, $1320 per year part-time. *Nonresident tuition:* $5400 full-time, $1782 per year part-time. *Full-time mandatory fees:* $100. *Books and supplies per academic year:* $500.

Financial Aid Institutionally sponsored need-based grants/scholarships, institutionally sponsored non-need grants/scholarships, Federal Nursing Student Loans, Federal Pell Grants, Federal Perkins Loans. *Application deadline:* 3/1.

RN Baccalaureate Program (BS)

Applying *Required:* TOEFL for nonnative speakers of English, NLN Mobility Profile II for diploma RNs, high school chemistry, RN license, diploma or AD in nursing. 60 prerequisite credits must be completed before admission to the nursing program. *Options:* Advanced standing available through credit by exam. Course work may be accelerated. May apply for transfer of up to 60 total credits. *Application deadlines:* 7/30 (fall), 12/1 (spring). *Application fee:* $25.

Degree Requirements 120 total credit hours, 33 in nursing.

MASTER'S PROGRAM

Contact Dr. Peggy Gerard, Associate Professor, Department of Nursing, Purdue University Calumet, Hammond, IN 46323-2094, 219-989-2821. *Fax:* 219-989-2848.

Areas of Study Clinical nurse specialist programs in adult health nursing, critical care nursing; nurse practitioner program in family health.

Expenses *State resident tuition:* $3400 full-time, $1122 per year part-time. *Nonresident tuition:* $6200 full-time, $2046 per year part-time. *Full-time mandatory fees:* $100–$299.

Financial Aid Graduate assistantships, nurse traineeships. *Application deadline:* 9/1.

MS Program

Applying *Required:* bachelor's degree in nursing, minimum GPA of 3.0, RN license, 1 year of clinical experience, physical assessment course, statistics course, professional liability/malpractice insurance, essay, interview, 3 letters of recommendation, transcript of college record. *Application deadlines:* 4/15 (fall), 9/15 (spring), 2/15 (summer). *Application fee:* $25.

Degree Requirements 36–44 total credit hours dependent upon track, 27–44 in nursing.

SAINT FRANCIS COLLEGE
Department of Nursing
Fort Wayne, Indiana

Programs • Generic Baccalaureate • RN Baccalaureate • Baccalaureate for Second Degree • LPN to Baccalaureate • MSN • Master's for Nurses with Non-Nursing Degrees • Continuing Education

The College Independent Roman Catholic comprehensive coed institution. Founded: 1890. *Primary accreditation:* regional. *Setting:* 73-acre suburban campus. *Total enrollment:* 964.

The Department of Nursing Founded in 1981. *Nursing program faculty:* 17 (6% with doctorates). *Off-campus program site:* Beech Grove.

Academic Facilities *Campus library:* 83,560 volumes (3,200 in health, 830 in nursing); 527 periodical subscriptions (101 health-care related). *Nursing school resources:* CAI, computer lab, nursing audiovisuals, interactive nursing skills videos, learning resource lab.

Student Life *Student services:* personal counseling, career counseling, institutionally sponsored work-study program, job placement, campus safety program, special assistance for disabled students, tutoring. *International student services:* counseling/support, special assistance for nonnative speakers of English, ESL courses. *Nursing student activities:* Sigma Theta Tau, student nurses association, student government association.

Calendar Semesters.

NURSING STUDENT PROFILE

Undergraduate **Enrollment:** 117
Women: 92%; **Men:** 8%; **Minority:** 8%; **International:** 3%; **Part-time:** 8%
Graduate **Enrollment:** 62
Women: 98%; **Men:** 2%; **Minority:** 7%; **International:** 0%; **Part-time:** 98%

BACCALAUREATE PROGRAMS

Contact Mr. Michael Wank, Dean of Admissions, Department of Admissions, Saint Francis College, 2701 Spring Street, Fort Wayne, IN 46808-3994, 219-434-3269. *Fax:* 219-434-3183.

Expenses *Tuition:* $9820 full-time, $310 per semester hour part-time. *Full-time mandatory fees:* $60–$200. *Part-time mandatory fees:* $46–$152. *Room and board:* $4070–$4894. *Books and supplies per academic year:* ranges from $100 to $275.

Financial Aid Institutionally sponsored need-based grants/scholarships, institutionally sponsored non-need grants/scholarships, Federal Direct Loans, Federal Pell Grants, Federal Perkins Loans, Federal Supplemental

Educational Opportunity Grants, Federal Work-Study. 91% of undergraduate students in nursing programs received some form of financial aid in 1995–96. *Application deadline:* 3/1.

Generic Baccalaureate Program (BSN)

Applying *Required:* SAT I, ACT, minimum high school GPA of 2.5, minimum college GPA of 2.5, high school chemistry, high school biology, high school transcript, written essay, transcript of college record, high school class rank: top 50%. 9 prerequisite credits must be completed before admission to the nursing program. *Options:* Advanced standing available through the following means: advanced placement exams, advanced placement without credit, credit by exam. May apply for transfer of up to 96 total credits. *Application deadlines:* 8/15 (fall), 12/15 (spring). *Application fee:* $20.

Degree Requirements 132 total credit hours, 62 in nursing.

RN Baccalaureate Program (BSN)

Applying *Required:* minimum college GPA of 2.5, RN license, diploma or AD in nursing, interview, transcript of college record, minimum 2.8 GPA in nursing. 30 prerequisite credits must be completed before admission to the nursing program. *Options:* Advanced standing available through the following means: advanced placement exams, advanced placement without credit, credit by exam. May apply for transfer of up to 96 total credits. *Application deadlines:* 8/15 (fall), 12/15 (spring). *Application fee:* $20.

Degree Requirements 132 total credit hours, 45 in nursing.

Baccalaureate for Second Degree Program (BSN)

Applying *Required:* minimum college GPA of 2.5, high school chemistry, high school biology, interview, transcript of college record. 30 prerequisite credits must be completed before admission to the nursing program. *Options:* Advanced standing available through credit by exam. May apply for transfer of up to 96 total credits. *Application deadlines:* 8/15 (fall), 12/15 (spring). *Application fee:* $20.

Degree Requirements 132 total credit hours, 62 in nursing.

LPN to Baccalaureate Program (BSN)

Applying *Required:* minimum college GPA of 2.5, high school chemistry, high school biology, interview, transcript of college record. *Options:* Advanced standing available through the following means: advanced placement exams, credit by exam. May apply for transfer of up to 30 total credits. *Application deadlines:* 8/15 (fall), 12/15 (spring). *Application fee:* $20.

Degree Requirements 132 total credit hours, 62 in nursing.

MASTER'S PROGRAMS

Contact Michael Wank, Dean of Admissions, 2701 Spring Street, Fort Wayne, IN 46808-3994, 219-434-3269. *Fax:* 219-434-3183.

Areas of Study Nursing administration; nurse practitioner program in family health.

Expenses *Tuition:* $320 per semester hour. *Full-time mandatory fees:* $215. *Part-time mandatory fees:* $138. *Room and board:* $4070–$4894. *Books and supplies per academic year:* ranges from $200 to $400.

Financial Aid Graduate assistantships, Federal Direct Loans, employment opportunities. 39% of master's level students in nursing programs received some form of financial aid in 1995-96. *Application deadline:* 3/1.

MSN Program

Applying *Required:* bachelor's degree in nursing, bachelor's degree, minimum GPA of 3.0, RN license, physical assessment course, statistics course, essay, interview, 3 letters of recommendation, transcript of college record. *Application deadlines:* 8/15 (fall), 12/15 (spring). *Application fee:* $20.

Degree Requirements 39–44 total credit hours dependent upon track, 39–44 in nursing, 9 in business.

Distance learning Courses provided through interactive television.

Master's for Nurses with Non-Nursing Degrees Program (MSN)

Applying *Required:* Miller Analogies Test, bachelor's degree, minimum GPA of 3.0, RN license, physical assessment course, statistics course, essay, interview, 3 letters of recommendation, transcript of college record. *Application deadlines:* 8/15 (fall), 12/15 (spring). *Application fee:* $20.

Degree Requirements 39–44 total credit hours dependent upon track, 30–44 in nursing, 9 in business.

Distance learning Courses provided through interactive television.

CONTINUING EDUCATION PROGRAM

Contact Dr. Nancy Nightingale Gillespie, Chair, Department of Nursing, Saint Francis College, 2701 Spring Street, Fort Wayne, IN 46808, 219-434-3239. *Fax:* 219-434-3183.

SAINT MARY'S COLLEGE

Department of Nursing
Notre Dame, Indiana

Programs • Generic Baccalaureate • Accelerated Baccalaureate for Second Degree

The College Independent Roman Catholic 4-year women's college. Founded: 1844. *Primary accreditation:* regional. *Setting:* 275-acre suburban campus. *Total enrollment:* 1,579.

The Department of Nursing Founded in 1971. *Nursing program faculty:* 9.

Academic Facilities *Campus library:* 198,729 volumes (9,787 in health, 5,149 in nursing); 1,077 periodical subscriptions (70 health-care related). *Nursing school resources:* nursing audiovisuals, interactive nursing skills videos, learning resource lab.

Student Life *Student services:* health clinic, child-care facilities, personal counseling, career counseling, institutionally sponsored work-study program, job placement, campus safety program, special assistance for disabled students. *International student services:* counseling/support. *Nursing student activities:* Sigma Theta Tau, student nurses association.

Calendar Semesters.

NURSING STUDENT PROFILE

Undergraduate **Enrollment:** 120
Women: 100%; **Part-time:** 0%

BACCALAUREATE PROGRAMS

Contact Denise Martin, Admissions Office, Le Mans Hall, Saint Mary's College, Notre Dame, IN 46556, 219-284-4587. *Fax:* 219-284-4716.

Expenses *Full-time mandatory fees:* $656–$856. *Room and board:* $3518–$5134. *Books and supplies per academic year:* ranges from $200 to $400.

Financial Aid Institutionally sponsored need-based grants/scholarships, Federal Supplemental Educational Opportunity Grants. *Application deadline:* 3/1.

Generic Baccalaureate Program (BS)

Applying *Required:* SAT I or ACT, minimum college GPA of 3.0, 4 years of high school math, high school foreign language, high school transcript, interview, 2 letters of recommendation, written essay, transcript of college record. 68 prerequisite credits must be completed before admission to the nursing program. *Application deadline:* rolling. *Application fee:* $30.

Degree Requirements 128 total credit hours, 54 in nursing.

Accelerated Baccalaureate for Second Degree Program (BS)

Applying *Required:* SAT I or ACT, minimum college GPA of 2.5, interview, 2 letters of recommendation, written essay, transcript of college record. *Application deadline:* 2/15 (summer). *Application fee:* $30.

Degree Requirements 56 total credit hours, 56 in nursing. 2 summer sessions.

UNIVERSITY OF EVANSVILLE

Department of Nursing and Health Sciences
Evansville, Indiana

Programs • Generic Baccalaureate • MSN

The University Independent comprehensive coed institution, affiliated with United Methodist Church. Founded: 1854. *Primary accreditation:* regional. *Setting:* 75-acre suburban campus. *Total enrollment:* 3,185.

The Department of Nursing and Health Sciences Founded in 1953. *Nursing program faculty:* 9 (33% with doctorates). *Off-campus program site:* Grantham, England.

Academic Facilities *Campus library:* 228,070 volumes (8,985 in health, 1,760 in nursing); 1,113 periodical subscriptions (144 health-care related). *Nursing school resources:* CAI, computer lab, nursing audiovisuals, interactive nursing skills videos, learning resource lab.

Student Life *Student services:* health clinic, personal counseling, career counseling, institutionally sponsored work-study program, job placement, campus safety program, special assistance for disabled students.

University of Evansville (continued)
International student services: counseling/support, special assistance for nonnative speakers of English, ESL courses. *Nursing student activities:* Sigma Theta Tau, nursing club.

Calendar Semesters.

NURSING STUDENT PROFILE

Undergraduate **Enrollment:** 134
Women: 93%; **Men:** 7%; **Minority:** 4%; **International:** 0%; **Part-time:** 0%
Graduate **Enrollment:** 29
Women: 100%; **Minority:** 0%; **International:** 0%; **Part-time:** 86%

BACCALAUREATE PROGRAM

Contact Dr. Rita S. Behnke, Chair, Department of Nursing and Health Sciences, University of Evansville, 1800 Lincoln Avenue, Evansville, IN 47722, 812-479-2343. *Fax:* 812-479-2717. *E-mail:* rb7@cedars.evansville.edu

Expenses *Tuition:* $12,990 full-time, $375 per credit hour part-time. *Full-time mandatory fees:* $230. *Room and board:* $3045–$11,710. *Room only:* $1980–$2420. *Books and supplies per academic year:* ranges from $400 to $526.

Financial Aid Institutionally sponsored need-based grants/scholarships, institutionally sponsored non-need grants/scholarships, Federal Direct Loans, Federal Nursing Student Loans, Federal Perkins Loans, Federal Supplemental Educational Opportunity Grants, Federal Work-Study. *Application deadline:* 3/1.

Generic Baccalaureate Program (BSN)

Applying *Required:* SAT I or ACT, TOEFL for nonnative speakers of English, high school chemistry, high school biology, high school transcript, written essay, transcript of college record, high school class rank: top 33%. *Options:* May apply for transfer of up to 60 total credits. *Application deadline:* 2/15. *Application fee:* $30.

Degree Requirements 128 total credit hours, 64 in nursing.

MASTER'S PROGRAM

Contact Dr. Rita S. Behnke, Chair, Department of Nursing and Health Sciences, University of Evansville, 1800 Lincoln Avenue, Evansville, IN 47722, 812-479-2347. *Fax:* 812-479-2717. *E-mail:* rb7@cedars.evansville.edu

Areas of Study Clinical nurse specialist programs in adult health nursing, gerontological nursing.

Expenses *Tuition:* $6300 full-time, $350 per credit hour part-time. *Books and supplies per academic year:* ranges from $200 to $400.

Financial Aid Nurse traineeships. 17% of master's level students in nursing programs received some form of financial aid in 1995-96. *Application deadline:* 6/1.

MSN Program

Applying *Required:* GRE General Test (minimum combined score of 1400 on three tests), TOEFL for nonnative speakers of English, bachelor's degree in nursing, minimum GPA of 3.0, RN license, statistics course, professional liability/malpractice insurance, interview, 2 letters of recommendation, transcript of college record. *Application deadline:* rolling. *Application fee:* $20.

Degree Requirements 36 total credit hours, 31 in nursing.

UNIVERSITY OF INDIANAPOLIS
School of Nursing
Indianapolis, Indiana

Programs • Generic Baccalaureate • RN Baccalaureate • BSN to Master's

The University Independent comprehensive coed institution, affiliated with United Methodist Church. Founded: 1902. *Primary accreditation:* regional. *Setting:* 60-acre suburban campus. *Total enrollment:* 3,891.

The School of Nursing Founded in 1959. *Nursing program faculty:* 41 (7% with doctorates).

Academic Facilities *Campus library:* 144,102 volumes (9,431 in health); 1,118 periodical subscriptions (123 health-care related). *Nursing school resources:* CAI, computer lab, nursing audiovisuals, interactive nursing skills videos, learning resource lab.

Student Life *Student services:* health clinic, personal counseling, career counseling, institutionally sponsored work-study program, job placement, campus safety program, special assistance for disabled students. *International student services:* counseling/support, special assistance for nonnative speakers of English, ESL courses. *Nursing student activities:* Sigma Theta Tau, student nurses association.

Calendar Semesters.

NURSING STUDENT PROFILE

Undergraduate **Enrollment:** 256
Women: 95%; **Men:** 5%; **Minority:** 12%; **International:** 1%; **Part-time:** 0%
Graduate **Enrollment:** 26
Women: 100%; **Minority:** 0%; **International:** 0%; **Part-time:** 60%

BACCALAUREATE PROGRAMS

Contact Mr. Mark Wiegand, Director of Admissions, School of Nursing, University of Indianapolis, 1400 East Hanna Avenue, Indianapolis, IN 46227-3697, 317-788-3350. *Fax:* 317-788-3300. *E-mail:* wiegand@gandlf.uindy.edu

Expenses *Tuition:* $12,350 full-time, $158 per credit hour part-time. *Full-time mandatory fees:* $25–$42. *Room and board:* $4330. *Books and supplies per academic year:* $250.

Financial Aid Institutionally sponsored need-based grants/scholarships, institutionally sponsored non-need grants/scholarships, Federal Supplemental Educational Opportunity Grants, Federal Work-Study. 89% of undergraduate students in nursing programs received some form of financial aid in 1995–96. *Application deadline:* 3/1.

Generic Baccalaureate Program (BSN)

Applying *Required:* SAT I or ACT, minimum high school GPA of 2.5, minimum college GPA of 2.5, 3 years of high school math, 3 years of high school science, high school chemistry, high school biology, high school foreign language, high school transcript. 34 prerequisite credits must be completed before admission to the nursing program. *Options:* Course work may be accelerated. May apply for transfer of up to 60 total credits. *Application deadlines:* 8/15 (fall), 1/1 (spring). *Application fee:* $20.

Degree Requirements 124 total credit hours, 52 in nursing.

RN Baccalaureate Program (BSN)

Applying *Required:* SAT or NLN Assessment Test, minimum college GPA of 2.5, RN license, diploma or AD in nursing, transcript of college record. 43 prerequisite credits must be completed before admission to the nursing program. *Options:* Course work may be accelerated. May apply for transfer of up to 60 total credits. *Application deadlines:* 8/15 (fall), 1/1 (spring). *Application fee:* $20.

Degree Requirements 101 total credit hours, 29 in nursing.

MASTER'S PROGRAM

Contact Dr. Martha Sparks, MSN Program Coordinator, School of Nursing, University of Indianapolis, 1400 East Hanna Avenue, Indianapolis, IN 46227-3697, 317-788-3471. *Fax:* 317-788-3569. *E-mail:* msparks@gandlf.uindy.edu

Areas of Study Nurse practitioner program in family health.

Expenses *Tuition:* $7200 full-time, $400 part-time. *Books and supplies per academic year:* ranges from $450 to $600.

Financial Aid Nurse traineeships. 15% of master's level students in nursing programs received some form of financial aid in 1995-96. *Application deadline:* 8/15.

BSN to Master's Program (MSN)

Applying *Required:* GRE General Test, bachelor's degree in nursing, minimum GPA of 3.0, RN license, 1 year of clinical experience, statistics course, essay, interview, 3 letters of recommendation, transcript of college record. *Application deadlines:* 8/15 (fall), 1/1 (spring). *Application fee:* $40.

Degree Requirements 45 total credit hours, 36 in nursing, 9 in biology, math.

UNIVERSITY OF SOUTHERN INDIANA
School of Nursing and Health Professions
Evansville, Indiana

Programs • Generic Baccalaureate • RN Baccalaureate • BSN to Master's • Continuing Education

The University State-supported comprehensive coed institution. Part of Indiana Commission for Higher Education. Founded: 1965. *Primary accreditation:* regional. *Setting:* 300-acre suburban campus. *Total enrollment:* 7,666.

The School of Nursing and Health Professions Founded in 1988. *Nursing program faculty:* 17 (24% with doctorates). *Off-campus program sites:* Vincennes, Jasper.

Academic Facilities *Campus library:* 196,419 volumes (5,919 in health, 2,130 in nursing); 1,536 periodical subscriptions (113 health-care related). *Nursing school resources:* CAI, computer lab, nursing audiovisuals, interactive nursing skills videos, learning resource lab.

Student Life *Student services:* health clinic, child-care facilities, personal counseling, career counseling, institutionally sponsored work-study program, job placement, campus safety program, special assistance for disabled students. *International student services:* counseling/support. *Nursing student activities:* Sigma Theta Tau, student nurses association.

Calendar Semesters.

NURSING STUDENT PROFILE

Undergraduate **Enrollment:** 258
Women: 94%; **Men:** 6%; **Minority:** 3%; **International:** 0%; **Part-time:** 49%
Graduate **Enrollment:** 54
Women: 100%; **Minority:** 4%; **International:** 1%; **Part-time:** 83%

BACCALAUREATE PROGRAMS

Contact Dr. Nadine A. Coudret, Dean, School of Nursing and Health Professions, University of Southern Indiana, 8600 University Boulevard, Evansville, IN 47712, 812-465-1151. *Fax:* 812-465-7092. *E-mail:* ncoudret.ucs@smtp.usi.edu

Expenses *State resident tuition:* $1280 full-time, $80 per hour part-time. *Nonresident tuition:* $1884 full-time, $118 per hour part-time. *Full-time mandatory fees:* $35–$50. *Part-time mandatory fees:* $35–$50. *Room only:* $1742–$4348. *Books and supplies per academic year:* ranges from $250 to $500.

Financial Aid Institutionally sponsored need-based grants/scholarships, institutionally sponsored non-need grants/scholarships, Federal Direct Loans, Federal Pell Grants, Federal Perkins Loans, Federal Supplemental Educational Opportunity Grants, Federal Work-Study. *Application deadline:* 3/1.

Generic Baccalaureate Program (BSN)

Applying *Required:* SAT I or ACT, Psychological Services Bureau Pre-Nursing Exam, minimum high school GPA of 3.0, minimum college GPA of 2.7, high school transcript, written essay, transcript of college record, high school class rank: top 33%. 25 prerequisite credits must be completed before admission to the nursing program. *Options:* Course work may be accelerated. May apply for transfer of up to 98 total credits. *Application deadline:* 1/15. *Application fee:* $25.

Degree Requirements 128 total credit hours, 70 in nursing.

Distance learning Courses provided through video, audio, computer-based media.

RN Baccalaureate Program (BS)

Applying *Required:* TOEFL for nonnative speakers of English, RN licensc, diploma or AD in nursing, transcript of college record. *Options:* Course work may be accelerated. May apply for transfer of up to 64 total credits. *Application deadline:* rolling.

Degree Requirements 128 total credit hours, 70 in nursing.

Distance learning Courses provided through video, audio, computer-based media.

MASTER'S PROGRAM

Contact Melissa Vaudeveer, Program Coordinator, Graduate Nursing, 8600 University Boulevard, Evansville, IN 47712, 812-465-1171. *Fax:* 812-465-7092. *E-mail:* mvaudeve.ucs@smtp.usi.edu

Areas of Study Clinical nurse specialist program in family health nursing; nurse practitioner program in family health.

Expenses *State resident tuition:* $118 per credit hour. *Nonresident tuition:* $235 per credit hour. *Full-time mandatory fees:* $25. *Room only:* $1920. *Books and supplies per academic year:* ranges from $300 to $400.

Financial Aid Graduate assistantships, Federal Direct Loans, employment opportunities, institutionally sponsored non-need-based grants/scholarships, Child of Employee benefits. 2% of master's level students in nursing programs received some form of financial aid in 1995-96. *Application deadline:* 3/1.

BSN to Master's Program (MSN)

Applying *Required:* TOEFL for nonnative speakers of English, bachelor's degree in nursing, bachelor's degree, minimum GPA of 3.0, RN license, 1 year of clinical experience, statistics course, professional liability/malpractice insurance, essay, 2 letters of recommendation, transcript of college record. *Application deadline:* rolling. *Application fee:* $25.

Degree Requirements 43 total credit hours, 43 in nursing.

CONTINUING EDUCATION PROGRAM

Contact Peggy Graul, Coordinator of Continuing Education for Nursing and Health Professions, University of Southern Indiana, 8600 University Boulevard, Evansville, IN 47712, 812-465-1164. *Fax:* 812-465-7092. *E-mail:* pgraul.ucs@smtp.usi.edu

VALPARAISO UNIVERSITY
College of Nursing
Valparaiso, Indiana

Programs • Generic Baccalaureate • Accelerated Baccalaureate • RN Baccalaureate • Baccalaureate for Second Degree • Accelerated Baccalaureate for Second Degree • MSN • Accelerated MSN • RN to Master's

The University Independent comprehensive coed institution, affiliated with Lutheran Church–Missouri Synod. Founded: 1859. *Primary accreditation:* regional. *Setting:* 310-acre small-town campus. *Total enrollment:* 3,524.

The College of Nursing Founded in 1968. *Nursing program faculty:* 20 (50% with doctorates).

▶ *NOTEWORTHY*

The Bachelor of Science in Nursing program at Valparaiso University incorporates a holistic approach to the concepts of person, environment, health, and nursing. It is a dynamic program preparing the professional nurse to function in all levels of preventative and acute care. A 10:1 student-faculty ratio in clinicals and classes taught exclusively by professors make the educational experience personal, challenging, and supportive. Students begin clinical experiences in the first semester of the sophomore year. A professional role practicum provides work experience, giving graduates an advantage in the employment market. Graduates are eligible for licensing in all 50 states.

Academic Facilities *Campus library:* 261,256 volumes; 972 periodical subscriptions (92 health-care related). *Nursing school resources:* CAI, computer lab, nursing audiovisuals, interactive nursing skills videos, learning resource lab.

Student Life *Student services:* health clinic, personal counseling, career counseling, institutionally sponsored work-study program, job placement, campus safety program, special assistance for disabled students.

Valparaiso University (continued)

International student services: counseling/support, special assistance for nonnative speakers of English. *Nursing student activities:* Sigma Theta Tau, student nurses association.

Calendar Semesters.

NURSING STUDENT PROFILE

Undergraduate **Enrollment:** 319

Women: 88%; **Men:** 12%; **Minority:** 14%; **International:** 1%; **Part-time:** 5%

Graduate **Enrollment:** 87

Women: 95%; **Men:** 5%; **Minority:** 10%; **International:** 1%; **Part-time:** 60%

BACCALAUREATE PROGRAMS

Contact Dr. Freda S. Scales, Dean, College of Nursing, Valparaiso University, Valparaiso, IN 46383-6493, 219-464-5289. *Fax:* 219-464-5425. *E-mail:* fscales@exodus.valpo.edu

Expenses *Tuition:* $13,510 full-time, $585 per credit hour part-time. *Full-time mandatory fees:* $470. *Room and board:* $3260. *Books and supplies per academic year:* $500.

Financial Aid Institutionally sponsored need-based grants/scholarships, institutionally sponsored non-need grants/scholarships, Federal Direct Loans, Federal Pell Grants, Federal Perkins Loans, Federal Supplemental Educational Opportunity Grants, Federal Work-Study. *Application deadline:* 5/1.

Generic Baccalaureate Program (BSN)

Applying *Required:* SAT I, ACT, TOEFL for nonnative speakers of English, minimum high school GPA of 2.0, 3 years of high school math, high school transcript, written essay. *Options:* Advanced standing available through the following means: advanced placement exams, advanced placement without credit, credit by exam. Course work may be accelerated. May apply for transfer of up to 93 total credits. *Application deadline:* rolling. *Application fee:* $30.

Degree Requirements 126 total credit hours, 57 in nursing.

Accelerated Baccalaureate Program (BSN)

Applying *Required:* minimum college GPA of 3.0, transcript of college record. *Options:* Advanced standing available through the following means: advanced placement exams, advanced placement without credit, credit by exam. May apply for transfer of up to 93 total credits. *Application deadline:* rolling. *Application fee:* $30.

Degree Requirements 126 total credit hours, 57 in nursing.

RN Baccalaureate Program (BSN)

Applying *Required:* minimum college GPA of 2.0, RN license, diploma or AD in nursing, transcript of college record. *Options:* Advanced standing available through the following means: advanced placement exams, advanced placement without credit, credit by exam. Course work may be accelerated. May apply for transfer of up to 93 total credits. *Application deadline:* rolling. *Application fee:* $30.

Degree Requirements 126 total credit hours, 57 in nursing.

Baccalaureate for Second Degree Program (BSN)

Applying *Required:* minimum college GPA of 2.0. *Options:* Advanced standing available through the following means: advanced placement exams, advanced placement without credit. Course work may be accelerated. May apply for transfer of up to 93 total credits. *Application deadline:* rolling. *Application fee:* $30.

Degree Requirements 126 total credit hours, 57 in nursing.

Accelerated Baccalaureate for Second Degree Program (BSN)

Applying *Required:* minimum college GPA of 3.0, transcript of college record. *Options:* Advanced standing available through the following means: advanced placement exams, advanced placement without credit. Course work may be accelerated. May apply for transfer of up to 93 total credits. *Application deadline:* rolling. *Application fee:* $30.

Degree Requirements 126 total credit hours, 57 in nursing.

MASTER'S PROGRAMS

Contact Dr. Freda S. Scales, Dean, College of Nursing, Valparaiso University, Valparaiso, IN 46383-6493, 219-464-5289. *Fax:* 219-464-5425. *E-mail:* fscales@exodus.valpo.edu

Areas of Study Clinical nurse specialist programs in adult health nursing, community health nursing, maternity-newborn nursing, pediatric nursing, psychiatric–mental health nursing; nursing administration; nurse practitioner program in family health.

Expenses *Tuition:* $5760 full-time, $240 per credit hour part-time. *Full-time mandatory fees:* $0.

Financial Aid Nurse traineeships, employment opportunities.

MSN Program

Applying *Required:* bachelor's degree in nursing, minimum GPA of 3.0, physical assessment course, statistics course, professional liability/malpractice insurance, essay, 3 letters of recommendation, transcript of college record. *Application fee:* $30.

Degree Requirements 36 total credit hours, 30 in nursing.

Accelerated MSN Program

Applying *Required:* bachelor's degree in nursing, minimum GPA of 3.0, physical assessment course, statistics course, professional liability/malpractice insurance, essay, 3 letters of recommendation, transcript of college record, all but 6 credits completed for BSN. *Application deadline:* rolling. *Application fee:* $30.

Degree Requirements 36 total credit hours, 30 in nursing.

RN to Master's Program (MSN)

Applying *Required:* minimum GPA of 3.0, RN license, physical assessment course, statistics course, professional liability/malpractice insurance, essay, 3 letters of recommendation, transcript of college record, all but 6 credits completed for BSN. *Application deadline:* rolling. *Application fee:* $30.

Degree Requirements 126 total credit hours, 36 in nursing.

IOWA

BRIAR CLIFF COLLEGE

Department of Nursing
Sioux City, Iowa

Programs • Generic Baccalaureate • RN Baccalaureate

The College Independent Roman Catholic 4-year coed college. Founded: 1930. *Primary accreditation:* regional. *Setting:* 70-acre suburban campus. *Total enrollment:* 1,144.

The Department of Nursing Founded in 1980. *Nursing program faculty:* 7 (17% with doctorates). *Off-campus program sites:* Storm Lake, Denison.

Academic Facilities *Campus library:* 99,000 volumes (3,221 in nursing); 645 periodical subscriptions (66 health-care related). *Nursing school resources:* CAI, computer lab, nursing audiovisuals, interactive nursing skills videos, learning resource lab, Internet.

Student Life *Student services:* health clinic, personal counseling, career counseling, institutionally sponsored work-study program, job placement, campus safety program, special assistance for disabled students. *International student services:* counseling/support, special assistance for nonnative speakers of English, ESL courses. *Nursing student activities:* Sigma Theta Tau, nursing club, student nurses association.

Calendar Trimesters.

NURSING STUDENT PROFILE

Undergraduate **Enrollment:** 171

Women: 95%; **Men:** 5%; **Minority:** 19%; **International:** 3%; **Part-time:** 94%

BACCALAUREATE PROGRAMS

Contact Sr. Patricia Miller, Professor and Chairperson, Department of Nursing, Briar Cliff College, 3303 Rebecca Street, PO Box 2100, Sioux City, IA 51104, 712-279-5497. *Fax:* 712-279-1698.

Expenses *Tuition:* $11,100 per academic year. *Full-time mandatory fees:* $150. *Room and board:* $3840.

Financial Aid Institutionally sponsored need-based grants/scholarships, institutionally sponsored non-need grants/scholarships, Federal Nursing Student Loans, Federal Work-Study. *Application deadline:* 2/1.

GENERIC BACCALAUREATE PROGRAM (BSN)

Applying *Required:* ACT, TOEFL for nonnative speakers of English, minimum high school GPA of 2.5, minimum college GPA of 2.5, 3 years of high school math, 3 years of high school science, high school chemistry, high school foreign language, high school transcript, written essay, transcript of college record. *Options:* May apply for transfer of up to 60 total credits. *Application deadline:* 4/1. *Application fee:* $20.

Degree Requirements 139 total credit hours, 57 in nursing.

RN BACCALAUREATE PROGRAM (BSN)

Applying *Required:* ACT, TOEFL for nonnative speakers of English, minimum high school GPA of 2.5, minimum college GPA of 2.5, high school chemistry, RN license, diploma or AD in nursing, high school transcript, interview, transcript of college record. *Options:* Course work may be accelerated. May apply for transfer of up to 57 total credits. *Application deadline:* rolling. *Application fee:* $20.

Degree Requirements 139 total credit hours.

CLARKE COLLEGE

Nursing Department
Dubuque, Iowa

Programs • Generic Baccalaureate • RN Baccalaureate • Accelerated RN Baccalaureate • Baccalaureate for Second Degree

The College Independent Roman Catholic comprehensive coed institution. Founded: 1843. *Primary accreditation:* regional. *Setting:* 55-acre urban campus. *Total enrollment:* 1,030.

The Nursing Department Founded in 1983.

Academic Facilities *Campus library:* 9,716 volumes (2,500 in health, 1,800 in nursing); 550 periodical subscriptions (30 health-care related).

Calendar Semesters.

NURSING STUDENT PROFILE

Undergraduate **Enrollment:** 155

Women: 99%; **Men:** 1%; **Minority:** 1%; **International:** 1%; **Part-time:** 21%

BACCALAUREATE PROGRAMS

Contact Director of Admissions, Nursing Department, Clarke College, 1550 Clarke Drive, Dubuque, IA 52001, 319-588-6361. *Fax:* 319-588-6789.

Expenses *Tuition:* $9300 full-time, ranges from $200 to $300 per credit hour part-time.

Financial Aid Institutionally sponsored need-based grants/scholarships, institutionally sponsored non-need grants/scholarships, Federal Perkins Loans, Federal Supplemental Educational Opportunity Grants, Federal Work-Study, Federal PLUS Loans, Federal Stafford Loans. *Application deadline:* 3/1.

GENERIC BACCALAUREATE PROGRAM (BS)

Applying *Required:* SAT I or ACT, TOEFL for nonnative speakers of English, minimum high school GPA of 2.0, minimum college GPA of 2.5, 3 years of high school math, 2 years of high school science, high school foreign language, high school transcript, letter of recommendation, written essay, high school class rank: top 50%. *Application deadline:* rolling. *Application fee:* $20.

RN BACCALAUREATE PROGRAM (BS)

Applying *Required:* SAT I or ACT, minimum college GPA of 2.5, RN license, diploma or AD in nursing, high school transcript, transcript of college record. *Options:* May apply for transfer of up to 64 total credits. *Application deadline:* rolling. *Application fee:* $20.

ACCELERATED RN BACCALAUREATE PROGRAM (BSN)

Applying *Required:* SAT I or ACT, minimum college GPA of 2.5.

BACCALAUREATE FOR SECOND DEGREE PROGRAM (BSN)

Applying *Required:* SAT I or ACT, minimum college GPA of 2.5.

COE COLLEGE

Department of Nursing Education
Cedar Rapids, Iowa

Programs • Generic Baccalaureate • RN Baccalaureate

The College Independent comprehensive coed institution, affiliated with Presbyterian Church. Founded: 1851. *Primary accreditation:* regional. *Setting:* 55-acre urban campus. *Total enrollment:* 1,359.

The Department of Nursing Education Founded in 1971. *Nursing program faculty:* 12 (25% with doctorates).

Academic Facilities *Campus library:* 200,000 volumes (8,000 in nursing); 835 periodical subscriptions (25 health-care related). *Nursing school resources:* computer lab, nursing audiovisuals, learning resource lab.

Student Life *Student services:* health clinic, personal counseling, career counseling, institutionally sponsored work-study program, job placement, special assistance for disabled students. *International student services:* counseling/support, special assistance for nonnative speakers of English, ESL courses. *Nursing student activities:* Sigma Theta Tau, nursing club, student nurses association.

Calendar 4-1-4.

NURSING STUDENT PROFILE

Undergraduate **Enrollment:** 80

Women: 91%; **Men:** 9%; **International:** 1%; **Part-time:** 88%

BACCALAUREATE PROGRAMS

Contact Dr. Evelyn J. Benda, Chair, Department of Nursing Education, Coe College, 1220 First Avenue, NE, Cedar Rapids, IA 52402, 319-369-8120. *Fax:* 319-399-8748.

Expenses *Tuition:* $15,500 full-time, $880 per courses part-time. *Full-time mandatory fees:* $125. *Room and board:* $4950. *Room only:* $1990. *Books and supplies per academic year:* $600.

Financial Aid Federal Direct Loans, Federal Perkins Loans, Federal Work-Study. 94% of undergraduate students in nursing programs received some form of financial aid in 1995–96. *Application deadline:* 2/1.

GENERIC BACCALAUREATE PROGRAM (BSN)

Applying *Required:* SAT I or ACT, TOEFL for nonnative speakers of English, minimum high school GPA of 2.0, minimum college GPA of 2.5, high school transcript. *Options:* Advanced standing available through advanced placement exams. May apply for transfer of up to 83 total credits. *Application deadlines:* 6/1 (fall), 12/1 (spring). *Application fee:* $25.

Degree Requirements 119 total credit hours, 59 in nursing.

RN BACCALAUREATE PROGRAM (BSN)

Applying *Required:* minimum college GPA of 2.5, RN license, diploma or AD in nursing, transcript of college record. *Options:* Course work may be accelerated. *Application deadline:* rolling. *Application fee:* $25.

Degree Requirements Minimum of 40 semester hours.

DRAKE UNIVERSITY

Department of Nursing
Des Moines, Iowa

Programs • RN Baccalaureate • BSN to Master's • Post-Master's

The University Independent coed university. Founded: 1881. *Primary accreditation:* regional. *Setting:* 120-acre suburban campus. *Total enrollment:* 5,639.

The Department of Nursing Founded in 1985. *Nursing program faculty:* 6 (85% with doctorates). *Off-campus program site:* Knoxville.

Drake University (continued)

Academic Facilities *Campus library:* 900,000 volumes (8,500 in health, 3,587 in nursing); 2,500 periodical subscriptions (72 health-care related). *Nursing school resources:* computer lab.

Calendar Semesters.

NURSING STUDENT PROFILE

Undergraduate **Enrollment:** 92
Women: 96%; **Men:** 4%; **Minority:** 2%; **Part-time:** 100%
Graduate **Enrollment:** 62
Women: 90%; **Men:** 10%; **Part-time:** 71%

BACCALAUREATE PROGRAM

Contact Dr. Linda H. Brady, Chair, Department of Nursing, Drake University, Des Moines, IA 50311, 515-271-2830. *Fax:* 515-271-4569. *E-mail:* lb7411r@drake.acad.edu

Expenses *Tuition:* $14,380 full-time, $225 per credit hour part-time. *Books and supplies per academic year:* ranges from $100 to $300.

Financial Aid Institutionally sponsored need-based grants/scholarships, institutionally sponsored non-need grants/scholarships. 7% of undergraduate students in nursing programs received some form of financial aid in 1995–96.

RN Baccalaureate Program (BSN)

Applying *Required:* TOEFL for nonnative speakers of English, minimum college GPA of 2.5, RN license, diploma or AD in nursing, transcript of college record. *Options:* Advanced standing available through credit by exam. May apply for transfer of up to 62 total credits. *Application deadlines:* 8/15 (fall), 1/10 (spring), 5/15 (summer). *Application fee:* $25.

Degree Requirements 124 total credit hours, 32 in nursing.

MASTER'S PROGRAMS

Contact Dr. Linda H. Brady, Chair, Department of Nursing, Drake University, Des Moines, IA 50311, 515-271-2830. *Fax:* 515-271-4569. *E-mail:* lb7411r@drake.acad.edu

Areas of Study Nursing administration; nursing education; nurse practitioner program in family health.

Expenses *Tuition:* $15,180 full-time, $335 per credit hour part-time. *Room and board:* $3720–$4855. *Room only:* $2570–$3590. *Books and supplies per academic year:* ranges from $300 to $500.

Financial Aid Federal Direct Loans. 19% of master's level students in nursing programs received some form of financial aid in 1995-96.

BSN to Master's Program (MSN)

Applying *Required:* GRE General Test (minimum combined score of 1500 on three tests), Miller Analogies Test, bachelor's degree in nursing, minimum GPA, RN license, physical assessment course, statistics course, professional liability/malpractice insurance, essay, 3 letters of recommendation, transcript of college record. *Application deadline:* 8/15. *Application fee:* $25.

Degree Requirements 36 total credit hours, 30 in nursing, 6 in thesis or graduate project required; part-time study.

Post-Master's Program

Applying *Required:* GRE General Test (minimum combined score of 1500 on three tests), Miller Analogies Test, bachelor's degree in nursing, minimum GPA of 3.0, RN license, 1 year of clinical experience, physical assessment course, statistics course, professional liability/malpractice insurance, essay, 3 letters of recommendation, transcript of college record, MSN or equivalent. *Application deadline:* 8/15. *Application fee:* $25.

Degree Requirements 30 total credit hours, 24 in nursing, 6 in pharmacotherapeutics; ethics.

See full description on page 442.

GRACELAND COLLEGE
Division of Nursing
Lamoni, Iowa

Programs • Generic Baccalaureate • RN Baccalaureate • MSN • Post-Master's

The College Independent Reorganized Latter Day Saints comprehensive coed institution. Founded: 1895. *Primary accreditation:* regional. *Setting:* 169-acre small-town campus. *Total enrollment:* 1,176.

The Division of Nursing Founded in 1969. *Nursing program faculty:* 20 (25% with doctorates). *Off-campus program site:* Independence, MO.

▶ *NOTEWORTHY*

Through Graceland's Outreach Program, RNs may earn an NLN-accredited BSN and BSNs may earn an MSN. The College offers self-paced independent study courses taught by Graceland faculty members, instructional videotapes for all courses, and student-instructor consultations via toll-free phone lines and e-mail. BSN students are not required to validate RN training via proficiency exams, may be awarded up to 32 semester hours of advanced placement credit, and may complete clinical courses in their own communities. Students interact with other RNs from across the country during the residencies held on campus (two 2-week sessions for the BSN and three 2- or 3-week sessions for the MSN).

Academic Facilities *Campus library:* 205,711 volumes (10,000 in health); 1,053 periodical subscriptions (370 health-care related). *Nursing school resources:* CAI, computer lab, nursing audiovisuals, interactive nursing skills videos, learning resource lab.

Student Life *Student services:* health clinic, personal counseling, career counseling, institutionally sponsored work-study program, job placement, special assistance for disabled students. *International student services:* counseling/support. *Nursing student activities:* Sigma Theta Tau, student nurses association.

Calendar Semesters.

NURSING STUDENT PROFILE

Undergraduate **Enrollment:** 73
Women: 89%; **Men:** 11%; **Minority:** 7%; **International:** 0%; **Part-time:** 3%
Graduate **Enrollment:** 38
Women: 88%; **Men:** 12%; **Part-time:** 100%

BACCALAUREATE PROGRAMS

Contact Ms. Jeanne Dennis, Public Relations Assistant, Division of Nursing, Graceland College, 221 West Lexington, Suite 110, Independence, MO 64050-3720, 816-833-0524. *Fax:* 816-833-2990. *E-mail:* jeanned@graceland.edu

Expenses *Tuition:* $10,230 full-time, ranges from $240 to $320 per semester hour part-time. *Full-time mandatory fees:* $300–$350. *Part-time mandatory fees:* $180–$230. *Room and board:* $3310. *Room only:* $1240. *Books and supplies per academic year:* ranges from $250 to $300.

Financial Aid Institutionally sponsored need-based grants/scholarships, institutionally sponsored non-need grants/scholarships, Federal Direct Loans, Federal Nursing Student Loans, Federal Pell Grants, Federal Perkins Loans, Federal Supplemental Educational Opportunity Grants, Federal Work-Study. *Application deadline:* 6/1.

Generic Baccalaureate Program (BSN)

Applying *Required:* ACT, TOEFL for nonnative speakers of English, minimum college GPA of 2.5, high school transcript, 2 letters of recommendation, written essay, transcript of college record. 56 prerequisite credits must be completed before admission to the nursing program. *Options:* Course work may be accelerated. May apply for transfer of up to 75 total credits. *Application deadline:* 6/30. *Application fee:* $20.

Degree Requirements 128 total credit hours, 52 in nursing.

RN Baccalaureate Program (BSN)

Applying *Required:* TOEFL for nonnative speakers of English, RN license, high school transcript, letter of recommendation, transcript of college record. 60 prerequisite credits must be completed before admission to the nursing program. *Options:* Advanced standing available through the following means: advanced placement exams, credit by exam. Course work may be accelerated. May apply for transfer of up to 75 total credits. *Application deadline:* rolling. *Application fee:* $60.

Degree Requirements 128 total credit hours, 54 in nursing.

Distance learning Courses provided through correspondence, video, on-line. Specific degree requirements include 2 two-week residencies.

MASTER'S PROGRAMS

Contact Karen Fernengel, Chair, MSN Program, 220 West Lexington, Independence, MO 64050, 816-833-0524. *Fax:* 816-833-2990. *E-mail:* karenf@graceland.edu

Areas of Study Clinical nurse specialist program in family health nursing; nursing administration; nurse practitioner program in family health.

Expenses *Tuition:* ranges from $320 to $398 per semester hour. *Books and supplies per academic year:* ranges from $500 to $700.

MSN Program

Applying *Required:* GRE General Test, TOEFL for nonnative speakers of English, bachelor's degree in nursing, minimum GPA of 3.0, RN license, 2 years of clinical experience, physical assessment course, statistics course, professional liability/malpractice insurance, essay, 2 letters of recommendation, transcript of college record. *Application deadline:* rolling. *Application fee:* $80.

Degree Requirements 41–47 total credit hours dependent upon track, 41–47 in nursing.

Distance learning Courses provided through correspondence, video, on-line. Specific degree requirements include 3 residencies of 2 to 3 weeks each.

Post-Master's Program

Applying *Required:* bachelor's degree in nursing, minimum GPA of 3.0, RN license, 2 years of clinical experience, physical assessment course, statistics course, professional liability/malpractice insurance, essay, 2 letters of recommendation, transcript of college record, MSN. *Application deadline:* rolling. *Application fee:* $80.

Degree Requirements 24–27 total credit hours dependent upon track, 24–27 in nursing.

Distance learning Courses provided through correspondence, video, on-line. Specific degree requirements include 3 residencies of 2 to 3 weeks each.

GRAND VIEW COLLEGE
Division of Nursing
Des Moines, Iowa

Programs • Generic Baccalaureate • RN Baccalaureate • Baccalaureate for Second Degree • LPN to Baccalaureate • Continuing Education

The College Independent 4-year coed college, affiliated with Evangelical Lutheran Church in America. Founded: 1896. *Primary accreditation:* regional. *Setting:* 25-acre urban campus. *Total enrollment:* 1,482.

The Division of Nursing Founded in 1975. *Nursing program faculty:* 26 (12% with doctorates).

Academic Facilities *Campus library:* 77,800 volumes (4,430 in health); 715 periodical subscriptions (100 health-care related). *Nursing school resources:* CAI, computer lab, nursing audiovisuals, learning resource lab.

Student Life *Student services:* health clinic, personal counseling, career counseling, institutionally sponsored work-study program, job placement, campus safety program. *Nursing student activities:* Sigma Theta Tau, nursing club, student nurses association.

Calendar Semesters.

NURSING STUDENT PROFILE

Undergraduate **Enrollment:** 259

Women: 92%; **Men:** 8%; **Minority:** 2%; **International:** 0%; **Part-time:** 27%

BACCALAUREATE PROGRAMS

Contact Dr. Ellen M. Strachota, Head, Division of Nursing, Grand View College, 1200 Grandview Avenue, Des Moines, IA 50316-1599, 515-263-2850. *Fax:* 515-263-6095. *E-mail:* estrachota@gvc.edu

Expenses *Tuition:* $10,900 full-time, $760 per year part-time. *Full-time mandatory fees:* $75–$292. *Room and board:* $3630. *Books and supplies per academic year:* $570.

Financial Aid Institutionally sponsored need-based grants/scholarships, institutionally sponsored non-need grants/scholarships, Federal Supplemental Educational Opportunity Grants, Federal Work-Study. 80% of undergraduate students in nursing programs received some form of financial aid in 1995–96. *Application deadline:* 4/1.

Generic Baccalaureate Program (BSN)

Applying *Required:* ACT, high school chemistry, high school transcript, 3 letters of recommendation, transcript of college record, immunizations. 32 prerequisite credits must be completed before admission to the nursing program. *Options:* Advanced standing available through the following means: advanced placement exams, credit by exam. Course work may be accelerated. May apply for transfer of up to 94 total credits. *Application deadlines:* 6/1 (fall), 11/1 (spring).

Degree Requirements 124 total credit hours, 50 in nursing.

RN Baccalaureate Program (BSN)

Applying *Required:* ACT PEP, minimum college GPA of 2.2, RN license, diploma or AD in nursing, 3 letters of recommendation, transcript of college record, immunizations. 32 prerequisite credits must be completed before admission to the nursing program. *Options:* Advanced standing available through the following means: advanced placement exams, advanced placement without credit, credit by exam. May apply for transfer of up to 94 total credits. *Application deadline:* rolling.

Degree Requirements 124 total credit hours, 50 in nursing.

Baccalaureate for Second Degree Program (BSN)

Applying *Required:* ACT, TOEFL for nonnative speakers of English, high school chemistry, high school transcript, interview, 3 letters of recommendation, transcript of college record. 32 prerequisite credits must be completed before admission to the nursing program. *Options:* Advanced standing available through the following means: advanced placement exams, credit by exam. Course work may be accelerated. May apply for transfer of up to 96 total credits. *Application deadlines:* 6/1 (fall), 11/1 (spring).

Degree Requirements 124 total credit hours, 50 in nursing.

LPN to Baccalaureate Program (BSN)

Applying *Required:* ACT PEP, minimum college GPA of 2.2, 3 letters of recommendation, transcript of college record, LPN license. 32 prerequisite credits must be completed before admission to the nursing program. *Options:* Advanced standing available through the following means: advanced placement exams, credit by exam. May apply for transfer of up to 94 total credits. *Application deadline:* rolling.

Degree Requirements 124 total credit hours, 50 in nursing.

CONTINUING EDUCATION PROGRAM

Contact Ms. Barbara Heck, Associate Professor, Division of Nursing, Grand View College, 1200 Grandview Avenue, Des Moines, IA 50316-1599, 515-263-2850. *Fax:* 515-263-6095. *E-mail:* bheck@gvc.edu

IOWA WESLEYAN COLLEGE
Division of Nursing
Mount Pleasant, Iowa

Programs • Generic Baccalaureate • RN Baccalaureate • Continuing Education

The College Independent United Methodist 4-year coed college. Founded: 1842. *Primary accreditation:* regional. *Setting:* 60-acre small-town campus. *Total enrollment:* 829.

The Division of Nursing Founded in 1972. *Nursing program faculty:* 8 (25% with doctorates).

Academic Facilities *Campus library:* 110,190 volumes; 547 periodical subscriptions (40 health-care related). *Nursing school resources:* CAI, computer lab, nursing audiovisuals, learning resource lab.

Iowa Wesleyan College (continued)

Student Life *Student services:* health clinic, personal counseling, career counseling, job placement. *International student services:* counseling/support, special assistance for nonnative speakers of English, ESL courses. *Nursing student activities:* student nurses association.

Calendar 4-1-4.

NURSING STUDENT PROFILE

Undergraduate **Enrollment:** 100

Women: 90%; **Men:** 10%; **Minority:** 0%; **International:** 0%; **Part-time:** 50%

BACCALAUREATE PROGRAMS

Contact Ms. Judith Hausner, Chairperson, Division of Nursing, Iowa Wesleyan College, 601 North Main Street, Mount Pleasant, IA 52641, 319-385-6323. *Fax:* 319-385-6296.

Expenses *Tuition:* $11,300 full-time, $255 per hour part-time. *Full-time mandatory fees:* $30.

Financial Aid Institutionally sponsored need-based grants/scholarships, institutionally sponsored non-need grants/scholarships, Federal Work-Study. *Application deadline:* 6/1.

Generic Baccalaureate Program (BSN)

Applying *Required:* ACT, minimum high school GPA of 2.0, minimum college GPA of 2.0, high school transcript. 25 prerequisite credits must be completed before admission to the nursing program. *Options:* May apply for transfer of up to 94 total credits. *Application deadline:* rolling. *Application fee:* $15.

Degree Requirements 124 total credit hours, 50 in nursing.

RN Baccalaureate Program (BSN)

Applying *Required:* ACT, minimum college GPA of 2.0, RN license, diploma or AD in nursing, transcript of college record. *Options:* May apply for transfer of up to 94 total credits. *Application deadline:* rolling.

Degree Requirements 124 total credit hours, 50 in nursing.

CONTINUING EDUCATION PROGRAM

Contact Ms. Judith Hausner, Chairperson, Division of Nursing, Iowa Wesleyan College, 601 North Main Street, Mount Pleasant, IA 52641, 319-385-6323. *Fax:* 319-385-6296.

LUTHER COLLEGE
Department of Nursing
Decorah, Iowa

Programs • Generic Baccalaureate • RN Baccalaureate • Continuing Education

The College Independent 4-year coed college, affiliated with Evangelical Lutheran Church in America. Founded: 1861. *Primary accreditation:* regional. *Setting:* 800-acre small-town campus. *Total enrollment:* 2,386.

The Department of Nursing Founded in 1974. *Nursing program faculty:* 14 (21% with doctorates). *Off-campus program site:* Rochester, MN.

Academic Facilities *Campus library:* 385,000 volumes (3,337 in nursing); 68 health-care related periodical subscriptions. *Nursing school resources:* CAI, computer lab, nursing audiovisuals, interactive nursing skills videos, learning resource lab.

Student Life *Student services:* health clinic, personal counseling, career counseling, institutionally sponsored work-study program, job placement, campus safety program, special assistance for disabled students. *International student services:* counseling/support, special assistance for nonnative speakers of English. *Nursing student activities:* Sigma Theta Tau, student nurses association.

Calendar 4-1-4.

NURSING STUDENT PROFILE

Undergraduate **Enrollment:** 147

Women: 93%; **Men:** 7%; **Minority:** 1%; **International:** 1%; **Part-time:** 2%

BACCALAUREATE PROGRAMS

Contact Ms. Ruth Green, Secretary, Department of Nursing, Luther College, 700 College Drive, Decorah, IA 52101, 319-387-1057. *Fax:* 319-387-2149. *E-mail:* greenru@luther.edu

Expenses *Tuition:* $14,900 full-time, $532 per hour part-time. *State resident tuition:* $14,900 full-time, $532 per hour part-time. *Nonresident tuition:* $14,900 full-time, $532 per hour part-time. *Room and board:* $3650. *Books and supplies per academic year:* ranges from $600 to $700.

Financial Aid Institutionally sponsored need-based grants/scholarships, institutionally sponsored non-need grants/scholarships, Federal Direct Loans, Federal Pell Grants, Federal Perkins Loans, Federal Supplemental Educational Opportunity Grants, Federal Work-Study. *Application deadline:* 3/1.

Generic Baccalaureate Program (BA)

Applying *Required:* SAT I or ACT, 3 years of high school math, 3 years of high school science, high school transcript, transcript of college record. *Options:* Advanced standing available through credit by exam. May apply for transfer of up to 64 total credits. *Application deadline:* rolling. *Application fee:* $20.

Degree Requirements 128 total credit hours, 45 in nursing.

RN Baccalaureate Program (BA)

Applying *Required:* SAT I or ACT, 3 years of high school math, 3 years of high school science, RN license, diploma or AD in nursing, high school transcript, transcript of college record. *Options:* Advanced standing available through the following means: advanced placement exams, credit by exam. May apply for transfer of up to 64 total credits. *Application deadline:* rolling. *Application fee:* $20.

Degree Requirements 128 total credit hours, 45 in nursing.

CONTINUING EDUCATION PROGRAM

Contact Ms. Ruth Green, Secretary, Department of Nursing, Luther College, 700 College Drive, Decorah, IA 52101, 319-387-1057. *Fax:* 319-387-2149. *E-mail:* greenru@luther.edu

See full description on page 474.

MORNINGSIDE COLLEGE
Department of Nursing Education
Sioux City, Iowa

Programs • Generic Baccalaureate • RN Baccalaureate • Continuing Education

The College Independent United Methodist comprehensive coed institution. Founded: 1894. *Primary accreditation:* regional. *Setting:* 27-acre suburban campus. *Total enrollment:* 1,117.

The Department of Nursing Education Founded in 1972. *Nursing program faculty:* 9 (22% with doctorates).

Academic Facilities *Campus library:* 120,500 volumes (650 in health, 650 in nursing); 158 health-care related periodical subscriptions. *Nursing school resources:* CAI, computer lab, nursing audiovisuals, learning resource lab.

Student Life *Student services:* health clinic, child-care facilities, personal counseling, career counseling, institutionally sponsored work-study program, job placement, campus safety program, special assistance for disabled students, learning center. *International student services:* counseling/support, ESL courses. *Nursing student activities:* nursing club, student nurses association.

Calendar Semesters.

NURSING STUDENT PROFILE

Undergraduate **Enrollment:** 55

Women: 95%; **Men:** 5%; **Minority:** 4%; **International:** 0%; **Part-time:** 24%

BACCALAUREATE PROGRAMS

Contact Dr. Kathy Buchheit, Chair, Department of Nursing Education, Morningside College, 1501 Morningside Avenue, Sioux City, IA 51106-1751, 712-274-5156. *Fax:* 712-274-5101.

Expenses *Tuition:* $11,226 full-time, ranges from $230 to $370 per hour part-time. *Full-time mandatory fees:* $293+. *Room and board:* $4130. *Room only:* $2000. *Books and supplies per academic year:* ranges from $150 to $400.

Financial Aid Institutionally sponsored need-based grants/scholarships, institutionally sponsored non-need grants/scholarships, Federal Pell Grants, Federal Perkins Loans, Federal Supplemental Educational Opportunity Grants, Federal Work-Study, Federal Stafford Loans, state grants. *Application deadline:* 3/1.

Generic Baccalaureate Program (BSN)

Applying *Required:* SAT I, ACT, TOEFL for nonnative speakers of English, minimum college GPA of 2.0, high school math, high school chemistry, high school biology, high school transcript, interview, transcript of college record. 26 prerequisite credits must be completed before admission to the nursing program. *Options:* Advanced standing available through credit by exam. May apply for transfer of up to 62 total credits. *Application deadline:* rolling. *Application fee:* $15.

Degree Requirements 124 total credit hours, 48 in nursing. Departmental writing endorsement, oral proficiency.

RN Baccalaureate Program (BSN)

Applying *Required:* SAT I, ACT, minimum college GPA of 2.0, RN license, diploma or AD in nursing, high school transcript, interview, transcript of college record. *Options:* Advanced standing available through credit by exam. May apply for transfer of up to 62 total credits. *Application deadline:* rolling. *Application fee:* $15.

Degree Requirements 124 total credit hours, 48 in nursing. Departmental writing endorsement, oral proficiency.

CONTINUING EDUCATION PROGRAM

Contact Ms. Sandra Mitchell, Director of Academic Services, Morningside College, 1501 Morningside Avenue, Sioux City, IA 51106-1751, 712-274-5333. *Fax:* 712-274-5101.

MOUNT MERCY COLLEGE
Department of Nursing
Cedar Rapids, Iowa

Programs • Generic Baccalaureate • RN Baccalaureate • Continuing Education

The College Independent Roman Catholic 4-year coed college. Founded: 1928. *Primary accreditation:* regional. *Setting:* 36-acre suburban campus. *Total enrollment:* 1,224.

The Department of Nursing Founded in 1969. *Nursing program faculty:* 18 (6% with doctorates).

Academic Facilities *Campus library:* 88,689 volumes (4,119 in health, 1,200 in nursing); 625 periodical subscriptions (104 health-care related). *Nursing school resources:* CAI, computer lab, nursing audiovisuals, learning resource lab.

Student Life *Student services:* health clinic, personal counseling, career counseling, institutionally sponsored work-study program, job placement, campus safety program, special assistance for disabled students. *International student services:* counseling/support, special assistance for nonnative speakers of English. *Nursing student activities:* Sigma Theta Tau, nursing club, student nurses association.

Calendar 4-1-4.

NURSING STUDENT PROFILE

Undergraduate **Enrollment:** 120

Women: 95%; **Men:** 5%; **Minority:** 1%; **International:** 1%; **Part-time:** 30%

BACCALAUREATE PROGRAMS

Contact Dr. Mary P. Tarbox, Chair, Department of Nursing, Mount Mercy College, 1330 Elmhurst Drive, NE, Cedar Rapids, IA 52402-4798, 319-368-6471. *Fax:* 319-368-6479.

Expenses *Tuition:* $11,370 full-time, $320 per credit hour part-time. *Full-time mandatory fees:* $115. *Part-time mandatory fees:* $115. *Room and board:* $3800–$4180. *Room only:* $1530–$1910. *Books and supplies per academic year:* ranges from $200 to $300.

Financial Aid Institutionally sponsored need-based grants/scholarships, institutionally sponsored non-need grants/scholarships, Federal Nursing Student Loans, Federal Supplemental Educational Opportunity Grants, Federal Work-Study. 90% of undergraduate students in nursing programs received some form of financial aid in 1995–96. *Application deadline:* 3/1.

Generic Baccalaureate Program (BS)

Applying *Required:* SAT I, ACT, TOEFL for nonnative speakers of English, minimum college GPA of 2.5, 3 years of high school math, 3 years of high school science, high school transcript, interview, transcript of college record, high school class rank: top 50%. 43 prerequisite credits must be completed before admission to the nursing program. *Options:* Advanced standing available through credit by exam. May apply for transfer of up to 89 total credits. *Application deadlines:* 6/1 (fall), 10/1 (spring). *Application fee:* $20.

Degree Requirements 123 total credit hours, 42 in nursing.

RN Baccalaureate Program (BS)

Applying *Required:* SAT I, ACT, TOEFL for nonnative speakers of English, minimum college GPA of 2.5, RN license, diploma or AD in nursing, high school transcript, interview, transcript of college record. 40 prerequisite credits must be completed before admission to the nursing program. *Options:* Advanced standing available through credit by exam. May apply for transfer of up to 89 total credits. *Application deadlines:* 6/1 (fall), 10/1 (spring). *Application fee:* $20.

Degree Requirements 123 total credit hours, 42 in nursing.

CONTINUING EDUCATION PROGRAM

Contact Dr. Mary P. Tarbox, Chair, Department of Nursing, Mount Mercy College, 1330 Elmhurst Drive, NE, Cedar Rapids, IA 52402-4798, 319-368-6471. *Fax:* 319-368-6479.

TEIKYO MARYCREST UNIVERSITY
Division of Nursing
Davenport, Iowa

Programs • Generic Baccalaureate • RN Baccalaureate

The University Independent comprehensive coed institution. Founded: 1939. *Primary accreditation:* regional. *Setting:* 30-acre urban campus. *Total enrollment:* 1,049.

The Division of Nursing Founded in 1963. *Nursing program faculty:* 8 (37% with doctorates). *Off-campus program site:* Ottumwa.

Academic Facilities *Campus library:* 109,622 volumes; 522 periodical subscriptions (44 health-care related). *Nursing school resources:* CAI, computer lab, nursing audiovisuals, learning resource lab.

Student Life *Student services:* personal counseling, institutionally sponsored work-study program, job placement, campus safety program. *International student services:* counseling/support, ESL courses. *Nursing student activities:* student nurses association, Student Government Association.

Calendar Semesters.

NURSING STUDENT PROFILE

Undergraduate **Enrollment:** 111

Women: 91%; **Men:** 9%; **Minority:** 11%; **International:** 1%; **Part-time:** 45%

BACCALAUREATE PROGRAMS

Contact Dr. Dolores Hilden, Chairperson, Division of Nursing, Teikyo Marycrest University, 1607 West 12th Street, Davenport, IA 52804-4096, 319-326-9278. *Fax:* 319-326-9250. *E-mail:* dhilden@acc.mcrest.edu

Expenses *Tuition:* $10,850 full-time, $364 per credit part-time. *Full-time mandatory fees:* $160–$235. *Room and board:* $3610–$4590. *Room only:* $1540–$2340.

Generic Baccalaureate Program (BSN)

Applying *Required:* SAT I, ACT, minimum high school GPA of 2.3, minimum college GPA of 2.3, 3 years of high school math, high school chemistry, high school transcript, interview, written essay. 30 prerequisite credits must be completed before admission to the nursing program. *Options:* Advanced standing available through the following means: advanced placement exams, advanced placement without credit, credit by exam. May apply for transfer of up to 66–94 total credits. *Application deadline:* rolling. *Application fee:* $25.

Degree Requirements 124 total credit hours, 50 in nursing.

RN Baccalaureate Program (BSN)

Applying *Required:* SAT I, ACT, minimum high school GPA of 2.3, minimum college GPA of 2.3, 3 years of high school math, high school chemistry, RN license, diploma or AD in nursing, interview, written essay, transcript of college record, professional liability/malpractice insurance. *Options:* Advanced standing available through the following means: advanced placement exams, advanced placement without credit, credit

Teikyo Marycrest University (continued)
by exam. Course work may be accelerated. May apply for transfer of up to 66–94 total credits. *Application deadline:* rolling. *Application fee:* $25.

Degree Requirements 124 total credit hours, 22 in nursing.

Distance learning Courses provided through video. Specific degree requirements include RN license.

THE UNIVERSITY OF IOWA
College of Nursing
Iowa City, Iowa

Programs • Generic Baccalaureate • RN Baccalaureate • MSN • Accelerated MSN • Master's for Nurses with Non-Nursing Degrees • MSN/MBA • PhD • Postdoctoral • Continuing Education

The University State-supported coed university. Founded: 1847. *Primary accreditation:* regional. *Setting:* 1,900-acre small-town campus. *Total enrollment:* 27,597.

The College of Nursing Founded in 1897. *Nursing program faculty:* 72 (56% with doctorates). *Off-campus program sites:* Mason City, Fort Dodge, Emmetsburg.

Academic Facilities *Campus library:* 2.7 million volumes (250,000 in health); 25,894 periodical subscriptions (2,500 health-care related). *Nursing school resources:* CAI, computer lab, nursing audiovisuals, interactive nursing skills videos, learning resource lab.

Student Life *Student services:* health clinic, personal counseling, career counseling, institutionally sponsored work-study program, job placement, campus safety program, special assistance for disabled students. *International student services:* ESL courses. *Nursing student activities:* Sigma Theta Tau, student nurses association.

Calendar Semesters.

NURSING STUDENT PROFILE

Undergraduate **Enrollment:** 417
Women: 92%; **Men:** 8%; **Minority:** 4%; **International:** 0%; **Part-time:** 9%

Graduate **Enrollment:** 256
Women: 96%; **Men:** 4%; **Minority:** 2%; **International:** 2%; **Part-time:** 80%

BACCALAUREATE PROGRAMS

Contact Ms. Laraine Carmichael, Director, Student Services, 101 Nursing Building, College of Nursing, University of Iowa, Iowa City, IA 52242, 319-335-7015. *Fax:* 319-335-9990. *E-mail:* laraine-carmichael@uiowa.edu

Expenses *State resident tuition:* $2470 per academic year. *Nonresident tuition:* $9068 per academic year. *Full-time mandatory fees:* $1000. *Room and board:* $3853. *Books and supplies per academic year:* $560.

Financial Aid Institutionally sponsored need-based grants/scholarships, institutionally sponsored non-need grants/scholarships, Federal Nursing Student Loans, Federal Pell Grants, Federal Supplemental Educational Opportunity Grants, Federal Work-Study.

Generic Baccalaureate Program (BSN)

Applying *Required:* SAT I, ACT, TOEFL for nonnative speakers of English, minimum college GPA of 2.5, 3 years of high school math, 3 years of high school science, high school foreign language, high school transcript, transcript of college record. 40 prerequisite credits must be completed before admission to the nursing program. *Options:* May apply for transfer of up to 98 total credits. *Application deadlines:* 10/1 (fall), 3/1 (spring). *Application fee:* $20.

Degree Requirements 128 total credit hours, 56 in nursing.

RN Baccalaureate Program (BSN)

Applying *Required:* TOEFL for nonnative speakers of English, minimum college GPA of 2.5, 3 years of high school math, 3 years of high school science, RN license, diploma or AD in nursing, high school foreign language, high school transcript, transcript of college record. 45 prerequisite credits must be completed before admission to the nursing program. *Options:* Course work may be accelerated. *Application deadlines:* 10/1 (fall), 3/1 (spring). *Application fee:* $20.

Degree Requirements 128 total credit hours, 25 in nursing.

MASTER'S PROGRAMS

Contact Ms. Lori Anderson, Program Assistant, 101 Nursing Building, College of Nursing, University of Iowa, Iowa City, IA 52242, 319-335-7021. *Fax:* 319-335-9990. *E-mail:* lori-anderson@uiowa.edu

Areas of Study Clinical nurse specialist programs in adult health nursing, community health nursing, gerontological nursing, pediatric nursing; nurse anesthesia; nursing administration; nursing education; nurse practitioner programs in child care/pediatrics, gerontology.

Expenses *State resident tuition:* $2934 full-time, $163 per credit hour part-time. *Nonresident tuition:* $9452 full-time, ranges from $163 to $525 per credit hour part-time. *Full-time mandatory fees:* $250. *Room and board:* $4000. *Books and supplies per academic year:* $800.

Financial Aid Graduate assistantships, nurse traineeships. *Application deadline:* 4/1.

MSN Program

Applying *Required:* GRE General Test, TOEFL for nonnative speakers of English, bachelor's degree in nursing, minimum GPA of 3.1, RN license, physical assessment course, statistics course, professional liability/malpractice insurance, 3 letters of recommendation, transcript of college record. *Application deadlines:* 5/1 (fall), 12/1 (spring). *Application fee:* $20.

Degree Requirements 40 total credit hours, 34–37 in nursing.

Accelerated MSN Program

Applying *Required:* GRE General Test, ACT PEP, bachelor's degree in nursing, minimum GPA of 3.0, RN license, physical assessment course, statistics course, professional liability/malpractice insurance, 3 letters of recommendation, transcript of college record. *Application deadlines:* 5/1 (fall), 12/1 (spring). *Application fee:* $20.

Degree Requirements 34 total credit hours, 28–31 in nursing.

Master's for Nurses with Non-Nursing Degrees Program (MSN)

Applying *Required:* GRE General Test, ACT PEP, bachelor's degree, minimum GPA of 3.0, RN license, physical assessment course, statistics course, professional liability/malpractice insurance, 3 letters of recommendation, transcript of college record, community health clinical course. *Application deadlines:* 5/1 (fall), 12/1 (spring). *Application fee:* $20.

Degree Requirements 40 total credit hours, 34–37 in nursing.

MSN/MBA Program

Applying *Required:* GRE General Test, GMAT, bachelor's degree in nursing, minimum GPA of 3.0, RN license, statistics course, professional liability/malpractice insurance, 3 letters of recommendation, transcript of college record. *Application deadlines:* 5/1 (fall), 12/1 (spring). *Application fee:* $20.

Degree Requirements 61 total credit hours, 22 in nursing, 45 in business.

DOCTORAL PROGRAM

Contact Ms. Lori Anderson, Program Assistant, 101 Nursing Building, College of Nursing, University of Iowa, Iowa City, IA 52242, 319-335-7021. *Fax:* 319-335-9990. *E-mail:* lori-anderson@uiowa.edu

Areas of Study Nursing administration, aging.

Expenses *State resident tuition:* $2934 full-time, $163 per credit hour part-time. *Nonresident tuition:* $9452 full-time, ranges from $163 to $525 per credit hour part-time. *Full-time mandatory fees:* $250. *Room and board:* $4000. *Books and supplies per academic year:* $800.

Financial Aid Graduate assistantships, nurse traineeships, fellowships, grants. *Application deadline:* 2/1.

PhD Program

Applying *Required:* GRE General Test, TOEFL for nonnative speakers of English, master's degree in nursing, statistics course, interview, 3 letters of recommendation, vitae, competitive review by faculty committee, goals statement. *Application deadline:* 2/1. *Application fee:* $20.

Degree Requirements 60 total credit hours; 9 semester hours each in research, statistics, and cognate minor; 12 semester hours each in nursing focal area and dissertation research; 18 semester hours in nursing core; dissertation; oral exam; written exam; defense of dissertation; residency.

POSTDOCTORAL PROGRAM

Contact Jen Clougherty, Program Associate, 492 Nursing Building, College of Nursing, University of Iowa, Iowa City, IA 52242, 319-335-7119. *Fax:* 319-335-9990. *E-mail:* jennifer-clougherty@uiowa.edu

Areas of Study Nursing interventions, outcomes, and effectiveness; research training.

CONTINUING EDUCATION PROGRAM

Contact Director, Continuing Nursing Education, 406 Nursing Building, College of Nursing, University of Iowa, Iowa City, IA 52242, 319-335-7077. *Fax:* 319-335-9990.

KANSAS

BAKER UNIVERSITY
School of Nursing/Stormont-Vail Campus
Topeka, Kansas

Programs • Generic Baccalaureate • RN Baccalaureate • Continuing Education

The University Independent United Methodist comprehensive coed institution. Founded: 1858. *Primary accreditation:* regional. *Setting:* 26-acre small-town campus. *Total enrollment:* 2,041.

The School of Nursing/Stormont-Vail Campus Founded in 1991. *Nursing program faculty:* 15 (1% with doctorates).

Academic Facilities *Campus library:* 60,000 volumes (4,700 in health, 2,666 in nursing); 361 periodical subscriptions (361 health-care related). *Nursing school resources:* CAI, computer lab, nursing audiovisuals, interactive nursing skills videos, learning resource lab, tutorial lab.

Student Life *Student services:* health clinic, personal counseling, career counseling, institutionally sponsored work-study program, job placement, campus safety program. *International student services:* counseling/support, special assistance for nonnative speakers of English, ESL courses. *Nursing student activities:* nursing club, student nurses association, Nursing Honor Society.

Calendar Semesters.

NURSING STUDENT PROFILE

Undergraduate

Women: 88%; **Men:** 12%; **Minority:** 6%; **International:** 0%; **Part-time:** 8%

BACCALAUREATE PROGRAMS

Contact Ms. Peggy Geier, Student Affairs Specialist, School of Nursing/Stormont-Vail Campus, Baker University, 1500 Southwest Tenth Street, Topeka, KS 66604-1353, 913-354-5851. *Fax:* 913-354-5832.

Expenses *Tuition:* $7600 full-time, $235 per credit part-time. *Full-time mandatory fees:* $30. *Part-time mandatory fees:* $30. *Books and supplies per academic year:* ranges from $300 to $500.

Financial Aid Institutionally sponsored need-based grants/scholarships, institutionally sponsored non-need grants/scholarships, Federal Nursing Student Loans, Federal Pell Grants, Federal Perkins Loans, Federal Supplemental Educational Opportunity Grants. *Application deadline:* 5/1.

Generic Baccalaureate Program (BSN)

Applying *Required:* ACT, TOEFL for nonnative speakers of English, minimum college GPA of 2.5, high school transcript, written essay, transcript of college record, high school transcript or GED certificate. 64 prerequisite credits must be completed before admission to the nursing program. *Options:* Advanced standing available through credit by exam. May apply for transfer of up to 98 total credits. *Application deadlines:* 3/1 (fall), 10/1 (spring). *Application fee:* $20.

Degree Requirements 128 total credit hours, 60 in nursing. 6 credits in critical thinking and writing courses.

RN Baccalaureate Program (BSN)

Applying *Required:* TOEFL for nonnative speakers of English, minimum college GPA of 2.5, RN license, diploma or AD in nursing, high school transcript, transcript of college record, high school transcript or GED certificate. 64 prerequisite credits must be completed before admission to the nursing program. *Options:* Advanced standing available through credit by exam. *Application deadlines:* 3/1 (fall), 10/1 (spring). *Application fee:* $20.

Degree Requirements 128 total credit hours, 32 in nursing. 6 credits in critical thinking and writing courses.

CONTINUING EDUCATION PROGRAM

Contact Ms. Joyce Lind Watkins, Coordinator, Continuing Education, Baker University School of Nursing/Stormont-Vail Campus, Baker University, 1500 Southwest Tenth Street, Topeka, KS 66604-1353, 913-354-5829. *Fax:* 913-354-5059.

BETHEL COLLEGE
Department of Nursing
North Newton, Kansas

Programs • Generic Baccalaureate • Accelerated RN Baccalaureate • Baccalaureate for Second Degree • LPN to Baccalaureate

The College Independent 4-year coed college, affiliated with General Conference Mennonite Church. Founded: 1887. *Primary accreditation:* regional. *Setting:* 60-acre small-town campus. *Total enrollment:* 620.

The Department of Nursing Founded in 1908.

Academic Facilities *Campus library:* 118,717 volumes (5,500 in health, 3,008 in nursing); 852 periodical subscriptions (49 health-care related).

Student Life *Student services:* health clinic, personal counseling, career counseling, campus safety program. *Nursing student activities:* student nurses association.

Calendar 4-1-4.

BACCALAUREATE PROGRAMS

Contact Chairperson, Department of Nursing, Bethel College, 300 East 27th Street, North Newton, KS 67117, 316-284-5307. *Fax:* 316-284-5286.

Financial Aid Federal Pell Grants, Federal Perkins Loans, Federal Supplemental Educational Opportunity Grants, Federal Work-Study, Federal PLUS Loans, Federal Stafford Loans.

Generic Baccalaureate Program (BSN)

Applying *Required:* SAT I or ACT, minimum college GPA of 2.5, high school transcript, 2 letters of recommendation. 57 prerequisite credits must be completed before admission to the nursing program. *Application deadline:* rolling.

Degree Requirements 124 total credit hours, 50 in nursing.

Accelerated RN Baccalaureate Program (BSN)

Applying *Required:* SAT I or ACT, minimum college GPA of 2.5, high school transcript, 2 letters of recommendation. 57 prerequisite credits must be completed before admission to the nursing program. *Application deadline:* rolling.

Baccalaureate for Second Degree Program (BSN)

Applying *Required:* SAT I or ACT, minimum college GPA of 2.5, high school transcript, 2 letters of recommendation. 57 prerequisite credits must be completed before admission to the nursing program. *Application deadline:* rolling.

Degree Requirements 124 total credit hours, 50 in nursing.

LPN to Baccalaureate Program (BSN)

Applying *Required:* SAT I or ACT, minimum college GPA of 2.5, high school transcript, 2 letters of recommendation. 57 prerequisite credits must be completed before admission to the nursing program. *Application deadline:* rolling.

See full description on page 418.

FORT HAYS STATE UNIVERSITY
Department of Nursing
Hays, Kansas

Programs • Generic Baccalaureate • RN Baccalaureate • LPN to Baccalaureate • MSN • Post-Master's

The University State-supported comprehensive coed institution. Part of Kansas Regents System. Founded: 1902. *Primary accreditation:* regional. *Setting:* 200-acre small-town campus. *Total enrollment:* 5,441.

The Department of Nursing Founded in 1968. *Nursing program faculty:* 21 (29% with doctorates).

Academic Facilities *Campus library:* 250,000 volumes; 2,364 periodical subscriptions.

Calendar Semesters.

BACCALAUREATE PROGRAMS

Contact Dr. Mary Hassett, Chair, Stroup Hall, Department of Nursing, Fort Hays State University, 600 Park Street, Hays, KS 67601, 913-628-4498. *Fax:* 913-628-4080. *E-mail:* numh@fhsuvm.fhsu.edu

Expenses *State resident tuition:* $2224 full-time, $64 per credit hour part-time. *Nonresident tuition:* $6985 full-time, $201 per credit hour part-time.

Financial Aid Federal Direct Loans, Federal Perkins Loans, Federal Supplemental Educational Opportunity Grants, Federal Work-Study. *Application deadline:* 3/1.

Generic Baccalaureate Program (BSN)

Applying *Required:* SAT I or ACT, TOEFL for nonnative speakers of English, minimum high school GPA of 2.5, minimum college GPA of 2.0, 3 letters of recommendation, transcript of college record, GED certificate or high school transcript. *Options:* Advanced standing available through credit by exam. *Application deadline:* rolling. *Application fee:* $15.

Degree Requirements 139 total credit hours, 64 in nursing.

RN Baccalaureate Program (BSN)

Applying *Required:* TOEFL for nonnative speakers of English, NLN qualifying exams; Commission on Graduates of Foreign Nursing Schools exam for foreign students, minimum high school GPA of 2.5, minimum college GPA of 2.0, RN license, 3 letters of recommendation, transcript of college record. *Options:* Advanced standing available through credit by exam. *Application deadline:* rolling. *Application fee:* $15.

Degree Requirements 139 total credit hours, 64 in nursing.

LPN to Baccalaureate Program (BSN)

Applying *Required:* TOEFL for nonnative speakers of English, minimum high school GPA of 2.5, minimum college GPA of 2.0, 3 letters of recommendation, transcript of college record, LPN license. *Options:* Advanced standing available through credit by exam. *Application deadline:* rolling. *Application fee:* $15.

Degree Requirements 139 total credit hours, 64 in nursing.

MASTER'S PROGRAMS

Contact Dr. Mary Hassett, Chair, Stroup Hall, Department of Nursing, Fort Hays State University, 600 Park Street, Hays, KS 67601, 913-628-4498. *Fax:* 913-628-4080. *E-mail:* numh@fhsuvm.fhsu.edu

Areas of Study Clinical nurse specialist program in adult health nursing; nursing administration; nursing education; nurse practitioner program in family health.

Expenses *State resident tuition:* $1513 full-time, $89 per credit part-time. *Nonresident tuition:* $3978 full-time, $234 per credit part-time.

MSN Program

Applying *Required:* Miller Analogies Test, TOEFL for nonnative speakers of English, bachelor's degree in nursing, 3 letters of recommendation, transcript of college record, undergraduate pathophysiology course for family nurse practitioner track. *Application fee:* $15.

Degree Requirements 34 total credit hours, 34 in nursing. Comprehensive exams; research project instead of a thesis for family nurse practitioner track. Thesis required.

Post-Master's Program

Applying *Required:* Miller Analogies Test, TOEFL for nonnative speakers of English, transcript of college record, master's degree in nursing. *Application fee:* $15.

Degree Requirements 16 total credit hours, 16 in nursing.

KANSAS NEWMAN COLLEGE
Division of Nursing
Wichita, Kansas

Programs • Generic Baccalaureate • RN Baccalaureate

The College Independent Roman Catholic comprehensive coed institution. Founded: 1933. *Primary accreditation:* regional. *Setting:* 53-acre urban campus. *Total enrollment:* 1,989.

The Division of Nursing Founded in 1979. *Nursing program faculty:* 14 (29% with doctorates). *Off-campus program sites:* Hutchison Liberal, Dodge City Garden City, Pratt Great Bend.

Academic Facilities *Campus library:* 100,000 volumes (7,000 in nursing); 400 periodical subscriptions (75 health-care related). *Nursing school resources:* CAI, computer lab, nursing audiovisuals, learning resource lab.

Student Life *Student services:* personal counseling, career counseling, institutionally sponsored work-study program, job placement, campus safety program. *International student services:* counseling/support. *Nursing student activities:* Sigma Theta Tau, nursing club, student nurses association.

Calendar Semesters.

NURSING STUDENT PROFILE

Undergraduate **Enrollment:** 175

Women: 92%; **Men:** 8%; **Minority:** 10%; **International:** 1%; **Part-time:** 45%

BACCALAUREATE PROGRAMS

Contact Mr. Tom Green, Dean of Enrollment Services, Division of Nursing, Kansas Newman College, 3100 McCormick Avenue, Wichita, KS 67213, 316-942-4291. *Fax:* 316-942-4483. *E-mail:* greent@ksnewman.edu

Expenses *Tuition:* $8500 full-time, $286 per credit hour part-time. *Full-time mandatory fees:* $32–$72. *Room and board:* $3626–$4628. *Room only:* $1654–$2512. *Books and supplies per academic year:* $1200.

Financial Aid Institutionally sponsored need-based grants/scholarships, institutionally sponsored non-need grants/scholarships, Federal Pell Grants, Federal Perkins Loans, Federal Supplemental Educational Opportunity Grants, Federal Work-Study, Federal Stafford Loans. *Application deadline:* 5/1.

Generic Baccalaureate Program (BSN)

Applying *Required:* SAT I or ACT, TOEFL for nonnative speakers of English, minimum college GPA of 2.0, interview, 2 letters of recommendation, written essay, transcript of college record. 61 prerequisite credits must be completed before admission to the nursing program. *Options:* May apply for transfer of up to 77 total credits. *Application deadlines:* 11/1 (fall), 5/1 (spring). *Application fee:* $15.

Degree Requirements 124 total credit hours, 61 in nursing. Pathophysiology, statistics courses.

RN Baccalaureate Program (BSN)

Applying *Required:* RN license, diploma or AD in nursing, transcript of college record. 71 prerequisite credits must be completed before admission to the nursing program. *Options:* Course work may be accelerated. May apply for transfer of up to 84 total credits. *Application deadline:* rolling. *Application fee:* $15.

Degree Requirements 124 total credit hours, 35 in nursing. Pathophysiology, statistics courses.

Distance learning Courses provided through video.

KANSAS WESLEYAN UNIVERSITY
Division of Nursing Education
Salina, Kansas

Program • RN Baccalaureate

The University Independent United Methodist comprehensive coed institution. Founded: 1886. *Primary accreditation:* regional. *Setting:* 28-acre suburban campus. *Total enrollment:* 704.

The Division of Nursing Education Founded in 1988. *Nursing program faculty:* 10 (30% with doctorates).

Academic Facilities *Campus library:* 60,548 volumes (3,310 in nursing); 364 periodical subscriptions (51 health-care related). *Nursing school resources:* CAI, computer lab, nursing audiovisuals.

Student Life *Student services:* personal counseling, career counseling, institutionally sponsored work-study program, job placement, special assistance for disabled students. *International student services:* counseling/support, ESL courses. *Nursing student activities:* nursing club, student nurses association.

Calendar Semesters.

NURSING STUDENT PROFILE

Undergraduate **Enrollment:** 100
Women: 97%; **Men:** 3%; **Minority:** 9%; **International:** 0%; **Part-time:** 30%

BACCALAUREATE PROGRAM

Contact Dr. Patricia Kissell, Director, Division of Nursing Education, Kansas Wesleyan University, 100 East Claflin, Salina, KS 67401-6196, 913-827-5541 Ext. 7212. *Fax:* 913-827-0927.

Expenses *Tuition:* $4900 full-time, $140 per credit hour part-time. *Room and board:* $1750–$1950. *Books and supplies per academic year:* ranges from $500 to $700.

Financial Aid Institutionally sponsored need-based grants/scholarships, Federal Direct Loans, Federal Nursing Student Loans, Federal Pell Grants, Federal Perkins Loans, Federal Supplemental Educational Opportunity Grants, Federal Work-Study. 97% of undergraduate students in nursing programs received some form of financial aid in 1995–96. *Application deadline:* 5/15.

RN Baccalaureate Program (BSN)

Applying *Required:* SAT I or ACT, TOEFL for nonnative speakers of English, minimum college GPA of 2.3, RN license, diploma or AD in nursing, 3 letters of recommendation, transcript of college record, high school class rank: top 50%. 68 prerequisite credits must be completed before admission to the nursing program. *Options:* Advanced standing available through the following means: advanced placement without credit, credit by exam. May apply for transfer of up to 63 total credits. *Application deadline:* rolling. *Application fee:* $15.

Degree Requirements 130 total credit hours, 69 in nursing.

MIDAMERICA NAZARENE COLLEGE
Division of Nursing
Olathe, Kansas

Programs • Generic Baccalaureate • Accelerated RN Baccalaureate • Continuing Education

The College Independent comprehensive coed institution, affiliated with Church of the Nazarene. Founded: 1966. *Primary accreditation:* regional. *Setting:* 112-acre suburban campus. *Total enrollment:* 1,453.

The Division of Nursing Founded in 1978. *Nursing program faculty:* 8 (25% with doctorates).

Academic Facilities *Campus library:* 87,118 volumes (2,524 in nursing); 225 periodical subscriptions (47 health-care related). *Nursing school resources:* CAI, computer lab, nursing audiovisuals, learning resource lab.

Student Life *Student services:* health clinic, personal counseling, career counseling, institutionally sponsored work-study program, special assistance for disabled students. *International student services:* counseling/support, special assistance for nonnative speakers of English, ESL courses. *Nursing student activities:* nursing club, student nurses association.

Calendar Semesters.

NURSING STUDENT PROFILE

Undergraduate **Enrollment:** 129
Women: 92%; **Men:** 8%; **Minority:** 7%; **International:** 3%; **Part-time:** 11%

BACCALAUREATE PROGRAMS

Contact Dr. Palma Smith, Chairperson, Division of Nursing, MidAmerica Nazarene College, 2030 East College Way, Olathe, KS 66062-1899, 913-782-3750 Ext. 290. *Fax:* 913-791-3408. *E-mail:* psmith@manc.edu

Expenses *Tuition:* $8840 full-time, $272 per credit hour part-time. *Full-time mandatory fees:* $975–$1300. *Part-time mandatory fees:* $163+. *Room and board:* $4012–$4202. *Books and supplies per academic year:* ranges from $300 to $380.

Financial Aid Institutionally sponsored need-based grants/scholarships, institutionally sponsored non-need grants/scholarships, Federal Nursing Student Loans, Federal Pell Grants, Federal Perkins Loans, Federal Supplemental Educational Opportunity Grants, Federal Work-Study. *Application deadline:* 3/1.

Generic Baccalaureate Program (BSN)

Applying *Required:* ACT, TOEFL for nonnative speakers of English, Nursing Entrance Test, minimum college GPA of 2.6, high school transcript, 2 letters of recommendation, written essay, transcript of college record. 47 prerequisite credits must be completed before admission to the nursing program. *Options:* Advanced standing available through credit by exam. Course work may be accelerated. *Application deadlines:* 10/1 (fall), 10/1 (summer). *Application fee:* $10.

Degree Requirements 130 total credit hours, 67 in nursing.

Accelerated RN Baccalaureate Program (BSN)

Applying *Required:* ACT, TOEFL for nonnative speakers of English, minimum college GPA of 2.6, RN license, diploma or AD in nursing, high school transcript, 2 letters of recommendation, written essay, transcript of college record. 41 prerequisite credits must be completed before admission to the nursing program. *Options:* Advanced standing available through the following means: advanced placement without credit, credit by exam. *Application deadlines:* 10/1 (fall), 10/1 (summer).

Degree Requirements 130 total credit hours, 38 in nursing.

CONTINUING EDUCATION PROGRAM

Contact Ms. Phylis Deisher, Continuing Education Coordinator, Division of Nursing, MidAmerica Nazarene College, 2030 East College Way, Olathe, KS 66062-1899, 913-782-3750. *Fax:* 913-791-3290.

PITTSBURG STATE UNIVERSITY
Department of Nursing
Pittsburg, Kansas

Programs • Generic Baccalaureate • MSN

The University State-supported comprehensive coed institution. Part of Kansas Board of Regents. Founded: 1903. *Primary accreditation:* regional. *Setting:* 140-acre small-town campus. *Total enrollment:* 6,565.

The Department of Nursing Founded in 1970. *Nursing program faculty:* 12.

Academic Facilities *Campus library:* 350,000 volumes (4,500 in nursing); 1,810 periodical subscriptions (140 health-care related).

Calendar Semesters.

BACCALAUREATE PROGRAM

Contact Chair, Department of Nursing, Pittsburg State University, 1700 South Broadway, Pittsburg, KS 66762, 316-235-4431. *Fax:* 316-235-4449.

Financial Aid Institutionally sponsored need-based grants/scholarships, Federal Nursing Student Loans, Federal Pell Grants, Federal Perkins Loans, Federal Supplemental Educational Opportunity Grants, Federal Work-Study, Federal PLUS Loans, Federal Stafford Loans. *Application deadline:* 2/1.

Pittsburg State University (continued)

Generic Baccalaureate Program (BSN)

Applying *Required:* ACT, TOEFL for nonnative speakers of English, high school transcript, high school class rank: , CPR certification. *Options:* Advanced standing available through the following means: advanced placement exams, credit by exam. *Application deadline:* 1/15. *Application fee:* $15.

Degree Requirements 125 total credit hours, 58 in nursing.

MASTER'S PROGRAM

Areas of Study Nursing administration; nursing education; nurse practitioner programs in family health, gerontology.

MSN Program

Applying *Required:* GRE General Test, bachelor's degree in nursing, minimum GPA of 3.0, RN license. *Application deadline:* 1/15.

Degree Requirements 40 total credit hours, 40 in nursing. Oral comprehensive exam; either a thesis or a research project.

SOUTHWESTERN COLLEGE
Department of Nursing
Winfield, Kansas

Program • Generic Baccalaureate

The College Independent United Methodist comprehensive coed institution. Founded: 1885. *Primary accreditation:* regional. *Setting:* 70-acre small-town campus. *Total enrollment:* 758.

The Department of Nursing Founded in 1986.

Academic Facilities *Campus library:* 57,000 volumes (2,910 in nursing); 381 periodical subscriptions (33 health-care related).

Calendar Semesters.

BACCALAUREATE PROGRAM

Contact Program Director, Department of Nursing, Southwestern College, 100 North College Street, Winfield, KS 67156, 316-221-8306. *Fax:* 316-221-8382.

UNIVERSITY OF KANSAS
School of Nursing
Kansas City, Kansas

Programs • Generic Baccalaureate • Accelerated RN Baccalaureate • RN to Master's • MS/MHSA • PhD • PhD/MBA • Continuing Education

The University State-supported coed university. Founded: 1866. *Primary accreditation:* regional. *Setting:* 1,000-acre suburban campus. *Total enrollment:* 27,639.

The School of Nursing Founded in 1905. *Nursing program faculty:* 58 (41% with doctorates). *Off-campus program site:* Topeka.

▶ ***NOTEWORTHY***

The University of Kansas School of Nursing is on the campus of the University of Kansas Medical Center in Kansas City. It is in the top 20% of nursing schools in the United States, according to March 1994 rankings in *U.S. News & World Report.* Bachelor's, master's, and doctoral degrees in nursing are offered. Master's degree tracks include CNS, nursing administration, and nurse practitioner. Areas of study include adult health, community health, pediatric health, psychiatric–mental health, women's health, and adult/gerontology CNS/NP. The School also offers a joint master's degree program with health services administration (MS/MHSA).

Academic Facilities *Campus library:* 3.0 million volumes (145,690 in health, 4,621 in nursing); 1,491 periodical subscriptions (1,491 health-care related). *Nursing school resources:* CAI, computer lab, nursing audiovisuals, interactive nursing skills videos, learning resource lab, World Wide Web.

Student Life *Student services:* health clinic, child-care facilities, personal counseling, institutionally sponsored work-study program, campus safety program, special assistance for disabled students. *International student services:* counseling/support, special assistance for nonnative speakers of English, ESL courses. *Nursing student activities:* Sigma Theta Tau, recruiter club, nursing club, student nurses association.

Calendar Semesters.

NURSING STUDENT PROFILE

Undergraduate **Enrollment:** 305
Women: 85%; **Men:** 15%; **Minority:** 11%; **International:** 5%; **Part-time:** 5%
Graduate **Enrollment:** 294
Women: 96%; **Men:** 4%; **Minority:** 9%; **International:** 1%; **Part-time:** 91%

BACCALAUREATE PROGRAMS

Contact Dr. Rita Clifford, Associate Dean, Student Affairs, School of Nursing, University of Kansas, 3901 Rainbow Boulevard, Kansas City, KS 66160-7501, 913-588-1619. *Fax:* 913-588-1660. *E-mail:* rcliffor@kumc.edu

Expenses *State resident tuition:* $1953 per academic year. *Nonresident tuition:* $8215 per academic year. *Full-time mandatory fees:* $21–$56. *Books and supplies per academic year:* $600.

Financial Aid Institutionally sponsored need-based grants/scholarships, institutionally sponsored non-need grants/scholarships, Federal Nursing Student Loans, Federal Supplemental Educational Opportunity Grants, Federal Work-Study. *Application deadline:* 4/15.

Generic Baccalaureate Program (BSN)

Applying *Required:* SAT I, ACT, TOEFL for nonnative speakers of English, minimum college GPA of 2.5, high school transcript, 3 letters of recommendation, written essay, transcript of college record. 62 prerequisite credits must be completed before admission to the nursing program. *Options:* Advanced standing available through advanced placement exams. May apply for transfer of up to 65 total credits. *Application deadline:* 10/15. *Application fee:* $25.

Degree Requirements 124 total credit hours, 62 in nursing.

Accelerated RN Baccalaureate Program (BSN)

Applying *Required:* SAT I, ACT, TOEFL for nonnative speakers of English, minimum college GPA of 2.5, RN license, diploma or AD in nursing, high school transcript, 3 letters of recommendation, written essay, transcript of college record. 62 prerequisite credits must be completed before admission to the nursing program. *Options:* Advanced standing available through the following means: advanced placement exams, credit by exam. May apply for transfer of up to 65 total credits. *Application deadline:* 10/15. *Application fee:* $25.

Degree Requirements 124 total credit hours, 62 in nursing.

MASTER'S PROGRAMS

Contact Dr. Rita Clifford, Associate Dean, Student Affairs, School of Nursing, University of Kansas, 3901 Rainbow Boulevard, Kansas City, KS 66160-7501, 913-588-1619. *Fax:* 913-588-1660. *E-mail:* rcliffor@kumc.edu

Areas of Study Clinical nurse specialist programs in adult health nursing, community health nursing, pediatric nursing, psychiatric–mental health nursing; nursing administration; nurse practitioner programs in adult health, family health, psychiatric–mental health, women's health.

Expenses *State resident tuition:* $1128 full-time, $94 per credit hour part-time. *Nonresident tuition:* $3708 full-time, $309 per credit hour part-time. *Full-time mandatory fees:* $21–$56. *Books and supplies per academic year:* $600.

Financial Aid Graduate assistantships, nurse traineeships, Federal Nursing Student Loans, institutionally sponsored loans, employment opportunities, institutionally sponsored non-need-based grants/scholarships. *Application deadline:* 4/15.

RN to Master's Program (MS)

Applying *Required:* GRE General Test, TOEFL for nonnative speakers of English, bachelor's degree in nursing, minimum GPA of 3.0, RN license, 1 year of clinical experience, physical assessment course, essay, interview, 3 letters of recommendation, transcript of college record, graduate level statistics course. *Application deadlines:* 7/1 (fall), 11/1 (spring), 4/1 (summer). *Application fee:* $25.

Degree Requirements 36–48 total credit hours dependent upon track, 29–43 in nursing, 16–20 in statistics and business or health service administration. Thesis or research project.

Distance learning Courses provided through on-line, compressed video. Specific degree requirements include ON LINE available only to Garden City area students currently.

MS/MHSA Program

Applying *Required:* GRE General Test, bachelor's degree in nursing, minimum GPA of 3.0, RN license, 2 years of clinical experience, physical assessment course, essay, interview, 3 letters of recommendation, transcript of college record. *Application deadlines:* 7/1 (fall), 11/1 (spring), 4/1 (summer). *Application fee:* $25.

Degree Requirements 75 total credit hours, 29–46 in nursing, 32–46 in business, health service administration, statistics. Thesis or research project.

DOCTORAL PROGRAMS

Contact Dr. Rita Clifford, Associate Dean, Student Affairs, School of Nursing, University of Kansas, 3901 Rainbow Boulevard, Kansas City, KS 66160-7501, 913-588-1619. *Fax:* 913-588-1660. *E-mail:* rcliffor@kumc.edu

Areas of Study Nursing education, nursing research.

Expenses *State resident tuition:* $94 per credit hour. *Nonresident tuition:* $309 per credit hour. *Full-time mandatory fees:* $21–$56. *Books and supplies per academic year:* $400.

Financial Aid Graduate assistantships, nurse traineeships, fellowships, dissertation grants, grants, Federal Nursing Student Loans, institutionally sponsored loans, opportunities for employment, institutionally sponsored non-need-based grants/scholarships. *Application deadline:* 4/15.

PhD Program

Applying *Required:* GRE General Test, TOEFL for nonnative speakers of English, master's degree in nursing, master's degree, statistics course, interview, 3 letters of recommendation, vitae, writing sample, competitive review by faculty committee. *Application deadlines:* 4/1 (fall), 9/1 (spring). *Application fee:* $25.

Degree Requirements 66 total credit hours; 24 hours in nursing, 12 hours in minor, 12 hours in support courses, 18 hours of dissertation research; dissertation; oral exam; written exam; defense of dissertation; residency.

PhD/MBA Program

Applying *Required:* GRE General Test, TOEFL for nonnative speakers of English, master's degree in nursing, master's degree, statistics course, interview, 3 letters of recommendation, vitae, writing sample, competitive review by faculty committee. *Application deadlines:* 4/1 (fall), 9/11 (spring). *Application fee:* $25.

Degree Requirements 122 total credit hours; 24 hours in nursing, 12 hours in minor, 12 hours in support courses, 18 hours dissertation research, 56 hours in business; dissertation; oral exam; written exam; defense of dissertation; residency.

CONTINUING EDUCATION PROGRAM

Contact Pat Wahlstedt, Director, School of Nursing, University of Kansas, 3901 Rainbow Boulevard, Kansas City, KS 66160-7504, 913-588-1610. *Fax:* 913-588-1660. *E-mail:* pwahlste@kumc.edu

WASHBURN UNIVERSITY OF TOPEKA

School of Nursing
Topeka, Kansas

Programs • Generic Baccalaureate • Accelerated RN Baccalaureate • LPN to Baccalaureate • Continuing Education

The University City-supported comprehensive coed institution. Founded: 1865. *Primary accreditation:* regional. *Setting:* 160-acre urban campus. *Total enrollment:* 6,314.

The School of Nursing Founded in 1974. *Nursing program faculty:* 25 (20% with doctorates).

Academic Facilities *Campus library:* 323,647 volumes (13,592 in health, 2,000 in nursing); 1,614 periodical subscriptions (79 health-care related). *Nursing school resources:* CAI, computer lab, nursing audiovisuals, interactive nursing skills videos, learning resource lab, Internet.

Student Life *Student services:* health clinic, child-care facilities, personal counseling, career counseling, institutionally sponsored work-study program, job placement, campus safety program, special assistance for disabled students, learning enhancement center, writing center. *International student services:* counseling/support, special assistance for nonnative speakers of English, ESL courses, international center. *Nursing student activities:* Sigma Theta Tau, student nurses association.

Calendar Semesters.

NURSING STUDENT PROFILE

Undergraduate **Enrollment:** 250

Women: 83%; **Men:** 17%; **Minority:** 11%; **International:** 1%; **Part-time:** 13%

BACCALAUREATE PROGRAMS

Contact Ms. Mary V. Allen, Nursing Adviser, School of Nursing, Washburn University of Topeka, 1700 College Avenue, Topeka, KS 66621, 913-231-1010 Ext. 1525. *Fax:* 913-231-1089. *E-mail:* zzalle@acc.wuacc.edu

Expenses *State resident tuition:* $2880 full-time, $96 per credit hour part-time. *Nonresident tuition:* $6330 full-time, $211 per credit hour part-time. *Full-time mandatory fees:* $32. *Part-time mandatory fees:* $16. *Room and board:* $3110. *Books and supplies per academic year:* ranges from $600 to $800.

Financial Aid Institutionally sponsored need-based grants/scholarships, institutionally sponsored non-need grants/scholarships, Federal Direct Loans, Federal Perkins Loans, Federal Supplemental Educational Opportunity Grants, Federal Work-Study, endowed nursing scholarships. *Application deadline:* 3/1.

Generic Baccalaureate Program (BSN)

Applying *Required:* ACT, TOEFL for nonnative speakers of English, minimum college GPA of 2.7, written essay, transcript of college record, 2 references. 30 prerequisite credits must be completed before admission to the nursing program. *Options:* Advanced standing available through advanced placement exams. Course work may be accelerated. May apply for transfer of up to 84 total credits. *Application deadlines:* 2/15 (fall), 10/15 (spring).

Degree Requirements 124 total credit hours, 59 in nursing.

Accelerated RN Baccalaureate Program (BSN)

Applying *Required:* TOEFL for nonnative speakers of English, Commission on Graduates of Foreign Nursing Schools exam, minimum college GPA of 2.5, RN license, diploma or AD in nursing, written essay, transcript of college record, 2 references. 30 prerequisite credits must be completed before admission to the nursing program. *Options:* Advanced standing available through the following means: advanced placement exams, credit by exam. May apply for transfer of up to 27 total credits. *Application deadlines:* 2/15 (fall), 10/15 (spring).

Degree Requirements 124 total credit hours, 59 in nursing.

LPN to Baccalaureate Program (BSN)

Applying *Required:* ACT, minimum college GPA of 2.5, high school transcript, written essay, transcript of college record, LPN license. 30 prerequisite credits must be completed before admission to the nursing program. *Options:* Advanced standing available through the following means: advanced placement without credit, credit by exam. Course work may be accelerated. *Application deadlines:* 2/15 (fall), 10/15 (spring).

Degree Requirements 124 total credit hours, 59 in nursing.

CONTINUING EDUCATION PROGRAM

Contact Dr. Lois Rimmer, Assistant Dean and Professor, School of Nursing, Washburn University of Topeka, 1700 College Avenue, Topeka, KS 66621, 913-231-1010 Ext. 1210. *Fax:* 913-231-1089.

See full description on page 568.

WICHITA STATE UNIVERSITY

School of Nursing
Wichita, Kansas

Programs • Generic Baccalaureate • Accelerated RN Baccalaureate • MSN • RN to Master's • Continuing Education

The University State-supported coed university. Founded: 1895. *Primary accreditation:* regional. *Setting:* 335-acre urban campus. *Total enrollment:* 14,568.

The School of Nursing Founded in 1968. *Nursing program faculty:* 38 (37% with doctorates).

▶ ***NOTEWORTHY***

Wichita State University School of Nursing is located in the largest urban area in Kansas. This metropolitan advantage provides students with high-quality and diverse clinical learning experiences and

Wichita State University (continued)

community outreach activities. Progression to the BSN degree is facilitated for both traditional and nontraditional students through two admission classes per year. At the graduate level, technology provides avenues for Internet courses in nursing informatics and collaborative teaching in the family nurse practitioner program. The resources of the largest health-care community in the region, serving both rural and urban needs, are available to the MSN/MBA dual-degree program.

Academic Facilities *Campus library:* 1.0 million volumes (30,720 in health, 2,680 in nursing); 3,755 periodical subscriptions (406 health-care related). *Nursing school resources:* CAI, computer lab, nursing audiovisuals, interactive nursing skills videos, learning resource lab.

Student Life *Student services:* health clinic, child-care facilities, personal counseling, career counseling, institutionally sponsored work-study program, job placement, campus safety program, special assistance for disabled students. *International student services:* counseling/support, special assistance for nonnative speakers of English, ESL courses. *Nursing student activities:* Sigma Theta Tau, nursing club, student nurses association.

Calendar Semesters.

NURSING STUDENT PROFILE

Undergraduate **Enrollment:** 222
Women: 90%; **Men:** 10%; **Minority:** 17%; **International:** 2%; **Part-time:** 16%
Graduate **Enrollment:** 199
Women: 94%; **Men:** 6%; **Minority:** 5%; **Part-time:** 85%

BACCALAUREATE PROGRAMS

Contact Dr. Pam Larsen, Director, School of Nursing, Wichita State University, Wichita, KS 67260-0041, 316-978-3978 Ext. 5741. *Fax:* 316-978-3094. *E-mail:* larsen@chp.twsu.edu

Expenses *State resident tuition:* $1903 full-time, $79 per credit hour part-time. *Nonresident tuition:* $6642 full-time, $277 per credit hour part-time. *Full-time mandatory fees:* $475–$785. *Room and board:* $2945–$3465. *Room only:* $1565–$3635. *Books and supplies per academic year:* ranges from $500 to $950.

Financial Aid Institutionally sponsored need-based grants/scholarships, institutionally sponsored non-need grants/scholarships, Federal Perkins Loans, Federal Supplemental Educational Opportunity Grants, Federal Work-Study. *Application deadline:* 3/15.

Generic Baccalaureate Program (BSN)

Applying *Required:* TOEFL for nonnative speakers of English, NET Test, minimum high school GPA of 2.0, minimum college GPA of 2.5, high school transcript, written essay, transcript of college record. 60 prerequisite credits must be completed before admission to the nursing program. *Application deadlines:* 2/1 (fall), 9/1 (spring). *Application fee:* $15.

Degree Requirements 124 total credit hours, 55 in nursing.

Accelerated RN Baccalaureate Program (BSN)

Applying *Required:* TOEFL for nonnative speakers of English, minimum high school GPA of 2.0, minimum college GPA of 2.5, RN license, diploma or AD in nursing, high school transcript, transcript of college record. 60 prerequisite credits must be completed before admission to the nursing program. *Options:* Advanced standing available through credit by exam. May apply for transfer of up to 23 total credits. *Application deadline:* rolling. *Application fee:* $15.

Degree Requirements 124 total credit hours, 55 in nursing.

MASTER'S PROGRAMS

Contact Dr. Donna Hawley, Director, Graduate Program, School of Nursing, Wichita State University, Wichita, KS 67260-0041, 316-978-3610. *Fax:* 316-978-3094. *E-mail:* hawley@chp.twsu.edu

Areas of Study Clinical nurse specialist programs in adult health nursing, community health nursing, gerontological nursing, maternity-newborn nursing, medical-surgical nursing, pediatric nursing, psychiatric–mental health nursing; nursing administration; nursing education; nurse practitioner programs in child care/pediatrics, family health.

Expenses *State resident tuition:* $2617 full-time, $109 per credit hour part-time. *Nonresident tuition:* $7781 full-time, $320 per credit hour part-time. *Full-time mandatory fees:* $485–$865. *Room and board:* $2945–$3465. *Room only:* $1565–$3635. *Books and supplies per academic year:* ranges from $300 to $1500.

Financial Aid Graduate assistantships, nurse traineeships, institutionally sponsored loans, employment opportunities. *Application deadline:* 3/15.

MSN Program

Applying *Required:* bachelor's degree in nursing, minimum GPA of 3.0, RN license, 1 year of clinical experience, statistics course, professional liability/malpractice insurance, transcript of college record.

Degree Requirements 42 total credit hours, 36–42 in nursing. Thesis or project.

RN to Master's Program (MSN)

Applying *Required:* minimum GPA of 3.5, RN license, 3 years of clinical experience, statistics course, professional liability/malpractice insurance, 3 letters of recommendation, transcript of college record, BSN earned concurrently.

CONTINUING EDUCATION PROGRAM

Contact Ms. MaryAnn Claypool, Non-credit Program Officer, Wichita State University, Division of Continuing Education, Wichita, KS 67260-0136, 316-689-3726. *Fax:* 316-689-3650.

KENTUCKY

BELLARMINE COLLEGE
Lansing School of Nursing
Louisville, Kentucky

Programs • Generic Baccalaureate • RN Baccalaureate • Accelerated Baccalaureate for Second Degree • Master's for Nurses with Non-Nursing Degrees • Continuing Education

The College Independent Roman Catholic comprehensive coed institution. Founded: 1950. *Primary accreditation:* regional. *Setting:* 120-acre suburban campus. *Total enrollment:* 2,359.

The Lansing School of Nursing Founded in 1976. *Nursing program faculty:* 37 (50% with doctorates). *Off-campus program site:* Ashland.

Academic Facilities *Campus library:* 115,730 volumes (27,000 in nursing); 615 periodical subscriptions (100 health-care related). *Nursing school resources:* CAI, computer lab, nursing audiovisuals, interactive nursing skills videos, learning resource lab.

Student Life *Student services:* health clinic, personal counseling, career counseling, institutionally sponsored work-study program, job placement, campus safety program, special assistance for disabled students. *International student services:* counseling/support, special assistance for nonnative speakers of English. *Nursing student activities:* Sigma Theta Tau, student nurses association.

Calendar Semesters.

NURSING STUDENT PROFILE

Undergraduate **Enrollment:** 297
Women: 85%; **Men:** 15%; **Minority:** 3%; **International:** 0%; **Part-time:** 51%
Graduate **Enrollment:** 123
Women: 98%; **Men:** 2%; **Minority:** 3%; **International:** 0%; **Part-time:** 100%

BACCALAUREATE PROGRAMS

Contact Admissions, Bellarmine College, Newburg Road, Louisville, KY 40205, 502-452-8131. *Fax:* 502-452-8038.

Expenses *Tuition:* $10,320 full-time, $305 part-time. *Full-time mandatory fees:* $15–$90+. *Room and board:* $1400–$3600. *Books and supplies per academic year:* $350.

Financial Aid Institutionally sponsored need-based grants/scholarships, institutionally sponsored non-need grants/scholarships, Federal Pell Grants, Federal Perkins Loans, Federal Supplemental Educational Opportunity Grants, Federal Work-Study. 29% of undergraduate students in nursing programs received some form of financial aid in 1995–96. *Application deadline:* 3/15.

Generic Baccalaureate Program (BSN)

Applying *Required:* SAT I, ACT, TOEFL for nonnative speakers of English, minimum high school GPA of 2.5, minimum college GPA of 2.0, high school chemistry, high school transcript, 2 letters of recommendation, written essay, transcript of college record. 33 prerequisite credits must be completed before admission to the nursing program. *Options:* Advanced standing available through the following means: advanced placement exams, credit by exam. May apply for transfer of up to 92 total credits. *Application deadline:* 3/15. *Application fee:* $25.

Degree Requirements 128 total credit hours, 54 in nursing.

RN Baccalaureate Program (BSN)

Applying *Required:* TOEFL for nonnative speakers of English, RN Mobility II Examinations for diploma graduates only, minimum high school GPA of 2.5, minimum college GPA of 2.5, high school chemistry, RN license, diploma or AD in nursing, high school transcript, 2 letters of recommendation, written essay, transcript of college record. 33 prerequisite credits must be completed before admission to the nursing program. *Options:* Advanced standing available through credit by exam. May apply for transfer of up to 92 total credits. *Application deadline:* 3/15. *Application fee:* $25.

Degree Requirements 128 total credit hours, 57 in nursing.

Accelerated Baccalaureate for Second Degree Program (BSN)

Applying *Required:* TOEFL for nonnative speakers of English, minimum college GPA of 2.5, 2 letters of recommendation, written essay, transcript of college record, verification of baccalaureate degree in another field. 27 prerequisite credits must be completed before admission to the nursing program. *Options:* Course work may be accelerated. *Application deadline:* rolling. *Application fee:* $25.

Degree Requirements 63 total credit hours, 56 in nursing.

MASTER'S PROGRAM

Contact Admission, Bellarmine College, Newburg Road, Louisville, KY 40205, 502-452-8131. *Fax:* 502-452-8038.

Areas of Study Nursing administration; nursing education.

Expenses *Tuition:* $5940 full-time, $330 part-time. *Books and supplies per academic year:* ranges from $200 to $250.

Financial Aid Graduate assistantships, institutionally sponsored need-based grants/scholarships.

Master's for Nurses with Non-Nursing Degrees Program (MSN)

Applying *Required:* GRE General Test, TOEFL for nonnative speakers of English, bachelor's degree, minimum GPA of 2.75, RN license, professional liability/malpractice insurance, essay, interview, 2 letters of recommendation, transcript of college record. *Application fee:* $25.

Degree Requirements 38–41 total credit hours dependent upon track, 22–34 in nursing. Thesis required.

CONTINUING EDUCATION PROGRAM

Contact Dr. Susan Hockenberger, Dean, Lansing School of Nursing, Bellarmine College, Newburg Road, Louisville, KY 40205, 502-452-8414. *Fax:* 502-452-8058.

BEREA COLLEGE
Department of Nursing
Berea, Kentucky

Programs • Generic Baccalaureate • Continuing Education

The College Independent 4-year coed college. Founded: 1855. *Primary accreditation:* regional. *Setting:* 140-acre small-town campus. *Total enrollment:* 1,559.

The Department of Nursing Founded in 1960. *Nursing program faculty:* 10 (40% with doctorates).

Academic Facilities *Campus library:* 296,272 volumes (4,776 in health); 1,366 periodical subscriptions (73 health-care related). *Nursing school resources:* CAI, computer lab, nursing audiovisuals, interactive nursing skills videos, learning resource lab.

Student Life *Student services:* health clinic, child-care facilities, personal counseling, career counseling, institutionally sponsored work-study program, job placement, campus safety program, special assistance for disabled students. *International student services:* counseling/support, special assistance for nonnative speakers of English, ESL courses. *Nursing student activities:* nursing club, student nurses association.

Calendar 4-1-4.

NURSING STUDENT PROFILE

Undergraduate **Enrollment:** 46
Women: 85%; **Men:** 15%; **Minority:** 20%; **International:** 13%

BACCALAUREATE PROGRAM

Contact Dr. Cora Newell-Withrow, Chairperson and Professor, Department of Nursing, Berea College, CPO 2290, Berea, KY 40404, 606-986-9341 Ext. 5382. *Fax:* 606-986-4506.

Expenses *Tuition:* $0 full-time, $0 part-time. *Full-time mandatory fees:* $250. *Room and board:* $2634. *Room only:* $1134. *Books and supplies per academic year:* $500. All students are required to work a minimum of 10 hours per week in lieu of tuition.

Financial Aid Institutionally sponsored need-based grants/scholarships, institutionally sponsored non-need grants/scholarships, Federal Pell Grants, Federal Perkins Loans, Federal Supplemental Educational Opportunity Grants, Federal Work-Study. 100% of undergraduate students in nursing programs received some form of financial aid in 1995–96. *Application deadline:* 3/1.

Generic Baccalaureate Program (BS)

Applying *Required:* SAT I, ACT, high school transcript, letter of recommendation, written essay, transcript of college record, high school class rank: top 20%. 15 prerequisite credits must be completed before admission to the nursing program. *Application deadline:* rolling. *Application fee:* $5.

Degree Requirements 34 total credit hours, 14 in nursing.

CONTINUING EDUCATION PROGRAM

Contact Dr. Pamela Farley, Associate Professor, Department of Nursing, Berea College, CPO 606, Berea, KY 40404, 606-986-9341 Ext. 5384. *Fax:* 606-986-4506.

EASTERN KENTUCKY UNIVERSITY
Department of Baccalaureate Nursing
Richmond, Kentucky

Programs • Generic Baccalaureate • RN Baccalaureate • BSN to Master's

The University State-supported comprehensive coed institution. Part of Kentucky Council on Higher Education. Founded: 1906. *Primary accreditation:* regional. *Setting:* 350-acre small-town campus. *Total enrollment:* 16,060.

The Department of Baccalaureate Nursing Founded in 1971.

Academic Facilities *Campus library:* 850,000 volumes (1,450 in nursing); 4,070 periodical subscriptions (60 health-care related).

Calendar Semesters.

NURSING STUDENT PROFILE

Undergraduate **Enrollment:** 350
Women: 80%; **Men:** 20%; **Minority:** 15%; **International:** 5%; **Part-time:** 40%

BACCALAUREATE PROGRAMS

Contact Dr. Deborah Whitehouse, Chair, Department of Baccalaureate Nursing, Eastern Kentucky University, Rowlett 223, Richmond, KY 40475, 606-622-1956. *Fax:* 606-622-1972.

Expenses *State resident tuition:* $1970 full-time, $82 per credit hour part-time. *Nonresident tuition:* $5450 per academic year.

Financial Aid Institutionally sponsored need-based grants/scholarships, institutionally sponsored non-need grants/scholarships, Federal Pell Grants, Federal Perkins Loans, Federal Supplemental Educational Opportunity Grants, Federal Work-Study, Federal PLUS Loans, Federal Stafford Loans.

Eastern Kentucky University (continued)

Generic Baccalaureate Program (BSN)

Applying *Required:* ACT, TOEFL for nonnative speakers of English, minimum college GPA of 2.5, 3 years of high school math, high school chemistry, high school biology.

Degree Requirements 131 total credit hours, 54 in nursing.

RN Baccalaureate Program (BSN)

Applying *Required:* minimum college GPA of 2.5, RN license, diploma or AD in nursing, transcript of college record.

Degree Requirements 131 total credit hours, 54 in nursing.

MASTER'S PROGRAM

Areas of Study Nursing administration; nurse practitioner programs in community health, rural health.

Expenses *State resident tuition:* $2150 full-time, $120 per credit hour part-time. *Nonresident tuition:* $5990 per academic year.

BSN to Master's Program (MSN)

Applying *Required:* GRE General Test (minimum combined score of 1000 on three tests), bachelor's degree in nursing, minimum GPA of 2.7, RN license, 3 letters of recommendation, transcript of college record. *Application deadline:* rolling.

Degree Requirements 39 total credit hours, 30–36 in nursing.

MIDWAY COLLEGE
Program in Nursing
Midway, Kentucky

Program • RN Baccalaureate

The College Independent 4-year women's college, affiliated with Christian Church (Disciples of Christ). Founded: 1847. *Primary accreditation:* regional. *Setting:* 116-acre small-town campus. *Total enrollment:* 930.

The Program in Nursing Founded in 1989. *Nursing program faculty:* 3 (33% with doctorates). *Off-campus program site:* Danville.

Academic Facilities *Campus library:* 38,600 volumes (600 in nursing); 425 periodical subscriptions (80 health-care related). *Nursing school resources:* CAI, computer lab, nursing audiovisuals, interactive nursing skills videos, learning resource lab, compressed video classroom.

Student Life *Student services:* health clinic, child-care facilities, personal counseling, career counseling, institutionally sponsored work-study program, job placement, campus safety program. *Nursing student activities:* student nurses association.

Calendar Semesters.

NURSING STUDENT PROFILE

Undergraduate **Enrollment:** 48
Women: 100%; **Minority:** 6%; **International:** 0%; **Part-time:** 51%

BACCALAUREATE PROGRAM

Contact Barbara Clark, Chair, BSN Program, Program in Nursing, Midway College, 512 East Stephens Street, Midway, KY 40347-1120, 606-846-5730. *Fax:* 606-846-5349.

Expenses *Tuition:* $8775 full-time, $270 per credit hour part-time. *Full-time mandatory fees:* $85–$100. *Part-time mandatory fees:* $25. *Room and board:* $4250. *Books and supplies per academic year:* ranges from $500 to $600.

Financial Aid Institutionally sponsored need-based grants/scholarships, institutionally sponsored non-need grants/scholarships, Federal Direct Loans, Federal Pell Grants, Federal Perkins Loans, Federal Supplemental Educational Opportunity Grants, Federal Work-Study. 31% of undergraduate students in nursing programs received some form of financial aid in 1995–96. *Application deadline:* 4/1.

RN Baccalaureate Program (BSN)

Applying *Required:* ACT, TOEFL for nonnative speakers of English, minimum college GPA of 2.3, RN license, diploma or AD in nursing, high school transcript, interview, transcript of college record, personal resume/vita. 60 prerequisite credits must be completed before admission to the nursing program. *Options:* Advanced standing available through the following means: advanced placement exams, advanced placement without credit, credit by exam. Course work may be accelerated. May apply for transfer of up to 90 total credits. *Application deadline:* rolling. *Application fee:* $20.

Degree Requirements 130 total credit hours, 69 in nursing. 60 hours from BSN completion program.

Distance learning Courses provided through interactive compressed video.

MOREHEAD STATE UNIVERSITY
Department of Nursing and Allied Health Sciences
Morehead, Kentucky

Programs • Generic Baccalaureate • RN Baccalaureate • Continuing Education

The University State-supported comprehensive coed institution. Founded: 1922. *Primary accreditation:* regional. *Setting:* 809-acre small-town campus. *Total enrollment:* 8,454.

The Department of Nursing and Allied Health Sciences Founded in 1986. *Nursing program faculty:* 12 (25% with doctorates). *Off-campus program sites:* Ashland, Prestonsburg.

Academic Facilities *Campus library:* 14,500 volumes in nursing; 75 health-care related periodical subscriptions. *Nursing school resources:* CAI, computer lab, nursing audiovisuals, interactive nursing skills videos, learning resource lab.

Student Life *Student services:* health clinic, personal counseling, career counseling, institutionally sponsored work-study program, job placement, campus safety program, special assistance for disabled students. *International student services:* counseling/support, special assistance for nonnative speakers of English. *Nursing student activities:* nursing club, student nurses association.

Calendar Semesters.

NURSING STUDENT PROFILE

Undergraduate **Enrollment:** 200
Women: 90%; **Men:** 10%; **Minority:** 1%; **International:** 0%; **Part-time:** 25%

BACCALAUREATE PROGRAMS

Contact Dr. Betty Porter, Chair, Reed Hall, Department of Nursing and Allied Health Sciences, Morehead State University, Morehead, KY 40351, 606-783-2296. *Fax:* 606-783-5039. *E-mail:* b.porter@morehead-st.edu

Expenses *State resident tuition:* $1045 full-time, $88 per credit hour part-time. *Nonresident tuition:* $2780 full-time, $237 per credit hour part-time. *Full-time mandatory fees:* $80–$120. *Room only:* $1500. *Books and supplies per academic year:* ranges from $100 to $350.

Financial Aid Institutionally sponsored need-based grants/scholarships, Federal Direct Loans, Federal Perkins Loans, Federal Supplemental Educational Opportunity Grants, Federal Work-Study. 70% of undergraduate students in nursing programs received some form of financial aid in 1995–96. *Application deadline:* 2/1.

Generic Baccalaureate Program (BSN)

Applying *Required:* ACT, minimum college GPA of 2.5, high school transcript, transcript of college record. 34 prerequisite credits must be completed before admission to the nursing program. *Options:* Advanced standing available through credit by exam. *Application deadline:* 3/1.

Degree Requirements 134 total credit hours, 63 in nursing.

RN Baccalaureate Program (BSN)

Applying *Required:* ACT, NLN Mobility Profile II, minimum college GPA of 2.0, RN license, diploma or AD in nursing, transcript of college record. *Options:* Advanced standing available through credit by exam. *Application deadlines:* 3/1 (fall), 9/1 (spring).

Degree Requirements 60 total credit hours, 32 in nursing.

Distance learning Courses provided through on-line, compressed interactive video.

CONTINUING EDUCATION PROGRAM

Contact Mrs. Gail Wise, Assistant Director, Continuing Education, Morehead State University, 108 Waterfield Hall, Morehead, KY 40351, 606-783-2635. *Fax:* 606-783-2678.

MURRAY STATE UNIVERSITY
Department of Nursing
Murray, Kentucky

Programs • Generic Baccalaureate • RN Baccalaureate • MSN • RN to Master's • Post-Master's

The University State-supported comprehensive coed institution. Part of Kentucky Council on Higher Education. Founded: 1922. *Primary accreditation:* regional. *Setting:* 238-acre small-town campus. *Total enrollment:* 8,166.

The Department of Nursing Founded in 1964.

Academic Facilities *Campus library:* 360,776 volumes (9,801 in health, 1,251 in nursing); 2,327 periodical subscriptions (64 health-care related).

Calendar Semesters.

BACCALAUREATE PROGRAMS

Contact Chair, Department of Nursing, Murray State University, 1 Murray Street, Murray, KY 42071-3306, 502-762-2193. *Fax:* 502-762-6662.

Expenses *State resident tuition:* $2060 per academic year. *Nonresident tuition:* $5440 per academic year.

GENERIC BACCALAUREATE PROGRAM (BSN)

Applying *Required:* ACT, minimum college GPA of 2.5, high school transcript, transcript of college record. *Application deadlines:* 3/15 (fall), 11/15 (spring). *Application fee:* $15.

Degree Requirements 130–132 total credit hours dependent upon track, 60 in nursing.

RN BACCALAUREATE PROGRAM (BSN)

Applying *Required:* ACT, minimum college GPA of 2.5, RN license, diploma or AD in nursing, high school transcript, transcript of college record. 21 prerequisite credits must be completed before admission to the nursing program. *Application deadline:* 3/15. *Application fee:* $15.

Degree Requirements 128 total credit hours, 59 in nursing.

MASTER'S PROGRAMS

Contact Chair, Department of Nursing, Murray State University, 1 Murray Street, Murray, KY 42071-3306, 502-762-2193. *Fax:* 502-762-6662.

Areas of Study Clinical nurse specialist program in adult health nursing; nurse anesthesia; nurse practitioner program in family health.

Expenses *State resident tuition:* $2240 per academic year. *Nonresident tuition:* $6080 per academic year.

MSN PROGRAM

Applying *Required:* GRE General Test (minimum combined score of 800 on verbal and quantitative sections), bachelor's degree in nursing, RN license, transcript of college record. *Application deadline:* 3/15. *Application fee:* $15.

RN TO MASTER'S PROGRAM (MSN)

Applying *Required:* GRE General Test (minimum combined score of 800 on verbal and quantitative sections), 3 letters of recommendation, transcript of college record. *Application deadline:* 4/15. *Application fee:* $15.

POST-MASTER'S PROGRAM

Applying *Required:* GRE General Test, bachelor's degree in nursing, RN license, transcript of college record. *Application deadline:* 3/15. *Application fee:* $15.

Degree Requirements 32 total credit hours, 29 in nursing.

NORTHERN KENTUCKY UNIVERSITY
Department of Nursing
Highland Heights, Kentucky

Programs • Accelerated RN Baccalaureate • BSN to Master's • Post-Master's

The University State-supported comprehensive coed institution. Founded: 1968. *Primary accreditation:* regional. *Setting:* 300-acre suburban campus. *Total enrollment:* 11,671.

The Department of Nursing Founded in 1964. *Nursing program faculty:* 8 (50% with doctorates).

Academic Facilities *Campus library:* 530,418 volumes (2,180 in health, 5,720 in nursing); 3,964 periodical subscriptions (90 health-care related). *Nursing school resources:* CAI, computer lab, nursing audiovisuals, interactive nursing skills videos, learning resource lab.

Student Life *Student services:* health clinic, child-care facilities, personal counseling, career counseling, institutionally sponsored work-study program, job placement, campus safety program, special assistance for disabled students. *International student services:* counseling/support, special assistance for nonnative speakers of English. *Nursing student activities:* student nurses association.

Calendar Semesters.

NURSING STUDENT PROFILE

Undergraduate **Enrollment:** 92
Women: 96%; **Men:** 4%; **Minority:** 1%; **International:** 0%; **Part-time:** 62%
Graduate **Enrollment:** 52
Women: 95%; **Men:** 5%; **Minority:** 1%; **International:** 0%; **Part-time:** 95%

BACCALAUREATE PROGRAM

Contact Margaret Anderson, Director, BSN Program for RN's, 303 Albright Health Center, Department of Nursing, Northern Kentucky University, Highland Heights, KY 41099, 606-572-5553. *Fax:* 606-572-6098. *E-mail:* manderson@nku.edu

Expenses *State resident tuition:* $2020 full-time, $86 per semester hour part-time. *Nonresident tuition:* $5500 full-time, $231 per semester hour part-time. *Full-time mandatory fees:* $78. *Part-time mandatory fees:* $96. *Room and board:* $3164–$5930. *Room only:* $3164–$4490. *Books and supplies per academic year:* ranges from $250 to $500.

Financial Aid Institutionally sponsored need-based grants/scholarships, institutionally sponsored non-need grants/scholarships, Federal Direct Loans, Federal Nursing Student Loans, Federal Work-Study. *Application deadline:* 4/1.

ACCELERATED RN BACCALAUREATE PROGRAM (BSN)

Applying *Required:* minimum college GPA of 2.5, RN license, diploma or AD in nursing, transcript of college record, CPR certification, health record. *Options:* Advanced standing available through credit by exam. May apply for transfer of up to 98 total credits. *Application deadlines:* 8/1 (fall), 1/1 (spring). *Application fee:* $25.

Degree Requirements 129–134 total credit hours dependent upon track, 45 in nursing.

MASTER'S PROGRAMS

Contact Dr. Denise Robinson, Director of Graduate Nursing Program, Department of Nursing, Northern Kentucky University, Highland Heights, KY 41099, 606-572-5178. *Fax:* 606-572-6098. *E-mail:* robinson@nku.edu

Areas of Study Clinical nurse specialist program in acute care nursing; nursing administration; nurse practitioner programs in adult health, family health.

Expenses *State resident tuition:* $2200 full-time, $120 per semester hour part-time. *Nonresident tuition:* $6040 full-time, $333 per semester hour part-time. *Full-time mandatory fees:* $96. *Room and board:* $3164–$5930. *Room only:* $3164–$4490. *Books and supplies per academic year:* ranges from $250 to $500.

Financial Aid Graduate assistantships, Federal Direct Loans, Federal Nursing Student Loans, Kentucky Board of Nursing Loan and Clinical Agency Tuition Reimbursement. 2% of master's level students in nursing programs received some form of financial aid in 1995-96. *Application deadline:* 4/1.

BSN TO MASTER'S PROGRAM (MSN)

Applying *Required:* GRE General Test, GPA x 200 + GRE =1800, bachelor's degree in nursing, minimum GPA of 3.0, RN license, physical assessment course, statistics course, professional liability/malpractice insurance, transcript of college record. *Application deadlines:* 1/31 (adult and family nurse practitioner track), rolling. *Application fee:* $25.

Degree Requirements 36–40 total credit hours dependent upon track, 29–34 in nursing, 3–7 in advanced statistics and advanced human physiology. Integrative project.

POST-MASTER'S PROGRAM

Applying *Required:* bachelor's degree in nursing, minimum GPA of 3.0, RN license, 1 year of clinical experience, physical assessment course,

Northern Kentucky University (continued)

statistics course, professional liability/malpractice insurance, transcript of college record, MSN or equivalent. *Application deadline:* 1/31. *Application fee:* $25.

Degree Requirements 20 total credit hours, 16 in nursing, 4 in advanced human physiology.

SPALDING UNIVERSITY
School of Nursing and Health Sciences
Louisville, Kentucky

Programs • Generic Baccalaureate • MSN

The University Independent comprehensive coed institution, affiliated with Roman Catholic Church. Founded: 1814. *Primary accreditation:* regional. *Setting:* 5-acre urban campus. *Total enrollment:* 1,342.

The School of Nursing and Health Sciences Founded in 1933. *Nursing program faculty:* 32 (25% with doctorates).

Academic Facilities *Campus library:* 160,000 volumes; 459 periodical subscriptions (90 health-care related). *Nursing school resources:* CAI, computer lab, nursing audiovisuals, learning resource lab, health assessment lab.

Student Life *Student services:* health clinic, personal counseling, career counseling, institutionally sponsored work-study program, campus safety program. *International student services:* counseling/support. *Nursing student activities:* Sigma Theta Tau, recruiter club, student nurses association.

Calendar Semesters.

NURSING STUDENT PROFILE

Undergraduate **Enrollment:** 178
Women: 94%; **Men:** 6%; **Minority:** 5%; **International:** 0%; **Part-time:** 0%
Graduate **Enrollment:** 60
Women: 97%; **Men:** 3%; **Minority:** 3%; **Part-time:** 55%

BACCALAUREATE PROGRAM

Contact Dr. Marjorie M. Perrin, Dean and Professor, School of Nursing and Health Sciences, Spalding University, Louisville, KY 40203-2188, 502-585-7125. *Fax:* 502-588-7175.

Expenses *Tuition:* $9600 full-time, $300 per credit hour part-time. *Full-time mandatory fees:* $290. *Room and board:* $2520–$3350. *Books and supplies per academic year:* ranges from $400 to $500.

Financial Aid Institutionally sponsored need-based grants/scholarships, institutionally sponsored non-need grants/scholarships, Federal Nursing Student Loans, Federal Pell Grants, Federal Perkins Loans, Federal Supplemental Educational Opportunity Grants, Federal Work-Study, Federal Stafford Loans, Kentucky Tuition Grants, College Access Grants, Kentucky Nursing Incentive Scholarship Fund. *Application deadline:* 3/1.

Generic Baccalaureate Program (BSN)

Applying *Required:* SAT I or ACT, SAT II Writing Test, TOEFL for nonnative speakers of English, College Board math test, minimum college GPA of 2.5, high school transcript, transcript of college record. 29 prerequisite credits must be completed before admission to the nursing program. *Options:* Advanced standing available through the following means: advanced placement exams, credit by exam. *Application deadline:* 2/16. *Application fee:* $50.

Degree Requirements 131 total credit hours, 50 in nursing.

MASTER'S PROGRAM

Contact Dr. Judy Dulin, Director, School of Nursing and Health Sciences, Spalding University, Louisville, KY 40203-2188, 502-585-7125. *Fax:* 502-585-7158.

Areas of Study Nurse practitioner program in family health.

Expenses *Tuition:* $6240 full-time, $320 per credit part-time. *Full-time mandatory fees:* $301. *Books and supplies per academic year:* ranges from $500 to $1000.

Financial Aid Graduate assistantships, nurse traineeships, Federal Direct Loans, institutionally sponsored cultural diversity scholarships. *Application deadline:* 8/1.

MSN Program

Applying *Required:* GRE General Test (minimum combined score of 1200 on three tests), bachelor's degree in nursing, bachelor's degree, minimum GPA of 2.7, RN license, 1 year of clinical experience, statistics course, professional liability/malpractice insurance, essay, interview, 2 letters of recommendation, transcript of college record, physical assessment course for family nurse practitioner track. *Application deadlines:* 3/1 (fall), 11/1 (spring). *Application fee:* $30.

Degree Requirements 39 total credit hours, 27–39 in nursing, 12 in business administration and electives.

THOMAS MORE COLLEGE
Department of Nursing
Crestview Hills, Kentucky

Programs • Generic Baccalaureate • RN Baccalaureate

The College Independent Roman Catholic comprehensive coed institution. Founded: 1921. *Primary accreditation:* regional. *Setting:* 120-acre suburban campus. *Total enrollment:* 1,345.

The Department of Nursing Founded in 1978.

Academic Facilities *Campus library:* 128,000 volumes; 600 periodical subscriptions.

Calendar Semesters.

BACCALAUREATE PROGRAMS

Contact Chair, Department of Nursing, Thomas More College, Crestview Hills, KY 41017, 606-341-5800. *Fax:* 606-344-3345.

Expenses *Tuition:* $10,450 full-time, ranges from $268 to $300 per semester credit part-time. *Room and board:* $4286–$4952. *Room only:* $905–$1238.

Generic Baccalaureate Program (BSN)

Applying *Required:* SAT I or ACT, TOEFL for nonnative speakers of English, minimum high school GPA of 2.0. *Application fee:* $15.

Degree Requirements 128 total credit hours.

RN Baccalaureate Program (BSN)

Applying *Required:* SAT I or ACT, minimum college GPA of 2.0. *Application fee:* $15.

Degree Requirements 128 total credit hours.

UNIVERSITY OF KENTUCKY
College of Nursing
Lexington, Kentucky

Programs • Generic Baccalaureate • RN Baccalaureate • MSN • RN to Master's • Post-Master's • PhD • Continuing Education

The University State-supported coed university. Founded: 1865. *Primary accreditation:* regional. *Setting:* 682-acre urban campus. *Total enrollment:* 23,794.

The College of Nursing Founded in 1960. *Nursing program faculty:* 75 (45% with doctorates). *Off-campus program sites:* Elizabethtown, Hazard, Morehead.

Academic Facilities *Campus library:* 2.5 million volumes (30,000 in health, 5,421 in nursing); 25,000 periodical subscriptions (2,000 health-care related). *Nursing school resources:* CAI, computer lab, nursing audiovisuals, interactive nursing skills videos, learning resource lab.

Student Life *Student services:* health clinic, personal counseling, career counseling, institutionally sponsored work-study program, job placement, campus safety program, special assistance for disabled students. *International student services:* counseling/support, special assistance for

nonnative speakers of English, ESL courses. *Nursing student activities:* Sigma Theta Tau, nursing club, student nurses association.

Calendar Semesters.

NURSING STUDENT PROFILE

Undergraduate **Enrollment:** 404
Women: 92%; **Men:** 8%; **Minority:** 4%; **International:** 0%; **Part-time:** 27%
Graduate **Enrollment:** 197
Women: 90%; **Men:** 10%; **Minority:** 2%; **International:** 1%; **Part-time:** 55%

BACCALAUREATE PROGRAMS

Contact Ms. Joanne Davis, Student Affairs Officer, Undergraduate Studies, College of Nursing, University of Kentucky, Room 309, Lexington, KY 40536-0232, 606-323-5108. *Fax:* 606-323-1057.

Expenses *State resident tuition:* $2676 full-time, $104 per credit hour part-time. *Nonresident tuition:* $7356 full-time, $299 per credit hour part-time. *Full-time mandatory fees:* $334. *Room and board:* $3078–$3200. *Books and supplies per academic year:* ranges from $300 to $550.

Financial Aid Institutionally sponsored need-based grants/scholarships, institutionally sponsored non-need grants/scholarships, Federal Direct Loans, Federal Nursing Student Loans, Federal Perkins Loans, Federal Supplemental Educational Opportunity Grants, Federal Work-Study. *Application deadline:* 4/1.

Generic Baccalaureate Program (BSN)

Applying *Required:* SAT I, ACT, TOEFL for nonnative speakers of English, minimum high school GPA of 2.5, minimum college GPA of 2.35, 3 years of high school math, high school biology, high school transcript, written essay, transcript of college record, 1 year of high school chemistry or physics. *Options:* Advanced standing available through the following means: advanced placement exams, credit by exam. May apply for transfer of up to 67 total credits. *Application deadlines:* 2/1 (fall), 6/1 (spring). *Application fee:* $20.

Degree Requirements 131 total credit hours, 66 in nursing.

RN Baccalaureate Program (BSN)

Applying *Required:* ACT PEP for diploma RNs, minimum college GPA of 2.5, RN license, diploma or AD in nursing, transcript of college record. 60 prerequisite credits must be completed before admission to the nursing program. *Options:* Advanced standing available through credit by exam. May apply for transfer of up to 67 total credits. *Application deadlines:* 2/1 (fall), 6/1 (spring). *Application fee:* $20.

Degree Requirements 131 total credit hours, 40 in nursing.

MASTER'S PROGRAMS

Contact Ms. Julie Wachal, Student Affairs Officer, Graduate Studies, College of Nursing, University of Kentucky, Room 309, Lexington, KY 40536-0232, 606-323-5624. *Fax:* 606-323-1057. *E-mail:* jwachal@pop.uky.edu

Areas of Study Clinical nurse specialist programs in adult health nursing, community health nursing, critical care nursing, family health nursing, gerontological nursing, oncology nursing, parent-child nursing, pediatric nursing, perinatal nursing, psychiatric–mental health nursing, neonatal nursing; nurse midwifery; nursing administration; nurse practitioner programs in acute care, adult health, child care/pediatrics, family health, gerontology, neonatal health, primary care.

Expenses *State resident tuition:* $2580 full-time, $144 per credit hour part-time. *Nonresident tuition:* $7740 full-time, $430 per credit hour part-time. *Full-time mandatory fees:* $336. *Part-time mandatory fees:* $6. *Room only:* $3220–$4030. *Books and supplies per academic year:* ranges from $250 to $350.

Financial Aid Graduate assistantships, nurse traineeships, fellowships, Federal Nursing Student Loans, institutionally sponsored loans. 20% of master's level students in nursing programs received some form of financial aid in 1995-96. *Application deadline:* 3/1.

MSN Program

Applying *Required:* GRE General Test, TOEFL for nonnative speakers of English, bachelor's degree in nursing, minimum GPA of 2.5, RN license, 1 year of clinical experience, physical assessment course, essay, interview, 3 letters of recommendation, transcript of college record, minimum of 2 years of labor and delivery clinical experience for nurse midwife track. *Application deadlines:* 3/1 (fall), 11/1 (spring). *Application fee:* $15–30.

Degree Requirements 33–51 total credit hours dependent upon track, 24 in nursing, 9 in statistics, advanced science, and other specified areas. Research project.

Distance learning Courses provided through video.

RN to Master's Program (MSN)

Applying *Required:* GRE General Test, NLN Mobility Profile II, minimum GPA of 2.5, RN license, 1 year of clinical experience, statistics course, essay, interview, 3 letters of recommendation, transcript of college record. *Application deadlines:* 3/1 (fall), 11/1 (spring). *Application fee:* $15–30.

Degree Requirements 145–158 total credit hours dependent upon track, 58 in nursing.

Distance learning Courses provided through video.

Post-Master's Program

Applying *Required:* minimum GPA of 3.0, RN license, physical assessment course, interview, 2 letters of recommendation, transcript of college record, MSN, letter from preceptor. *Application deadlines:* 3/1 (fall), 11/1 (spring). *Application fee:* $30.

Degree Requirements 28–42 total credit hours dependent upon track, 22–36 in nursing, 6 in pharmacology, elective science.

DOCTORAL PROGRAM

Contact Ms. Julie Wachal, Student Affairs Officer, Graduate Studies, College of Nursing, University of Kentucky, Room 309, Lexington, KY 40536-0232, 606-323-5108. *Fax:* 606-323-1057. *E-mail:* jwachal@pop.uky.edu

Areas of Study Nursing research.

Expenses *State resident tuition:* $2580 full-time, $144 per credit hour part-time. *Nonresident tuition:* $7740 full-time, $144 per credit hour part-time. *Full-time mandatory fees:* $334. *Part-time mandatory fees:* $6. *Room only:* $3220–$4030.

Financial Aid Graduate assistantships, nurse traineeships, fellowships, dissertation grants. *Application deadline:* 2/15.

PhD Program

Applying *Required:* GRE General Test (minimum combined score of 1500 on three tests), TOEFL for nonnative speakers of English, master's degree in nursing, statistics course, interview, 3 letters of recommendation, writing sample, competitive review by faculty committee. *Application deadlines:* 2/15 (fall), 9/15 (spring). *Application fee:* $20.

Degree Requirements 63 total credit hours; 45 hours of coursework, 18 hours of residency credit for dissertation; dissertation; oral exam; written exam; defense of dissertation; residency.

CONTINUING EDUCATION PROGRAM

Contact Dr. Kay Robinson, Director for Continuing Education, College of Nursing, University of Kentucky, Room 315, Lexington, KY 40536-0232, 606-323-5237. *Fax:* 606-323-1057. *E-mail:* mkrobi00@pop.uky.edu

See full description on page 536.

UNIVERSITY OF LOUISVILLE
School of Nursing
Louisville, Kentucky

Programs • Generic Baccalaureate • RN Baccalaureate • MSN • RN to Master's

The University State-supported coed university. Founded: 1798. *Primary accreditation:* regional. *Setting:* 169-acre urban campus. *Total enrollment:* 21,218.

The School of Nursing Founded in 1974. *Nursing program faculty:* 23 (70% with doctorates).

Academic Facilities *Campus library:* 1.3 million volumes (188,856 in health, 4,100 in nursing); 12,263 periodical subscriptions (2,100 health-care related). *Nursing school resources:* CAI, computer lab, nursing audiovisuals, interactive nursing skills videos, learning resource lab.

Student Life *Student services:* health clinic, child-care facilities, personal counseling, career counseling, institutionally sponsored work-study program, job placement, campus safety program, special assistance for

University of Louisville (continued)

disabled students. *International student services:* counseling/support, ESL courses. *Nursing student activities:* Sigma Theta Tau, student nurses association, Nursing Student Council Association.

Calendar Semesters.

NURSING STUDENT PROFILE

Undergraduate **Enrollment:** 333

Women: 85%; **Men:** 15%; **Minority:** 12%; **International:** 0%; **Part-time:** 43%

Graduate **Enrollment:** 108

Women: 96%; **Men:** 4%; **Minority:** 15%; **International:** 0%; **Part-time:** 90%

BACCALAUREATE PROGRAMS

Contact Dr. Deborah Scott, Acting Assistant Dean, Undergraduate Program, School of Nursing, University of Louisville, Louisville, KY 40292, 502-852-5366. *Fax:* 502-852-8783.

Expenses *State resident tuition:* $2570 full-time, $107 per credit hour part-time. *Nonresident tuition:* $7250 full-time, $302 per credit hour part-time. *Full-time mandatory fees:* $30. *Part-time mandatory fees:* $15. *Room only:* $1880–$2480. *Books and supplies per academic year:* ranges from $200 to $600.

Financial Aid Institutionally sponsored need-based grants/scholarships, institutionally sponsored non-need grants/scholarships, Federal Direct Loans, Federal Nursing Student Loans, Federal Pell Grants, Federal Perkins Loans, Federal Supplemental Educational Opportunity Grants, Federal Work-Study. *Application deadline:* 4/15.

Generic Baccalaureate Program (BSN)

Applying *Required:* ACT, TOEFL for nonnative speakers of English, minimum college GPA of 2.5, 3 years of high school math, 3 years of high school science, high school transcript, transcript of college record. 31 prerequisite credits must be completed before admission to the nursing program. *Options:* Course work may be accelerated. May apply for transfer of up to 60 total credits. *Application deadline:* 2/1. *Application fee:* $25.

Degree Requirements 126 total credit hours, 64 in nursing.

RN Baccalaureate Program (BSN)

Applying *Required:* minimum college GPA of 2.5, RN license, transcript of college record. 37 prerequisite credits must be completed before admission to the nursing program. *Options:* Course work may be accelerated. May apply for transfer of up to 60 total credits. *Application deadline:* 2/1. *Application fee:* $25.

Degree Requirements 126 total credit hours, 64 in nursing.

MASTER'S PROGRAMS

Contact Dr. Patricia Lacefield, Acting Dean, Graduate Program, School of Nursing, University of Louisville, Louisville, KY 40292, 502-852-5366. *Fax:* 502-852-8783.

Areas of Study Clinical nurse specialist program in psychiatric–mental health nursing; nurse practitioner programs in adult health, gerontology, neonatal health, women's health.

Expenses *State resident tuition:* $2810 full-time, $155 per credit hour part-time. *Nonresident tuition:* $7970 full-time, $442 per credit hour part-time. *Full-time mandatory fees:* $30. *Part-time mandatory fees:* $15. *Room only:* $1880–$2480. *Books and supplies per academic year:* ranges from $200 to $600.

Financial Aid Nurse traineeships, Federal Nursing Student Loans. *Application deadline:* 4/15.

MSN Program

Applying *Required:* GRE General Test, bachelor's degree in nursing, minimum GPA of 3.0, RN license, 2 letters of recommendation, transcript of college record. *Application deadlines:* 8/1 (fall), 12/1 (spring), 5/1 (summer). *Application fee:* $25.

Degree Requirements 42–45 total credit hours dependent upon track, 39 in nursing, 3 in pharmacology. Thesis or research project.

RN to Master's Program (MSN)

Applying *Required:* GRE General Test, minimum GPA of 2.5, RN license, physical assessment course, statistics course, professional liability/malpractice insurance, transcript of college record. *Application deadline:* 2/1. *Application fee:* $25.

Degree Requirements 123 total credit hours, 62 in nursing.

WESTERN KENTUCKY UNIVERSITY

Department of Nursing
Bowling Green, Kentucky

Programs • Generic Baccalaureate • RN Baccalaureate • BSN to Master's • Continuing Education

The University State-supported comprehensive coed institution. Founded: 1906. *Primary accreditation:* regional. *Setting:* 223-acre suburban campus. *Total enrollment:* 14,721.

The Department of Nursing Founded in 1964. *Nursing program faculty:* 21 (24% with doctorates). *Off-campus program site:* Owensboro.

Academic Facilities *Campus library:* 869,085 volumes (13,426 in health, 1,321 in nursing); 11,314 periodical subscriptions (67 health-care related). *Nursing school resources:* CAI, computer lab, nursing audiovisuals, interactive nursing skills videos, learning resource lab.

Student Life *Student services:* health clinic, child-care facilities, personal counseling, career counseling, institutionally sponsored work-study program, job placement, campus safety program, special assistance for disabled students. *International student services:* counseling/support, special assistance for nonnative speakers of English. *Nursing student activities:* Sigma Theta Tau, student nurses association.

Calendar Semesters.

NURSING STUDENT PROFILE

Undergraduate **Enrollment:** 306

Women: 90%; **Men:** 10%; **Minority:** 5%; **International:** 1%; **Part-time:** 30%

Graduate **Enrollment:** 16

Women: 99%; **Men:** 1%; **Minority:** 0%; **International:** 0%; **Part-time:** 100%

BACCALAUREATE PROGRAMS

Contact Dr. Kay Carr, Interim Head, Academic Complex, Department of Nursing, Western Kentucky University, Bowling Green, KY 42101-3576, 502-745-3391. *Fax:* 502-745-3392. *E-mail:* kay.carr@wku.edu

Expenses *State resident tuition:* $1910 full-time, $78 per hour part-time. *Nonresident tuition:* $5270 full-time, $218 per hour part-time. *Full-time mandatory fees:* $52–$90. *Room and board:* $1300–$1600. *Books and supplies per academic year:* $600.

Financial Aid Institutionally sponsored need-based grants/scholarships, institutionally sponsored non-need grants/scholarships, Federal Supplemental Educational Opportunity Grants, Federal Work-Study. *Application deadline:* 3/1.

Generic Baccalaureate Program (BSN)

Applying *Required:* ACT, TOEFL for nonnative speakers of English, minimum college GPA of 2.75, 3 years of high school math, 3 years of high school science, high school transcript, written essay, transcript of college record. 30 prerequisite credits must be completed before admission to the nursing program. *Options:* May apply for transfer of up to 67 total credits. *Application deadline:* 1/15.

Degree Requirements 131 total credit hours, 66 in nursing.

RN Baccalaureate Program (BSN)

Applying *Required:* minimum college GPA of 2.75, RN license, diploma or AD in nursing, transcript of college record. 30 prerequisite credits must be completed before admission to the nursing program. *Options:* Course work may be accelerated. May apply for transfer of up to 67 total credits. *Application deadline:* 1/15.

Degree Requirements 131 total credit hours, 66 in nursing.

MASTER'S PROGRAM

Contact Dr. Kay Carr, Interim Head, Academic Complex, Department of Nursing, Western Kentucky University, Bowling Green, KY 42101-3576, 502-745-3391. *Fax:* 502-745-3392. *E-mail:* kay.carr@wku.edu

Areas of Study Nursing education; nurse practitioner program in primary care.

Expenses *State resident tuition:* $2070 full-time, $112 per hour part-time. *Nonresident tuition:* $5750 full-time, $317 per hour part-time.

Financial Aid Nurse traineeships. 19% of master's level students in nursing programs received some form of financial aid in 1995-96.

BSN to Master's Program (MS)

Applying *Required:* GRE General Test (minimum combined score of 1350 on three tests), bachelor's degree in nursing, minimum GPA of 2.75, RN license, essay, interview, 3 letters of recommendation, transcript of college record.

Degree Requirements Thesis or project.

CONTINUING EDUCATION PROGRAM

Contact Ms. Angela Drexler, Continuing Nursing Education, Academic Complex, Department of Nursing, Western Kentucky University, Bowling Green, KY 42101-3576, 502-745-3762. *Fax:* 502-745-3392.

LOUISIANA

DILLARD UNIVERSITY
Division of Nursing
New Orleans, Louisiana

Program • Generic Baccalaureate

The University Independent interdenominational 4-year coed college. Founded: 1869. *Primary accreditation:* regional. *Setting:* 46-acre urban campus. *Total enrollment:* 1,570.

The Division of Nursing Founded in 1942. *Nursing program faculty:* 13 (23% with doctorates).

Academic Facilities *Campus library:* 95,688 volumes (3,070 in health, 4,622 in nursing); 370 periodical subscriptions (56 health-care related). *Nursing school resources:* CAI, computer lab, nursing audiovisuals, interactive nursing skills videos, learning resource lab.

Student Life *Student services:* health clinic, personal counseling, career counseling, institutionally sponsored work-study program. *International student services:* counseling/support, special assistance for nonnative speakers of English. *Nursing student activities:* student nurses association.

Calendar Semesters.

NURSING STUDENT PROFILE

Undergraduate **Enrollment:** 156

Women: 90%; **Men:** 10%; **Minority:** 97%; **International:** 0%; **Part-time:** 3%

BACCALAUREATE PROGRAM

Contact Dr. Enrica K. Singleton, Chair, Division of Nursing, Dillard University, 2601 Gentilly Boulevard, New Orleans, LA 70122, 504-286-4718. *Fax:* 504-286-4861.

Expenses *Tuition:* $7500 per academic year. *Full-time mandatory fees:* $600. *Room and board:* $3950. *Books and supplies per academic year:* $300.

Financial Aid Institutionally sponsored need-based grants/scholarships, institutionally sponsored non-need grants/scholarships, Federal Nursing Student Loans, Federal Pell Grants, Federal Perkins Loans, Federal Supplemental Educational Opportunity Grants, Federal Work-Study. *Application deadline:* 3/1.

Generic Baccalaureate Program (BSN)

Applying *Required:* SAT I or ACT, TOEFL for nonnative speakers of English, NLN Preadmission Examination, minimum high school GPA of 2.0, minimum college GPA of 2.5, high school math, high school science, high school biology, high school transcript, 2 letters of recommendation, written essay, transcript of college record. 38 prerequisite credits must be completed before admission to the nursing program. *Options:* May apply for transfer of up to 60 total credits. *Application deadline:* 4/15. *Application fee:* $10.

Degree Requirements 133 total credit hours, 52 in nursing.

GRAMBLING STATE UNIVERSITY
School of Nursing
Grambling, Louisiana

Programs • Generic Baccalaureate • RN Baccalaureate • LPN to Baccalaureate

The University State-supported comprehensive coed institution. Founded: 1901. *Primary accreditation:* regional. *Setting:* 340-acre small-town campus. *Total enrollment:* 8,000.

The School of Nursing Founded in 1984.

Academic Facilities *Campus library:* 272,997 volumes.

Calendar Semesters.

BACCALAUREATE PROGRAMS

Contact Dean, School of Nursing, Grambling State University, PO Box 4272, Grambling, LA 71245, 318-274-2672.

Expenses *State resident tuition:* $4724 full-time, $2100 per year part-time. *Nonresident tuition:* $6874 full-time, $4976 per year part-time.

Financial Aid Institutionally sponsored need-based grants/scholarships, institutionally sponsored non-need grants/scholarships, Federal Pell Grants, Federal Perkins Loans, Federal Work-Study, Federal Stafford Loans.

Generic Baccalaureate Program (BSN)

Applying *Required:* SAT I or ACT, TOEFL for nonnative speakers of English, psychological pre-entrance exam, minimum high school GPA of 2.0, minimum college GPA of 2.0, high school transcript, transcript of college record. *Options:* Advanced standing available through credit by exam. *Application deadlines:* 6/15 (fall), 11/1 (spring). *Application fee:* $5.

Degree Requirements 141 total credit hours, 71 in nursing.

RN Baccalaureate Program (BSN)

Applying *Required:* psychological pre-entrance exam, RN license, diploma or AD in nursing, high school transcript, transcript of college record. *Application deadlines:* 6/15 (fall), 11/1 (spring). *Application fee:* $5.

Degree Requirements 141 total credit hours, 71 in nursing.

LPN to Baccalaureate Program (BSN)

Applying *Required:* psychological pre-entrance exam, high school transcript. *Application deadlines:* 6/15 (fall), 11/1 (spring). *Application fee:* $5.

Degree Requirements 141 total credit hours, 71 in nursing.

LOUISIANA COLLEGE
Division of Nursing
Pineville, Louisiana

Programs • Generic Baccalaureate • RN Baccalaureate

The College Independent Southern Baptist 4-year coed college. Founded: 1906. *Primary accreditation:* regional. *Setting:* 81-acre small-town campus. *Total enrollment:* 1,024.

The Division of Nursing Founded in 1984. *Nursing program faculty:* 8 (13% with doctorates).

Academic Facilities *Campus library:* 131,622 volumes (5,550 in health, 1,500 in nursing); 554 periodical subscriptions (56 health-care related). *Nursing school resources:* CAI, computer lab, nursing audiovisuals, learning resource lab.

Student Life *Student services:* health clinic, personal counseling, career counseling, institutionally sponsored work-study program, job placement, campus safety program, special assistance for disabled students. *International student services:* counseling/support, special assistance for

Louisiana College (continued)
nonnative speakers of English, ESL courses. *Nursing student activities:* Sigma Theta Tau, student nurses association, Baptist nursing fellowship.

Calendar Semesters.

NURSING STUDENT PROFILE

Undergraduate **Enrollment:** 127
Women: 76%; **Men:** 24%; **Minority:** 8%; **International:** 3%

BACCALAUREATE PROGRAMS

Contact Dr. Anne Fortenberry, Chair, Division of Nursing, Louisiana College, 1140 College Drive, Pineville, LA 71359-0556, 318-487-7127. *Fax:* 318-487-7488. *E-mail:* fortenb@andria.lacollege.edu

Expenses *Full-time mandatory fees:* $200. *Room and board:* $2810–$3737. *Room only:* $1300–$1950. *Books and supplies per academic year:* ranges from $1000 to $1200.

Financial Aid Institutionally sponsored need-based grants/scholarships, institutionally sponsored non-need grants/scholarships, Federal Nursing Student Loans, Federal Pell Grants, Federal Supplemental Educational Opportunity Grants, Federal Work-Study. 95% of undergraduate students in nursing programs received some form of financial aid in 1995–96. *Application deadline:* 3/15.

Generic Baccalaureate Program (BSN)

Applying *Required:* ACT, TOEFL for nonnative speakers of English, minimum high school GPA of 2.0, minimum college GPA of 2.6, high school transcript, interview, letter of recommendation, transcript of college record. 79 prerequisite credits must be completed before admission to the nursing program. *Options:* Advanced standing available through the following means: advanced placement exams, credit by exam. *Application deadline:* 3/1.

Degree Requirements 136 total credit hours, 57 in nursing.

RN Baccalaureate Program (BSN)

Applying *Required:* ACT, TOEFL for nonnative speakers of English, minimum high school GPA of 2.0, minimum college GPA of 2.5, RN license, diploma or AD in nursing, interview, letter of recommendation, transcript of college record. 79 prerequisite credits must be completed before admission to the nursing program. *Options:* Advanced standing available through the following means: advanced placement exams, credit by exam. *Application deadline:* 3/15.

Degree Requirements 136 total credit hours, 57 in nursing.

LOUISIANA STATE UNIVERSITY MEDICAL CENTER

School of Nursing
New Orleans, Louisiana

Programs • Generic Baccalaureate • Accelerated RN Baccalaureate • BSN to Master's • DNS • Continuing Education

The University State-supported coed university. Part of Louisiana State University System. Founded: 1931. *Primary accreditation:* regional. *Total enrollment:* 3,059.

The School of Nursing Founded in 1933. *Nursing program faculty:* 82 (29% with doctorates).

Academic Facilities *Campus library:* 181,235 volumes (181,235 in health); 1,964 periodical subscriptions (1,964 health-care related). *Nursing school resources:* CAI, computer lab, nursing audiovisuals, interactive nursing skills videos, learning resource lab, IV mini-lab.

Student Life *Student services:* health clinic, personal counseling, institutionally sponsored work-study program, campus safety program, special assistance for disabled students. *International student services:* counseling/support. *Nursing student activities:* Sigma Theta Tau, student nurses association, student government association.

Calendar Semesters.

NURSING STUDENT PROFILE

Undergraduate **Enrollment:** 531
Women: 81%; **Men:** 19%; **Minority:** 13%; **International:** 0%; **Part-time:** 18%
Graduate **Enrollment:** 169
Women: 92%; **Men:** 8%; **Minority:** 25%; **International:** 0%; **Part-time:** 70%

BACCALAUREATE PROGRAMS

Contact Ms. Sylvia Toval, Admissions Analyst II, School of Nursing, Louisiana State University Medical College, 1900 Gravier Street, New Orleans, LA 70112, 504-568-4200. *Fax:* 504-568-5853. *E-mail:* stoval@nomvs.lsumc.edu

Expenses *State resident tuition:* $1896 full-time, ranges from $711 to $742 per semester part-time. *Nonresident tuition:* $3596 full-time, ranges from $1285 to $1316 per semester part-time.

Financial Aid Institutionally sponsored need-based grants/scholarships, institutionally sponsored non-need grants/scholarships, Federal Nursing Student Loans, Federal Pell Grants, Federal Supplemental Educational Opportunity Grants, Federal Work-Study.

Generic Baccalaureate Program (BSN)

Applying *Required:* NLN Preadmission Examination-RN, minimum college GPA of 2.8, interview, transcript of college record, basic life support certificate, computer literacy. 35 prerequisite credits must be completed before admission to the nursing program. *Options:* Advanced standing available through credit by exam. May apply for transfer of up to 60 total credits. *Application deadlines:* 3/17 (fall), 9/5 (spring). *Application fee:* $50.

Degree Requirements 130 total credit hours, 62 in nursing.

Accelerated RN Baccalaureate Program (BSN)

Applying *Required:* minimum college GPA of 2.8, RN license, diploma or AD in nursing, basic life support certificate, computer literacy. 35 prerequisite credits must be completed before admission to the nursing program. *Options:* Advanced standing available through credit by exam. May apply for transfer of up to 100 total credits. *Application deadlines:* 3/17 (fall), 9/5 (spring). *Application fee:* $50.

Degree Requirements 130 total credit hours, 62 in nursing.

MASTER'S PROGRAM

Contact Dr. Barbara Donlon, Acting Director, Graduate Nursing Program, School of Nursing, Louisiana State University Medical Center, 1900 Gravier Street, New Orleans, LA 70112, 504-568-4141. *Fax:* 504-568-3308. *E-mail:* bdonlo@lsumc.edu

Areas of Study Clinical nurse specialist programs in adult health nursing, community health nursing, parent-child nursing, psychiatric–mental health nursing, public health nursing; nursing administration; nurse practitioner programs in adult health, neonatal health, primary care.

Expenses *State resident tuition:* $2222 full-time, $762 per semester part-time. *Nonresident tuition:* $4722 full-time, $1595 per semester part-time.

Financial Aid Graduate assistantships, nurse traineeships, Federal Nursing Student Loans. *Application deadline:* 10/1.

BSN to Master's Program (MN)

Applying *Required:* GRE General Test, Miller Analogies Test, TOEFL for nonnative speakers of English, bachelor's degree in nursing, minimum GPA of 3.0, RN license, 2 years of clinical experience, statistics course, 3 letters of recommendation, transcript of college record, documentation of physical assessment skills. *Application deadline:* 3/17. *Application fee:* $50.

Degree Requirements 39 total credit hours, 30 in nursing.

DOCTORAL PROGRAM

Contact Dr. Barbara Donlon, Acting Director, Graduate Nursing Program, School of Nursing, Louisiana State University Medical Center, 1900 Gravier Street, New Orleans, LA 70112, 504-568-4141. *Fax:* 504-568-3308. *E-mail:* bdonlo@lsumc.edu

Areas of Study Nursing administration, nursing education.

Expenses *State resident tuition:* $2222 full-time, $762 per semester part-time. *Nonresident tuition:* $4722 full-time, $1595 per semester part-time.

Financial Aid Nurse traineeships.

DNS PROGRAM

Applying *Required:* GRE General Test, Miller Analogies Test, TOEFL for nonnative speakers of English, master's degree in nursing, 2 years of clinical experience, 1 scholarly paper, 3 letters of recommendation, competitive review by faculty committee, licensed or eligibility for licensure in Louisiana. *Application deadline:* 10/1. *Application fee:* $50.

Degree Requirements 54 total credit hours; dissertation; written exam; defense of dissertation.

CONTINUING EDUCATION PROGRAM

Contact Ms. Susan Seifert, Acting Director, Faculty Development, School of Nursing, Louisiana State University Medical Center, 1900 Gravier Street, New Orleans, LA 70112, 504-568-4202. *Fax:* 504-568-3308.

LOYOLA UNIVERSITY, NEW ORLEANS
Department of Nursing
New Orleans, Louisiana

Programs • RN Baccalaureate • Accelerated MSN

The University Independent Roman Catholic (Jesuit) comprehensive coed institution. Founded: 1912. *Primary accreditation:* regional. *Setting:* 26-acre urban campus. *Total enrollment:* 5,234.

The Department of Nursing Founded in 1978. *Nursing program faculty:* 10 (80% with doctorates). *Off-campus program site:* Baton Rouge.

Academic Facilities *Campus library:* 390,000 volumes (10,534 in health, 2,500 in nursing); 2,186 periodical subscriptions (150 health-care related). *Nursing school resources:* CAI, computer lab, nursing audiovisuals, learning resource lab.

Student Life *Student services:* health clinic, child-care facilities, personal counseling, career counseling, institutionally sponsored work-study program, job placement, campus safety program, special assistance for disabled students. *International student services:* counseling/support, special assistance for nonnative speakers of English, ESL courses. *Nursing student activities:* Sigma Theta Tau, Nursing Honor Society.

Calendar Semesters.

NURSING STUDENT PROFILE

Undergraduate **Enrollment:** 300
Women: 91%; **Men:** 9%; **Minority:** 13%; **International:** 0%; **Part-time:** 99%

BACCALAUREATE PROGRAM

Contact Dr. Billie Ann Wilson, Department Chair, Nursing Department, Loyola University, New Orleans, 6363 St. Charles Avenue, New Orleans, LA 70118, 504-865-3142. *Fax:* 504-865-3883.

Expenses *Tuition:* $190 per credit.

Financial Aid Institutionally sponsored need-based grants/scholarships, Federal Direct Loans.

RN BACCALAUREATE PROGRAM (BSN)

Applying *Required:* minimum college GPA of 2.25, RN license, diploma or AD in nursing. *Options:* Advanced standing available through the following means: advanced placement exams, credit by exam. Course work may be accelerated. May apply for transfer of up to 97 total credits. *Application deadline:* rolling. *Application fee:* $20.

Degree Requirements 129 total credit hours, 50 in nursing.

Distance learning Courses provided through video, on-line.

MASTER'S PROGRAM

Contact Dr. Billie Ann Wilson, Department Chair, Loyola University, New Orleans, Box 14, 6363 St. Charles Avenue, New Orleans, LA 70118, 504-865-3142. *Fax:* 504-865-3254.

Areas of Study Nurse practitioner program in family health.

Expenses *Tuition:* $475 per credit.

Financial Aid Federal Direct Loans, institutionally sponsored need-based grants/scholarships.

ACCELERATED MSN PROGRAM

Applying *Required:* GRE General Test, bachelor's degree in nursing, minimum GPA of 3.0, RN license, 1 year of clinical experience, statistics course, professional liability/malpractice insurance, essay, interview, 3 letters of recommendation, transcript of college record, 10 hours of biological science, 6 hours of chemistry/physics. *Application deadline:* 2/15. *Application fee:* $20.

Degree Requirements 45 total credit hours, 45 in nursing.

MCNEESE STATE UNIVERSITY
College of Nursing
Lake Charles, Louisiana

Programs • Generic Baccalaureate • RN Baccalaureate • LPN to Baccalaureate • MSN

The University State-supported comprehensive coed institution. Founded: 1939. *Primary accreditation:* regional. *Setting:* 580-acre suburban campus. *Total enrollment:* 8,444.

The College of Nursing Founded in 1954.

Academic Facilities *Campus library:* 300,000 volumes (5,000 in health, 1,400 in nursing); 1,557 periodical subscriptions (192 health-care related).

Calendar Semesters.

BACCALAUREATE PROGRAMS

Contact Ms. Kathy Roan, Coordinator, BSN Program, College of Nursing, McNeese State University, PO Box 90415, Lake Charles, LA 70609-0415, 318-475-5820. *Fax:* 318-475-5702.

Expenses *State resident tuition:* $0 per academic year. *Nonresident tuition:* $3530 full-time, $148 per hour part-time. *Full-time mandatory fees:* $2012. *Part-time mandatory fees:* $330–$1779.

Financial Aid Federal Pell Grants. *Application deadline:* 5/1.

GENERIC BACCALAUREATE PROGRAM (BSN)

Applying *Required:* ACT, TOEFL for nonnative speakers of English, score in 50th percentile in reading/math composite and critical thinking on Nursing Entrance Test, minimum college GPA of 2.7, high school transcript. *Application deadlines:* 5/15 (fall), 10/15 (spring), 3/15 (summer). *Application fee:* $10.

Degree Requirements 130 total credit hours, 61 in nursing.

RN BACCALAUREATE PROGRAM (BSN)

Applying *Required:* minimum college GPA of 2.7, interview, transcript of college record. 57 prerequisite credits must be completed before admission to the nursing program. *Application deadlines:* 5/15 (fall), 10/15 (spring), 3/15 (summer). *Application fee:* $10.

Degree Requirements 130 total credit hours, 61 in nursing.

LPN TO BACCALAUREATE PROGRAM (BSN)

Applying *Required:* ACT, TOEFL for nonnative speakers of English, minimum college GPA of 2.7, high school transcript, interview, transcript of college record. *Application deadlines:* 5/15 (fall), 10/15 (spring), 3/15 (summer). *Application fee:* $10.

Degree Requirements 130 total credit hours, 61 in nursing.

MASTER'S PROGRAM

Contact Dr. Anita Fields, Dean, College of Nursing, McNeese State University, PO Box 90415, Lake Charles, LA 70609-0415, 318-475-5822. *Fax:* 318-475-5824.

Areas of Study Clinical nurse specialist programs in cardiovascular nursing, gerontological nursing, oncology nursing, emergency nursing; nursing administration; nursing education; nurse practitioner program in adult health.

Expenses *State resident tuition:* $0 per academic year. *Nonresident tuition:* $3530 full-time, ranges from $146 to $588 per hour part-time. *Full-time mandatory fees:* $1906. *Part-time mandatory fees:* $330–$1356.

MSN PROGRAM

Applying *Required:* GRE General Test, bachelor's degree in nursing, minimum GPA of 2.7, RN license, 1 year of clinical experience, physical assessment course, statistics course. *Application deadlines:* 5/1 (fall), 10/1 (spring), 3/1 (summer). *Application fee:* $10.

Degree Requirements 42 total credit hours, 42 in nursing. Thesis required.

McNeese State University (continued)

NICHOLLS STATE UNIVERSITY
Department of Nursing
Thibodaux, Louisiana

Programs • Generic Baccalaureate • RN Baccalaureate • LPN to Baccalaureate

The University State-supported comprehensive coed institution. Part of Louisiana State University System. Founded: 1948. *Primary accreditation:* regional. *Setting:* 210-acre small-town campus. *Total enrollment:* 7,366.

The Department of Nursing Founded in 1981. *Nursing program faculty:* 24.

Academic Facilities *Campus library:* 400,000 volumes (10,950 in nursing); 3,000 periodical subscriptions (159 health-care related).

Calendar Semesters.

BACCALAUREATE PROGRAMS

Contact BSN Program Director, Department of Nursing, Nicholls State University, PO Box 2143, Thibodaux, LA 70310, 504-448-4694. *Fax:* 504-448-4923.

Expenses *State resident tuition:* $2016 full-time, $69 per hour part-time. *Nonresident tuition:* $4609 full-time, $177 per hour part-time.

Financial Aid Institutionally sponsored need-based grants/scholarships, institutionally sponsored non-need grants/scholarships, Federal Pell Grants, Federal Perkins Loans, Federal Supplemental Educational Opportunity Grants, Federal Work-Study, Federal PLUS Loans, Federal Stafford Loans, state aid. *Application deadline:* 3/29.

Generic Baccalaureate Program (BSN)

Applying *Required:* ACT, TOEFL for nonnative speakers of English, minimum college GPA of 2.75. 38 prerequisite credits must be completed before admission to the nursing program. *Options:* Advanced standing available through credit by exam. Course work may be accelerated. *Application fee:* $10.

Degree Requirements 138 total credit hours, 54 in nursing.

RN Baccalaureate Program (BSN)

Applying *Required:* minimum college GPA of 2.75, RN license, diploma or AD in nursing, transcript of college record. 38 prerequisite credits must be completed before admission to the nursing program. *Options:* Advanced standing available through credit by exam. Course work may be accelerated. *Application fee:* $10.

Degree Requirements 138 total credit hours, 54 in nursing.

LPN to Baccalaureate Program (BSN)

Applying *Required:* ACT, NLN Mobility Profile I, minimum college GPA of 2.75, diploma or AD in nursing, transcript of college record, 2 years of clinical experience, LPN license. *Options:* Advanced standing available through credit by exam. *Application fee:* $10.

Degree Requirements 138 total credit hours, 54 in nursing.

NORTHEAST LOUISIANA UNIVERSITY
School of Nursing
Monroe, Louisiana

Programs • Generic Baccalaureate • RN Baccalaureate • LPN to Baccalaureate

The University State-supported comprehensive coed institution. Founded: 1931. *Primary accreditation:* regional. *Setting:* 238-acre urban campus. *Total enrollment:* 11,553.

The School of Nursing Founded in 1960. *Nursing program faculty:* 24 (13% with doctorates).

Academic Facilities *Campus library:* 532,940 volumes (16,690 in health, 2,513 in nursing); 2,935 periodical subscriptions (400 health-care related).

Calendar Semesters.

BACCALAUREATE PROGRAMS

Contact Director, School of Nursing, Northeast Louisiana University, 700 University Avenue, Monroe, LA 71209-0460, 318-342-1644. *Fax:* 318-342-1606.

Financial Aid Institutionally sponsored need-based grants/scholarships, institutionally sponsored non-need grants/scholarships, Federal Pell Grants, Federal Supplemental Educational Opportunity Grants, Federal Work-Study, Federal PLUS Loans, Federal Stafford Loans, state aid. *Application deadline:* 4/1.

Generic Baccalaureate Program (BSN)

Applying *Required:* ACT, TOEFL for nonnative speakers of English, minimum college GPA of 2.5, high school math, high school science, high school chemistry, high school foreign language. *Options:* Advanced standing available through the following means: advanced placement exams, credit by exam. *Application deadline:* rolling.

Degree Requirements 131 total credit hours, 62 in nursing.

RN Baccalaureate Program (BSN)

Applying *Required:* ACT, TOEFL for nonnative speakers of English, RN license, diploma or AD in nursing. 57 prerequisite credits must be completed before admission to the nursing program. *Options:* Advanced standing available through credit by exam. *Application deadline:* rolling.

Degree Requirements 62 total credit hours in nursing.

LPN to Baccalaureate Program (BSN)

Applying *Required:* ACT, TOEFL for nonnative speakers of English, diploma or AD in nursing, transcript of college record, LPN license. *Options:* Advanced standing available through credit by exam. *Application deadline:* rolling.

Degree Requirements 131 total credit hours, 62 in nursing.

NORTHWESTERN STATE UNIVERSITY OF LOUISIANA
Division of Nursing
Natchitoches, Louisiana

Programs • Generic Baccalaureate • RN Baccalaureate • LPN to Baccalaureate • MSN

The University State-supported comprehensive coed institution. Founded: 1884. *Primary accreditation:* regional. *Setting:* 1,000-acre small-town campus. *Total enrollment:* 9,040.

The Division of Nursing Founded in 1949. *Nursing program faculty:* 34.

Academic Facilities *Campus library:* 310,000 volumes; 2,500 periodical subscriptions.

BACCALAUREATE PROGRAMS

Contact Norann Planchock, Acting Director, Division of Nursing, Northwestern State University of Louisiana, Natchitoches, LA 71497, 318-487-5298. *Fax:* 318-677-3127.

Expenses *State resident tuition:* $0 per academic year. *Nonresident tuition:* $2430 full-time, $101 per credit hour part-time. *Full-time mandatory fees:* $642–$2018. *Part-time mandatory fees:* $321+. *Room and board:* $1186–$1909. *Room only:* $980–$1240.

Financial Aid Institutionally sponsored non-need grants/scholarships, Federal Pell Grants, Federal Perkins Loans, Federal Supplemental Educational Opportunity Grants, Federal Work-Study, Federal Family Education Loan Program (FFELP). *Application deadline:* 5/1.

Generic Baccalaureate Program (BSN)

Applying *Required:* SAT I or ACT, TOEFL for nonnative speakers of English, minimum college GPA of 2.0, high school transcript, letter of recommendation. *Options:* Advanced standing available through credit by exam. *Application deadlines:* 7/25 (fall), 12/1 (spring), 4/15 (summer). *Application fee:* $15.

Degree Requirements 122 total credit hours, 54 in nursing.

RN Baccalaureate Program (BSN)

Applying *Required:* RN license, diploma or AD in nursing, interview, transcript of college record, 1 year of practice as an RN, CPR certification. *Application deadlines:* 7/25 (fall), 12/1 (spring), 4/15 (summer). *Application fee:* $15.

Degree Requirements 122 total credit hours, 54 in nursing.

LPN to Baccalaureate Program (BSN)

Applying *Required:* 1 year of experience as a nurse, LPN license. *Application deadlines:* 7/15 (fall), 12/1 (spring), 4/15 (summer). *Application fee:* $15.

Degree Requirements 122 total credit hours, 54 in nursing.

MASTER'S PROGRAM

Contact Norann Planchock, Acting Director, Division of Nursing, Northwestern State University of Louisiana, Natchitoches, LA 71497, 318-487-5298. *Fax:* 318-677-3127.

Areas of Study Clinical nurse specialist programs in adult health nursing, critical care nursing, maternity-newborn nursing, psychiatric–mental health nursing.

Expenses *State resident tuition:* $0 per academic year. *Nonresident tuition:* $2430 full-time, $101 per credit hour part-time. *Full-time mandatory fees:* $642–$1607. *Part-time mandatory fees:* $321+. *Room and board:* $1186–$1909. *Room only:* $980–$1240.

MSN Program

Applying *Required:* bachelor's degree in nursing, RN license, physical assessment course, statistics course, transcript of college record. *Application deadline:* rolling.

Degree Requirements 39+ total credit hours dependent upon track, 39+ in nursing. Research project instead of thesis for family nurse practitioner track. Thesis required.

OUR LADY OF HOLY CROSS COLLEGE

Division of Nursing
New Orleans, Louisiana

Program • Generic Baccalaureate

The College Independent Roman Catholic comprehensive coed institution. Founded: 1916. *Primary accreditation:* regional. *Setting:* 40-acre suburban campus. *Total enrollment:* 1,367.

The Division of Nursing Founded in 1983. *Nursing program faculty:* 16 (25% with doctorates).

Academic Facilities *Campus library:* 43,988 volumes (3,800 in nursing); 779 periodical subscriptions (50 health-care related).

Calendar Semesters.

NURSING STUDENT PROFILE

Undergraduate **Enrollment:** 140

Women: 89%; **Men:** 11%; **Minority:** 16%; **International:** 0%; **Part-time:** 57%

BACCALAUREATE PROGRAM

Contact Mr. Stanton McNeely, Admissions and Recruitment Office, Our Lady of Holy Cross College, 4123 Woodland Drive, New Orleans, LA 70131, 504-394-7744 Ext. 213. *Fax:* 504-391-2421.

Expenses *Tuition:* $3840 full-time, $160 per credit part-time.

Generic Baccalaureate Program (BSN)

Applying *Required:* ACT, NLN Preadmission Examination-RN, minimum college GPA of 2.5, 3 letters of recommendation, written essay, transcript of college record, formal application. 31 prerequisite credits must be completed before admission to the nursing program. *Options:* Advanced standing available through credit by exam. *Application deadline:* 12/19.

Degree Requirements 134 total credit hours, 53 in nursing.

SOUTHEASTERN LOUISIANA UNIVERSITY

School of Nursing
Hammon, Louisiana

Programs • Generic Baccalaureate • RN Baccalaureate • LPN to Baccalaureate • MSN

The University State-supported comprehensive coed institution. Founded: 1925. *Primary accreditation:* regional. *Setting:* 365-acre small-town campus. *Total enrollment:* 14,344.

The School of Nursing Founded in 1964. *Nursing program faculty:* 50 (22% with doctorates). *Off-campus program site:* Baton Rouge.

Academic Facilities *Campus library:* 292,542 volumes (16,000 in nursing); 1,960 periodical subscriptions (80 health-care related). *Nursing school resources:* CAI, computer lab, nursing audiovisuals, interactive nursing skills videos, learning resource lab.

Student Life *Student services:* health clinic, personal counseling, career counseling, institutionally sponsored work-study program, job placement, campus safety program, special assistance for disabled students. *International student services:* counseling/support, special assistance for nonnative speakers of English. *Nursing student activities:* student nurses association.

Calendar Semesters.

NURSING STUDENT PROFILE

Undergraduate **Enrollment:** 400

Women: 85%; **Men:** 15%

Graduate **Enrollment:** 46

Women: 100%; **Minority:** 2%; **International:** 0%; **Part-time:** 89%

BACCALAUREATE PROGRAMS

Contact Dr. Donnie M. Booth, Director, School of Nursing, Southeastern Louisiana University, Hammond, LA 70402, 504-549-2000.

Expenses *State resident tuition:* $1920 per academic year. *Nonresident tuition:* $2232 per academic year. *Full-time mandatory fees:* $52–$480.

Financial Aid Institutionally sponsored need-based grants/scholarships, institutionally sponsored non-need grants/scholarships, Federal Supplemental Educational Opportunity Grants, Federal Work-Study. *Application deadline:* 5/13.

Generic Baccalaureate Program (BS)

Applying *Required:* ACT, minimum college GPA of 2.0, 3 years of high school math, 3 years of high school science, high school transcript. 42 prerequisite credits must be completed before admission to the nursing program. *Application deadlines:* 5/15 (fall), 10/15 (spring), 5/1 (summer). *Application fee:* $50.

Degree Requirements 133 total credit hours, 68 in nursing. Half of major hours at Southeastern Louisiana University.

RN Baccalaureate Program (BS)

Applying *Required:* ACT PEP, NLN Achievement Tests, minimum college GPA of 2.0, RN license, transcript of college record. *Options:* May apply for transfer of up to 68 total credits. *Application deadlines:* 7/15 (fall), 12/1 (spring), 5/1 (summer). *Application fee:* $50.

Degree Requirements 133 total credit hours, 68 in nursing. Half of major hours at Southeastern Louisiana University.

LPN to Baccalaureate Program (BS)

Applying *Required:* ACT, Louisiana LPN license. 30 prerequisite credits must be completed before admission to the nursing program. *Options:* Advanced standing available through the following means: advanced placement exams, credit by exam. Course work may be accelerated. *Application deadlines:* 5/15 (fall), 10/15 (spring). *Application fee:* $50.

Degree Requirements 133 total credit hours, 68 in nursing.

MASTER'S PROGRAM

Contact Dr. Carole H. Lund, RN, Director of Graduate Nursing, School of Nursing, Southwestern Louisiana University 448, Hammond, LA 70402, 504-549-5045. *Fax:* 504-549-5087. *E-mail:* clund@selu.edu

Areas of Study Clinical nurse specialist programs in community health nursing, psychiatric–mental health nursing; nursing administration; nursing education; nurse practitioner program in primary care.

Expenses *State resident tuition:* $1920 per academic year. *Nonresident tuition:* $2232 per academic year.

Financial Aid Institutionally sponsored loans, institutionally sponsored need-based grants/scholarships, institutionally sponsored non-need-based grants/scholarships. *Application deadline:* 5/13.

MSN Program

Applying *Required:* GRE General Test, TOEFL for nonnative speakers of English, bachelor's degree in nursing, minimum GPA of 2.7, RN license, 1 year of clinical experience, physical assessment course, statistics course, transcript of college record. *Application deadline:* rolling. *Application fee:* $10.

Degree Requirements 42 total credit hours, 39 in nursing, 3 in non-nursing elective. Thesis required.

SOUTHERN UNIVERSITY AND AGRICULTURAL AND MECHANICAL COLLEGE
School of Nursing
Baton Rouge, Louisiana

Programs • Generic Baccalaureate • Master's

The University State-supported comprehensive coed institution. Part of Southern University System. Founded: 1880. *Primary accreditation:* regional. *Setting:* 512-acre suburban campus. *Total enrollment:* 9,800.

The School of Nursing Founded in 1985.

Academic Facilities *Campus library:* 719,930 volumes; 1,989 periodical subscriptions.

Calendar Semesters.

BACCALAUREATE PROGRAM

Contact Dr. Janet Rami, Dean, School of Nursing, Southern University and Agricultural and Mechanical College, PO Box 11794, Baton Rouge, LA 70813, 504-771-2166.

Expenses *Tuition:* $2028 full-time, $287 per 3 credit hours part-time.

Financial Aid Institutionally sponsored need-based grants/scholarships, institutionally sponsored non-need grants/scholarships, Federal Pell Grants, Federal Supplemental Educational Opportunity Grants, Federal Work-Study, state student incentive grants.

Generic Baccalaureate Program (BSN)

Applying *Required:* SAT I or ACT, TOEFL for nonnative speakers of English, minimum college GPA of 2.5, high school transcript. *Options:* Advanced standing available through the following means: advanced placement exams, credit by exam. *Application deadlines:* 7/1 (fall), 11/1 (spring), 5/1 (summer). *Application fee:* $5.

Degree Requirements 139 total credit hours, 66 in nursing. Comprehensive exam.

MASTER'S PROGRAMS

Areas of Study Nurse practitioner program in family health.

Expenses *Tuition:* $2046 full-time, $252 per 3 credit hours part-time.

UNIVERSITY OF SOUTHWESTERN LOUISIANA
College of Nursing
Lafayette, Louisiana

Programs • Generic Baccalaureate • RN Baccalaureate • LPN to Baccalaureate

The University State-supported coed university. Founded: 1898. *Primary accreditation:* regional. *Setting:* 1,375-acre urban campus. *Total enrollment:* 16,902.

The College of Nursing Founded in 1951.

Academic Facilities *Campus library:* 687,142 volumes (2,523 in health, 3,664 in nursing); 6,850 periodical subscriptions (209 health-care related).

Calendar Semesters.

BACCALAUREATE PROGRAMS

Contact Director of Nursing Student Services, College of Nursing, University of Southwestern Louisiana, PO Box 43810, Lafayette, LA 70592, 318-482-5604. *Fax:* 318-231-5649.

Expenses *State resident tuition:* $1896 full-time, $69 per credit hour part-time. *Nonresident tuition:* $5496 full-time, $150 per credit hour part-time.

Financial Aid Institutionally sponsored non-need grants/scholarships, Federal Nursing Student Loans, Federal Pell Grants, Federal Perkins Loans, Federal Supplemental Educational Opportunity Grants, Federal Work-Study, Federal PLUS Loans, Federal Stafford Loans, state aid.

Generic Baccalaureate Program (BSN)

Applying *Required:* ACT, TOEFL for nonnative speakers of English, minimum college GPA of 2.5, 3 years of high school math, 3 years of high school science. *Application deadline:* rolling. *Application fee:* $5.

Degree Requirements 137 total credit hours, 70 in nursing.

RN Baccalaureate Program (BSN)

Applying *Required:* RN license, diploma or AD in nursing. *Options:* Advanced standing available through credit by exam. *Application deadline:* rolling. *Application fee:* $5.

Degree Requirements 137 total credit hours, 70 in nursing.

LPN to Baccalaureate Program (BSN)

Applying *Required:* diploma or AD in nursing, LPN license. *Options:* Advanced standing available through credit by exam. *Application deadline:* rolling. *Application fee:* $5.

Degree Requirements 137 total credit hours, 70 in nursing.

MAINE

HUSSON COLLEGE
Husson College and Eastern Maine Medical Center School of Nursing
Bangor, Maine

Programs • Generic Baccalaureate • RN Baccalaureate

The College Independent comprehensive coed institution. Founded: 1898. *Primary accreditation:* regional. *Setting:* 170-acre suburban campus. *Total enrollment:* 2,036.

The School of Nursing Founded in 1983.

▶ ***NOTEWORTHY***

Reflecting Husson's ongoing commitment to educate nurses for the challenges of the 21st century, the family and community nurse practitioner program was developed to educate advanced practice nurses at the master's level to provide cost-effective improved access to family health care. The nursing program is designed to equip students for the best and broadest careers possible as are the physical therapy and RN-completion programs. The programs' success is attributed to the fact that Husson offers twice the number of clinical hours as most programs with a wide variety of clinical experiences, ranging from hospital to community settings.

Academic Facilities *Campus library:* 34,500 volumes (1,125 in health, 1,050 in nursing); 387 periodical subscriptions (70 health-care related).

Calendar Semesters.

BACCALAUREATE PROGRAMS

Contact Dr. Elizabeth Burns, Dean of Nursing and Health Professions, Husson College and Eastern Maine Medical Center School of Nursing, Husson College, One College Circle, Bangor, ME 04401, 207-941-7182. *Fax:* 207-941-7750.

Expenses *Tuition:* $16,080 full-time, $268 per credit hour part-time.

Financial Aid Institutionally sponsored need-based grants/scholarships, institutionally sponsored non-need grants/scholarships, Federal Direct Loans, Federal Perkins Loans, Federal Supplemental Educational Opportunity Grants, Federal Work-Study, Federal Family Education Loan Program (FFELP), state scholarships and grants.

Generic Baccalaureate Program (BS)

Applying *Required:* SAT I or ACT, TOEFL for nonnative speakers of English, 2 years of high school math, 2 years of high school science, high school transcript, 2 letters of recommendation, written essay, transcript of college record, 4 years of high school English. *Options:* Advanced standing available through credit by exam. *Application fee:* $25.

Degree Requirements 126 total credit hours, 61 in nursing.

RN Baccalaureate Program (BS)

Applying *Required:* 2 years of high school math, 2 years of high school science, high school chemistry, RN license, diploma or AD in nursing, 2 letters of recommendation, written essay, transcript of college record. *Options:* Advanced standing available through credit by exam. *Application fee:* $25.

Degree Requirements 125 total credit hours, 57 in nursing.

See full description on page 458.

SAINT JOSEPH'S COLLEGE
Department of Nursing
Standish, Maine

Programs • Generic Baccalaureate • RN Baccalaureate • LPN to Baccalaureate • BSN to Master's

The College Independent comprehensive coed institution, affiliated with Roman Catholic Church. Founded: 1912. *Primary accreditation:* regional. *Setting:* 328-acre rural campus. *Total enrollment:* 1,087.

The Department of Nursing Founded in 1974. *Nursing program faculty:* 15 (7% with doctorates). *Off-campus program site:* Portland.

▶ *NOTEWORTHY*

Saint Joseph's College in Maine offers both on-campus and distance education instruction in its nursing programs. The 4-year BSN is a traditional campus-based program with more than 700 hours of clinical and laboratory experience. Students may attend on a full- or part-time basis. Clinicals have a 6:1 student-faculty ratio, lower than the Board of Nursing requirement. The LPN-BSN, RN-BSN, and the MS in nursing programs are offered on a part-time basis through a combination of distance education instruction and on-campus summer residencies.

Academic Facilities *Campus library:* 69,200 volumes (13,148 in health, 4,152 in nursing); 450 periodical subscriptions (90 health-care related). *Nursing school resources:* CAI, computer lab, nursing audiovisuals, learning resource lab.

Student Life *Student services:* health clinic, personal counseling, career counseling, institutionally sponsored work-study program, campus safety program. *International student services:* counseling/support. *Nursing student activities:* Sigma Theta Tau, student nurses association.

Calendar Semesters.

NURSING STUDENT PROFILE

Undergraduate **Enrollment:** 372
Women: 93%; **Men:** 7%; **Minority:** 1%; **International:** 0%; **Part-time:** 52%

BACCALAUREATE PROGRAMS

Contact Admissions Office, Department of Nursing, Saint Joseph's College, Standish, ME 04084-5263, 800-338-7057. *Fax:* 207-892-7746.

Expenses *Tuition:* $10,990 full-time, $190 per credit part-time. *Full-time mandatory fees:* $395. *Part-time mandatory fees:* $200–$395. *Room and board:* $5380. *Books and supplies per academic year:* ranges from $200 to $500.

Financial Aid Institutionally sponsored need-based grants/scholarships, institutionally sponsored non-need grants/scholarships, Federal Nursing Student Loans, Federal Pell Grants, Federal Perkins Loans, Federal Supplemental Educational Opportunity Grants, Federal Work-Study. *Application deadline:* 3/1.

Generic Baccalaureate Program (BSN)

Applying *Required:* SAT I, minimum high school GPA of 2.0, minimum college GPA of 2.0, high school math, 3 years of high school science, high school chemistry, high school biology, high school transcript, letter of recommendation, written essay, transcript of college record. *Options:* Advanced standing available through the following means: advanced placement exams, credit by exam. May apply for transfer of up to 97 total credits. *Application deadline:* rolling. *Application fee:* $25.

Degree Requirements 129 total credit hours, 52 in nursing.

RN Baccalaureate Program (BSN)

Applying *Required:* RN license, diploma or AD in nursing, 3 letters of recommendation, written essay, transcript of college record, nursing school transcript, telephone interview. *Options:* Advanced standing available through credit by exam. Course work may be accelerated. May apply for transfer of up to 97 total credits. *Application deadline:* rolling. *Application fee:* $50.

Degree Requirements 129 total credit hours, 52 in nursing.

Distance learning Courses provided through correspondence. Specific degree requirements include two- to three-week on-campus summer residencies.

LPN to Baccalaureate Program (BSN)

Applying *Required:* interview, 3 letters of recommendation, written essay, LPN license, nursing school transcript. *Options:* Advanced standing available through credit by exam. Course work may be accelerated. May apply for transfer of up to 57 total credits. *Application deadline:* rolling. *Application fee:* $50.

Degree Requirements 129 total credit hours, 52 in nursing.

Distance learning Courses provided through correspondence. Specific degree requirements include two- to three-week on-campus summer residencies.

MASTER'S PROGRAM

Contact Dr. Linda Conover, Graduate Adviser, Saint Joseph's College, 278 Whites Bridge Road, Standish, ME 04084-5263, 207-893-7961. *Fax:* 207-892-7423.

Areas of Study Nursing administration; nursing education.

Expenses *Tuition:* $3780 full-time, ranges from $210 to $225 per credit hour part-time.

BSN to Master's Program (MS)

Applying *Required:* GRE General Test, Miller Analogies Test, TOEFL for nonnative speakers of English, bachelor's degree in nursing, bachelor's degree, minimum GPA of 3.0, RN license, 2 years of clinical experience, statistics course, professional liability/malpractice insurance, essay, interview, 3 letters of recommendation, transcript of college record, nurses with non-nursing baccalaureate degrees may be admitted, but must take upper division baccalaureate nursing courses as a prerequisite. *Application deadline:* rolling. *Application fee:* $50.

Degree Requirements 42 total credit hours, 33 in nursing. Thesis or professional paper.

Distance learning Courses provided through Specific degree requirements include on-campus summer residency.

See full description on page 498.

UNIVERSITY OF MAINE
School of Nursing
Orono, Maine

Programs • Generic Baccalaureate • RN Baccalaureate • BSN to Master's • RN to Master's • Post-Master's

The University State-supported coed university. Part of University of Maine System. Founded: 1865. *Primary accreditation:* regional. *Setting:* 3,298-acre small-town campus. *Total enrollment:* 9,996.

The School of Nursing Founded in 1958. *Nursing program faculty:* 13 (80% with doctorates). *Off-campus program sites:* Ellsworth, Augusta, Waterville.

Academic Facilities *Campus library:* 826,648 volumes; 5,400 periodical subscriptions. *Nursing school resources:* CAI, computer lab, nursing audiovisuals, interactive nursing skills videos, learning resource lab.

Student Life *Student services:* health clinic, child-care facilities, personal counseling, career counseling, institutionally sponsored work-study program, job placement, campus safety program, special assistance for

University of Maine (continued)

disabled students. *International student services:* counseling/support, special assistance for nonnative speakers of English, ESL courses. *Nursing student activities:* Sigma Theta Tau, nursing club, student nurses association.

Calendar Semesters.

NURSING STUDENT PROFILE

Undergraduate **Enrollment:** 600
Women: 92%; **Men:** 8%; **Minority:** 7%; **International:** 3%; **Part-time:** 12%

Graduate **Enrollment:** 37
Women: 97%; **Men:** 3%; **Minority:** 0%; **International:** 0%; **Part-time:** 50%

BACCALAUREATE PROGRAMS

Contact Ms. Joan M. Brissette, Assistant to the Director and Coordinator of Student Services, 214 Dunn Hall, School of Nursing, University of Maine, Orono, ME 04469, 207-581-2600. *Fax:* 207-581-2585. *E-mail:* jaybee@maine.maine.edu

Expenses *State resident tuition:* $3528 full-time, $112 per credit hour part-time. *Nonresident tuition:* $9986 full-time, $317 per credit hour part-time. *Full-time mandatory fees:* $461. *Room and board:* $4842–$4906. *Room only:* $2390–$2516. *Books and supplies per academic year:* ranges from $500 to $700.

Financial Aid Institutionally sponsored need-based grants/scholarships, institutionally sponsored non-need grants/scholarships, Federal Perkins Loans, Federal Supplemental Educational Opportunity Grants, Federal Work-Study. 52% of undergraduate students in nursing programs received some form of financial aid in 1995–96. *Application deadline:* 3/1.

Generic Baccalaureate Program (BSN)

Applying *Required:* SAT I, 2 College Board Achievements, SAT II Writing Test, TOEFL for nonnative speakers of English, minimum college GPA of 2.6, 3 years of high school math, 3 years of high school science, high school chemistry, high school biology, high school transcript, transcript of college record, high school class rank: top 30%. *Options:* Advanced standing available through the following means: advanced placement exams, credit by exam. May apply for transfer of up to 90 total credits. *Application deadline:* rolling. *Application fee:* $25.

Degree Requirements 126 total credit hours, 54 in nursing.

RN Baccalaureate Program (BSN)

Applying *Required:* SAT I, ACT, 2 College Board Achievements, SAT II Writing Test, TOEFL for nonnative speakers of English, 3 years of high school math, 3 years of high school science, high school chemistry, high school biology, RN license, diploma or AD in nursing, high school transcript, transcript of college record. *Options:* Advanced standing available through the following means: advanced placement exams, credit by exam. May apply for transfer of up to 90 total credits. *Application fee:* $25.

Degree Requirements 126 total credit hours, 54 in nursing.

MASTER'S PROGRAMS

Contact Dr. Carol Wood, Coordinator, 218 Dunn Hall, School of Nursing, University of Maine, Orono, ME 04469, 207-581-2605. *Fax:* 207-581-2585. *E-mail:* cwood@maine.maine.edu

Areas of Study Nurse practitioner program in family health.

Expenses *State resident tuition:* $3222 full-time, $179 per credit hour part-time. *Nonresident tuition:* $9108 full-time, $506 per credit hour part-time. *Full-time mandatory fees:* $400–$450. *Room and board:* $5006. *Books and supplies per academic year:* ranges from $300 to $500.

Financial Aid Nurse traineeships, Federal Direct Loans, institutionally sponsored loans, institutionally sponsored need-based grants/scholarships, institutionally sponsored non-need-based grants/scholarships. 100% of master's level students in nursing programs received some form of financial aid in 1995-96. *Application deadline:* 3/1.

BSN to Master's Program (MSN)

Applying *Required:* GRE General Test or Miller Analogies Test, TOEFL for nonnative speakers of English, bachelor's degree in nursing, minimum GPA of 3.0, RN license, 2 years of clinical experience, physical assessment course, statistics course, essay, interview, 3 letters of recommendation, transcript of college record. *Application deadline:* 12/1. *Application fee:* $50.

Degree Requirements 45 total credit hours, 45 in nursing. Scholarly project or identified special courses.

RN to Master's Program (MSN)

Applying *Required:* GRE General Test or Miller Analogies Test, TOEFL for nonnative speakers of English, bachelor's degree in nursing, minimum GPA of 3.0, RN license, 1 year of clinical experience, physical assessment course, statistics course, essay, interview, 3 letters of recommendation, transcript of college record, a minimum of 95 undergraduate credits. *Application deadline:* 12/1. *Application fee:* $50.

Degree Requirements 45 total credit hours, 45 in nursing. Study must be completed within a six-year period.

Post-Master's Program

Applying *Required:* GRE General Test or Miller Analogies Test, TOEFL for nonnative speakers of English, bachelor's degree in nursing, minimum GPA of 3.0, RN license, 1 year of clinical experience, physical assessment course, statistics course, essay, interview, 3 letters of recommendation, transcript of college record, MSN. *Application deadline:* 12/1. *Application fee:* $50.

Degree Requirements 45 total credit hours, 45 in nursing.

UNIVERSITY OF MAINE AT FORT KENT
Nursing Department
Fort Kent, Maine

Programs • Generic Baccalaureate • RN Baccalaureate • Continuing Education

The University State-supported 4-year coed college. Part of University of Maine System. Founded: 1878. *Primary accreditation:* regional. *Setting:* 52-acre rural campus. *Total enrollment:* 731.

The Nursing Department Founded in 1985. *Nursing program faculty:* 5 (20% with doctorates).

▶ *NOTEWORTHY*

The University's location in the scenic St. John River Valley on the United States–Canada border provides a unique opportunity for study in a bilingual, multicultural environment. Focusing on rural community health, the BSN program takes advantage of several cooperative associations with U.S. and Canadian regional health facilities. This can include the option of completing clinical experience at a hospital in French-speaking Canada. University emphasis on knowledgeable, critical thinking blends a solid liberal arts education with an extensive professional program. The very low student-faculty ratio allows classes to be small and makes the faculty readily available for guidance and support.

Academic Facilities *Campus library:* 55,000 volumes (190 in health, 450 in nursing); 314 periodical subscriptions (35 health-care related). *Nursing school resources:* CAI, computer lab, nursing audiovisuals, learning resource lab.

Student Life *Student services:* child-care facilities, personal counseling, career counseling, institutionally sponsored work-study program, special assistance for disabled students. *International student services:* counseling/support. *Nursing student activities:* student nurses association.

Calendar Semesters.

NURSING STUDENT PROFILE

Undergraduate **Enrollment:** 136
Women: 85%; **Men:** 15%; **Minority:** 0%; **International:** 10%; **Part-time:** 19%

BACCALAUREATE PROGRAMS

Contact Ms. Kelly Goudreau, Chair, Advisement and Advancement Committee, Nursing Department, University of Maine at Fort Kent, 25 Pleasant Street, Fort Kent, ME 04743-1292, 207-834-7582. *Fax:* 207-834-7577. *E-mail:* goudreau@maine.maine.edu

Expenses *State resident tuition:* $5520 full-time, $92 per credit part-time. *Nonresident tuition:* $13,440 full-time, $224 per credit part-time. *Full-time mandatory fees:* $90–$120. *Room and board:* $3550–$3600. *Room only:* $1825. *Books and supplies per academic year:* ranges from $200 to $250.

Financial Aid Institutionally sponsored need-based grants/scholarships, institutionally sponsored non-need grants/scholarships, Federal Nursing

Student Loans, Federal Work-Study. 79% of undergraduate students in nursing programs received some form of financial aid in 1995–96. *Application deadline:* 3/15.

Generic Baccalaureate Program (BSN)

Applying *Required:* SAT I, minimum college GPA of 2.5, high school transcript, interview, 2 letters of recommendation, written essay, transcript of college record. 73 prerequisite credits must be completed before admission to the nursing program. *Application deadlines:* 8/15 (fall), 1/10 (spring). *Application fee:* $25.

Degree Requirements 123 total credit hours, 50 in nursing.

RN Baccalaureate Program (BSN)

Applying *Required:* SAT I, minimum college GPA of 2.5, RN license, diploma or AD in nursing, high school transcript, interview, 2 letters of recommendation, written essay, transcript of college record. *Options:* Advanced standing available through credit by exam. *Application deadlines:* 8/15 (fall), 1/10 (spring). *Application fee:* $25.

Degree Requirements 123 total credit hours, 50 in nursing.

Distance learning Courses provided through interactive television system.

CONTINUING EDUCATION PROGRAM

Contact Rachel Albert, Assistant Professor of Nursing, University of Maine at Fort Kent, 25 Pleasant Street, Fort Kent, ME 04743, 207-834-7584. *Fax:* 207-834-7577. *E-mail:* realbert@maine.maine.edu

UNIVERSITY OF NEW ENGLAND–UNIVERSITY CAMPUS

Department of Nursing
Biddeford, Maine

Programs • Accelerated RN Baccalaureate • RN to Master's

The University Independent comprehensive coed institution. Founded: 1953. *Primary accreditation:* regional. *Setting:* 410-acre small-town campus. *Total enrollment:* 1,782.

The Department of Nursing Founded in 1986. *Nursing program faculty:* 11 (10% with doctorates).

Academic Facilities *Campus library:* 45,075 volumes (9,440 in health, 3,115 in nursing); 886 periodical subscriptions (575 health-care related). *Nursing school resources:* CAI, computer lab, nursing audiovisuals, learning resource lab.

Student Life *Student services:* health clinic, personal counseling, career counseling, institutionally sponsored work-study program, job placement, campus safety program, special assistance for disabled students. *International student services:* counseling/support, ESL courses. *Nursing student activities:* nursing club, student nurses association.

Calendar Semesters.

NURSING STUDENT PROFILE

Undergraduate **Enrollment:** 118
Women: 85%; **Men:** 15%; **Minority:** 1%; **International:** 0%; **Part-time:** 20%

Graduate **Enrollment:** 68
Women: 75%; **Men:** 25%; **Minority:** 19%; **International:** 0%; **Part-time:** 0%

BACCALAUREATE PROGRAM

Contact Barbara Teague, Chair, Department of Nursing, University of New England-University Campus, 11 Hills Beach Road, Biddeford, ME 04005, 207-283-0171. *Fax:* 207-282-6379. *E-mail:* bteague@mailbox.une.edu

Expenses *Tuition:* $13,050 full-time, $415 per credit hour part-time. *Full-time mandatory fees:* $510. *Room and board:* $5495. *Books and supplies per academic year:* ranges from $300 to $500.

Financial Aid Institutionally sponsored need-based grants/scholarships, institutionally sponsored non-need grants/scholarships, Federal Direct Loans, Federal Nursing Student Loans, Federal Pell Grants, Federal Perkins Loans, Federal Supplemental Educational Opportunity Grants, Federal Work-Study. 95% of undergraduate students in nursing programs received some form of financial aid in 1995–96. *Application deadline:* 4/1.

Accelerated RN Baccalaureate Program (BSN)

Applying *Required:* SAT I or ACT, TOEFL for nonnative speakers of English, minimum college GPA of 2.5, high school chemistry, high school biology, RN license, diploma or AD in nursing, interview, 2 letters of recommendation, written essay, transcript of college record. 60 prerequisite credits must be completed before admission to the nursing program. *Options:* Advanced standing available through the following means: advanced placement exams, credit by exam. May apply for transfer of up to 85 total credits. *Application deadline:* rolling. *Application fee:* $40.

Degree Requirements 124 total credit hours, 39 in nursing.

MASTER'S PROGRAM

Contact Dr. Carl Spirito, Nurse Anesthesia Program Director, University of New England-University Campus, 11 Hills Beach Road, Biddeford, ME 04005, 207-283-0171. *Fax:* 207-282-6379. *E-mail:* cspirito@mailbox.une.edu

Areas of Study Nurse anesthesia.

Expenses *Tuition:* $5670 full-time, $315 per credit hour part-time. *Full-time mandatory fees:* $260. *Books and supplies per academic year:* ranges from $300 to $600.

Financial Aid Federal Direct Loans, Federal Nursing Student Loans, institutionally sponsored need-based grants/scholarships. 97% of master's level students in nursing programs received some form of financial aid in 1995-96. *Application deadline:* 5/1.

RN to Master's Program (MS)

Applying *Required:* GRE General Test, TOEFL for nonnative speakers of English, bachelor's degree in nursing, bachelor's degree, minimum GPA of 2.75, RN license, professional liability/malpractice insurance, essay, interview, 3 letters of recommendation, transcript of college record, ACLS certification. *Application deadline:* 1/15. *Application fee:* $35.

Degree Requirements 54 total credit hours, 22 in nursing, 32 in basic sciences.

See full description on page 546.

UNIVERSITY OF NEW ENGLAND–WESTBROOK COLLEGE CAMPUS

Nursing Program
Portland, Maine

Programs • Generic Baccalaureate • RN Baccalaureate • Accelerated MS • RN to Master's • Master's for Nurses with Non-Nursing Degrees

The University Independent 4-year coed college. Founded: 1831. *Primary accreditation:* regional. *Setting:* 40-acre urban campus. *Total enrollment:* 261.

The Nursing Program Founded in 1964. *Nursing program faculty:* 7 (28% with doctorates).

Academic Facilities *Campus library:* 62,046 volumes (9,000 in health, 4,981 in nursing); 599 periodical subscriptions (170 health-care related). *Nursing school resources:* CAI, computer lab, nursing audiovisuals, interactive nursing skills videos, learning resource lab.

Student Life *Student services:* health clinic, child-care facilities, personal counseling, career counseling, institutionally sponsored work-study program, job placement, campus safety program. *Nursing student activities:* student nurses association, Nursing Honor Society.

Calendar Semesters.

NURSING STUDENT PROFILE

Undergraduate **Enrollment:** 56
Women: 94%; **Men:** 6%; **Minority:** 3%; **International:** 1%; **Part-time:** 5%

Graduate **Enrollment:** 71
Women: 96%; **Men:** 4%; **Minority:** 0%; **International:** 0%; **Part-time:** 25%

BACCALAUREATE PROGRAMS

Contact Dr. Catherine Berardelli, Director, Nursing Program, Department of Nursing, University of New England-Westbrook College Campus, Stevens Avenue, Portland, ME 04103, 207-797-7261. *Fax:* 207-797-7225. *E-mail:* berardel@saturn.caps.maine.edu

University of New England–Westbrook College Campus (continued)

Expenses *Tuition:* $13,050 full-time, $415 per credit hour part-time. *Full-time mandatory fees:* $250. *Room and board:* $5495. *Books and supplies per academic year:* ranges from $300 to $600.

Financial Aid Institutionally sponsored need-based grants/scholarships, institutionally sponsored non-need grants/scholarships, Federal Direct Loans, Federal Nursing Student Loans, Federal Pell Grants, Federal Perkins Loans, Federal Supplemental Educational Opportunity Grants, Federal Work-Study. 100% of undergraduate students in nursing programs received some form of financial aid in 1995–96. *Application deadline:* 5/1.

Generic Baccalaureate Program (BSN)

Applying *Required:* SAT I or ACT, TOEFL for nonnative speakers of English, minimum high school GPA of 2.5, minimum college GPA of 2.5, 3 years of high school math, 3 years of high school science, high school chemistry, high school biology, high school transcript, 2 letters of recommendation, written essay, transcript of college record. *Options:* May apply for transfer of up to 60 total credits. *Application deadline:* rolling. *Application fee:* $40.

Degree Requirements 123 total credit hours, 58 in nursing.

RN Baccalaureate Program (BSN)

Applying *Required:* NLN Mobility Profile II, minimum high school GPA of 2.5, minimum college GPA of 2.5, high school math, high school science, high school chemistry, high school biology, RN license, diploma or AD in nursing, transcript of college record. *Options:* Course work may be accelerated. *Application deadline:* rolling. *Application fee:* $40.

Degree Requirements 123 total credit hours, 62 in nursing.

MASTER'S PROGRAMS

Contact Catherine M. Berardelli, Director, Nursing Programs, Department of Nursing, University of New England-Westbrook College Campus, 716 Stevens Avenue, Portland, ME 04103, 207-797-7261. *Fax:* 207-797-6894. *E-mail:* berardel@saturn.caps.maine.edu

Areas of Study Nurse practitioner programs in adult health, child care/pediatrics, family health.

Expenses *Tuition:* $9828 full-time, $546 per credit hour part-time. *Full-time mandatory fees:* $260.

Financial Aid Nurse traineeships, Federal Direct Loans, Federal Nursing Student Loans.

Accelerated MS Program

Applying *Required:* GRE General Test, minimum GPA of 3.0, 1 year of clinical experience, physical assessment course, statistics course, professional liability/malpractice insurance, essay, 3 letters of recommendation, transcript of college record, minimum grade of "B" in human physiology course. *Application deadline:* 3/1. *Application fee:* $50.

Degree Requirements 44 total credit hours. Thesis required.

RN to Master's Program (MS)

Applying *Required:* GRE General Test, minimum GPA of 3.0, RN license, 1 year of clinical experience, physical assessment course, statistics course, professional liability/malpractice insurance, essay, 3 letters of recommendation, transcript of college record, minimum grade of "B" in human physiology course. *Application deadline:* 3/1. *Application fee:* $50.

Degree Requirements 44 total credit hours. Thesis required.

Master's for Nurses with Non-Nursing Degrees Program (MS)

Applying *Required:* GRE General Test, minimum GPA of 3.0, 1 year of clinical experience, physical assessment course, statistics course, professional liability/malpractice insurance, essay, 3 letters of recommendation, transcript of college record, minimum grade of "B" in human physiology course. *Application deadline:* 3/1. *Application fee:* $50.

Degree Requirements 44 total credit hours. Thesis required.

See full description on page 546.

UNIVERSITY OF SOUTHERN MAINE
College of Nursing and the School of Health Professions
Portland, Maine

Programs • Generic Baccalaureate • RN Baccalaureate • MS • RN to Master's • Accelerated Master's for Non-Nursing College Graduates • Post-Master's • Continuing Education

The University State-supported comprehensive coed institution. Part of University of Maine System. Founded: 1878. *Primary accreditation:* regional. *Setting:* 120-acre urban campus. *Total enrollment:* 9,721.

The College of Nursing and the School of Health Professions Founded in 1968. *Nursing program faculty:* 22 (77% with doctorates). *Off-campus program site:* Lewiston.

Academic Facilities *Campus library:* 347,575 volumes (1,552 in health, 20,073 in nursing); 1,878 periodical subscriptions (250 health-care related). *Nursing school resources:* CAI, computer lab, nursing audiovisuals, interactive nursing skills videos, learning resource lab.

Student Life *Student services:* health clinic, child-care facilities, personal counseling, career counseling, institutionally sponsored work-study program, job placement, campus safety program, special assistance for disabled students. *International student services:* counseling/support, special assistance for nonnative speakers of English, ESL courses. *Nursing student activities:* Sigma Theta Tau, student nurses association, Maine Student Nurse Association.

Calendar Semesters.

NURSING STUDENT PROFILE

Undergraduate **Enrollment:** 327
Women: 90%; **Men:** 10%; **Minority:** 3%; **International:** 0%; **Part-time:** 66%
Graduate **Enrollment:** 116
Women: 94%; **Men:** 6%; **Minority:** 3%; **International:** 1%; **Part-time:** 66%

BACCALAUREATE PROGRAMS

Contact Ms. Elizabeth K. Elliott, Coordinator of Advising, School of Nursing, University of Southern Maine, PO Box 9300, Portland, ME 04104-9300, 207-780-4130. *Fax:* 207-780-4997.

Expenses *State resident tuition:* ranges from $3386 to $3497 full-time, $111 per credit part-time. *Nonresident tuition:* ranges from $9577 to $9891 full-time, $314 per credit part-time. *Full-time mandatory fees:* $155. *Part-time mandatory fees:* $110. *Room and board:* $2358–$2808. *Room only:* $1065–$1098. *Books and supplies per academic year:* ranges from $200 to $400.

Financial Aid Institutionally sponsored need-based grants/scholarships, institutionally sponsored non-need grants/scholarships, Federal Nursing Student Loans, Federal Perkins Loans, Federal Supplemental Educational Opportunity Grants, Federal Work-Study. 84% of undergraduate students in nursing programs received some form of financial aid in 1995–96. *Application deadline:* 2/1.

Generic Baccalaureate Program (BS)

Applying *Required:* SAT I, TOEFL for nonnative speakers of English, minimum college GPA of 2.5, high school chemistry, high school biology, high school transcript, letter of recommendation, written essay, transcript of college record, high school class rank: top 25%. 30 prerequisite credits must be completed before admission to the nursing program. *Options:* Advanced standing available through credit by exam. Course work may be accelerated. *Application deadlines:* 2/1 (fall), 3/1 (transfers). *Application fee:* $25.

Degree Requirements 122–126 total credit hours dependent upon track, 53 in nursing.

RN Baccalaureate Program (BS)

Applying *Required:* TOEFL for nonnative speakers of English, RN license, diploma or AD in nursing, transcript of college record. *Options:* Advanced standing available through credit by exam. Course work may be accelerated. *Application deadline:* rolling. *Application fee:* $25.

Degree Requirements 122 total credit hours, 51 in nursing.

Distance learning Courses provided through video, audio, interactive television.

MASTER'S PROGRAMS

Contact Ms. Mary Sloan, Assistant Director, Office of Graduate Affairs, University of Southern Maine, 96 Falmouth Street, PO Box 9300, Portland, ME 04104-9300, 207-780-4386. *Fax:* 207-780-4969.

Areas of Study Clinical nurse specialist programs in adult health nursing, community health nursing, psychiatric–mental health nursing; nursing administration; nurse practitioner programs in adult health, family health.

Expenses *State resident tuition:* $4088 full-time, $167 per credit part-time. *Nonresident tuition:* $10,598 full-time, $471 per credit part-time. *Full-time mandatory fees:* $97. *Books and supplies per academic year:* ranges from $100 to $400.

Financial Aid Graduate assistantships, nurse traineeships, Federal Nursing Student Loans. *Application deadline:* 2/1.

MS Program

Applying *Required:* GRE General Test (minimum combined score of 1500 on three tests), Miller Analogies Test, TOEFL for nonnative speakers of English, bachelor's degree in nursing, minimum GPA of 3.0, RN license, physical assessment course, statistics course, essay, 2 letters of recommendation, transcript of college record. *Application deadline:* 3/1. *Application fee:* $25.

Degree Requirements 48 total credit hours, 45 in nursing.

RN to Master's Program (MS)

Applying *Required:* GRE General Test (minimum combined score of 1500 on three tests), Miller Analogies Test, TOEFL for nonnative speakers of English, minimum GPA of 3.0, RN license, essay, 2 letters of recommendation, transcript of college record. *Application deadline:* 3/1. *Application fee:* $25.

Degree Requirements 132 total credit hours, 62 in nursing.

Accelerated Master's for Non-Nursing College Graduates Program (MS)

Applying *Required:* GRE General Test (minimum combined score of 1500 on three tests), Miller Analogies Test, bachelor's degree, minimum GPA of 3.0, statistics course, essay, 2 letters of recommendation, transcript of college record. *Application deadline:* 12/1. *Application fee:* $25.

Degree Requirements 88 total credit hours, 85 in nursing.

Post-Master's Program

Applying *Required:* RN license, essay, 2 letters of recommendation, transcript of college record, master's degree in nursing. *Application deadline:* 3/1. *Application fee:* $25.

Degree Requirements 24 total credit hours, 21–24 in nursing, 3 in mental-health related areas.

CONTINUING EDUCATION PROGRAM

Contact Ms. Mary Ann Rost, RN, Director of Health Professions, Center for Continuing Education - PO Box 9300, Portland, ME 04104, 207-780-5951. *Fax:* 207-780-5925.

MARYLAND

BOWIE STATE UNIVERSITY
Department of Nursing
Bowie, Maryland

Programs • RN Baccalaureate • RN to Master's • Continuing Education

The University State-supported comprehensive coed institution. Part of University of Maryland System. Founded: 1865. *Primary accreditation:* regional. *Setting:* 267-acre small-town campus. *Total enrollment:* 5,258.

The Department of Nursing Founded in 1979. *Nursing program faculty:* 7 (57% with doctorates).

Academic Facilities *Campus library:* 175,000 volumes (3,289 in health, 5,700 in nursing); 1,333 periodical subscriptions (255 health-care related). *Nursing school resources:* computer lab, nursing audiovisuals, learning resource lab.

Student Life *Student services:* health clinic, child-care facilities, personal counseling, career counseling, institutionally sponsored work-study program, job placement, campus safety program, special assistance for disabled students. *International student services:* counseling/support, ESL courses, assistance with immigration matters. *Nursing student activities:* nursing club.

Calendar Semesters.

NURSING STUDENT PROFILE

Undergraduate **Enrollment:** 81
Women: 95%; **Men:** 5%; **Minority:** 65%; **International:** 29%; **Part-time:** 92%
Graduate **Enrollment:** 73
Women: 92%; **Men:** 8%; **Minority:** 63%; **International:** 6%; **Part-time:** 3%

BACCALAUREATE PROGRAM

Contact Mrs. Nethelyne Coleman, Admissions, Progressions, and Graduation Coordinator, Department of Nursing, Bowie State University, Bowie, MD 20715, 301-464-6551. *Fax:* 301-464-7569.

Expenses *State resident tuition:* $2381 full-time, $104 per credit part-time. *Nonresident tuition:* $6304 full-time, $280 per credit part-time. *Full-time mandatory fees:* $361. *Part-time mandatory fees:* $88. *Room and board:* $3871–$5204. *Room only:* $1123–$1705.

Financial Aid Institutionally sponsored need-based grants/scholarships, institutionally sponsored non-need grants/scholarships, Federal Direct Loans, Federal Perkins Loans, Federal Supplemental Educational Opportunity Grants, Federal Work-Study. *Application deadline:* 5/1.

RN Baccalaureate Program (BSN)

Applying *Required:* ACT, TOEFL for nonnative speakers of English, nursing transition courses, minimum college GPA of 2.0, RN license, diploma or AD in nursing, 3 letters of recommendation, written essay, transcript of college record, CPR certification, resume, medical history/physical examination, and NET test. 34 prerequisite credits must be completed before admission to the nursing program. *Options:* Advanced standing available through credit by exam. May apply for transfer of up to 87 total credits. *Application deadlines:* 4/15 (fall), 10/15 (spring).

Degree Requirements 120 total credit hours, 33 in nursing. English proficiency exam.

MASTER'S PROGRAM

Contact Mrs. Nethelyne Coleman, Admissions, Progressions, and Graduation Coordinator, Department of Nursing, Bowie State University, Bowie, MD 20715, 301-464-6551. *Fax:* 301-464-7569. *E-mail:* ncoleman@bowiestate.edu

Areas of Study Nursing administration; nursing education; nurse practitioner program in family health.

Expenses *State resident tuition:* $2592 full-time, $144 per credit part-time. *Nonresident tuition:* $4392 full-time, $244 per credit part-time. *Full-time mandatory fees:* $82.

Financial Aid Graduate assistantships, nurse traineeships, Federal Direct Loans, Federal Nursing Student Loans. *Application deadline:* 5/1.

RN to Master's Program (MSN)

Applying *Required:* TOEFL for nonnative speakers of English, minimum GPA of 2.5, RN license, 1 year of clinical experience, physical assessment course, statistics course, professional liability/malpractice insurance, essay, interview, 3 letters of recommendation, transcript of college record. *Application deadline:* rolling. *Application fee:* $30.

Degree Requirements 149–156 total credit hours dependent upon track, 91–98 in nursing, 58 in education, management, information systems. Comprehensive exam.

CONTINUING EDUCATION PROGRAM

Contact Mrs. Carolyn Velga, Coordinator, Continuing Education, Department of Nursing, Bowie State University, Bowie, MD 20715, 301-464-7273.

Bowie State University (continued)

Generic Baccalaureate Program (BSN)

Applying *Required:* SAT I, ACT, Nelson-Denny Reading Test, self-concept and critical thinking scales, minimum high school GPA of 2.5, minimum college GPA of 2.5, 3 years of high school math, 3 years of high school science, high school transcript, interview, 2 letters of recommendation, written essay, transcript of college record. 27 prerequisite credits must be completed before admission to the nursing program. *Options:* Course work may be accelerated. May apply for transfer of up to 70 total credits. *Application deadline:* 2/1. *Application fee:* $20.

Degree Requirements 128 total credit hours, 53 in nursing. Skills workshop.

RN Baccalaureate Program (BSN)

Applying *Required:* SAT I, ACT, Nelson-Denny Reading Test, minimum college GPA of 2.5, RN license, diploma or AD in nursing, high school transcript, interview, 2 letters of recommendation, written essay, transcript of college record. 42 prerequisite credits must be completed before admission to the nursing program. *Options:* Course work may be accelerated. May apply for transfer of up to 70 total credits. *Application deadline:* rolling. *Application fee:* $20.

Degree Requirements 120 total credit hours, 33 in nursing.

COLLEGE OF NOTRE DAME OF MARYLAND
Department of Nursing
Baltimore, Maryland

Program • RN Baccalaureate

The College Independent Roman Catholic comprehensive women's institution. Founded: 1873. *Primary accreditation:* regional. *Setting:* 58-acre suburban campus. *Total enrollment:* 2,205.

The Department of Nursing Founded in 1979.

Academic Facilities *Campus library:* 290,000 volumes (850 in health, 341 in nursing); 2,000 periodical subscriptions (61 health-care related). *Nursing school resources:* CAI, computer lab, nursing audiovisuals.

Calendar Semesters.

BACCALAUREATE PROGRAM

Contact Chair and Associate Professor, Department of Nursing, College of Notre Dame of Maryland, 4701 North Charles Street, Baltimore, MD 21210-2476, 410-532-5526. *Fax:* 410-435-5937.

RN Baccalaureate Program (BSN)

Applying *Required:* SAT I, TOEFL for nonnative speakers of English, RN license, diploma or AD in nursing, high school transcript, letter of recommendation, written essay, transcript of college record. 36 prerequisite credits must be completed before admission to the nursing program. *Application deadlines:* 2/15 (fall), 12/15 (spring). *Application fee:* $25.

COLUMBIA UNION COLLEGE
Department of Nursing
Takoma Park, Maryland

Programs • Generic Baccalaureate • RN Baccalaureate • Continuing Education

The College Independent Seventh-day Adventist 4-year coed college. Founded: 1904. *Primary accreditation:* regional. *Setting:* 19-acre suburban campus. *Total enrollment:* 1,141.

The Department of Nursing Founded in 1904. *Nursing program faculty:* 14 (20% with doctorates).

Academic Facilities *Campus library:* 124,000 volumes (300 in nursing); 431 periodical subscriptions (87 health-care related). *Nursing school resources:* CAI, computer lab, nursing audiovisuals, interactive nursing skills videos, learning resource lab.

Student Life *Student services:* health clinic, personal counseling, career counseling, institutionally sponsored work-study program, job placement, campus safety program. *International student services:* counseling/support, ESL courses. *Nursing student activities:* nursing club, student nurses association.

Calendar Semesters.

NURSING STUDENT PROFILE

Undergraduate **Enrollment:** 132

Women: 89%; **Men:** 11%; **Minority:** 48%; **International:** 13%; **Part-time:** 20%

BACCALAUREATE PROGRAMS

Contact Dr. Shirley Wilson-Anderson, Chair, Department of Nursing, Columbia Union College, 7600 Flower Avenue, Takoma Park, MD 20912, 301-891-4144. *Fax:* 301-891-4191.

Expenses *Tuition:* $10,950 full-time, $460 per credit hour part-time. *Full-time mandatory fees:* $153–$426. *Room and board:* $3990. *Room only:* $2150. *Books and supplies per academic year:* $1400.

Financial Aid Institutionally sponsored need-based grants/scholarships, institutionally sponsored non-need grants/scholarships, Federal Nursing Student Loans, Federal Pell Grants, Federal Perkins Loans, Federal Supplemental Educational Opportunity Grants, Federal Work-Study. *Application deadline:* 3/31.

CONTINUING EDUCATION PROGRAM

Contact Dr. Shirley Wilson-Anderson, Chair, Department of Nursing, Columbia Union College, 7600 Flower Avenue, Takoma Park, MD 20912, 301-891-4144. *Fax:* 301-891-4191.

COPPIN STATE COLLEGE
Helene Fuld School of Nursing
Baltimore, Maryland

Programs • Generic Baccalaureate • RN Baccalaureate

The College State-supported comprehensive coed institution. Part of University of Maryland System. Founded: 1900. *Primary accreditation:* regional. *Setting:* 33-acre urban campus. *Total enrollment:* 3,540.

The Helene Fuld School of Nursing Founded in 1974. *Nursing program faculty:* 14 (36% with doctorates).

Academic Facilities *Nursing school resources:* CAI, computer lab, nursing audiovisuals, interactive nursing skills videos, learning resource lab.

Student Life *Student services:* health clinic, personal counseling, career counseling, institutionally sponsored work-study program, job placement, campus safety program. *International student services:* counseling/support. *Nursing student activities:* student nurses association, Chi Eta Phi.

Calendar Semesters.

NURSING STUDENT PROFILE

Undergraduate **Enrollment:** 320

Women: 97%; **Men:** 3%; **Minority:** 99%; **International:** 5%; **Part-time:** 25%

BACCALAUREATE PROGRAMS

Contact Mr. Darryl A. Boyd, Nursing Recruiter and Admission Counselor, Helene Fuld School of Nursing, Coppin State College, 2500 West North Avenue, Baltimore, MD 21215-3698, 410-383-5740. *Fax:* 410-462-3032. *E-mail:* d6pcboy@coppin.umd.edu

Expenses *State resident tuition:* $2867 full-time, $99 per credit hour part-time. *Nonresident tuition:* $6872 full-time, $198 per credit hour part-time. *Full-time mandatory fees:* $64–$727. *Room and board:* $4850–$5050. *Room only:* $3150–$3350. *Books and supplies per academic year:* $250.

Financial Aid Institutionally sponsored need-based grants/scholarships, institutionally sponsored non-need grants/scholarships, Federal Supplemental Educational Opportunity Grants, Federal Work-Study. *Application deadline:* 7/15.

Generic Baccalaureate Program (BSN)

Applying *Required:* SAT I, ACT, Nursing Entrance Test, New Jersey Placement Exam for freshmen or transfer students with fewer than 25 credits, minimum high school GPA of 2.5, minimum college GPA of 2.5, 3 years of high school math, high school foreign language, high school transcript, 3 letters of recommendation, transcript of college record, 2 years of high school lab science. *Application deadlines:* 7/15 (fall), 12/15 (spring). *Application fee:* $25.

Degree Requirements 124 total credit hours, 69 in nursing.

RN Baccalaureate Program (BSN)

Applying *Required:* minimum high school GPA of 2.5, minimum college GPA of 2.5, 3 years of high school math, RN license, diploma or AD in nursing, high school foreign language, high school transcript, 3 letters of recommendation, transcript of college record, 2 years of high school lab science. 60 prerequisite credits must be completed before admission to the nursing program. *Application deadlines:* 7/15 (fall), 12/15 (spring). *Application fee:* $25.

Degree Requirements 121 total credit hours, 29 in nursing.

JOHNS HOPKINS UNIVERSITY
School of Nursing
Baltimore, Maryland

Programs • Generic Baccalaureate • RN Baccalaureate • Accelerated Baccalaureate for Second Degree • MSN • MSN/MSBA • MSN/MPH • Post-Master's • PhD • Postdoctoral

The University Independent coed university. Founded: 1876. *Primary accreditation:* regional. *Setting:* 140-acre urban campus. *Total enrollment:* 4,847.

The School of Nursing Founded in 1983. *Nursing program faculty:* 49 (55% with doctorates).

▶ ***NOTEWORTHY***

The Johns Hopkins University School of Nursing is committed to the education of nurse leaders and provides a unique combination of academic, clinical, and research opportunities that have earned it international recognition. The MSN/MS in business is offered with the School of Continuing Studies and the MSN/MPH with the School of Hygiene and Public Health. Postdoctoral fellowships are offered in infection prevention and wound healing. Special programs include the Institute for Johns Hopkins Nursing, a joint venture with the Johns Hopkins Hospital Department of Nursing, and the Peace Corps Preparatory Program and the Peace Corps Fellows/AmeriCorps Health and Housing Program, in collaboration with the Peace Corps of the United States.

Academic Facilities *Campus library:* 367,000 volumes; 3,400 periodical subscriptions. *Nursing school resources:* CAI, computer lab, nursing audiovisuals, interactive nursing skills videos, learning resource lab.

Student Life *Student services:* health clinic, personal counseling, career counseling, institutionally sponsored work-study program, campus safety program, special assistance for disabled students. *International student services:* counseling/support, special assistance for nonnative speakers of English. *Nursing student activities:* Sigma Theta Tau, student nurses association, Multicultural Students Organization, Undergraduate Student Government Association, Graduate Student Organization, RN/BS Organization.

Calendar Semesters.

NURSING STUDENT PROFILE

Undergraduate **Enrollment:** 286
Women: 87%; **Men:** 13%; **Minority:** 12%; **International:** 0%; **Part-time:** 7%
Graduate **Enrollment:** 133
Women: 96%; **Men:** 4%; **Minority:** 13%; **International:** 3%; **Part-time:** 87%

BACCALAUREATE PROGRAMS

Contact Ms. Mary F. Herlihy, Director of Admissions and Student Services, School of Nursing, Johns Hopkins University, 1830 East Monument Street, Suite 200, Baltimore, MD 21205, 410-955-7548. *Fax:* 410-955-9177. *E-mail:* mherlihy@sonnet.nsg.jhu.edu

Expenses *Tuition:* $15,750 full-time, $656 per semester credit hour part-time. *Full-time mandatory fees:* $500–$1500. *Room and board:* $5000–$6500. *Room only:* $3000–$5000. *Books and supplies per academic year:* ranges from $650 to $800.

Financial Aid Institutionally sponsored need-based grants/scholarships, institutionally sponsored non-need grants/scholarships, Federal Direct Loans, Federal Nursing Student Loans, Federal Pell Grants, Federal Perkins Loans, Federal Supplemental Educational Opportunity Grants, Federal Work-Study. 84% of undergraduate students in nursing programs received some form of financial aid in 1995–96. *Application deadline:* 2/15.

Generic Baccalaureate Program (BS)

Applying *Required:* SAT I or ACT, TOEFL for nonnative speakers of English, minimum college GPA of 3.0, high school transcript, interview, 3 letters of recommendation, written essay, transcript of college record. 60 prerequisite credits must be completed before admission to the nursing program. *Options:* Course work may be accelerated. May apply for transfer of up to 60 total credits. *Application deadlines:* 2/15 (fall), 11/1 (early decision). *Application fee:* $40.

Degree Requirements 120 total credit hours, 54 in nursing.

RN Baccalaureate Program (BS)

Applying *Required:* TOEFL for nonnative speakers of English, minimum college GPA of 3.0, RN license, diploma or AD in nursing, interview, 3 letters of recommendation, written essay, transcript of college record. 60 prerequisite credits must be completed before admission to the nursing program. *Options:* Advanced standing available through credit by exam. Course work may be accelerated. May apply for transfer of up to 60 total credits. *Application deadlines:* 2/15 (fall), 11/15 (spring). *Application fee:* $40.

Degree Requirements 120 total credit hours, 54 in nursing.

Accelerated Baccalaureate for Second Degree Program (BS)

Applying *Required:* TOEFL for nonnative speakers of English, minimum college GPA of 3.0, interview, 3 letters of recommendation, written essay, transcript of college record, courses in human anatomy, physiology, and microbiology, previous baccalaureate degree or higher in field other than nursing. 60 prerequisite credits must be completed before admission to the nursing program. *Options:* Course work may be accelerated. May apply for transfer of up to 60 total credits. *Application deadline:* 12/15 (early decision - 11/1, summer). *Application fee:* $40.

Degree Requirements 54 total credit hours, 54 in nursing.

MASTER'S PROGRAMS

Contact Ms. Mary F. Herlihy, Director of Admissions and Student Services, School of Nursing, Johns Hopkins University, 1830 East Monument Street, Suite 200, Baltimore, MD 21205, 410-955-7548. *Fax:* 410-955-9177. *E-mail:* mherlihy@sonnet.nsg.jhu.edu

Areas of Study Clinical nurse specialist programs in adult health nursing, community health nursing, oncology nursing, HIV/AIDS nursing; nursing administration; nurse practitioner programs in acute care, adult health, child care/pediatrics, primary care.

Expenses *Tuition:* $15,750 full-time, $656 per semester credit hour part-time. *Full-time mandatory fees:* $500–$1500. *Room and board:* $3000–$6000. *Books and supplies per academic year:* ranges from $650 to $800.

Financial Aid Nurse traineeships, Federal Direct Loans, Federal Nursing Student Loans, institutionally sponsored loans, employment opportunities, institutionally sponsored non-need-based grants/scholarships. 25% of master's level students in nursing programs received some form of financial aid in 1995-96. *Application deadline:* 2/15.

MSN Program

Applying *Required:* GRE General Test, TOEFL for nonnative speakers of English, bachelor's degree in nursing, minimum GPA of 3.0, RN license, 1 year of clinical experience, physical assessment course, statistics course, essay, interview, 3 letters of recommendation, transcript of college record. *Application deadline:* 3/1. *Application fee:* $40.

Degree Requirements 35–55 total credit hours dependent upon track.

MSN/MSBA Program

Applying *Required:* GRE General Test, TOEFL for nonnative speakers of English, bachelor's degree in nursing, minimum GPA of 3.0, RN license, essay, interview, 3 letters of recommendation, transcript of college record. *Application deadline:* rolling.

Degree Requirements 50 total credit hours, 23 in nursing, 27 in business.

MSN/MPH Program

Applying *Required:* GRE General Test, TOEFL for nonnative speakers of English, bachelor's degree in nursing, minimum GPA of 3.0, RN license, 2 years of clinical experience, physical assessment course, statistics course, essay, interview, 3 letters of recommendation, transcript of college record, college-level course work in algebra, biology, chemistry, or physics. *Application deadline:* 1/31 (summer). *Application fee:* $40.

Degree Requirements 60–65 total credit hours dependent upon track, 30 in nursing, 30–35 in public health.

Johns Hopkins University (continued)

POST-MASTER'S PROGRAM

Applying *Required:* minimum GPA of 3.0, RN license, 2 years of clinical experience, physical assessment course, interview, 2 letters of recommendation, transcript of college record, master's degree in nursing with clinical major or 2 years of recent clinical experience. *Application deadlines:* 3/1 (fall), 11/1 (spring). *Application fee:* $40.

Degree Requirements 18 total credit hours, 18 in nursing.

DOCTORAL PROGRAM

Contact Ms. Mary F. Herlihy, Director of Admissions and Student Services, School of Nursing, Johns Hopkins University, 1830 East Monument Street, Suite 200, Baltimore, MD 21205, 410-955-7548. *Fax:* 410-955-9177. *E-mail:* mherlihy@sonnet.nsg.jhu.edu

Areas of Study Selected areas congruent with applicant's goals and expertise of the faculty.

Expenses *Tuition:* $20,740 full-time, $864 per semester credit hour part-time. *Full-time mandatory fees:* $500–$1500. *Room and board:* $6800. *Books and supplies per academic year:* ranges from $600 to $800.

Financial Aid Graduate assistantships, nurse traineeships, fellowships, Federal Direct Loans, institutionally sponsored non-need-based grants/scholarships. *Application deadline:* 2/15.

PHD PROGRAM

Applying *Required:* GRE General Test, TOEFL for nonnative speakers of English, master's degree, year of clinical experience, year in proposed area of specialization, statistics course, interview, 3 letters of recommendation, writing sample, competitive review by faculty committee, BSN or MSN, RN license, transcripts, proof of immunization required upon acceptance. *Application deadline:* 3/1. *Application fee:* $40.

Degree Requirements 63 total credit hours; dissertation; oral exam; written exam; defense of dissertation; residency; minimum of 9 credit hours of course work must be taken outside the School of Nursing.

POSTDOCTORAL PROGRAM

Contact Dr. Martha Hill, Director of the Center for Nursing Research, School of Nursing, Johns Hopkins University, 1830 East Monument Street, Baltimore, MD 21205, 410-614-1422. *Fax:* 410-614-1446.

Areas of Study Infection prevention/skin care, health promotion/health behavior.

See full description on page 464.

SALISBURY STATE UNIVERSITY

Department of Nursing
Salisbury, Maryland

Programs • Generic Baccalaureate • RN Baccalaureate • MS • Accelerated Master's for Non-Nursing College Graduates • Post-Master's

The University State-supported comprehensive coed institution. Part of University of Maryland System. Founded: 1925. *Primary accreditation:* regional. *Setting:* 140-acre small-town campus. *Total enrollment:* 6,010.

The Department of Nursing Founded in 1977. *Nursing program faculty:* 17 (35% with doctorates).

Academic Facilities *Campus library:* 1,652 periodical subscriptions (146 health-care related). *Nursing school resources:* CAI, computer lab, nursing audiovisuals, interactive nursing skills videos, learning resource lab.

Student Life *Student services:* health clinic, personal counseling, career counseling, institutionally sponsored work-study program, job placement, campus safety program, special assistance for disabled students. *International student services:* counseling/support, ESL courses. *Nursing student activities:* Sigma Theta Tau, student nurses association.

Calendar Semesters.

NURSING STUDENT PROFILE

Undergraduate **Enrollment:** 180
Women: 92%; **Men:** 8%; **Minority:** 11%; **International:** 11%; **Part-time:** 11%
Graduate **Enrollment:** 65
Women: 88%; **Men:** 12%; **Minority:** 8%; **International:** 12%

BACCALAUREATE PROGRAMS

Contact Dr. Lisa A. Seldomridge, Chair, Department of Nursing, Salisbury State University, 1101 Camden Avenue, Salisbury, MD 21801, 410-543-6413. *Fax:* 410-548-3313. *E-mail:* laseldomridge@ssu.edu

Expenses *State resident tuition:* $3608 full-time, $105 per credit part-time. *Nonresident tuition:* $6918 full-time, $190 per credit part-time. *Full-time mandatory fees:* $90. *Room only:* $5000–$5300. *Books and supplies per academic year:* ranges from $300 to $400.

Financial Aid Institutionally sponsored need-based grants/scholarships, Federal Nursing Student Loans, Federal Supplemental Educational Opportunity Grants, Federal Work-Study. *Application deadline:* 3/1.

GENERIC BACCALAUREATE PROGRAM (BS)

Applying *Required:* SAT I, TOEFL for nonnative speakers of English, 3 years of high school math, high school chemistry, high school biology, high school foreign language, high school transcript. 39 prerequisite credits must be completed before admission to the nursing program. *Options:* May apply for transfer of up to 50 total credits. *Application deadlines:* 3/1 (fall), 1/15 (spring). *Application fee:* $30.

Degree Requirements 123 total credit hours, 51 in nursing.

RN BACCALAUREATE PROGRAM (BS)

Applying *Required:* TOEFL for nonnative speakers of English, RN license, diploma or AD in nursing, transcript of college record. *Options:* Advanced standing available through credit by exam. *Application deadlines:* 3/1 (fall), 1/15 (spring). *Application fee:* $30.

Degree Requirements 123 total credit hours, 51 in nursing.

MASTER'S PROGRAMS

Contact Dr. Karen Badros, Director, Graduate Program, Department of Nursing, Salisbury State University, 1101 Camden Avenue, Salisbury, MD 21801, 410-543-6402. *Fax:* 410-548-3313. *E-mail:* kkbadros@ssu.edu

Areas of Study Clinical nurse specialist programs in family health nursing, rural health nursing; nursing administration; nurse practitioner program in family health.

Expenses *State resident tuition:* $140 per credit. *Nonresident tuition:* $210 per credit. *Full-time mandatory fees:* $20–$90. *Books and supplies per academic year:* ranges from $150 to $300.

Financial Aid Graduate assistantships, nurse traineeships, Federal Nursing Student Loans, employment opportunities. *Application deadline:* 3/1.

MS PROGRAM

Applying *Required:* bachelor's degree in nursing, minimum GPA of 3.0, RN license, essay, 2 letters of recommendation, transcript of college record. *Application fee:* $35.

Degree Requirements 39 total credit hours, 33 in nursing, 6 in statistics, business, education, or physiology. Thesis required.

ACCELERATED MASTER'S FOR NON-NURSING COLLEGE GRADUATES PROGRAM (MS)

Applying *Required:* bachelor's degree, minimum GPA of 2.75, interview, 2 letters of recommendation, transcript of college record, BSN earned concurrently. *Application fee:* $35.

Degree Requirements 83 total credit hours, 71 in nursing, 12 in pathophysiology, statistics, education, or business or physiology. Thesis required.

POST-MASTER'S PROGRAM

Applying *Required:* bachelor's degree in nursing, RN license, 2 years of clinical experience, physical assessment course, professional liability/malpractice insurance, essay, interview, 2 letters of recommendation, transcript of college record, MS or MSN. *Application fee:* $35.

Degree Requirements 42 total credit hours, 33 in nursing, 9 in math, biology, education, business. Thesis required.

TOWSON STATE UNIVERSITY
Department of Nursing
Towson, Maryland

Programs • Generic Baccalaureate • RN Baccalaureate • Baccalaureate for Second Degree

The University State-supported comprehensive coed institution. Part of University of Maryland System. Founded: 1866. *Primary accreditation:* regional. *Setting:* 321-acre suburban campus. *Total enrollment:* 14,643.

The Department of Nursing Founded in 1972. *Nursing program faculty:* 15 (87% with doctorates).

Academic Facilities *Campus library:* 545,439 volumes (23,000 in health, 3,700 in nursing); 2,126 periodical subscriptions (136 health-care related). *Nursing school resources:* CAI, computer lab, nursing audiovisuals, interactive nursing skills videos, learning resource lab.

Student Life *Student services:* health clinic, child-care facilities, personal counseling, career counseling, institutionally sponsored work-study program, job placement, campus safety program, special assistance for disabled students. *International student services:* counseling/support, special assistance for nonnative speakers of English, ESL courses. *Nursing student activities:* Sigma Theta Tau, student nurses association, nursing class groups.

Calendar Semesters.

NURSING STUDENT PROFILE

Undergraduate **Enrollment:** 209

Women: 92%; **Men:** 8%; **Minority:** 14%; **International:** 6%; **Part-time:** 20%

BACCALAUREATE PROGRAMS

Contact Dr. Elizabeth Keenen, Coordinator for Admission and Progression, Burdick Hall 121, Department of Nursing, Towson State University, Towson, MD 21252-7097, 410-830-4207. *Fax:* 410-830-4325.

Expenses *State resident tuition:* $2878 full-time, $123 per credit part-time. *Nonresident tuition:* $6980 full-time, $265 per credit part-time. *Full-time mandatory fees:* $898–$1100. *Room and board:* $4540. *Books and supplies per academic year:* ranges from $200 to $300.

Financial Aid Institutionally sponsored need-based grants/scholarships, Federal Work-Study. *Application deadline:* 3/15.

Generic Baccalaureate Program (BS)

Applying *Required:* SAT I, TOEFL for nonnative speakers of English, minimum high school GPA of 2.5, minimum college GPA of 2.5, 3 years of high school math, 3 years of high school science, high school chemistry, high school biology, high school transcript, transcript of college record. 42 prerequisite credits must be completed before admission to the nursing program. *Options:* Advanced standing available through the following means: advanced placement exams, credit by exam. May apply for transfer of up to 90 total credits. *Application deadlines:* 1/15 (fall), 8/15 (spring). *Application fee:* $25.

Degree Requirements 123 total credit hours, 58 in nursing.

RN Baccalaureate Program (BS)

Applying *Required:* TOEFL for nonnative speakers of English, minimum college GPA of 2.5, RN license, diploma or AD in nursing, transcript of college record, Maryland Statewide Articulation Model. 60 prerequisite credits must be completed before admission to the nursing program. *Options:* Advanced standing available through the following means: advanced placement exams, credit by exam. May apply for transfer of up to 90 total credits. *Application deadlines:* 1/15 (fall), 8/15 (spring). *Application fee:* $25.

Degree Requirements 120 total credit hours, 26 in nursing.

Baccalaureate for Second Degree Program (BS)

Applying *Required:* SAT I, TOEFL for nonnative speakers of English, minimum college GPA of 2.5, transcript of college record. 42 prerequisite credits must be completed before admission to the nursing program. *Options:* Advanced standing available through the following means: advanced placement exams, credit by exam. May apply for transfer of up to 90 total credits. *Application deadlines:* 1/15 (fall), 8/15 (spring). *Application fee:* $25.

Degree Requirements 120 total credit hours, 58 in nursing.

UNIVERSITY OF MARYLAND AT BALTIMORE
School of Nursing
Baltimore, Maryland

Programs • Generic Baccalaureate • RN Baccalaureate • Accelerated Baccalaureate for Second Degree • RN to Master's • Master's for Nurses with Non-Nursing Degrees • MS/MBA • Post-Master's • Generic Doctorate • Postbaccalaureate Doctorate • PhD/MBA • Continuing Education

The University State-supported upper-level coed institution. Part of University of Maryland System. Founded: 1807. *Primary accreditation:* regional. *Setting:* 30-acre urban campus. *Total enrollment:* 4,982.

The School of Nursing Founded in 1889. *Nursing program faculty:* 115 (83% with doctorates).

Academic Facilities *Campus library:* 172,495 volumes (172,495 in health); 2,000 periodical subscriptions (2,000 health-care related). *Nursing school resources:* CAI, computer lab, nursing audiovisuals, interactive nursing skills videos, learning resource lab, clinical simulation lab.

Student Life *Student services:* health clinic, personal counseling, career counseling, institutionally sponsored work-study program, job placement, campus safety program, special assistance for disabled students. *International student services:* counseling/support, special assistance for nonnative speakers of English, ESL courses. *Nursing student activities:* Sigma Theta Tau, student nurses association, nursing student government, Black Student Nurses Association, Graduates in Nursing.

Calendar 4-1-4.

NURSING STUDENT PROFILE

Undergraduate **Enrollment:** 777

Women: 90%; **Men:** 10%; **Minority:** 25%; **International:** 1%; **Part-time:** 41%

Graduate **Enrollment:** 783

Women: 94%; **Men:** 6%; **Minority:** 17%; **International:** 4%; **Part-time:** 80%

BACCALAUREATE PROGRAMS

Contact Debra Dehn, Undergraduate Admissions Coordinator, School of Nursing, University of Maryland at Baltimore, 655 West Lombard Street, Room 402, Baltimore, MD 21201-1579, 410-706-0491. *Fax:* 410-706-7238. *E-mail:* dehn@nurse-1.ab.umd.edu

Expenses *State resident tuition:* $1928 full-time, $168 per credit part-time. *Nonresident tuition:* $4893 full-time, $252 per credit part-time. *Full-time mandatory fees:* $456–$910. *Part-time mandatory fees:* $178–$318. *Room only:* $1683–$5000. *Books and supplies per academic year:* ranges from $650 to $1000.

Financial Aid Institutionally sponsored need-based grants/scholarships, institutionally sponsored non-need grants/scholarships, Federal Direct Loans, Federal Nursing Student Loans, Federal Pell Grants, Federal Perkins Loans, Federal Supplemental Educational Opportunity Grants, Federal Work-Study. 44% of undergraduate students in nursing programs received some form of financial aid in 1995–96.

Generic Baccalaureate Program (BSN)

Applying *Required:* TOEFL for nonnative speakers of English, minimum college GPA of 2.0, written essay, transcript of college record. 59 prerequisite credits must be completed before admission to the nursing program. *Options:* Advanced standing available through credit by exam. May apply for transfer of up to 89 total credits. *Application deadline:* 4/15. *Application fee:* $42.

Degree Requirements 122 total credit hours, 63 in nursing. 59 additional credits in various health, science, and liberal arts classes.

RN Baccalaureate Program (BSN)

Applying *Required:* ACT PEP for diploma RNs, minimum college GPA of 2.0, written essay, transcript of college record. 59 prerequisite credits must be completed before admission to the nursing program. *Options:* Advanced standing available through credit by exam. May apply for transfer of up to 89 total credits. *Application deadlines:* 7/1 (fall), 12/1 (spring), 4/15 (summer). *Application fee:* $42.

Degree Requirements 122 total credit hours, 63 in nursing. 59 additional credits in various health, science, and liberal arts classes.

Distance learning Courses provided through interactive video. Specific degree requirements include a mandatory 2-day workshop on campus.

University of Maryland at Baltimore (continued)

Accelerated Baccalaureate for Second Degree Program (BSN)

Applying *Required:* TOEFL for nonnative speakers of English, minimum college GPA of 3.0, 2 letters of recommendation, written essay, transcript of college record. 120 prerequisite credits must be completed before admission to the nursing program. *Options:* Advanced standing available through the following means: advanced placement exams, credit by exam. Course work may be accelerated. May apply for transfer of up to 90 total credits. *Application deadline:* 4/15. *Application fee:* $42.

Degree Requirements 122 total credit hours, 59 in nursing. 22 additional credits in various health, science, and liberal arts classes.

MASTER'S PROGRAMS

Contact Cassandra Smith Moore, Graduate Admissions Coordinator, School of Nursing, University of Maryland at Baltimore, 655 West Lombard Street, Room 402, Baltimore, MD 21201-1579, 410-706-0489. *Fax:* 410-706-7238. *E-mail:* moore@nurse-1.ab.umd.edu

Areas of Study Clinical nurse specialist programs in community health nursing, gerontological nursing, medical-surgical nursing, oncology nursing, psychiatric–mental health nursing, women's health nursing; nursing administration; nursing education; nurse practitioner programs in acute care, adult health, family health, gerontology, neonatal health, women's health.

Expenses *State resident tuition:* $4851 full-time, $231 per credit part-time. *Nonresident tuition:* $8736 full-time, $416 per credit part-time. *Full-time mandatory fees:* $288. *Part-time mandatory fees:* $288. *Room only:* $1683–$5000. *Books and supplies per academic year:* ranges from $650 to $1000.

Financial Aid Graduate assistantships, nurse traineeships, Federal Direct Loans, Federal Nursing Student Loans, employment opportunities, institutionally sponsored need-based grants/scholarships, institutionally sponsored non-need-based grants/scholarships. 13% of master's level students in nursing programs received some form of financial aid in 1995-96.

RN to Master's Program (MS)

Applying *Required:* GRE General Test, minimum GPA of 3.0, RN license, 1 year of clinical experience, physical assessment course, statistics course, essay, interview, 2 letters of recommendation, transcript of college record. *Application deadlines:* 7/15 (fall), 12/1 (spring), 5/15 (summer). *Application fee:* $42.

Degree Requirements 150–153 total credit hours dependent upon track, 91–94 in nursing, 59 in liberal arts, science, and social sciences.

Master's for Nurses with Non-Nursing Degrees Program (MS)

Applying *Required:* GRE General Test, TOEFL for nonnative speakers of English, minimum GPA of 3.0, RN license, physical assessment course, statistics course, essay, 2 letters of recommendation, transcript of college record. *Application deadlines:* 4/15 (fall), 11/1 (spring). *Application fee:* $42.

Degree Requirements 39–42 total credit hours dependent upon track, 39–42 in nursing.

MS/MBA Program

Applying *Required:* GRE General Test, TOEFL for nonnative speakers of English, bachelor's degree in nursing, minimum GPA of 3.0, RN license, statistics course, essay, 2 letters of recommendation, transcript of college record. *Application deadlines:* 7/15 (fall), 12/1 (spring), 5/15 (summer). *Application fee:* $42.

Degree Requirements 66 total credit hours, 30 in nursing, 36 in economics, marketing, management, finance, accounting, operations research.

Post-Master's Program

Applying *Required:* GRE General Test, bachelor's degree in nursing, minimum GPA of 3.0, RN license, 2 years of clinical experience, physical assessment course, statistics course, essay, 2 letters of recommendation, transcript of college record. *Application deadlines:* 7/15 (fall), 12/1 (spring). *Application fee:* $42.

DOCTORAL PROGRAMS

Contact Cassandra Smith Moore, Graduate Admissions Coordinator, School of Nursing, University of Maryland at Baltimore, 655 West Lombard Street, Baltimore, MD 21201-1579, 410-706-0489. *Fax:* 410-706-7238. *E-mail:* moore@nurse-1.ab.umd.edu

Areas of Study Nursing administration, nursing education, nursing research, clinical practice, nursing policy, information systems.

Expenses *State resident tuition:* $4851 full-time, $231 per credit part-time. *Nonresident tuition:* $8736 full-time, $416 per credit part-time. *Full-time mandatory fees:* $288. *Part-time mandatory fees:* $288. *Room only:* $1683–$5000. *Books and supplies per academic year:* ranges from $650 to $1000.

Financial Aid Graduate assistantships, nurse traineeships, Federal Direct Loans, opportunities for employment, institutionally sponsored need-based grants/scholarships, institutionally sponsored non-need-based grants/scholarships.

Generic Doctorate Program (PhD)

Applying *Required:* GRE General Test, TOEFL for nonnative speakers of English, master's degree in nursing, statistics course, interview, 3 letters of recommendation, vitae, writing sample, competitive review by faculty committee. *Application deadline:* 3/1. *Application fee:* $42.

Degree Requirements 60 total credit hours; dissertation; oral exam; written exam; defense of dissertation.

Postbaccalaureate Doctorate (PhD)

Applying *Required:* GRE General Test, TOEFL for nonnative speakers of English, master's degree in nursing, statistics course, interview, 3 letters of recommendation, vitae, writing sample, competitive review by faculty committee. *Application deadline:* 3/1. *Application fee:* $42.

Degree Requirements 84–87 total credit hours dependent upon track; dissertation; oral exam; written exam; defense of dissertation.

PhD/MBA Program

Applying *Required:* GRE General Test, TOEFL for nonnative speakers of English, master's degree in nursing, statistics course, interview, letter of recommendation, vitae, writing sample, competitive review by faculty committee. *Application deadline:* 3/1. *Application fee:* $42.

Degree Requirements 82 total credit hours; dissertation; oral exam; written exam; defense of dissertation.

CONTINUING EDUCATION PROGRAM

Contact Dr. Carol Allen, Acting Assistant Dean, Office of Professional Development, School of Nursing, University of Maryland at Baltimore, 655 West Lombard Street, Baltimore, MD 21201-1579, 410-706-3767. *Fax:* 410-706-0018. *E-mail:* callen@nurse-1.ab.umd.edu

See full description on page 538.

VILLA JULIE COLLEGE

Villa Julie College-Union Memorial Hospital Nursing Program
Stevenson, Maryland

Programs • Generic Baccalaureate • Baccalaureate for Second Degree

The College Independent 4-year coed college. Founded: 1952. *Primary accreditation:* regional. *Setting:* 60-acre suburban campus. *Total enrollment:* 1,804.

The Villa Julie College-Union Memorial Hospital Nursing Program Founded in 1991. *Nursing program faculty:* 38 (8% with doctorates). *Off-campus program site:* Baltimore.

▶ *NOTEWORTHY*

The Villa Julie/Union Memorial Hospital Nursing Program is designed to prepare graduates with the education to creatively meet the challenges and demands of nursing in the 21st century. This program combines the best of both worlds, with Villa Julie College's outstanding liberal arts program and Union Memorial Hospital's excellence in nursing education. One important feature of this program is the fact that nursing courses begin in the first semester. This bachelor's degree program can be completed on a full-time or part-time basis and has both day and evening/weekend classes and clinical experience.

Academic Facilities *Campus library:* 102,789 volumes (10,682 in health, 2,957 in nursing); 945 periodical subscriptions (420 health-care related). *Nursing school resources:* CAI, computer lab, nursing audiovisuals, interactive nursing skills videos, learning resource lab.

Student Life *Student services:* personal counseling, career counseling, institutionally sponsored work-study program, job placement, campus safety program, special assistance for disabled students. *Nursing student activities:* student nurses association.

Calendar Semesters.

NURSING STUDENT PROFILE

Undergraduate **Enrollment:** 303
Women: 92%; **Men:** 8%; **Minority:** 17%; **Part-time:** 39%

BACCALAUREATE PROGRAMS

Contact Mrs. Kathryn Betta, Admissions Coordinator, School of Nursing, Villa Julie College, Greenspring Valley Road, Stevenson, MD 21153, 410-602-6524. *Fax:* 410-486-3552.

Expenses *Tuition:* $8510 full-time, $250 per credit hour part-time. *Full-time mandatory fees:* $100. *Room only:* $3000. *Books and supplies per academic year:* ranges from $300 to $600.

Financial Aid Institutionally sponsored need-based grants/scholarships, institutionally sponsored non-need grants/scholarships, Federal Perkins Loans, Federal Supplemental Educational Opportunity Grants, Federal Work-Study, Maryland State Nursing Scholarship, Educational Assistance Grants, Senator's Delegate Scholarships. *Application deadline:* 3/1.

Generic Baccalaureate Program (BS)

Applying *Required:* SAT I, TOEFL for nonnative speakers of English, minimum college GPA of 3.0, 2 years of high school math, 2 years of high school science, high school chemistry, high school biology, high school transcript, interview, 2 letters of recommendation, written essay, transcript of college record. *Options:* Advanced standing available through the following means: advanced placement exams, advanced placement without credit, credit by exam. May apply for transfer of up to 90 total credits. *Application deadlines:* 3/1 (fall), 10/1 (spring). *Application fee:* $25.

Degree Requirements 136 total credit hours, 60 in nursing.

Baccalaureate for Second Degree Program (BS)

Applying *Required:* SAT I, TOEFL for nonnative speakers of English, minimum college GPA of 3.0, 2 years of high school math, 2 years of high school science, high school chemistry, high school biology, high school transcript, interview, 2 letters of recommendation, written essay, transcript of college record. *Options:* Advanced standing available through the following means: advanced placement exams, advanced placement without credit, credit by exam. May apply for transfer of up to 90 total credits. *Application deadlines:* 3/1 (fall), 10/1 (spring). *Application fee:* $25.

Degree Requirements 136 total credit hours, 60 in nursing.

MASSACHUSETTS

AMERICAN INTERNATIONAL COLLEGE
Division of Nursing
Springfield, Massachusetts

Programs • Generic Baccalaureate • RN Baccalaureate

The College Independent comprehensive coed institution. Founded: 1885. *Primary accreditation:* regional. *Setting:* 58-acre urban campus. *Total enrollment:* 1,913.

The Division of Nursing Founded in 1977. *Nursing program faculty:* 10 (30% with doctorates).

▶ ***NOTEWORTHY***

American International College in Springfield, Massachusetts, offers a 4-year program in nursing leading to a Bachelor of Science in Nursing degree. The program, founded in 1977, offers students the solid foundation of knowledge and skills that expert professional nursing requires. The program goal is for graduates to be competent, caring nurses capable of dealing intelligently, effectively, and humanely with clients, families, and professional colleagues. Students have a variety of clinical experiences in the Springfield area at such high-quality health-care facilities as Baystate Medical Center, Springfield Municipal Hospital, the Springfield Visiting Nurses Association, and others.

Academic Facilities *Campus library:* 104,000 volumes (10,000 in health); 450 periodical subscriptions (50 health-care related). *Nursing school resources:* computer lab, nursing audiovisuals, learning resource lab.

Student Life *Student services:* health clinic, personal counseling, career counseling, institutionally sponsored work-study program, job placement, campus safety program, special assistance for disabled students. *International student services:* counseling/support, ESL courses. *Nursing student activities:* nursing club, student nurses association, Nursing Honor Society.

Calendar Semesters.

NURSING STUDENT PROFILE

Undergraduate **Enrollment:** 150
Women: 93%; **Men:** 7%; **Minority:** 8%; **International:** 2%; **Part-time:** 4%

BACCALAUREATE PROGRAMS

Contact Dr. Anne R. Glanovsky, Director, Division of Nursing, American International College, 100 State Street, Springfield, MA 01109, 413-747-6361. *Fax:* 413-737-2803.

Expenses *Tuition:* $10,400 full-time, $325 per credit hour part-time. *Full-time mandatory fees:* $652. *Room and board:* $5062–$5310. *Books and supplies per academic year:* $500.

Financial Aid Institutionally sponsored need-based grants/scholarships, institutionally sponsored non-need grants/scholarships, Federal Perkins Loans, Federal Supplemental Educational Opportunity Grants, Federal Work-Study. 70% of undergraduate students in nursing programs received some form of financial aid in 1995–96. *Application deadline:* 4/15.

Generic Baccalaureate Program (BSN)

Applying *Required:* SAT I, TOEFL for nonnative speakers of English, minimum college GPA of 2.5, 2 years of high school science, high school chemistry, high school biology, high school transcript, letter of recommendation, transcript of college record. *Application deadline:* rolling. *Application fee:* $20.

Degree Requirements 121 total credit hours, 59 in nursing.

RN Baccalaureate Program (BSN)

Applying *Required:* TOEFL for nonnative speakers of English, RN license, diploma or AD in nursing, interview, transcript of college record. *Application deadline:* rolling. *Application fee:* $20.

Degree Requirements 121 total credit hours, 59 in nursing.

ANNA MARIA COLLEGE
Department of Nursing
Paxton, Massachusetts

Programs • RN Baccalaureate • Baccalaureate for Second Degree

The College Independent Roman Catholic comprehensive coed institution. Founded: 1946. *Primary accreditation:* regional. *Setting:* 180-acre rural campus. *Total enrollment:* 1,611.

The Department of Nursing Founded in 1979. *Nursing program faculty:* 5.

Academic Facilities *Campus library:* 120,000 volumes; 40 health-care related periodical subscriptions. *Nursing school resources:* CAI, computer lab, nursing audiovisuals, learning resource lab, Internet, Medline.

Student Life *Student services:* health clinic, personal counseling, career counseling, institutionally sponsored work-study program, job placement, campus safety program, special assistance for disabled students.

Anna Maria College (continued)

International student services: counseling/support, special assistance for nonnative speakers of English, ESL courses. *Nursing student activities:* nursing club.

Calendar Semesters.

NURSING STUDENT PROFILE

Undergraduate **Enrollment:** 89
Women: 99%; **Men:** 1%; **Minority:** 1%; **International:** 0%; **Part-time:** 100%

BACCALAUREATE PROGRAMS

Contact Ms. Evelyn D. Murphy, Chair, Department of Nursing, Anna Maria College, 10 Sunset Lane, Paxton, MA 01612-1198, 508-849-3354. *Fax:* 508-849-3362.

Expenses *Tuition:* ranges from $165 to $244 per credit. *Part-time mandatory fees:* $30–$105. *Books and supplies per academic year:* ranges from $300 to $400.

Financial Aid Institutionally sponsored need-based grants/scholarships, Federal Nursing Student Loans, Federal Supplemental Educational Opportunity Grants, Federal Work-Study. *Application deadline:* 3/1.

RN Baccalaureate Program (BSN)

Applying *Required:* RN license, diploma or AD in nursing, high school transcript, interview, 2 letters of recommendation, transcript of college record, professional liability insurance. *Options:* Advanced standing available through the following means: advanced placement exams, credit by exam. May apply for transfer of up to 75 total credits. *Application deadline:* rolling. *Application fee:* $35.

Degree Requirements 120 total credit hours, 30 in nursing.

Baccalaureate for Second Degree Program (BSN)

Applying *Required:* high school transcript, interview, 2 letters of recommendation, transcript of college record. *Options:* May apply for transfer of up to 75 total credits. *Application deadline:* rolling. *Application fee:* $35.

Degree Requirements 30 total credit hours, 30 in nursing.

ATLANTIC UNION COLLEGE
Department of Nursing
South Lancaster, Massachusetts

Program • RN Baccalaureate

The College Independent Seventh-day Adventist comprehensive coed institution. Founded: 1882. *Primary accreditation:* regional. *Setting:* 314-acre small-town campus. *Total enrollment:* 500.

The Department of Nursing Founded in 1964. *Nursing program faculty:* 10 (1% with doctorates). *Off-campus program site:* Stoneham.

Academic Facilities *Campus library:* 100,001 volumes (107 in health, 395 in nursing); 845 periodical subscriptions (99 health-care related). *Nursing school resources:* computer lab, nursing audiovisuals, interactive nursing skills videos, learning resource lab.

Student Life *Student services:* health clinic, personal counseling, career counseling, institutionally sponsored work-study program, job placement. *International student services:* counseling/support, ESL courses. *Nursing student activities:* Sigma Theta Tau.

Calendar Semesters.

NURSING STUDENT PROFILE

Undergraduate **Enrollment:** 225
Women: 91%; **Men:** 9%; **Minority:** 26%; **International:** 3%; **Part-time:** 66%

BACCALAUREATE PROGRAM

Contact Ms. Vera B. Davis, Program Director, Department of Nursing, Atlantic Union College, Main Street, South Lancaster, MA 01561, 508-368-2410. *Fax:* 508-368-2015.

Expenses *Tuition:* $13,064 full-time, $150 per semester credit part-time. *Full-time mandatory fees:* $1970. *Room and board:* $3600. *Books and supplies per academic year:* ranges from $600 to $700.

Financial Aid Institutionally sponsored need-based grants/scholarships, institutionally sponsored non-need grants/scholarships, Federal Direct Loans, Federal Nursing Student Loans, Federal Perkins Loans, Federal Supplemental Educational Opportunity Grants, Federal Work-Study. 33% of undergraduate students in nursing programs received some form of financial aid in 1995–96. *Application deadline:* 5/1.

RN Baccalaureate Program (BS)

Applying *Required:* TOEFL for nonnative speakers of English, RN license, diploma or AD in nursing, high school foreign language, interview, 2 letters of recommendation, transcript of college record. 54 prerequisite credits must be completed before admission to the nursing program. *Application deadline:* rolling. *Application fee:* $15.

Degree Requirements 128 total credit hours, 59 in nursing.

BOSTON COLLEGE
School of Nursing
Chestnut Hill, Massachusetts

Programs • Generic Baccalaureate • RN Baccalaureate • Accelerated RN Baccalaureate • Baccalaureate for Second Degree • MS • RN to Master's • MS/MBA • Continuing Education

The College Independent Roman Catholic (Jesuit) coed university. Founded: 1863. *Primary accreditation:* regional. *Setting:* 240-acre suburban campus. *Total enrollment:* 14,695.

The School of Nursing Founded in 1947. *Nursing program faculty:* 60 (93% with doctorates).

Academic Facilities *Campus library:* 1.3 million volumes (33,615 in health, 7,435 in nursing); 9,000 periodical subscriptions (1,027 health-care related). *Nursing school resources:* computer lab, nursing audiovisuals, interactive nursing skills videos, learning resource lab, nursing simulation lab.

Student Life *Student services:* health clinic, child-care facilities, personal counseling, career counseling, institutionally sponsored work-study program, job placement, campus safety program, special assistance for disabled students, academic counseling center. *International student services:* counseling/support, special assistance for nonnative speakers of English, ESL courses, tutoring. *Nursing student activities:* Sigma Theta Tau, nursing club, student nurses association.

Calendar Semesters.

NURSING STUDENT PROFILE

Undergraduate **Enrollment:** 325
Women: 98%; **Men:** 2%; **Minority:** 11%; **Part-time:** 1%
Graduate **Enrollment:** 239
Women: 97%; **Men:** 3%; **Minority:** 3%; **International:** 2%; **Part-time:** 80%

BACCALAUREATE PROGRAMS

Contact Ms. Cally Wein, Receptionist, School of Nursing, Boston College, 140 Commonwealth Avenue, Chestnut Hill, MA 02167, 617-552-4250. *Fax:* 617-552-0745.

Expenses *Tuition:* $18,820 per academic year. *Full-time mandatory fees:* $600. *Room and board:* $8015. *Books and supplies per academic year:* $600.

Financial Aid Institutionally sponsored need-based grants/scholarships, institutionally sponsored non-need grants/scholarships, Federal Nursing Student Loans, Federal Supplemental Educational Opportunity Grants, Federal Work-Study. 74% of undergraduate students in nursing programs received some form of financial aid in 1995–96. *Application deadline:* 2/1.

Generic Baccalaureate Program (BS)

Applying *Required:* SAT I, ACT, 3 College Board Achievements, minimum high school GPA, minimum college GPA, 3 years of high school math, 3 years of high school science, high school chemistry, high school biology, high school foreign language, high school transcript, 2 letters of recommendation, written essay, transcript of college record. *Options:* Advanced standing available through the following means: advanced placement exams, advanced placement without credit. May apply for transfer of up to 60 total credits. *Application deadlines:* 5/15 (fall), 11/15 (spring). *Application fee:* $50.

Degree Requirements 121 total credit hours, 61 in nursing. University core curriculum.

RN Baccalaureate Program (BS)

Applying *Required:* SAT I, ACT, high school chemistry, high school biology, RN license, diploma or AD in nursing, high school transcript, 2

letters of recommendation, written essay, transcript of college record. *Options:* Course work may be accelerated. May apply for transfer of up to 60 total credits. *Application deadlines:* 5/15 (fall), 11/15 (spring). *Application fee:* $50.

Degree Requirements 121 total credit hours.

Accelerated RN Baccalaureate Program (BS)

Applying *Required:* SAT I, ACT, high school chemistry, high school biology, RN license, diploma or AD in nursing, high school transcript, 2 letters of recommendation, written essay, transcript of college record. *Options:* Course work may be accelerated. *Application deadlines:* 5/15 (fall), 11/15 (spring). *Application fee:* $50.

Degree Requirements 121 total credit hours.

Baccalaureate for Second Degree Program (BS)

Applying *Required:* SAT I, ACT, high school chemistry, high school biology, high school foreign language, high school transcript, 2 letters of recommendation, transcript of college record. *Application deadlines:* 5/15 (fall), 11/15 (spring). *Application fee:* $50.

Degree Requirements 121 total credit hours.

MASTER'S PROGRAMS

Contact Ms. Ellen Robidoux, Administrative Secretary, Graduate Programs, School of Nursing, Boston College, Chestnut Hill, MA 02167, 617-552-4928. *Fax:* 617-552-0745.

Areas of Study Clinical nurse specialist programs in community health nursing, critical care nursing, psychiatric–mental health nursing, public health nursing; nurse practitioner programs in adult health, child care/pediatrics, community health, family health, gerontology, women's health.

Expenses *Tuition:* $566 per semester hour. *Full-time mandatory fees:* $368.

Financial Aid Graduate assistantships, nurse traineeships, Federal Nursing Student Loans, employment opportunities. *Application deadline:* 4/30.

MS Program

Applying *Required:* GRE General Test, bachelor's degree in nursing, minimum GPA of 3.0, RN license, 1 year of clinical experience, physical assessment course, statistics course, professional liability/malpractice insurance, essay, interview, 3 letters of recommendation, transcript of college record. *Application deadlines:* 2/1 (fall), 10/15 (spring). *Application fee:* $40.

Degree Requirements 45 total credit hours, 42 in nursing, 3 in other specified areas.

RN to Master's Program (MS)

Applying *Required:* GRE General Test (minimum combined score of 1350 on three tests), NLN Mobility Profile exam, bachelor's degree in nursing, minimum GPA of 3.0, RN license, 1 year of clinical experience, physical assessment course, statistics course, professional liability/malpractice insurance, essay, 3 letters of recommendation, transcript of college record, completion of BSN equivalence. *Application deadlines:* 2/1 (fall), 10/15 (winter term). *Application fee:* $40.

Degree Requirements 45 total credit hours, 42 in nursing, 3 in elective. Thesis or comprehensive exam.

MS/MBA Program

Applying *Required:* GRE General Test, bachelor's degree in nursing, minimum GPA of 3.0, 1 year of clinical experience, statistics course, essay, interview, 3 letters of recommendation, transcript of college record, 1 year nursing management experience. *Application deadlines:* 2/1 (fall), 10/15 (spring). *Application fee:* $40.

Degree Requirements 82 total credit hours, 42 in nursing.

DOCTORAL PROGRAM

Contact Dr. DeLois Weekes, Associate Dean of Graduate Programs, School of Nursing, Boston College, Chestnut Hill, MA 02167, 617-552-4928. *Fax:* 617-552-0745.

Areas of Study Nursing research.

Expenses *Tuition:* $566 per semester hour. *Full-time mandatory fees:* $368. *Books and supplies per academic year:* $500.

Financial Aid Graduate assistantships, nurse traineeships, fellowships, dissertation grants, grants, opportunities for employment. *Application deadline:* 1/31.

Generic Doctorate Program (PhD)

Applying *Required:* GRE General Test, master's degree in nursing, 1 scholarly paper, statistics course, interview, 3 letters of recommendation, vitae, writing sample, competitive review by faculty committee. *Application deadline:* 1/31. *Application fee:* $40.

Degree Requirements 46 total credit hours; dissertation; oral exam; written exam; defense of dissertation.

CONTINUING EDUCATION PROGRAM

Contact Dr. Jean Weyman, Director of Continuing Education, School of Nursing, Boston College, Chestnut Hill, MA 02167, 617-552-4256. *Fax:* 617-552-0745.

See full description on page 420.

COLLEGE OF OUR LADY OF THE ELMS
Department of Nursing
Chicopee, Massachusetts

Programs • Generic Baccalaureate • RN Baccalaureate

The College Independent Roman Catholic comprehensive women's institution. Founded: 1928. *Primary accreditation:* regional. *Setting:* 32-acre suburban campus. *Total enrollment:* 1,257.

The Department of Nursing Founded in 1979.

Academic Facilities *Campus library:* 97,207 volumes (3,550 in nursing); 500 periodical subscriptions (88 health-care related).

Calendar Semesters.

BACCALAUREATE PROGRAMS

Contact Admissions Department, Department of Nursing, Elms College, 291 Springfield Street, Chicopee, MA 01013, 413-594-2761. *Fax:* 413-592-4871.

Expenses *Tuition:* $12,450 full-time, $278 per credit hour part-time.

Financial Aid Institutionally sponsored need-based grants/scholarships, institutionally sponsored non-need grants/scholarships, Federal Perkins Loans, Federal Work-Study, Federal PLUS Loans, Federal Stafford Loans. *Application deadline:* 2/15.

Generic Baccalaureate Program (BS)

Applying *Required:* SAT I or ACT, minimum high school GPA of 2.0, 2 years of high school math, 4 years of high school science, high school chemistry, high school transcript, 2 letters of recommendation. *Options:* Advanced standing available through credit by exam. May apply for transfer of up to 75 total credits. *Application fee:* $30.

Degree Requirements 127 total credit hours, 61 in nursing. 66 core credits.

RN Baccalaureate Program (BS)

Applying *Required:* SAT I, TOEFL for nonnative speakers of English, RN license, diploma or AD in nursing, high school transcript, interview, 2 letters of recommendation, written essay, transcript of college record. *Options:* Advanced standing available through credit by exam. May apply for transfer of up to 75 total credits.

Degree Requirements 123 total credit hours, 61 in nursing. 62 core credits.

CURRY COLLEGE
Division of Nursing Studies
Milton, Massachusetts

Programs • Generic Baccalaureate • RN Baccalaureate • Baccalaureate for Second Degree • Continuing Education

The College Independent comprehensive coed institution. Founded: 1879. *Primary accreditation:* regional. *Setting:* 120-acre suburban campus. *Total enrollment:* 1,433.

The Division of Nursing Studies Founded in 1977. *Nursing program faculty:* 16 (38% with doctorates). *Off-campus program site:* Plymouth.

▶ ***NOTEWORTHY***

Clinical experience begins in the sophomore year at Curry College. Boston and metropolitan hospitals and community agencies provide Curry students with a wide range of clinical exposure and the latest

Curry College (continued)

in nursing techniques and methodology to enhance potential for employment. Boston clinical practice sites include Beth Israel Hospital, University Hospital, and the Children's Hospital. The hallmark of a Curry education is personalized attention and respect for the individuality of every student. The College's commitment to the liberal arts and developmental learning, in combination with an intense professional clinical program, gives Curry nursing students the advantage in synthesizing knowledge and applying practice skills.

Academic Facilities *Campus library:* 80,000 volumes; 600 periodical subscriptions. *Nursing school resources:* CAI, computer lab, nursing audiovisuals, interactive nursing skills videos, learning resource lab.

Student Life *Student services:* health clinic, personal counseling, career counseling, institutionally sponsored work-study program, job placement, campus safety program, special assistance for disabled students, program for advancement of learning for students with dyslexia. *Nursing student activities:* Sigma Theta Tau, student nurses association.

Calendar Semesters.

NURSING STUDENT PROFILE

Undergraduate **Enrollment:** 203

Women: 96%; **Men:** 4%; **Minority:** 14%; **International:** 0%; **Part-time:** 27%

BACCALAUREATE PROGRAMS

Contact Ms. Janet Kelly, Dean of Admissions and Financial Aid, Admissions Office, Curry College, 1071 Blue Hill Avenue, Milton, MA 02186, 617-333-2210. *Fax:* 617-333-6860.

Expenses *Tuition:* $14,805 per academic year. *Full-time mandatory fees:* $400–$700. *Room and board:* $5740. *Room only:* $3140. *Books and supplies per academic year:* ranges from $800 to $900.

Financial Aid Institutionally sponsored need-based grants/scholarships, Federal Pell Grants, Federal Perkins Loans, Federal Supplemental Educational Opportunity Grants, Federal Work-Study. 57% of undergraduate students in nursing programs received some form of financial aid in 1995–96. *Application deadline:* 3/1.

Generic Baccalaureate Program (BSN)

Applying *Required:* SAT I or ACT, TOEFL for nonnative speakers of English, minimum high school GPA of 2.0, minimum college GPA of 2.0, 3 years of high school math, 3 years of high school science, high school chemistry, high school biology, high school transcript, letter of recommendation, written essay. *Application deadlines:* 4/1 (fall), 12/1 (spring). *Application fee:* $40.

Degree Requirements 122 total credit hours, 59 in nursing. General education distribution.

RN Baccalaureate Program (BSN)

Applying *Required:* SAT I, minimum high school GPA of 2.0, minimum college GPA of 2.0, 3 years of high school math, 3 years of high school science, high school chemistry, high school biology, RN license, diploma or AD in nursing, high school transcript, letter of recommendation, written essay, transcript of college record. *Options:* Course work may be accelerated. *Application deadlines:* 4/1 (fall), 12/1 (spring). *Application fee:* $40.

Degree Requirements 122 total credit hours, 30 in nursing. General education distribution.

Baccalaureate for Second Degree Program (BSN)

Applying *Required:* minimum high school GPA of 2.0, minimum college GPA of 2.0, 3 years of high school math, 3 years of high school science, high school chemistry, high school biology, high school transcript, letter of recommendation, written essay, transcript of college record. *Application deadlines:* 4/1 (fall), 12/1 (spring). *Application fee:* $40.

Degree Requirements 122 total credit hours, 59 in nursing.

CONTINUING EDUCATION PROGRAM

Contact Ms. Gerri Luke, Director, Continuing Education, Division of Nursing Studies, Curry College, 1071 Blue Hill Avenue, Milton, MA 02186, 617-333-9674. *Fax:* 617-333-6860.

EMMANUEL COLLEGE
Department of Nursing
Boston, Massachusetts

Program • RN Baccalaureate

The College Independent Roman Catholic comprehensive women's institution. Founded: 1919. *Primary accreditation:* regional. *Setting:* 16-acre urban campus. *Total enrollment:* 1,553.

The Department of Nursing Founded in 1981. *Nursing program faculty:* 8 (40% with doctorates). *Off-campus program site:* Leominster.

▶ *NOTEWORTHY*

The Emmanuel College nursing program is designed specifically for the registered nurse. The faculty subscribes to a philosophy of values-centered education that acknowledges the needs of adults and recognizes the educational and clinical background of registered nurses. The College also offers advanced placement through a liberal transfer-credit policy that includes the option of several challenge examinations. Courses, registration, and advising are offered at times designed to meet the needs of working nurses. Evening, weekend, and Saturday morning courses are available. Clinical courses use the Partnership Model and may be taken in a variety of community-based settings. The Emmanuel College nursing program truly works for the registered nurse.

Academic Facilities *Campus library:* 89,626 volumes (2,169 in health, 286 in nursing); 673 periodical subscriptions (97 health-care related). *Nursing school resources:* CAI, computer lab, nursing audiovisuals.

Student Life *Student services:* health clinic, personal counseling, career counseling, institutionally sponsored work-study program, campus safety program. *International student services:* counseling/support, special assistance for nonnative speakers of English, ESL courses. *Nursing student activities:* Nursing Honor Society.

Calendar Semesters.

NURSING STUDENT PROFILE

Undergraduate **Enrollment:** 150

Women: 94%; **Men:** 6%; **Minority:** 5%; **International:** 0%; **Part-time:** 94%

BACCALAUREATE PROGRAM

Contact Dr. Joan Riley, Chair and Associate Professor, Department of Nursing, Emmanuel College, 400 The Fenway, Boston, MA 02115, 617-735-9700. *Fax:* 617-735-9797. *E-mail:* riley@emmanuel.edu

Expenses *Tuition:* $995 per course. *Full-time mandatory fees:* $30. *Books and supplies per academic year:* ranges from $250 to $500.

Financial Aid Institutionally sponsored need-based grants/scholarships, Federal Nursing Student Loans, Federal Supplemental Educational Opportunity Grants, Federal Work-Study.

RN Baccalaureate Program (BSN)

Applying *Required:* ACT, TOEFL for nonnative speakers of English, RN license, diploma or AD in nursing, interview, 2 letters of recommendation. 28 prerequisite credits must be completed before admission to the nursing program. *Options:* Advanced standing available through advanced placement exams. May apply for transfer of up to 80 total credits. *Application deadline:* rolling. *Application fee:* $30.

Degree Requirements 128 total credit hours, 68 in nursing.

FITCHBURG STATE COLLEGE
Department of Nursing
Fitchburg, Massachusetts

Programs • Generic Baccalaureate • RN Baccalaureate • RN to Master's

The College State-supported comprehensive coed institution. Part of Massachusetts Public Higher Education System. Founded: 1894. *Primary accreditation:* regional. *Setting:* 45-acre small-town campus. *Total enrollment:* 4,351.

The Department of Nursing Founded in 1962. *Nursing program faculty:* 32 (20% with doctorates).

Academic Facilities *Campus library:* 176,256 volumes; 31,199 periodical subscriptions. *Nursing school resources:* CAI, computer lab, nursing audiovisuals, interactive nursing skills videos, learning resource lab.

Student Life *Student services:* health clinic, child-care facilities, personal counseling, career counseling, institutionally sponsored work-study program, campus safety program, special assistance for disabled students. *International student services:* counseling/support. *Nursing student activities:* Sigma Theta Tau, student nurses association.

Calendar Semesters.

NURSING STUDENT PROFILE

Undergraduate **Enrollment:** 370
Women: 94%; **Men:** 6%; **Minority:** 4%; **International:** 1%; **Part-time:** 9%
Graduate **Enrollment:** 22
Women: 100%; **Part-time:** 100%

BACCALAUREATE PROGRAMS

Contact Dr. Sophia Harrell, Chairperson, Department of Nursing, Fitchburg State College, 160 Pearl Street, Fitchburg, MA 01420-2697, 508-665-3221. *Fax:* 508-665-4501. *E-mail:* sharrell@fsc.edu

Expenses *State resident tuition:* $1338 per academic year. *Nonresident tuition:* $5726 per academic year. *Full-time mandatory fees:* $1908. *Room and board:* $2340.

Financial Aid Institutionally sponsored need-based grants/scholarships, institutionally sponsored non-need grants/scholarships, Federal Nursing Student Loans, Federal Supplemental Educational Opportunity Grants, Federal Work-Study. *Application deadline:* 3/30.

Generic Baccalaureate Program (BS)

Applying *Required:* SAT I, TOEFL for nonnative speakers of English, 2 years of high school science, high school chemistry, high school transcript. *Options:* Advanced standing available through advanced placement exams. May apply for transfer of up to 45 total credits. *Application deadline:* rolling. *Application fee:* $10–20.

Degree Requirements 126 total credit hours, 63 in nursing.

RN Baccalaureate Program (BS)

Applying *Required:* NLN Mobility Profile II, NCLEX, RN license, diploma or AD in nursing, interview, transcript of college record. *Options:* Advanced standing available through the following means: advanced placement exams, advanced placement without credit, credit by exam. Course work may be accelerated. May apply for transfer of up to 45–62 total credits. *Application deadline:* rolling. *Application fee:* $10–20.

Degree Requirements 123 total credit hours, 64 in nursing.

MASTER'S PROGRAM

Contact Barbara P. Madden, Chair, Master's in Nursing, Graduate and Continuing Education, 160 Pearl Street, Fitchburg, MA 01420, 508-665-3181. *Fax:* 508-665-3658.

Expenses *State resident tuition:* $140 per semester hour. *Nonresident tuition:* $140 per semester hour.

Financial Aid Graduate assistantships, Federal Nursing Student Loans, employment opportunities, institutionally sponsored need-based grants/scholarships, veteran's education.

RN to Master's Program (MS)

Applying *Required:* GRE General Test, bachelor's degree in nursing, bachelor's degree, minimum GPA of 2.8, RN license, 1 year of clinical experience, 3 letters of recommendation, transcript of college record. *Application deadline:* rolling. *Application fee:* $10.

Degree Requirements 39 total credit hours.

FRAMINGHAM STATE COLLEGE

Nursing Department
Framingham, Massachusetts

Program • RN Baccalaureate

The College State-supported comprehensive coed institution. Founded: 1839. *Primary accreditation:* regional. *Setting:* 73-acre suburban campus. *Total enrollment:* 4,972.

The Nursing Department Founded in 1983. *Nursing program faculty:* 6 (50% with doctorates).

Academic Facilities *Campus library:* 198,000 volumes; 1,370 periodical subscriptions. *Nursing school resources:* CAI, computer lab, nursing audiovisuals, learning resource lab.

Student Life *Student services:* health clinic, child-care facilities, personal counseling, career counseling, institutionally sponsored work-study program, job placement, campus safety program, special assistance for disabled students. *International student services:* counseling/support, special assistance for nonnative speakers of English, ESL courses. *Nursing student activities:* nursing club.

Calendar Semesters.

NURSING STUDENT PROFILE

Undergraduate **Enrollment:** 100
Women: 98%; **Men:** 2%; **Minority:** 2%; **International:** 0%; **Part-time:** 85%

BACCALAUREATE PROGRAM

Contact Dr. Dolores Rojas Torti, Chairperson and Professor, Nursing Department, Framingham State College, 100 State Street, Framingham, MA 01701, 508-626-4715. *Fax:* 508-626-4746. *E-mail:* dtorti@frc.mass.edu

Expenses *State resident tuition:* $1338 full-time, $225 per 4-credit course part-time. *Nonresident tuition:* $5726 full-time, $955 per 4- part-time. *Full-time mandatory fees:* $1900. *Room and board:* $3900. *Room only:* $2499. *Books and supplies per academic year:* ranges from $475 to $600.

Financial Aid Institutionally sponsored need-based grants/scholarships, institutionally sponsored non-need grants/scholarships, Federal Nursing Student Loans, Federal Supplemental Educational Opportunity Grants, Federal Work-Study. *Application deadline:* 3/1.

RN Baccalaureate Program (BS)

Applying *Required:* NLN Mobility Profile II or Articulation from AD or Diploma Program, RN license, diploma or AD in nursing. 52 prerequisite credits must be completed before admission to the nursing program. *Options:* Advanced standing available through the following means: advanced placement exams, credit by exam. May apply for transfer of up to 92 total credits. *Application deadline:* rolling. *Application fee:* $10.

Degree Requirements 128 total credit hours, 36 in nursing.

MASSACHUSETTS COLLEGE OF PHARMACY AND ALLIED HEALTH SCIENCES

Department of Nursing
Boston, Massachusetts

Program • RN Baccalaureate

The College Independent specialized coed university. Founded: 1823. *Primary accreditation:* regional. *Setting:* 2-acre urban campus. *Total enrollment:* 1,451.

The Department of Nursing Founded in 1982.

Academic Facilities *Campus library:* 70,000 volumes (56,000 in health, 7,000 in nursing); 800 periodical subscriptions (713 health-care related). *Nursing school resources:* computer lab.

Student Life *Student services:* health clinic, campus safety program. *International student services:* counseling/support. *Nursing student activities:* student nurses association.

Calendar Quarters.

Massachusetts College of Pharmacy and Allied Health Sciences (continued)

BACCALAUREATE PROGRAM

Contact Director of Nursing Development, Department of Nursing, Massachusetts College of Pharmacy and Allied Health Sciences, 179 Longwood Avenue, Boston, MA 02115, 617-732-2966. *Fax:* 617-732-2801.

Financial Aid Institutionally sponsored need-based grants/scholarships, Federal Nursing Student Loans, Federal Pell Grants, Federal Perkins Loans, Federal Supplemental Educational Opportunity Grants, Federal Work-Study, Federal Family Education Loan Program (FFELP). *Application deadline:* 4/1.

RN Baccalaureate Program (BSN)

Applying *Required:* TOEFL for nonnative speakers of English, minimum college GPA of 2.0, RN license, diploma or AD in nursing, interview, 3 letters of recommendation, transcript of college record. *Options:* Advanced standing available through the following means: advanced placement exams, credit by exam. May apply for transfer of up to 41 total credits. *Application deadline:* 3/1. *Application fee:* $25.

Degree Requirements 175 total credit hours, 52 in nursing. Nursing symposium, transition course for validation of prior learning.

MGH INSTITUTE OF HEALTH PROFESSIONS

Graduate Program in Nursing
Boston, Massachusetts

Programs • MSN • Master's for Nurses with Non-Nursing Degrees • Master's for Non-Nursing College Graduates • Post-Master's

The Institution Independent graduate specialized coed institution. Founded: 1977. *Primary accreditation:* regional. *Total enrollment:* 385.

The Graduate Program in Nursing Founded in 1977. *Nursing program faculty:* 23 (70% with doctorates).

Academic Facilities *Campus library:* 53,100 volumes (2,180 in nursing); 957 periodical subscriptions. *Nursing school resources:* CAI, computer lab, nursing audiovisuals, interactive nursing skills videos, learning resource lab.

Student Life *Student services:* personal counseling, career counseling, campus safety program, special assistance for disabled students. *International student services:* counseling/support, ESL courses. *Nursing student activities:* student nurses association.

Calendar Semesters.

NURSING STUDENT PROFILE

Graduate **Enrollment:** 172
Women: 90%; **Men:** 10%; **Minority:** 5%; **International:** 0%; **Part-time:** 15%

MASTER'S PROGRAMS

Contact Ms. Vonda Bradbury, Director, Student Affairs, Graduate Program in Nursing, MGH Institute of Health Professions, 101 Merrimac Street, Boston, MA 02114, 617-726-3140. *Fax:* 617-726-8010.

Areas of Study Nurse practitioner programs in adult health, child care/pediatrics, family health, gerontology, primary care, women's health, HIV/AIDS.

Expenses *Tuition:* $15,100 full-time, $455 per credit part-time. *Full-time mandatory fees:* $0.

Financial Aid Graduate assistantships, nurse traineeships, Federal Nursing Student Loans, institutionally sponsored need-based grants/scholarships. 28% of master's level students in nursing programs received some form of financial aid in 1995-96. *Application deadline:* 3/1.

MSN Program

Applying *Required:* GRE General Test, TOEFL for nonnative speakers of English, bachelor's degree in nursing, minimum GPA of 3.0, RN license, essay, 3 letters of recommendation, transcript of college record. *Application deadlines:* 4/1 (fall), 10/15 (spring), 2/15 (summer). *Application fee:* $50.

Degree Requirements 46–62 total credit hours dependent upon track, 31 in nursing.

Master's for Nurses with Non-Nursing Degrees Program (MSN)

Applying *Required:* GRE General Test, TOEFL for nonnative speakers of English, NLN Mobility Profile II, bachelor's degree, minimum GPA of 3.0, RN license, essay, 3 letters of recommendation, transcript of college record. *Application deadlines:* 4/18 (fall), 3/21 (spring), 2/15 (summer). *Application fee:* $50.

Degree Requirements 46–62 total credit hours dependent upon track, 45 in nursing.

Master's for Non-Nursing College Graduates Program (MSN)

Applying *Required:* GRE General Test, TOEFL for nonnative speakers of English, minimum GPA of 3.0, essay, 3 letters of recommendation, transcript of college record, computer literacy. *Application deadline:* 1/24. *Application fee:* $50.

Degree Requirements 94–100 total credit hours dependent upon track, 77 in nursing.

Post-Master's Program

Applying *Required:* RN license, essay, 2 letters of recommendation, transcript of college record. *Application deadlines:* 4/15 (fall), 11/11 (spring), 3/21 (summer). *Application fee:* $50.

Degree Requirements 26 total credit hours, 26 in nursing.

NORTHEASTERN UNIVERSITY

College of Nursing
Boston, Massachusetts

Programs • Generic Baccalaureate • RN Baccalaureate • Baccalaureate for Second Degree • MS • RN to Master's • MS/MBA • Post-Master's

The University Independent coed university. Founded: 1898. *Primary accreditation:* regional. *Setting:* 57-acre urban campus. *Total enrollment:* 24,605.

The College of Nursing Founded in 1964. *Nursing program faculty:* 32 (75% with doctorates).

Academic Facilities *Campus library:* 725,000 volumes (48,250 in health, 2,350 in nursing); 8,000 periodical subscriptions (1,372 health-care related). *Nursing school resources:* CAI, computer lab, nursing audiovisuals, learning resource lab.

Student Life *Student services:* health clinic, child-care facilities, personal counseling, career counseling, institutionally sponsored work-study program, job placement, campus safety program, special assistance for disabled students, cooperative education. *International student services:* counseling/support, ESL courses. *Nursing student activities:* Sigma Theta Tau, student nurses association.

Calendar Quarters.

NURSING STUDENT PROFILE

Undergraduate **Enrollment:** 570
Women: 90%; **Men:** 10%; **Minority:** 10%; **International:** 1%; **Part-time:** 0%
Graduate **Enrollment:** 317
Women: 95%; **Men:** 5%; **Minority:** 8%; **International:** 2%; **Part-time:** 84%

BACCALAUREATE PROGRAMS

Contact Ms. Christine Letzeiser, Assistant Dean of Student Affairs, 211 Robinson Hall, College of Nursing, Northeastern University, 360 Huntington Avenue, Boston, MA 02115, 617-373-3610. *Fax:* 617-373-8672. *E-mail:* cletzeiser@lynx.neu.edu

Expenses *Tuition:* ranges from $13,370 to $15,045 per academic year. *Full-time mandatory fees:* $597. *Room and board:* $4825–$7195. *Room only:* $3825–$6195. *Books and supplies per academic year:* ranges from $900 to $1500.

Financial Aid Institutionally sponsored need-based grants/scholarships, institutionally sponsored non-need grants/scholarships, Federal Nursing Student Loans, Federal Supplemental Educational Opportunity Grants, Federal Work-Study. *Application deadline:* 3/1.

Generic Baccalaureate Program (BSN)

Applying *Required:* SAT I, TOEFL for nonnative speakers of English, minimum high school GPA of 2.4, high school math, 3 years of high school science, high school chemistry, high school biology, high school transcript, 2 letters of recommendation, written essay, transcript of college record, high school class rank: top 10%. 45 prerequisite credits must be completed before admission to the nursing program. *Options:* Course work may be accelerated. May apply for transfer of up to 50 total credits. *Application deadline:* rolling. *Application fee:* $40.

Degree Requirements 177 total credit hours, 91 in nursing.

RN Baccalaureate Program (BSN)

Applying *Required:* SAT I, TOEFL for nonnative speakers of English, 3 years of high school math, 3 years of high school science, high school chemistry, high school biology, diploma or AD in nursing, transcript of college record, transcript from RN nursing program, Massachusetts RN license. *Options:* Course work may be accelerated. May apply for transfer of up to 50 total credits. *Application deadline:* rolling.

Degree Requirements 177 total credit hours, 91 in nursing.

Baccalaureate for Second Degree Program (BSN)

Applying *Required:* SAT I, TOEFL for nonnative speakers of English, minimum high school GPA of 2.4, minimum college GPA of 2.5, 3 years of high school science, high school chemistry, high school biology, high school transcript, letter of recommendation, written essay, transcript of college record, high school class rank: top 10%, college-level chemistry I and II, anatomy and physiology I and II with lab component. 45 prerequisite credits must be completed before admission to the nursing program. *Options:* Advanced standing available through advanced placement exams. Course work may be accelerated. May apply for transfer of up to 100 total credits. *Application deadline:* rolling. *Application fee:* $40.

Degree Requirements 177 total credit hours, 91 in nursing.

MASTER'S PROGRAMS

Contact Ms. Ann Kellner, Assistant Director, 205 Robinson Hall, College of Nursing, Northeastern University, 360 Huntington Avenue, Boston, MA 02115, 617-373-3590. *Fax:* 617-373-8672.

Areas of Study Clinical nurse specialist programs in adult health nursing, community health nursing, critical care nursing, family health nursing, pediatric nursing, psychiatric–mental health nursing, public health nursing; nurse anesthesia; nursing administration; nurse practitioner programs in acute care, adult health, child care/pediatrics, community health, family health, gerontology, neonatal health, primary care, home health care.

Expenses *Tuition:* $14,040 full-time, $390 per quarter hour part-time. *Full-time mandatory fees:* $506–$1292. *Room and board:* $9300. *Books and supplies per academic year:* ranges from $750 to $800.

Financial Aid Graduate assistantships, nurse traineeships, fellowships, Federal Nursing Student Loans, employment opportunities. *Application deadline:* 3/1.

MS Program

Applying *Required:* GRE General Test, TOEFL for nonnative speakers of English, bachelor's degree in nursing, minimum GPA of 3.0, RN license, 1 year of clinical experience, statistics course, professional liability/malpractice insurance, essay, interview, 3 letters of recommendation, transcript of college record. *Application deadlines:* 4/1 (fall), 2/1 (spring), 10/1 (nurse anesthesia track). *Application fee:* $50.

Degree Requirements 52–54 total credit hours dependent upon track, 46–48 in nursing. Research practicum or thesis.

RN to Master's Program (MS)

Applying *Required:* TOEFL for nonnative speakers of English, minimum GPA of 3.0, RN license, 5 years of clinical experience, statistics course, professional liability/malpractice insurance, essay, interview, 3 letters of recommendation, transcript of college record. *Application deadlines:* 4/1 (fall), 10/1 (spring). *Application fee:* $50.

Degree Requirements 85 total credit hours, 79 in nursing. Research practicum or thesis.

MS/MBA Program

Applying *Required:* GMAT, bachelor's degree in nursing, minimum GPA of 3.0, RN license, 2 years of clinical experience, statistics course, professional liability/malpractice insurance, 3 letters of recommendation, transcript of college record, goal statement. *Application deadline:* 4/1. *Application fee:* $50.

Degree Requirements 88 total credit hours. Research practicum and management practicum.

Post-Master's Program

Applying *Required:* bachelor's degree in nursing, minimum GPA of 3.3, RN license, 1 year of clinical experience, professional liability/malpractice insurance, essay, 3 letters of recommendation, transcript of college record. *Application deadline:* rolling. *Application fee:* $50.

Degree Requirements 30–32 total credit hours dependent upon track, 30–32 in nursing.

See full description on page 486.

REGIS COLLEGE

Division of Nursing
Weston, Massachusetts

Programs • RN Baccalaureate • MS • Master's for Non-Nursing College Graduates • Post-Master's • Continuing Education

The College Independent Roman Catholic comprehensive women's institution. Founded: 1927. *Primary accreditation:* regional. *Setting:* 168-acre small-town campus. *Total enrollment:* 1,336.

The Division of Nursing Founded in 1983. *Nursing program faculty:* 25 (28% with doctorates).

▶ *NOTEWORTHY*

The Division of Nursing at Regis College offers a bachelor's in nursing degree, a master's degree in nursing administration, a master's degree in advanced practice nursing with a choice of pediatric nurse practitioner or family nurse practitioner, and a post-master's certificate nurse practitioner program. The master's program in nursing administration has 2 tracks, one for the RN with a bachelor's degree in nursing and one for the RN with a non-nursing baccalaureate degree. All nursing programs are accredited by the National League for Nursing. The nursing program subscribes to and functions within the stated mission and goals of Regis College, a liberal arts institution. Financial aid is available.

Academic Facilities *Campus library:* 147,400 volumes (6,300 in health, 3,554 in nursing); 826 periodical subscriptions (228 health-care related). *Nursing school resources:* CAI, computer lab, nursing audiovisuals, interactive nursing skills videos, learning resource lab.

Student Life *Student services:* health clinic, child-care facilities, personal counseling, career counseling, institutionally sponsored work-study program, job placement, campus safety program, special assistance for disabled students. *International student services:* counseling/support, special assistance for nonnative speakers of English, ESL courses. *Nursing student activities:* student nurses association, Nursing Honor Society.

Calendar Semesters.

NURSING STUDENT PROFILE

Undergraduate **Enrollment:** 127
Women: 99%; **Men:** 1%; **Minority:** 1%; **Part-time:** 94%
Graduate **Enrollment:** 158
Women: 99%; **Men:** 1%; **Minority:** 1%; **Part-time:** 70%

BACCALAUREATE PROGRAM

Contact Patricia Andaloro, Nurse Recruiter, Division of Nursing, Regis College, 235 Wellesley Street, Weston, MA 02193, 617-768-7188. *Fax:* 617-768-8339.

Expenses *Tuition:* $14,500 full-time, ranges from $185 to $270 per credit part-time. *Full-time mandatory fees:* $70–$170. *Part-time mandatory fees:* $70. *Room and board:* $6900. *Books and supplies per academic year:* ranges from $200 to $300.

Financial Aid Institutionally sponsored need-based grants/scholarships, Federal Nursing Student Loans, Federal Perkins Loans, Federal Supplemental Educational Opportunity Grants, Federal Work-Study, tuition remission. 19% of undergraduate students in nursing programs received some form of financial aid in 1995–96. *Application deadline:* 4/1.

RN Baccalaureate Program (BSN)

Applying *Required:* minimum college GPA of 2.0, RN license, diploma or AD in nursing, interview, 2 letters of recommendation, transcript of college record. *Options:* Advanced standing available through credit by

Regis College (continued)

exam. Course work may be accelerated. May apply for transfer of up to 66 total credits. *Application deadline:* rolling. *Application fee:* $30.

Degree Requirements 44–88 total credit hours dependent upon track, 36–60 in nursing.

MASTER'S PROGRAMS

Contact Patricia Andaloro, Nurse Recruiter, 235 Wellesley Street, Weston, MA 02193, 617-768-7188. *Fax:* 617-768-8339.

Areas of Study Nurse practitioner programs in child care/pediatrics, family health.

Expenses *Tuition:* $14,500 full-time, $350 per credit part-time. *Full-time mandatory fees:* $200–$300. *Part-time mandatory fees:* $70–$150. *Room and board:* $6900. *Books and supplies per academic year:* ranges from $200 to $300.

Financial Aid Federal Direct Loans, tuition remission. 13% of master's level students in nursing programs received some form of financial aid in 1995-96. *Application deadline:* 4/1.

Nurse Practitioner (MS)

Applying *Required:* Miller Analogies Test, bachelor's degree in nursing, minimum GPA of 3.0, RN license, physical assessment course, statistics course, professional liability/malpractice insurance, essay, interview, 3 letters of recommendation, transcript of college record. *Application deadline:* 2/1. *Application fee:* $30.

Degree Requirements 44 total credit hours, 41 in nursing, 3 in biology. Thesis required.

Master's for Non-Nursing College Graduates Program (MS)

Applying *Required:* Miller Analogies Test, bachelor's degree, minimum GPA of 3.0, statistics course, essay, interview, 3 letters of recommendation, transcript of college record. *Application deadline:* 2/1. *Application fee:* $30.

Degree Requirements 100 total credit hours, 3 in advanced pathophysiology, biology. Thesis required.

Post-Master's Program

Applying *Required:* bachelor's degree in nursing, minimum GPA of 3.0, RN license, statistics course, professional liability/malpractice insurance, essay, interview, 3 letters of recommendation, transcript of college record, MS in nursing. *Application deadline:* 2/1. *Application fee:* $30.

Degree Requirements 29 total credit hours, 27 in nursing including three hours in biology.

CONTINUING EDUCATION PROGRAM

Contact Dr. Amelia Anderson, Chairperson, Division of Nursing, Regis College, 235 Wellesley Street, Weston, MA 02193, 617-768-7090. *Fax:* 617-768-8339.

SALEM STATE COLLEGE
School of Nursing
Salem, Massachusetts

Programs • Generic Baccalaureate • RN Baccalaureate • Baccalaureate for Second Degree • LPN to Baccalaureate • MSN

The College State-supported comprehensive coed institution. Part of Massachusetts Public Higher Education System. Founded: 1854. *Primary accreditation:* regional. *Setting:* 62-acre small-town campus. *Total enrollment:* 10,132.

The School of Nursing Founded in 1970. *Nursing program faculty:* 31.

Academic Facilities *Campus library:* 1,400 periodical subscriptions.

Calendar Semesters.

BACCALAUREATE PROGRAMS

Contact Director of Admissions, School of Nursing, Salem State College, Salem, MA 01970, 508-741-6200. *Fax:* 508-741-6818.

Expenses *State resident tuition:* $1408 full-time, $59 per credit hour part-time. *Nonresident tuition:* $5726 full-time, $239 per credit hour part-time. *Full-time mandatory fees:* $210. *Room and board:* $2952–$3864. *Room only:* $2310.

Financial Aid Institutionally sponsored need-based grants/scholarships, institutionally sponsored non-need grants/scholarships, Federal Direct Loans, Federal Nursing Student Loans, Federal Perkins Loans, Federal Supplemental Educational Opportunity Grants, Federal Work-Study, Federal PLUS Loans.

Generic Baccalaureate Program (BS)

Applying *Required:* SAT I or ACT, TOEFL for nonnative speakers of English, high school transcript, transcript of college record. *Options:* Advanced standing available through the following means: advanced placement exams, credit by exam. *Application fee:* $10–40.

Degree Requirements 125 total credit hours, 55 in nursing.

RN Baccalaureate Program (BS)

Applying *Required:* SAT I or ACT, TOEFL for nonnative speakers of English, high school transcript, transcript of college record. *Options:* Advanced standing available through the following means: advanced placement exams, credit by exam. *Application fee:* $10–40.

Degree Requirements 125 total credit hours, 55 in nursing.

Baccalaureate for Second Degree Program (BS)

Applying *Required:* SAT I or ACT, TOEFL for nonnative speakers of English, high school transcript, transcript of college record. *Options:* Advanced standing available through the following means: advanced placement exams, credit by exam. *Application fee:* $10–40.

Degree Requirements 125 total credit hours, 55 in nursing.

LPN to Baccalaureate Program (BS)

Applying *Required:* SAT I or ACT, TOEFL for nonnative speakers of English, high school transcript, transcript of college record. *Options:* Advanced standing available through the following means: advanced placement exams, credit by exam. *Application fee:* $10–40.

Degree Requirements 125 total credit hours, 55 in nursing.

MASTER'S PROGRAM

Contact Coordinator, Graduate Program, Division of Graduate and Continuing Education, Salem State College, Salem, MA 01970, 508-741-6306. *Fax:* 508-741-6818.

Expenses *State resident tuition:* $140 per credit hour. *Nonresident tuition:* $230 per credit hour.

MSN Program

SIMMONS COLLEGE
Department of Nursing
Boston, Massachusetts

Programs • Generic Baccalaureate • RN Baccalaureate • Baccalaureate for Second Degree • RN to Master's • Post-Master's

The College Independent comprehensive women's institution. Founded: 1899. *Primary accreditation:* regional. *Setting:* 12-acre urban campus. *Total enrollment:* 3,614.

The Department of Nursing Founded in 1934.

Academic Facilities *Campus library:* 260,000 volumes (4,605 in health, 1,129 in nursing); 2,000 periodical subscriptions (109 health-care related).

Student Life *Student services:* health clinic, personal counseling, career counseling, job placement, campus safety program, student activities center, sports center, Institute on Women: Work, Family, and Social Change. *Nursing student activities:* Sigma Theta Tau.

Calendar Semesters.

NURSING STUDENT PROFILE
Undergraduate
Women: 100%

BACCALAUREATE PROGRAMS

Contact Dean of Admissions, Department of Nursing, Simmons College, 300 The Fenway, Boston, MA 02115, 617-521-2051. *Fax:* 617-521-3190.

Expenses *Tuition:* $546 per semester hour. *Full-time mandatory fees:* $500. *Room and board:* $7228. *Books and supplies per academic year:* $600.

Generic Baccalaureate Program (BS)

Applying *Required:* SAT I or ACT, high school transcript, 2 letters of recommendation. *Application deadline:* 2/1. *Application fee:* $35.

RN Baccalaureate Program (BS)

Applying *Required:* SAT I or ACT, TOEFL for nonnative speakers of English, NLN Mobility Profile II, high school transcript, 2 letters of recommendation. *Application deadline:* 2/1. *Application fee:* $35.

Baccalaureate for Second Degree Program (BS)

Applying *Required:* SAT I or ACT, TOEFL for nonnative speakers of English, high school transcript, 2 letters of recommendation. *Application deadline:* 2/1. *Application fee:* $35.

MASTER'S PROGRAMS

Contact Director, Graduate Program in Primary Health Care Nursing, Department of Nursing, Simmons College, 300 The Fenway, Boston, MA 02115, 617-521-2141. *Fax:* 617-521-3199.

Areas of Study Nurse practitioner programs in adult health, child care/pediatrics, family health, gerontology, occupational health, school health, women's health.

Expenses *Tuition:* $546 per semester hour. *Full-time mandatory fees:* $500. *Books and supplies per academic year:* $1200.

RN to Master's Program (MS)

Applying *Required:* GRE General Test, TOEFL for nonnative speakers of English, RN license, 3 letters of recommendation, transcript of college record. *Application deadline:* 1/15. *Application fee:* $50.

Degree Requirements 44 total credit hours, 44 in nursing.

Post-Master's Program

Applying *Required:* MSN. *Application deadline:* 1/31. *Application fee:* $50.

See full description on pages 504 and 506.

UNIVERSITY OF MASSACHUSETTS AMHERST
School of Nursing
Amherst, Massachusetts

Programs • Generic Baccalaureate • Accelerated RN Baccalaureate • Accelerated Baccalaureate for Second Degree • MS • PhD • Continuing Education

The University State-supported coed university. Part of University of Massachusetts. Founded: 1863. *Primary accreditation:* regional. *Setting:* 1,405-acre small-town campus. *Total enrollment:* 22,916.

The School of Nursing Founded in 1954. *Nursing program faculty:* 34 (54% with doctorates). *Off-campus program site:* Pittsfield.

▶ ***NOTEWORTHY***

The University of Massachusetts Amherst is located in the picturesque and historic Pioneer Valley and is the flagship school of a five-campus system. The School of Nursing has a reputation for excellence in preparing nurses to be leaders in health care. Faculty commitment to educational excellence and career mobility is evident in special programs such as the bachelor's degree for registered nurses, the BS in nursing as a second degree, advanced nurse practitioner graduate programs, and the PhD in nursing, which is offered collaboratively with the Worcester campus. The School of Nursing serves society and the commonwealth by functioning as a center for development and dissemination of nursing knowledge and research.

Academic Facilities *Campus library:* 4.0 million volumes (61,365 in health). *Nursing school resources:* CAI, computer lab, nursing audiovisuals, interactive nursing skills videos, learning resource lab.

Student Life *Student services:* health clinic, child-care facilities, personal counseling, career counseling, institutionally sponsored work-study program, job placement, campus safety program, special assistance for disabled students. *International student services:* counseling/support, special assistance for nonnative speakers of English, ESL courses. *Nursing student activities:* Sigma Theta Tau, student nurses association.

Calendar Semesters.

NURSING STUDENT PROFILE

Undergraduate **Enrollment:** 295
Women: 93%; **Men:** 7%; **Minority:** 10%; **International:** 0%; **Part-time:** 2%
Graduate **Enrollment:** 136
Women: 93%; **Men:** 7%; **Minority:** 7%; **International:** 1%; **Part-time:** 64%

BACCALAUREATE PROGRAMS

Contact Dr. Leda M. McKenry, Undergraduate Program Director, School of Nursing, University of Massachusetts at Amherst, Box 30420, Amherst, MA 01003-0420, 413-545-2703. *Fax:* 413-545-0086. *E-mail:* lmckenry@nursing.umass.edu

Expenses *State resident tuition:* $2109 per academic year. *Nonresident tuition:* $8842 per academic year. *Full-time mandatory fees:* $3304. *Room and board:* $4028. *Room only:* $2266. *Books and supplies per academic year:* $600.

Financial Aid Institutionally sponsored need-based grants/scholarships, institutionally sponsored non-need grants/scholarships, Federal Supplemental Educational Opportunity Grants, Federal Work-Study. *Application deadline:* 3/1.

Generic Baccalaureate Program (BS)

Applying *Required:* SAT I, TOEFL for nonnative speakers of English, 3 years of high school math, 3 years of high school science, high school foreign language, high school transcript, written essay. *Application deadline:* 2/15. *Application fee:* $20.

Degree Requirements 120 total credit hours, 57 in nursing.

Accelerated RN Baccalaureate Program (BS)

Applying *Required:* NLN Mobility Profile II, minimum college GPA of 2.5, RN license, diploma or AD in nursing, transcript of college record. 63 prerequisite credits must be completed before admission to the nursing program. *Options:* May apply for transfer of up to 45 total credits. *Application deadline:* 2/1 (summer). *Application fee:* $65.

Degree Requirements 120 total credit hours, 57 in nursing. University's general education requirements.

Distance learning Courses provided through picturetel.

Accelerated Baccalaureate for Second Degree Program (BS)

Applying *Required:* TOEFL for nonnative speakers of English, GRE General Test, minimum college GPA of 3.0, interview, 3 letters of recommendation, written essay, transcript of college record. 18 prerequisite credits must be completed before admission to the nursing program. *Options:* May apply for transfer of up to 0 total credits. *Application deadline:* 10/1. *Application fee:* $15.

Degree Requirements 54 total credit hours, 54 in nursing. Internship.

MASTER'S PROGRAM

Contact Dr. Sally Hardin, Graduate Program Director, 230 Arnold House, School of Nursing, University of Massachusetts at Amherst, Box 30420, Amherst, MA 01003-0420, 413-545-5088. *Fax:* 413-545-0086.

Areas of Study Clinical nurse specialist programs in gerontological nursing, psychiatric–mental health nursing; nursing education; nurse practitioner programs in child care/pediatrics, family health, primary care.

Expenses *State resident tuition:* $2778 full-time, $116 per credit part-time. *Nonresident tuition:* $8842 full-time, $369 per credit part-time. *Full-time mandatory fees:* $2816. *Room and board:* $4326. *Room only:* $2376.

Financial Aid Graduate assistantships, nurse traineeships. *Application deadline:* 3/1.

MS Program

Applying *Required:* GRE General Test, bachelor's degree in nursing, minimum GPA of 3.0, RN license, physical assessment course, statistics course, professional liability/malpractice insurance, interview, 2 letters of recommendation, transcript of college record, two samples of scholarly writing. *Application deadline:* 3/1. *Application fee:* $20–35.

Degree Requirements 36–45 total credit hours dependent upon track, 30–40 in nursing.

University of Massachusetts Amherst (continued)

DOCTORAL PROGRAM

Contact Dr. Sally Hardin, Graduate Program Director, 231 Arnold House, School of Nursing, University of Massachusetts at Amherst, Box 30420, Amherst, MA 01003-0420, 413-545-1302. *Fax:* 413-545-0086.

Areas of Study Nursing education, nursing research.

Expenses *State resident tuition:* $2778 full-time, $116 per credit part-time. *Nonresident tuition:* $8842 full-time, $369 per credit part-time. *Full-time mandatory fees:* $2816. *Room and board:* $4326. *Room only:* $2376.

Financial Aid Graduate assistantships, nurse traineeships, dissertation grants, Federal Direct Loans, Federal Nursing Student Loans. *Application deadline:* 3/1.

PhD Program

Applying *Required:* GRE General Test, TOEFL for nonnative speakers of English, master's degree in nursing, 2 years of clinical experience, 2 scholarly papers, statistics course, interview, 2 letters of recommendation, vitae, writing sample, competitive review by faculty committee. *Application deadline:* 3/1. *Application fee:* $35.

Degree Requirements 57 total credit hours; dissertation; oral exam; written exam; defense of dissertation; residency.

CONTINUING EDUCATION PROGRAM

Contact Dr. Genevieve Chandler, Coordinator of Nursing, Continuing Education Programs, Arnold House, School of Nursing, University of Massachusetts at Amherst, Box 30420, Amherst, MA 01003-0420, 413-545-1343. *Fax:* 413-545-0086.

UNIVERSITY OF MASSACHUSETTS BOSTON

College of Nursing
Boston, Massachusetts

Programs • Generic Baccalaureate • RN Baccalaureate • MS • RN to Master's • MS/MBA • PhD

The University State-supported coed university. Part of University of Massachusetts. Founded: 1964. *Primary accreditation:* regional. *Setting:* 177-acre urban campus. *Total enrollment:* 10,109.

The College of Nursing Founded in 1974. *Nursing program faculty:* 31 (87% with doctorates).

Academic Facilities *Campus library:* 525,000 volumes (9,252 in health, 1,260 in nursing); 3,000 periodical subscriptions (126 health-care related). *Nursing school resources:* CAI, computer lab, nursing audiovisuals, interactive nursing skills videos, learning resource lab.

Student Life *Student services:* health clinic, child-care facilities, personal counseling, career counseling, institutionally sponsored work-study program, job placement, campus safety program, special assistance for disabled students. *International student services:* counseling/support, special assistance for nonnative speakers of English, ESL courses. *Nursing student activities:* Sigma Theta Tau, student nurses association.

Calendar Semesters.

NURSING STUDENT PROFILE

Undergraduate **Enrollment:** 751
Women: 86%; **Men:** 14%; **Minority:** 22%; **Part-time:** 56%
Graduate **Enrollment:** 132
Women: 94%; **Men:** 6%; **Minority:** 7%; **International:** 1%; **Part-time:** 62%

BACCALAUREATE PROGRAMS

Contact Ms. Kay Walsh, Director, Admissions Information, College of Nursing, University of Massachusetts at Boston, 100 Morrissey Boulevard, Boston, MA 02125, 617-287-6000. *Fax:* 617-287-6242. *E-mail:* umb.registrar@umass_p.edu

Expenses *State resident tuition:* $2108 full-time, $88 per credit part-time. *Nonresident tuition:* $8842 full-time, $369 per credit part-time. *Full-time mandatory fees:* $1069+. *Books and supplies per academic year:* ranges from $300 to $400.

Financial Aid Institutionally sponsored need-based grants/scholarships, Federal Direct Loans, Federal Nursing Student Loans, Federal Pell Grants, Federal Perkins Loans, Federal Supplemental Educational Opportunity Grants, Federal Work-Study. *Application deadline:* 3/1.

Generic Baccalaureate Program (BS)

Applying *Required:* SAT I, TOEFL for nonnative speakers of English, minimum high school GPA of 2.75, minimum college GPA of 2.75, 3 years of high school math, high school chemistry, high school biology, high school foreign language, high school transcript, written essay, transcript of college record. *Options:* May apply for transfer of up to 90 total credits. *Application deadline:* 3/1. *Application fee:* $20.

Degree Requirements 123 total credit hours, 63 in nursing. Writing proficiency exam.

RN Baccalaureate Program (BS)

Applying *Required:* TOEFL for nonnative speakers of English, minimum high school GPA of 2.75, minimum college GPA of 2.75, RN license, diploma or AD in nursing, high school transcript, written essay, transcript of college record, diploma program transcript. *Options:* May apply for transfer of up to 90 total credits. *Application fee:* $20.

Degree Requirements 123 total credit hours, 63 in nursing. Writing proficiency exam.

MASTER'S PROGRAMS

Contact Dr. Diane Arathuzik, Graduate Program Director, College of Nursing, University of Massachusetts at Boston, 100 Morrissey Boulevard, Boston, MA 02125, 617-287-7500. *Fax:* 617-287-7527. *E-mail:* arathuzik@umbksy.cc.umb.edu

Areas of Study Clinical nurse specialist programs in critical care nursing, family health nursing, gerontological nursing; nursing administration; nursing education; nurse practitioner programs in adult health, family health, gerontology.

Expenses *State resident tuition:* $2778 full-time, $116 per credit part-time. *Nonresident tuition:* $8842 full-time, $369 per credit part-time. *Full-time mandatory fees:* $1069+. *Books and supplies per academic year:* ranges from $500 to $700.

Financial Aid Graduate assistantships, nurse traineeships, Federal Direct Loans, institutionally sponsored need-based grants/scholarships, institutionally sponsored non-need-based grants/scholarships. *Application deadline:* 3/1.

MS Program

Applying *Required:* GRE General Test, bachelor's degree in nursing, minimum GPA of 2.75, RN license, 1 year of clinical experience, physical assessment course, statistics course, essay, 3 letters of recommendation, transcript of college record. *Application deadlines:* 6/1 (fall), 11/1 (spring), 3/1 (early admission). *Application fee:* $20–35.

Degree Requirements 42–45 total credit hours dependent upon track, 36–42 in nursing.

RN to Master's Program (MS)

Applying *Required:* GRE General Test, minimum GPA of 3.0, RN license, 1 year of clinical experience, physical assessment course, statistics course, essay, interview, 3 letters of recommendation, transcript of college record. *Application deadlines:* 4/1 (fall), 11/1 (spring), 3/1 (early admission). *Application fee:* $20–35.

Degree Requirements 67 total credit hours, 61 in nursing.

MS/MBA Program

Applying *Required:* GMAT, bachelor's degree in nursing, minimum GPA of 2.75, RN license, 1 year of clinical experience, physical assessment course, statistics course, essay, 3 letters of recommendation, transcript of college record. *Application deadlines:* 6/1 (fall), 11/1 (spring). *Application fee:* $20–35.

DOCTORAL PROGRAM

Contact Dr. Frances Portnoy, Doctoral Program Director, College of Nursing, University of Massachusetts at Boston, 100 Morrissey Boulevard, Boston, MA 02125, 617-287-7500. *Fax:* 617-287-7527. *E-mail:* portnoy@umbsky.cc.umb.edu

Areas of Study Nursing research, nursing policy, health promotion and disease prevention, urban family and aging population.

Expenses *State resident tuition:* $2778 full-time, $116 per credit part-time. *Nonresident tuition:* $8842 full-time, $369 per credit part-time. *Full-time mandatory fees:* $1069+. *Books and supplies per academic year:* ranges from $250 to $300.

Financial Aid Graduate assistantships, fellowships, Federal Direct Loans.

PhD Program

Applying *Required:* GRE General Test, TOEFL for nonnative speakers of English, master's degree in nursing, 2 years of clinical experience, 3 letters of recommendation, vitae, competitive review by faculty committee, minimum 3.3 GPA. *Application deadlines:* 4/1 (fall), 3/1 (early admission). *Application fee:* $35.

Degree Requirements 60 total credit hours; dissertation; oral exam; written exam; defense of dissertation.

UNIVERSITY OF MASSACHUSETTS DARTMOUTH

College of Nursing
North Dartmouth, Massachusetts

Programs • Generic Baccalaureate • RN Baccalaureate • MSN • Master's for Nurses with Non-Nursing Degrees • Continuing Education

The University State-supported comprehensive coed institution. Part of University of Massachusetts. Founded: 1895. *Primary accreditation:* regional. *Setting:* 710-acre suburban campus. *Total enrollment:* 5,443.

The College of Nursing Founded in 1969. *Nursing program faculty:* 40 (40% with doctorates). *Off-campus program sites:* Buzzards Bay, Hyannis.

▶ ***NOTEWORTHY***

The graduate of the University of Massachusetts Dartmouth will understand the forces that impact the health-care system, as well as how these forces affect the delivery of nursing care to persons in the community. Critical judgment, the ability to apply research to practice, and therapeutic, communication, and leadership skills are fostered throughout the program of study. The commitment to humanism and the promotion of optimal levels of function for all members of society are important goals for the graduate of this college.

Academic Facilities *Campus library:* 390,000 volumes (10,000 in nursing); 2,000 periodical subscriptions. *Nursing school resources:* CAI, computer lab, nursing audiovisuals, interactive nursing skills videos, learning resource lab, therapeutic simulation lab.

Student Life *Student services:* health clinic, child-care facilities, personal counseling, career counseling, institutionally sponsored work-study program, job placement, campus safety program, special assistance for disabled students. *International student services:* counseling/support. *Nursing student activities:* Sigma Theta Tau, student nurses association.

Calendar Semesters.

NURSING STUDENT PROFILE

Undergraduate **Enrollment:** 374

Women: 92%; **Men:** 8%; **Minority:** 16%; **International:** 0%; **Part-time:** 36%

Graduate **Enrollment:** 85

Women: 97%; **Men:** 3%; **Minority:** 10%; **International:** 0%; **Part-time:** 89%

BACCALAUREATE PROGRAMS

Contact Dr. Richard Burke, Admission Office, University of Massachusetts Dartmouth, North Dartmouth, MA 02747-2300, 508-999-8605. *Fax:* 508-999-8755.

Expenses *State resident tuition:* $4151 per academic year. *Nonresident tuition:* $10,733 per academic year. *Full-time mandatory fees:* $2000–$2500. *Room and board:* $4600–$5100. *Books and supplies per academic year:* ranges from $100 to $500.

Financial Aid Institutionally sponsored need-based grants/scholarships, institutionally sponsored non-need grants/scholarships, Federal Nursing Student Loans, Federal Supplemental Educational Opportunity Grants, Federal Work-Study. *Application deadline:* 10/1.

Generic Baccalaureate Program (BSN)

Applying *Required:* SAT I, ACT, TOEFL for nonnative speakers of English, 3 years of high school math, 3 years of high school science, high school chemistry, high school biology, high school transcript, written essay, high school class rank: top 33%. *Options:* Advanced standing available through the following means: advanced placement exams, credit by exam. May apply for transfer of up to 61 total credits. *Application deadline:* rolling. *Application fee:* $20.

Degree Requirements 122 total credit hours, 68 in nursing.

RN Baccalaureate Program (BSN)

Applying *Required:* RN license, diploma or AD in nursing, transcript of college record, transfer or challenge credits. 64 prerequisite credits must be completed before admission to the nursing program. *Options:* Advanced standing available through credit by exam. May apply for transfer of up to 77 total credits. *Application deadline:* rolling. *Application fee:* $20.

Degree Requirements 122 total credit hours, 66 in nursing.

MASTER'S PROGRAMS

Contact Dr. Nancy Dluhy, Director, Graduate Program, College of Nursing, University of Massachusetts Dartmouth, North Dartmouth, MA 02747-2300, 508-999-8159. *Fax:* 508-999-9127.

Areas of Study Clinical nurse specialist programs in adult health nursing, community health nursing; nurse practitioner program in adult health.

Expenses *State resident tuition:* $667 per 3 credits. *Full-time mandatory fees:* $160–$225. *Books and supplies per academic year:* ranges from $500 to $700.

Financial Aid Graduate assistantships, Federal Nursing Student Loans. *Application deadline:* 2/15.

MSN Program

Applying *Required:* GRE General Test, bachelor's degree in nursing, minimum GPA of 3.0, RN license, physical assessment course, statistics course, professional liability/malpractice insurance, interview, 3 letters of recommendation, transcript of college record. *Application deadline:* rolling. *Application fee:* $20.

Degree Requirements 39 total credit hours, 39 in nursing. Thesis required.

Master's for Nurses with Non-Nursing Degrees Program (MSN)

Applying *Required:* GRE General Test, bachelor's degree, minimum GPA of 3.0, RN license, physical assessment course, professional liability/malpractice insurance, interview, 3 letters of recommendation, transcript of college record. *Application deadline:* rolling. *Application fee:* $20.

Degree Requirements 45 total credit hours, 45 in nursing. Thesis required.

CONTINUING EDUCATION PROGRAM

Contact Lorraine Fisher, Director, Division of Continuing Education-Nursing, College of Nursing, University of Massachusetts, Dartmouth, 285 Old Westport Road, North Dartmouth, MA 02747-2300, 508-999-8749. *Fax:* 508-999-9127.

UNIVERSITY OF MASSACHUSETTS LOWELL

Department of Nursing
Lowell, Massachusetts

Programs • Generic Baccalaureate • MS • PhD

The University State-supported coed university. Part of University of Massachusetts. Founded: 1894. *Primary accreditation:* regional. *Setting:* 100-acre urban campus. *Total enrollment:* 12,731.

The Department of Nursing Founded in 1968. *Nursing program faculty:* 22 (55% with doctorates).

Academic Facilities *Campus library:* 433,084 volumes (33,776 in health, 21,557 in nursing); 3,500 periodical subscriptions. *Nursing school resources:* CAI, computer lab, nursing audiovisuals, interactive nursing skills videos, learning resource lab.

Student Life *Student services:* health clinic, personal counseling, career counseling, institutionally sponsored work-study program, job placement, campus safety program, special assistance for disabled students.

University of Massachusetts Lowell (continued)
International student services: counseling/support, ESL courses. *Nursing student activities:* Sigma Theta Tau, student nurses association.

Calendar Semesters.

NURSING STUDENT PROFILE

Undergraduate **Enrollment:** 203
Women: 86%; **Men:** 14%; **Minority:** 5%; **International:** 3%; **Part-time:** 5%
Graduate **Enrollment:** 100
Women: 90%; **Men:** 10%; **Minority:** 10%; **International:** 1%; **Part-time:** 60%

BACCALAUREATE PROGRAM

Contact Dr. May Futrell, Chair and Professor, Department of Nursing, University of Massachusetts Lowell, Lowell, MA 01854, 508-934-4467. *Fax:* 508-934-3006.

Expenses *State resident tuition:* $1790 full-time, $75 per credit part-time. *Nonresident tuition:* $7253 full-time, $302 per credit part-time. *Full-time mandatory fees:* $2722. *Room and board:* $5260. *Room only:* $2610. *Books and supplies per academic year:* ranges from $400 to $600.

Financial Aid Institutionally sponsored need-based grants/scholarships, institutionally sponsored non-need grants/scholarships, Federal Supplemental Educational Opportunity Grants, Federal Work-Study. 78% of undergraduate students in nursing programs received some form of financial aid in 1995–96. *Application deadline:* 3/1.

Generic Baccalaureate Program (BS)

Applying *Required:* SAT I, TOEFL for nonnative speakers of English, minimum high school GPA of 2.5, minimum college GPA of 2.5, 3 years of high school math, 3 years of high school science, high school chemistry, high school biology, high school foreign language, high school transcript, letter of recommendation, transcript of college record. *Options:* Advanced standing available through advanced placement exams. Course work may be accelerated. May apply for transfer of up to 66 total credits. *Application deadlines:* 4/1 (fall), 11/15 (spring). *Application fee:* $20–35.

Degree Requirements 120 total credit hours, 58 in nursing.

MASTER'S PROGRAM

Contact Dr. May Futrell, Chair and Professor, Department of Nursing, University of Massachusetts Lowell, Lowell, MA 01854, 508-934-4467. *Fax:* 508-934-3006.

Areas of Study Nurse practitioner programs in family health, gerontology, psychiatric–mental health.

Expenses *State resident tuition:* $1695 full-time, $94 per credit part-time. *Nonresident tuition:* $5440 full-time, $302 per credit part-time. *Full-time mandatory fees:* $2046. *Room and board:* $5260. *Books and supplies per academic year:* ranges from $400 to $600.

Financial Aid Graduate assistantships, nurse traineeships, employment opportunities. 45% of master's level students in nursing programs received some form of financial aid in 1995-96. *Application deadline:* 6/1.

MS Program

Applying *Required:* GRE General Test, TOEFL for nonnative speakers of English, bachelor's degree in nursing, minimum GPA of 3.0, RN license, statistics course, professional liability/malpractice insurance, interview, 3 letters of recommendation, transcript of college record. *Application deadline:* 4/19. *Application fee:* $30.

Degree Requirements 42 total credit hours. Thesis or research project.

DOCTORAL PROGRAM

Contact Dr. May Futrell, Chair and Professor, Department of Nursing, University of Massachusetts Lowell, Lowell, MA 01854, 508-934-4467. *Fax:* 508-934-3006.

Areas of Study Health promotion.

Expenses *State resident tuition:* $1695 full-time, $94 per credit part-time. *Nonresident tuition:* $5440 full-time, $302 per credit part-time. *Full-time mandatory fees:* $2046. *Room and board:* $5260. *Books and supplies per academic year:* up to $500+.

Financial Aid Graduate assistantships, nurse traineeships, opportunities for employment. *Application deadline:* 6/1.

PhD Program

Applying *Required:* GRE General Test, TOEFL for nonnative speakers of English, master's degree in nursing, statistics course, 3 letters of recommendation. *Application deadline:* 4/19. *Application fee:* $30.

Degree Requirements 60 total credit hours; dissertation; oral exam; written exam; defense of dissertation; residency.

UNIVERSITY OF MASSACHUSETTS WORCESTER
Graduate School of Nursing
Worcester, Massachusetts

Programs • BSN to Master's • Post-Master's • PhD • Continuing Education

The University State-supported graduate specialized coed institution. Part of University of Massachusetts. Founded: 1962. *Primary accreditation:* specialized. *Total enrollment:* 609.

The Graduate School of Nursing Founded in 1985. *Nursing program faculty:* 12 (60% with doctorates). *Off-campus program site:* Amherst.

▶ *NOTEWORTHY*

The Graduate School of Nursing, which offers master's, post-master's, and doctoral degrees, educates advanced practice nurses within two specialties: adult acute/critical care nurse practitioner and adult ambulatory/community care nurse practitioner. The School's interdisciplinary programs prepare nurses to be leaders capable of responding to the health-care needs of society. The newly instituted collaborative doctoral program between the University of Massachusetts Amherst and Worcester campuses prepares nurse scientists for faculty, research, and other nursing leadership positions. The School is located on the University of Massachusetts Worcester campus, which is rich in excellent practitioners, clinical resources, and library, computer, and research facilities.

Academic Facilities *Campus library:* 226,056 volumes (162,840 in health); 2,100 periodical subscriptions (2,100 health-care related). *Nursing school resources:* CAI, computer lab, nursing audiovisuals.

Student Life *Student services:* health clinic, child-care facilities, personal counseling, campus safety program, special assistance for disabled students. *International student services:* counseling/support. *Nursing student activities:* Sigma Theta Tau.

Calendar Semesters.

NURSING STUDENT PROFILE

Graduate **Enrollment:** 95
Women: 93%; **Men:** 7%; **Minority:** 3%; **International:** 1%; **Part-time:** 82%

MASTER'S PROGRAMS

Contact Ms. Mary Garabedian, Coordinator, Student Affairs, Graduate School of Nursing, University of Massachusetts Worcester, 55 Lake Avenue North, Worcester, MA 01655-0115, 508-856-5801. *Fax:* 508-856-6552.

Areas of Study Nurse practitioner programs in acute care, adult health, gerontology, adult ambulatory/community care.

Expenses *State resident tuition:* $4107 full-time, $2399 per year part-time. *Nonresident tuition:* $21,483 full-time, $7497 per year part-time. *Full-time mandatory fees:* $1775–$2393. *Part-time mandatory fees:* $937–$1367. *Books and supplies per academic year:* ranges from $300 to $500.

Financial Aid Nurse traineeships, institutionally sponsored loans, federal family education loans. 17% of master's level students in nursing programs received some form of financial aid in 1995-96. *Application deadline:* 4/22.

BSN to Master's Program (MS)

Applying *Required:* GRE General Test, TOEFL for nonnative speakers of English, bachelor's degree in nursing, minimum GPA of 3.0, RN license, 1 year of clinical experience, physical assessment course, statistics course, professional liability/malpractice insurance, essay, interview, 3 letters of recommendation, transcript of college record. *Application deadline:* 3/15. *Application fee:* $18–25.

Degree Requirements 39 total credit hours, 36 in nursing.

Post-Master's Program

Applying *Required:* minimum GPA of 3.0, RN license, 1 year of clinical experience, physical assessment course, statistics course, professional liability/malpractice insurance, essay, interview, 3 letters of recommendation, transcript of college record. *Application deadline:* 3/15. *Application fee:* $18–25.

Degree Requirements 24 total credit hours, 24 in nursing.

DOCTORAL PROGRAM

Contact Dr. James Fain, Coordinator, Collaborative PhD Program and Associate Professor, Graduate School of Nursing, University of Massachusetts Worcester, 55 Lake Avenue North, Worcester, MA 01655-0115, 508-856-5661. *Fax:* 508-856-6552. *E-mail:* jfain@bangate1.ummed.edu

Areas of Study Nursing education, nursing research, clinical practice.

Expenses *State resident tuition:* $5462 full-time, $2273 per year part-time. *Nonresident tuition:* $14,618 full-time, $5324 per year part-time. *Full-time mandatory fees:* $500–$600. *Books and supplies per academic year:* ranges from $500 to $800.

Financial Aid Graduate assistantships, nurse traineeships, opportunities for employment. *Application deadline:* 4/1.

PhD Program

Applying *Required:* GRE General Test, master's degree in nursing, 2 scholarly papers, 2 letters of recommendation, vitae, competitive review by faculty committee. *Application deadline:* 3/1. *Application fee:* $18.

Degree Requirements 54 total credit hours; dissertation; oral exam; written exam; defense of dissertation; residency.

CONTINUING EDUCATION PROGRAM

Contact Ms. Carol Shustak, Assistant Director, Nursing Program, Graduate School of Nursing, University of Massachusetts Medical Center at Worcester, 55 Lake Avenue, North, Worcester, MA 01655-0115, 508-856-3043.

WORCESTER STATE COLLEGE
Department of Nursing
Worcester, Massachusetts

Programs • Generic Baccalaureate • Accelerated RN Baccalaureate

The College State-supported comprehensive coed institution. Founded: 1874. *Primary accreditation:* regional. *Setting:* 58-acre urban campus. *Total enrollment:* 5,505.

The Department of Nursing Founded in 1974. *Nursing program faculty:* 8 (63% with doctorates).

Academic Facilities *Campus library:* 133,000 volumes (5,400 in health, 500 in nursing); 985 periodical subscriptions (85 health-care related).

Student Life *Student services:* health clinic, campus safety program. *Nursing student activities:* Sigma Theta Tau.

Calendar Semesters.

BACCALAUREATE PROGRAMS

Contact Dr. Anne Brown, Chair, Department of Nursing, Worcester State College, 486 Chandler Street, Worcester, MA 01602, 508-793-8129. *Fax:* 508-793-8191.

Expenses *State resident tuition:* $1338 full-time, $56 per credit part-time. *Nonresident tuition:* $5726 full-time, $239 per credit part-time. *Full-time mandatory fees:* $1344. *Part-time mandatory fees:* $56+.

Financial Aid Institutionally sponsored need-based grants/scholarships, institutionally sponsored non-need grants/scholarships, Federal Pell Grants, Federal Perkins Loans, Federal Supplemental Educational Opportunity Grants, Federal Work-Study, Federal PLUS Loans, Federal Stafford Loans, state aid. *Application deadline:* 3/1.

Generic Baccalaureate Program (BSN)

Applying *Required:* SAT I or ACT, SAT II Writing Test, minimum college GPA of 2.6, high school math, 3 years of high school science, high school chemistry, high school foreign language, high school transcript, interview, written essay, immunizations. 30 prerequisite credits must be completed before admission to the nursing program. *Options:* Advanced standing available through advanced placement exams. *Application fee:* $10–40.

Degree Requirements 120 total credit hours, 48 in nursing.

Accelerated RN Baccalaureate Program (BSN)

Applying *Required:* minimum college GPA of 2.0, RN license, diploma or AD in nursing, interview, transcript of college record. 68 prerequisite credits must be completed before admission to the nursing program. *Application fee:* $10–40.

Degree Requirements 120 total credit hours, 48 in nursing.

MICHIGAN

ANDREWS UNIVERSITY
Department of Nursing
Berrien Springs, Michigan

Programs • Generic Baccalaureate • RN Baccalaureate • Baccalaureate for Second Degree • MS

The University Independent Seventh-day Adventist coed university. Founded: 1874. *Primary accreditation:* regional. *Setting:* 1,650-acre small-town campus. *Total enrollment:* 3,014.

The Department of Nursing Founded in 1970.

▶ ***NOTEWORTHY***

Andrews University is committed to providing high-quality Christian education and welcomes students from all nations and faiths who meet entrance qualifications and who subscribe to the ideals of the University. The Department of Nursing offers a part-time, 3-year master's degree program on off-campus sites in Florida, Illinois, Michigan, Nebraska, and Ohio. Intensive classes are offered in 2-week blocks, Monday through Thursday. Clinical practica are arranged with local preceptors. Students may transfer 12 credit hours from another university. Two weeks residence required second summer. New sites are opened at the request of hospitals or communities (minimum 25 students).

Academic Facilities *Campus library:* 570,000 volumes (20,210 in health, 1,728 in nursing); 2,828 periodical subscriptions (248 health-care related).

Calendar Quarters.

BACCALAUREATE PROGRAMS

Contact Director, BS Program, Department of Nursing, Andrews University, Berrien Springs, MI 49104, 616-471-3311.

Expenses *Tuition:* $10,896 per academic year.

Financial Aid Institutionally sponsored long-term loans, Federal Perkins Loans, Federal Work-Study, Federal PLUS Loans, Federal Stafford Loans. *Application deadline:* 3/31.

Generic Baccalaureate Program (BS)

Degree Requirements 190 total credit hours, 87 in nursing.

RN Baccalaureate Program (BS)

Applying *Options:* May apply for transfer of up to 40 total credits.

Baccalaureate for Second Degree Program (BS)

Degree Requirements 87 total credit hours in nursing.

MASTER'S PROGRAM

Contact Chair, Department of Nursing, Andrews University, Berrien Springs, MI 49104, 616-471-3311. *Fax:* 616-471-3454.

Areas of Study Nursing administration; nurse practitioner program in adult health.

Expenses *Tuition:* $15,600 full-time, $260 per quarter hour part-time.

Financial Aid Federal Direct Loans.

Andrews University (continued)

MS Program

Applying *Required:* GRE General Test, TOEFL for nonnative speakers of English, bachelor's degree in nursing, minimum GPA of 2.75, RN license, 1 year of clinical experience, professional liability/malpractice insurance, essay, 2 letters of recommendation, transcript of college record. *Application deadline:* rolling. *Application fee:* $30.

Degree Requirements 60 total credit hours, 60 in nursing. Research project.

CALVIN COLLEGE
Hope-Calvin Department of Nursing
Grand Rapids, Michigan

Program • Generic Baccalaureate

The College Independent comprehensive coed institution, affiliated with Christian Reformed Church. Founded: 1876. *Primary accreditation:* regional. *Setting:* 370-acre suburban campus. *Total enrollment:* 3,963.

The Hope-Calvin Department of Nursing Founded in 1984. *Nursing program faculty:* 18 (16% with doctorates).

Academic Facilities *Campus library:* 393,477 volumes (6,411 in health, 652 in nursing); 2,848 periodical subscriptions (70 health-care related). *Nursing school resources:* CAI, computer lab, nursing audiovisuals, interactive nursing skills videos, learning resource lab.

Student Life *Student services:* health clinic, personal counseling, career counseling, institutionally sponsored work-study program, job placement, campus safety program, special assistance for disabled students. *International student services:* counseling/support, special assistance for nonnative speakers of English. *Nursing student activities:* Sigma Theta Tau, student nurses association.

Calendar 4-1-4.

NURSING STUDENT PROFILE

Undergraduate **Enrollment:** 131

Women: 92%; **Men:** 8%; **Minority:** 5%; **International:** 0%; **Part-time:** 1%

BACCALAUREATE PROGRAM

Contact Ms. Sharon Kyser, Secretary, Hope-Calvin Department of Nursing, Calvin College, 3201 Burton Street, SE, Grand Rapids, MI 49546-4388, 616-957-7076. *Fax:* 616-957-6501. *E-mail:* skyser@calvin.edu

Expenses *Tuition:* $11,655 full-time, $440 per semester hour part-time. *Full-time mandatory fees:* $50. *Room and board:* $3850–$4040. *Books and supplies per academic year:* ranges from $620 to $750.

Financial Aid Institutionally sponsored need-based grants/scholarships, institutionally sponsored non-need grants/scholarships, Federal Work-Study. *Application deadline:* 3/1.

Generic Baccalaureate Program (BSN)

Applying *Required:* SAT I or ACT, TOEFL for nonnative speakers of English, minimum high school GPA of 2.5, minimum college GPA of 2.3, 3 years of high school math, high school chemistry, high school biology, 2 letters of recommendation, transcript of college record. *Application deadline:* 1/15. *Application fee:* $100.

Degree Requirements 124 total credit hours, 50–54 in nursing.

EASTERN MICHIGAN UNIVERSITY
Department of Nursing
Ypsilanti, Michigan

Programs • Generic Baccalaureate • RN Baccalaureate • BSN to Master's

The University State-supported comprehensive coed institution. Founded: 1849. *Primary accreditation:* regional. *Setting:* 460-acre suburban campus. *Total enrollment:* 23,142.

The Department of Nursing Founded in 1972. *Nursing program faculty:* 18 (44% with doctorates). *Off-campus program site:* Jackson.

Academic Facilities *Campus library:* 549,511 volumes (2,048 in nursing); 4,096 periodical subscriptions (275 health-care related). *Nursing school resources:* computer lab, nursing audiovisuals, learning resource lab, health assessment lab.

Student Life *Student services:* health clinic, personal counseling, career counseling, institutionally sponsored work-study program, job placement, campus safety program. *International student services:* counseling/support, special assistance for nonnative speakers of English, ESL courses. *Nursing student activities:* Sigma Theta Tau, student nurses association.

Calendar Semesters.

NURSING STUDENT PROFILE

Undergraduate **Enrollment:** 307

Women: 87%; **Men:** 13%; **Minority:** 14%; **International:** 1%; **Part-time:** 17%

BACCALAUREATE PROGRAMS

Contact Dr. Regina M. Williams, Head and Professor, Department of Nursing, Eastern Michigan University, 228 King Hall, Ypsilanti, MI 48197, 313-487-2310. *Fax:* 313-487-6946.

Expenses *State resident tuition:* $2295 full-time, ranges from $91 to $99 per credit part-time. *Nonresident tuition:* $5880 full-time, ranges from $237 to $253 per credit part-time. *Full-time mandatory fees:* $350. *Room and board:* $4170–$5459. *Books and supplies per academic year:* ranges from $200 to $400.

Financial Aid Institutionally sponsored need-based grants/scholarships, institutionally sponsored non-need grants/scholarships, Federal Perkins Loans, Federal Supplemental Educational Opportunity Grants, Federal Work-Study. *Application deadline:* 3/15.

Generic Baccalaureate Program (BSN)

Applying *Required:* SAT I, ACT, TOEFL for nonnative speakers of English, minimum college GPA of 2.8, high school transcript, transcript of college record. 26 prerequisite credits must be completed before admission to the nursing program. *Options:* Advanced standing available through credit by exam. May apply for transfer of up to 75 total credits. *Application deadline:* 5/15.

Degree Requirements 124 total credit hours, 60 in nursing.

RN Baccalaureate Program (BSN)

Applying *Required:* SAT I or ACT, TOEFL for nonnative speakers of English, minimum college GPA of 2.8, RN license, high school transcript, transcript of college record. 26 prerequisite credits must be completed before admission to the nursing program. *Options:* Advanced standing available through credit by exam. May apply for transfer of up to 75 total credits. *Application deadlines:* 8/5 (fall), 12/9 (spring), 6/6 (spring; 4/15 summer).

Degree Requirements 124 total credit hours, 60 in nursing.

MASTER'S PROGRAM

Contact Dr. Lorraine Wilson, Coordinator, Department of Nursing, Eastern Michigan University, 228 King Hall, Ypsilanti, MI 48197, 313-487-3274. *Fax:* 313-487-6946.

Areas of Study Clinical nurse specialist program in adult health nursing; nursing administration; nursing education.

Expenses *State resident tuition:* $136 per credit. *Nonresident tuition:* $317 per credit.

Financial Aid Graduate assistantships, Federal Direct Loans, institutionally sponsored loans, institutionally sponsored need-based grants/scholarships, institutionally sponsored non-need-based grants/scholarships.

BSN to Master's Program (MSN)

Applying *Required:* GRE General Test, TOEFL for nonnative speakers of English, bachelor's degree in nursing, minimum GPA of 3.0, RN license, physical assessment course, statistics course, professional liability/malpractice insurance, essay, interview, 3 letters of recommendation, transcript of college record. *Application deadline:* rolling. *Application fee:* $25.

Degree Requirements 39–41 total credit hours dependent upon track, 33–35 in nursing, 6 in cognate of choice.

Distance learning Courses provided through video.

FERRIS STATE UNIVERSITY
Department of Nursing
Big Rapids, Michigan

Program • RN Baccalaureate

The University State-supported comprehensive coed institution. Founded: 1884. *Primary accreditation:* regional. *Setting:* 650-acre small-town campus. *Total enrollment:* 9,767.

The Department of Nursing Founded in 1968.

Academic Facilities *Campus library:* 235,224 volumes (22,247 in health, 1,137 in nursing); 3,500 periodical subscriptions (344 health-care related).

Calendar Semesters.

BACCALAUREATE PROGRAM

Contact Head, Birkam Health Center Room 227, Department of Nursing, Ferris State University, 1019 Campus Drive, Big Rapids, MI 49307-2280, 616-592-2267. *Fax:* 616-592-5970.

Financial Aid Institutionally sponsored need-based grants/scholarships, institutionally sponsored non-need grants/scholarships, Federal Direct Loans, Federal Perkins Loans. *Application deadline:* 4/1.

RN Baccalaureate Program (BSN)

Applying *Required:* minimum college GPA of 2.0, RN license, diploma or AD in nursing.

Degree Requirements 60 total credit hours, 30 in nursing.

GRAND VALLEY STATE UNIVERSITY
Kirkhof School of Nursing
Allendale, Michigan

Programs • Generic Baccalaureate • RN Baccalaureate • Baccalaureate for Second Degree • MSN • Accelerated MSN • RN to Master's • Continuing Education

The University State-supported comprehensive coed institution. Founded: 1960. *Primary accreditation:* regional. *Setting:* 900-acre small-town campus. *Total enrollment:* 13,887.

The Kirkhof School of Nursing Founded in 1974. *Nursing program faculty:* 43 (33% with doctorates). *Off-campus program sites:* Benton Harbor, Traverse City, Kalamazoo.

Academic Facilities *Campus library:* 290,083 volumes (15,000 in health, 3,000 in nursing); 2,471 periodical subscriptions (292 health-care related). *Nursing school resources:* CAI, computer lab, nursing audiovisuals, interactive nursing skills videos, learning resource lab.

Student Life *Student services:* health clinic, child-care facilities, personal counseling, career counseling, institutionally sponsored work-study program, job placement, campus safety program, special assistance for disabled students. *International student services:* counseling/support, ESL courses, academic support services. *Nursing student activities:* Sigma Theta Tau, nursing club, student nurses association, student ambassadors.

Calendar Semesters.

NURSING STUDENT PROFILE

Undergraduate **Enrollment:** 235
Women: 88%; **Men:** 12%; **Minority:** 5%; **International:** 2%; **Part-time:** 1%

Graduate **Enrollment:** 208
Women: 98%; **Men:** 2%; **Minority:** 3%; **International:** 0%; **Part-time:** 95%

BACCALAUREATE PROGRAMS

Contact Dr. Linda Bond, Assistant Dean for Academic Affairs, 206 Henry Hall, Kirkhof School of Nursing, Grand Valley State University, Allendale, MI 49401-9403, 616-895-3558. *Fax:* 616-895-2510. *E-mail:* bondl@gvsu.edu

Expenses *State resident tuition:* $2866 full-time, $128 per credit part-time. *Nonresident tuition:* $6650 full-time, $287 per credit part-time. *Full-time mandatory fees:* $206–$238. *Room and board:* $1860–$5780. *Room only:* $1860. *Books and supplies per academic year:* ranges from $1000 to $1500.

Financial Aid Institutionally sponsored need-based grants/scholarships, institutionally sponsored non-need grants/scholarships, Federal Direct Loans, Federal Nursing Student Loans, Federal Pell Grants, Federal Perkins Loans, Federal Work-Study. *Application deadline:* 2/15.

Generic Baccalaureate Program (BSN)

Applying *Required:* SAT I, ACT, minimum high school GPA of 2.7. 51 prerequisite credits must be completed before admission to the nursing program. *Application deadlines:* 2/28 (fall), 9/30 (spring). *Application fee:* $20.

Degree Requirements 120 total credit hours, 42 in nursing.

RN Baccalaureate Program (BSN)

Applying *Required:* minimum college GPA of 2.7, RN license, transcript of college record. *Options:* Advanced standing available through credit by exam. *Application deadline:* 2/28. *Application fee:* $20.

Degree Requirements 120 total credit hours, 46 in nursing.

Distance learning Courses provided through computer-based media, interactive video.

Baccalaureate for Second Degree Program (BSN)

Applying *Required:* minimum college GPA of 2.7, transcript of college record. *Options:* Course work may be accelerated. *Application deadlines:* 9/30 (fall), 9/30 (spring). *Application fee:* $20.

Degree Requirements 120 total credit hours, 44 in nursing.

MASTER'S PROGRAMS

Contact Dr. Linda Bond, Assistant Dean for Academic Affairs, 206 Henry Hall, Kirkhof School of Nursing, Grand Valley State University, Allendale, MI 49401-9403, 616-895-3558. *Fax:* 616-895-2510. *E-mail:* bondl@gvsu.edu

Areas of Study Clinical nurse specialist programs in adult health nursing, gerontological nursing, pediatric nursing, psychiatric–mental health nursing; nursing administration; nursing education; nurse practitioner programs in adult health, child care/pediatrics, family health, gerontology, psychiatric–mental health, women's health.

Expenses *State resident tuition:* $1206 full-time, $134 per credit part-time. *Nonresident tuition:* $2628 full-time, $292 per Credit part-time. *Full-time mandatory fees:* $139.

Financial Aid Graduate assistantships, nurse traineeships. *Application deadline:* 8/30.

MSN Program

Applying *Required:* GRE General Test, bachelor's degree in nursing, minimum GPA of 3.0, RN license, 1 year of clinical experience, physical assessment course, statistics course, essay, 3 letters of recommendation, transcript of college record. *Application deadline:* rolling. *Application fee:* $20.

Degree Requirements 40 total credit hours, 33 in nursing, 7–9 in pathophysiology/neuroscience and other specified areas. Thesis required.

Accelerated MSN Program

Applying *Required:* GRE General Test, bachelor's degree in nursing, minimum GPA of 3.0, 1 year of clinical experience, physical assessment course, statistics course, essay, 3 letters of recommendation, transcript of college record. *Application deadline:* rolling. *Application fee:* $20.

Degree Requirements 40 total credit hours, 33 in nursing, 7–9 in pathophysiology/neuroscience and other specified areas. Thesis required.

RN to Master's Program (MSN)

Applying *Required:* GRE General Test, bachelor's degree in nursing, minimum GPA of 3.0, RN license, 1 year of clinical experience, physical assessment course, statistics course, essay, 3 letters of recommendation, transcript of college record. *Application deadline:* rolling. *Application fee:* $20.

Degree Requirements 40 total credit hours, 33 in nursing, 7–9 in pathophysiology/neuroscience and other specified areas. Thesis required.

CONTINUING EDUCATION PROGRAM

Contact Dr. Linda Bond, Assistant Dean for Academic Affairs, 206 Henry Hall, Kirkhof School of Nursing, Grand Valley State University, Allendale, MI 49401-9403, 616-895-3558. *Fax:* 616-895-2510.

HOPE COLLEGE
Hope-Calvin Department of Nursing
Holland, Michigan

Program • Generic Baccalaureate

The College Independent 4-year coed college, affiliated with Reformed Church in America. Founded: 1866. *Primary accreditation:* regional. *Setting:* 45-acre small-town campus. *Total enrollment:* 2,919.

The Hope-Calvin Department of Nursing Founded in 1984. *Nursing program faculty:* 18 (16% with doctorates).

Academic Facilities *Campus library:* 275,000 volumes; 1,600 periodical subscriptions. *Nursing school resources:* CAI, computer lab, nursing audiovisuals, interactive nursing skills videos, learning resource lab.

Student Life *Student services:* health clinic, personal counseling, career counseling, special assistance for disabled students. *International student services:* counseling/support, special assistance for nonnative speakers of English. *Nursing student activities:* Sigma Theta Tau, student nurses association.

Calendar 4-1-4.

NURSING STUDENT PROFILE

Undergraduate **Enrollment:** 137
Women: 92%; **Men:** 8%; **Minority:** 5%; **International:** 0%; **Part-time:** 1%

BACCALAUREATE PROGRAM

Contact Ms. Sharon Kyser, Secretary, Hope-Calvin Department of Nursing, Hope College, 3201 Burton Street, SE, Grand Rapids, MI 49546-4388, 616-957-7076. *Fax:* 616-957-6501. *E-mail:* skyser@calvin.edu

Expenses *Tuition:* $18,826 full-time, $490 per credit hour part-time. *Full-time mandatory fees:* $50. *Room and board:* $2456. *Room only:* $2060. *Books and supplies per academic year:* ranges from $620 to $750.

Financial Aid Institutionally sponsored need-based grants/scholarships, institutionally sponsored non-need grants/scholarships, Federal Work-Study. *Application deadline:* 3/1.

Generic Baccalaureate Program (BSN)

Applying *Required:* SAT I or ACT, TOEFL for nonnative speakers of English, minimum high school GPA of 2.5, minimum college GPA of 2.3, high school chemistry, high school biology, 2 letters of recommendation, transcript of college record. *Options:* Advanced standing available through the following means: advanced placement exams, credit by exam. *Application deadline:* 1/27. *Application fee:* $100.

Degree Requirements 126 total credit hours, 50–54 in nursing.

LAKE SUPERIOR STATE UNIVERSITY
Department of Nursing
Sault Sainte Marie, Michigan

Programs • Generic Baccalaureate • RN Baccalaureate • Continuing Education

The University State-supported comprehensive coed institution. Founded: 1946. *Primary accreditation:* regional. *Setting:* 121-acre small-town campus. *Total enrollment:* 3,437.

The Department of Nursing Founded in 1974. *Nursing program faculty:* 11 (27% with doctorates). *Off-campus program sites:* Petoskey, Alpena, Escanaba.

Academic Facilities *Campus library:* 126,000 volumes (5,114 in health); 917 periodical subscriptions (72 health-care related). *Nursing school resources:* CAI, computer lab, nursing audiovisuals, interactive nursing skills videos, learning resource lab.

Student Life *Student services:* health clinic, child-care facilities, personal counseling, career counseling, institutionally sponsored work-study program, job placement, campus safety program, special assistance for disabled students. *Nursing student activities:* Sigma Theta Tau, nursing club, student nurses association.

Calendar Semesters.

NURSING STUDENT PROFILE

Undergraduate **Enrollment:** 225
Women: 83%; **Men:** 17%; **Minority:** 8%; **International:** 23%; **Part-time:** 20%

BACCALAUREATE PROGRAMS

Contact Dr. Judith Sadler, Associate Professor and Chair, Department of Nursing, Lake Superior State University, 650 West Easterday Avenue, Sault Sainte Marie, MI 49783, 906-635-2446. *Fax:* 906-635-6663. *E-mail:* jsadler@lakers.lssu.edu

Expenses *State resident tuition:* $3534 full-time, $147 per credit hour part-time. *Nonresident tuition:* $6948 full-time, $289 per credit hour part-time. *Full-time mandatory fees:* $543. *Part-time mandatory fees:* $543. *Room and board:* $4464. *Books and supplies per academic year:* ranges from $1000 to $1400.

Financial Aid Institutionally sponsored need-based grants/scholarships, institutionally sponsored non-need grants/scholarships, Federal Nursing Student Loans, Federal Work-Study. *Application deadline:* 3/31.

Generic Baccalaureate Program (BS)

Applying *Required:* ACT, minimum high school GPA of 2.0, minimum college GPA of 2.5, high school chemistry, high school biology, high school transcript, transcript of college record. *Options:* Advanced standing available through credit by exam. Course work may be accelerated. *Application deadlines:* 8/1 (fall), 12/1 (spring). *Application fee:* $20.

Degree Requirements 127 total credit hours, 57 in nursing. Writing, math competency.

RN Baccalaureate Program (BS)

Applying *Required:* minimum college GPA of 2.5, RN license, diploma or AD in nursing, college-supplied work experience and reference list. 32 prerequisite credits must be completed before admission to the nursing program. *Options:* Advanced standing available through credit by exam. *Application deadline:* 9/1. *Application fee:* $20.

Degree Requirements 127 total credit hours, 57 in nursing. Writing, math competency.

Distance learning Courses provided through video.

CONTINUING EDUCATION PROGRAM

Contact Ms. Susan Camp, Director of Continuing Education, Lake Superior State University, Sault Sainte Marie, MI 49783, 906-635-2554. *Fax:* 906-635-2111.

MADONNA UNIVERSITY
College of Nursing and Health
Livonia, Michigan

Programs • Generic Baccalaureate • RN Baccalaureate • LPN to Baccalaureate • MSN • MSN/MSA • Continuing Education

The University Independent Roman Catholic comprehensive coed institution. Founded: 1947. *Primary accreditation:* regional. *Setting:* 49-acre suburban campus. *Total enrollment:* 4,109.

The College of Nursing and Health Founded in 1962. *Nursing program faculty:* 51 (16% with doctorates).

Academic Facilities *Campus library:* 118,632 volumes (18,000 in health, 6,692 in nursing); 1,250 periodical subscriptions (142 health-care related). *Nursing school resources:* CAI, computer lab, nursing audiovisuals, interactive nursing skills videos, learning resource lab.

Student Life *Student services:* personal counseling, career counseling, institutionally sponsored work-study program, job placement, campus safety program, special assistance for disabled students, tutoring. *International*

student services: counseling/support, special assistance for nonnative speakers of English, ESL courses. *Nursing student activities:* Sigma Theta Tau, student nurses association.

Calendar Semesters.

NURSING STUDENT PROFILE

Undergraduate **Enrollment:** 600
Women: 90%; **Men:** 10%; **Minority:** 13%; **Part-time:** 41%
Graduate **Enrollment:** 90
Women: 98%; **Men:** 2%; **Minority:** 8%; **Part-time:** 100%

BACCALAUREATE PROGRAMS

Contact Ms. Delores Santana, Nursing Admissions Counselor, College of Nursing and Health, Madonna University, 36600 Schoolcraft Road, Livonia, MI 48150-1173, 313-432-5718. *Fax:* 313-432-5463. *E-mail:* santana@smtp.munet.edu

Expenses *Tuition:* $2947 full-time, $238 per credit part-time. *Full-time mandatory fees:* $80. *Room and board:* $2130–$2180. *Room only:* $1908–$2164. *Books and supplies per academic year:* $240.

Financial Aid Institutionally sponsored need-based grants/scholarships, institutionally sponsored non-need grants/scholarships, Federal Nursing Student Loans, Federal Supplemental Educational Opportunity Grants, Federal Work-Study. *Application deadline:* 8/1.

Generic Baccalaureate Program (BSN)

Applying *Required:* ACT, TOEFL for nonnative speakers of English, minimum high school GPA of 2.75, minimum college GPA of 2.5, high school chemistry, high school biology, high school transcript, transcript of college record. *Options:* Advanced standing available through the following means: advanced placement exams, credit by exam. May apply for transfer of up to 64 total credits. *Application deadline:* rolling. *Application fee:* $25.

Degree Requirements 124 total credit hours, 50 in nursing.

RN Baccalaureate Program (BSN)

Applying *Required:* ACT, minimum college GPA of 2.5, high school chemistry, high school biology, RN license, diploma or AD in nursing, high school transcript, interview, transcript of college record, high school algebra. *Options:* Advanced standing available through credit by exam. May apply for transfer of up to 64 total credits. *Application deadline:* rolling. *Application fee:* $25.

Degree Requirements 120 total credit hours, 53 in nursing.

LPN to Baccalaureate Program (BSN)

Applying *Required:* ACT, minimum high school GPA of 2.5, high school chemistry, high school biology, high school transcript, transcript of college record, 1 year of high school algebra. *Options:* Advanced standing available through credit by exam. May apply for transfer of up to 39 total credits. *Application deadline:* rolling. *Application fee:* $25.

Degree Requirements 120 total credit hours, 53 in nursing.

MASTER'S PROGRAMS

Contact Dr. Mary Eddy, Coordinator, Graduate Level Nursing, College of Nursing and Health, Madonna University, 36600 Schoolcraft Road, Livonia, MI 48150-1173, 313-432-5461. *Fax:* 313-432-5463. *E-mail:* eddy@smtp.munet.edu

Areas of Study Clinical nurse specialist program in adult health nursing; nursing administration.

Expenses *Tuition:* $240 per credit hour. *Full-time mandatory fees:* $65–$75. *Books and supplies per academic year:* ranges from $100 to $150.

Financial Aid Federal Nursing Student Loans, employment opportunities, Michigan tuition grant. *Application deadline:* 8/1.

MSN Program

Applying *Required:* GRE General Test, TOEFL for Adult Health-Chronic Health Track, bachelor's degree in nursing, minimum GPA of 3.0, RN license, physical assessment course, professional liability/malpractice insurance, essay, interview, 2 letters of recommendation, transcript of college record. *Application deadline:* rolling. *Application fee:* $25.

Degree Requirements 36–37 total credit hours dependent upon track, 23–35 in nursing, 16 in social science, biology, administration. Thesis required.

MSN/MSA Program

Applying *Required:* GRE General Test, bachelor's degree in nursing, minimum GPA of 3.0, RN license, physical assessment course, professional liability/malpractice insurance, essay, interview, 2 letters of recommendation, transcript of college record. *Application deadline:* rolling. *Application fee:* $25.

Degree Requirements 60 total credit hours, 19 in nursing, 41 in business and research. Thesis required.

CONTINUING EDUCATION PROGRAM

Contact Marilyn Harton, RN, Continuing Education Coordinator, 36600 Schoolcraft Road, Livonia, MI 48150-1173, 313-432-5482. *Fax:* 313-432-5463. *E-mail:* harton@smtp.munet.edu

MICHIGAN STATE UNIVERSITY
College of Nursing
East Lansing, Michigan

Programs • Generic Baccalaureate • RN Baccalaureate • MSN • Master's for Nurses with Non-Nursing Degrees • Continuing Education

The University State-supported coed university. Founded: 1855. *Primary accreditation:* regional. *Setting:* 5,000-acre small-town campus. *Total enrollment:* 40,647.

The College of Nursing Founded in 1950. *Nursing program faculty:* 53 (40% with doctorates). *Off-campus program sites:* Battle Creek, Lansing, Muskegon.

Academic Facilities *Campus library:* 2.9 million volumes (122,541 in health, 4,500 in nursing); 8,964 periodical subscriptions (1,015 health-care related). *Nursing school resources:* CAI, computer lab, nursing audiovisuals, interactive nursing skills videos, learning resource lab.

Student Life *Student services:* health clinic, child-care facilities, personal counseling, career counseling, institutionally sponsored work-study program, job placement, campus safety program, special assistance for disabled students. *International student services:* counseling/support, special assistance for nonnative speakers of English, ESL courses. *Nursing student activities:* Sigma Theta Tau, student nurses association.

Calendar Semesters.

NURSING STUDENT PROFILE

Undergraduate **Enrollment:** 274
Women: 88%; **Men:** 12%; **Minority:** 16%; **International:** 1%; **Part-time:** 45%
Graduate **Enrollment:** 207
Women: 96%; **Men:** 4%; **Minority:** 5%; **Part-time:** 82%

BACCALAUREATE PROGRAMS

Contact Ms. Sharon Graver, Adviser, A-230 Life Sciences, College of Nursing, Michigan State University, East Lansing, MI 48824, 517-353-4827. *Fax:* 517-353-9553.

Expenses *State resident tuition:* $4644 full-time, $152 per credit part-time. *Nonresident tuition:* $6718 full-time, $386 per credit part-time. *Full-time mandatory fees:* $278. *Room and board:* $3664–$3700. *Books and supplies per academic year:* ranges from $400 to $600.

Financial Aid Institutionally sponsored need-based grants/scholarships, institutionally sponsored non-need grants/scholarships, Federal Nursing Student Loans, Federal Supplemental Educational Opportunity Grants, Federal Work-Study. *Application deadline:* 1/8.

Generic Baccalaureate Program (BSN)

Applying *Required:* ACT, TOEFL for nonnative speakers of English, minimum college GPA of 2.5, letter of recommendation, transcript of college record. 30 prerequisite credits must be completed before admission to the nursing program. *Options:* Advanced standing available through credit by exam. May apply for transfer of up to 60 total credits. *Application deadline:* 4/1. *Application fee:* $30.

Degree Requirements 120 total credit hours, 47 in nursing.

RN Baccalaureate Program (BSN)

Applying *Required:* ACT, TOEFL for nonnative speakers of English, minimum college GPA of 2.5, RN license, diploma or AD in nursing, letter of recommendation, transcript of college record. 30 prerequisite credits

Michigan State University (continued)

must be completed before admission to the nursing program. *Options:* May apply for transfer of up to 60 total credits. *Application deadline:* 4/1. *Application fee:* $30.

Degree Requirements 120 total credit hours.

Distance learning Courses provided through classroom instruction CODEC.

MASTER'S PROGRAMS

Contact Ms. Renee B. Canady, Director, Office of Student Affairs, A-230 Life Sciences Building, College of Nursing, Michigan State University, East Lansing, MI 48824, 517-353-4827. *Fax:* 517-353-9553. *E-mail:* nuro7@msu.edu

Areas of Study Nurse practitioner programs in family health, gerontology.

Expenses *State resident tuition:* $2189 full-time, $210 per credit part-time. *Nonresident tuition:* $3260 full-time, $424 per credit part-time. *Full-time mandatory fees:* $278. *Room and board:* $3644–$3700. *Books and supplies per academic year:* ranges from $600 to $1000.

Financial Aid Graduate assistantships, nurse traineeships, Federal Nursing Student Loans, employment opportunities, institutionally sponsored non-need-based grants/scholarships. *Application deadline:* 1/8.

MSN Program

Applying *Required:* GRE General Test, TOEFL for nonnative speakers of English, bachelor's degree in nursing, minimum GPA of 3.0, RN license, 1 year of clinical experience, statistics course, essay, 3 letters of recommendation, transcript of college record. *Application deadline:* 2/1. *Application fee:* $30.

Degree Requirements 40 total credit hours, 36 in nursing, 4 in other specified areas. Thesis or scholarly project.

Distance learning Courses provided through video, classroom instruction CODEC.

Master's for Nurses with Non-Nursing Degrees Program (MSN)

Applying *Required:* GRE General Test, TOEFL for nonnative speakers of English, bachelor's degree, minimum GPA of 3.0, RN license, 1 year of clinical experience, statistics course, essay, 3 letters of recommendation, transcript of college record. *Application deadline:* 2/1. *Application fee:* $30.

Degree Requirements 40 total credit hours, 36 in nursing, 4 in other specified areas. Thesis or scholarly project.

CONTINUING EDUCATION PROGRAM

Contact Dr. Joan Predko, Director of Outreach, A-214 Life Sciences Building, College of Nursing, Michigan State University, East Lansing, MI 48824, 517-355-6525. *Fax:* 517-353-9553.

NORTHERN MICHIGAN UNIVERSITY

College of Nursing and Allied Health Sciences
Marquette, Michigan

Programs • Generic Baccalaureate • RN Baccalaureate • MSN • Continuing Education

The University State-supported comprehensive coed institution. Part of Michigan Department of Education. Founded: 1899. *Primary accreditation:* regional. *Setting:* 300-acre small-town campus. *Total enrollment:* 7,442.

The College of Nursing and Allied Health Sciences Founded in 1968. *Nursing program faculty:* 19 (50% with doctorates). *Off-campus program sites:* Escanaba, Sault St. Marie, Iron Mountain.

Academic Facilities *Campus library:* 500,730 volumes (10,920 in health, 2,960 in nursing); 1,926 periodical subscriptions (150 health-care related). *Nursing school resources:* CAI, computer lab, nursing audiovisuals, interactive nursing skills videos, learning resource lab.

Student Life *Student services:* health clinic, personal counseling, career counseling, institutionally sponsored work-study program, job placement, campus safety program, special assistance for disabled students. *International student services:* counseling/support, special assistance for nonnative speakers of English. *Nursing student activities:* Sigma Theta Tau, student nurses association.

Calendar Semesters.

NURSING STUDENT PROFILE

Undergraduate **Enrollment:** 362
Women: 96%; **Men:** 4%; **Minority:** 1%; **International:** 1%; **Part-time:** 25%
Graduate **Enrollment:** 64
Women: 100%; **Minority:** 1%; **International:** 0%; **Part-time:** 75%

BACCALAUREATE PROGRAMS

Contact Dr. Elmer Moisio, Department Head, 222 Magers Hall, College of Nursing and Allied Health Sciences, Northern Michigan University, Marquette, MI 49855, 906-227-2834. *Fax:* 906-227-1658.

Expenses *State resident tuition:* $2952 full-time, $92 per credit hour part-time. *Nonresident tuition:* $5459 full-time, $171 per credit hour part-time. *Full-time mandatory fees:* $93–$114. *Part-time mandatory fees:* $93. *Books and supplies per academic year:* ranges from $200 to $400.

Financial Aid Institutionally sponsored need-based grants/scholarships, institutionally sponsored non-need grants/scholarships, Federal Direct Loans, Federal Nursing Student Loans, Federal Pell Grants, Federal Perkins Loans, Federal Supplemental Educational Opportunity Grants, Federal Work-Study. *Application deadline:* 6/1.

Generic Baccalaureate Program (BSN)

Applying *Required:* SAT I or ACT, minimum college GPA of 2.6, high school chemistry, high school biology, high school transcript, transcript of college record, immunizations. 24 prerequisite credits must be completed before admission to the nursing program. *Options:* Advanced standing available through the following means: advanced placement exams, credit by exam. May apply for transfer of up to 64 total credits. *Application deadlines:* 10/1 (fall), 2/1 (spring).

Degree Requirements 131 total credit hours, 56 in nursing.

RN Baccalaureate Program (BSN)

Applying *Required:* NLN Mobility Profile II, minimum college GPA of 2.6, high school chemistry, high school biology, RN license, diploma or AD in nursing, high school transcript, transcript of college record, immunizations. *Options:* May apply for transfer of up to 64 total credits. *Application deadline:* rolling.

Degree Requirements 131 total credit hours, 56 in nursing.

MASTER'S PROGRAM

Contact Dr. Sara Doubledee, Coordinator of MSN Program, 219 Magers Hall, College of Nursing and Allied Health Sciences, Northern Michigan University, Marquette, MI 49855, 906-227-2486. *Fax:* 906-227-1658.

Areas of Study Clinical nurse specialist program in adult health nursing; nursing administration; nurse practitioner program in family health.

Expenses *State resident tuition:* $1914 full-time, $120 per credit hour part-time. *Nonresident tuition:* $2730 full-time, $171 per credit hour part-time. *Full-time mandatory fees:* $70–$77. *Books and supplies per academic year:* ranges from $500 to $800.

Financial Aid Graduate assistantships. *Application deadline:* 6/1.

MSN Program

Applying *Required:* GRE General Test or Miller Analogies Test, bachelor's degree in nursing, minimum GPA of 3.0, RN license, 2 years of clinical experience, physical assessment course, professional liability/malpractice insurance, interview, transcript of college record, immunizations. *Application deadline:* 8/1.

Degree Requirements 36 total credit hours, 30–32 in nursing, 4–6 in other specified areas. Thesis required.

CONTINUING EDUCATION PROGRAM

Contact Mr. Perrin Fenske, Director of Research Development, Academic Outreach, and Sponsored Programs, 309 Cohodas Administration Center, Northern Michigan University, Marquette, MI 49855, 906-227-2301.

OAKLAND UNIVERSITY
School of Nursing
Rochester, Michigan

Programs • Generic Baccalaureate • RN Baccalaureate • MSN • Post-Master's

The University State-supported coed university. Founded: 1957. *Primary accreditation:* regional. *Setting:* 1,444-acre suburban campus. *Total enrollment:* 13,600.

The School of Nursing Founded in 1974. *Nursing program faculty:* 44 (25% with doctorates). *Off-campus program sites:* Detroit, Royal Oak, Southfield.

Academic Facilities *Campus library:* 375,000 volumes; 24,000 periodical subscriptions. *Nursing school resources:* CAI, computer lab, nursing audiovisuals, interactive nursing skills videos, learning resource lab.

Student Life *Student services:* health clinic, child-care facilities, personal counseling, career counseling, institutionally sponsored work-study program, job placement, campus safety program, special assistance for disabled students. *International student services:* counseling/support, special assistance for nonnative speakers of English. *Nursing student activities:* Sigma Theta Tau, student nurses association.

Calendar Semesters.

NURSING STUDENT PROFILE

Undergraduate **Enrollment:** 544
Women: 91%; **Men:** 9%; **Minority:** 13%; **International:** 2%; **Part-time:** 62%
Graduate **Enrollment:** 129
Women: 91%; **Men:** 9%; **Minority:** 7%; **International:** 0%; **Part-time:** 88%

BACCALAUREATE PROGRAMS

Contact Ms. Sue Lindberg, Coordinator, Academic Advising, School of Nursing, Oakland University, Rochester, MI 48309-4401, 810-370-4253. *Fax:* 810-370-4279.

Expenses *State resident tuition:* $3792 full-time, $119 per credit part-time. *Nonresident tuition:* $10,944 full-time, $342 per credit part-time. *Full-time mandatory fees:* $274–$537. *Room and board:* $4250–$4970. *Books and supplies per academic year:* $400.

Financial Aid Institutionally sponsored need-based grants/scholarships, institutionally sponsored non-need grants/scholarships, Federal Supplemental Educational Opportunity Grants, Federal Work-Study. *Application deadline:* 5/1.

Generic Baccalaureate Program (BSN)

Applying *Required:* ACT, TOEFL for nonnative speakers of English, minimum high school GPA of 2.8, minimum college GPA of 3.0, high school chemistry, high school biology, high school transcript, transcript of college record. 28 prerequisite credits must be completed before admission to the nursing program. *Options:* Advanced standing available through the following means: advanced placement exams, advanced placement without credit, credit by exam. May apply for transfer of up to 63 total credits. *Application deadlines:* 7/15 (fall), 11/15 (winter). *Application fee:* $25.

Degree Requirements 125 total credit hours, 60 in nursing. 32 credits of general education, 8 credits of English composition, 33 credits in specific science and social science courses.

RN Baccalaureate Program (BSN)

Applying *Required:* ACT, TOEFL for nonnative speakers of English, minimum college GPA of 2.8, RN license, diploma or AD in nursing. *Options:* Advanced standing available through the following means: advanced placement exams, advanced placement without credit, credit by exam. May apply for transfer of up to 63 total credits. *Application deadlines:* 7/15 (fall), 11/15 (winter). *Application fee:* $25.

Degree Requirements 125 total credit hours, 60 in nursing. 32 credits of general education, 8 credits of English composition, 33 credits in specific science and social science courses.

MASTER'S PROGRAMS

Contact Ms. Sue Lindberg, Coordinator, Academic Advising, School of Nursing, Oakland University, Rochester, MI 48309-4401, 810-370-4073. *Fax:* 810-370-4259.

Areas of Study Clinical nurse specialist program in adult health nursing; nurse anesthesia; nursing administration; nurse practitioner program in family health.

Expenses *State resident tuition:* $3204 full-time, $200 per credit part-time. *Nonresident tuition:* $7096 full-time, $444 per credit part-time. *Full-time mandatory fees:* $254. *Room and board:* $4250–$4970. *Books and supplies per academic year:* $400.

Financial Aid Graduate assistantships, nurse traineeships, employment opportunities. *Application deadline:* 5/1.

MSN Program

Applying *Required:* GRE General Test, TOEFL for nonnative speakers of English, bachelor's degree in nursing, minimum GPA of 3.0, RN license, 1 year of clinical experience, professional liability/malpractice insurance, essay, interview, 3 letters of recommendation, transcript of college record. *Application deadlines:* 7/1 (fall), 11/1 (winter). *Application fee:* $30.

Degree Requirements 36–50 total credit hours dependent upon track, 28–39 in nursing, 2–11 in business and other specified areas. Thesis or project.

Post-Master's Program

Applying *Required:* TOEFL for nonnative speakers of English, RN license, 2 years of clinical experience, physical assessment course, professional liability/malpractice insurance, interview, 3 letters of recommendation, transcript of college record, MSN or equivalent, 3.3 GPA in MSN, graduate pathophysiology course. *Application deadline:* 7/1. *Application fee:* $30.

Degree Requirements 24 total credit hours, 24 in nursing.

SAGINAW VALLEY STATE UNIVERSITY
College of Nursing and Allied Health Sciences
University Center, Michigan

Programs • Generic Baccalaureate • RN Baccalaureate • MSN • Continuing Education

The University State-supported comprehensive coed institution. Part of Michigan Department of Education. Founded: 1963. *Primary accreditation:* regional. *Setting:* 782-acre rural campus. *Total enrollment:* 7,300.

The College of Nursing and Allied Health Sciences Founded in 1976. *Nursing program faculty:* 14 (43% with doctorates). *Off-campus program sites:* Caro, Tawas.

Academic Facilities *Campus library:* 212,876 volumes (41,659 in nursing); 1,075 periodical subscriptions (80 health-care related). *Nursing school resources:* CAI, computer lab, nursing audiovisuals, learning resource lab.

Student Life *Student services:* health clinic, child-care facilities, personal counseling, career counseling, institutionally sponsored work-study program, job placement, campus safety program, special assistance for disabled students. *International student services:* counseling/support, special assistance for nonnative speakers of English, ESL courses. *Nursing student activities:* Sigma Theta Tau, nursing club, student nurses association.

Calendar Semesters.

NURSING STUDENT PROFILE

Undergraduate **Enrollment:** 175
Women: 85%; **Men:** 15%; **Minority:** 5%; **International:** 1%; **Part-time:** 1%
Graduate **Enrollment:** 52
Women: 100%; **Minority:** 6%; **International:** 2%; **Part-time:** 0%

BACCALAUREATE PROGRAMS

Contact Mr. James Dwyer, Director, Admissions, 178 Wickes Hall, College of Nursing and Allied Health Sciences, Saginaw Valley State University, University Center, MI 48710, 517-790-4200.

Expenses *State resident tuition:* $5636 full-time, $117 per credit hour part-time. *Nonresident tuition:* $10,896 full-time, $227 per credit hour

Saginaw Valley State University (continued)

part-time. *Full-time mandatory fees:* $400–$600. *Books and supplies per academic year:* ranges from $500 to $800.

Financial Aid Institutionally sponsored need-based grants/scholarships, institutionally sponsored non-need grants/scholarships, Federal Nursing Student Loans, Federal Supplemental Educational Opportunity Grants, Federal Work-Study. 23% of undergraduate students in nursing programs received some form of financial aid in 1995–96. *Application deadline:* 3/1.

Generic Baccalaureate Program (BSN)

Applying *Required:* SAT I, ACT, TOEFL for nonnative speakers of English, minimum high school GPA of 2.0, minimum college GPA of 2.5, high school transcript, interview, written essay, transcript of college record. 36 prerequisite credits must be completed before admission to the nursing program. *Options:* Course work may be accelerated. May apply for transfer of up to 92 total credits. *Application deadlines:* 7/1 (fall), 10/1 (spring). *Application fee:* $25.

Degree Requirements 124 total credit hours, 57 in nursing.

RN Baccalaureate Program (BSN)

Applying *Required:* TOEFL for nonnative speakers of English, minimum college GPA of 2.5, RN license, diploma or AD in nursing, transcript of college record. *Options:* Course work may be accelerated. May apply for transfer of up to 62 total credits. *Application deadlines:* 7/1 (fall), 10/1 (spring). *Application fee:* $25.

Degree Requirements 124 total credit hours, 24 in nursing.

MASTER'S PROGRAM

Contact Dr. Janalou Blecke, Assistant Dean and Professor, College of Nursing and Allied Health Sciences, Saginaw Valley State University, University Center, MI 48710, 517-790-4145.

Areas of Study Clinical nurse specialist programs in adult health nursing, cardiovascular nursing, community health nursing, family health nursing, gerontological nursing, medical-surgical nursing, pediatric nursing, psychiatric–mental health nursing; nursing administration; nursing education; nurse practitioner program in family health.

Expenses *State resident tuition:* $2797 full-time, $155 per credit hour part-time. *Nonresident tuition:* $5346 full-time, $297 per credit hour part-time. *Full-time mandatory fees:* $300–$500. *Books and supplies per academic year:* ranges from $200 to $500.

Financial Aid Institutionally sponsored loans. *Application deadline:* 3/1.

MSN Program

Applying *Required:* GRE General Test, bachelor's degree in nursing, minimum GPA of 3.0, RN license, 2 years of clinical experience, physical assessment course, statistics course, professional liability/malpractice insurance, essay, interview, 2 letters of recommendation, transcript of college record. *Application deadlines:* 7/1 (fall), 10/1 (spring). *Application fee:* $25.

Degree Requirements 39 total credit hours, 33 in nursing, 6 in education or business. Thesis or field study.

CONTINUING EDUCATION PROGRAM

Contact Dr. Janalou Blecke, Assistant Dean, Director of Continuing Education, College of Nursing and Allied Health Services, Saginaw Valley State University, University Center, MI 48710, 517-790-4145.

UNIVERSITY OF DETROIT MERCY
McAuley School of Nursing
Detroit, Michigan

Programs • Generic Baccalaureate • RN Baccalaureate • Baccalaureate for Second Degree

The University Independent Roman Catholic (Jesuit) coed university. Founded: 1877. *Primary accreditation:* regional. *Setting:* 70-acre urban campus. *Total enrollment:* 7,524.

The McAuley School of Nursing Founded in 1946.

Academic Facilities *Campus library:* 500,000 volumes (11,880 in health, 4,168 in nursing); 3,100 periodical subscriptions (511 health-care related). *Nursing school resources:* computer lab.

Student Life *Student services:* health clinic. *Nursing student activities:* Sigma Theta Tau.

Calendar Semesters.

Contact Admissions Office, University of Detroit Mercy, 8200 West Outer Drive, PO Box 19900, Detroit, MI 48219-0900, 313-993-6030. *Fax:* 313-993-3317. *E-mail:* admissions@udmercy.edu

Expenses *Tuition:* $12,216 full-time, $303 per credit part-time.

Financial Aid Institutionally sponsored need-based grants/scholarships, institutionally sponsored non-need grants/scholarships, Federal Perkins Loans, Federal Supplemental Educational Opportunity Grants, Federal PLUS Loans, Federal Stafford Loans.

Generic Baccalaureate Program (BSN)

Applying *Required:* SAT I or ACT, minimum high school GPA of 2.5, 2 years of high school math, 2 years of high school science, high school chemistry, high school biology, high school transcript. *Options:* Advanced standing available through advanced placement exams. *Application deadline:* rolling. *Application fee:* $25.

Degree Requirements 134 total credit hours, 55 in nursing.

RN Baccalaureate Program (BSN)

Applying *Required:* NLN Mobility Profile II, minimum college GPA of 2.5, RN license, diploma or AD in nursing. *Options:* Advanced standing available through credit by exam. *Application deadline:* rolling. *Application fee:* $25.

Degree Requirements 134 total credit hours, 52 in nursing.

Baccalaureate for Second Degree Program (BSN)

Applying *Required:* Nursing Entrance Test, minimum college GPA of 3.0. *Application deadline:* rolling. *Application fee:* $25.

Degree Requirements 134 total credit hours, 52 in nursing.

UNIVERSITY OF MICHIGAN
School of Nursing
Ann Arbor, Michigan

Programs • Generic Baccalaureate • RN Baccalaureate • Baccalaureate for Second Degree • BSN to Master's • MS • MSN/MBA • PhD • Postdoctoral

The University State-supported coed university. Founded: 1817. *Primary accreditation:* regional. *Setting:* 2,871-acre suburban campus. *Total enrollment:* 36,687.

The School of Nursing Founded in 1891. *Nursing program faculty:* 105 (54% with doctorates). *Off-campus program sites:* Kalamazoo, Traverse City.

Academic Facilities *Campus library:* 6.8 million volumes (411,491 in nursing). *Nursing school resources:* CAI, computer lab, nursing audiovisuals, learning resource lab, clinical simulation lab.

Student Life *Student services:* health clinic, personal counseling, career counseling, institutionally sponsored work-study program, job placement, campus safety program, special assistance for disabled students. *International student services:* counseling/support, special assistance for

nonnative speakers of English, ESL courses, international center. *Nursing student activities:* Sigma Theta Tau, student nurses association.

Calendar Semesters.

NURSING STUDENT PROFILE

Undergraduate **Enrollment:** 573
Women: 93%; **Men:** 7%; **Minority:** 16%; **International:** 1%; **Part-time:** 21%
Graduate **Enrollment:** 301
Women: 95%; **Men:** 5%; **Minority:** 11%; **International:** 14%; **Part-time:** 55%

BACCALAUREATE PROGRAMS

Contact Undergraduate Admissions, Office of Academic Affairs, 400 North Ingalls Building, Room 1160, College of Nursing, University of Michigan, Ann Arbor, MI 48109-0482, 313-763-9438. *Fax:* 313-936-3644.

Expenses *State resident tuition:* $2766 per academic year. *Nonresident tuition:* $8869 per academic year. *Full-time mandatory fees:* $185. *Room and board:* $4700. *Books and supplies per academic year:* $500.

Financial Aid Institutionally sponsored need-based grants/scholarships, institutionally sponsored non-need grants/scholarships, Federal Direct Loans, Federal Nursing Student Loans, Federal Perkins Loans, Federal Supplemental Educational Opportunity Grants, Federal Work-Study. 73% of undergraduate students in nursing programs received some form of financial aid in 1995–96. *Application deadline:* 4/15.

Generic Baccalaureate Program (BSN)

Applying *Required:* SAT I or ACT, TOEFL for nonnative speakers of English, placement portfolio by English Composition Board, minimum high school GPA of 3.0, minimum college GPA of 3.0, 3 years of high school math, high school chemistry, high school transcript, written essay, transcript of college record, 2 units of lab science, 3 years of English. *Options:* Advanced standing available through advanced placement exams. May apply for transfer of up to 60 total credits. *Application deadline:* 2/1. *Application fee:* $40.

Degree Requirements 124 total credit hours, 90 in nursing.

RN Baccalaureate Program (BSN)

Applying *Required:* NLN Mobility Profile II, minimum high school GPA of 3.0, minimum college GPA of 3.0, RN license, diploma or AD in nursing, written essay, transcript of college record, minimum 6 months employment as RN. 15 prerequisite credits must be completed before admission to the nursing program. *Options:* Advanced standing available through the following means: advanced placement exams, credit by exam. May apply for transfer of up to 54 total credits. *Application deadline:* 2/1. *Application fee:* $40.

Degree Requirements 124 total credit hours, 90 in nursing.

Baccalaureate for Second Degree Program (BSN)

Applying *Required:* minimum college GPA of 3.0, written essay, transcript of college record. *Options:* Advanced standing available through credit by exam. May apply for transfer of up to 57 total credits. *Application deadlines:* 5/1 (fall), 6/15 (winter). *Application fee:* $40.

Degree Requirements 124 total credit hours, 90 in nursing.

MASTER'S PROGRAMS

Contact Academic Affairs Office, 400 North Ingalls Building, Room 1160, School of Nursing, University of Michigan, Ann Arbor, MI 48109-0482, 313-763-9438. *Fax:* 313-936-3644.

Areas of Study Clinical nurse specialist programs in community health nursing, gerontological nursing, medical-surgical nursing, occupational health nursing, pediatric nursing, psychiatric–mental health nursing, home health care, nurse midwifery; nursing administration; nurse practitioner programs in acute care, adult health, family health, gerontology, primary care, psychiatric–mental health, women's health.

Expenses *State resident tuition:* $9322 full-time, ranges from $486 to $776 per hour part-time. *Nonresident tuition:* $18,940 full-time, ranges from $1020 to $1310 per hour part-time. *Full-time mandatory fees:* $178. *Room and board:* $9000–$10,000. *Books and supplies per academic year:* ranges from $300 to $500.

Financial Aid Graduate assistantships, nurse traineeships, Federal Nursing Student Loans, institutionally sponsored loans, employment opportunities, merit award for underrepresented minorities. 37% of master's level students in nursing programs received some form of financial aid in 1995-96. *Application deadline:* 4/15.

BSN to Master's Program (MSN)

Applying *Required:* GRE General Test, bachelor's degree in nursing, minimum GPA of 3.0, RN license, interview, 3 letters of recommendation. *Application deadlines:* 2/1 (fall), 11/1 (winter). *Application fee:* $55.

Degree Requirements 24+ total credit hours dependent upon track, 24+ in nursing, 4–6 in other specified areas. 25 undergraduate hours at the University of Michigan plus transfer and test credits.

MS Program

Applying *Required:* GRE General Test, TOEFL for nonnative speakers of English, bachelor's degree in nursing, minimum GPA of 3.0, RN license, statistics course, essay, interview, 3 letters of recommendation, transcript of college record, computer literacy. *Application deadlines:* 2/1 (fall), 11/1 (winter). *Application fee:* $55.

Degree Requirements 36–46 total credit hours dependent upon track, 30 in nursing, 6 in other specified areas. Project.

MSN/MBA Program

Applying *Required:* GRE General Test, GMAT, bachelor's degree in nursing, minimum GPA of 3.5, RN license, 1 year of clinical experience, statistics course, essay, interview, 3 letters of recommendation, transcript of college record. *Application deadline:* 3/1. *Application fee:* $55.

Degree Requirements 70 total credit hours, 25 in nursing, 45 in business.

DOCTORAL PROGRAM

Contact Doctoral and Postdoctoral Studies, 400 North Ingalls Building, Room 1305, School of Nursing, University of Michigan, Ann Arbor, MI 48109-0482, 313-764-9454. *Fax:* 313-936-3644.

Areas of Study Nursing administration, nursing research, nursing policy, information systems, health promotion/risk reduction, neuro-behavior, women's health.

Expenses *State resident tuition:* $9322 full-time, ranges from $486 to $776 per hour part-time. *Nonresident tuition:* $18,940 full-time, ranges from $1020 to $1310 per hour part-time. *Full-time mandatory fees:* $178. *Room and board:* $9500–$10,500. *Books and supplies per academic year:* ranges from $600 to $900.

Financial Aid Graduate assistantships, nurse traineeships, fellowships, dissertation grants, grants, Federal Direct Loans, Federal Nursing Student Loans, institutionally sponsored loans, opportunities for employment, institutionally sponsored need-based grants/scholarships, institutionally sponsored non-need-based grants/scholarships, merit award for underrepresented minorities. *Application deadline:* 7/31.

PhD Program

Applying *Required:* GRE General Test, TOEFL or Michigan English Language Assessment Battery for nonnative speakers of English, 2 scholarly papers, statistics course, interview, 3 letters of recommendation, vitae, writing sample, competitive review by faculty committee, BSN and/or MSN, RN license, transcript of college records. *Application deadline:* 12/1. *Application fee:* $55.

Degree Requirements 50–68 total credit hours dependent upon track; dissertation; oral exam; written exam; defense of dissertation; residency; work and research experience.

POSTDOCTORAL PROGRAM

Contact Doctoral and Postdoctoral Studies, 400 North Ingalls Building, Room 1305, School of Nursing, University of Michigan, Ann Arbor, MI 48109-0482, 313-764-9454. *Fax:* 313-936-3644.

Areas of Study Health promotion/risk reduction, neuro-behavior.

See full description on page 542.

UNIVERSITY OF MICHIGAN–FLINT

Department of Nursing
Flint, Michigan

Programs • Generic Baccalaureate • RN Baccalaureate

The University State-supported comprehensive coed institution. Part of University of Michigan System. Founded: 1956. *Primary accreditation:* regional. *Setting:* 42-acre urban campus. *Total enrollment:* 6,236.

The Department of Nursing Founded in 1989. *Nursing program faculty:* 32 (31% with doctorates).

Academic Facilities *Campus library:* 185,000 volumes (2,500 in health, 4,500 in nursing); 1,143 periodical subscriptions (231 health-care related).

University of Michigan–Flint (continued)

Nursing school resources: CAI, computer lab, nursing audiovisuals, interactive nursing skills videos, learning resource lab.

Student Life *Student services:* child-care facilities, personal counseling, career counseling, institutionally sponsored work-study program, job placement, campus safety program, special assistance for disabled students. *International student services:* counseling/support, ESL courses, minority student services. *Nursing student activities:* Sigma Theta Tau, student nurses association, student support group.

Calendar Semesters.

NURSING STUDENT PROFILE

Undergraduate **Enrollment:** 204

Women: 91%; **Men:** 9%; **Minority:** 13%; **International:** 0%; **Part-time:** 19%

BACCALAUREATE PROGRAMS

Contact Andrew Flagel, Director of Admissions, Admissions Department, University of Michigan-Flint, 303 East Kearsley, Flint, MI 48502-2186, 810-762-3300. *Fax:* 810-762-3446. *E-mail:* davis_m@pavilion.flint.umich.edu

Expenses *State resident tuition:* $1900 full-time, ranges from $158 to $200 per credit hour part-time. *Nonresident tuition:* $5230 full-time, ranges from $433 to $474 per credit hour part-time. *Full-time mandatory fees:* $450–$500. *Books and supplies per academic year:* ranges from $250 to $400.

Financial Aid Institutionally sponsored need-based grants/scholarships, institutionally sponsored non-need grants/scholarships, Federal Direct Loans, Federal Nursing Student Loans, Federal Perkins Loans, Federal Work-Study. 55% of undergraduate students in nursing programs received some form of financial aid in 1995–96. *Application deadline:* 3/15.

Generic Baccalaureate Program (BSN)

Applying *Required:* SAT I or ACT, minimum college GPA of 2.75, 2 letters of recommendation, written essay, transcript of college record. 29 prerequisite credits must be completed before admission to the nursing program. *Options:* Advanced standing available through advanced placement exams. May apply for transfer of up to 62–75 total credits. *Application deadlines:* 2/1 (fall), 9/1 (spring).

Degree Requirements 125 total credit hours, 73 in nursing.

RN Baccalaureate Program (BSN)

Applying *Required:* NLN Mobility Profile II for graduates of non-NLN accredited RN programs, minimum college GPA of 2.75, RN license, diploma or AD in nursing, transcript of college record. 39 prerequisite credits must be completed before admission to the nursing program. *Options:* Advanced standing available through the following means: advanced placement exams, credit by exam. May apply for transfer of up to 62–75 total credits. *Application deadline:* rolling. *Application fee:* $30.

Degree Requirements 125 total credit hours, 74–76 in nursing.

WAYNE STATE UNIVERSITY
College of Nursing
Detroit, Michigan

Programs • Generic Baccalaureate • RN Baccalaureate • Baccalaureate for Second Degree • MSN • Accelerated AD/RN to Master's • PhD • Postdoctoral

The University State-supported coed university. Founded: 1868. *Primary accreditation:* regional. *Setting:* 201-acre urban campus. *Total enrollment:* 32,149.

The College of Nursing Founded in 1945. *Nursing program faculty:* 58 (55% with doctorates). *Off-campus program sites:* Clinton Township, Farmington Hills.

Academic Facilities *Campus library:* 2.2 million volumes (400,000 in health, 15,000 in nursing); 12,500 periodical subscriptions (2,500 health-care related). *Nursing school resources:* CAI, computer lab, nursing audiovisuals, interactive nursing skills videos, learning resource lab, center for health research.

Student Life *Student services:* child-care facilities, personal counseling, career counseling, institutionally sponsored work-study program, job placement, campus safety program, special assistance for disabled students, minority and women's resource center. *International student services:* counseling/support, special assistance for nonnative speakers of English, ESL courses. *Nursing student activities:* Sigma Theta Tau, student nurses association, College of Nursing Council, Chi Eta Phi.

Calendar Semesters.

NURSING STUDENT PROFILE

Undergraduate **Enrollment:** 473

Women: 85%; **Men:** 15%; **Minority:** 23%; **International:** 1%; **Part-time:** 43%

Graduate **Enrollment:** 232

Women: 98%; **Men:** 2%; **Minority:** 14%; **International:** 1%; **Part-time:** 76%

BACCALAUREATE PROGRAMS

Contact Ms. Vickie Radoye, Administrative Assistant Dean for Student Affairs, Office of Student Affairs, 10 Cohn Building, College of Nursing, Wayne State University, 5557 Cass Avenue, Detroit, MI 48202, 313-577-4082. *Fax:* 313-577-6949. *E-mail:* vradoye@cms.cc.wayne.edu

Expenses *State resident tuition:* ranges from $2448 to $2880 full-time, ranges from $102 to $120 per credit hour part-time. *Nonresident tuition:* ranges from $5448 to $6480 full-time, ranges from $227 to $270 per credit hour part-time. *Full-time mandatory fees:* $92–$102. *Books and supplies per academic year:* ranges from $250 to $400.

Financial Aid Institutionally sponsored need-based grants/scholarships, institutionally sponsored non-need grants/scholarships, Federal Direct Loans, Federal Nursing Student Loans, Federal Pell Grants, Federal Perkins Loans, Federal Supplemental Educational Opportunity Grants, Federal Work-Study. 80% of undergraduate students in nursing programs received some form of financial aid in 1995–96. *Application deadline:* 5/1.

Generic Baccalaureate Program (BSN)

Applying *Required:* ACT, TOEFL for nonnative speakers of English, minimum high school GPA of 2.8, minimum college GPA of 2.0, high school transcript, transcript of college record, minimum 2.5 GPA in prerequisite courses. 30 prerequisite credits must be completed before admission to the nursing program. *Options:* Advanced standing available through the following means: advanced placement exams, credit by exam. May apply for transfer of up to 64 total credits. *Application deadline:* 3/1. *Application fee:* $20.

Degree Requirements 127 total credit hours, 66 in nursing.

RN Baccalaureate Program (BSN)

Applying *Required:* TOEFL for nonnative speakers of English, minimum college GPA of 2.0, RN license, diploma or AD in nursing, transcript of college record. *Options:* Advanced standing available through the following means: advanced placement exams, credit by exam. May apply for transfer of up to 64 total credits. *Application deadlines:* 8/1 (fall), 4/1 (spring), 12/1 (winter). *Application fee:* $20.

Degree Requirements 127 total credit hours, 66 in nursing.

Baccalaureate for Second Degree Program (BSN)

Applying *Required:* TOEFL for nonnative speakers of English, transcript of college record, baccalaureate degree from an accredited institution, minimum 2.5 GPA in prerequisite courses. 33 prerequisite credits must be completed before admission to the nursing program. *Options:* Advanced standing available through credit by exam. *Application deadline:* 3/31. *Application fee:* $20.

Degree Requirements 65 total credit hours, 62 in nursing.

MASTER'S PROGRAMS

Contact Ms. Vickie Radoye, Administrative Assistant Dean, Office of Student Affairs, 10 Cohn Building, College of Nursing, Wayne State University, 5557 Cass Avenue, Detroit, MI 48202, 313-577-4082. *Fax:* 313-577-6949. *E-mail:* vradoye@cms.cc.wayne.edu

Areas of Study Clinical nurse specialist programs in community health nursing, psychiatric–mental health nursing; nursing administration; nursing education; nurse practitioner programs in acute care, child care/pediatrics, gerontology, neonatal health, primary care, women's health, critical care.

Expenses *State resident tuition:* $2368 full-time, $148 per credit hour part-time. *Nonresident tuition:* $5104 full-time, $319 per credit hour part-time. *Full-time mandatory fees:* $72–$142. *Books and supplies per academic year:* ranges from $300 to $400.

Financial Aid Nurse traineeships, Federal Direct Loans, Federal Nursing Student Loans, institutionally sponsored loans, institutionally sponsored non-need-based grants/scholarships. 14% of master's level students in nursing programs received some form of financial aid in 1995-96. *Application deadline:* 5/1.

MSN Program

Applying *Required:* GRE General Test, TOEFL for nonnative speakers of English, bachelor's degree in nursing, minimum GPA of 2.8, RN license, essay, 3 letters of recommendation, transcript of college record. *Application deadlines:* 7/1 (fall), 3/15 (spring), 11/1 (winter). *Application fee:* $20.

Degree Requirements 38–52 total credit hours dependent upon track, 32–46 in nursing, 6 in cognate courses. Master's research project.

Accelerated AD/RN to Master's Program (MSN)

Applying *Required:* GRE General Test, TOEFL for nonnative speakers of English, minimum GPA of 3.3, RN license, essay, letter of recommendation, transcript of college record, AD in nursing, BSN work must be completed prior to admission to master's program. *Application deadlines:* 7/1 (fall), 3/15 (spring), 11/1 (winter). *Application fee:* $20.

Degree Requirements 167 total credit hours, 100 in nursing, 67 in general education, cognate courses. Master's research project.

DOCTORAL PROGRAM

Contact Dr. Marjorie A. Isenberg, Associate Dean for Academic Affairs, 230 Cohn Building, College of Nursing, Wayne State University, 5557 Cass Avenue, Detroit, MI 48202, 313-577-4138. *Fax:* 313-577-0414. *E-mail:* misenbe@cms.cc.wayne.edu

Areas of Study Nursing research.

Expenses *State resident tuition:* $2368 full-time, $148 per credit hour part-time. *Nonresident tuition:* $5104 full-time, $319 per credit hour part-time. *Full-time mandatory fees:* $72. *Books and supplies per academic year:* ranges from $250 to $500.

Financial Aid Graduate assistantships, fellowships, dissertation grants, grants, Federal Direct Loans, institutionally sponsored loans, institutionally sponsored non-need-based grants/scholarships, college private scholarships. *Application deadline:* 5/1.

PhD Program

Applying *Required:* GRE General Test, TOEFL for nonnative speakers of English, 1 year of clinical experience, 2 scholarly papers, 3 letters of recommendation, writing sample, competitive review by faculty committee, 3.5 BSN or 3.3 MSN honor point average, goals statement. *Application deadline:* 12/1. *Application fee:* $20.

Degree Requirements 90 total credit hours; 60 credits of course work, 30 credits for dissertation; dissertation; oral exam; written exam; defense of dissertation; residency.

POSTDOCTORAL PROGRAM

Contact Dr. Marjorie A. Isenberg, Associate Dean for Academic Affairs, 230 Cohn Building, College of Nursing, Wayne State University, 5557 Cass Avenue, Detroit, MI 48202, 313-577-4138. *Fax:* 313-577-0414. *E-mail:* misenbe@cms.cc.wayne.edu

Areas of Study Self-care research.

See full description on page 570.

MINNESOTA

AUGSBURG COLLEGE
Department of Nursing
Minneapolis, Minnesota

Program • Accelerated RN Baccalaureate

The College Independent Lutheran comprehensive coed institution. Founded: 1869. *Primary accreditation:* regional. *Setting:* 23-acre urban campus. *Total enrollment:* 2,858.

The Department of Nursing Founded in 1976. *Nursing program faculty:* 6 (100% with doctorates).

Academic Facilities *Campus library:* 135,000 volumes (1,550 in health, 200 in nursing); 800 periodical subscriptions (70 health-care related). *Nursing school resources:* CAI, computer lab, nursing audiovisuals, learning resource lab.

Student Life *Student services:* health clinic, personal counseling, career counseling, institutionally sponsored work-study program, job placement, campus safety program, special assistance for disabled students. *International student services:* counseling/support, special assistance for nonnative speakers of English, ESL courses. *Nursing student activities:* Augsburg Nurses Alumni Association.

Calendar Trimesters.

NURSING STUDENT PROFILE

Undergraduate **Enrollment:** 49
Women: 100%; **Minority:** 8%; **International:** 2%; **Part-time:** 80%

BACCALAUREATE PROGRAM

Contact Ms. Luann Watson, Adviser for New Students, Department of Nursing, Augsburg College, 2211 Riverside Avenue South, Minneapolis, MN 55454, 612-330-1204. *Fax:* 612-330-1649. *E-mail:* watson@augsburg.edu

Expenses *Tuition:* $8852 full-time, $1073 per course part-time. *Full-time mandatory fees:* $715. *Room only:* $2234.

Financial Aid Institutionally sponsored need-based grants/scholarships, institutionally sponsored non-need grants/scholarships, Federal Nursing Student Loans, Federal Work-Study.

Accelerated RN Baccalaureate Program (BS)

Applying *Required:* SAT I, TOEFL for nonnative speakers of English, minimum college GPA of 2.5, RN license, diploma or AD in nursing, high school transcript, written essay, transcript of college record. 36 prerequisite credits must be completed before admission to the nursing program. *Options:* May apply for transfer of up to 96 total credits. *Application deadlines:* 8/23 (fall), 3/24 (spring), 12/6 (winter). *Application fee:* $20.

Degree Requirements 132 total credit hours, 36 in nursing. Upper division biomedical ethics course.

BEMIDJI STATE UNIVERSITY
Department of Nursing
Bemidji, Minnesota

Program • RN Baccalaureate

The University State-supported comprehensive coed institution. Part of Minnesota State College and University System. Founded: 1919. *Primary accreditation:* regional. *Setting:* 83-acre small-town campus. *Total enrollment:* 4,122.

The Department of Nursing Founded in 1983. *Nursing program faculty:* 4 (50% with doctorates). *Off-campus program sites:* Hibbing, Virginia.

Academic Facilities *Campus library:* 200,000 volumes (6,000 in health, 600 in nursing); 800 periodical subscriptions (200 health-care related). *Nursing school resources:* computer lab.

Calendar Quarters.

NURSING STUDENT PROFILE

Undergraduate **Enrollment:** 58
Women: 98%; **Men:** 2%; **Minority:** 2%; **Part-time:** 96%

BACCALAUREATE PROGRAM

Contact Dr. Ranae Womack, Chair, D-10, Department of Nursing, Bemidji State University, Bemidji, MN 56601, 218-755-3860. *Fax:* 218-755-4402. *E-mail:* rwomack@vax1.bemidji.msas.edu

Expenses *State resident tuition:* $2784 full-time, $58 per credit part-time. *Nonresident tuition:* $3840 full-time, $80 per credit part-time. *Full-time mandatory fees:* $21–$620.

Financial Aid Institutionally sponsored need-based grants/scholarships, institutionally sponsored non-need grants/scholarships, Federal Nursing Student Loans, Federal Supplemental Educational Opportunity Grants, Federal Work-Study.

RN Baccalaureate Program (BS)

Applying *Required:* RN license, diploma or AD in nursing, transcript of college record. 30 prerequisite credits must be completed before admission to the nursing program. *Application deadline:* 3/1. *Application fee:* $20.

Degree Requirements 192 total credit hours, 66 in nursing.

BETHEL COLLEGE
Department of Nursing
St. Paul, Minnesota

Programs • Generic Baccalaureate • Accelerated RN Baccalaureate

The College Independent comprehensive coed institution, affiliated with Baptist General Conference. Founded: 1871. *Primary accreditation:* regional. *Setting:* 231-acre suburban campus. *Total enrollment:* 2,348.

The Department of Nursing Founded in 1981. *Nursing program faculty:* 21 (20% with doctorates).

Academic Facilities *Campus library:* 129,000 volumes; 690 periodical subscriptions. *Nursing school resources:* CAI, computer lab, nursing audiovisuals, interactive nursing skills videos, learning resource lab.

Student Life *Student services:* health clinic, child-care facilities, personal counseling, career counseling, institutionally sponsored work-study program, job placement, campus safety program, special assistance for disabled students. *International student services:* counseling/support, special assistance for nonnative speakers of English. *Nursing student activities:* nursing club, student nurses association, Nurses Christian Fellowship.

Calendar 4-1-4.

NURSING STUDENT PROFILE

Undergraduate **Enrollment:** 175
Women: 85%; **Men:** 15%; **Minority:** 5%; **Part-time:** 10%

BACCALAUREATE PROGRAMS

Contact Dr. Sagrid E. Edman, Chair, Department of Nursing, Bethel College, St. Paul, MN 55116, 612-638-6199. *Fax:* 612-638-6001.

Expenses *Tuition:* $13,180 full-time, $500 per credit part-time. *Full-time mandatory fees:* $35–$95. *Part-time mandatory fees:* $35+. *Room and board:* $4690. *Room only:* $2640.

Financial Aid Institutionally sponsored need-based grants/scholarships, institutionally sponsored non-need grants/scholarships, Federal Direct Loans, Federal Perkins Loans, Federal Supplemental Educational Opportunity Grants, Federal Work-Study. 80% of undergraduate students in nursing programs received some form of financial aid in 1995–96.

Generic Baccalaureate Program (BSN)

Applying *Required:* SAT I, ACT, minimum college GPA of 2.5, high school transcript, interview, 2 letters of recommendation, written essay, transcript of college record, minimum 2.3 GPA required in prerequisite science courses. 60 prerequisite credits must be completed before admission to the nursing program. *Application deadline:* 2/1. *Application fee:* $20.

Degree Requirements 122 total credit hours, 44 in nursing.

Accelerated RN Baccalaureate Program (BS)

Applying *Required:* NLN Mobility Profile II, minimum college GPA of 2.25, RN license, diploma or AD in nursing, high school transcript, interview, 2 letters of recommendation, written essay, transcript of college record, minimum 2.25 GPA in science courses. 61 prerequisite credits must be completed before admission to the nursing program. *Options:* Advanced standing available through advanced placement exams. May apply for transfer of up to 85 total credits. *Application deadline:* rolling. *Application fee:* $20.

Degree Requirements 122 total credit hours, 23 in nursing.

COLLEGE OF SAINT BENEDICT
College of Saint Benedict/Saint John's University, Department of Nursing
Saint Joseph, Minnesota

Programs • Generic Baccalaureate • RN Baccalaureate

The College Independent Roman Catholic 4-year women's college, coordinate with Saint John's University (MN). Founded: 1913. *Primary accreditation:* regional. *Setting:* 700-acre small-town campus. *Total enrollment:* 1,897.

The College of Saint Benedict/Saint John's University, Department of Nursing Founded in 1971. *Nursing program faculty:* 15 (20% with doctorates).

Academic Facilities *Campus library:* 500,000 volumes (725 in nursing); 1,200 periodical subscriptions (103 health-care related). *Nursing school resources:* CAI, computer lab, nursing audiovisuals, interactive nursing skills videos, learning resource lab.

Student Life *Student services:* personal counseling, career counseling, institutionally sponsored work-study program, job placement, campus safety program, special assistance for disabled students. *International student services:* counseling/support. *Nursing student activities:* Sigma Theta Tau, nursing club, student nurses association.

Calendar 4-1-4.

NURSING STUDENT PROFILE

Undergraduate **Enrollment:** 103
Women: 90%; **Men:** 10%; **Minority:** 4%; **International:** 2%; **Part-time:** 16%

BACCALAUREATE PROGRAMS

Contact Dr. Joann P. Wessman, Chair and Professor, Department of Nursing, College of Saint Benedict, 37 South College Avenue, Saint Joseph, MN 56374, 320-363-5469. *Fax:* 320-363-6099. *E-mail:* jwessman@csbsju.edu

Expenses *Tuition:* $13,858 full-time, $208 per credit part-time. *Full-time mandatory fees:* $188. *Room only:* $2590–$2700. *Books and supplies per academic year:* ranges from $500 to $1200.

Financial Aid Institutionally sponsored need-based grants/scholarships, institutionally sponsored non-need grants/scholarships, Federal Pell Grants, Federal Perkins Loans, Federal Supplemental Educational Opportunity Grants, Federal Work-Study. 88% of undergraduate students in nursing programs received some form of financial aid in 1995–96. *Application deadline:* 8/15.

Generic Baccalaureate Program (BS)

Applying *Required:* SAT I, ACT, TOEFL for nonnative speakers of English, 3 years of high school math, 2 years of high school science, high school transcript, written essay. 32 prerequisite credits must be completed before admission to the nursing program. *Application deadline:* 5/1. *Application fee:* $20.

Degree Requirements 124 total credit hours, 44 in nursing.

RN Baccalaureate Program (BS)

Applying *Required:* minimum college GPA of 2.5, RN license, diploma or AD in nursing, 3 letters of recommendation, written essay, transcript of college record. 36 prerequisite credits must be completed before admission to the nursing program. *Options:* Advanced standing available through credit by exam. *Application deadline:* 6/1. *Application fee:* $20.

Degree Requirements 124 total credit hours, 44 in nursing.

COLLEGE OF ST. CATHERINE
Department of Nursing
St. Paul, Minnesota

Programs • Generic Baccalaureate • RN Baccalaureate • MA • Post-Master's

The College Independent Roman Catholic comprehensive women's institution. Founded: 1905. *Primary accreditation:* regional. *Setting:* 110-acre urban campus. *Total enrollment:* 2,728.

The Department of Nursing Founded in 1952. *Nursing program faculty:* 30 (23% with doctorates).

Academic Facilities *Campus library:* 200,000 volumes (7,400 in health, 600 in nursing); 1,000 periodical subscriptions (173 health-care related). *Nursing school resources:* computer lab, nursing audiovisuals, learning resource lab.

Student Life *Student services:* health clinic, child-care facilities, personal counseling, career counseling, institutionally sponsored work-study program, campus safety program, special assistance for disabled students. *International student services:* counseling/support, special assistance for nonnative speakers of English, ESL courses. *Nursing student activities:* Sigma Theta Tau, nursing club, student nurses association.

Calendar 4-1-4, Trimesters.

NURSING STUDENT PROFILE

Undergraduate **Enrollment:** 208
Women: 99%; **Men:** 1%; **Minority:** 6%; **International:** 0%; **Part-time:** 0%
Graduate **Enrollment:** 50
Women: 96%; **Men:** 4%; **Minority:** 0%; **International:** 0%; **Part-time:** 0%

BACCALAUREATE PROGRAMS

Contact Ms. Vicki Schug, Assistant Professor, Department of Nursing, College of St. Catherine, 2004 Randolph Avenue, St. Paul, MN 55105, 612-690-6940. *Fax:* 612-690-6024. *E-mail:* vlschug@alex.stkate.edu

Expenses *Tuition:* $13,683 full-time, $421 per credit part-time. *Full-time mandatory fees:* $525. *Room and board:* $2000. *Books and supplies per academic year:* $300.

Financial Aid Institutionally sponsored need-based grants/scholarships, institutionally sponsored non-need grants/scholarships, Federal Nursing Student Loans, Federal Supplemental Educational Opportunity Grants, Federal Work-Study. 41% of undergraduate students in nursing programs received some form of financial aid in 1995–96. *Application deadline:* 4/1.

Generic Baccalaureate Program (BS)

Applying *Required:* SAT I, ACT, TOEFL for nonnative speakers of English, minimum college GPA of 2.75, 3 years of high school math, 2 years of high school science, high school transcript, transcript of college record, high school class rank: top 22%. 64 prerequisite credits must be completed before admission to the nursing program. *Options:* May apply for transfer of up to 82 total credits. *Application deadline:* rolling. *Application fee:* $20.

Degree Requirements 130 total credit hours, 40 in nursing.

RN Baccalaureate Program (BS)

Applying *Required:* SAT I, ACT, TOEFL for nonnative speakers of English, minimum college GPA of 2.75, 3 years of high school math, 2 years of high school science, RN license, diploma or AD in nursing, high school transcript, transcript of college record, readiness assessment. 64 prerequisite credits must be completed before admission to the nursing program. *Options:* May apply for transfer of up to 82 total credits. *Application deadline:* rolling. *Application fee:* $20.

Degree Requirements 130 total credit hours, 32 in nursing.

MASTER'S PROGRAMS

Contact Dr. Brenda Canedy, Graduate Program Director, Department of Nursing, College of St. Catherine, 2004 Randolph Avenue, St. Paul, MN 55105, 612-690-6539. *Fax:* 612-690-6024. *E-mail:* bhcanedy@alex.stkate.edu

Areas of Study Nurse practitioner programs in adult health, child care/pediatrics, gerontology, neonatal health.

Expenses *Tuition:* $8700 full-time, $435 per credit part-time. *Full-time mandatory fees:* $0. *Books and supplies per academic year:* $400.

Financial Aid Nurse traineeships, Federal Nursing Student Loans, family-based, need-based loans. 170% of master's level students in nursing programs received some form of financial aid in 1995-96. *Application deadline:* 2/1.

MA Program

Applying *Required:* GRE General Test, bachelor's degree in nursing, minimum GPA of 3.0, RN license, 2 years of clinical experience, physical assessment course, statistics course, professional liability/malpractice insurance, essay, interview, 3 letters of recommendation, transcript of college record. *Application deadline:* 2/1. *Application fee:* $20.

Degree Requirements 40 total credit hours, 40 in nursing. Thesis required.

Post-Master's Program

Applying *Required:* GRE General Test, minimum GPA of 3.0, RN license, statistics course, professional liability/malpractice insurance, essay, interview, 3 letters of recommendation, transcript of college record. *Application deadline:* 2/1. *Application fee:* $20.

Degree Requirements 26 total credit hours, 26 in nursing. Thesis required.

THE COLLEGE OF ST. SCHOLASTICA

Department of Nursing
Duluth, Minnesota

Programs • Generic Baccalaureate • Accelerated RN Baccalaureate • MA • RN to Master's • Continuing Education

The College Independent comprehensive coed institution, affiliated with Roman Catholic Church. Founded: 1912. *Primary accreditation:* regional. *Setting:* 160-acre suburban campus. *Total enrollment:* 1,895.

The Department of Nursing Founded in 1930. *Nursing program faculty:* 27 (30% with doctorates).

Academic Facilities *Campus library:* 127,355 volumes (7,280 in health, 1,150 in nursing); 1,000 periodical subscriptions (291 health-care related). *Nursing school resources:* CAI, computer lab, nursing audiovisuals, interactive nursing skills videos, learning resource lab, nursing skills lab.

Student Life *Student services:* health clinic, child-care facilities, personal counseling, career counseling, institutionally sponsored work-study program, job placement, campus safety program, special assistance for disabled students, crisis intervention, learning assistance center. *International student services:* counseling/support. *Nursing student activities:* Sigma Theta Tau, nursing club, student nurses association, Nurses Christian Fellowship.

Calendar Quarters.

NURSING STUDENT PROFILE

Undergraduate **Enrollment:** 114
Women: 86%; **Men:** 14%; **Minority:** 4%; **International:** 0%; **Part-time:** 3%
Graduate **Enrollment:** 75
Women: 96%; **Men:** 4%; **Minority:** 0%; **International:** 0%; **Part-time:** 52%

BACCALAUREATE PROGRAMS

Contact Dr. Mary Wright, Director, Undergraduate Program in Nursing, Department of Nursing, The College of St. Scholastica, 1200 Kenwood Avenue, Duluth, MN 55811, 218-723-6296. *Fax:* 218-723-6472. *E-mail:* mwright@css1.css.edu

Expenses *Tuition:* $13,056 full-time, $272 per credit part-time. *Full-time mandatory fees:* $283–$305. *Room and board:* $3807–$4005. *Room only:* $1860–$2193. *Books and supplies per academic year:* ranges from $500 to $600.

Financial Aid Institutionally sponsored need-based grants/scholarships, institutionally sponsored non-need grants/scholarships, Federal Direct Loans, Federal Nursing Student Loans, Federal Pell Grants, Federal Perkins Loans, Federal Supplemental Educational Opportunity Grants, Federal Work-Study. 95% of undergraduate students in nursing programs received some form of financial aid in 1995–96. *Application deadline:* 3/1.

Generic Baccalaureate Program (BA)

Applying *Required:* SAT I or ACT, TOEFL for nonnative speakers of English, minimum college GPA of 3.0, high school transcript, interview, written essay, transcript of college record, minimum 2.0 GPA for transfer students. 96 prerequisite credits must be completed before admission to the nursing program. *Options:* May apply for transfer of up to 86 total credits. *Application deadline:* rolling. *Application fee:* $25.

Degree Requirements 192 total credit hours, 71 in nursing.

Accelerated RN Baccalaureate Program (BA)

Applying *Required:* TOEFL for nonnative speakers of English, minimum college GPA of 3.0, RN license, diploma or AD in nursing, high school transcript, transcript of college record. 124 prerequisite credits must be completed before admission to the nursing program. *Options:* Advanced standing available through credit by exam. May apply for transfer of up to 124 total credits. *Application deadline:* rolling. *Application fee:* $25.

Degree Requirements 192 total credit hours, 68 in nursing.

The College of St. Scholastica (continued)

MASTER'S PROGRAMS

Contact Dr. Frances M. Schall, Director, Graduate Program in Nursing, Department of Nursing, The College of St. Scholastica, 1200 Kenwood Avenue, Duluth, MN 55811, 218-723-6024. *Fax:* 218-723-6472. *E-mail:* fschall@css1.css.edu

Areas of Study Clinical nurse specialist program in adult health nursing; nurse practitioner program in family health.

Expenses *Tuition:* $10,500 full-time, $292 per credit part-time. *Full-time mandatory fees:* $75. *Books and supplies per academic year:* ranges from $200 to $400.

Financial Aid Graduate assistantships, nurse traineeships, Federal Nursing Student Loans, employment opportunities. 95% of master's level students in nursing programs received some form of financial aid in 1995-96. *Application deadline:* 3/15.

MA Program

Applying *Required:* GRE General Test, Miller Analogies Test, TOEFL for nonnative speakers of English, bachelor's degree in nursing, minimum GPA of 3.0, RN license, 1 year of clinical experience, physical assessment course, statistics course, professional liability/malpractice insurance, essay, interview, transcript of college record, CPR certification. *Application deadline:* 5/1. *Application fee:* $50.

Degree Requirements 52–71 total credit hours dependent upon track, 33–50 in nursing, 7–19 in biology, psychology. Research study or project.

RN to Master's Program (MA)

Applying *Required:* TOEFL for nonnative speakers of English, minimum GPA of 3.2, RN license, 1 year of clinical experience, physical assessment course, statistics course, professional liability/malpractice insurance, essay, interview, transcript of college record, CPR certification. *Application deadline:* 8/1. *Application fee:* $50.

Degree Requirements 52–71 total credit hours dependent upon track, 33–45 in nursing, 7–19 in biology, psychology. Research study or project.

CONTINUING EDUCATION PROGRAM

Contact Patricia Michals, Director, Nursing Continuing Education, Department of Nursing, The College of St. Scholastica, 1200 Kenwood Avenue, Duluth, MN 55811, 218-723-5913. *Fax:* 218-723-6472. *E-mail:* pmichals@css1.css.edu

CONCORDIA COLLEGE

Tri-College University Nursing Consortium
Moorhead, Minnesota

Program • Generic Baccalaureate

The College Independent 4-year coed college, affiliated with Evangelical Lutheran Church in America. Founded: 1891. *Primary accreditation:* regional. *Setting:* 120-acre suburban campus. *Total enrollment:* 2,958.

The Tri-College University Nursing Consortium Founded in 1986. *Nursing program faculty:* 7 (14% with doctorates). *Off-campus program site:* Fargo, ND.

Academic Facilities *Campus library:* 288,736 volumes (654 in health, 604 in nursing); 1,500 periodical subscriptions (123 health-care related). *Nursing school resources:* CAI, computer lab, nursing audiovisuals, learning resource lab.

Student Life *Student services:* health clinic, child-care facilities, personal counseling, career counseling, institutionally sponsored work-study program, job placement, campus safety program, special assistance for disabled students. *International student services:* counseling/support, ESL courses. *Nursing student activities:* Sigma Theta Tau, student nurses association.

Calendar Semesters.

NURSING STUDENT PROFILE	
Undergraduate	**Enrollment:** 52
Women: 94%; **Men:** 6%; **Minority:** 2%; **International:** 0%; **Part-time:** 2%	

BACCALAUREATE PROGRAM

Contact Dr. Lois F. Nelson, Chair, Tri-College University Nursing Consortium, Concordia College, 901 South 8th Street, Moorhead, MN 56562, 218-299-3879. *Fax:* 218-299-3947. *E-mail:* lnelson@cord.edu

Expenses *Tuition:* $11,470 per academic year. *Full-time mandatory fees:* $130–$155. *Room and board:* $3400. *Room only:* $1500. *Books and supplies per academic year:* ranges from $150 to $550.

Financial Aid Institutionally sponsored need-based grants/scholarships, institutionally sponsored non-need grants/scholarships, Federal Nursing Student Loans, Federal Supplemental Educational Opportunity Grants, Federal Work-Study. *Application deadline:* 4/1.

Generic Baccalaureate Program (BA)

Applying *Required:* ACT, TOEFL for nonnative speakers of English, minimum college GPA of 2.5. 60 prerequisite credits must be completed before admission to the nursing program. *Options:* Advanced standing available through the following means: advanced placement exams, advanced placement without credit, credit by exam. *Application deadline:* 2/1.

Degree Requirements 126 total credit hours, 48 in nursing.

GUSTAVUS ADOLPHUS COLLEGE

Minnesota Intercollegiate Nursing Consortium
St. Peter, Minnesota

Programs • Generic Baccalaureate • RN Baccalaureate

The College Independent 4-year coed college, affiliated with Evangelical Lutheran Church in America. Founded: 1862. *Primary accreditation:* regional. *Setting:* 309-acre small-town campus. *Total enrollment:* 2,361.

The Minnesota Intercollegiate Nursing Consortium Founded in 1956. *Nursing program faculty:* 9 (22% with doctorates). *Off-campus program sites:* Minneapolis, Gaylord.

Academic Facilities *Campus library:* 200,000 volumes (300 in nursing); 1,300 periodical subscriptions (100 health-care related). *Nursing school resources:* CAI, computer lab, nursing audiovisuals, learning resource lab.

Student Life *Student services:* health clinic, personal counseling, career counseling, institutionally sponsored work-study program, job placement, campus safety program, special assistance for disabled students. *International student services:* counseling/support, ESL courses. *Nursing student activities:* Sigma Theta Tau, nursing club, student nurses association.

Calendar 4-1-4.

NURSING STUDENT PROFILE	
Undergraduate	**Enrollment:** 69
Women: 84%; **Men:** 16%; **Minority:** 3%; **International:** 2%; **Part-time:** 0%	

BACCALAUREATE PROGRAMS

Contact Ms. Kay Wold, Chair of Nursing Department, Minnesota Intercollegiate Nursing Consortium, Gustavus Adolphus College, 800 West College Avenue, St. Peter, MN 56082, 507-933-7317. *Fax:* 507-933-7041. *E-mail:* kaywold@gac.edu

Expenses *Tuition:* $19,250 full-time, $1700 per course part-time.

Financial Aid Institutionally sponsored need-based grants/scholarships, institutionally sponsored non-need grants/scholarships, Federal Direct Loans, Federal Nursing Student Loans, Federal Pell Grants. 13% of undergraduate students in nursing programs received some form of financial aid in 1995–96. *Application deadline:* 3/30.

Generic Baccalaureate Program (BA)

Applying *Required:* PSAT, SAT, or ACT, minimum college GPA of 2.7, high school transcript, 2 letters of recommendation, written essay. *Options:* Advanced standing available through advanced placement exams. Course work may be accelerated. *Application deadline:* rolling. *Application fee:* $25.

Degree Requirements 35 courses, including 10 in nursing.

RN Baccalaureate Program (BA)

Applying *Required:* PSAT, SAT, or ACT, minimum college GPA of 2.7, RN license, diploma or AD in nursing, high school transcript, 2 letters of recommendation, transcript of college record. *Application deadline:* rolling.

Degree Requirements 35 total credit hours, 10 in nursing.

MANKATO STATE UNIVERSITY
School of Nursing
Mankato, Minnesota

Programs • Generic Baccalaureate • RN Baccalaureate • LPN to Baccalaureate • BSN to Master's • Master's for Nurses with Non-Nursing Degrees • Continuing Education

The University State-supported comprehensive coed institution. Part of Minnesota State College and University System. Founded: 1868. *Primary accreditation:* regional. *Setting:* 303-acre small-town campus. *Total enrollment:* 13,175.

The School of Nursing Founded in 1953. *Nursing program faculty:* 32 (31% with doctorates). *Off-campus program site:* Minneapolis/St. Paul.

Academic Facilities *Campus library:* 900,000 volumes (2,000 in health, 1,500 in nursing); 3,200 periodical subscriptions (100 health-care related). *Nursing school resources:* CAI, computer lab, nursing audiovisuals, interactive nursing skills videos, learning resource lab.

Student Life *Student services:* health clinic, child-care facilities, personal counseling, career counseling, institutionally sponsored work-study program, job placement, campus safety program, special assistance for disabled students. *International student services:* counseling/support, special assistance for nonnative speakers of English, ESL courses. *Nursing student activities:* Sigma Theta Tau, student nurses association.

Calendar Quarters.

NURSING STUDENT PROFILE

Undergraduate **Enrollment:** 242

Women: 84%; **Men:** 16%; **Minority:** 5%; **International:** 0%; **Part-time:** 9%

Graduate **Enrollment:** 46

Women: 96%; **Men:** 4%; **Minority:** 0%; **International:** 0%

BACCALAUREATE PROGRAMS

Contact Ms. Candice Mentele, Student Relations Coordinator, School of Nursing, Mankato State University, PO Box 8400, MSU 27, Mankato, MN 56002-8400, 507-389-6022. *Fax:* 507-389-6516. *E-mail:* candice_mentele@ms1.mankato.msus.edu

Expenses *State resident tuition:* $3023 full-time, $63 per credit part-time. *Nonresident tuition:* $6131 full-time, $128 per credit part-time. *Full-time mandatory fees:* $500. *Books and supplies per academic year:* ranges from $200 to $300.

Financial Aid Institutionally sponsored need-based grants/scholarships, institutionally sponsored non-need grants/scholarships, Federal Nursing Student Loans, Federal Supplemental Educational Opportunity Grants, Federal Work-Study. 90% of undergraduate students in nursing programs received some form of financial aid in 1995–96. *Application deadline:* 4/1.

Generic Baccalaureate Program (BS)

Applying *Required:* ACT, minimum high school GPA of 2.0, minimum college GPA of 2.5, high school transcript, transcript of college record. 45 prerequisite credits must be completed before admission to the nursing program. *Options:* May apply for transfer of up to 96 total credits. *Application deadlines:* 1/15 (spring), 9/30 (winter). *Application fee:* $20.

Degree Requirements 192 total credit hours, 91 in nursing.

RN Baccalaureate Program (BS)

Applying *Required:* ACT, minimum high school GPA of 2.0, minimum college GPA of 2.5, RN license, diploma or AD in nursing, high school transcript, 2 letters of recommendation, transcript of college record. 45 prerequisite credits must be completed before admission to the nursing program. *Options:* May apply for transfer of up to 44 total credits. *Application deadlines:* 1/15 (spring), 9/30 (winter). *Application fee:* $20.

Degree Requirements 192 total credit hours, 91 in nursing.

Distance learning Courses provided through correspondence, audio, on-line.

LPN to Baccalaureate Program (BS)

Applying *Required:* ACT, minimum high school GPA of 2.0, minimum college GPA of 2.5, high school transcript, letter of recommendation, transcript of college record, LPN license. *Options:* May apply for transfer of up to 11 total credits. *Application deadline:* 1/15. *Application fee:* $20.

Degree Requirements 192 total credit hours, 91 in nursing. 17 credit hours transferred.

MASTER'S PROGRAMS

Contact Dr. Linda Rosenbaum, Graduate Program Director, School of Nursing, Mankato State University, PO Box 8400, MSU 27, Manlcato, MN 56002-8400, 507-389-6022. *Fax:* 507-389-6516. *E-mail:* linda_rosenbaum@ms1.mankato.msus.edu

Areas of Study Clinical nurse specialist program in family health nursing; nurse practitioner program in family health.

Expenses *State resident tuition:* $2901 full-time, $91 per credit part-time. *Nonresident tuition:* $4399 full-time, $137 per credit part-time. *Full-time mandatory fees:* $0–$15. *Books and supplies per academic year:* $800.

Financial Aid Graduate assistantships, Federal Nursing Student Loans. 17% of master's level students in nursing programs received some form of financial aid in 1995-96. *Application deadline:* 4/1.

BSN to Master's Program (MSN)

Applying *Required:* GRE General Test (minimum combined score of 1350 on three tests), Miller Analogies Test, bachelor's degree in nursing, bachelor's degree, minimum GPA of 3.0, RN license, 2 years of clinical experience, statistics course, professional liability/malpractice insurance, essay, 3 letters of recommendation, transcript of college record. *Application deadline:* 2/15. *Application fee:* $20.

Degree Requirements 48–64 total credit hours dependent upon track, 48–61 in nursing, 3 in advanced pharmacology for FNP track. Thesis or clinical project as culminating experience.

Distance learning Courses provided through ITV. Specific degree requirements include travel to closest of 3 sites.

Master's for Nurses with Non-Nursing Degrees Program (MSN)

Applying *Required:* GRE General Test (minimum combined score of 1350 on three tests), Miller Analogies Test, bachelor's degree, minimum GPA of 3.0, RN license, 2 years of clinical experience, statistics course, professional liability/malpractice insurance, essay, 3 letters of recommendation, transcript of college record, undergraduate research course, leadership and management course, and public health or community health nursing course, both theoretical and practical components. *Application deadline:* 2/15. *Application fee:* $20.

Degree Requirements 48–64 total credit hours dependent upon track, 48–61 in nursing, 3 in advanced pharmacology for FNP track. Thesis or clinical project as culminating experience.

Distance learning Courses provided through ITV. Specific degree requirements include travel to closest of 3 sites.

CONTINUING EDUCATION PROGRAM

Contact Pat Priem, Continuing Nursing Education Program Secretary, School of Nursing, Mankato State University, PO Box 8400, MSU 27, Mankato, MN 56002-8400, 507-389-6826. *Fax:* 507-389-6516. *E-mail:* pat_priem@ms1.mankato.msus.edu

METROPOLITAN STATE UNIVERSITY
School of Nursing
St. Paul, Minnesota

Programs • RN Baccalaureate • MSN

The University State-supported comprehensive coed institution. Part of Minnesota State University System. Founded: 1971. *Primary accreditation:* regional. *Total enrollment:* 5,175.

The School of Nursing Founded in 1981. *Nursing program faculty:* 7 (57% with doctorates).

Academic Facilities *Nursing school resources:* computer lab, nursing audiovisuals, learning resource lab, ITV.

Calendar Quarters.

NURSING STUDENT PROFILE

Undergraduate **Enrollment:** 254
Women: 95%; **Men:** 5%; **Minority:** 3%; **International:** 0%; **Part-time:** 90%
Graduate **Enrollment:** 35
Women: 97%; **Men:** 3%; **Minority:** 7%; **International:** 0%; **Part-time:** 66%

BACCALAUREATE PROGRAM

Contact Admissions Office, Metropolitan State University, 700 East 7th Street, St. Paul, MN 55106-5000, 612-772-7600. *Fax:* 612-772-7738.

Expenses *State resident tuition:* $1908 full-time, $53 per credit part-time. *Nonresident tuition:* $4224 full-time, $117 per credit part-time. *Full-time mandatory fees:* $26. *Part-time mandatory fees:* $9.

Financial Aid Institutionally sponsored need-based grants/scholarships, institutionally sponsored non-need grants/scholarships, Federal Pell Grants, Federal Supplemental Educational Opportunity Grants, Federal Work-Study. 11% of undergraduate students in nursing programs received some form of financial aid in 1995–96. *Application deadline:* 7/1.

RN Baccalaureate Program (BSN)

Applying *Required:* TOEFL for nonnative speakers of English, minimum college GPA of 2.5, RN license, diploma or AD in nursing, transcript of college record. 99 prerequisite credits must be completed before admission to the nursing program. *Options:* May apply for transfer of up to 99 total credits. *Application deadline:* rolling. *Application fee:* $20.

Degree Requirements 186 total credit hours, 48 in nursing.

MASTER'S PROGRAM

Contact Admissions Office, Metropolitan State University, 700 East 7th Street, St. Paul, MN 55106-5000, 612-772-7600. *Fax:* 612-772-7738.

Areas of Study Clinical nurse specialist program in community health nursing; nurse practitioner program in family health.

Expenses *State resident tuition:* $2885 full-time, $80 per credit part-time. *Nonresident tuition:* $4570 full-time, $127 per credit part-time. *Full-time mandatory fees:* $78. *Part-time mandatory fees:* $7.

Financial Aid Institutionally sponsored loans, institutionally sponsored need-based grants/scholarships, institutionally sponsored non-need-based grants/scholarships. *Application deadline:* 7/1.

MSN Program

Applying *Required:* GRE General Test (minimum combined score of 1350 on three tests), Miller Analogies Test, TOEFL for nonnative speakers of English, bachelor's degree in nursing, minimum GPA of 3.0, RN license, 2 years of clinical experience, statistics course, essay, 3 letters of recommendation, transcript of college record, validation of computer competencies in word processing, database management, spreadsheet development. *Application deadline:* 2/15. *Application fee:* $20.

Degree Requirements 63 total credit hours, 63 in nursing. Thesis or clinical project.

MOORHEAD STATE UNIVERSITY
Nursing Department
Moorhead, Minnesota

Program • RN Baccalaureate

The University State-supported comprehensive coed institution. Part of Minnesota State Colleges and Universities System. Founded: 1885. *Primary accreditation:* regional. *Setting:* 104-acre urban campus. *Total enrollment:* 6,268.

The Nursing Department Founded in 1976.

Academic Facilities *Campus library:* 360,000 volumes; 1,500 periodical subscriptions (50 health-care related).

Calendar Quarters.

BACCALAUREATE PROGRAM

Contact Dr. Rhoda T. Hooper, Director, Nursing Department, Moorhead State University, Moorhead, MN 56563, 218-236-2693. *Fax:* 218-299-5990. *E-mail:* hooper@mhd.1.moorhead.msus.edu

Expenses *State resident tuition:* ranges from $1848 to $2256 full-time, ranges from $77 to $94 per credit hour part-time. *Nonresident tuition:* $4176 full-time, $174 per credit hour part-time.

Financial Aid Federal Pell Grants, Federal Perkins Loans, Federal Supplemental Educational Opportunity Grants, Federal Work-Study, Federal PLUS Loans, Federal Stafford Loans, state aid. *Application deadline:* 3/1.

RN Baccalaureate Program (BSN)

Applying *Required:* RN license, diploma or AD in nursing, high school transcript, transcript of college record. *Application fee:* $15.

Degree Requirements 128 total credit hours, 41 in nursing.

ST. OLAF COLLEGE
Department of Nursing
Northfield, Minnesota

Programs • Generic Baccalaureate • RN Baccalaureate • Continuing Education

The College Independent Lutheran 4-year coed college. Founded: 1874. *Primary accreditation:* regional. *Setting:* 350-acre small-town campus. *Total enrollment:* 2,936.

The Department of Nursing Founded in 1952. *Nursing program faculty:* 9 (22% with doctorates). *Off-campus program site:* Minneapolis.

Academic Facilities *Campus library:* 365,000 volumes (7,300 in nursing); 1,650 periodical subscriptions (100 health-care related). *Nursing school resources:* CAI, computer lab, nursing audiovisuals, learning resource lab.

Student Life *Student services:* health clinic, personal counseling, career counseling, institutionally sponsored work-study program, job placement, campus safety program, special assistance for disabled students. *International student services:* counseling/support, special assistance for nonnative speakers of English. *Nursing student activities:* Sigma Theta Tau, student nurses association.

Calendar 4-1-4.

NURSING STUDENT PROFILE

Undergraduate **Enrollment:** 72
Women: 96%; **Men:** 4%; **Minority:** 1%; **International:** 0%; **Part-time:** 0%

BACCALAUREATE PROGRAMS

Contact Dr. Rita S. Glazebrook, Director, Minnesota Intercollegiate Nursing Consortium, St. Olaf College, 1520 St. Olaf Avenue, Northfield, MN 55057-1098, 507-646-3265. *Fax:* 507-646-3733. *E-mail:* glazebro@stolaf.edu

Expenses *Tuition:* $15,700 per academic year. *Full-time mandatory fees:* $0. *Room and board:* $3850. *Books and supplies per academic year:* $550.

Financial Aid Institutionally sponsored need-based grants/scholarships, institutionally sponsored non-need grants/scholarships, Federal Direct Loans, Federal Nursing Student Loans, Federal Pell Grants, Federal Perkins Loans, Federal Supplemental Educational Opportunity Grants, Federal Work-Study.

Generic Baccalaureate Program (BA)

Applying *Required:* PSAT, SAT, or ACT, minimum college GPA of 2.7, high school transcript, 2 letters of recommendation, written essay, transcript of college record. 32 prerequisite credits must be completed before admission to the nursing program. *Application deadline:* rolling. *Application fee:* $25.

Degree Requirements 140 total credit hours, 40 in nursing.

RN Baccalaureate Program (BA)

Applying *Required:* PSAT, SAT, or ACT, minimum college GPA of 2.7, RN license, diploma or AD in nursing, high school transcript, 2 letters of recommendation, written essay, transcript of college record. *Application deadline:* rolling. *Application fee:* $25.

Degree Requirements 140 total credit hours, 40 in nursing.

CONTINUING EDUCATION PROGRAM

Contact Ms. Susan Hamerski, Director, Continuing Education and Academic Outreach, Minnesota Intercollegiate Nursing Consortium, St. Olaf College, 1520 St. Olaf Avenue, Northfield, MN 55057-1098, 507-646-3066. *Fax:* 507-646-3549. *E-mail:* hamerski@stolaf.edu

UNIVERSITY OF MINNESOTA, TWIN CITIES CAMPUS

School of Nursing
Minneapolis, Minnesota

Programs • Generic Baccalaureate • RN Baccalaureate • RN to Master's • PhD • Continuing Education

The University State-supported coed university. Part of University of Minnesota System. Founded: 1851. *Primary accreditation:* regional. *Setting:* 2,000-acre urban campus. *Total enrollment:* 36,995.

The School of Nursing Founded in 1909. *Nursing program faculty:* 69 (52% with doctorates). *Off-campus program sites:* Moorhead, Rochester.

Academic Facilities *Campus library:* 4.0 million volumes (4,000 in health, 1,500 in nursing); 39,000 periodical subscriptions (4,800 health-care related). *Nursing school resources:* computer lab, learning resource lab.

Student Life *Student services:* health clinic, child-care facilities, personal counseling, career counseling, institutionally sponsored work-study program, campus safety program, special assistance for disabled students, student unions, Minnesota Women's Center, Student Diversity Institute, student cultural centers. *International student services:* counseling/support, special assistance for nonnative speakers of English, ESL courses. *Nursing student activities:* Sigma Theta Tau, nursing club, student nurses association.

Calendar Quarters.

NURSING STUDENT PROFILE

Undergraduate **Enrollment:** 210
Women: 85%; **Men:** 15%; **Minority:** 10%; **International:** 1%; **Part-time:** 10%
Graduate **Enrollment:** 333
Women: 97%; **Men:** 3%; **Minority:** 7%; **International:** 0%; **Part-time:** 64%

BACCALAUREATE PROGRAMS

Contact Ms. Kate Hanson, Nursing Recruiter, 5-160 Health Sciences Unit F, School of Nursing, University of Minnesota, 308 Harvard Street, SE, Minneapolis, MN 55455-0213, 612-624-9494. *Fax:* 612-626-2359. *E-mail:* hanso041@maroon.tc.umn.edu

Expenses *State resident tuition:* $4054 per academic year. *Nonresident tuition:* $11,460 per academic year. *Full-time mandatory fees:* $470. *Room and board:* $4119. *Books and supplies per academic year:* ranges from $600 to $1000.

Financial Aid Institutionally sponsored need-based grants/scholarships, institutionally sponsored non-need grants/scholarships, Federal Nursing Student Loans, Federal Perkins Loans. 31% of undergraduate students in nursing programs received some form of financial aid in 1995–96. *Application deadline:* 9/20.

Generic Baccalaureate Program (BS)

Applying *Required:* TOEFL for nonnative speakers of English, minimum college GPA of 2.8, 3 years of high school math, 3 years of high school science, high school chemistry, high school biology, high school foreign language, high school transcript, written essay, transcript of college record. 64 prerequisite credits must be completed before admission to the nursing program. *Options:* May apply for transfer of up to 145 total credits. *Application deadline:* 4/1. *Application fee:* $25.

Degree Requirements 188 total credit hours, 98 in nursing.

RN Baccalaureate Program (BS)

Applying *Required:* minimum college GPA of 2.8, RN license, diploma or AD in nursing, 3 letters of recommendation, written essay, transcript of college record. *Options:* May apply for transfer of up to 145 total credits. *Application deadline:* 4/1. *Application fee:* $25.

Degree Requirements 180 total credit hours, 90 in nursing.

MASTER'S PROGRAM

Contact Ms. Kate Hanson, Student Recruiter, 5-160 Weaver-Densford Hall, School of Nursing, University of Minnesota, 308 Harvard Street SE, Minneapolis, MN 55455-0213, 612-624-9494. *Fax:* 612-626-2359. *E-mail:* hanso041@maroon.tc.umn.edu

Areas of Study Clinical nurse specialist programs in adult health nursing, family health nursing, gerontological nursing, medical-surgical nursing, oncology nursing, pediatric nursing, psychiatric–mental health nursing, public health nursing, children with special health care needs nursing; nurse midwifery; nursing administration; nursing education; nurse practitioner programs in child care/pediatrics, family health, gerontology, women's health.

Expenses *State resident tuition:* $5820 full-time, $275 per credit part-time. *Nonresident tuition:* $11,670 full-time, $473 per credit part-time. *Full-time mandatory fees:* $470. *Room and board:* $4119. *Books and supplies per academic year:* ranges from $200 to $600.

Financial Aid Graduate assistantships, nurse traineeships, fellowships, Federal Nursing Student Loans, employment opportunities. 30% of master's level students in nursing programs received some form of financial aid in 1995-96. *Application deadline:* 9/20.

RN to Master's Program (MS)

Applying *Required:* GRE General Test, completion of RN/BSN Undergraduate program, minimum GPA of 3.0, RN license, essay, 3 letters of recommendation, transcript of college record, completion of RN/BSN undergraduate program. *Application deadlines:* 4/15 (fall), 1/15 (spring), 10/25 (winter). *Application fee:* $40.

Degree Requirements 44 total credit hours, 32 in nursing, 12 in related field or minor. Thesis or course work.

DOCTORAL PROGRAM

Contact Ms. Kate Hanson, Student Recruiter, 5-160 Weaver-Densford Hall, School of Nursing, University of Minnesota, 308 Harvard Street SE, Minneapolis, MN 55455-0213, 612-624-9494. *Fax:* 612-626-2359. *E-mail:* hanso041@maroon.tc.umn.edu

Areas of Study Nursing research.

Expenses *State resident tuition:* $5820 full-time, $275 per credit part-time. *Nonresident tuition:* $11,670 full-time, $473 per credit part-time. *Full-time mandatory fees:* $470. *Room and board:* $4119. *Books and supplies per academic year:* ranges from $200 to $600.

Financial Aid Graduate assistantships, fellowships, grants. *Application deadline:* 9/20.

PhD Program

Applying *Required:* GRE General Test, interview, 2 letters of recommendation, competitive review by faculty committee, profile statement, BA/BS. *Application deadline:* 1/25. *Application fee:* $40.

Degree Requirements 36 thesis credits; dissertation; oral exam; written exam; defense of dissertation; residency.

CONTINUING EDUCATION PROGRAM

Contact Ms. Rachel Christensen, Associate Continuing Education Specialist, 202 Wesbrook Hall, Extension Classes, School of Nursing, University of Minnesota, 308 Harvard Street SE, Minneapolis, MN 55455-0213, 612-624-0540.

See full description on page 544.

WINONA STATE UNIVERSITY
College of Nursing and Health Sciences
Winona, Minnesota

Programs • Generic Baccalaureate • RN Baccalaureate • MSN • Post-Master's

The University State-supported comprehensive coed institution. Part of Minnesota State Colleges and Universities System. Founded: 1858. *Primary accreditation:* regional. *Setting:* 40-acre small-town campus. *Total enrollment:* 7,500.

The College of Nursing and Health Sciences Founded in 1964. *Nursing program faculty:* 35 (29% with doctorates). *Off-campus program site:* Rochester, MN.

Academic Facilities *Campus library:* 240,000 volumes (35,000 in nursing); 2,200 periodical subscriptions (200 health-care related). *Nursing school resources:* CAI, computer lab, nursing audiovisuals, interactive nursing skills videos, learning resource lab.

Student Life *Student services:* health clinic, child-care facilities, personal counseling, career counseling, institutionally sponsored work-study program, job placement, campus safety program, special assistance for disabled students. *International student services:* counseling/support, special assistance for nonnative speakers of English, ESL courses. *Nursing student activities:* Sigma Theta Tau, recruiter club, student nurses association.

Calendar Quarters.

NURSING STUDENT PROFILE

Undergraduate **Enrollment:** 633
Women: 91%; **Men:** 9%; **Minority:** 3%; **International:** 1%; **Part-time:** 12%
Graduate **Enrollment:** 92
Women: 97%; **Men:** 3%; **Minority:** 1%; **International:** 1%; **Part-time:** 81%

BACCALAUREATE PROGRAMS

Contact Stark Hall, Room 303, College of Nursing and Health Sciences, Winona State University, PO Box 5838, Winona, MN 55987-5838, 507-457-5120. *Fax:* 507-457-5550.

Expenses *State resident tuition:* $53 per credit hour. *Nonresident tuition:* $114 per credit hour. *Full-time mandatory fees:* $10–$397.

Financial Aid Institutionally sponsored need-based grants/scholarships, institutionally sponsored non-need grants/scholarships, Federal Supplemental Educational Opportunity Grants, Federal Work-Study.

Generic Baccalaureate Program (BSN)

Applying *Required:* SAT I, ACT, minimum college GPA of 2.75, transcript of college record. 66 prerequisite credits must be completed before admission to the nursing program. *Options:* May apply for transfer of up to 96 total credits. *Application deadline:* 3/28. *Application fee:* $15.

Degree Requirements 192 total credit hours, 78 in nursing.

RN Baccalaureate Program (BSN)

Applying *Required:* SAT I, ACT, minimum college GPA of 2.75, RN license, diploma or AD in nursing, transcript of college record. 66 prerequisite credits must be completed before admission to the nursing program. *Options:* May apply for transfer of up to 96 total credits. *Application deadline:* 3/28. *Application fee:* $15.

Degree Requirements 192 total credit hours, 78 in nursing.

MASTER'S PROGRAMS

Contact Dr. Marjorie Smith, Director, College of Nursing and Health Sciences, Winona State University, 859 Southeast 30th Avenue, Rochester, MN 55904, 507-285-7489. *Fax:* 507-285-7170. *E-mail:* mjs@vax2.winona.msus.edu

Areas of Study Clinical nurse specialist program in adult health nursing; nursing administration; nursing education; nurse practitioner programs in adult health, family health.

Expenses *State resident tuition:* $2124 full-time, $78 per credit part-time. *Nonresident tuition:* $3363 full-time, $125 per credit part-time. *Full-time mandatory fees:* $10–$397. *Books and supplies per academic year:* $500.

Financial Aid Graduate assistantships, nurse traineeships, National Health Service Corps Scholarships, Minnesota Center for Rural Health loan repayment program. 16% of master's level students in nursing programs received some form of financial aid in 1995-96. *Application deadline:* 3/1.

MSN Program

Applying *Required:* GRE General Test (minimum combined score of 1350 on three tests), bachelor's degree in nursing, minimum GPA of 3.0, RN license, 1 year of clinical experience, physical assessment course, statistics course, professional liability/malpractice insurance, essay, interview, 3 letters of recommendation, transcript of college record, computer literacy in word processing, spreadsheet, and database programs; 2 years of clinical experience, interview for nurse practitioner program. *Application deadline:* 2/1. *Application fee:* $20.

Degree Requirements 51–58 total credit hours dependent upon track, 48–55 in nursing, 3 in statistics. Optional thesis or professional study.

Post-Master's Program

Applying *Required:* bachelor's degree in nursing, minimum GPA of 3.0, RN license, physical assessment course, statistics course, professional liability/malpractice insurance, 3 letters of recommendation, transcript of college record, computer literacy in word processing, spreadsheet, and database programs; 2 years of clinical experience, interview for nurse practitioner program. *Application deadline:* 2/1. *Application fee:* $20.

Degree Requirements 33–41 total credit hours dependent upon track.

MISSISSIPPI

ALCORN STATE UNIVERSITY
School of Nursing
Natchez, Mississippi

Programs • Generic Baccalaureate • RN Baccalaureate

The University State-supported comprehensive coed institution. Part of Mississippi Institutions of Higher Learning. Founded: 1871. *Primary accreditation:* regional. *Setting:* 1,700-acre rural campus. *Total enrollment:* 3,033.

The School of Nursing Founded in 1979.

Calendar Semesters.

BACCALAUREATE PROGRAMS

Contact Chairperson, Department of Baccalaureate Nursing, School of Nursing, Alcorn State University, Natchez, MS 39122, 601-442-3901. *Fax:* 601-446-5942.

Financial Aid Federal Nursing Student Loans, Federal Pell Grants, Federal Perkins Loans, Federal Supplemental Educational Opportunity Grants, Federal Work-Study, Federal PLUS Loans, Mississippi Guaranteed Student Loan Program.

Generic Baccalaureate Program (BS)

Applying *Required:* SAT I or ACT, TOEFL for nonnative speakers of English, minimum college GPA of 2.5, 3 years of high school math, 3 years of high school science, high school transcript. *Options:* May apply for transfer of up to 56 total credits. *Application deadline:* 12/15.

Degree Requirements 129–133 total credit hours dependent upon track, 73 in nursing.

RN Baccalaureate Program (BS)

Applying *Required:* ACT. *Options:* May apply for transfer of up to 56 total credits. *Application deadline:* 12/15.

Degree Requirements 129–133 total credit hours dependent upon track, 73 in nursing.

DELTA STATE UNIVERSITY
School of Nursing
Cleveland, Mississippi

Programs • Generic Baccalaureate • RN Baccalaureate • BSN to Master's • Post-Master's

The University State-supported comprehensive coed institution. Part of Mississippi Institutions of Higher Learning. Founded: 1925. *Primary accreditation:* regional. *Setting:* 274-acre small-town campus. *Total enrollment:* 3,887.

The School of Nursing Founded in 1977. *Nursing program faculty:* 20 (20% with doctorates).

Academic Facilities *Campus library:* 353,361 volumes (5,000 in health, 1,000 in nursing); 100 health-care related periodical subscriptions. *Nursing school resources:* CAI, computer lab, nursing audiovisuals, learning resource lab.

Student Life *Student services:* health clinic, personal counseling, career counseling, institutionally sponsored work-study program, job placement. *International student services:* counseling/support. *Nursing student activities:* student nurses association, honor society.

Calendar Semesters.

NURSING STUDENT PROFILE

Undergraduate **Enrollment:** 62
Women: 80%; **Men:** 20%; **Minority:** 12%; **International:** 0%; **Part-time:** 7%

Graduate **Enrollment:** 28
Women: 85%; **Men:** 15%; **Minority:** 22%; **International:** 0%; **Part-time:** 40%

BACCALAUREATE PROGRAMS

Contact Dr. Barbara Powell, Dean, School of Nursing, Delta State University, Box 3343, Cleveland, MS 38733, 601-846-4268. *Fax:* 601-846-4267. *E-mail:* bpowell@dsu.deltast.edu

Expenses *State resident tuition:* $2294 full-time, $83 per semester hour part-time. *Nonresident tuition:* $4888 full-time, $191 per semester hour part-time. *Full-time mandatory fees:* $50–$80. *Room and board:* $1090. *Books and supplies per academic year:* ranges from $300 to $700.

Financial Aid Institutionally sponsored need-based grants/scholarships, Federal Supplemental Educational Opportunity Grants, Federal Work-Study. 95% of undergraduate students in nursing programs received some form of financial aid in 1995–96.

Generic Baccalaureate Program (BSN)

Applying *Required:* ACT, minimum college GPA of 2.5, 3 letters of recommendation, transcript of college record. 71 prerequisite credits must be completed before admission to the nursing program. *Options:* May apply for transfer of up to 71 total credits. *Application deadlines:* 10/1 (spring), 3/15 (summer).

Degree Requirements 136 total credit hours, 66 in nursing.

RN Baccalaureate Program (BSN)

Applying *Required:* minimum college GPA of 2.5, RN license, diploma or AD in nursing, 3 letters of recommendation, transcript of college record. 71 prerequisite credits must be completed before admission to the nursing program. *Options:* Advanced standing available through advanced placement without credit. May apply for transfer of up to 71 total credits. *Application deadline:* 3/15 (summer).

Degree Requirements 135 total credit hours, 65 in nursing.

MASTER'S PROGRAMS

Contact Dr. Katherine Riffle, Coordinator, Graduate Nursing Program, School of Nursing, Delta State University, Box 3343, Cleveland, MS 38733, 601-846-4273. *Fax:* 601-846-4267.

Areas of Study Nursing administration; nursing education; nurse practitioner program in family health.

Expenses *State resident tuition:* $2294 full-time, $110 per semester hour part-time. *Nonresident tuition:* $4888 full-time, $254 per semester hour part-time. *Full-time mandatory fees:* $500–$600. *Room and board:* $1090. *Books and supplies per academic year:* ranges from $1600 to $2000.

Financial Aid Graduate assistantships, state nurse education funds.

BSN to Master's Program (MSN)

Applying *Required:* GRE General Test, Miller Analogies Test, bachelor's degree in nursing, bachelor's degree, minimum GPA of 3.0, RN license, 1 year of clinical experience, physical assessment course, statistics course, professional liability/malpractice insurance, essay, letter of recommendation, transcript of college record. *Application deadline:* 4/1.

Degree Requirements 46 total credit hours, 43 in nursing, 3–6 in electives.

Post-Master's Program

Applying *Required:* GRE General Test, Miller Analogies Test, bachelor's degree in nursing, bachelor's degree, minimum GPA of 3.0, RN license, 1 year of clinical experience, physical assessment course, statistics course, professional liability/malpractice insurance, essay, letter of recommendation, transcript of college record, MSN. *Application deadline:* 4/1.

Degree Requirements 25 total credit hours, 25 in nursing.

MISSISSIPPI COLLEGE
School of Nursing
Clinton, Mississippi

Programs • Generic Baccalaureate • RN Baccalaureate

The College Independent Southern Baptist comprehensive coed institution. Founded: 1826. *Primary accreditation:* regional. *Setting:* 320-acre small-town campus. *Total enrollment:* 3,238.

The School of Nursing Founded in 1969. *Nursing program faculty:* 17 (35% with doctorates).

Academic Facilities *Campus library:* 350,000 volumes (4,000 in health, 8,000 in nursing); 1,000 periodical subscriptions (110 health-care related). *Nursing school resources:* CAI, computer lab, nursing audiovisuals, interactive nursing skills videos, learning resource lab.

Student Life *Student services:* health clinic, personal counseling, career counseling, institutionally sponsored work-study program, job placement, campus safety program, special assistance for disabled students. *International student services:* counseling/support, special assistance for nonnative speakers of English, ESL courses. *Nursing student activities:* student nurses association, Baptist Nursing Fellowship, Nursing Honor Society.

Calendar Semesters.

NURSING STUDENT PROFILE

Undergraduate **Enrollment:** 139
Women: 83%; **Men:** 17%; **Minority:** 12%; **International:** 0%; **Part-time:** 17%

BACCALAUREATE PROGRAMS

Contact Dr. Mary Jean Padgett, Dean, School of Nursing, Mississippi College, Clinton, MS 39058, 601-925-3278. *Fax:* 601-925-3379. *E-mail:* padgett@mc.edu

Expenses *Tuition:* $6570 full-time, $219 per hour part-time. *Full-time mandatory fees:* $190. *Part-time mandatory fees:* $190. *Room and board:* $2840–$3040. *Room only:* $1270–$1360.

Financial Aid Institutionally sponsored need-based grants/scholarships, institutionally sponsored non-need grants/scholarships, Federal Nursing Student Loans, Federal Pell Grants, Federal Supplemental Educational Opportunity Grants, Federal Work-Study, Federal Stafford Loans. 86% of undergraduate students in nursing programs received some form of financial aid in 1995–96. *Application deadline:* 4/1.

Generic Baccalaureate Program (BSN)

Applying *Required:* SAT I or ACT, College English Proficiency Exam, NLN Preadmission Examination, Nelson-Denny Reading Test, California Critical Thinking Disposition Inventory, minimum college GPA of 2.5, high school chemistry, high school biology, high school transcript, 2 letters of recommendation, transcript of college record. 70 prerequisite credits must be completed before admission to the nursing program. *Options:* May apply for transfer of up to 65 total credits. *Application deadlines:* 6/1 (fall), 10/1 (spring). *Application fee:* $15.

Degree Requirements 131 total credit hours, 61 in nursing.

RN Baccalaureate Program (BSN)

Applying *Required:* NLN Mobility Profile II, English proficiency exam, minimum college GPA of 2.5, RN license, diploma or AD in nursing, 2 letters of recommendation, transcript of college record. 70 prerequisite credits must be completed before admission to the nursing program. *Options:* May apply for transfer of up to 65 total credits. *Application deadline:* 6/1 (summer). *Application fee:* $15.

Degree Requirements 131 total credit hours, 60 in nursing.

MISSISSIPPI UNIVERSITY FOR WOMEN
Division of Nursing
Columbus, Mississippi

Programs • Generic Baccalaureate • RN Baccalaureate • MSN

The University State-supported comprehensive primarily women's institution. Part of Mississippi Institutions of Higher Learning. Founded: 1884. *Primary accreditation:* regional. *Setting:* 110-acre small-town campus. *Total enrollment:* 3,071.

The Division of Nursing Founded in 1971. *Nursing program faculty:* 34 (20% with doctorates). *Off-campus program site:* Tupelo.

Academic Facilities *Nursing school resources:* CAI, computer lab, nursing audiovisuals, interactive nursing skills videos, learning resource lab.

Student Life *Student services:* health clinic, child-care facilities, personal counseling, career counseling, institutionally sponsored work-study program, job placement, campus safety program, special assistance for disabled students. *International student services:* counseling/support, special assistance for nonnative speakers of English. *Nursing student activities:* Sigma Theta Tau, nursing club, student nurses association.

Calendar Semesters.

NURSING STUDENT PROFILE

Undergraduate **Enrollment:** 235
Women: 90%; **Men:** 10%; **Minority:** 15%; **International:** 1%; **Part-time:** 0%
Graduate **Enrollment:** 40
Women: 90%; **Men:** 10%; **Minority:** 8%; **International:** 0%; **Part-time:** 30%

BACCALAUREATE PROGRAMS

Contact Janice Gialliouvakis, Interim Director of the Baccalaureate Program, Division of Nursing, Mississippi University for Women, Box W-910, Columbus, MS 39701, 601-329-7299. *Fax:* 601-329-8555.

Expenses *Tuition:* $2244 full-time, $72 per semester hour part-time. *Full-time mandatory fees:* $25–$100. *Room and board:* $2367. *Books and supplies per academic year:* ranges from $100 to $500.

Financial Aid Institutionally sponsored need-based grants/scholarships, institutionally sponsored non-need grants/scholarships, Federal Pell Grants, Federal Perkins Loans, Federal Supplemental Educational Opportunity Grants, Federal Work-Study. *Application deadline:* 4/1.

Generic Baccalaureate Program (BSN)

Applying *Required:* ACT, NLN Preadmission Examination-RN, minimum college GPA of 2.5, high school transcript, transcript of college record. *Application deadline:* 5/15.

Degree Requirements 133 total credit hours, 65 in nursing.

RN Baccalaureate Program (BSN)

Applying *Required:* ACT, minimum college GPA of 2.5, RN license, diploma or AD in nursing, transcript of college record. 71 prerequisite credits must be completed before admission to the nursing program. *Options:* Advanced standing available through advanced placement exams. *Application deadline:* rolling.

Degree Requirements 133 total credit hours, 35 in nursing.

Distance learning Courses provided through video, computer-based media, on-line.

MASTER'S PROGRAM

Contact Dr. Mary Pat Curtis, Director of Graduate Programs, Division of Nursing, Mississippi University for Women, Box W-910, Columbus, MS 39701, 601-329-7323. *Fax:* 601-329-7372.

Areas of Study Nurse practitioner programs in child care/pediatrics, family health, gerontology.

Expenses *Tuition:* $2244 full-time, $97 per semester hours part-time. *Full-time mandatory fees:* $25–$100. *Books and supplies per academic year:* ranges from $200 to $500.

Financial Aid Nurse traineeships, institutionally sponsored non-need-based grants/scholarships. *Application deadline:* 4/1.

MSN Program

Applying *Required:* GRE General Test, English proficiency exam, bachelor's degree in nursing, minimum GPA of 3.0, RN license, 1 year of clinical experience, professional liability/malpractice insurance, interview, transcript of college record. *Application deadline:* 4/1.

Degree Requirements 36 total credit hours, 32 in nursing. Thesis required.

UNIVERSITY OF MISSISSIPPI MEDICAL CENTER
School of Nursing
Jackson, Mississippi

Programs • Generic Baccalaureate • Accelerated RN Baccalaureate • MSN • Post-Master's • PhD • Continuing Education

The University State-supported upper-level coed institution. Part of University of Mississippi. Founded: 1955. *Primary accreditation:* regional. *Setting:* 164-acre urban campus. *Total enrollment:* 1,817.

The School of Nursing Founded in 1948. *Nursing program faculty:* 38 (42% with doctorates).

Academic Facilities *Campus library:* 174,341 volumes; 2,393 periodical subscriptions. *Nursing school resources:* CAI, computer lab, nursing audiovisuals, interactive nursing skills videos, learning resource lab.

Student Life *Student services:* health clinic, personal counseling, career counseling, institutionally sponsored work-study program, job placement, campus safety program, special assistance for disabled students. *Nursing student activities:* Sigma Theta Tau, student nurses association.

Calendar Semesters.

NURSING STUDENT PROFILE

Undergraduate **Enrollment:** 265
Women: 83%; **Men:** 17%; **Minority:** 14%; **Part-time:** 2%
Graduate **Enrollment:** 20
Women: 90%; **Men:** 10%; **Minority:** 10%; **Part-time:** 73%

BACCALAUREATE PROGRAMS

Contact Debbie MacSherry, Recruiter, School of Nursing, University of Mississippi Medical Center, 2500 North State Street, Jackson, MS 39216-4505, 601-984-6251. *Fax:* 601-984-6214.

Expenses *State resident tuition:* $1996 full-time, $83 per hour part-time. *Nonresident tuition:* $2819 full-time, $117 per hour part-time. *Full-time mandatory fees:* $130. *Room only:* $1340–$1960. *Books and supplies per academic year:* $1200.

Financial Aid Institutionally sponsored need-based grants/scholarships, institutionally sponsored non-need grants/scholarships, Federal Nursing Student Loans, Federal Supplemental Educational Opportunity Grants, Federal Work-Study. 82% of undergraduate students in nursing programs received some form of financial aid in 1995–96. *Application deadline:* 6/1.

Generic Baccalaureate Program (BSN)

Applying *Required:* ACT, minimum college GPA of 2.5, 3 letters of recommendation, transcript of college record. 62 prerequisite credits must be completed before admission to the nursing program. *Options:* May apply for transfer of up to 67 total credits. *Application deadline:* 4/1. *Application fee:* $10.

Degree Requirements 132 total credit hours, 70 in nursing.

Accelerated RN Baccalaureate Program (BSN)

Applying *Required:* minimum college GPA of 2.5, RN license, diploma or AD in nursing, 3 letters of recommendation, transcript of college record. 62 prerequisite credits must be completed before admission to the nursing program. *Options:* May apply for transfer of up to 102 total credits. *Application deadlines:* 7/1 (fall), 11/1 (spring), 4/1 (summer). *Application fee:* $10.

Degree Requirements 132 total credit hours, 30 in nursing.

MASTER'S PROGRAMS

Contact Debbie MacSherry, Recruiter, School of Nursing, University of Mississippi Medical Center, 2500 North State Street, Jackson, MS 39216-4505, 601-984-6251. *Fax:* 601-984-6214.

Areas of Study Clinical nurse specialist program in student-selected role focus; nursing administration; nursing education; nurse practitioner programs in adult health, family health, neonatal health.

Expenses *State resident tuition:* $1996 full-time, $111 per hour part-time. *Nonresident tuition:* $2319 full-time, $129 per hour part-time. *Full-time mandatory fees:* $110. *Room only:* $1340–$1960. *Books and supplies per academic year:* $600.

Financial Aid Nurse traineeships, Federal Nursing Student Loans, institutionally sponsored loans, employment opportunities. 85% of master's level students in nursing programs received some form of financial aid in 1995-96. *Application deadline:* 6/1.

MSN Program

Applying *Required:* GRE General Test, bachelor's degree in nursing, minimum GPA of 2.75, RN license, 1 year of clinical experience, statistics course, professional liability/malpractice insurance, 3 letters of recommendation, transcript of college record. *Application deadlines:* 4/1 (fall), 10/1 (spring), 4/1 (summer). *Application fee:* $10.

Degree Requirements 40 total credit hours, 31 in nursing.

Post-Master's Program

Applying *Required:* minimum GPA of 2.75, RN license, transcript of college record. *Application fee:* $10.

Degree Requirements 22 total credit hours, 22 in nursing.

DOCTORAL PROGRAM

Contact Debbie MacSherry, Recruiter, School of Nursing, University of Mississippi Medical Center, 2500 North State Street, Jackson, MS 39216-4505, 601-984-6251. *Fax:* 601-984-6214.

Areas of Study Clinical health sciences.

Expenses *State resident tuition:* $1996 full-time, $111 part-time. *Nonresident tuition:* $2319 full-time, $129 part-time. *Full-time mandatory fees:* $75+.

Financial Aid Opportunities for employment. *Application deadline:* 6/1.

PhD Program

Applying *Required:* GRE General Test, master's degree, year of clinical experience, interview, vitae, writing sample, competitive review by faculty committee. *Application deadline:* 3/1. *Application fee:* $10.

Degree Requirements 56 total credit hours; dissertation; oral exam; written exam; defense of dissertation.

CONTINUING EDUCATION PROGRAM

Contact Ms. Bobbie Ward, Chair, Continuing Education Committee, School of Nursing, University of Mississippi Medical Center, 2500 North State Street, Jackson, MS 39216-4505, 601-984-6208. *Fax:* 601-984-6214.

UNIVERSITY OF SOUTHERN MISSISSIPPI

School of Nursing
Hattiesburg, Mississippi

Programs • Generic Baccalaureate • RN Baccalaureate • MSN • RN to Master's

The University State-supported coed university. Founded: 1910. *Primary accreditation:* regional. *Setting:* 840-acre suburban campus. *Total enrollment:* 12,113.

The School of Nursing Founded in 1965. *Nursing program faculty:* 43 (47% with doctorates). *Off-campus program sites:* Meridian, Long Beach.

Academic Facilities *Campus library:* 791,450 volumes; 5,250 periodical subscriptions (150 health-care related). *Nursing school resources:* CAI, computer lab, nursing audiovisuals, interactive nursing skills videos, learning resource lab, Internet.

Student Life *Student services:* health clinic, child-care facilities, personal counseling, career counseling, institutionally sponsored work-study program, job placement, campus safety program, special assistance for disabled students. *International student services:* counseling/support, special assistance for nonnative speakers of English, ESL courses. *Nursing student activities:* Sigma Theta Tau, student nurses association.

Calendar Semesters.

NURSING STUDENT PROFILE

Undergraduate **Enrollment:** 335
Women: 87%; **Men:** 13%; **Minority:** 9%; **International:** 0%; **Part-time:** 10%

Graduate **Enrollment:** 137
Women: 92%; **Men:** 8%; **Minority:** 16%; **International:** 0%; **Part-time:** 60%

BACCALAUREATE PROGRAMS

Contact Dr. Gerry Cadenhead, Interim Director, School of Nursing, University of Southern Mississippi, Southern Station Box 5095, Hattiesburg, MS 39406-5095, 601-266-5639. *Fax:* 601-266-5927. *E-mail:* cadenhead@nursing.usm.edu

Expenses *State resident tuition:* $2468 full-time, $88 per semester hour part-time. *Nonresident tuition:* $5288 full-time, $205 per semester hour part-time. *Full-time mandatory fees:* $55–$65. *Room and board:* $2330–$2600. *Room only:* $625–$700. *Books and supplies per academic year:* ranges from $300 to $600.

Financial Aid Institutionally sponsored need-based grants/scholarships, institutionally sponsored non-need grants/scholarships, Federal Nursing Student Loans, Federal Pell Grants, Federal Perkins Loans, Federal Supplemental Educational Opportunity Grants, Federal Work-Study, Federal Stafford Loans. 90% of undergraduate students in nursing programs received some form of financial aid in 1995–96. *Application deadline:* 3/1.

Generic Baccalaureate Program (BSN)

Applying *Required:* ACT, minimum high school GPA of 2.0, minimum college GPA of 2.5, transcript of college record. 64 prerequisite credits must be completed before admission to the nursing program. *Options:* May apply for transfer of up to 64 total credits. *Application deadlines:* 10/1 (fall), 3/1 (spring). *Application fee:* $20.

Degree Requirements 131 total credit hours, 67 in nursing.

RN Baccalaureate Program (BSN)

Applying *Required:* minimum high school GPA of 2.0, minimum college GPA of 2.5, RN license, diploma or AD in nursing, transcript of college record. 64 prerequisite credits must be completed before admission to the nursing program. *Options:* May apply for transfer of up to 64 total credits. *Application deadline:* rolling.

Degree Requirements 128 total credit hours, 64 in nursing.

MASTER'S PROGRAMS

Contact Dr. Pat Kurtz, Acting Assistant Director, School of Nursing, University of Southern Mississippi, Southern Station Box 5095, Hattiesburg, MS 39406-5095, 601-266-5639. *Fax:* 601-266-5927. *E-mail:* kurtz@nursing.usm.edu

Areas of Study Clinical nurse specialist programs in adult health nursing, community health nursing, psychiatric–mental health nursing; nursing administration; nursing education; nurse practitioner program in family health.

Expenses *State resident tuition:* $2468 full-time, $116 per semester hour part-time. *Nonresident tuition:* $5288 full-time, $273 per semester hour part-time. *Full-time mandatory fees:* $45–$100. *Room and board:* $2330–$2600. *Books and supplies per academic year:* ranges from $300 to $600.

Financial Aid Graduate assistantships, nurse traineeships, Federal Nursing Student Loans, employment opportunities. 36% of master's level students in nursing programs received some form of financial aid in 1995-96. *Application deadline:* 6/1.

MSN Program

Applying *Required:* GRE General Test, bachelor's degree in nursing, minimum GPA of 3.0, RN license, 2 years of clinical experience, physical assessment course, statistics course, professional liability/malpractice insurance, 2 letters of recommendation, transcript of college record. *Application deadlines:* 3/1 (family nurse practitioner track), rolling. *Application fee:* $20.

Degree Requirements 42 total credit hours, 36 in nursing, 6 in other specified areas. Thesis or project.

University of Southern Mississippi (continued)

RN TO MASTER'S PROGRAM (MSN)

Applying *Required:* GRE General Test, minimum GPA of 3.0, RN license, 1 year of clinical experience, physical assessment course, statistics course, professional liability/malpractice insurance, transcript of college record. *Application deadline:* rolling.

Degree Requirements 159 total credit hours, 95 in nursing, 64 in prerequisite courses. Thesis or project.

WILLIAM CAREY COLLEGE
School of Nursing
Hattiesburg, Mississippi

Program • Generic Baccalaureate

The College Independent Southern Baptist comprehensive coed institution. Founded: 1906. *Primary accreditation:* regional. *Setting:* 64-acre small-town campus. *Total enrollment:* 2,172.

The School of Nursing Founded in 1968.

Academic Facilities *Campus library:* 133,993 volumes (6,239 in health); 587 periodical subscriptions (45 health-care related).

Calendar Trimesters.

BACCALAUREATE PROGRAM

Contact Office of Admissions, School of Nursing, William Carey College, Hattiesburg, MS 39401, 800-962-5991. *Fax:* 601-586-6454.

Expenses *Tuition:* $5280 full-time, $165 per semester hour part-time. *Room and board:* $2175–$2835. *Room only:* $735–$1185.

GENERIC BACCALAUREATE PROGRAM (BSN)

Applying *Required:* English proficiency test, minimum 100 on NLN Preadmission Examination-RN, minimum college GPA of 2.5, high school transcript, transcript of college record. *Application fee:* $10.

Degree Requirements 128 total credit hours.

MISSOURI

AVILA COLLEGE
Department of Nursing
Kansas City, Missouri

Programs • Generic Baccalaureate • RN Baccalaureate • Continuing Education

The College Independent Roman Catholic comprehensive coed institution. Founded: 1916. *Primary accreditation:* regional. *Setting:* 50-acre suburban campus. *Total enrollment:* 1,404.

The Department of Nursing Founded in 1948. *Nursing program faculty:* 9 (11% with doctorates).

Academic Facilities *Campus library:* 68,366 volumes; 493 periodical subscriptions (55 health-care related). *Nursing school resources:* CAI, computer lab, nursing audiovisuals, interactive nursing skills videos, learning resource lab.

Student Life *Student services:* health clinic, child-care facilities, personal counseling, career counseling, institutionally sponsored work-study program, job placement, campus safety program, special assistance for disabled students. *International student services:* counseling/support, special assistance for nonnative speakers of English, ESL courses, special transportation, orientation. *Nursing student activities:* Sigma Theta Tau, nursing club, student nurses association.

Calendar Semesters.

NURSING STUDENT PROFILE

Undergraduate **Enrollment:** 63
Women: 95%; **Men:** 5%; **Minority:** 19%; **International:** 0%; **Part-time:** 3%

BACCALAUREATE PROGRAMS

Contact Admissions Office, Avila College, 11901 Wornall Road, Kansas City, MO 64145-1698, 816-942-8400 Ext. 3500. *Fax:* 816-942-3362. *E-mail:* admissions@mail.avila.edu

Expenses *Tuition:* $10,100 full-time, $220 per credit hour part-time. *Full-time mandatory fees:* $360+. *Room and board:* $4150–$5000. *Books and supplies per academic year:* ranges from $150 to $500.

Financial Aid Institutionally sponsored need-based grants/scholarships, institutionally sponsored non-need grants/scholarships, Federal Pell Grants, Federal Perkins Loans, Federal Supplemental Educational Opportunity Grants, Federal Work-Study. *Application deadline:* 7/1.

GENERIC BACCALAUREATE PROGRAM (BSN)

Applying *Required:* ACT, TOEFL for nonnative speakers of English, math and English placement exams, minimum high school GPA of 2.5, minimum college GPA of 2.0, high school transcript, written essay. 47 prerequisite credits must be completed before admission to the nursing program. *Options:* Advanced standing available through the following means: advanced placement exams, credit by exam. May apply for transfer of up to 64 total credits. *Application deadlines:* 1/15 (nursing applications), rolling.

Degree Requirements 128 total credit hours, 55 in nursing. College core curriculum, nursing prerequisite and program requirements.

RN BACCALAUREATE PROGRAM (BSN)

Applying *Required:* TOEFL for nonnative speakers of English, math and English placement exams if not transferring credit, ACT if transferring fewer than 24 hours, minimum college GPA of 2.0, RN license, diploma or AD in nursing, written essay, transcript of college record, high school transcript if transferring fewer than 24 hours. *Options:* Advanced standing available through the following means: advanced placement exams, credit by exam. May apply for transfer of up to 64 total credits. *Application deadlines:* 1/15 (nursing), rolling.

Degree Requirements 128 total credit hours, 55 in nursing.

CONTINUING EDUCATION PROGRAM

Contact Shiloh Garies, Director of Re-Entry Program, Avila College, 11901 Wornall Road, Kansas City, MO 64145-1698, 816-942-8400 Ext. 2271. *Fax:* 816-942-3362. *E-mail:* gariessa@mail.avila.edu

CENTRAL MISSOURI STATE UNIVERSITY
Department of Nursing
Warrensburg, Missouri

Programs • Generic Baccalaureate • RN Baccalaureate

The University State-supported comprehensive coed institution. Founded: 1871. *Primary accreditation:* regional. *Setting:* 1,166-acre small-town campus. *Total enrollment:* 10,951.

The Department of Nursing Founded in 1960.

Academic Facilities *Campus library:* 805,000 volumes; 2,603 periodical subscriptions. *Nursing school resources:* computer lab.

BACCALAUREATE PROGRAMS

Contact Dr. Elaine Frank-Ragan, Chair, Student Health Center 106, Department of Nursing, Central Missouri, Warrensburg, MO 64093, 816-543-4775.

Expenses *State resident tuition:* $2520 full-time, $84 per credit hour part-time. *Nonresident tuition:* $5040 full-time, $168 per credit hour part-time.

Financial Aid Institutionally sponsored need-based grants/scholarships, institutionally sponsored non-need grants/scholarships, Federal Pell Grants, Federal Supplemental Educational Opportunity Grants, Federal Work-Study.

GENERIC BACCALAUREATE PROGRAM (BS)

Applying *Required:* ACT, TOEFL for nonnative speakers of English, Nelson-Denny Reading Tests, minimum college GPA of 2.0, high school math, high school foreign language, transcript of college record, high school class rank: , physical exam, immunizations. *Options:* Advanced standing available through the following means: advanced placement exams, credit by exam. May apply for transfer of up to 30 total credits. *Application deadline:* rolling. *Application fee:* $25.

Degree Requirements 124 total credit hours, 83 in nursing.

RN BACCALAUREATE PROGRAM (BS)

Applying *Required:* ACT, TOEFL for nonnative speakers of English, minimum college GPA of 2.0, RN license, transcript of college record, physical exam, immunizations. *Options:* May apply for transfer of up to 64 total credits. *Application deadline:* rolling. *Application fee:* $25.

Degree Requirements 124 total credit hours, 83 in nursing.

CULVER-STOCKTON COLLEGE

Blessing-Rieman College of Nursing
Canton, Missouri / Quincy, Illinois

Programs • Generic Baccalaureate • RN Baccalaureate

The College Independent 4-year coed college, affiliated with Christian Church (Disciples of Christ). Founded: 1853. *Primary accreditation:* regional. *Setting:* 143-acre rural campus. *Total enrollment:* 1,001.

The Blessing-Rieman College of Nursing Founded in 1985. *Nursing program faculty:* 13 (8% with doctorates).

Academic Facilities *Campus library:* 4,000 volumes (1,000 in health, 3,000 in nursing); 111 periodical subscriptions (103 health-care related). *Nursing school resources:* CAI, computer lab, nursing audiovisuals, interactive nursing skills videos, learning resource lab.

Student Life *Student services:* child-care facilities, personal counseling, career counseling, job placement. *Nursing student activities:* student nurses association, honor society.

Calendar Semesters.

NURSING STUDENT PROFILE

Undergraduate **Enrollment:** 183
Women: 90%; **Men:** 10%; **Minority:** 4%; **International:** 0%; **Part-time:** 16%

BACCALAUREATE PROGRAMS

Contact Ms. Sharon Wharton, Director of Admissions, Blessing-Rieman College of Nursing, Broadway at 11th Street, Box 7005, Quincy, IL 62305-7005, 217-223-5220 Ext. 6961. *Fax:* 217-223-6400. *E-mail:* swharton@culver.edu

Expenses *Tuition:* $8800 full-time, $370 per credit hour part-time. *Full-time mandatory fees:* $100–$200. *Part-time mandatory fees:* $100–$200. *Room and board:* $3800. *Room only:* $1800.

Financial Aid Institutionally sponsored need-based grants/scholarships, institutionally sponsored non-need grants/scholarships, Federal Nursing Student Loans, Federal Pell Grants, Federal Family Education Loan Program (FFELP). 56% of undergraduate students in nursing programs received some form of financial aid in 1995–96. *Application deadline:* 6/1.

GENERIC BACCALAUREATE PROGRAM (BSN)

Applying *Required:* SAT I or ACT, TOEFL for nonnative speakers of English, minimum high school GPA of 3.0, minimum college GPA of 2.0, high school chemistry, high school biology, high school transcript, transcript of college record, high school class rank: top 50%, high school transcript or GED certificate. *Options:* Advanced standing available through advanced placement exams. *Application deadline:* rolling.

Degree Requirements 128 total credit hours, 32 in nursing.

RN BACCALAUREATE PROGRAM (BSN)

Applying *Required:* TOEFL for nonnative speakers of English, RN license, diploma or AD in nursing, transcript of college record, copy of current licensure. *Options:* Advanced standing available through advanced placement exams. *Application deadline:* rolling.

Degree Requirements 128 total credit hours, 32 in nursing.

See full description on page 434.

DEACONESS COLLEGE OF NURSING

St. Louis, Missouri

Program • Generic Baccalaureate

The College Independent 4-year specialized coed college, affiliated with United Church of Christ. Founded: 1889. *Primary accreditation:* regional. *Setting:* 15-acre urban campus. *Total enrollment:* 380. Founded in 1898. *Nursing program faculty:* 24 (30% with doctorates).

► *NOTEWORTHY*

Deaconess College of Nursing offers a fully accredited Bachelor of Science in Nursing degree program and Associate Degree in Nursing program. Deaconess combines a liberal arts background with an extensive hands-on clinical component, resulting in professional nurses well-equipped to work in today's health-care industry. Students' placement in clinicals is guaranteed from day one with satisfactory academic progress. Deaconess College of Nursing boasts a 100% passing rate on state boards for the past 10 years. The College is centrally located in St. Louis, Missouri, and is affiliated with a dynamic health organization that includes a 527-bed community-teaching hospital.

Academic Facilities *Campus library:* 7,896 volumes; 225 periodical subscriptions (225 health-care related). *Nursing school resources:* CAI, computer lab, nursing audiovisuals, interactive nursing skills videos, learning resource lab.

Student Life *Student services:* health clinic, child-care facilities, personal counseling, career counseling, institutionally sponsored work-study program, campus safety program, special assistance for disabled students. *International student services:* counseling/support. *Nursing student activities:* student nurses association.

Calendar Semesters.

NURSING STUDENT PROFILE

Undergraduate **Enrollment:** 391
Women: 92%; **Men:** 8%; **Minority:** 10%; **International:** 0%; **Part-time:** 20%

BACCALAUREATE PROGRAM

Contact Ms. Amy Storey, Admissions Coordinator, Deaconess College of Nursing, 6150 Oakland Avenue, St. Louis, MO 63139, 314-768-3044. *Fax:* 314-768-5673.

Expenses *Tuition:* $7170 full-time, $257 per credit hour part-time. *Full-time mandatory fees:* $160. *Room and board:* $2866–$3748. *Books and supplies per academic year:* $866.

Financial Aid Institutionally sponsored need-based grants/scholarships, institutionally sponsored non-need grants/scholarships, Federal Direct Loans, Federal Nursing Student Loans, Federal Pell Grants, Federal Supplemental Educational Opportunity Grants, Federal Work-Study. 79% of undergraduate students in nursing programs received some form of financial aid in 1995–96. *Application deadline:* 6/15.

GENERIC BACCALAUREATE PROGRAM (BSN)

Applying *Required:* SAT I or ACT, TOEFL for nonnative speakers of English, minimum high school GPA of 2.5, minimum college GPA of 2.5, 3 years of high school math, 3 years of high school science, high school transcript, written essay, transcript of college record, high school class rank: top 33%. 34 prerequisite credits must be completed before admission to the nursing program. *Options:* Advanced standing available through advanced placement exams. May apply for transfer of up to 48 total credits. *Application deadline:* rolling. *Application fee:* $30.

Degree Requirements 128 total credit hours, 62 in nursing.

MARYVILLE UNIVERSITY OF SAINT LOUIS
Department of Nursing
St. Louis, Missouri

Programs • Generic Baccalaureate • RN Baccalaureate

The University Independent comprehensive coed institution. Founded: 1872. *Primary accreditation:* regional. *Setting:* 130-acre suburban campus. *Total enrollment:* 3,378.

The Department of Nursing Founded in 1970. *Nursing program faculty:* 27 (11% with doctorates). *Off-campus program site:* O'Fallon.

Academic Facilities *Campus library:* 140,000 volumes. *Nursing school resources:* CAI, computer lab, nursing audiovisuals, interactive nursing skills videos, learning resource lab.

Student Life *Student services:* health clinic, personal counseling, career counseling, institutionally sponsored work-study program, campus safety program, special assistance for disabled students. *International student services:* counseling/support, special assistance for nonnative speakers of English, ESL courses. *Nursing student activities:* student nurses association, Nursing Honor Society.

Calendar Semesters.

NURSING STUDENT PROFILE

Undergraduate **Enrollment:** 205
Women: 91%; **Men:** 9%; **Minority:** 14%; **International:** 1%; **Part-time:** 75%

BACCALAUREATE PROGRAMS

Contact Dr. Mary Margaret Mooney, Director, Department of Nursing, Maryville University of Saint Louis, 13550 Conway Road, St. Louis, MO 63141-7299, 314-529-9479. *Fax:* 314-542-9085.

Expenses *Tuition:* $10,280 full-time, $293 per credit hour part-time. *Full-time mandatory fees:* $170–$200. *Room and board:* $5700. *Room only:* $4800–$5700. *Books and supplies per academic year:* ranges from $300 to $500.

Financial Aid Institutionally sponsored need-based grants/scholarships, institutionally sponsored non-need grants/scholarships, Federal Nursing Student Loans, Federal Supplemental Educational Opportunity Grants, Federal Work-Study. *Application deadline:* 2/1.

GENERIC BACCALAUREATE PROGRAM (BSN)

Applying *Required:* SAT I or ACT, TOEFL for nonnative speakers of English, minimum high school GPA of 2.0, minimum college GPA of 2.75, high school chemistry, high school biology, high school transcript, interview, written essay, transcript of college record. 24 prerequisite credits must be completed before admission to the nursing program. *Options:* Advanced standing available through the following means: advanced placement exams, credit by exam. May apply for transfer of up to 98 total credits. *Application deadline:* rolling. *Application fee:* $20.

Degree Requirements 128 total credit hours, 58 in nursing.

RN BACCALAUREATE PROGRAM (BSN)

Applying *Required:* TOEFL for nonnative speakers of English, minimum college GPA of 2.5, RN license, diploma or AD in nursing, high school transcript, interview, written essay, transcript of college record. 30 prerequisite credits must be completed before admission to the nursing program. *Options:* Advanced standing available through the following means: advanced placement exams, credit by exam. May apply for transfer of up to 98 total credits. *Application deadline:* rolling. *Application fee:* $20.

Degree Requirements 128 total credit hours, 58 in nursing.

MISSOURI SOUTHERN STATE COLLEGE
Department of Nursing
Joplin, Missouri

Programs • Generic Baccalaureate • RN Baccalaureate • LPN to Baccalaureate

The College State-supported 4-year coed college. Part of Missouri Coordinating Board for Higher Education. Founded: 1937. *Primary accreditation:* regional. *Setting:* 350-acre small-town campus. *Total enrollment:* 5,461.

The Department of Nursing Founded in 1966.

Academic Facilities *Campus library:* 238,000 volumes; 1,248 periodical subscriptions.

BACCALAUREATE PROGRAMS

Contact Kuhn Hall, Department of Nursing, Missouri Southern State College, 3950 Newman Road, Joplin, MO 64801-1595, 417-625-9322.

Expenses *State resident tuition:* $2240 full-time, $70 per credit hour part-time. *Nonresident tuition:* $4480 full-time, $140 per credit hour part-time. *Full-time mandatory fees:* $80. *Part-time mandatory fees:* $40. *Room only:* $3170.

Financial Aid Institutionally sponsored need-based grants/scholarships, institutionally sponsored non-need grants/scholarships, Federal Pell Grants, Federal Perkins Loans, Federal Supplemental Educational Opportunity Grants, Federal Work-Study, Federal PLUS Loans, Federal Stafford Loans. *Application deadline:* 2/15.

GENERIC BACCALAUREATE PROGRAM (BSN)

Applying *Required:* ACT, TOEFL for nonnative speakers of English, minimum college GPA of 2.5, high school transcript, interview, 2 letters of recommendation. *Application deadlines:* 3/1 (fall), 11/15 (spring). *Application fee:* $15.

Degree Requirements 134 total credit hours, 83 in nursing.

RN BACCALAUREATE PROGRAM (BSN)

Applying *Required:* minimum college GPA of 2.5, RN license, diploma or AD in nursing, high school transcript, interview, 3 letters of recommendation. *Application deadlines:* 3/1 (fall), 11/15 (spring). *Application fee:* $15.

Degree Requirements 134 total credit hours, 83 in nursing.

LPN TO BACCALAUREATE PROGRAM (BSN)

Applying *Required:* ACT, TOEFL for nonnative speakers of English, minimum college GPA of 2.5, high school transcript, interview, 2 letters of recommendation. *Application deadlines:* 3/1 (fall), 11/15 (spring). *Application fee:* $15.

Degree Requirements 134 total credit hours, 83 in nursing.

MISSOURI WESTERN STATE COLLEGE
Department of Nursing
St. Joseph, Missouri

Programs • Generic Baccalaureate • RN Baccalaureate • Continuing Education

The College State-supported 4-year coed college. Founded: 1915. *Primary accreditation:* regional. *Setting:* 744-acre suburban campus. *Total enrollment:* 5,167.

The Department of Nursing Founded in 1985. *Nursing program faculty:* 13 (23% with doctorates).

Academic Facilities *Campus library:* 182,000 volumes (6,397 in nursing); 1,250 periodical subscriptions (97 health-care related). *Nursing school resources:* CAI, computer lab, nursing audiovisuals, interactive nursing skills videos, learning resource lab, CINAHL, Dialog, InLex System, OCLC, Internet.

Student Life *Student services:* health clinic, child-care facilities, personal counseling, career counseling, institutionally sponsored work-study program, job placement, campus safety program, special assistance for disabled students, tutoring. *International student services:* counseling/support. *Nursing student activities:* student nurses association, Nursing Honor Society.

Calendar Semesters.

NURSING STUDENT PROFILE

Undergraduate **Enrollment:** 250
Women: 85%; **Men:** 15%; **Minority:** 5%; **International:** 2%; **Part-time:** 20%

BACCALAUREATE PROGRAMS

Contact Dr. Jeanne M. Daffron, Associate Professor and Chairperson, Department of Nursing, Missouri Western State College, 4525 Downs Drive, St. Joseph, MO 64507, 816-271-4415. *Fax:* 816-271-5849. *E-mail:* daffron@griffon.mwsc.edu

Expenses *State resident tuition:* $2300 full-time, $98 per credit hour part-time. *Nonresident tuition:* $3928 full-time, $164 per credit hour part-time. *Full-time mandatory fees:* $40–$80. *Room and board:* $2810. *Books and supplies per academic year:* $500.

Financial Aid Institutionally sponsored need-based grants/scholarships, institutionally sponsored non-need grants/scholarships, Federal Direct

Loans, Federal Nursing Student Loans, Federal Pell Grants, Federal Perkins Loans, Federal Supplemental Educational Opportunity Grants, Federal Work-Study. 60% of undergraduate students in nursing programs received some form of financial aid in 1995–96. *Application deadline:* 2/1.

Generic Baccalaureate Program (BSN)

Applying *Required:* ACT, minimum college GPA of 2.5, high school transcript, 3 letters of recommendation, written essay, transcript of college record. 45 prerequisite credits must be completed before admission to the nursing program. *Options:* Advanced standing available through credit by exam. May apply for transfer of up to 60 total credits. *Application deadlines:* 1/15 (fall), 8/31 (spring). *Application fee:* $30.

Degree Requirements 124 total credit hours, 59 in nursing.

RN Baccalaureate Program (BSN)

Applying *Required:* ACT, minimum college GPA of 2.5, RN license, diploma or AD in nursing, high school transcript, 3 letters of recommendation, written essay, transcript of college record. 60 prerequisite credits must be completed before admission to the nursing program. *Options:* Advanced standing available through the following means: advanced placement exams, credit by exam. May apply for transfer of up to 90 total credits. *Application deadline:* rolling. *Application fee:* $30.

Degree Requirements 124 total credit hours, 59 in nursing.

CONTINUING EDUCATION PROGRAM

Contact Dr. Ed Gorsky, Dean, Continuing Education, Department of Nursing, Missouri Western State College, 4525 Downs Drive, St. Joseph, MO 64507, 816-271-4218. *Fax:* 816-271-4574.

RESEARCH COLLEGE OF NURSING–ROCKHURST COLLEGE

Kansas City, Missouri

Programs • Generic Baccalaureate • Baccalaureate for Second Degree • Accelerated Baccalaureate for Second Degree • BSN to Master's

The College Independent 4-year specialized coed college. Founded: 1980. *Primary accreditation:* regional. *Setting:* 66-acre urban campus. *Total enrollment:* 2,140. Founded in 1980. *Nursing program faculty:* 43 (20% with doctorates).

Academic Facilities *Campus library:* 122,548 volumes (13,500 in health, 6,700 in nursing); 1,094 periodical subscriptions (490 health-care related). *Nursing school resources:* CAI, computer lab, nursing audiovisuals, interactive nursing skills videos, learning resource lab.

Student Life *Student services:* health clinic, child-care facilities, personal counseling, career counseling, institutionally sponsored work-study program, job placement, campus safety program, special assistance for disabled students. *International student services:* counseling/support. *Nursing student activities:* nursing club, student nurses association.

Calendar Semesters.

NURSING STUDENT PROFILE

Undergraduate **Enrollment:** 268

Women: 92%; **Men:** 8%; **Minority:** 9%; **International:** 1%; **Part-time:** 20%

BACCALAUREATE PROGRAMS

Contact Mrs. Leslie Mendenhall, Assistant Director of Admission, Research College of Nursing-Rockhurst College, 1100 Rockhurst Road, Kansas City, MO 64110-2508, 816-501-4100. *Fax:* 816-501-4588. *E-mail:* mendenhall@vax2.rockhurst.edu

Expenses *Tuition:* $11,000 full-time, $365 per credit hour part-time. *Full-time mandatory fees:* $550–$600. *Part-time mandatory fees:* $80–$100. *Room and board:* $4350–$4490. *Room only:* $2130. *Books and supplies per academic year:* ranges from $500 to $600.

Financial Aid Institutionally sponsored need-based grants/scholarships, institutionally sponsored non-need grants/scholarships, Federal Nursing Student Loans, Federal Pell Grants, Federal Perkins Loans, Federal Supplemental Educational Opportunity Grants, Federal Work-Study. *Application deadline:* 3/15.

Generic Baccalaureate Program (BSN)

Applying *Required:* SAT I, ACT, TOEFL for nonnative speakers of English, minimum high school GPA of 2.5, minimum college GPA of 2.5, 3 years of high school math, 3 years of high school science, high school chemistry, high school biology, high school transcript, letter of recommendation, transcript of college record, high school class rank: top 50%. *Options:* Advanced standing available through the following means: advanced placement exams, advanced placement without credit. *Application deadlines:* 1/31 (transfer), rolling. *Application fee:* $20.

Degree Requirements 128 total credit hours, 57 in nursing.

Baccalaureate for Second Degree Program (BSN)

Applying *Required:* TOEFL for nonnative speakers of English, minimum college GPA of 2.5, interview, transcript of college record. 24 prerequisite credits must be completed before admission to the nursing program. *Application deadline:* 1/31. *Application fee:* $20.

Degree Requirements 128 total credit hours, 57 in nursing.

Accelerated Baccalaureate for Second Degree Program (BSN)

Applying *Required:* TOEFL for nonnative speakers of English, minimum college GPA of 2.8, interview, 2 letters of recommendation, transcript of college record. *Options:* Course work may be accelerated. *Application deadline:* 1/31. *Application fee:* $20.

Degree Requirements 128 total credit hours, 57 in nursing.

MASTER'S PROGRAM

Contact Dr. Charles Dorlac, Associate Dean for Administrative and Student Affairs, Research College of Nursing-Rockhurst College, 2316 East Meyer Boulevard, Kansas City, MO 64132, 816-276-4729. *Fax:* 816-276-3526.

Areas of Study Nurse practitioner program in family health.

Expenses *Tuition:* $300 per credit hour. *Part-time mandatory fees:* $0. *Books and supplies per academic year:* ranges from $500 to $1000.

BSN to Master's Program (MSN)

Applying *Required:* GRE General Test (minimum combined score of 1000 on three tests), TOEFL for nonnative speakers of English, bachelor's degree in nursing, minimum GPA of 3.0, RN license, 2 years of clinical experience, physical assessment course, statistics course, professional liability/malpractice insurance, essay, interview, 3 letters of recommendation, transcript of college record. *Application deadline:* 10/31. *Application fee:* $50.

Degree Requirements 45 total credit hours, 45 in nursing.

SAINT LOUIS UNIVERSITY

School of Nursing
St. Louis, Missouri

Programs • Generic Baccalaureate • RN Baccalaureate • Baccalaureate for Second Degree • MSN • RN to Master's • MSN/MPH • Post-Master's • PhD • Continuing Education

The University Independent Roman Catholic (Jesuit) coed university. Founded: 1818. *Primary accreditation:* regional. *Setting:* 250-acre urban campus. *Total enrollment:* 10,719.

The School of Nursing Founded in 1928.

Academic Facilities *Campus library:* 1.4 million volumes (122,749 in health); 12,800 periodical subscriptions (6,427 health-care related).

Calendar Semesters.

BACCALAUREATE PROGRAMS

Contact Dr. Judith Lewis, Director, Baccalaureate Programs, School of Nursing, Saint Louis University, 3525 Caroline Street, St. Louis, MO 63104, 314-577-8915. *Fax:* 314-577-8949.

Expenses *Tuition:* $14,940 per academic year.

Financial Aid Institutionally sponsored need-based grants/scholarships, institutionally sponsored non-need grants/scholarships, Federal Nursing Student Loans, Federal Pell Grants, Federal Perkins Loans, Federal Supplemental Educational Opportunity Grants, Federal Work-Study, Federal PLUS Loans, Federal Stafford Loans, state aid. *Application deadline:* 3/1.

Saint Louis University (continued)

Generic Baccalaureate Program (BSN)

Applying *Required:* SAT I or ACT, TOEFL for nonnative speakers of English, minimum college GPA of 2.5, high school chemistry, high school transcript, transcript of college record, CPR certification. *Application fee:* $25.

Degree Requirements 120 total credit hours, 50 in nursing.

RN Baccalaureate Program (BSN)

Applying *Required:* minimum college GPA of 2.0, RN license, diploma or AD in nursing, transcript of college record, CPR certification. *Options:* Advanced standing available through credit by exam. *Application fee:* $25.

Degree Requirements 120 total credit hours, 50 in nursing.

Baccalaureate for Second Degree Program (BSN)

Applying *Required:* minimum college GPA of 3.0, 2 letters of recommendation, transcript of college record, specific prerequisites, CPR certification, baccalaureate degree. *Options:* Course work may be accelerated. *Application fee:* $25.

Degree Requirements 52 total credit hours, 52 in nursing.

MASTER'S PROGRAMS

Contact Dr. Janice A. Noack, Director, Master's Program in Nursing, School of Nursing, Saint Louis University, 3525 Caroline Street, St. Louis, MO 63104, 314-577-8912. *Fax:* 314-577-8949.

Expenses *Tuition:* ranges from $18,540 to $22,660 full-time, $515 per credit hour part-time.

MSN Program

RN to Master's Program (MSN)

MSN/MPH Program

Post-Master's Program

DOCTORAL PROGRAM

Contact Dr. Irene I. Riddle, Director, Doctoral Program, School of Nursing, Saint Louis University, 3525 Caroline Street, St. Louis, MO 63104, 314-577-8971. *Fax:* 314-577-8949.

CONTINUING EDUCATION PROGRAM

Contact Dr. Irene Kalnins, Director, Continuing Education, School of Nursing, Saint Louis University, 3525 Caroline Street, St. Louis, MO 63104, 314-577-8920. *Fax:* 314-577-8949.

SAINT LUKE'S COLLEGE
Kansas City, Missouri

Programs • Generic Baccalaureate • RN Baccalaureate

The College Independent Episcopal upper-level coed institution. *Primary accreditation:* regional. *Setting:* 3-acre urban campus. *Total enrollment:* 103. Founded in 1991. *Nursing program faculty:* 18 (6% with doctorates).

Academic Facilities *Nursing school resources:* CAI, computer lab, nursing audiovisuals, interactive nursing skills videos, learning resource lab.

Student Life *Student services:* health clinic, personal counseling, career counseling, institutionally sponsored work-study program, campus safety program. *International student services:* counseling/support. *Nursing student activities:* student nurses association.

Calendar Semesters.

NURSING STUDENT PROFILE

Undergraduate **Enrollment:** 108

Women: 88%; **Men:** 12%; **Minority:** 9%; **International:** 0%; **Part-time:** 11%

BACCALAUREATE PROGRAMS

Contact Marsha Thomas, Director, Admissions and Records, Saint Luke's College, 4426 Wornall Road, Kansas City, MO 64111, 816-932-2073. *Fax:* 816-932-3831. *E-mail:* mjthomas@saint-lukes.org

Expenses *Tuition:* $7500 full-time, $250 per credit hour part-time. *Full-time mandatory fees:* $240. *Room only:* $1200–$3400. *Books and supplies per academic year:* ranges from $600 to $900.

Financial Aid Institutionally sponsored need-based grants/scholarships, institutionally sponsored non-need grants/scholarships, Federal Nursing Student Loans, Federal Pell Grants, Federal Perkins Loans, Federal Supplemental Educational Opportunity Grants, Federal Work-Study, Missouri Student Grants. 86% of undergraduate students in nursing programs received some form of financial aid in 1995–96. *Application deadline:* 2/28.

Generic Baccalaureate Program (BSN)

Applying *Required:* TOEFL for nonnative speakers of English, minimum college GPA of 2.5, high school transcript, interview, letter of recommendation, written essay, transcript of college record, health insurance, physical examination. 67 prerequisite credits must be completed before admission to the nursing program. *Options:* Advanced standing available through credit by exam. *Application deadline:* 12/15. *Application fee:* $20.

Degree Requirements 124 total credit hours, 57 in nursing.

RN Baccalaureate Program (BSN)

Applying *Required:* TOEFL for nonnative speakers of English, minimum college GPA of 2.5, RN license, diploma or AD in nursing, high school transcript, interview, letter of recommendation, written essay, transcript of college record, health insurance, physical examination. 67 prerequisite credits must be completed before admission to the nursing program. *Options:* Advanced standing available through credit by exam. *Application deadline:* 12/15. *Application fee:* $20.

Degree Requirements 124 total credit hours, 57 in nursing.

SOUTHEAST MISSOURI STATE UNIVERSITY
Department of Nursing
Cape Girardeau, Missouri

Programs • Generic Baccalaureate • RN Baccalaureate • MSN

The University State-supported comprehensive coed institution. Part of Missouri Coordinating Board for Higher Education. Founded: 1873. *Primary accreditation:* regional. *Setting:* 800-acre small-town campus. *Total enrollment:* 8,118.

The Department of Nursing Founded in 1958. *Nursing program faculty:* 18 (63% with doctorates).

Academic Facilities *Campus library:* 397,000 volumes (6,500 in health, 14,000 in nursing); 2,400 periodical subscriptions (165 health-care related).

Calendar Semesters.

BACCALAUREATE PROGRAMS

Contact Chairperson, Student Affairs Committee, Department of Nursing, Southeast Missouri State University, One University Plaza, Cape Girardeau, MO 63701, 314-651-2867. *Fax:* 314-651-5113.

Expenses *State resident tuition:* $2790 full-time, $90 per hour part-time. *Nonresident tuition:* $5177 full-time, $167 per hour part-time.

Financial Aid Institutionally sponsored need-based grants/scholarships, institutionally sponsored non-need grants/scholarships, Federal Nursing Student Loans, Federal Perkins Loans, Federal Supplemental Educational Opportunity Grants, Federal Work-Study, Federal PLUS Loans, Federal Stafford Loans, Mission State Grant. *Application deadline:* 3/1.

Generic Baccalaureate Program (BSN)

Applying *Required:* SAT I or ACT, minimum college GPA of 2.5, high school math, 2 years of high school science, high school chemistry, high school biology, high school transcript, transcript of college record, high school class rank: top 50%. 21 prerequisite credits must be completed before admission to the nursing program. *Options:* Advanced standing available through the following means: advanced placement exams, credit by exam. *Application deadline:* 1/30. *Application fee:* $20.

Degree Requirements 124 total credit hours, 54 in nursing.

RN Baccalaureate Program (BSN)

Applying *Required:* SAT I or ACT, TOEFL for nonnative speakers of English, minimum college GPA of 2.5, RN license, diploma or AD in nursing, transcript of college record. *Options:* Advanced standing available through the following means: advanced placement exams, credit by exam. Course work may be accelerated. *Application deadline:* 4/1. *Application fee:* $20.

Degree Requirements 124 total credit hours, 54 in nursing.

MASTER'S PROGRAM

Areas of Study Clinical nurse specialist programs in family health nursing, rural area nursing; nursing administration; nursing education.

Expenses *State resident tuition:* $96 per hour. *Nonresident tuition:* $178 per hour.

Financial Aid Graduate assistantships, institutionally sponsored non-need-based grants/scholarships.

MSN Program

Applying *Required:* bachelor's degree in nursing, minimum GPA of 3.0, RN license, physical assessment course, statistics course, essay, 2 letters of recommendation, CPR certification.

Degree Requirements 37 total credit hours, 31 in nursing, 6 in elective. Thesis required.

SOUTHWEST BAPTIST UNIVERSITY

Department of Nursing
Springfield, Missouri

Program • RN Baccalaureate

The University Independent Southern Baptist comprehensive coed institution. Founded: 1878. *Primary accreditation:* regional. *Setting:* 123-acre small-town campus. *Total enrollment:* 3,072.

The Department of Nursing Founded in 1982.

Calendar Semesters.

NURSING STUDENT PROFILE

Undergraduate **Enrollment:** 249
Women: 90%; **Men:** 10%

BACCALAUREATE PROGRAM

Contact Dr. Marilyn Meinert, Chair, Department of Nursing, Southwest Baptist University, 1211 South Glenstone, Suite 502, Springfield, MO 65804, 417-863-2210. *Fax:* 417-866-8897.

Expenses *Tuition:* $97 per credit hour.

RN Baccalaureate Program (BSN)

Applying *Required:* NLN Mobility Profile II, RN license. *Options:* Advanced standing available through credit by exam. *Application deadline:* rolling. *Application fee:* $25.

Degree Requirements 128 total credit hours, 64 in nursing.

SOUTHWEST MISSOURI STATE UNIVERSITY

Department of Nursing
Springfield, Missouri

Programs • RN Baccalaureate • Master's for Non-Nursing College Graduates

The University State-supported comprehensive coed institution. Founded: 1905. *Primary accreditation:* regional. *Setting:* 183-acre suburban campus. *Total enrollment:* 16,439.

The Department of Nursing Founded in 1977. *Nursing program faculty:* 4 (50% with doctorates). *Off-campus program site:* West Plains.

Academic Facilities *Campus library:* 535,000 volumes (17,689 in nursing); 4,700 periodical subscriptions. *Nursing school resources:* computer lab, nursing audiovisuals, learning resource lab.

Student Life *Student services:* health clinic, child-care facilities, personal counseling, career counseling, institutionally sponsored work-study program, job placement, campus safety program, special assistance for disabled students. *Nursing student activities:* Sigma Theta Tau, student nurses association.

Calendar Semesters.

NURSING STUDENT PROFILE

Undergraduate **Enrollment:** 362
Women: 90%; **Men:** 10%; **Minority:** 3%; **International:** 1%; **Part-time:** 49%
Graduate
Women: 90%; **Men:** 10%; **Minority:** 0%; **International:** 0%; **Part-time:** 65%

BACCALAUREATE PROGRAM

Contact Dr. Sherry Mustapha, Head, Department of Nursing, Southwest Missouri State University, 901 South National, Springfield, MO 65804, 417-836-5310. *Fax:* 417-836-5484. *E-mail:* shm274f@vma.smsu.edu

Expenses *State resident tuition:* $1124 full-time, $85 per credit hour part-time. *Nonresident tuition:* $2144 per academic year. *Full-time mandatory fees:* $0.

Financial Aid Institutionally sponsored need-based grants/scholarships, institutionally sponsored non-need grants/scholarships, Federal Nursing Student Loans, Federal Supplemental Educational Opportunity Grants, Federal Work-Study. *Application deadline:* 3/31.

RN Baccalaureate Program (BSN)

Applying *Required:* NLN Achievement Tests, minimum college GPA of 2.5, diploma or AD in nursing, interview, 2 letters of recommendation, transcript of college record, Missouri RN license. 60 prerequisite credits must be completed before admission to the nursing program. *Options:* May apply for transfer of up to 64 total credits. *Application deadline:* rolling. *Application fee:* $15.

Degree Requirements 124 total credit hours, 61 in nursing.

MASTER'S PROGRAM

Contact Dr. Sherry L. Mustapha, RN, Head, Department of Nursing, Southwest Missouri State University, 901 South National, Springfield, MO 65804, 417-836-5310. *Fax:* 417-836-5484. *E-mail:* shm274f@vma.smsu.edu

Areas of Study Clinical nurse specialist program in nurse case management; nursing education; nurse practitioner programs in family health, gerontology.

Expenses *State resident tuition:* $95 per credit hour. *Nonresident tuition:* $2004 per academic year.

Master's for Non-Nursing College Graduates Program (MSN)

Applying *Required:* GRE General Test, bachelor's degree in nursing, minimum GPA of 3.0, RN license, physical assessment course, statistics course, professional liability/malpractice insurance, transcript of college record, nursing research course, evidence of vaccination of vaccine-preventable diseases.

Degree Requirements 37–49 total credit hours dependent upon track.

TRUMAN STATE UNIVERSITY

Nursing Program
Kirksville, Missouri

Program • Generic Baccalaureate

The University State-supported comprehensive coed institution. Founded: 1867. *Primary accreditation:* regional. *Setting:* 140-acre small-town campus. *Total enrollment:* 6,287.

The Nursing Program Founded in 1960.

Academic Facilities *Campus library:* 470,161 volumes (8,268 in health, 1,129 in nursing); 1,943 periodical subscriptions (66 health-care related).

Calendar Semesters.

BACCALAUREATE PROGRAM

Contact Director, BT 222, Nursing Program, Truman State University, Kirksville, MO 63501, 816-785-4557. *Fax:* 816-785-7424.

Expenses *State resident tuition:* $308 full-time, $125 per hour part-time. *Nonresident tuition:* $5416 full-time, $225 per hour part-time. *Room and board:* $1480–$4440.

Financial Aid Institutionally sponsored need-based grants/scholarships, institutionally sponsored non-need grants/scholarships, Federal Direct

Truman State University (continued)

Loans, Federal Nursing Student Loans, Federal Pell Grants, Federal Perkins Loans, Federal Supplemental Educational Opportunity Grants, Federal Work-Study, Federal PLUS Loans, Federal Stafford Loans.

Generic Baccalaureate Program (BSN)

Applying *Required:* SAT I or ACT, TOEFL for nonnative speakers of English, minimum high school GPA, high school transcript, written essay, transcript of college record, high school class rank: . *Options:* May apply for transfer of up to 60 total credits. *Application deadline:* rolling.

Degree Requirements 129 total credit hours, 50 in nursing.

UNIVERSITY OF MISSOURI–COLUMBIA

Sinclair School of Nursing
Columbia, Missouri

Programs • Generic Baccalaureate • RN Baccalaureate • MS • PhD • Continuing Education

The University State-supported coed university. Part of University of Missouri System. Founded: 1839. *Primary accreditation:* regional. *Setting:* 1,342-acre small-town campus. *Total enrollment:* 22,313.

The Sinclair School of Nursing Founded in 1901. *Nursing program faculty:* 46 (41% with doctorates). *Off-campus program site:* Kirksville.

▶ ***NOTEWORTHY***

The University of Missouri–Columbia School of Nursing is located within a health sciences center on a comprehensive university campus of almost 25,000 students. The baccalaureate degree offered starts graduates on the path to careers as leaders in the nursing field. Nurses who are graduates of ADN or diploma programs have options that recognize prior learning and experience. The Master of Science and PhD programs are designed to prepare specialists (including nurse practitioners and midwives) who will be the future nurse leaders. Their areas of study include health promotion and protection, health restoration and support, and health-care systems.

Academic Facilities *Campus library:* 2.6 million volumes (190,000 in health, 12,000 in nursing); 13,000 periodical subscriptions (1,823 health-care related). *Nursing school resources:* CAI, computer lab, nursing audiovisuals, interactive nursing skills videos, learning resource lab.

Student Life *Student services:* health clinic, child-care facilities, personal counseling, career counseling, institutionally sponsored work-study program, job placement, campus safety program, special assistance for disabled students. *International student services:* counseling/support, special assistance for nonnative speakers of English, ESL courses. *Nursing student activities:* Sigma Theta Tau, student nurses association.

Calendar Semesters.

NURSING STUDENT PROFILE

Undergraduate **Enrollment:** 242
Women: 88%; **Men:** 12%; **Minority:** 2%; **International:** 2%; **Part-time:** 13%
Graduate **Enrollment:** 142
Women: 96%; **Men:** 4%; **Minority:** 3%; **International:** 2%; **Part-time:** 73%

BACCALAUREATE PROGRAMS

Contact Mr. Jerry Griffith, Academic Adviser, S235, School of Nursing, University of Missouri-Columbia, Columbia, MO 65211, 800-437-4339. *Fax:* 314-884-4544. *E-mail:* nursgrif@showme.missouri.edu

Expenses *State resident tuition:* $3388 full-time, $121 per credit hour part-time. *Nonresident tuition:* $6740 full-time, $362 per credit hour part-time. *Full-time mandatory fees:* $240. *Room and board:* $3812. *Books and supplies per academic year:* $600.

Financial Aid Institutionally sponsored need-based grants/scholarships, institutionally sponsored non-need grants/scholarships, Federal Direct Loans, Federal Nursing Student Loans, Federal Perkins Loans, Federal Supplemental Educational Opportunity Grants, Federal Work-Study. *Application deadline:* 3/1.

Generic Baccalaureate Program (BSN)

Applying *Required:* ACT, TOEFL for nonnative speakers of English, TWE, TSE for nonnative speakers of English, minimum college GPA of 3.0, 3 years of high school math, 3 years of high school science, high school chemistry, high school biology, high school transcript, transcript of college record, for freshmen: combination of high school curriculum, class rank, and ACT score. 45 prerequisite credits must be completed before admission to the nursing program. *Options:* Advanced standing available through the following means: advanced placement exams, credit by exam. May apply for transfer of up to 56 total credits. *Application deadlines:* 2/1 (fall), 9/15 (spring). *Application fee:* $25.

Degree Requirements 120 total credit hours, 64 in nursing.

RN Baccalaureate Program (BSN)

Applying *Required:* TOEFL for nonnative speakers of English, TWE, TSE for nonnative speakers of English, minimum college GPA of 2.5, high school chemistry, RN license, diploma or AD in nursing, transcript of college record. 45 prerequisite credits must be completed before admission to the nursing program. *Options:* Advanced standing available through the following means: advanced placement exams, credit by exam. May apply for transfer of up to 56 total credits. *Application deadlines:* 2/1 (fall), 9/15 (spring). *Application fee:* $25.

Degree Requirements 120 total credit hours, 64 in nursing.

Distance learning Courses provided through video, audio.

MASTER'S PROGRAM

Contact Ms. Nancy Johnson, Coordinator of Student Affairs, S240, School of Nursing, University of Missouri-Columbia, Columbia, MO 65211, 800-437-4399. *Fax:* 314-884-4544. *E-mail:* nursjohn@showme.missouri.edu

Areas of Study Clinical nurse specialist programs in adult health nursing, psychiatric–mental health nursing, public health nursing; nurse midwifery; nursing administration; nursing education; nurse practitioner programs in family health, gerontology.

Expenses *State resident tuition:* $1379 full-time, $153 per credit hour part-time. *Nonresident tuition:* $2767 full-time, $307 per credit hour part-time. *Full-time mandatory fees:* $184–$228. *Part-time mandatory fees:* $15–$117. *Books and supplies per academic year:* ranges from $300 to $800.

Financial Aid Graduate assistantships, nurse traineeships, Federal Nursing Student Loans, institutionally sponsored loans, employment opportunities. *Application deadline:* 2/28.

MS Program

Applying *Required:* GRE General Test, TOEFL for nonnative speakers of English, TWE, TSE for nonnative speakers of English, bachelor's degree in nursing, minimum GPA of 3.0, RN license, interview, 2 letters of recommendation, transcript of college record. *Application deadlines:* 7/1 (fall), 11/1 (spring), 4/1 (summer). *Application fee:* $25.

Degree Requirements 36–42 total credit hours dependent upon track, 30–36 in nursing, 6 in other specified areas. Thesis, research practicum, or project.

Distance learning Courses provided through telecommunications.

DOCTORAL PROGRAM

Contact Ms. Nancy Johnson, Coordinator of Student Affairs, S240, School of Nursing, University of Missouri-Columbia, Columbia, MO 65211, 800-437-4399. *Fax:* 314-884-4544.

Areas of Study Nursing administration, nursing research, clinical practice, nursing policy.

Expenses *State resident tuition:* $1379 full-time, $153 per credit hour part-time. *Nonresident tuition:* $2767 full-time, $307 per credit hour part-time. *Full-time mandatory fees:* $184–$228. *Part-time mandatory fees:* $15–$117. *Books and supplies per academic year:* ranges from $300 to $800.

Financial Aid Graduate assistantships, nurse traineeships, fellowships, institutionally sponsored loans, opportunities for employment. *Application deadline:* 2/28.

PhD Program

Applying *Required:* GRE General Test (minimum combined score of 1500 on three tests), TWE, TSE for nonnative speakers of English, master's degree in nursing, interview, 3 letters of recommendation, vitae, writing sample, competitive review by faculty committee. *Application deadline:* 1/1. *Application fee:* $25.

Degree Requirements 72 total credit hours; dissertation; oral exam; written exam; defense of dissertation; residency.

CONTINUING EDUCATION PROGRAM

Contact Ms. Shirley Farrah, Director of Continuing Nursing Education, S266B, School of Nursing, University of Missouri-Columbia, Columbia, MO 65211, 314-882-0215. *Fax:* 314-884-4544. *E-mail:* farrahs@ext.missouri.edu

UNIVERSITY OF MISSOURI–KANSAS CITY
School of Nursing
Kansas City, Missouri

Programs • RN Baccalaureate • MSN • RN to Master's • PhD

The University State-supported coed university. Part of University of Missouri System. Founded: 1929. *Primary accreditation:* regional. *Setting:* 191-acre urban campus. *Total enrollment:* 10,209.

The School of Nursing Founded in 1979. *Nursing program faculty:* 17 (80% with doctorates). *Off-campus program sites:* St. Louis, St. Joseph, Joplin.

▶ ***NOTEWORTHY***

The University of Missouri–Kansas City School of Nursing is dedicated to high-quality education. The School offers 3 degree programs. The BSN completion program provides registered nurses with the opportunity to obtain a Bachelor of Science in Nursing degree without repeating course content or clinical experience. The MSN program offers a clinical specialty in nursing care of adults, women, or children and functional role options through nurse educator, administrator, clinical nurse specialist, and nurse practitioner tracks. The nurse practitioner role also has a family option. The PhD program is designed for study in one of 3 substantive areas: health promotion, health restoration, and health-care systems.

Academic Facilities *Campus library:* 800,000 volumes (69,200 in health, 2,700 in nursing); 10,000 periodical subscriptions (50 health-care related). *Nursing school resources:* computer lab, nursing audiovisuals, interactive nursing skills videos, learning resource lab.

Student Life *Student services:* child-care facilities, personal counseling, career counseling, institutionally sponsored work-study program, job placement, campus safety program, special assistance for disabled students. *International student services:* counseling/support, special assistance for nonnative speakers of English, ESL courses, post-degree job training. *Nursing student activities:* Sigma Theta Tau, student nurses association.

Calendar Semesters.

NURSING STUDENT PROFILE

Undergraduate **Enrollment:** 70
Women: 93%; **Men:** 7%; **Minority:** 15%; **International:** 0%; **Part-time:** 93%

Graduate **Enrollment:** 277
Women: 95%; **Men:** 5%; **Minority:** 6%; **International:** 0%; **Part-time:** 93%

BACCALAUREATE PROGRAM

Contact Ms. Judy Jellison, Coordinator, Nursing Student Services, School of Nursing, University of Missouri-Kansas City, 2220 Holmes Street, Kansas City, MO 64108, 816-235-1740. *Fax:* 816-235-1701. *E-mail:* jellisoj@smptgate.umkc.edu

Expenses *State resident tuition:* $3204 full-time, $138 per credit hour part-time. *Nonresident tuition:* $9005 full-time, $378 per credit hour part-time. *Books and supplies per academic year:* ranges from $1000 to $1500.

Financial Aid Institutionally sponsored need-based grants/scholarships, Federal Direct Loans, Federal Nursing Student Loans, Federal Perkins Loans, Federal Supplemental Educational Opportunity Grants, Federal Work-Study. *Application deadline:* 7/1.

RN Baccalaureate Program (BSN)

Applying *Required:* TOEFL for nonnative speakers of English, ACT PEP for non-NLN-accredited or diploma program graduates, minimum college GPA of 2.5, RN license, diploma or AD in nursing, transcript of college record. 60 prerequisite credits must be completed before admission to the nursing program. *Options:* Advanced standing available through the following means: advanced placement exams, credit by exam. Course work may be accelerated. May apply for transfer of up to 61 total credits. *Application deadlines:* 7/15 (fall), 11/15 (spring). *Application fee:* $25.

Degree Requirements 121 total credit hours, 61 in nursing.

Distance learning Courses provided through video.

MASTER'S PROGRAMS

Contact Ms. Judy Jellison, Coordinator, Nursing Student Services, School of Nursing, University of Missouri-Kansas City, 2220 Holmes Street, Kansas City, MO 64108, 816-235-1740. *Fax:* 816-235-1701. *E-mail:* jellisoj@smptgate.umkc.edu

Areas of Study Clinical nurse specialist programs in adult health nursing, pediatric nursing, women's health nursing; nursing administration; nursing education; nurse practitioner programs in adult health, child care/pediatrics, family health, women's health.

Expenses *State resident tuition:* $3415 full-time, $170 per credit hour part-time. *Nonresident tuition:* $8948 full-time, $477 per credit hour part-time. *Books and supplies per academic year:* ranges from $1000 to $1500.

Financial Aid Graduate assistantships, nurse traineeships, Federal Direct Loans, Federal Nursing Student Loans, institutionally sponsored loans, institutionally sponsored need-based grants/scholarships. *Application deadline:* 7/1.

MSN Program

Applying *Required:* TOEFL for nonnative speakers of English, bachelor's degree in nursing, minimum GPA of 3.0, RN license, 1 year of clinical experience, physical assessment course, statistics course, essay, 2 letters of recommendation, transcript of college record. *Application deadlines:* 2/1 (fall), 9/1 (spring). *Application fee:* $25.

Degree Requirements 36–43 total credit hours dependent upon track, 36–43 in nursing. Thesis or research project.

Distance learning Courses provided through video.

RN to Master's Program (MSN)

Applying *Required:* TOEFL for nonnative speakers of English, ACT PEP for non-NLN accredited or diploma program graduates, minimum GPA of 3.0, RN license, transcript of college record. *Application deadlines:* 2/1 (fall), 9/1 (spring). *Application fee:* $25.

Degree Requirements 150 total credit hours, 90 in nursing. Thesis or project.

Distance learning Courses provided through video.

DOCTORAL PROGRAM

Contact Ms. Judy Jellison, Coordinator, Nursing Student Services, School of Nursing, University of Missouri-Kansas City, 2220 Holmes Street, Kansas City, MO 64108, 816-235-1740. *Fax:* 816-235-1701. *E-mail:* jellisoj@smptgate.umkc.edu

Areas of Study Nursing administration, nursing research, health promotion/disease prevention, health restoration/maintenance.

Expenses *State resident tuition:* $3115 full-time, $170 per credit hour part-time. *Nonresident tuition:* $8648 full-time, $477 per credit hour part-time. *Books and supplies per academic year:* ranges from $1000 to $1500.

Financial Aid Graduate assistantships, nurse traineeships, Federal Nursing Student Loans, institutionally sponsored need-based grants/scholarships. *Application deadline:* 7/1.

PhD Program

Applying *Required:* GRE General Test, TOEFL for nonnative speakers of English, master's degree in nursing, interview, 2 letters of recommendation, vitae, writing sample, competitive review by faculty committee, goals statement. *Application deadline:* 2/1. *Application fee:* $25.

Degree Requirements 72+ total credit hours dependent upon track; dissertation; oral exam; written exam; defense of dissertation; residency.

UNIVERSITY OF MISSOURI–ST. LOUIS

Barnes College of Nursing
St. Louis, Missouri

Programs • Generic Baccalaureate • RN Baccalaureate • MS • Post-Master's • PhD

The University State-supported coed university. Part of University of Missouri System. Founded: 1963. *Primary accreditation:* regional. *Setting:* 230-acre suburban campus. *Total enrollment:* 12,223.

The Barnes College of Nursing Founded in 1981. *Nursing program faculty:* 66 (55% with doctorates). *Off-campus program sites:* Rolla, Poplar Bluff, St. Charles.

Academic Facilities *Campus library:* 625,249 volumes (14,767 in health, 8,300 in nursing); 5,828 periodical subscriptions (477 health-care related). *Nursing school resources:* CAI, computer lab, nursing audiovisuals, interactive nursing skills videos, learning resource lab.

Student Life *Student services:* health clinic, child-care facilities, personal counseling, career counseling, institutionally sponsored work-study program, job placement, campus safety program, special assistance for disabled students. *International student services:* counseling/support, special assistance for nonnative speakers of English, ESL courses. *Nursing student activities:* Sigma Theta Tau, nursing club, student nurses association.

Calendar Semesters.

NURSING STUDENT PROFILE

Undergraduate **Enrollment:** 628
Women: 92%; **Men:** 8%; **Minority:** 18%; **International:** 0%; **Part-time:** 41%
Graduate **Enrollment:** 323
Women: 94%; **Men:** 6%; **Minority:** 13%; **International:** 0%; **Part-time:** 85%

BACCALAUREATE PROGRAMS

Contact Ms. Tina Saunders, Academic Adviser, Barnes College of Nursing, University of Missouri-St. Louis, 8001 Natural Bridge Road, St. Louis, MO 63121-4499, 314-516-6066. *Fax:* 314-516-6730.

Expenses *State resident tuition:* $3872 full-time, $121 per semester credit part-time. *Nonresident tuition:* $11,574 full-time, $362 per semester credit part-time. *Full-time mandatory fees:* $150. *Part-time mandatory fees:* $150. *Room and board:* $3848–$4048. *Room only:* $2448–$2648. *Books and supplies per academic year:* $600.

Financial Aid Institutionally sponsored need-based grants/scholarships, institutionally sponsored non-need grants/scholarships, Federal Direct Loans, Federal Nursing Student Loans, Federal Pell Grants, Federal Perkins Loans, Federal Supplemental Educational Opportunity Grants, Federal Work-Study. 81% of undergraduate students in nursing programs received some form of financial aid in 1995–96. *Application deadline:* 10/31.

Generic Baccalaureate Program (BSN)

Applying *Required:* ACT, minimum high school GPA of 2.5, 3 years of high school math, 3 years of high school science, high school chemistry, high school biology, high school transcript, high school class rank: top 33%. *Options:* Advanced standing available through credit by exam. May apply for transfer of up to 30 total credits. *Application deadline:* rolling.

Degree Requirements 124 total credit hours, 72 in nursing.

RN Baccalaureate Program (BSN)

Applying *Required:* minimum college GPA of 2.5, RN license, diploma or AD in nursing, transcript of college record. 30 prerequisite credits must be completed before admission to the nursing program. *Options:* Advanced standing available through credit by exam. May apply for transfer of up to 64 total credits. *Application deadline:* rolling.

Degree Requirements 120 total credit hours, 32 in nursing.

Distance learning Courses provided through interactive telecommunication.

MASTER'S PROGRAMS

Contact Dr. Shirley A. Martin, Dean, Barnes College of Nursing, University of Missouri-St. Louis, 8001 Natural Bridge Road, St. Louis, MO 63121-4499, 314-516-6067. *Fax:* 314-516-6730.

Areas of Study Clinical nurse specialist programs in adult health nursing, pediatric nursing, women's health nursing; nursing administration; nursing education; nurse practitioner programs in adult health, child care/pediatrics, family health, women's health.

Expenses *State resident tuition:* $2451 full-time, $153 per semester hour part-time. *Nonresident tuition:* $7370 full-time, $461 per semester hour part-time. *Full-time mandatory fees:* $25–$29. *Part-time mandatory fees:* $25–$29. *Room and board:* $3848–$4048. *Room only:* $2448–$2648. *Books and supplies per academic year:* $400.

Financial Aid Nurse traineeships. 65% of master's level students in nursing programs received some form of financial aid in 1995-96. *Application deadline:* 5/30.

MS Program

Applying *Required:* bachelor's degree in nursing, minimum GPA of 3.0, RN license, 1 year of clinical experience, physical assessment course, statistics course, 2 letters of recommendation, transcript of college record, minimum 2 years clinical experience in past 5 years for practitioner programs. *Application deadlines:* 4/1 (fall), 10/30 (spring).

Degree Requirements 36–43 total credit hours dependent upon track, 30–37 in nursing.

Distance learning Courses provided through interactive telecommunication.

Post-Master's Program

Applying *Required:* minimum GPA of 3.0, RN license, 2 years of clinical experience, essay, 2 letters of recommendation, transcript of college record. *Application deadline:* 7/1.

Degree Requirements 19 total credit hours, 19 in nursing.

DOCTORAL PROGRAMS

Contact Dr. Shirley A. Martin, Dean, Barnes College of Nursing, University of Missouri-St. Louis, 8001 Natural Bridge Road, St. Louis, MO 63121-4499, 314-516-6066. *Fax:* 314-516-6730.

Areas of Study Nursing administration, nursing education, nursing research, clinical practice, nursing policy.

Expenses *State resident tuition:* $2451 full-time, $153 per semester hour part-time. *Nonresident tuition:* $7370 full-time, $461 per semester hour part-time. *Full-time mandatory fees:* $25–$29. *Part-time mandatory fees:* $25–$29. *Room and board:* $3848–$4048. *Room only:* $2448–$2648. *Books and supplies per academic year:* $400.

Financial Aid Graduate assistantships, nurse traineeships, opportunities for employment. *Application deadline:* 6/1.

PhD Program

Applying *Required:* GRE General Test (minimum combined score of 1500 on three tests), TOEFL for nonnative speakers of English, master's degree in nursing, interview, 3 letters of recommendation, vitae, writing sample, competitive review by faculty committee. *Application deadline:* 2/1.

Degree Requirements 42 total credit hours; dissertation; oral exam; written exam; defense of dissertation; residency.

Postbaccalaureate Doctorate (PhD)

Applying *Required:* GRE General Test (minimum combined score of 1500 on three tests), TOEFL for nonnative speakers of English, interview, 3 letters of recommendation, vitae, writing sample, competitive review by faculty committee, BSN. *Application deadline:* 2/1.

Degree Requirements 72 total credit hours; dissertation; oral exam; written exam; defense of dissertation; residency.

WEBSTER UNIVERSITY
Nursing Department
St. Louis, Missouri

Programs • RN Baccalaureate • Accelerated MSN

The University Independent comprehensive coed institution. Founded: 1915. *Primary accreditation:* regional. *Setting:* 47-acre suburban campus. *Total enrollment:* 11,246.

The Nursing Department Founded in 1983. *Nursing program faculty:* 13 (54% with doctorates). *Off-campus program site:* Kansas City.

Academic Facilities *Campus library:* 204,421 volumes (7,030 in health, 3,114 in nursing); 1,232 periodical subscriptions (108 health-care related). *Nursing school resources:* computer lab, nursing audiovisuals, learning resource lab.

Calendar Semesters.

NURSING STUDENT PROFILE

Undergraduate **Enrollment:** 375
Women: 94%; **Men:** 6%; **Minority:** 12%; **International:** 0%; **Part-time:** 99%
Graduate **Enrollment:** 28
Women: 96%; **Men:** 4%; **Minority:** 0%; **International:** 0%; **Part-time:** 100%

BACCALAUREATE PROGRAM

Contact Dr. Janice I. Hooper, Chair, Nursing Department, Webster University, 470 East Lockwood Avenue, St. Louis, MO 63119-3194, 314-968-7488. *Fax:* 314-963-6101. *E-mail:* hooperji@websteruniv.edu

Expenses *Tuition:* $5146 full-time, $315 per credit hour part-time. *Full-time mandatory fees:* $0. *Books and supplies per academic year:* ranges from $150 to $300.

Financial Aid Institutionally sponsored need-based grants/scholarships, institutionally sponsored non-need grants/scholarships. 2% of undergraduate students in nursing programs received some form of financial aid in 1995–96. *Application deadline:* 4/1.

RN Baccalaureate Program (BSN)

Applying *Required:* TOEFL for nonnative speakers of English, minimum college GPA of 2.5, RN license, diploma or AD in nursing, interview, written essay, transcript of college record. 17 prerequisite credits must be completed before admission to the nursing program. *Options:* May apply for transfer of up to 98 total credits. *Application deadlines:* 8/1 (fall), 12/1 (spring). *Application fee:* $25.

Degree Requirements 128 total credit hours, 65 in nursing. Advanced physiology, statistics.

MASTER'S PROGRAM

Contact Susan Heady, RN, Coordinator, MSN Program, 470 East Lockwood Avenue, St. Louis, MO 63119, 314-968-7176. *Fax:* 314-963-6101.

Areas of Study Clinical nurse specialist program in family health nursing; nursing education.

Expenses *Tuition:* $315 per credit hour. *Books and supplies per academic year:* ranges from $150 to $250.

Accelerated MSN Program

Applying *Required:* bachelor's degree in nursing, bachelor's degree, minimum GPA of 3.0, RN license, 1 year of clinical experience, physical assessment course, statistics course, professional liability/malpractice insurance, essay, interview, 3 letters of recommendation, transcript of college record. *Application deadlines:* 7/1 (fall), 12/1 (spring). *Application fee:* $25.

Degree Requirements 36 total credit hours, 30 in nursing. Case study.

WILLIAM JEWELL COLLEGE
Department of Nursing
Liberty, Missouri

Programs • Generic Baccalaureate • RN Baccalaureate

The College Independent Baptist 4-year coed college. Founded: 1849. *Primary accreditation:* regional. *Setting:* 700-acre small-town campus. *Total enrollment:* 1,250.

The Department of Nursing Founded in 1970. *Nursing program faculty:* 14 (14% with doctorates).

Academic Facilities *Campus library:* 233,084 volumes (4,000 in health, 10,000 in nursing); 914 periodical subscriptions (81 health-care related). *Nursing school resources:* CAI, computer lab, nursing audiovisuals, learning resource lab.

Student Life *Student services:* health clinic, personal counseling, career counseling, institutionally sponsored work-study program, job placement. *International student services:* counseling/support. *Nursing student activities:* Sigma Theta Tau, student nurses association.

Calendar Semesters.

NURSING STUDENT PROFILE

Undergraduate **Enrollment:** 115
Women: 93%; **Men:** 7%; **Minority:** 3%; **International:** 2%; **Part-time:** 0%

BACCALAUREATE PROGRAMS

Contact Dr. Joanne Kersten, Chair and Professor, Department of Nursing, William Jewell College, 500 College Hill, Liberty, MO 64068, 816-781-7700 Ext. 5453. *Fax:* 816-415-5027. *E-mail:* kerstenj@william.jewell.edu

Expenses *Tuition:* $11,130 per academic year. *Full-time mandatory fees:* $50. *Room and board:* $3270. *Room only:* $1370. *Books and supplies per academic year:* $400.

Financial Aid Institutionally sponsored need-based grants/scholarships, institutionally sponsored non-need grants/scholarships, Federal Direct Loans, Federal Nursing Student Loans, Federal Perkins Loans, Federal Supplemental Educational Opportunity Grants, Federal Work-Study. *Application deadline:* 3/15.

Generic Baccalaureate Program (BS)

Applying *Required:* ACT, TOEFL for nonnative speakers of English, minimum college GPA of 2.0, high school transcript, letter of recommendation, written essay, transcript of college record, high school class rank: top 50%. 37 prerequisite credits must be completed before admission to the nursing program. *Application deadline:* 6/1. *Application fee:* $50.

Degree Requirements 124 total credit hours, 51 in nursing.

RN Baccalaureate Program (BS)

Applying *Required:* minimum college GPA of 2.5, RN license, diploma or AD in nursing, written essay. 32 prerequisite credits must be completed before admission to the nursing program. *Options:* Advanced standing available through credit by exam. *Application deadline:* 6/1. *Application fee:* $25.

Degree Requirements 124 total credit hours, 53 in nursing.

MONTANA

CARROLL COLLEGE
Department of Nursing
Helena, Montana

Programs • Generic Baccalaureate • RN Baccalaureate

The College Independent Roman Catholic 4-year coed college. Founded: 1909. *Primary accreditation:* regional. *Setting:* 64-acre small-town campus. *Total enrollment:* 1,412.

The Department of Nursing Founded in 1973.

Academic Facilities *Campus library:* 94,000 volumes (1,950 in health); 430 periodical subscriptions. *Nursing school resources:* computer lab.

Calendar Semesters.

Carroll College (continued)

BACCALAUREATE PROGRAMS

Contact Director, Department of Admissions, Department of Nursing, Carroll College, 1610 North Benton Avenue, Helena, MT 59625, 406-447-4388. *Fax:* 406-447-4533.

Financial Aid Institutionally sponsored need-based grants/scholarships, institutionally sponsored non-need grants/scholarships, Federal Pell Grants, Federal Perkins Loans, Federal Work-Study, Federal PLUS Loans, Federal Stafford Loans. *Application deadline:* 3/1.

GENERIC BACCALAUREATE PROGRAM (BA)

Applying *Required:* SAT I or ACT, TOEFL for nonnative speakers of English, minimum college GPA of 2.5, high school transcript, letter of recommendation. 65 prerequisite credits must be completed before admission to the nursing program. *Application deadline:* rolling. *Application fee:* $25.

Degree Requirements 122 total credit hours, 60 in nursing.

RN BACCALAUREATE PROGRAM (BA)

Applying *Required:* minimum college GPA of 2.5, RN license, diploma or AD in nursing, transcript of college record. *Options:* Advanced standing available through credit by exam. *Application deadline:* rolling. *Application fee:* $25.

Degree Requirements 122 total credit hours, 60 in nursing.

MONTANA STATE UNIVERSITY–BOZEMAN

College of Nursing
Bozeman, Montana

Programs • Generic Baccalaureate • RN Baccalaureate • MN

The University State-supported coed university. Part of Montana University System. Founded: 1893. *Primary accreditation:* regional. *Setting:* 1,170-acre small-town campus. *Total enrollment:* 11,267.

The College of Nursing Founded in 1937. *Nursing program faculty:* 59 (24% with doctorates). *Off-campus program sites:* Billings, Great Falls, Missoula.

Academic Facilities *Campus library:* 569,866 volumes (75,999 in health, 10,857 in nursing); 5,078 periodical subscriptions (761 health-care related). *Nursing school resources:* CAI, computer lab, nursing audiovisuals, interactive nursing skills videos, learning resource lab.

Student Life *Student services:* health clinic, child-care facilities, personal counseling, career counseling, institutionally sponsored work-study program, job placement, campus safety program, special assistance for disabled students, alcohol education program, tutoring, Return to Learn (reentry support service). *International student services:* counseling/support, special assistance for nonnative speakers of English, intensive English language institute. *Nursing student activities:* Sigma Theta Tau, student nurses association, Student Forum.

Calendar Semesters.

NURSING STUDENT PROFILE

Undergraduate **Enrollment:** 538
Women: 85%; **Men:** 15%; **Minority:** 5%; **International:** 0%; **Part-time:** 10%
Graduate **Enrollment:** 19
Women: 100%; **Minority:** 0%; **International:** 0%; **Part-time:** 37%

BACCALAUREATE PROGRAMS

Contact Dr. Vonna Koehler, Acting Assistant Dean, College of Nursing, Montana State University-Bozeman, Bozeman, MT 59717, 406-994-3785. *Fax:* 406-994-6020. *E-mail:* unuvk@msu.oscs.montana.edu

Expenses *State resident tuition:* $1831 full-time, $65 per credit part-time. *Nonresident tuition:* $4637 full-time, $166 per credit part-time. *Full-time mandatory fees:* $2195–$3194. *Part-time mandatory fees:* $39+. *Books and supplies per academic year:* ranges from $1000 to $1200.

Financial Aid Institutionally sponsored need-based grants/scholarships, institutionally sponsored non-need grants/scholarships, Federal Direct Loans, Federal Nursing Student Loans, Federal Pell Grants, Federal Perkins Loans, Federal Supplemental Educational Opportunity Grants, Federal Work-Study. *Application deadline:* 3/1.

GENERIC BACCALAUREATE PROGRAM (BSN)

Applying *Required:* SAT I, ACT, TOEFL for nonnative speakers of English, minimum high school GPA of 2.5, minimum college GPA of 2.5, high school transcript, transcript of college record, high school class rank: top 50%. *Application deadlines:* 7/1 (fall), 12/1 (spring). *Application fee:* $30.

Degree Requirements 120 total credit hours, 68 in nursing.

RN BACCALAUREATE PROGRAM (BSN)

Applying *Required:* TOEFL for nonnative speakers of English, minimum college GPA of 2.5, RN license, diploma or AD in nursing, transcript of college record. *Options:* Advanced standing available through credit by exam. Course work may be accelerated. *Application deadlines:* 7/1 (fall), 12/1 (spring). *Application fee:* $30.

Degree Requirements 120 total credit hours.

MASTER'S PROGRAM

Contact Dr. Kathleen Chafey, Acting Associate Dean, College of Nursing, Montana State University, Bozeman, MT 59717, 406-994-3500. *Fax:* 406-994-6020. *E-mail:* unukc@msu.oscs.montana.edu

Areas of Study Nursing administration; nurse practitioner program in family health.

Expenses *State resident tuition:* $1413 full-time, $79 per credit part-time. *Nonresident tuition:* $2980 full-time, $166 per credit part-time. *Full-time mandatory fees:* $1177–$2644. *Part-time mandatory fees:* $39+.

Financial Aid Graduate assistantships, nurse traineeships, Federal Direct Loans, institutionally sponsored need-based grants/scholarships, institutionally sponsored non-need-based grants/scholarships. *Application deadline:* 3/1.

MN PROGRAM

Applying *Required:* GRE General Test, TOEFL for nonnative speakers of English, bachelor's degree in nursing, minimum GPA of 3.0, RN license, 1 year of clinical experience, physical assessment course, statistics course, professional liability/malpractice insurance, essay, interview, 3 letters of recommendation, transcript of college record. *Application deadline:* 2/15. *Application fee:* $50.

Degree Requirements 66 total credit hours, 62 in nursing, 4 in other specified areas. Thesis/professional project.

MONTANA STATE UNIVERSITY–NORTHERN

Department of Nursing
Havre, Montana

Program • RN Baccalaureate

The University State-supported comprehensive coed institution. Part of Montana University System. Founded: 1929. *Primary accreditation:* regional. *Setting:* 105-acre small-town campus. *Total enrollment:* 1,680.

The Department of Nursing Founded in 1966. *Nursing program faculty:* 12 (12% with doctorates). *Off-campus program sites:* Great Falls, Butte.

Academic Facilities *Campus library:* 6,336 volumes; 606 periodical subscriptions (63 health-care related). *Nursing school resources:* CAI, computer lab, nursing audiovisuals, interactive nursing skills videos, learning resource lab.

Student Life *Student services:* health clinic, personal counseling, career counseling, institutionally sponsored work-study program, job placement, campus safety program, special assistance for disabled students. *International student services:* counseling/support, international student club and international student adviser. *Nursing student activities:* nursing club, student nurses association.

Calendar Semesters.

NURSING STUDENT PROFILE

Undergraduate **Enrollment:** 217
Women: 90%; **Men:** 10%; **Minority:** 10%; **International:** 2%; **Part-time:** 10%

BACCALAUREATE PROGRAM

Contact Dr. Jackie Swanson, Chair, Department of Nursing, Montana State University-Northern, Box 7751, Havre, MT 59501, 406-265-3788. *Fax:* 406-265-3777.

Expenses *State resident tuition:* $2350 full-time, $198 per 2-credit course part-time. *Nonresident tuition:* $6662 full-time, $506 per 2-credit course part-time. *Room and board:* $3480–$3880. *Room only:* $1340–$1650.

Financial Aid Institutionally sponsored need-based grants/scholarships, institutionally sponsored non-need grants/scholarships, Federal Direct

Loans, Federal Nursing Student Loans, Federal Pell Grants, Federal Perkins Loans, Federal Work-Study, Indian health service scholarships. 90% of undergraduate students in nursing programs received some form of financial aid in 1995–96.

RN Baccalaureate Program (BSN)

Applying *Required:* minimum college GPA of 2.5, RN license, diploma or AD in nursing, high school transcript, transcript of college record. *Options:* Advanced standing available through advanced placement exams. *Application deadline:* 4/1.

Degree Requirements 120–121 total credit hours dependent upon track, 73 in nursing.

NEBRASKA

CLARKSON COLLEGE
Department of Nursing, Health Services Management and Allied Health
Omaha, Nebraska

Programs • Generic Baccalaureate • Accelerated Baccalaureate • RN Baccalaureate • BSN to Master's • Post-Master's • Continuing Education

The College Independent comprehensive coed institution. Founded: 1888. *Primary accreditation:* regional. *Setting:* 3-acre urban campus. *Total enrollment:* 569.

The Department of Nursing, Health Services Management and Allied Health Founded in 1981. *Nursing program faculty:* 28 (18% with doctorates).

Academic Facilities *Campus library:* 6,439 volumes; 441 periodical subscriptions. *Nursing school resources:* CAI, computer lab, nursing audiovisuals, interactive nursing skills videos, learning resource lab.

Student Life *Student services:* health clinic, child-care facilities, personal counseling, career counseling, institutionally sponsored work-study program, job placement, campus safety program, special assistance for disabled students. *Nursing student activities:* student nurses association.

Calendar Semesters.

NURSING STUDENT PROFILE

Undergraduate **Enrollment:** 325
Women: 90%; **Men:** 10%; **Minority:** 10%; **Part-time:** 7%
Graduate **Enrollment:** 133
Women: 93%; **Men:** 7%; **Part-time:** 46%

BACCALAUREATE PROGRAMS

Contact Mr. Jeff Beals, Director of Enrollment Services, Clarkson College, 101 South 42nd Street, Omaha, NE 68131-2739, 800-647-5500. *Fax:* 402-552-6057. *E-mail:* beals@clrkcol.crhsnet.edu

Expenses *Tuition:* $8384 full-time, $262 per credit hour part-time. *Full-time mandatory fees:* $215. *Room only:* $1850. *Books and supplies per academic year:* $150.

Financial Aid Institutionally sponsored need-based grants/scholarships, institutionally sponsored non-need grants/scholarships, Federal Nursing Student Loans, Federal Supplemental Educational Opportunity Grants, Federal Work-Study. *Application deadline:* 5/1.

Generic Baccalaureate Program (BSN)

Applying *Required:* ACT, TOEFL for nonnative speakers of English, minimum high school GPA of 2.0, 3 years of high school math, 3 years of high school science, high school transcript, transcript of college record, health exam, immunizations, basic life support certification, health insurance, professional liability/malpractice insurance. *Options:* Advanced standing available through advanced placement exams. Course work may be accelerated. May apply for transfer of up to 90 total credits. *Application deadline:* rolling. *Application fee:* $15.

Degree Requirements 128 total credit hours, 68 in nursing.

Distance learning Courses provided through video, audio, computer-based media.

Accelerated Baccalaureate Program (BSN)

Applying *Required:* ACT, TOEFL for nonnative speakers of English, minimum high school GPA of 2.0, high school math, high school science, high school transcript, transcript of college record, health exam, immunizations, basic life support certification, health insurance, professional liability/malpractice insurance. *Options:* Advanced standing available through advanced placement exams. Course work may be accelerated. May apply for transfer of up to 90 total credits. *Application deadline:* rolling. *Application fee:* $15.

Degree Requirements 128 total credit hours, 68 in nursing.

Distance learning Courses provided through video, audio, computer-based media.

RN Baccalaureate Program (BSN)

Applying *Required:* ACT, TOEFL for nonnative speakers of English, minimum high school GPA of 2.0, high school math, high school science, RN license, high school transcript, transcript of college record, health exam, immunizations, basic life support certification, health insurance, professional liability/malpractice insurance. *Options:* Advanced standing available through advanced placement exams. Course work may be accelerated. May apply for transfer of up to 90 total credits. *Application deadline:* rolling. *Application fee:* $15.

Degree Requirements 128 total credit hours, 68 in nursing.

Distance learning Courses provided through video, audio, computer-based media.

MASTER'S PROGRAMS

Contact Mr. Jeff Beals, Director of Enrollment Services, Clarkson College, 101 South 42nd Street, Omaha, NE 68131-2739, 800-647-5500. *Fax:* 402-552-6057. *E-mail:* beals@clrkcol.crhsnet.edu

Areas of Study Nursing administration; nursing education; nurse practitioner program in family health.

BSN to Master's Program (MSN)

Applying *Required:* bachelor's degree in nursing, bachelor's degree, minimum GPA of 3.0, RN license, statistics course, professional liability/malpractice insurance, essay, 2 letters of recommendation, transcript of college record. *Application deadline:* rolling. *Application fee:* $15.

Degree Requirements 36 total credit hours, 36 in nursing. Thesis required.

Distance learning Courses provided through video, audio, computer-based media.

Post-Master's Program

Applying *Required:* bachelor's degree in nursing, bachelor's degree, minimum GPA of 3.0, RN license, statistics course, professional liability/malpractice insurance, essay, 2 letters of recommendation, transcript of college record. *Application deadline:* rolling. *Application fee:* $15.

Degree Requirements 45 total credit hours, 45 in nursing. Thesis required.

Distance learning Courses provided through video, audio, computer-based media.

CONTINUING EDUCATION PROGRAM

Contact Dr. Charles J. Beauchamp, Dean of Nursing, Health Service Management, and Allied Health, Clarkson College, 101 South 42nd Street, Omaha, NE 68131-2739, 800-647-5500. *Fax:* 402-552-6058.

COLLEGE OF SAINT MARY
Division of Nursing
Omaha, Nebraska

Program • RN Baccalaureate

The College Independent Roman Catholic 4-year women's college. Founded: 1923. *Primary accreditation:* regional. *Setting:* 25-acre suburban campus. *Total enrollment:* 1,096.

The Division of Nursing Founded in 1970. *Nursing program faculty:* 23 (13% with doctorates).

Academic Facilities *Campus library:* 68,000 volumes; 500 periodical subscriptions (100 health-care related). *Nursing school resources:* CAI, computer lab, nursing audiovisuals, learning resource lab, nursing skills lab.

Student Life *Student services:* health clinic, personal counseling, career counseling, institutionally sponsored work-study program, campus safety

College of Saint Mary (continued)

program, special assistance for disabled students, campus ministry, volunteer center. *International student services:* counseling/support, special assistance for nonnative speakers of English. *Nursing student activities:* nursing club, student nurses association.

Calendar Semesters.

NURSING STUDENT PROFILE

Undergraduate

Women: 100%; **Minority:** 5%; **International:** 1%; **Part-time:** 40%

BACCALAUREATE PROGRAM

Contact Dr. Mary E. Partusch, Baccalaureate Program Director, Division of Nursing, College of Saint Mary, 1901 South 72nd Street, Omaha, NE 68124, 402-399-2653. *Fax:* 402-399-2654.

Expenses *Tuition:* $10,994 full-time, $361 per credit hour part-time.

Financial Aid Institutionally sponsored need-based grants/scholarships, institutionally sponsored non-need grants/scholarships, Federal Nursing Student Loans, Federal Supplemental Educational Opportunity Grants, Federal Work-Study. *Application deadline:* 3/15.

RN Baccalaureate Program (BSN)

Applying *Required:* ACT, minimum college GPA of 2.5, RN license, diploma or AD in nursing, high school transcript, 2 letters of recommendation, transcript of college record. *Options:* Advanced standing available through credit by exam. Course work may be accelerated. May apply for transfer of up to 98 total credits. *Application deadlines:* 8/15 (fall), 1/10 (spring). *Application fee:* $20.

Degree Requirements 128 total credit hours, 60 in nursing. 47 semester hours of general education.

CREIGHTON UNIVERSITY

School of Nursing
Omaha, Nebraska

Programs • Generic Baccalaureate • RN Baccalaureate • Baccalaureate for Second Degree • RN to Master's • Master's for Nurses with Non-Nursing Degrees

The University Independent Roman Catholic coed university. Founded: 1878. *Primary accreditation:* regional. *Setting:* 85-acre urban campus. *Total enrollment:* 6,069.

The School of Nursing Founded in 1928. *Nursing program faculty:* 46 (26% with doctorates). *Off-campus program site:* Hastings.

Academic Facilities *Campus library:* 594,819 volumes (117,648 in health); 7,415 periodical subscriptions (1,606 health-care related). *Nursing school resources:* CAI, computer lab, nursing audiovisuals, interactive nursing skills videos, learning resource lab.

Student Life *Student services:* health clinic, child-care facilities, personal counseling, career counseling, institutionally sponsored work-study program, job placement, campus safety program, special assistance for disabled students. *International student services:* counseling/support, special assistance for nonnative speakers of English, ESL courses. *Nursing student activities:* Sigma Theta Tau, student nurses association, Nursing Student Senate.

Calendar Semesters.

NURSING STUDENT PROFILE

Undergraduate **Enrollment:** 324

Women: 90%; **Men:** 10%; **Minority:** 8%; **International:** 0%; **Part-time:** 8%

Graduate **Enrollment:** 81

Women: 95%; **Men:** 5%; **Minority:** 3%; **International:** 0%; **Part-time:** 83%

BACCALAUREATE PROGRAMS

Contact Recruitment Counselor, School of Nursing, Creighton University, 2500 California Plaza, Omaha, NE 68178, 800-544-5071. *Fax:* 402-280-2045.

Expenses *Tuition:* $11,746 full-time, $366 per credit hour part-time. *Full-time mandatory fees:* $477. *Room and board:* $4406–$7109. *Room only:* $2514–$4995. *Books and supplies per academic year:* ranges from $200 to $300.

Financial Aid Institutionally sponsored need-based grants/scholarships, institutionally sponsored non-need grants/scholarships, Federal Nursing Student Loans, Federal Supplemental Educational Opportunity Grants, Federal Work-Study. *Application deadline:* 6/30.

Generic Baccalaureate Program (BSN)

Applying *Required:* SAT I, ACT, TOEFL for nonnative speakers of English, high school transcript, letter of recommendation, transcript of college record. *Options:* Course work may be accelerated. May apply for transfer of up to 80 total credits. *Application deadline:* rolling. *Application fee:* $30.

Degree Requirements 128 total credit hours, 57 in nursing. Pharmacology, ethics courses.

RN Baccalaureate Program (BSN)

Applying *Required:* TOEFL for nonnative speakers of English, RN license, diploma or AD in nursing, high school transcript, 2 letters of recommendation, transcript of college record. *Options:* Advanced standing available through the following means: advanced placement exams, credit by exam. Course work may be accelerated. May apply for transfer of up to 80 total credits. *Application deadline:* rolling. *Application fee:* $30.

Degree Requirements 128 total credit hours, 57 in nursing. Pharmacology, ethics courses.

Baccalaureate for Second Degree Program (BSN)

Applying *Required:* TOEFL for nonnative speakers of English, minimum college GPA of 2.5, high school transcript, 4 letters of recommendation, written essay, transcript of college record. 70 prerequisite credits must be completed before admission to the nursing program. *Options:* May apply for transfer of up to 80 total credits. *Application deadline:* rolling. *Application fee:* $30.

Degree Requirements 128 total credit hours, 57 in nursing. Pharmacology, ethics courses.

MASTER'S PROGRAMS

Contact Dr. Sheila Ciciulla, Associate Dean for Academic Affairs, School of Nursing, Creighton University, 2500 California Plaza, Omaha, NE 68178, 402-280-2000. *Fax:* 402-280-2334.

Areas of Study Clinical nurse specialist programs in adult health nursing, family health nursing, family focused psychiatric-mental health nursing; nursing administration; nursing education; nurse practitioner programs in adult health, family health, gerontology.

Expenses *Tuition:* $366 per semester hour. *Full-time mandatory fees:* $21–$201. *Books and supplies per academic year:* ranges from $80 to $250.

Financial Aid Nurse traineeships, Federal Nursing Student Loans, employment opportunities. *Application deadline:* 2/1.

RN to Master's Program (MS)

Applying *Required:* GRE General Test, TOEFL for nonnative speakers of English, bachelor's degree in nursing, minimum GPA of 2.5, RN license, physical assessment course, statistics course, professional liability/malpractice insurance, 3 letters of recommendation, transcript of college record. *Application deadline:* rolling. *Application fee:* $20.

Degree Requirements 164–167 total credit hours dependent upon track, 84 in nursing.

Master's for Nurses with Non-Nursing Degrees Program (MS)

Applying *Required:* GRE General Test, TOEFL for nonnative speakers of English, bachelor's degree in nursing, bachelor's degree, minimum GPA of 2.5, RN license, physical assessment course, statistics course, professional liability/malpractice insurance, 3 letters of recommendation, transcript of college record. *Application deadline:* rolling. *Application fee:* $30.

Degree Requirements 103 total credit hours, 97 in nursing.

MIDLAND LUTHERAN COLLEGE
Division of Nursing
Fremont, Nebraska

Programs • Generic Baccalaureate • Accelerated RN Baccalaureate • LPN to Baccalaureate • Continuing Education

The College Independent Lutheran 4-year coed college. Founded: 1883. *Primary accreditation:* regional. *Setting:* 27-acre small-town campus. *Total enrollment:* 1,030.

The Division of Nursing Founded in 1974. *Nursing program faculty:* 15 (20% with doctorates). *Off-campus program sites:* Omaha, Council Bluffs, IA.

Academic Facilities *Campus library:* 111,000 volumes (4,800 in health, 1,800 in nursing); 640 periodical subscriptions (78 health-care related). *Nursing school resources:* CAI, computer lab, nursing audiovisuals, learning resource lab.

Student Life *Student services:* health clinic, personal counseling, career counseling, institutionally sponsored work-study program, job placement, special assistance for disabled students. *International student services:* counseling/support, special assistance for nonnative speakers of English. *Nursing student activities:* Sigma Theta Tau, student nurses association.

Calendar 4-1-4.

NURSING STUDENT PROFILE

Undergraduate **Enrollment:** 190
Women: 95%; **Men:** 5%; **Minority:** 1%; **International:** 0%; **Part-time:** 48%

BACCALAUREATE PROGRAMS

Contact Mr. Roland R. Kahnk, Vice President for Admissions and Financial Aid, Midland Lutheran College, 900 North Clarkson, Fremont, NE 68025, 402-721-5480. *Fax:* 402-721-0250. *E-mail:* rkahnk@admin.mlc.edu

Expenses *Tuition:* $11,650 full-time, $260 per credit hour part-time. *Full-time mandatory fees:* $50–$66. *Room and board:* $3160. *Room only:* $1300. *Books and supplies per academic year:* $500.

Financial Aid Institutionally sponsored need-based grants/scholarships, institutionally sponsored non-need grants/scholarships, Federal Supplemental Educational Opportunity Grants, Federal Work-Study. 91% of undergraduate students in nursing programs received some form of financial aid in 1995–96.

Generic Baccalaureate Program (BSN)

Applying *Required:* ACT, minimum college GPA of 2.5, 3 years of high school math, 2 years of high school science, high school chemistry, high school biology, high school transcript, interview, 2 letters of recommendation, written essay, transcript of college record, high school class rank: top 25%. 26 prerequisite credits must be completed before admission to the nursing program. *Options:* May apply for transfer of up to 96 total credits. *Application deadline:* rolling. *Application fee:* $20.

Degree Requirements 128 total credit hours, 55 in nursing.

Accelerated RN Baccalaureate Program (BSN)

Applying *Required:* minimum college GPA of 2.5, RN license, diploma or AD in nursing, high school transcript, interview, 2 letters of recommendation, transcript of college record. *Options:* Advanced standing available through credit by exam. May apply for transfer of up to 96 total credits. *Application deadline:* rolling. *Application fee:* $20.

Degree Requirements 128 total credit hours, 55 in nursing.

Distance learning Courses provided through video. Specific degree requirements include possible need to be on campus for "testing out" of various courses including all clinical nursing courses, except community health nursing.

LPN to Baccalaureate Program (BSN)

Applying *Required:* minimum college GPA of 2.5, high school transcript, interview, 2 letters of recommendation, transcript of college record, LPN license. 42 prerequisite credits must be completed before admission to the nursing program. *Options:* Advanced standing available through credit by exam. Course work may be accelerated. May apply for transfer of up to 96 total credits. *Application deadline:* rolling. *Application fee:* $20.

Degree Requirements 128 total credit hours, 55 in nursing.

CONTINUING EDUCATION PROGRAM

Contact Dr. Nancy A. Harms, Chair, Division of Nursing, Midland Lutheran College, 900 North Clarkson, Fremont, NE 68025, 402-721-5480. *Fax:* 402-721-0250. *E-mail:* harms@admin.mlc.edu

NEBRASKA METHODIST COLLEGE OF NURSING AND ALLIED HEALTH
Omaha, Nebraska

Program • Generic Baccalaureate

The College Independent 4-year primarily women's college. Founded: 1891. *Primary accreditation:* regional. *Setting:* 5-acre urban campus. *Total enrollment:* 357. Founded in 1891.

Academic Facilities *Campus library:* 13,461 volumes (8,077 in health, 4,038 in nursing); 392 periodical subscriptions (361 health-care related).

Calendar Semesters.

BACCALAUREATE PROGRAM

Contact Coordinator of Admissions, Nebraska Methodist College of Nursing and Allied Health, 8501 West Dodge Road, Omaha, NE 68114, 402-354-4922. *Fax:* 402-354-8875.

NEBRASKA WESLEYAN UNIVERSITY
Department of Nursing
Lincoln, Nebraska

Program • RN Baccalaureate

The University Independent United Methodist 4-year coed college. Founded: 1887. *Primary accreditation:* regional. *Setting:* 50-acre suburban campus. *Total enrollment:* 1,584.

The Department of Nursing Founded in 1981. *Nursing program faculty:* 3 (67% with doctorates).

Calendar Semesters.

BACCALAUREATE PROGRAM

Contact Dr. Patricia Jean Morin, Chair, Department of Nursing, Nebraska Wesleyan University, Lincoln, NE 68504, 402-466-2371.

Expenses *Tuition:* $10,284 full-time, $142 per credit hour part-time.

Financial Aid Institutionally sponsored need-based grants/scholarships, institutionally sponsored non-need grants/scholarships, Federal Pell Grants, Federal Perkins Loans, Federal Supplemental Educational Opportunity Grants, Federal PLUS Loans, Federal Stafford Loans, state aid.

RN Baccalaureate Program (BSN)

Applying *Required:* SAT I or ACT, ACT PEP, RN license, diploma or AD in nursing, high school transcript. *Application fee:* $20.

UNION COLLEGE
Division of Health Sciences - Nursing Program
Lincoln, Nebraska

Programs • Generic Baccalaureate • RN Baccalaureate • LPN to Baccalaureate

The College Independent Seventh-day Adventist 4-year coed college. Founded: 1891. *Primary accreditation:* regional. *Setting:* 26-acre suburban campus. *Total enrollment:* 576.

The Division of Health Sciences - Nursing Program Founded in 1946. *Nursing program faculty:* 6 (33% with doctorates).

Academic Facilities *Campus library:* 140,381 volumes; 636 periodical subscriptions (79 health-care related). *Nursing school resources:* CAI, computer lab, nursing audiovisuals, interactive nursing skills videos, learning resource lab.

Student Life *Student services:* health clinic, personal counseling, career counseling, institutionally sponsored work-study program, job placement, special assistance for disabled students. *International student services:*

Union College (continued)

counseling/support, special assistance for nonnative speakers of English, ESL courses. *Nursing student activities:* Sigma Theta Tau, nursing club, student nurses association.

Calendar Semesters.

NURSING STUDENT PROFILE

Undergraduate **Enrollment:** 86
Women: 88%; **Men:** 12%; **Minority:** 10%; **International:** 3%; **Part-time:** 10%

BACCALAUREATE PROGRAMS

Contact Ms. Pamela Chambers, Office Manager, Division of Health Sciences - Nursing Program, Union College, 3800 South 48, Lincoln, NE 68506, 402-486-2524. *Fax:* 402-486-2895. *E-mail:* pachambe@ucollege.edu

Expenses *Tuition:* $9550 full-time, $398 per credit hour part-time. *Full-time mandatory fees:* $112–$120. *Room and board:* $2850–$3550. *Room only:* $1750–$2200. *Books and supplies per academic year:* ranges from $500 to $750.

Financial Aid Institutionally sponsored need-based grants/scholarships, institutionally sponsored non-need grants/scholarships, Federal Nursing Student Loans, Federal Perkins Loans, Federal Supplemental Educational Opportunity Grants, Federal Work-Study. *Application deadline:* 6/15.

Generic Baccalaureate Program (BSN)

Applying *Required:* ACT, TOEFL for nonnative speakers of English, TOEFL or Michigan English Language Assessment Battery for nonnative speakers of English, math placement test, minimum college GPA of 2.5, high school transcript, 3 letters of recommendation, written essay, transcript of college record. *Options:* Advanced standing available through credit by exam. *Application deadlines:* 4/1 (fall), 11/1 (spring).

Degree Requirements 128 total credit hours, 55 in nursing.

RN Baccalaureate Program (BSN)

Applying *Required:* ACT, TOEFL for nonnative speakers of English, TOEFL or Michigan English Language Assessment Battery for nonnative speakers of English, math placement test, minimum college GPA of 2.5, RN license, diploma or AD in nursing, high school transcript, 3 letters of recommendation, written essay, transcript of college record. *Options:* Advanced standing available through credit by exam. *Application deadlines:* 4/1 (fall), 11/1 (spring).

Degree Requirements 128 total credit hours, 55 in nursing.

LPN to Baccalaureate Program (BSN)

Applying *Required:* ACT, TOEFL for nonnative speakers of English, TOEFL or Michigan English Language Assessment Battery for nonnative speakers of English, math placement test, minimum college GPA of 2.5, high school transcript, 3 letters of recommendation, written essay, transcript of college record, LPN license. *Options:* Advanced standing available through credit by exam. *Application deadlines:* 4/1 (fall), 11/1 (spring).

Degree Requirements 128 total credit hours, 55 in nursing.

UNIVERSITY OF NEBRASKA MEDICAL CENTER
College of Nursing
Omaha, Nebraska

Programs • Generic Baccalaureate • RN Baccalaureate • MSN • PhD • Continuing Education

The University State-supported upper-level coed institution. Part of University of Nebraska System. Founded: 1869. *Primary accreditation:* regional. *Setting:* 51-acre urban campus. *Total enrollment:* 2,765.

The College of Nursing Founded in 1917. *Nursing program faculty:* 104 (53% with doctorates). *Off-campus program sites:* Lincoln, Kearney, Scottsbluff.

Academic Facilities *Campus library:* 237,470 volumes (237,470 in health, 3,500 in nursing); 2,174 periodical subscriptions (2,174 health-care related). *Nursing school resources:* CAI, computer lab, nursing audiovisuals, interactive nursing skills videos, learning resource lab.

Student Life *Student services:* health clinic, child-care facilities, personal counseling, career counseling, institutionally sponsored work-study program, campus safety program, special assistance for disabled students. *International student services:* counseling/support, ESL courses. *Nursing student activities:* Sigma Theta Tau, student nurses association.

Calendar Semesters.

NURSING STUDENT PROFILE

Undergraduate **Enrollment:** 592
Women: 88%; **Men:** 12%; **Minority:** 6%; **International:** 1%; **Part-time:** 8%
Graduate **Enrollment:** 189
Women: 98%; **Men:** 2%; **Minority:** 1%; **International:** 0%; **Part-time:** 73%

BACCALAUREATE PROGRAMS

Contact Mr. Larry Hewitt, Student Services Coordinator, College of Nursing, University of Nebraska Medical Center, 600 South 42nd Street, PO Box 985330, Omaha, NE 68198-5330, 402-559-5102. *Fax:* 402-559-6379. *E-mail:* lhewitt@unmc.edu

Expenses *State resident tuition:* $2667 full-time, $95 per credit hour part-time. *Nonresident tuition:* $7140 full-time, $255 per credit hour part-time. *Full-time mandatory fees:* $340–$817. *Part-time mandatory fees:* $200–$817. *Books and supplies per academic year:* ranges from $400 to $600.

Financial Aid Institutionally sponsored need-based grants/scholarships, institutionally sponsored non-need grants/scholarships, Federal Nursing Student Loans, Federal Pell Grants, Federal Perkins Loans, Federal Supplemental Educational Opportunity Grants, Federal Work-Study. 76% of undergraduate students in nursing programs received some form of financial aid in 1995–96. *Application deadline:* 2/1.

Generic Baccalaureate Program (BSN)

Applying *Required:* TOEFL and TSE for nonnative speakers of English, minimum college GPA of 3.0, high school transcript, 2 letters of recommendation, transcript of college record. 55 prerequisite credits must be completed before admission to the nursing program. *Options:* Advanced standing available through the following means: advanced placement exams, credit by exam. May apply for transfer of up to 64 total credits. *Application deadlines:* 12/31 (fall), 6/30 (spring). *Application fee:* $25.

Degree Requirements 128 total credit hours, 64 in nursing.

RN Baccalaureate Program (BSN)

Applying *Required:* TOEFL and TSE for nonnative speakers of English, minimum college GPA of 3.0, RN license, diploma or AD in nursing, letter of recommendation, transcript of college record. 64 prerequisite credits must be completed before admission to the nursing program. *Options:* Advanced standing available through the following means: advanced placement exams, advanced placement without credit, credit by exam. Course work may be accelerated. May apply for transfer of up to 64 total credits. *Application deadlines:* 12/31 (fall), 6/30 (spring). *Application fee:* $25.

Degree Requirements 128 total credit hours, 64 in nursing.

MASTER'S PROGRAM

Contact Dr. Nancy Bergstrom, Interim Associate Dean, Graduate Nursing, College of Nursing, University of Nebraska Medical Center, 600 South 42nd Street, PO Box 985330, Omaha, NE 68198-5330, 402-559-7457. *Fax:* 402-559-4303. *E-mail:* nbergstr@unmc.edu

Areas of Study Clinical nurse specialist programs in adult health nursing, community health nursing, critical care nursing, gerontological nursing, oncology nursing, pediatric nursing, psychiatric–mental health nursing, women's health nursing, geropsychiatric nursing; nursing administration; nursing education; nurse practitioner programs in adult health, child care/pediatrics, family health, gerontology, primary care, women's health.

Expenses *State resident tuition:* $108 per credit hour. *Nonresident tuition:* $275 per credit hour. *Full-time mandatory fees:* $69. *Part-time mandatory fees:* $69. *Books and supplies per academic year:* $400.

Financial Aid Graduate assistantships, nurse traineeships, Federal Nursing Student Loans, institutionally sponsored need-based grants/scholarships, institutionally sponsored non-need-based grants/scholarships. *Application deadline:* 2/1.

MSN Program

Applying *Required:* GRE General Test, TOEFL for nonnative speakers of English, bachelor's degree in nursing, minimum GPA of 3.0, RN license,

physical assessment course, statistics course, interview, 3 letters of recommendation, transcript of college record, research course. *Application deadlines:* 5/1 (fall), 10/1 (spring). *Application fee:* $25.

Degree Requirements 36–44 total credit hours dependent upon track, 36–44 in nursing.

DOCTORAL PROGRAM

Contact Dr. Nancy Bergstrom, Interim Associate Dean, Graduate Nursing, College of Nursing, University of Nebraska Medical Center, 600 42nd Street, PO Box 985330, Omaha, NE 68198-5330, 402-559-4286. *Fax:* 402-559-4303.

Areas of Study Nursing research.

Expenses *State resident tuition:* $108 per credit hour. *Nonresident tuition:* $275 per credit hour.

Financial Aid Graduate assistantships, fellowships, grants, opportunities for employment.

PhD Program

Applying *Required:* GRE General Test, TOEFL for nonnative speakers of English, master's degree in nursing, master's degree, 2 scholarly papers, interview, 3 letters of recommendation, vitae, writing sample. *Application deadlines:* 3/1 (fall), 3/1 (spring). *Application fee:* $25.

Degree Requirements 71 total credit hours; dissertation; oral exam; defense of dissertation; residency; proof of manuscript submitted to a journal reporting dissertation.

CONTINUING EDUCATION PROGRAM

Contact College of Nursing, University of Nebraska Medical Center, 600 South 42nd Street, PO Box 985330, Omaha, NE 68198-5330, 402-559-7487. *Fax:* 402-559-7570.

NEVADA

UNIVERSITY OF NEVADA, LAS VEGAS
Department of Nursing
Las Vegas, Nevada

Programs • Generic Baccalaureate • RN Baccalaureate • MSN • Continuing Education

The University State-supported coed university. Part of University and Community College System of Nevada. Founded: 1957. *Primary accreditation:* regional. *Setting:* 335-acre urban campus. *Total enrollment:* 20,257.

The Department of Nursing Founded in 1964. *Nursing program faculty:* 25 (28% with doctorates). *Off-campus program site:* Elko.

Academic Facilities *Campus library:* 497,972 volumes (19,051 in health, 2,040 in nursing); 6,680 periodical subscriptions (305 health-care related). *Nursing school resources:* CAI, computer lab, interactive nursing skills videos.

Student Life *Student services:* health clinic, child-care facilities, personal counseling, career counseling, institutionally sponsored work-study program, job placement, campus safety program, special assistance for disabled students. *International student services:* counseling/support, ESL courses. *Nursing student activities:* Sigma Theta Tau, student nurses association.

Calendar Semesters.

NURSING STUDENT PROFILE

Undergraduate **Enrollment:** 188
Women: 85%; **Men:** 15%; **Minority:** 26%; **International:** 4%; **Part-time:** 1%

Graduate **Enrollment:** 50
Women: 92%; **Men:** 8%; **Minority:** 10%; **International:** 0%; **Part-time:** 64%

BACCALAUREATE PROGRAMS

Contact Dr. Myrlene LaMancusa, Pre-Nursing Adviser, Department of Nursing, University of Nevada, Las Vegas, 4505 Maryland Parkway, Las Vegas, NV 89154, 702-895-3360. *Fax:* 702-895-4807.

Expenses *State resident tuition:* $2200 full-time, $64 per credit part-time. *Nonresident tuition:* $7300 full-time, $64 per credit part-time. *Full-time mandatory fees:* $500–$550. *Room and board:* $4230–$5642. *Room only:* $3470. *Books and supplies per academic year:* ranges from $200 to $300.

Financial Aid Institutionally sponsored need-based grants/scholarships, institutionally sponsored non-need grants/scholarships, Federal Direct Loans, Federal Pell Grants, Federal Supplemental Educational Opportunity Grants. 50% of undergraduate students in nursing programs received some form of financial aid in 1995–96. *Application deadline:* 4/1.

Generic Baccalaureate Program (BSN)

Applying *Required:* ACT, TOEFL for nonnative speakers of English, minimum high school GPA of 2.5, minimum college GPA of 3.0, 3 years of high school math, 3 years of high school science, high school chemistry, high school biology, high school transcript, transcript of college record, computer literacy. 65 prerequisite credits must be completed before admission to the nursing program. *Options:* Advanced standing available through credit by exam. May apply for transfer of up to 64 total credits. *Application deadlines:* 7/15 (fall), 12/15 (spring), 5/13 (summer). *Application fee:* $40.

Degree Requirements 132 total credit hours, 67 in nursing.

RN Baccalaureate Program (BSN)

Applying *Required:* TOEFL for nonnative speakers of English, graduation from NLN-accredited associate degree program or minimum of 100 on NLN Mobility Profile II, minimum college GPA of 3.0, RN license, diploma or AD in nursing, transcript of college record. 64 prerequisite credits must be completed before admission to the nursing program. *Options:* Advanced standing available through credit by exam. May apply for transfer of up to 64 total credits. *Application deadlines:* 7/15 (fall), 12/15 (spring), 5/13 (summer). *Application fee:* $40.

Degree Requirements 130 total credit hours, 34 in nursing.

Distance learning Courses provided through video.

MASTER'S PROGRAM

Contact Dr. Margaret Louis, Coordinator, Graduate Programs, Department of Nursing, University of Nevada, Las Vegas, 4505 Maryland Parkway, Las Vegas, NV 89154, 702-895-3360. *Fax:* 702-895-4807.

Areas of Study Nurse practitioner program in family health.

Expenses *State resident tuition:* $1960 full-time, $87 per credit part-time. *Nonresident tuition:* $7060 full-time, $87 per credit part-time. *Full-time mandatory fees:* $500–$650. *Room and board:* $4230–$5642. *Room only:* $3470. *Books and supplies per academic year:* ranges from $300 to $400.

Financial Aid Graduate assistantships, employment opportunities, institutionally sponsored need-based grants/scholarships, institutionally sponsored non-need-based grants/scholarships. 20% of master's level students in nursing programs received some form of financial aid in 1995-96. *Application deadline:* 4/1.

MSN Program

Applying *Required:* GRE General Test, TOEFL for nonnative speakers of English, bachelor's degree in nursing, minimum GPA of 3.0, RN license, 1 year of clinical experience, physical assessment course, statistics course, professional liability/malpractice insurance, essay, 2 letters of recommendation, transcript of college record, 2 years of clinical experience for family nurse practitioner track. *Application deadlines:* 4/15 (fall), 11/1 (spring).

Degree Requirements 43–48 total credit hours dependent upon track, 37–45 in nursing, 6 in management, education, or family dynamics. Thesis or professional paper.

CONTINUING EDUCATION PROGRAM

Contact Dr. Myrlene LaMancusa, Pre-Nursing Adviser, Department of Nursing, University of Nevada, Las Vegas, 4505 Maryland Parkway, Las Vegas, NV 89154, 702-895-3360. *Fax:* 702-895-4807.

UNIVERSITY OF NEVADA, RENO
Orvis School of Nursing
Reno, Nevada

Programs • Generic Baccalaureate • RN Baccalaureate • MSN • Post-Master's

The University State-supported coed university. Part of University and Community College System of Nevada. Founded: 1874. *Primary accreditation:* regional. *Setting:* 200-acre urban campus. *Total enrollment:* 11,459.

The Orvis School of Nursing Founded in 1957. *Nursing program faculty:* 20 (48% with doctorates).

Academic Facilities *Campus library:* 810,000 volumes; 6,500 periodical subscriptions (172 health-care related). *Nursing school resources:* CAI, computer lab, nursing audiovisuals, interactive nursing skills videos, learning resource lab.

Student Life *Student services:* health clinic, personal counseling, career counseling, institutionally sponsored work-study program, job placement, campus safety program, special assistance for disabled students. *International student services:* counseling/support, ESL courses. *Nursing student activities:* Sigma Theta Tau, student nurses association.

Calendar Semesters.

NURSING STUDENT PROFILE

Undergraduate **Enrollment:** 120

Women: 80%; **Men:** 20%; **Minority:** 16%; **International:** 0%; **Part-time:** 20%

Graduate **Enrollment:** 36

Women: 90%; **Men:** 10%; **Minority:** 0%; **International:** 0%; **Part-time:** 85%

BACCALAUREATE PROGRAMS

Contact Dr. Julie E. Johnson, Director, Orvis School of Nursing, University of Nevada, Reno, Mail Stop #134, Reno, NV 89557, 702-784-6841. *Fax:* 702-784-4262. *E-mail:* jej@equinox.unr.edu

Expenses *State resident tuition:* $1920 full-time, $384 per semester part-time. *Nonresident tuition:* $7020 full-time, $2934 per semester part-time. *Full-time mandatory fees:* $58–$1856. *Books and supplies per academic year:* ranges from $200 to $300.

Financial Aid Institutionally sponsored need-based grants/scholarships, Federal Nursing Student Loans, Federal Work-Study. 42% of undergraduate students in nursing programs received some form of financial aid in 1995–96. *Application deadline:* 3/1.

Generic Baccalaureate Program (BSN)

Applying *Required:* SAT I, ACT, TOEFL for nonnative speakers of English, Watson-Glaser Critical Thinking Test, minimum high school GPA of 2.5, 3 years of high school math, 3 years of high school science, high school chemistry, high school biology, high school transcript, immunizations, fingerprints. 65 prerequisite credits must be completed before admission to the nursing program. *Options:* May apply for transfer of up to 60 total credits. *Application fee:* $20.

Degree Requirements 128 total credit hours.

RN Baccalaureate Program (BSN)

Applying *Required:* RN license, diploma or AD in nursing. 65 prerequisite credits must be completed before admission to the nursing program. *Options:* Advanced standing available through credit by exam. Course work may be accelerated. May apply for transfer of up to 60 total credits. *Application deadline:* 11/4.

Degree Requirements 128 total credit hours.

MASTER'S PROGRAMS

Contact Dr. Julie E. Johnson, Director, Orvis School of Nursing, University of Nevada, Reno, Mail Stop 134, Reno, NV 89557, 702-784-6841. *Fax:* 702-784-4262. *E-mail:* jej@equinox.unr.edu

Areas of Study Clinical nurse specialist programs in community health nursing, high-risk population nursing; nursing administration; nurse practitioner program in family health.

Expenses *State resident tuition:* $1566 full-time, $522 per semester part-time. *Nonresident tuition:* $6840 full-time, $3072 per semester part-time. *Full-time mandatory fees:* $81–$1782. *Books and supplies per academic year:* ranges from $500 to $700.

Financial Aid Graduate assistantships, nurse traineeships. 25% of master's level students in nursing programs received some form of financial aid in 1995-96. *Application deadline:* 3/1.

MSN Program

Applying *Required:* GRE General Test or Miller Analogies Test, bachelor's degree in nursing, minimum GPA of 3.0, RN license, physical assessment course, statistics course, essay, interview, 3 letters of recommendation, transcript of college record. *Application deadline:* 3/1. *Application fee:* $20.

Degree Requirements 36 total credit hours. Thesis or research project.

Post-Master's Program

Applying *Required:* GRE General Test, Miller Analogies Test, TOEFL for nonnative speakers of English, bachelor's degree in nursing, minimum GPA of 3.0, RN license, physical assessment course, statistics course, professional liability/malpractice insurance, essay, interview, 3 letters of recommendation, transcript of college record. *Application deadline:* 3/1. *Application fee:* $20.

Degree Requirements 52 total credit hours.

NEW HAMPSHIRE

COLBY-SAWYER COLLEGE
Department of Nursing
New London, New Hampshire

Programs • Generic Baccalaureate • RN Baccalaureate

The College Independent 4-year coed college. Founded: 1837. *Primary accreditation:* regional. *Setting:* 188-acre small-town campus. *Total enrollment:* 712.

The Department of Nursing Founded in 1981. *Nursing program faculty:* 6. *Off-campus program sites:* Concord, Lebanon.

Academic Facilities *Campus library:* 73,726 volumes (2,343 in health, 815 in nursing); 906 periodical subscriptions (75 health-care related). *Nursing school resources:* CAI, computer lab, nursing audiovisuals, interactive nursing skills videos, learning resource lab.

Student Life *Student services:* health clinic, personal counseling, career counseling, institutionally sponsored work-study program, campus safety program, special assistance for disabled students. *International student services:* counseling/support, special assistance for nonnative speakers of English, ESL courses. *Nursing student activities:* student nurses association.

Calendar Semesters.

NURSING STUDENT PROFILE

Undergraduate **Enrollment:** 91

Women: 93%; **Men:** 7%; **Minority:** 3%; **International:** 0%; **Part-time:** 11%

BACCALAUREATE PROGRAMS

Contact Ms. Mary K. Colvin, Chair, Department of Nursing, Colby-Sawyer College, 100 Main Street, New London, NH 03257, 603-526-3647. *Fax:* 603-526-2135. *E-mail:* mcolvin@colby-sawyer.edu

Expenses *Tuition:* $15,530 full-time, $520 per credit hour part-time. *Room and board:* $5950. *Books and supplies per academic year:* $600.

Financial Aid Institutionally sponsored need-based grants/scholarships, institutionally sponsored non-need grants/scholarships, Federal Pell Grants, Federal Perkins Loans, Federal Supplemental Educational Opportunity Grants, Federal Work-Study. 69% of undergraduate students in nursing programs received some form of financial aid in 1995–96. *Application deadline:* 3/1.

Generic Baccalaureate Program (BS)

Applying *Required:* SAT I or ACT, TOEFL for nonnative speakers of English, 3 years of high school math, 3 years of high school science, high school chemistry, high school biology, high school transcript, 2 letters of recommendation, written essay, transcript of college record. 40 prerequisite credits must be completed before admission to the nursing program. *Options:* Advanced standing available through the following means: advanced placement exams, credit by exam. Course work may be accelerated. May apply for transfer of up to 90 total credits. *Application deadline:* rolling. *Application fee:* $40.

Degree Requirements 120 total credit hours, 48 in nursing.

RN Baccalaureate Program (BS)

Applying *Required:* SAT I or ACT, TOEFL for nonnative speakers of English, 3 years of high school math, 3 years of high school science, high school chemistry, high school biology, RN license, diploma or AD in nursing, high school transcript, interview, 2 letters of recommendation, written essay, transcript of college record. 40 prerequisite credits must be completed before admission to the nursing program. *Options:* Advanced standing available through the following means: advanced placement exams, credit by exam. Course work may be accelerated. May apply for transfer of up to 90 total credits. *Application deadline:* rolling. *Application fee:* $40.

Degree Requirements 120 total credit hours, 52 in nursing.

See full description on page 428.

RIVIER COLLEGE
School of Nursing and Health Sciences
Nashua, New Hampshire

Programs • RN Baccalaureate • Master's for Nurses with Non-Nursing Degrees

The College Independent Roman Catholic comprehensive coed institution. Founded: 1933. *Primary accreditation:* regional. *Setting:* 60-acre suburban campus. *Total enrollment:* 2,798.

The School of Nursing and Health Sciences Founded in 1983. *Nursing program faculty:* 23 (26% with doctorates). *Off-campus program site:* Keene.

Academic Facilities *Campus library:* 133,256 volumes; 928 periodical subscriptions (77 health-care related). *Nursing school resources:* CAI, computer lab, nursing audiovisuals, interactive nursing skills videos, learning resource lab.

Student Life *Student services:* health clinic, child-care facilities, personal counseling, career counseling, institutionally sponsored work-study program, job placement, campus safety program, special assistance for disabled students. *International student services:* counseling/support, ESL courses. *Nursing student activities:* student nurses association.

Calendar Semesters.

NURSING STUDENT PROFILE

Undergraduate **Enrollment:** 555
Women: 97%; **Men:** 3%; **Minority:** 3%; **International:** 0%; **Part-time:** 71%
Graduate **Enrollment:** 110
Women: 98%; **Men:** 2%; **Minority:** 2%; **International:** 1%; **Part-time:** 75%

BACCALAUREATE PROGRAM

Contact Ms. Maureen E. Karr, Associate Director of Admissions for Nursing, School of Nursing and Health Sciences, Rivier College, 420 Main Street, Nashua, NH 03060-5086, 603-888-1311 Ext. 8515. *Fax:* 603-891-1799. *E-mail:* mkarr@mighty.riv.edu

Expenses *Tuition:* $11,160 full-time, ranges from $184 to $390 per credit part-time. *Full-time mandatory fees:* $75. *Part-time mandatory fees:* $75. *Room and board:* $5250. *Books and supplies per academic year:* ranges from $400 to $500.

Financial Aid Institutionally sponsored need-based grants/scholarships, institutionally sponsored non-need grants/scholarships, Federal Direct Loans, Federal Pell Grants, Federal Supplemental Educational Opportunity Grants, Federal Work-Study. 81% of undergraduate students in nursing programs received some form of financial aid in 1995–96. *Application deadline:* 4/1.

RN Baccalaureate Program (BS)

Applying *Required:* TOEFL for nonnative speakers of English, RN license, letter of recommendation, written essay, transcript of college record. 60 prerequisite credits must be completed before admission to the nursing program. *Options:* Advanced standing available through credit by exam. May apply for transfer of up to 90 total credits. *Application deadline:* rolling. *Application fee:* $25.

Degree Requirements 60 total credit hours, 24 in nursing.

MASTER'S PROGRAM

Contact Dr. Joan Lewis, Chairperson, Baccalaureate and Graduate Programs, School of Nursing and Health Sciences, Rivier College, 420 Main Street, Nashua, NH 03060-5086, 603-888-1311 Ext. 8529. *Fax:* 603-891-0378. *E-mail:* jlewis@mighty.riv.edu

Areas of Study Nurse practitioner programs in family health, psychiatric–mental health.

Expenses *Tuition:* $8580 full-time, $390 per credit part-time. *Full-time mandatory fees:* $60. *Part-time mandatory fees:* $60. *Room and board:* $5250. *Books and supplies per academic year:* ranges from $600 to $700.

Financial Aid Nurse traineeships, Federal Direct Loans, employment opportunities. 32% of master's level students in nursing programs received some form of financial aid in 1995-96.

Master's for Nurses with Non-Nursing Degrees Program (MS)

Applying *Required:* GRE General Test, Miller Analogies Test, TOEFL for nonnative speakers of English, bachelor's degree, RN license, essay, interview, 2 letters of recommendation, transcript of college record. *Application deadline:* rolling. *Application fee:* $25.

Degree Requirements 43 total credit hours.

See full description on page 494.

SAINT ANSELM COLLEGE
Nursing Department
Manchester, New Hampshire

Programs • Generic Baccalaureate • Continuing Education

The College Independent Roman Catholic 4-year coed college. Founded: 1889. *Primary accreditation:* regional. *Setting:* 450-acre suburban campus. *Total enrollment:* 1,910.

The Nursing Department Founded in 1952. *Nursing program faculty:* 20 (44% with doctorates).

Academic Facilities *Campus library:* 136,500 volumes (4,000 in health, 1,000 in nursing); 1,162 periodical subscriptions (165 health-care related). *Nursing school resources:* CAI, computer lab, nursing audiovisuals, interactive nursing skills videos, learning resource lab, simulated ICU lab.

Student Life *Student services:* health clinic, personal counseling, career counseling, institutionally sponsored work-study program, job placement, campus safety program, special assistance for disabled students. *International student services:* counseling/support, special assistance for nonnative speakers of English. *Nursing student activities:* Sigma Theta Tau, student nurses association.

Calendar Semesters.

NURSING STUDENT PROFILE

Undergraduate **Enrollment:** 278
Women: 94%; **Men:** 6%; **Minority:** 2%; **International:** 0%; **Part-time:** 3%

BACCALAUREATE PROGRAM

Contact Dr. Joanne K. Farley, Director, Nursing Program, Nursing Department, Saint Anselm College, 100 Saint Anselm Drive #1745, Manchester, NH 03102-1310, 603-641-7084. *Fax:* 603-641-7377. *E-mail:* jfarley@anselm.edu

Expenses *Tuition:* $14,550 full-time, $1455 per course part-time. *Full-time mandatory fees:* $900–$1000. *Room and board:* $5710. *Books and supplies per academic year:* ranges from $200 to $300.

Financial Aid Institutionally sponsored need-based grants/scholarships, institutionally sponsored non-need grants/scholarships, Federal Nursing Student Loans, Federal Pell Grants, Federal Perkins Loans, Federal

Saint Anselm College (continued)

Supplemental Educational Opportunity Grants, Federal Work-Study. 81% of undergraduate students in nursing programs received some form of financial aid in 1995–96. *Application deadline:* 4/15.

Generic Baccalaureate Program (BSN)

Applying *Required:* SAT I, 3 years of high school math, 3 years of high school science, high school chemistry, high school foreign language, high school transcript, 2 letters of recommendation. *Options:* Advanced standing available through advanced placement exams. *Application deadline:* 4/15. *Application fee:* $25.

Degree Requirements 143 total credit hours, 58 in nursing.

CONTINUING EDUCATION PROGRAM

Contact Dr. Patricia Fay, Director, Continuing Nursing Education, Nursing Department, Saint Anselm College, 100 Saint Anselm Drive #1745, Manchester, NH 03102-1310, 603-641-7083. *Fax:* 603-641-7089. *E-mail:* patfay@anselm.edu

UNIVERSITY OF NEW HAMPSHIRE
Department of Nursing
Durham, New Hampshire

Programs • Generic Baccalaureate • RN Baccalaureate • MS

The University State-supported coed university. Part of University System of New Hampshire. Founded: 1866. *Primary accreditation:* regional. *Setting:* 200-acre small-town campus. *Total enrollment:* 12,414.

The Department of Nursing Founded in 1965. *Nursing program faculty:* 27 (50% with doctorates). *Off-campus program sites:* Keene, Manchester, Twin Mountain.

Academic Facilities *Campus library:* 1.1 million volumes (25,090 in health, 2,090 in nursing); 7,000 periodical subscriptions (339 health-care related). *Nursing school resources:* CAI, computer lab, nursing audiovisuals, interactive nursing skills videos, learning resource lab, Internet.

Student Life *Student services:* health clinic, child-care facilities, personal counseling, career counseling, institutionally sponsored work-study program, job placement, campus safety program, special assistance for disabled students. *International student services:* counseling/support, special assistance for nonnative speakers of English, ESL courses. *Nursing student activities:* Sigma Theta Tau, student nurses association.

Calendar Semesters.

NURSING STUDENT PROFILE

Undergraduate **Enrollment:** 751

Women: 96%; **Men:** 4%; **Minority:** 2%; **International:** 0%; **Part-time:** 63%

Graduate **Enrollment:** 71

Women: 99%; **Men:** 1%; **Minority:** 0%; **International:** 0%; **Part-time:** 84%

BACCALAUREATE PROGRAMS

Contact Ms. Ann Kelley, Chairperson, Hewitt Hall, Department of Nursing, University of New Hampshire, 4 Library Way, Durham, NH 03824-3563, 603-862-2260. *Fax:* 603-862-4771. *E-mail:* akelley@hopper.unh.edu

Expenses *State resident tuition:* $12,100 per academic year. *Nonresident tuition:* $20,950 per academic year. *Full-time mandatory fees:* $1171–$1406. *Room and board:* $4150. *Books and supplies per academic year:* ranges from $250 to $400.

Financial Aid Institutionally sponsored need-based grants/scholarships, institutionally sponsored non-need grants/scholarships, Federal Nursing Student Loans, Federal Supplemental Educational Opportunity Grants, Federal Work-Study. *Application deadline:* 3/1.

Generic Baccalaureate Program (BS)

Applying *Required:* SAT I or ACT, TOEFL for nonnative speakers of English, 4 years of high school math, 4 years of high school science, high school chemistry, high school biology, high school foreign language, high school transcript, letter of recommendation, written essay, transcript of college record. *Options:* Advanced standing available through advanced placement exams. May apply for transfer of up to 96 total credits. *Application deadlines:* 3/1 (fall), 11/1 (spring). *Application fee:* $25–40.

Degree Requirements 128 total credit hours, 56 in nursing.

Distance learning Courses provided through ITV.

RN Baccalaureate Program (BS)

Applying *Required:* minimum college GPA of 2.5, RN license, diploma or AD in nursing, high school transcript, letter of recommendation, transcript of college record. *Options:* Course work may be accelerated. May apply for transfer of up to 96 total credits. *Application deadlines:* 6/1 (fall), 11/1 (spring). *Application fee:* $25–40.

Degree Requirements 128 total credit hours, 56 in nursing.

Distance learning Courses provided through ITV.

MASTER'S PROGRAM

Contact Jane Dufresne, Graduate Secretary, Hewitt Hall, Department of Nursing, University of New Hampshire, 4 Library Way, Durham, NH 03824-3563, 603-862-2299. *Fax:* 603-862-4771. *E-mail:* janed@christa.unh.edu

Areas of Study Clinical nurse specialist program in adult health nursing; nursing administration; nurse practitioner programs in adult health, family health.

Expenses *State resident tuition:* $4320 full-time, $240 per credit hour part-time. *Nonresident tuition:* $13,290 full-time, $541 per credit hour part-time. *Full-time mandatory fees:* $763. *Part-time mandatory fees:* $30+. *Books and supplies per academic year:* ranges from $300 to $400.

Financial Aid Graduate assistantships, nurse traineeships, Federal Nursing Student Loans, institutionally sponsored loans, employment opportunities, institutionally sponsored need-based grants/scholarships, institutionally sponsored non-need-based grants/scholarships. 14% of master's level students in nursing programs received some form of financial aid in 1995-96. *Application deadline:* 3/1.

MS Program

Applying *Required:* GRE General Test or Miller Analogies Test, bachelor's degree, RN license, 1 year of clinical experience, statistics course, professional liability/malpractice insurance, essay, 3 letters of recommendation, transcript of college record, research course. *Application deadline:* 4/1. *Application fee:* $50.

Degree Requirements 39–45 total credit hours dependent upon track. Thesis or project.

NEW JERSEY

BLOOMFIELD COLLEGE
Presbyterian Division of Nursing
Bloomfield, New Jersey

Programs • Generic Baccalaureate • RN Baccalaureate

The College Independent 4-year coed college, affiliated with Presbyterian Church (U.S.A.). Founded: 1868. *Primary accreditation:* regional. *Setting:* 12-acre suburban campus. *Total enrollment:* 2,173.

The Presbyterian Division of Nursing Founded in 1968. *Nursing program faculty:* 14 (36% with doctorates). *Off-campus program site:* Lakewood.

Academic Facilities *Campus library:* 65,000 volumes (2,050 in health, 1,000 in nursing); 375 periodical subscriptions (45 health-care related). *Nursing school resources:* CAI, computer lab, nursing audiovisuals, interactive nursing skills videos, learning resource lab.

Student Life *Student services:* health clinic, personal counseling, career counseling, institutionally sponsored work-study program, job placement.

International student services: counseling/support, special assistance for nonnative speakers of English, ESL courses. *Nursing student activities:* student nurses association.

Calendar Semesters.

NURSING STUDENT PROFILE

Undergraduate **Enrollment:** 181
Women: 97%; **Men:** 3%; **Minority:** 43%; **International:** 1%; **Part-time:** 47%

BACCALAUREATE PROGRAMS

Contact Mr. Warner Smith, Associate Director of Admission, Office of Admission, Bloomfield College, 1 Park Place, Bloomfield, NJ 07003, 201-748-9000 Ext. 230. *Fax:* 201-748-0916.

Expenses *Tuition:* $9100 full-time, $920 per course part-time. *Full-time mandatory fees:* $600. *Part-time mandatory fees:* $50. *Room and board:* $4650. *Books and supplies per academic year:* $1000.

Financial Aid Institutionally sponsored need-based grants/scholarships, institutionally sponsored non-need grants/scholarships, Federal Pell Grants, Federal Supplemental Educational Opportunity Grants, Federal Work-Study. 41% of undergraduate students in nursing programs received some form of financial aid in 1995–96. *Application deadline:* 6/1.

Generic Baccalaureate Program (BSN)

Applying *Required:* SAT I or ACT, TOEFL for nonnative speakers of English, NLN Preadmission Examination-RN, minimum high school GPA of 2.5, minimum college GPA of 2.5, 2 years of high school math, high school chemistry, high school biology, high school transcript, 2 letters of recommendation, transcript of college record, high school class rank: top 50%. 32 prerequisite credits must be completed before admission to the nursing program. *Options:* Advanced standing available through credit by exam. May apply for transfer of up to 60 total credits. *Application deadline:* rolling. *Application fee:* $25.

Degree Requirements 132 total credit hours, 52 in nursing.

RN Baccalaureate Program (BSN)

Applying *Required:* minimum college GPA of 2.5, RN license, diploma or AD in nursing, 3 letters of recommendation, transcript of college record, professional liability/malpractice insurance. 20 prerequisite credits must be completed before admission to the nursing program. *Options:* Advanced standing available through credit by exam. May apply for transfer of up to 60 total credits. *Application deadline:* rolling. *Application fee:* $25.

Degree Requirements 132 total credit hours, 52 in nursing.

THE COLLEGE OF NEW JERSEY
School of Nursing
Trenton, New Jersey

Programs • Generic Baccalaureate • RN Baccalaureate • MSN

The College State-supported comprehensive coed institution. Founded: 1855. *Primary accreditation:* regional. *Setting:* 250-acre suburban campus. *Total enrollment:* 6,666.

The School of Nursing Founded in 1966. *Nursing program faculty:* 13 (77% with doctorates).

Academic Facilities *Campus library:* 500,000 volumes (30,000 in health, 18,800 in nursing); 1,500 periodical subscriptions (228 health-care related).

Calendar Semesters.

BACCALAUREATE PROGRAMS

Contact Ms. Lovena Haumann, Assistant Professor, School of Nursing, The College of New Jersey, Hillwood Lakes, CN 4700, Trenton, NJ 08650-4700, 609-771-2591. *Fax:* 609-530-7619.

Expenses *State resident tuition:* $10,239 full-time, $141 per credit hour part-time. *Nonresident tuition:* $12,825 full-time, $225 per credit hour part-time.

Generic Baccalaureate Program (BSN)

Applying *Required:* SAT I or ACT, 2 years of high school math, 2 years of high school science, high school chemistry, high school biology, high school transcript. *Application deadlines:* 3/1 (fall), 11/1 (spring), 11/15 (early decision). *Application fee:* $50.

Degree Requirements 127–129 total credit hours dependent upon track, 67–69 in nursing. Comprehensive exam.

RN Baccalaureate Program (BSN)

Applying *Required:* RN license, diploma or AD in nursing. *Options:* May apply for transfer of up to 64 total credits. *Application deadlines:* 3/1 (fall), 11/1 (spring), 11/15 (early decision). *Application fee:* $50.

Degree Requirements 128 total credit hours, 69 in nursing.

MASTER'S PROGRAM

Contact MSN Coordinator, School of Nursing, The College of New Jersey, Hillwood Lakes, CN 4700, Trenton, NJ 08650-4700, 609-771-2591. *Fax:* 609-530-7619.

Areas of Study Clinical nurse specialist program in family health nursing; nursing administration; nurse practitioner program in family health.

Expenses *State resident tuition:* $5732 full-time, $239 per credit hour part-time. *Nonresident tuition:* $7986 full-time, $333 per credit hour part-time. *Full-time mandatory fees:* $500–$600.

Financial Aid Federal Direct Loans, educational opportunity fund.

MSN Program

Applying *Required:* TOEFL for nonnative speakers of English, bachelor's degree in nursing, minimum GPA of 3.0, RN license, physical assessment course, statistics course, professional liability/malpractice insurance. *Application fee:* $50.

Degree Requirements 36–39 total credit hours dependent upon track, 36–39 in nursing. Comprehensive exam.

COLLEGE OF SAINT ELIZABETH
Nursing Department
Morristown, New Jersey

Programs • RN Baccalaureate • Continuing Education

The College Independent Roman Catholic comprehensive primarily women's institution. Founded: 1899. *Primary accreditation:* regional. *Setting:* 188-acre suburban campus. *Total enrollment:* 1,763.

The Nursing Department *Nursing program faculty:* 6 (33% with doctorates). *Off-campus program sites:* Orange, Passaic, Randolph.

Academic Facilities *Campus library:* 210,474 volumes (3,924 in health, 542 in nursing); 828 periodical subscriptions (183 health-care related). *Nursing school resources:* CAI, computer lab, nursing audiovisuals, learning resource lab, CINAHL.

Student Life *Student services:* health clinic, personal counseling, career counseling, institutionally sponsored work-study program, job placement, campus safety program, special assistance for disabled students. *International student services:* counseling/support, special assistance for nonnative speakers of English, ESL courses. *Nursing student activities:* Sigma Theta Tau, nursing club.

Calendar Trimesters.

NURSING STUDENT PROFILE

Undergraduate **Enrollment:** 152
Women: 99%; **Men:** 1%; **Minority:** 19%; **International:** 0%; **Part-time:** 99%

BACCALAUREATE PROGRAM

Contact Sr. Anita Marcellis, Assistant Director, Adult Undergraduate Degree Program, College of Saint Elizabeth, 2 Convent Road, Morristown, NJ 07960-6989, 201-605-7124. *Fax:* 201-605-7676.

Expenses *Tuition:* $11,904 full-time, $372 per credit part-time. *Full-time mandatory fees:* $160. *Part-time mandatory fees:* $40–$160. *Books and supplies per academic year:* ranges from $100 to $250.

Financial Aid Institutionally sponsored need-based grants/scholarships, institutionally sponsored non-need grants/scholarships, Federal Pell

College of Saint Elizabeth (continued)
Grants, Federal Perkins Loans, Federal Supplemental Educational Opportunity Grants, Federal Work-Study. *Application deadline:* 9/1.

RN Baccalaureate Program (BSN)

Applying *Required:* RN license, diploma or AD in nursing, transcript of college record. 56 prerequisite credits must be completed before admission to the nursing program. *Options:* Advanced standing available through credit by exam. Course work may be accelerated. May apply for transfer of up to 64–68 total credits. *Application deadline:* rolling. *Application fee:* $35.

Degree Requirements 128 total credit hours, 30 in nursing. Comprehensive exams.

CONTINUING EDUCATION PROGRAM

Contact Mrs. Karen D'Alonzo, Assistant Professor, Nursing Department, College of Saint Elizabeth, 2 Convent Road, Morristown, NJ 07960-6989, 201-605-7074. *Fax:* 201-605-7177. *E-mail:* dalonzo@liza.st-elizabeth.edu

FAIRLEIGH DICKINSON UNIVERSITY, TEANECK-HACKENSACK CAMPUS
Henry P. Becton School of Nursing and Allied Health
Teaneck, New Jersey

Programs • Generic Baccalaureate • Accelerated Baccalaureate for Second Degree • MSN

The University Independent comprehensive coed institution. Founded: 1942. *Primary accreditation:* regional. *Setting:* 125-acre suburban campus. *Total enrollment:* 6,830.

The Henry P. Becton School of Nursing and Allied Health Founded in 1951. *Nursing program faculty:* 10 (60% with doctorates).

Academic Facilities *Nursing school resources:* CAI, computer lab, nursing audiovisuals, interactive nursing skills videos, learning resource lab.

Student Life *Student services:* health clinic, personal counseling, career counseling, institutionally sponsored work-study program, job placement, campus safety program, special assistance for disabled students. *International student services:* counseling/support, special assistance for nonnative speakers of English, ESL courses, English language institute. *Nursing student activities:* Sigma Theta Tau, student nurses association.

Calendar Semesters.

NURSING STUDENT PROFILE

Undergraduate **Enrollment:** 200
Women: 82%; **Men:** 18%; **Minority:** 50%; **Part-time:** 38%
Graduate **Enrollment:** 20
Women: 100%; **Minority:** 20%; **Part-time:** 100%

BACCALAUREATE PROGRAMS

Contact Dr. Caroline Jordet, Director, Dickinson Hall, School of Nursing, Fairleigh Dickinson University, 1000 River Road, Teaneck, NJ 07666, 201-692-2888. *Fax:* 201-692-2388.

Expenses *Tuition:* $12,600 full-time, $409 per credit part-time. *Full-time mandatory fees:* $804–$1049. *Part-time mandatory fees:* $174–$419. *Room and board:* $5864–$7264. *Room only:* $3458–$4458. *Books and supplies per academic year:* ranges from $492 to $983.

Financial Aid Institutionally sponsored need-based grants/scholarships, institutionally sponsored non-need grants/scholarships, Federal Direct Loans, Federal Nursing Student Loans, Federal Pell Grants, Federal Perkins Loans, Federal Supplemental Educational Opportunity Grants, Federal Work-Study, nursing scholarships. 60% of undergraduate students in nursing programs received some form of financial aid in 1995–96. *Application deadline:* 3/15.

Generic Baccalaureate Program (BSN)

Applying *Required:* SAT I, ACT, TOEFL for nonnative speakers of English, minimum college GPA of 2.5, 2 years of high school math, high school chemistry, high school biology, high school transcript, interview, transcript of college record. *Options:* Advanced standing available through the following means: advanced placement exams, credit by exam. Course work may be accelerated. May apply for transfer of up to 75 total credits. *Application deadline:* rolling. *Application fee:* $35.

Degree Requirements 128 total credit hours, 54 in nursing.

Accelerated Baccalaureate for Second Degree Program (BSN)

Applying *Required:* minimum college GPA of 2.5, transcript of college record, 25 credits of specified prerequisites. 71 prerequisite credits must be completed before admission to the nursing program. *Options:* Advanced standing available through the following means: advanced placement exams, credit by exam. Course work may be accelerated. May apply for transfer of up to 71 total credits. *Application deadline:* rolling. *Application fee:* $35.

Degree Requirements 128 total credit hours, 54 in nursing. 25 credits of specified prerequisites.

MASTER'S PROGRAM

Contact Ann B. Tritak, Associate Director, Graduate Program, 1000 River Road, Teaneck, NJ 07666, 201-692-2882. *Fax:* 201-692-2388. *E-mail:* tritak@alpha.fdu.edu

Areas of Study Nursing administration; nursing education; nurse practitioner program in adult health.

Expenses *Tuition:* $8478 full-time, $471 per credit part-time. *Full-time mandatory fees:* $280. *Part-time mandatory fees:* $132. *Room and board:* $5864–$7264. *Room only:* $3458–$4458. *Books and supplies per academic year:* ranges from $492 to $983.

Financial Aid Federal Direct Loans. *Application deadline:* 3/15.

MSN Program

Applying *Required:* GRE General Test, bachelor's degree in nursing, minimum GPA of 3.0, RN license, physical assessment course, statistics course, professional liability/malpractice insurance, essay, interview, 3 letters of recommendation, transcript of college record. *Application deadline:* rolling. *Application fee:* $35.

Degree Requirements 45 total credit hours, 42 in nursing. Thesis required.

See full description on page 446.

JERSEY CITY STATE COLLEGE
Department of Nursing
Jersey City, New Jersey

Programs • RN Baccalaureate • Continuing Education

The College State-supported comprehensive coed institution. Founded: 1927. *Primary accreditation:* regional. *Setting:* 17-acre urban campus. *Total enrollment:* 7,356.

The Department of Nursing Founded in 1974. *Nursing program faculty:* 9 (22% with doctorates). *Off-campus program sites:* Montclair, Newark.

Academic Facilities *Campus library:* 235,683 volumes (6,100 in health, 750 in nursing); 1,445 periodical subscriptions (125 health-care related). *Nursing school resources:* CAI, computer lab, nursing audiovisuals, learning resource lab.

Student Life *Student services:* health clinic, child-care facilities, personal counseling, career counseling, institutionally sponsored work-study program, job placement, campus safety program. *International student services:* counseling/support, special assistance for nonnative speakers of English, ESL courses, orientation. *Nursing student activities:* Sigma Theta Tau, nursing club.

Calendar Semesters.

NURSING STUDENT PROFILE

Undergraduate **Enrollment:** 301
Women: 89%; **Men:** 11%; **Minority:** 59%; **International:** 1%; **Part-time:** 92%

BACCALAUREATE PROGRAM

Contact Dr. Eileen K. Gardner, Chairperson, Department of Nursing, Jersey City State College, 2039 Kennedy Boulevard, Jersey City, NJ 07305, 201-200-3157. *Fax:* 201-200-3141. *E-mail:* gardner@jcs1.jcstate.edu

Expenses *State resident tuition:* $2610 full-time, $87 per credit part-time. *Nonresident tuition:* $4080 full-time, $136 per credit part-time. *Full-time mandatory fees:* $918. *Part-time mandatory fees:* $60+.

Financial Aid Institutionally sponsored need-based grants/scholarships, institutionally sponsored non-need grants/scholarships, Federal Nursing

Student Loans, Federal Supplemental Educational Opportunity Grants, Federal Work-Study. 2% of undergraduate students in nursing programs received some form of financial aid in 1995–96. *Application deadline:* 4/15.

RN Baccalaureate Program (BSN)

Applying *Required:* minimum college GPA of 2.5, RN license, diploma or AD in nursing, transcript of college record. *Options:* Advanced standing available through credit by exam. Course work may be accelerated. May apply for transfer of up to 96 total credits. *Application deadlines:* 5/1 (fall), 12/1 (spring). *Application fee:* $35.

Degree Requirements 128 total credit hours, 53 in nursing.

CONTINUING EDUCATION PROGRAM

Contact Dr. Barbara Anne Collett, Chair, Continuing Education, Department of Nursing, Jersey City State College, 2039 Kennedy Boulevard, Jersey City, NJ 07305, 201-200-3157. *Fax:* 201-200-3141. *E-mail:* collett@jcsl.jcstate.edu

KEAN COLLEGE OF NEW JERSEY
Nursing Department
Union, New Jersey

Programs • RN Baccalaureate • Accelerated MSN

The College State-supported comprehensive coed institution. Part of New Jersey State College System. Founded: 1855. *Primary accreditation:* regional. *Setting:* 151-acre urban campus. *Total enrollment:* 11,746.

The Nursing Department Founded in 1981. *Nursing program faculty:* 7 (100% with doctorates). *Off-campus program sites:* Elizabeth, Plainfield.

Academic Facilities *Campus library:* 80,000 volumes (6,000 in health, 3,200 in nursing); 142 periodical subscriptions (30 health-care related). *Nursing school resources:* CAI, computer lab, nursing audiovisuals, interactive nursing skills videos, learning resource lab.

Student Life *Student services:* health clinic, child-care facilities, personal counseling, career counseling, institutionally sponsored work-study program, job placement, campus safety program, special assistance for disabled students. *International student services:* counseling/support, special assistance for nonnative speakers of English, ESL courses. *Nursing student activities:* Sigma Theta Tau, nursing club.

Calendar Semesters.

NURSING STUDENT PROFILE

Undergraduate **Enrollment:** 202
Women: 98%; **Men:** 2%; **Minority:** 16%; **International:** 1%; **Part-time:** 85%
Graduate **Enrollment:** 36
Women: 100%; **Minority:** 18%; **International:** 1%; **Part-time:** 100%

BACCALAUREATE PROGRAM

Contact Dr. Virginia Fitzsimons, Chairperson, Nursing Department, Kean College of New Jersey, 1000 Morris Street, Union, NJ 07083, 908-527-2608. *Fax:* 908-352-6427.

Expenses *State resident tuition:* $2400 full-time, $82 per credit part-time. *Nonresident tuition:* $3900 full-time, $96 per credit part-time. *Full-time mandatory fees:* $18–$22. *Books and supplies per academic year:* ranges from $280 to $310.

Financial Aid Institutionally sponsored need-based grants/scholarships, Federal Nursing Student Loans. *Application deadline:* 3/30.

RN Baccalaureate Program (BSN)

Applying *Required:* nursing department exam, minimum college GPA of 2.0, RN license, diploma or AD in nursing, transcript of college record. 26 prerequisite credits must be completed before admission to the nursing program. *Options:* Advanced standing available through credit by exam. Course work may be accelerated. May apply for transfer of up to 72 total credits. *Application deadline:* 3/30. *Application fee:* $20.

Degree Requirements 132 total credit hours, 26 in nursing.

MASTER'S PROGRAM

Contact Susan Salmond, Coordinator, Graduate Program, Kean College, Union, NJ 07083, 908-527-2608. *Fax:* 908-352-6427.

Areas of Study Nursing administration.

Expenses *State resident tuition:* $96 per credit. *Nonresident tuition:* $107 per credit. *Part-time mandatory fees:* $82. *Books and supplies per academic year:* ranges from $270 to $400.

Financial Aid Graduate assistantships, Federal Direct Loans. 100% of master's level students in nursing programs received some form of financial aid in 1995-96.

Accelerated MSN Program

Applying *Required:* GRE General Test, RN license, interview, transcript of college record. *Application deadline:* rolling. *Application fee:* $30.

Degree Requirements 34 total credit hours, 28 in nursing.

MONMOUTH UNIVERSITY
Department of Nursing
West Long Branch, New Jersey

Programs • RN Baccalaureate • RN to Master's

The University Independent comprehensive coed institution. Founded: 1933. *Primary accreditation:* regional. *Setting:* 138-acre suburban campus. *Total enrollment:* 4,482.

The Department of Nursing Founded in 1981. *Nursing program faculty:* 9 (44% with doctorates).

Academic Facilities *Campus library:* 248,000 volumes (56 in health, 35 in nursing); 1,300 periodical subscriptions (91 health-care related). *Nursing school resources:* computer lab, nursing audiovisuals, learning resource lab.

Student Life *Student services:* health clinic, personal counseling, career counseling, institutionally sponsored work-study program, job placement, campus safety program, special assistance for disabled students. *International student services:* counseling/support. *Nursing student activities:* Sigma Theta Tau, student nurses association.

Calendar Semesters.

NURSING STUDENT PROFILE

Undergraduate **Enrollment:** 142
Women: 99%; **Men:** 1%; **Minority:** 7%; **Part-time:** 97%
Graduate **Enrollment:** 54
Women: 98%; **Men:** 2%; **Minority:** 6%; **Part-time:** 96%

BACCALAUREATE PROGRAM

Contact Dr. Emily S. Tompkins, Chairperson and Associate Professor, Department of Nursing, Monmouth University, West Long Branch, NJ 07764, 908-571-3443. *Fax:* 908-263-5131. *E-mail:* tompki@mondec.monmouth.edu

Expenses *Tuition:* $13,270 full-time, $384 per credit part-time. *Full-time mandatory fees:* $354. *Part-time mandatory fees:* $219. *Room and board:* $5264–$6826. *Room only:* $2224–$3786. *Books and supplies per academic year:* $400.

Financial Aid Institutionally sponsored need-based grants/scholarships, institutionally sponsored non-need grants/scholarships, Federal Work-Study. 15% of undergraduate students in nursing programs received some form of financial aid in 1995–96. *Application deadline:* 5/1.

RN Baccalaureate Program (BSN)

Applying *Required:* ACT for diploma graduates, RN license, diploma or AD in nursing, interview, 2 letters of recommendation, transcript of college record. *Options:* Advanced standing available through credit by exam. May apply for transfer of up to 96 total credits. *Application deadlines:* 8/30 (fall), 1/30 (spring). *Application fee:* $30.

Degree Requirements 131 total credit hours, 34 in nursing. 30-33 credits in core, 25 in sciences, 6 of guided electives, 6 of free electives.

Monmouth University (continued)

MASTER'S PROGRAM

Contact Dr. Marilyn Lauria, Associate Professor and Director of MSN program, Monmouth University, West Long Branch, NJ 07764, 908-571-4494. *Fax:* 908-263-5131. *E-mail:* lauria@mondec.monmouth.edu

Areas of Study Nurse practitioner programs in acute care, adult health, family health, gerontology.

Expenses *Tuition:* $419 per credit. *Full-time mandatory fees:* $265. *Part-time mandatory fees:* $130. *Room and board:* $5264–$6826. *Room only:* $2224–$3786. *Books and supplies per academic year:* $400.

Financial Aid Institutionally sponsored need-based grants/scholarships, institutionally sponsored non-need-based grants/scholarships. 35% of master's level students in nursing programs received some form of financial aid in 1995-96. *Application deadline:* 5/1.

RN to Master's Program (MSN)

Applying *Required:* GRE General Test (minimum combined score of 1350 on three tests), bachelor's degree, RN license, physical assessment course, professional liability/malpractice insurance, interview, letter of recommendation, transcript of college record.

Degree Requirements 40 total credit hours, 31 in nursing, 9 in histology/pathophysiology, pharmacology, economics. Thesis required.

THE RICHARD STOCKTON COLLEGE OF NEW JERSEY

Nursing Program
Pomona, New Jersey

Program • RN Baccalaureate

The College State-supported 4-year coed college. Part of New Jersey State College System. Founded: 1971. *Primary accreditation:* regional. *Setting:* 1,600-acre suburban campus. *Total enrollment:* 5,367.

The Nursing Program Founded in 1975. *Nursing program faculty:* 5 (80% with doctorates).

Academic Facilities *Campus library:* 160,000 volumes (7,069 in health, 626 in nursing). *Nursing school resources:* CAI, computer lab, nursing audiovisuals, learning resource lab.

Student Life *Student services:* health clinic, child-care facilities, personal counseling, career counseling, institutionally sponsored work-study program, campus safety program, special assistance for disabled students. *International student services:* counseling/support. *Nursing student activities:* Sigma Theta Tau.

Calendar Semesters.

NURSING STUDENT PROFILE

Undergraduate **Enrollment:** 105

Women: 96%; **Men:** 4%; **Minority:** 7%; **International:** 0%; **Part-time:** 80%

BACCALAUREATE PROGRAM

Contact Dr. Linda Aaronson, Coordinator, Nursing Program, Division of Professional Studies, Richard Stockton College of New Jersey, Pomona, NJ 08240, 609-652-4250. *Fax:* 609-652-4858.

Expenses *State resident tuition:* $3532 full-time, $82 per credit part-time. *Nonresident tuition:* $5072 full-time, $132 per credit part-time. *Room and board:* $1063–$3125. *Books and supplies per academic year:* ranges from $350 to $600.

Financial Aid Institutionally sponsored need-based grants/scholarships, institutionally sponsored non-need grants/scholarships, Federal Direct Loans, Federal Pell Grants, Federal Perkins Loans, Federal Supplemental Educational Opportunity Grants, Federal Work-Study. 5% of undergraduate students in nursing programs received some form of financial aid in 1995–96. *Application deadline:* 3/1.

RN Baccalaureate Program (BSN)

Applying *Required:* minimum college GPA of 2.5, RN license, diploma or AD in nursing, written essay, transcript of college record, CPR certification. 50 prerequisite credits must be completed before admission to the nursing program. *Options:* May apply for transfer of up to 96 total credits. *Application deadlines:* 6/1 (fall), 12/1 (spring). *Application fee:* $35.

Degree Requirements 128 total credit hours, 80 in nursing.

RUTGERS, THE STATE UNIVERSITY OF NEW JERSEY, CAMDEN COLLEGE OF ARTS AND SCIENCES

Department of Nursing
Camden, New Jersey

Programs • Generic Baccalaureate • Accelerated RN Baccalaureate • MS

The University State-supported 4-year coed college. Part of Rutgers, The State University of New Jersey. Founded: 1927. *Primary accreditation:* regional. *Setting:* 25-acre urban campus. *Total enrollment:* 48,135.

The Department of Nursing Founded in 1973. *Nursing program faculty:* 8 (90% with doctorates).

Academic Facilities *Campus library:* 347,545 volumes (8,323 in health); 2,107 periodical subscriptions (70 health-care related). *Nursing school resources:* CAI, computer lab, nursing audiovisuals, interactive nursing skills videos, learning resource lab.

Student Life *Student services:* health clinic, personal counseling, career counseling, institutionally sponsored work-study program, job placement, campus safety program, special assistance for disabled students. *International student services:* counseling/support, special assistance for nonnative speakers of English. *Nursing student activities:* Sigma Theta Tau, nursing club, student nurses association.

Calendar Semesters.

NURSING STUDENT PROFILE

Undergraduate **Enrollment:** 90

Women: 89%; **Men:** 11%; **Minority:** 15%

BACCALAUREATE PROGRAMS

Contact Dr. Mary E. Greipp, Chairperson and Associate Professor, Department of Nursing, Rutgers, The State University of New Jersey, Camden College of Arts and Sciences, 311 North Fifth Street, Camden, NJ 08102, 609-225-6226. *Fax:* 609-225-6541.

Expenses *State resident tuition:* $4028 full-time, $130 per credit part-time. *Nonresident tuition:* $8200 full-time, $266 per credit part-time. *Full-time mandatory fees:* $84–$101. *Room and board:* $4253.

Financial Aid Institutionally sponsored need-based grants/scholarships, institutionally sponsored non-need grants/scholarships, Federal Supplemental Educational Opportunity Grants, Federal Work-Study. *Application deadline:* 3/1.

Generic Baccalaureate Program (BS)

Applying *Required:* SAT I, ACT, 3 years of high school math, high school foreign language, high school transcript, transcript of college record. 62 prerequisite credits must be completed before admission to the nursing program. *Options:* May apply for transfer of up to 64 total credits. *Application deadline:* 12/1. *Application fee:* $40.

Degree Requirements 120 total credit hours, 49 in nursing.

Accelerated RN Baccalaureate Program (BS)

Applying *Required:* SAT I, ACT, 3 years of high school math, RN license, diploma or AD in nursing, high school foreign language, high school transcript, transcript of college record. 62 prerequisite credits must be completed before admission to the nursing program. *Options:* May apply for transfer of up to 64 total credits. *Application deadline:* 12/1. *Application fee:* $40.

Degree Requirements 120 total credit hours, 49 in nursing.

MASTER'S PROGRAM

Contact Dr. Martha Pollick, Program Coordinator, Rutgers, The State University of New Jersey, Camden College of Arts and Science, 311 North Fifth Street, Camden, NJ 08102, 609-225-6526. *Fax:* 609-225-6541.

Areas of Study Clinical nurse specialist programs in adult health nursing, community health nursing; nurse practitioner programs in adult health, community health.

Expenses *State resident tuition:* $5734 full-time, $329 per credit part-time. *Nonresident tuition:* $8406 full-time, $492 per credit part-time. *Full-time mandatory fees:* $330–$348. *Room and board:* $4500–$5500. *Room only:* $2400. *Books and supplies per academic year:* $500.

MS Program

Applying *Required:* GRE General Test (minimum combined score of 1500 on three tests), bachelor's degree in nursing, minimum GPA of 3.0, RN license, physical assessment course, statistics course, professional liability/ malpractice insurance, essay, 3 letters of recommendation, transcript of college record. *Application deadlines:* 8/15 (fall), 12/15 (spring). *Application fee:* $40.

Degree Requirements 36 total credit hours, 12–18 in nursing, 15 in other specified areas.

RUTGERS, THE STATE UNIVERSITY OF NEW JERSEY, COLLEGE OF NURSING

Newark, New Jersey

Programs • Generic Baccalaureate • RN Baccalaureate • Baccalaureate for Second Degree • MS • PhD • Continuing Education

The University State-supported 4-year specialized coed college. Part of Rutgers, The State University of New Jersey. Founded: 1956. *Primary accreditation:* regional. *Setting:* 34-acre urban campus. *Total enrollment:* 48,135. Founded in 1956. *Nursing program faculty:* 59 (54% with doctorates). *Off-campus program sites:* Camden, New Brunswick.

Academic Facilities *Campus library:* 550,000 volumes; 2,400 periodical subscriptions. *Nursing school resources:* CAI, computer lab, nursing audiovisuals, interactive nursing skills videos, learning resource lab.

Student Life *Student services:* health clinic, personal counseling, career counseling, institutionally sponsored work-study program, job placement, campus safety program, special assistance for disabled students. *International student services:* counseling/support, ESL courses. *Nursing student activities:* Sigma Theta Tau, student nurses association.

Calendar Semesters.

NURSING STUDENT PROFILE

Undergraduate **Enrollment:** 400
Women: 89%; **Men:** 11%; **Minority:** 51%; **Part-time:** 9%
Graduate **Enrollment:** 275
Women: 98%; **Men:** 2%; **Minority:** 10%; **International:** 1%; **Part-time:** 95%

BACCALAUREATE PROGRAMS

Contact Mr. John Scott, Director, Newark Admission Office, Rutgers, The State University of New Jersey, College of Nursing, 180 University Avenue, Newark, NJ 07102-1803, 201-648-5205. *E-mail:* scott@asb_ugadm.rutgers.edu

Expenses *State resident tuition:* $4028 full-time, $130 per credit part-time. *Nonresident tuition:* $8200 full-time, $266 per credit part-time. *Full-time mandatory fees:* $852. *Part-time mandatory fees:* $184. *Room and board:* $4253. *Books and supplies per academic year:* ranges from $250 to $500.

Financial Aid Institutionally sponsored need-based grants/scholarships, institutionally sponsored non-need grants/scholarships, Federal Nursing Student Loans, Federal Work-Study. 60% of undergraduate students in nursing programs received some form of financial aid in 1995–96. *Application deadline:* 3/1.

Generic Baccalaureate Program (BS)

Applying *Required:* SAT I, ACT, TOEFL for nonnative speakers of English, minimum high school GPA of 3.0, 3 years of high school math, high school chemistry, high school biology, high school transcript, high school class rank: top 15%. *Application deadline:* 1/15. *Application fee:* $40.

Degree Requirements 125 total credit hours, 67 in nursing.

RN Baccalaureate Program (BS)

Applying *Required:* TOEFL for nonnative speakers of English, minimum college GPA of 3.0, RN license, diploma or AD in nursing, transcript of college record. *Options:* Advanced standing available through credit by exam. Course work may be accelerated. *Application deadline:* 1/15. *Application fee:* $40.

Degree Requirements 125 total credit hours, 67 in nursing.

Baccalaureate for Second Degree Program (BS)

Applying *Required:* TOEFL for nonnative speakers of English, minimum college GPA of 3.0, transcript of college record. *Options:* Advanced standing available through credit by exam. Course work may be accelerated. *Application deadline:* 1/15. *Application fee:* $40.

Degree Requirements 125 total credit hours, 67 in nursing.

MASTER'S PROGRAM

Contact Dr. Elaine Dolinsky, Associate Dean for Student Life and Services, Rutgers, The State University of New Jersey, College of Nursing, 180 University Avenue, Newark, NJ 07102-1803, 201-648-5060. *Fax:* 201-648-1277. *E-mail:* dolinsky@nightingale.rutgers.edu

Areas of Study Clinical nurse specialist programs in adult health nursing, community health nursing, critical care nursing, pediatric nursing, psychiatric–mental health nursing; nurse practitioner programs in acute care, adult health, child care/pediatrics, family health, primary care.

Expenses *State resident tuition:* $5734 full-time, $236 per credit part-time. *Nonresident tuition:* $8506 full-time, $349 per credit part-time. *Full-time mandatory fees:* $706. *Part-time mandatory fees:* $170. *Room and board:* $4500–$5500. *Room only:* $2700. *Books and supplies per academic year:* $500.

Financial Aid Graduate assistantships, nurse traineeships, employment opportunities. 15% of master's level students in nursing programs received some form of financial aid in 1995-96. *Application deadline:* 3/1.

MS Program

Applying *Required:* GRE General Test (minimum combined score of 1500 on three tests), bachelor's degree in nursing, minimum GPA of 3.0, RN license, physical assessment course, statistics course, professional liability/ malpractice insurance, essay, 3 letters of recommendation, transcript of college record. *Application deadlines:* 8/15 (fall), 12/15 (spring). *Application fee:* $40.

Degree Requirements 42–48 total credit hours dependent upon track, 12–18 in nursing, 15 in other specified areas.

DOCTORAL PROGRAM

Contact Dr. Adela Yarcheski, Graduate Program Director, Rutgers, The State University of New Jersey, College of Nursing, 180 University Avenue, Newark, NJ 07102-1803, 201-648-5022. *Fax:* 201-648-1277. *E-mail:* yarcheski@nightingale.rutgers.edu

Areas of Study Nursing research.

Expenses *State resident tuition:* $5734 full-time, $236 per credit part-time. *Nonresident tuition:* $8506 full-time, $349 per credit part-time. *Full-time mandatory fees:* $706. *Part-time mandatory fees:* $170. *Room and board:* $4500–$5500. *Room only:* $2700. *Books and supplies per academic year:* ranges from $200 to $500.

Financial Aid Nurse traineeships, fellowships, opportunities for employment. *Application deadline:* 3/15.

PhD Program

Applying *Required:* GRE General Test (minimum combined score of 1500 on three tests), master's degree in nursing, 2 scholarly papers, statistics course, interview, 3 letters of recommendation, vitae, writing sample, competitive review by faculty committee. *Application deadlines:* 3/15 (fall), 8/15 (spring). *Application fee:* $40.

Degree Requirements 59 total credit hours; dissertation; oral exam; written exam; defense of dissertation; residency.

CONTINUING EDUCATION PROGRAM

Contact Dr. Gayle Pearson, Director, Continuing Education Program, Rutgers, The State University of New Jersey, College of Nursing, 180 University Avenue, Newark, NJ 07102-1803, 201-648-5895. *Fax:* 201-648-1277. *E-mail:* pearson@nightingale.rutgers.edu

SAINT PETER'S COLLEGE

Nursing Department

Jersey City, New Jersey

Programs • RN Baccalaureate • Continuing Education

Saint Peter's College (continued)

The College Independent Roman Catholic (Jesuit) comprehensive coed institution. Founded: 1872. *Primary accreditation:* regional. *Setting:* 10-acre urban campus. *Total enrollment:* 3,654.

The Nursing Department Founded in 1981. *Nursing program faculty:* 11 (60% with doctorates). *Off-campus program sites:* Englewood Cliffs, Hoboken, West Orange.

▶ *NOTEWORTHY*

Saint Peter's College offers an upper-division BSN program for registered nurses at the main campus in Jersey City and the branch campus in Englewood Cliffs. The program, geared for the working nurse, is offered on a trimester calendar. Day and evening courses are available, including selected required liberal arts courses on a once-a-week schedule. Students may attend on a full- or part-time basis. The clinical experiences include on-site assignments with various community agencies. An option for international study is available to students in the final clinical course. The major electives offered afford students various perspectives on holistic healing, multiculturalism, and education for better health.

Academic Facilities *Campus library:* 27,835 volumes; 1,700 periodical subscriptions (88 health-care related). *Nursing school resources:* CAI, computer lab, nursing audiovisuals, learning resource lab.

Student Life *Student services:* personal counseling, career counseling. *International student services:* ESL courses. *Nursing student activities:* Sigma Theta Tau, Registered Nurses Association.

Calendar Trimesters.

NURSING STUDENT PROFILE

Undergraduate **Enrollment:** 203
Women: 98%; **Men:** 2%; **Minority:** 20%; **Part-time:** 94%

BACCALAUREATE PROGRAM

Contact Dr. Doris L. Collins, Chairperson, Nursing Department, Saint Peter's College, Jersey City, NJ 07306, 201-915-9412. *Fax:* 201-915-9062. *E-mail:* nudept@spcvxa.spc.edu

Expenses *Tuition:* $14,436 full-time, $401 per credit part-time. *Full-time mandatory fees:* $115. *Part-time mandatory fees:* $55. *Books and supplies per academic year:* ranges from $500 to $700.

Financial Aid Institutionally sponsored need-based grants/scholarships, institutionally sponsored non-need grants/scholarships, institutionally sponsored short-term loans. *Application deadline:* 6/1.

RN Baccalaureate Program (BSN)

Applying *Required:* minimum college GPA of 2.0, RN license, diploma or AD in nursing, transcript of college record, professional liability/malpractice insurance. *Options:* Advanced standing available through advanced placement exams. May apply for transfer of up to 102 total credits. *Application deadlines:* 8/19 (fall), 2/11 (spring), 11/13 (winter). *Application fee:* $40.

Degree Requirements 133 total credit hours, 61 in nursing.

CONTINUING EDUCATION PROGRAM

Contact Dr. Doris L. Collins, Chairperson, Nursing Department, Saint Peter's College, Jersey City, NJ 07306, 201-915-9412. *Fax:* 201-915-9062. *E-mail:* nudept@spcvxa.spc.edu

SETON HALL UNIVERSITY
College of Nursing
South Orange, New Jersey

Programs • Generic Baccalaureate • RN Baccalaureate • Baccalaureate for Second Degree • Accelerated Baccalaureate for Second Degree • MA • MSN • Post-Master's

The University Independent Roman Catholic coed university. Founded: 1856. *Primary accreditation:* regional. *Setting:* 58-acre suburban campus. *Total enrollment:* 8,693.

The College of Nursing Founded in 1937. *Nursing program faculty:* 52 (37% with doctorates). *Off-campus program sites:* Point Pleasant, Trenton, Somerville.

Academic Facilities *Campus library:* 518,137 volumes (25,250 in health, 4,750 in nursing); 2,600 periodical subscriptions (322 health-care related). *Nursing school resources:* CAI, computer lab, nursing audiovisuals, interactive nursing skills videos, learning resource lab.

Student Life *Student services:* health clinic, personal counseling, career counseling, institutionally sponsored work-study program, job placement, campus safety program, special assistance for disabled students. *International student services:* counseling/support, special assistance for nonnative speakers of English, ESL courses. *Nursing student activities:* Sigma Theta Tau, student nurses association.

Calendar Semesters.

NURSING STUDENT PROFILE

Undergraduate **Enrollment:** 495
Women: 94%; **Men:** 6%; **Minority:** 33%; **International:** 0%; **Part-time:** 36%
Graduate **Enrollment:** 202
Women: 98%; **Men:** 2%; **Minority:** 8%; **International:** 0%; **Part-time:** 99%

BACCALAUREATE PROGRAMS

Contact Ms. Kathleen Enge, Director of Recruitment, College of Nursing, Seton Hall University, 400 South Orange Avenue, South Orange, NJ 07079-2693, 201-761-9285. *Fax:* 201-761-9607. *E-mail:* engekath@lanmail.shu.edu

Expenses *Tuition:* $13,200 full-time, $410 per credit part-time. *Full-time mandatory fees:* $275–$450. *Part-time mandatory fees:* $85–$200. *Room and board:* $6960–$7700. *Books and supplies per academic year:* ranges from $300 to $500.

Financial Aid Institutionally sponsored need-based grants/scholarships, institutionally sponsored non-need grants/scholarships, Federal Nursing Student Loans, Federal Perkins Loans, Federal Supplemental Educational Opportunity Grants, Federal Work-Study, ROTC scholarships, New Jersey Tuition Aid Grants.

Generic Baccalaureate Program (BSN)

Applying *Required:* SAT I, ACT, TOEFL for nonnative speakers of English, minimum high school GPA of 2.5, minimum college GPA of 2.5, 3 years of high school math, 3 years of high school science, high school chemistry, high school biology, high school foreign language, high school transcript, interview, written essay, transcript of college record, high school class rank: top 50%. *Options:* Advanced standing available through the following means: advanced placement exams, credit by exam. May apply for transfer of up to 62 total credits. *Application deadlines:* 3/1 (fall), 12/1 (spring). *Application fee:* $25.

Degree Requirements 130 total credit hours, 58 in nursing.

RN Baccalaureate Program (BSN)

Applying *Required:* NLN Mobility Profile II, minimum college GPA of 2.5, RN license, diploma or AD in nursing, high school transcript, transcript of college record. *Options:* Advanced standing available through credit by exam. May apply for transfer of up to 62 total credits. *Application deadlines:* 6/1 (fall), 12/1 (spring). *Application fee:* $25.

Degree Requirements 130 total credit hours, 58 in nursing.

Baccalaureate for Second Degree Program (BSN)

Applying *Required:* minimum college GPA of 2.5, high school transcript, interview, written essay, transcript of college record, baccalaureate degree, 41 credits of specified prerequisites in science, math, and social science. *Options:* Advanced standing available through the following means: advanced placement exams, credit by exam. *Application deadlines:* 6/1 (fall), 12/1 (spring). *Application fee:* $25.

Degree Requirements 58 total credit hours, 58 in nursing.

Accelerated Baccalaureate for Second Degree Program (BSN)

Applying *Required:* minimum college GPA of 2.5, high school transcript, interview, written essay, transcript of college record, baccalaureate degree, 41 credits of specified prerequisites in science, math, and social science. *Application deadline:* 10/31 (summer). *Application fee:* $25.

Degree Requirements 58 total credit hours, 58 in nursing.

MASTER'S PROGRAMS

Contact Ms. Kathleen Enge, Director of Recruitment, College of Nursing, Seton Hall University, 400 South Orange Avenue, South Orange, NJ 07079-2693, 201-761-9285. *Fax:* 201-761-9607. *E-mail:* engekath@lanmail.shu.edu

Areas of Study Clinical nurse specialist program in critical care nursing; nursing administration; nursing education; nurse practitioner programs in adult health, child care/pediatrics, gerontology, school health, women's health.

Expenses *Tuition:* $437 per credit. *Full-time mandatory fees:* $85–$450. *Room and board:* $7600–$8600. *Room only:* $5800. *Books and supplies per academic year:* ranges from $700 to $1500.

Financial Aid Graduate assistantships, nurse traineeships, Federal Nursing Student Loans, institutionally sponsored loans, employment opportunities. 17% of master's level students in nursing programs received some form of financial aid in 1995-96. *Application deadline:* 8/30.

MA Program

Applying *Required:* bachelor's degree in nursing, minimum GPA of 3.0, RN license, professional liability/malpractice insurance, interview, 2 letters of recommendation, transcript of college record, master's degree in a clinical specialization. *Application deadlines:* 5/1 (fall), 11/1 (spring). *Application fee:* $50.

Degree Requirements 30 total credit hours, 12 in nursing, 18 in education.

MSN Program

Applying *Required:* Miller Analogies Test, bachelor's degree in nursing, minimum GPA of 3.0, RN license, statistics course, professional liability/malpractice insurance, essay, interview, 2 letters of recommendation, transcript of college record, nursing research course. *Application deadlines:* 5/1 (fall), 11/1 (spring). *Application fee:* $50.

Degree Requirements 42 total credit hours, 30–42 in nursing, up to 12 in counseling, education, public administration, business administration. Thesis required.

Post-Master's Program

Applying *Required:* bachelor's degree in nursing, minimum GPA of 3.0, RN license, professional liability/malpractice insurance, essay, interview, letter of recommendation, transcript of college record, master's in nursing. *Application deadline:* 12/1. *Application fee:* $50.

Degree Requirements 21–27 total credit hours dependent upon track, 21–27 in nursing.

THOMAS EDISON STATE COLLEGE
Nursing Program
Trenton, New Jersey

Program • RN Baccalaureate

The College State-supported comprehensive coed institution. Founded: 1972. *Primary accreditation:* regional. *Setting:* 2-acre urban campus. *Total enrollment:* 8,500.

The Nursing Program Founded in 1983. *Nursing program faculty:* 12 (42% with doctorates).

Academic Facilities *Nursing school resources:* CAI, nursing audiovisuals, learning resource lab.

Student Life *Student services:* special assistance for disabled students, student/graduate directory, study groups. *Nursing student activities:* BSN newsletter.

Calendar Open enrollment.

NURSING STUDENT PROFILE

Undergraduate **Enrollment:** 230

Women: 92%; **Men:** 8%; **Minority:** 15%; **International:** 0%; **Part-time:** 100%

BACCALAUREATE PROGRAM

Contact Admissions Office, Thomas Edison State College, 101 West State Street, Trenton, NJ 08625, 609-984-1150. *Fax:* 609-984-8447.

Expenses *Books and supplies per academic year:* $50.

RN Baccalaureate Program (BSN)

Applying *Required:* RN license, residence or employment in New Jersey. *Options:* Course work may be accelerated. May apply for transfer of up to 22 total credits. *Application deadline:* rolling. *Application fee:* $75.

Degree Requirements 120 total credit hours, 48 in nursing.

UNIVERSITY OF MEDICINE AND DENTISTRY OF NEW JERSEY
School of Nursing
Newark, New Jersey

Programs • Master's for Nurses with Non-Nursing Degrees • Post-Master's • Continuing Education

The University State-supported graduate specialized coed institution. Founded: 1954. *Primary accreditation:* regional. *Total enrollment:* 4,032.

The School of Nursing Founded in 1990. *Nursing program faculty:* 48 (25% with doctorates). *Off-campus program sites:* Mahwah, Edison, Stratford.

Academic Facilities *Campus library:* 100,000 volumes (100,000 in health); 2,200 periodical subscriptions (2,200 health-care related). *Nursing school resources:* CAI, computer lab, nursing audiovisuals, interactive nursing skills videos, learning resource lab.

Student Life *Student services:* health clinic, child-care facilities, personal counseling, career counseling, institutionally sponsored work-study program, job placement, campus safety program, special assistance for disabled students. *International student services:* counseling/support, special assistance for nonnative speakers of English, ESL courses. *Nursing student activities:* student nurses association, Nursing Honor Society.

Calendar Semesters.

NURSING STUDENT PROFILE

Graduate **Enrollment:** 145

Women: 92%; **Men:** 8%; **Minority:** 20%; **International:** 0%; **Part-time:** 77%

MASTER'S PROGRAMS

Contact Mr. Peter Falk, Registrar, School of Nursing, University of Medicine and Dentistry of New Jersey, 30 Bergen Street, Room 118, Newark, NJ 07107-3001, 201-982-6012. *Fax:* 201-982-7453.

Areas of Study Nurse anesthesia; nurse practitioner programs in adult health, family health, occupational health, psychiatric–mental health, women's health.

Expenses *State resident tuition:* $4840 full-time, $242 per credit part-time. *Nonresident tuition:* $6440 full-time, $322 per credit part-time. *Full-time mandatory fees:* $195–$245. *Part-time mandatory fees:* $180–$230. *Books and supplies per academic year:* ranges from $700 to $825.

Financial Aid Graduate assistantships, nurse traineeships, Federal Nursing Student Loans, institutionally sponsored loans, institutionally sponsored non-need-based grants/scholarships.

Master's for Nurses with Non-Nursing Degrees Program (MSN)

Applying *Required:* TOEFL for nonnative speakers of English, admissions evaluation essay (in-house administration), bachelor's degree, minimum GPA of 3.0, RN license, 1 year of clinical experience, physical assessment course, statistics course, professional liability/malpractice insurance, 3 letters of recommendation, transcript of college record. *Application deadline:* 4/15. *Application fee:* $30.

Degree Requirements 40 total credit hours, 40 in nursing. 600-700 clinical hours, 408-552 didactic hours.

Post-Master's Program

Applying *Required:* minimum GPA of 3.0, RN license, physical assessment course, professional liability/malpractice insurance, interview, 2 letters of recommendation, transcript of college record. *Application deadline:* 4/15. *Application fee:* $30.

Degree Requirements 346 clinical hours, 255 didactic hours.

CONTINUING EDUCATION PROGRAM

Contact Kathleen Donnelly, Academic Support Services Coordinator, School of Nursing, University of Medicine and Dentistry, 30 Bergen Street, Room 118, Newark, NJ 07107, 201-982-6012. *Fax:* 201-982-7453.

See full description on page 540.

WILLIAM PATERSON COLLEGE OF NEW JERSEY
Department of Nursing
Wayne, New Jersey

Programs • Generic Baccalaureate • RN Baccalaureate • RN to Master's

The College State-supported comprehensive coed institution. Part of New Jersey State College System. Founded: 1855. *Primary accreditation:* regional. *Setting:* 250-acre small-town campus. *Total enrollment:* 9,090.

The Department of Nursing Founded in 1966. *Nursing program faculty:* 26 (50% with doctorates).

Academic Facilities *Campus library:* 300,000 volumes (12,700 in nursing); 2,500 periodical subscriptions (120 health-care related). *Nursing school resources:* CAI, computer lab, nursing audiovisuals, interactive nursing skills videos, learning resource lab.

Student Life *Student services:* health clinic, child-care facilities, personal counseling, career counseling, institutionally sponsored work-study program, campus safety program, special assistance for disabled students. *International student services:* counseling/support, ESL courses. *Nursing student activities:* Sigma Theta Tau, nursing club, student nurses association.

Calendar Semesters.

NURSING STUDENT PROFILE

Undergraduate **Enrollment:** 360
Women: 90%; **Men:** 10%; **Minority:** 25%; **International:** 1%; **Part-time:** 15%
Graduate **Enrollment:** 49
Women: 98%; **Men:** 2%; **Minority:** 8%; **Part-time:** 95%

BACCALAUREATE PROGRAMS

Contact Dr. Sandra DeYoung, Chairperson, Department of Nursing, William Paterson College of New Jersey, 300 Pompton Road, Wayne, NJ 07470, 201-595-2286. *Fax:* 201-595-2668. *E-mail:* deyoung@frontier.wilpaterson.edu

Expenses *State resident tuition:* $2530 per academic year. *Nonresident tuition:* $4510 per academic year. *Full-time mandatory fees:* $848. *Room and board:* $3900–$4160. *Room only:* $3100–$3360. *Books and supplies per academic year:* $400.

Financial Aid Institutionally sponsored need-based grants/scholarships, institutionally sponsored non-need grants/scholarships, Federal Direct Loans, Federal Nursing Student Loans, Federal Perkins Loans, Federal Supplemental Educational Opportunity Grants. *Application deadline:* 4/1.

GENERIC BACCALAUREATE PROGRAM (BSN)

Applying *Required:* SAT I, TOEFL for nonnative speakers of English, minimum college GPA of 2.5, 3 years of high school math, 3 years of high school science, high school chemistry, high school biology, high school transcript, transcript of college record, high school class rank: top 50%. *Options:* May apply for transfer of up to 90 total credits. *Application deadline:* 3/1. *Application fee:* $35.

Degree Requirements 128 total credit hours, 56 in nursing.

RN BACCALAUREATE PROGRAM (BSN)

Applying *Required:* TOEFL for nonnative speakers of English, minimum college GPA of 2.5, 3 years of high school math, 3 years of high school science, high school chemistry, high school biology, RN license, diploma or AD in nursing, high school transcript, transcript of college record. *Options:* May apply for transfer of up to 90 total credits. *Application deadline:* 3/1. *Application fee:* $35.

Degree Requirements 128 total credit hours, 56 in nursing.

MASTER'S PROGRAM

Contact Dr. Barbara Bohny, Graduate Coordinator, 300 Pompton Road, Wayne, NJ 07470, 201-595-2452. *Fax:* 201-595-2668.

Areas of Study Clinical nurse specialist program in community health nursing; nursing administration; nursing education; nurse practitioner program in adult health.

Expenses *State resident tuition:* $163 per credit. *Nonresident tuition:* $242 per credit. *Full-time mandatory fees:* $24. *Part-time mandatory fees:* $24. *Books and supplies per academic year:* $200.

Financial Aid Graduate assistantships, employment opportunities.

RN TO MASTER'S PROGRAM (MS)

Applying *Required:* GRE General Test or Miller Analogies Test, TOEFL for nonnative speakers of English, bachelor's degree in nursing, minimum GPA of 3.0, RN license, 1 year of clinical experience, physical assessment course, statistics course, professional liability/malpractice insurance, essay, 3 letters of recommendation, transcript of college record. *Application deadlines:* 4/1 (fall), 9/15 (spring). *Application fee:* $35.

Degree Requirements 36–40 total credit hours dependent upon track, 30 in nursing, 6 in pathophysiology. Thesis required.

NEW MEXICO

NEW MEXICO STATE UNIVERSITY
Department of Nursing
Las Cruces, New Mexico

Programs • Generic Baccalaureate • RN Baccalaureate • MSN • Master's for Nurses with Non-Nursing Degrees

The University State-supported coed university. Part of New Mexico State University System. Founded: 1888. *Primary accreditation:* regional. *Setting:* 5,800-acre suburban campus. *Total enrollment:* 15,127.

The Department of Nursing Founded in 1972. *Nursing program faculty:* 15 (40% with doctorates).

Academic Facilities *Campus library:* 953,352 volumes (28,615 in health, 17,539 in nursing); 7,528 periodical subscriptions (619 health-care related). *Nursing school resources:* CAI, nursing audiovisuals, learning resource lab.

Student Life *Student services:* health clinic, child-care facilities, personal counseling, career counseling, institutionally sponsored work-study program, job placement, campus safety program, special assistance for disabled students. *International student services:* counseling/support, special assistance for nonnative speakers of English, ESL courses. *Nursing student activities:* student nurses association, honor society.

Calendar Semesters.

NURSING STUDENT PROFILE

Undergraduate **Enrollment:** 157
Women: 85%; **Men:** 15%; **Minority:** 40%; **Part-time:** 28%
Graduate **Enrollment:** 23
Women: 88%; **Men:** 12%; **Minority:** 28%; **Part-time:** 72%

BACCALAUREATE PROGRAMS

Contact Dr. Judith Karshmer, Academic Department Head, Department of Nursing, New Mexico State University, PO Box 30001/Department 3185, Las Cruces, NM 88003-8001, 505-646-3812. *Fax:* 505-646-2167. *E-mail:* jkarshme@nmsu.edu

Expenses *State resident tuition:* $1098 full-time, $92 per credit part-time. *Nonresident tuition:* $3576 full-time, $298 per credit part-time. *Full-time mandatory fees:* $105–$130. *Room and board:* $2548–$3680. *Room only:* $1650–$2042. *Books and supplies per academic year:* $500.

Financial Aid Institutionally sponsored need-based grants/scholarships, institutionally sponsored non-need grants/scholarships, Federal Direct Loans, Federal Nursing Student Loans, Federal Pell Grants, Federal Perkins Loans, Federal Supplemental Educational Opportunity Grants, Federal Work-Study, Federal Stafford Loans, state-sponsored nursing student loans. 70% of undergraduate students in nursing programs received some form of financial aid in 1995–96. *Application deadline:* 3/1.

GENERIC BACCALAUREATE PROGRAM (BSN)

Applying *Required:* ACT, TOEFL for nonnative speakers of English, minimum college GPA of 2.0, high school math, high school science, high school transcript, transcript of college record, either minimum high school GPA of 2.0 and ACT (minimum score of 18) or 2.5 GPA. 49 prerequisite credits must be completed before admission to the nursing program. *Options:* Advanced standing available through advanced placement exams. *Application deadlines:* 3/1 (fall), 9/1 (spring). *Application fee:* $10.

Degree Requirements 138 total credit hours, 77 in nursing. Completion of general education requirements and 55 upper division credits.

Distance learning Courses provided through video, computer-based media.

RN Baccalaureate Program (BSN)

Applying *Required:* ACT, TOEFL for nonnative speakers of English, minimum college GPA of 2.5, RN license, diploma or AD in nursing, transcript of college record. 29 prerequisite credits must be completed before admission to the nursing program. *Options:* Course work may be accelerated. *Application deadlines:* 7/31 (fall), 11/1 (spring), 5/1 (summer). *Application fee:* $10.

Degree Requirements 128 total credit hours, 35 in nursing. Completion of general education requirements and 55 upper division credits plus a minimum of 66 credits counting toward BSN.

Distance learning Courses provided through video, computer-based media.

MASTER'S PROGRAMS

Contact Dr. Judith Karshmer, Academic Department Head, Department of Nursing, New Mexico University, PO Box 30001/Dept. 3185, Las Cruces, NM 88003, 505-646-3812. *Fax:* 505-646-2167.

Areas of Study Clinical nurse specialist programs in community health nursing, medical-surgical nursing, psychiatric–mental health nursing; nursing administration; nursing education.

Expenses *State resident tuition:* $1176 full-time, $98 per credit part-time. *Nonresident tuition:* $3672 full-time, $306 per credit part-time. *Full-time mandatory fees:* $98. *Room and board:* $2548–$3680. *Room only:* $1650–$2042. *Books and supplies per academic year:* $500.

Financial Aid Graduate assistantships, nurse traineeships, Federal Nursing Student Loans, employment opportunities, institutionally sponsored non-need-based grants/scholarships, State sponsored Nursing Student Loans. *Application deadline:* 3/1.

MSN Program

Applying *Required:* TOEFL for nonnative speakers of English, bachelor's degree, minimum GPA of 3.0, RN license, statistics course, 3 letters of recommendation, transcript of college record. *Application deadlines:* 7/1 (fall), 11/1 (spring), 4/1 (summer).

Degree Requirements 42 total credit hours, 33 in nursing. Comprehensive exam.

Master's for Nurses with Non-Nursing Degrees Program (MSN)

Applying *Required:* TOEFL for nonnative speakers of English, bachelor's degree, minimum GPA of 3.0, RN license, statistics course, 3 letters of recommendation, transcript of college record. *Application deadlines:* 7/1 (fall), 11/1 (spring), 4/1 (summer).

Degree Requirements 42 total credit hours, 33 in nursing. Comprehensive exam.

Distance learning Courses provided through video, computer-based media.

UNIVERSITY OF NEW MEXICO
College of Nursing
Albuquerque, New Mexico

Programs • Generic Baccalaureate • RN Baccalaureate • Accelerated MSN • Master's for Nurses with Non-Nursing Degrees • MSN/Master's in Latin American Studies • Post-Master's • Continuing Education

The University State-supported coed university. Founded: 1889. *Primary accreditation:* regional. *Setting:* 625-acre urban campus. *Total enrollment:* 24,431.

The College of Nursing Founded in 1955. *Nursing program faculty:* 70 (44% with doctorates). *Off-campus program site:* 23 rural New Mexico locations.

Academic Facilities *Campus library:* 1.9 million volumes (154,264 in health, 3,084 in nursing); 21,910 periodical subscriptions (1,836 health-care related). *Nursing school resources:* CAI, computer lab, interactive nursing skills videos.

Student Life *Student services:* health clinic, child-care facilities, personal counseling, career counseling, institutionally sponsored work-study program, job placement, campus safety program, special assistance for disabled students. *International student services:* counseling/support, special assistance for nonnative speakers of English, ESL courses. *Nursing student activities:* Sigma Theta Tau, student nurses association, Phi Kappa Phi.

Calendar Semesters.

NURSING STUDENT PROFILE

Undergraduate **Enrollment:** 519
Women: 88%; **Men:** 12%; **Minority:** 29%; **International:** 0%; **Part-time:** 41%
Graduate **Enrollment:** 113
Women: 92%; **Men:** 8%; **Minority:** 15%; **International:** 0%; **Part-time:** 70%

BACCALAUREATE PROGRAMS

Contact Ms. Ann Marie Oechsler, Student Adviser, College of Nursing, University of New Mexico, Albuquerque, NM 87131-1061, 505-277-4223. *Fax:* 505-277-3970.

Expenses *State resident tuition:* $1035 full-time, $86 per credit hour part-time. *Nonresident tuition:* $3911 full-time, $86 per credit hour part-time. *Full-time mandatory fees:* $550–$650. *Room and board:* $4000–$4500. *Books and supplies per academic year:* ranges from $750 to $900.

Financial Aid Institutionally sponsored need-based grants/scholarships, institutionally sponsored non-need grants/scholarships, Federal Nursing Student Loans, Federal Supplemental Educational Opportunity Grants, Federal Work-Study. *Application deadline:* 3/1.

Generic Baccalaureate Program (BSN)

Applying *Required:* ACT, TOEFL for nonnative speakers of English, minimum high school GPA of 2.0, minimum college GPA of 2.5, transcript of college record. 30 prerequisite credits must be completed before admission to the nursing program. *Application deadline:* 6/15. *Application fee:* $15.

Degree Requirements 136 total credit hours, 70 in nursing.

Distance learning Courses provided through correspondence, video, computer-based media. Specific degree requirements include on-campus clinical applications course (2 credits).

RN Baccalaureate Program (BSN)

Applying *Required:* minimum college GPA of 2.5, RN license, diploma or AD in nursing, transcript of college record. 26 prerequisite credits must be completed before admission to the nursing program. *Options:* Advanced standing available through the following means: advanced placement exams, advanced placement without credit, credit by exam. Course work may be accelerated. May apply for transfer of up to 72 total credits. *Application deadlines:* 7/1 (fall), 11/1 (spring), 3/1 (summer). *Application fee:* $15.

Degree Requirements 136 total credit hours, 36 in nursing.

MASTER'S PROGRAMS

Contact Dr. Jeannette Cochran, Interim Associate Dean for Graduate Program, College of Nursing, University of New Mexico, Albuquerque, NM 87131-1061, 505-277-0849. *Fax:* 505-277-3970.

Areas of Study Clinical nurse specialist programs in community health nursing, gerontological nursing, medical-surgical nursing, parent-child nursing, psychiatric–mental health nursing; nurse midwifery; nursing administration; nurse practitioner programs in family health, primary care.

Expenses *State resident tuition:* $1123 full-time, $95 per credit hour part-time. *Nonresident tuition:* $4012 full-time, $334 per credit hour part-time. *Full-time mandatory fees:* $32. *Books and supplies per academic year:* ranges from $50 to $100.

Financial Aid Graduate assistantships, nurse traineeships, graduate tuition fellowships. *Application deadline:* 6/1.

Accelerated MSN Program

Applying *Required:* GRE General Test, bachelor's degree in nursing, minimum GPA of 3.0, RN license, 1 year of clinical experience, essay, 3 letters of recommendation, transcript of college record. *Application deadlines:* 6/15 (fall), 10/15 (spring), 2/1 (primary care). *Application fee:* $25.

Degree Requirements 39–50 total credit hours dependent upon track. 49-50 total credit hours for primary care track.

Master's for Nurses with Non-Nursing Degrees Program (MSN)

Applying *Required:* GRE General Test, NLN Community Health Baccalaureate Test, bachelor's degree, minimum GPA of 3.0, RN license, 1 year of

University of New Mexico (continued)
clinical experience, essay, 3 letters of recommendation, transcript of college record. *Application deadlines:* 6/15 (fall), 10/15 (spring), 2/1 (primary care). *Application fee:* $25.

Degree Requirements 39–50 total credit hours dependent upon track. 49-50 total credit hours for primary care track.

MSN/Master's in Latin American Studies Program

Applying *Required:* GRE General Test, bachelor's degree in nursing, bachelor's degree, minimum GPA of 3.0, RN license, 1 year of clinical experience, essay, 3 letters of recommendation, transcript of college record. *Application deadlines:* 6/15 (fall), 10/15 (spring), 2/1 (primary care). *Application fee:* $25.

Degree Requirements 42–50 total credit hours dependent upon track, 23 in Latin American studies. 49-50 total credit hours for primary care track.

Post-Master's Program

Applying *Required:* minimum GPA of 3.0, RN license, 1 year of clinical experience, essay, 3 letters of recommendation, transcript of college record. *Application deadlines:* 6/15 (fall), 10/15 (spring), 2/1 (primary care). *Application fee:* $25.

Degree Requirements 15–41 total credit hours dependent upon track.

CONTINUING EDUCATION PROGRAM

Contact Ms. Carol L'Esperance, Program Manager, Nursing Continuing Education, University of New Mexico, 1634 University Boulevard, NE, Albuquerque, NM 87131-4006, 505-277-3905. *Fax:* 505-277-8975.

NEW YORK

ADELPHI UNIVERSITY
School of Nursing
Garden City, New York

Programs • Generic Baccalaureate • RN Baccalaureate • MSN

The University Independent coed university. Founded: 1896. *Primary accreditation:* regional. *Setting:* 75-acre suburban campus. *Total enrollment:* 7,003.

The School of Nursing Founded in 1943. *Nursing program faculty:* 13 (92% with doctorates).

Academic Facilities *Campus library:* 458,595 volumes (18,669 in health, 2,111 in nursing); 1,651 periodical subscriptions (84 health-care related). *Nursing school resources:* CAI, computer lab, nursing audiovisuals, interactive nursing skills videos, learning resource lab.

Student Life *Student services:* health clinic, child-care facilities, personal counseling, career counseling, institutionally sponsored work-study program, job placement, special assistance for disabled students. *International student services:* counseling/support, special assistance for nonnative speakers of English, ESL courses. *Nursing student activities:* Sigma Theta Tau, nursing club, student nurses association.

Calendar Semesters.

NURSING STUDENT PROFILE

Undergraduate **Enrollment:** 370
Women: 90%; **Men:** 10%; **Minority:** 21%; **Part-time:** 34%
Graduate **Enrollment:** 347
Women: 98%; **Men:** 2%; **Minority:** 26%; **Part-time:** 98%

BACCALAUREATE PROGRAMS

Contact Esther Goodcuff, Associate Director of Admissions, Admissions and Recruitment, Levermore Hall, Garden City, NY 11530, 516-877-3050. *Fax:* 516-877-3039.

Expenses *Tuition:* $14,970 full-time, $440 per credit part-time. *Full-time mandatory fees:* $150–$400. *Part-time mandatory fees:* $150–$400. *Room only:* $3310–$4180. *Books and supplies per academic year:* ranges from $700 to $1000.

Financial Aid Institutionally sponsored need-based grants/scholarships, institutionally sponsored non-need grants/scholarships, Federal Nursing Student Loans, Federal Pell Grants, Federal Perkins Loans, Federal Work-Study. 58% of undergraduate students in nursing programs received some form of financial aid in 1995–96. *Application deadline:* 2/15.

Generic Baccalaureate Program (BS)

Applying *Required:* SAT I, ACT, TOEFL for nonnative speakers of English, minimum college GPA of 2.8, high school transcript, interview, written essay, transcript of college record. *Options:* May apply for transfer of up to 90 total credits. *Application deadline:* rolling. *Application fee:* $35.

Degree Requirements 123 total credit hours, 57 in nursing.

RN Baccalaureate Program (BS)

Applying *Required:* TOEFL for nonnative speakers of English, minimum college GPA of 2.5, RN license, diploma or AD in nursing, high school transcript, interview, letter of recommendation, written essay, transcript of college record. *Options:* Course work may be accelerated. May apply for transfer of up to 90 total credits. *Application deadline:* rolling. *Application fee:* $35.

Degree Requirements 123 total credit hours, 57 in nursing.

MASTER'S PROGRAM

Contact Esther Goodcuff, Associate Director of Admissions, Admissions and Recruitment, Levermore Hall, Garden City, NY 11530, 516-877-3050. *Fax:* 516-877-3039.

Areas of Study Clinical nurse specialist programs in adult health nursing, maternity-newborn nursing, pediatric nursing, perinatal nursing, psychiatric–mental health nursing; nursing administration; nursing education; nurse practitioner programs in adult health, child care/pediatrics, family health, gerontology, psychiatric–mental health.

Expenses *Tuition:* $14,850 full-time, $445 per credit part-time. *Full-time mandatory fees:* $50–$75. *Part-time mandatory fees:* $50–$75. *Room only:* $3310–$4180. *Books and supplies per academic year:* ranges from $700 to $1000.

Financial Aid Federal Nursing Student Loans, institutionally sponsored loans, employment opportunities. *Application deadline:* 2/15.

MSN Program

Applying *Required:* bachelor's degree in nursing, minimum GPA of 3.0, RN license, 1 year of clinical experience, statistics course, essay, interview, 2 letters of recommendation, transcript of college record. *Application deadline:* rolling. *Application fee:* $50.

Degree Requirements 43 total credit hours. Thesis required.

See full description on page 414.

COLLEGE OF MOUNT SAINT VINCENT
Department of Nursing
Riverdale, New York

Programs • Generic Baccalaureate • RN Baccalaureate • MS • Master's for Nurses with Non-Nursing Degrees • Continuing Education

The College Independent comprehensive coed institution. Founded: 1911. *Primary accreditation:* regional. *Setting:* 70-acre suburban campus. *Total enrollment:* 1,454.

The Department of Nursing Founded in 1974. *Nursing program faculty:* 17 (59% with doctorates). *Off-campus program sites:* Bronx, Manhattan, Staten Island.

▶ ***NOTEWORTHY***

The College of Mount Saint Vincent, a 4-year, coeducational liberal arts college, is a private, independent institution with an enrollment of approximately 1,500 full-time and part-time students representing diverse backgrounds. The Department of Nursing offers baccalaureate programs for adult and traditional students, a flexible program for registered nurses, and an RN to MS program. Graduate students may prepare for advanced practice in any one of 4 areas of concentration: adult nurse practitioner (including post-master's advanced certificate), administration, or clinical specialist in addictions nursing or nursing of the adult and aged. Graduate and undergraduate students may enroll in interdisciplinary courses with health-care and business majors.

Academic Facilities *Campus library:* 149,748 volumes (883 in health, 5,304 in nursing); 620 periodical subscriptions. *Nursing school resources:* CAI, computer lab, nursing audiovisuals, interactive nursing skills videos, learning resource lab.

Student Life *Student services:* health clinic, personal counseling, career counseling, institutionally sponsored work-study program, job placement. *International student services:* counseling/support. *Nursing student activities:* Sigma Theta Tau, nursing club, student nurses association.

Calendar Semesters.

NURSING STUDENT PROFILE

Undergraduate **Enrollment:** 455
Women: 95%; **Men:** 5%; **Minority:** 43%; **International:** 2%; **Part-time:** 28%
Graduate **Enrollment:** 186
Women: 95%; **Men:** 5%; **Minority:** 50%; **International:** 5%; **Part-time:** 96%

BACCALAUREATE PROGRAMS

Contact Dr. Carol Vicino, Chairperson, Baccalaureate Program, Department of Nursing, College of Mount Saint Vincent, 6301 Riverdale Avenue, Riverdale, NY 10471-1093, 718-405-3362. *Fax:* 718-601-6392.

Expenses *Tuition:* $13,000 full-time, $380 per credit hour part-time. *Full-time mandatory fees:* $125–$250. *Room and board:* $6250. *Books and supplies per academic year:* $500.

Financial Aid Institutionally sponsored need-based grants/scholarships, institutionally sponsored non-need grants/scholarships, Federal Direct Loans, Federal Nursing Student Loans, Federal Pell Grants, Federal Perkins Loans, Federal Work-Study, New York State Tuition Assistance Program (TAP), Veterans Administration Educational Benefits.

Generic Baccalaureate Program (BS)

Applying *Required:* SAT I or ACT, minimum high school GPA of 2.0, minimum college GPA of 2.0, 3 years of high school math, 3 years of high school science, high school chemistry, high school biology, high school transcript. *Options:* May apply for transfer of up to 65–75 total credits. *Application deadlines:* 8/15 (fall), 12/15 (spring). *Application fee:* $25.

Degree Requirements 126 total credit hours, 46 in nursing.

RN Baccalaureate Program (BS)

Applying *Required:* NLN Mobility Profile II for diploma graduates, minimum college GPA of 2.5, RN license, diploma or AD in nursing, transcript of college record. *Options:* May apply for transfer of up to 75 total credits. *Application deadlines:* 8/15 (fall), 12/15 (spring). *Application fee:* $25.

Degree Requirements 126 total credit hours, 19 in nursing.

MASTER'S PROGRAMS

Contact Dr. Kem Louie, Chairperson, Graduate Program, Department of Nursing, College of Mount Saint Vincent, 6301 Riverdale Avenue, Riverdale, NY 10471-1093, 718-405-3354. *Fax:* 718-601-6392.

Areas of Study Clinical nurse specialist programs in adult health nursing, gerontological nursing, addictions nursing; nursing administration; nurse practitioner program in adult health.

Expenses *Tuition:* $7920 full-time, $440 per credit part-time. *Full-time mandatory fees:* $100. *Room and board:* $6250. *Books and supplies per academic year:* ranges from $400 to $500.

Financial Aid Graduate assistantships, nurse traineeships, employment opportunities. 5% of master's level students in nursing programs received some form of financial aid in 1995-96.

MS Program

Applying *Required:* English writing exam, bachelor's degree in nursing, minimum GPA of 3.0, RN license, physical assessment course, statistics course, professional liability/malpractice insurance, interview, 2 letters of recommendation, transcript of college record, computer literacy. *Application deadlines:* 6/15 (fall), 12/1 (spring). *Application fee:* $50.

Degree Requirements 42 total credit hours, 27–42 in nursing. Project, 9 hours in business for nurse administration students.

Master's for Nurses with Non-Nursing Degrees Program (MS)

Applying *Required:* nursing validation exam, English writing exam, NLN achievement test for baccalaureate nurses, bachelor's degree, minimum GPA of 3.0, RN license, statistics course, professional liability/malpractice insurance, essay, interview, 2 letters of recommendation, transcript of college record, BA or BS must be in health-related field, computer literacy, transition course. *Application deadlines:* 6/15 (fall), 12/1 (spring). *Application fee:* $50.

Degree Requirements 48 total credit hours, 27–48 in nursing. Project, 9 hours in business for nurse administration students.

CONTINUING EDUCATION PROGRAM

Contact Ms. Lisa Fermicoli, Director, Department of Adult and Continuing Education, College of Mount Saint Vincent, 6301 Riverdale Avenue, Riverdale, NY 10471-1093, 718-405-3319. *Fax:* 718-601-6392.

COLLEGE OF NEW ROCHELLE
School of Nursing
New Rochelle, New York

Programs • Generic Baccalaureate • Accelerated RN Baccalaureate • Baccalaureate for Second Degree • Accelerated Baccalaureate for Second Degree • MS • Post-Master's • Continuing Education

The College Independent comprehensive primarily women's institution. Founded: 1904. *Primary accreditation:* regional. *Setting:* 20-acre suburban campus. *Total enrollment:* 2,612.

The School of Nursing Founded in 1976. *Nursing program faculty:* 46 (35% with doctorates).

► ***NOTEWORTHY***

The College of New Rochelle School of Nursing, located in the New York metropolitan area, offers 4 programs: generic baccalaureate, RN to BSN, BSN for non-nursing degree graduates, and MS in nursing, including family nurse practitioner, acute-care nurse practitioner, holistic clinical specialist, and administrator. Offering one of the first graduate holistic programs in the country, the School of Nursing integrates holistic nursing concepts throughout all curricula. Clinical learning takes place in acute and community-based health-care facilities throughout metropolitan New York. The Learning Center for Nursing, an on-campus multipurpose resource, consists of nursing laboratories, a computer center, multimedia laboratory, and interactive instruction area.

Academic Facilities *Campus library:* 189,800 volumes (5,550 in health, 5,900 in nursing); 1,441 periodical subscriptions (193 health-care related). *Nursing school resources:* CAI, computer lab, nursing audiovisuals, interactive nursing skills videos, learning resource lab, CINAHL on CD-ROM, COMAS on-line.

Student Life *Student services:* health clinic, personal counseling, career counseling, institutionally sponsored work-study program, job placement, campus safety program, special assistance for disabled students. *International student services:* counseling/support, ESL courses. *Nursing student activities:* Sigma Theta Tau, nursing club, student nurses association, Nursing Honors Program, Nursing Mentor Program.

Calendar Semesters.

NURSING STUDENT PROFILE

Undergraduate **Enrollment:** 535
Women: 95%; **Men:** 5%; **Minority:** 59%; **International:** 1%; **Part-time:** 59%
Graduate **Enrollment:** 120
Women: 99%; **Men:** 1%; **Minority:** 40%; **International:** 0%; **Part-time:** 97%

BACCALAUREATE PROGRAMS

Contact Dr. Geraldine Valencia-Go, Chairperson, School of Nursing, College of New Rochelle, New Rochelle, NY 10805-2308, 800-948-4766. *Fax:* 914-654-5994.

Expenses *Tuition:* $11,000 full-time, $370 per credit part-time. *Full-time mandatory fees:* $155–$365. *Room and board:* $5550–$6350. *Books and supplies per academic year:* ranges from $500 to $600.

Financial Aid Institutionally sponsored need-based grants/scholarships, institutionally sponsored non-need grants/scholarships, Federal Direct Loans, Federal Nursing Student Loans, Federal Pell Grants, Federal Perkins Loans, Federal Supplemental Educational Opportunity Grants, Federal Work-Study. 80% of undergraduate students in nursing programs received some form of financial aid in 1995–96.

College of New Rochelle (continued)

Generic Baccalaureate Program (BSN)

Applying *Required:* SAT I, ACT, TOEFL for nonnative speakers of English, minimum college GPA of 2.0, 3 years of high school math, 3 years of high school science, high school chemistry, high school biology, high school transcript, 2 letters of recommendation, written essay. *Options:* Advanced standing available through advanced placement exams. Course work may be accelerated. May apply for transfer of up to 60 total credits. *Application deadline:* rolling. *Application fee:* $20.

Degree Requirements 120 total credit hours, 61 in nursing. CPR certification, child abuse certification, infection control.

Accelerated RN Baccalaureate Program (BSN)

Applying *Required:* RN license, diploma or AD in nursing, high school transcript, interview, transcript of college record, employer recommendation. *Options:* Advanced standing available through credit by exam. Course work may be accelerated. May apply for transfer of up to 90 total credits. *Application deadline:* rolling. *Application fee:* $15.

Degree Requirements 120 total credit hours, 61 in nursing.

Baccalaureate for Second Degree Program (BSN)

Applying *Required:* minimum high school GPA of 2.5, interview, transcript of college record, associate or baccalaureate degree. 59 prerequisite credits must be completed before admission to the nursing program. *Options:* Advanced standing available through credit by exam. Course work may be accelerated. May apply for transfer of up to 59 total credits. *Application deadline:* rolling. *Application fee:* $15.

Degree Requirements 120 total credit hours, 61 in nursing. CPR certification, child abuse certification, infection control.

Accelerated Baccalaureate for Second Degree Program (BSN)

Applying *Required:* minimum college GPA of 2.5, associate or baccalaureate degree. 59 prerequisite credits must be completed before admission to the nursing program. *Options:* Advanced standing available through credit by exam. Course work may be accelerated. May apply for transfer of up to 59 total credits. *Application deadline:* rolling. *Application fee:* $15.

Degree Requirements 120 total credit hours, 61 in nursing. CPR certification, child abuse certification, infection control.

MASTER'S PROGRAMS

Contact Dr. Mary N. Moore, Chairperson, School of Nursing, College of New Rochelle, New Rochelle, NY 10805-2308, 800-948-4766. *Fax:* 914-654-5994.

Areas of Study Clinical nurse specialist program in holistic nursing; nursing administration; nurse practitioner programs in acute care, family health.

Expenses *Tuition:* $9120 full-time, $380 per credit part-time. *Books and supplies per academic year:* ranges from $800 to $1000.

Financial Aid Nurse traineeships. 3% of master's level students in nursing programs received some form of financial aid in 1995-96. *Application deadline:* 12/17.

MS Program

Applying *Required:* GRE General Test, Miller Analogies Test, TOEFL for nonnative speakers of English, bachelor's degree in nursing, minimum GPA of 3.0, RN license, 2 years of clinical experience, physical assessment course, statistics course, professional liability/malpractice insurance, essay, interview, 2 letters of recommendation, transcript of college record, resume. *Application deadline:* rolling. *Application fee:* $30.

Degree Requirements 45 total credit hours, 45 in nursing. Project.

Post-Master's Program

Applying *Required:* TOEFL for nonnative speakers of English, minimum GPA of 3.0, RN license, 2 years of clinical experience, physical assessment course, statistics course, professional liability/malpractice insurance, transcript of college record, college health service clearance, New York RN license, resume for HIV/AIDS nursing certificate, statistics, physical assessment, BSN for nurse practitioner track. *Application deadline:* rolling. *Application fee:* $30.

Degree Requirements 17–31 total credit hours dependent upon track, 17–31 in nursing.

CONTINUING EDUCATION PROGRAM

Contact Dr. Connie Vance, Dean, School of Nursing, College of New Rochelle, New Rochelle, NY 10805-2308, 800-948-4766. *Fax:* 914-654-5994. *E-mail:* cvancern@aol.com

COLLEGE OF STATEN ISLAND OF THE CITY UNIVERSITY OF NEW YORK

Department of Nursing
Staten Island, New York

Programs • RN Baccalaureate • Continuing Education

The University State and locally supported comprehensive coed institution. Part of City University of New York System. Founded: 1955. *Primary accreditation:* regional. *Setting:* 204-acre urban campus. *Total enrollment:* 12,196.

The Department of Nursing Founded in 1965. *Nursing program faculty:* 20 (50% with doctorates).

Academic Facilities *Campus library:* 50,000 volumes (1,500 in health, 1,000 in nursing); 400 periodical subscriptions (75 health-care related). *Nursing school resources:* CAI, computer lab, nursing audiovisuals, learning resource lab.

Student Life *Student services:* health clinic, child-care facilities, personal counseling, career counseling, institutionally sponsored work-study program, job placement, campus safety program, special assistance for disabled students. *International student services:* counseling/support, special assistance for nonnative speakers of English, ESL courses. *Nursing student activities:* Sigma Theta Tau, nursing club, student nurses association.

Calendar Semesters.

NURSING STUDENT PROFILE

Undergraduate **Enrollment:** 400
Women: 85%; **Men:** 15%; **Minority:** 20%; **International:** 10%; **Part-time:** 10%

BACCALAUREATE PROGRAM

Contact Dr. Louise M. Malarkey, Chair, Room 5S-213, Marcus Hall, Department of Nursing, College of Staten Island of the City University of New York, 2800 Victory Boulevard, Staten Island, NY 10314, 718-982-3810. *Fax:* 718-982-3813.

Expenses *State resident tuition:* $2950 full-time, $125 per credit part-time. *Nonresident tuition:* $6550 full-time, $275 per credit part-time. *Full-time mandatory fees:* $100. *Books and supplies per academic year:* $500.

Financial Aid Institutionally sponsored need-based grants/scholarships, institutionally sponsored non-need grants/scholarships, Federal Direct Loans, Federal Nursing Student Loans, Federal Pell Grants, Federal Perkins Loans, Federal Supplemental Educational Opportunity Grants, Federal Work-Study.

RN Baccalaureate Program (BS)

Applying *Required:* TOEFL for nonnative speakers of English, minimum college GPA of 2.0, RN license, diploma or AD in nursing, high school transcript, transcript of college record. *Options:* Advanced standing available through the following means: advanced placement exams, credit by exam. May apply for transfer of up to 90 total credits. *Application deadline:* rolling. *Application fee:* $20.

Degree Requirements 120 total credit hours, 33 in nursing. 25 nursing credits from AAS or diploma education.

CONTINUING EDUCATION PROGRAM

Contact Patricia Miele, Continuing Education Officer, Continuing Education Department 2A-201, College of Staten Island of the City University of New York, 2800 Victory Boulevard, Staten Island, NY 10314, 718-982-2182.

COLUMBIA UNIVERSITY

School of Nursing
New York, New York

Programs • Accelerated RN Baccalaureate • Baccalaureate for Second Degree • MSN • MS/MBA • MS/MPH • DNSc • Continuing Education

The University Independent coed university. Founded: 1754. *Primary accreditation:* regional. *Total enrollment:* 19,000.

The School of Nursing Founded in 1892. *Nursing program faculty:* 190 (33% with doctorates). *Off-campus program site:* Bronx.

▶ *NOTEWORTHY*

Columbia University School of Nursing was founded in 1892 with Anna C. Maxwell as its first director. From its inception, the mission of the School has been to prepare clinically excellent nursing practitioners, clinical nurse specialists, and scholars. The School of Nursing was the first in the country to award a master's degree in a clinical nursing specialty (1956). The emphasis on clinical scholarship at Columbia University is particularly appropriate because of the interdisciplinary collaboration of the School of Nursing with the other professional schools within its environs. The graduates of the School are one of its major strengths and are recruited for leadership positions in practice, education, and management.

Academic Facilities *Campus library:* 469,000 volumes (469,000 in health); 4,352 periodical subscriptions (4,352 health-care related). *Nursing school resources:* computer lab, nursing audiovisuals, learning resource lab.

Student Life *Student services:* health clinic, child-care facilities, personal counseling, career counseling, institutionally sponsored work-study program, campus safety program, special assistance for disabled students. *Nursing student activities:* Sigma Theta Tau.

Calendar Semesters.

NURSING STUDENT PROFILE

Undergraduate **Enrollment:** 160
Women: 91%; **Men:** 9%; **Minority:** 18%; **International:** 1%; **Part-time:** 41%

Graduate **Enrollment:** 459
Women: 94%; **Men:** 6%; **Minority:** 30%; **International:** 1%; **Part-time:** 87%

BACCALAUREATE PROGRAMS

Contact Dr. Theresa Doddato, Associate Dean, School of Nursing, Columbia University, 630 West 168th Street, New York, NY 10032, 212-305-5756. *Fax:* 212-305-6937. *E-mail:* tmd3@columbia.edu

Expenses *Tuition:* $28,305 full-time, $629 per credit part-time. *Full-time mandatory fees:* $1596. *Part-time mandatory fees:* $150. *Room and board:* $11,550–$13,043. *Room only:* $5472–$11,400. *Books and supplies per academic year:* $1800.

Financial Aid Institutionally sponsored need-based grants/scholarships, Federal Nursing Student Loans, Federal Perkins Loans, Federal Work-Study. 87% of undergraduate students in nursing programs received some form of financial aid in 1995–96. *Application deadline:* 3/15.

Accelerated RN Baccalaureate Program (BS)

Applying *Required:* TOEFL for nonnative speakers of English, GRE, minimum college GPA of 3.0, RN license, diploma or AD in nursing, interview, 3 letters of recommendation, written essay, transcript of college record. *Options:* Advanced standing available through the following means: advanced placement exams, credit by exam. May apply for transfer of up to 0 total credits. *Application deadlines:* 4/1 (fall), 10/1 (spring), 2/1 (summer). *Application fee:* $60.

Degree Requirements 60 total credit hours, 60 in nursing. NLN Mobility Profile II exam.

Baccalaureate for Second Degree Program (BSN)

Applying *Required:* GRE, minimum college GPA of 3.0, interview, 3 letters of recommendation, written essay, transcript of college record, baccalaureate degree. 12 prerequisite credits must be completed before admission to the nursing program. *Options:* Advanced standing available through advanced placement exams. *Application deadline:* rolling. *Application fee:* $60.

Degree Requirements 60 total credit hours, 60 in nursing.

MASTER'S PROGRAMS

Contact Dr. Theresa Doddato, Associate Dean, School of Nursing, Columbia University, 630 West 168th Street, New York, NY 10032, 212-305-5756. *Fax:* 212-305-6937. *E-mail:* tmd3@columbia.edu

Areas of Study Clinical nurse specialist programs in critical care nursing, oncology nursing, psychiatric–mental health nursing; nurse anesthesia; nurse midwifery; nurse practitioner programs in adult health, child care/pediatrics, emergency care, family health, gerontology, women's health.

Expenses *Tuition:* $15,096+ full-time, $629 per credit part-time. *Full-time mandatory fees:* $1596. *Part-time mandatory fees:* $150. *Room and board:* $11,500–$13,043. *Room only:* $5472–$11,400. *Books and supplies per academic year:* $1600.

Financial Aid Graduate assistantships, nurse traineeships, Federal Nursing Student Loans, institutionally sponsored loans, employment opportunities, institutionally sponsored need-based grants/scholarships. 27% of master's level students in nursing programs received some form of financial aid in 1995-96. *Application deadline:* 3/15.

MSN Program

Applying *Required:* GRE General Test or Miller Analogies Test, bachelor's degree in nursing, minimum GPA of 3.0, RN license, 1 year of clinical experience, physical assessment course, statistics course, professional liability/malpractice insurance, essay, interview, 3 letters of recommendation, transcript of college record. *Application deadlines:* 4/1 (fall), 10/1 (spring), 2/1 (summer). *Application fee:* $60.

Degree Requirements 45 total credit hours, 45 in nursing.

MS/MBA Program

Applying *Required:* GMAT, bachelor's degree in nursing, minimum GPA of 3.0, RN license, 1 year of clinical experience, physical assessment course, statistics course, professional liability/malpractice insurance, essay, interview, 3 letters of recommendation, transcript of college record. *Application deadlines:* 4/1 (fall), 10/1 (spring), 2/1 (summer). *Application fee:* $60.

MS/MPH Program

Applying *Required:* GRE General Test, bachelor's degree in nursing, minimum GPA of 3.0, RN license, 1 year of clinical experience, physical assessment course, statistics course, professional liability/malpractice insurance, essay, interview, 3 letters of recommendation, transcript of college record. *Application deadlines:* 4/1 (fall), 10/1 (spring), 2/1 (summer). *Application fee:* $60.

DOCTORAL PROGRAM

Contact Dr. Theresa Doddato, Associate Dean, School of Nursing, Columbia University, 630 West 168th Street, New York, NY 10032, 212-305-5756. *Fax:* 212-305-6937. *E-mail:* tmd3@columbia.edu

Areas of Study Health policy.

Expenses *Tuition:* $20,472+ full-time, $853 per credit part-time. *Full-time mandatory fees:* $300. *Part-time mandatory fees:* $150.

Financial Aid Nurse traineeships, fellowships, grants, opportunities for employment. *Application deadline:* 3/1.

DNSc Program

Applying *Required:* GRE General Test, master's degree in nursing, master's degree, year of clinical experience, scholarly paper, statistics course, interview, 3 letters of recommendation, vitae, writing sample, competitive review by faculty committee. *Application deadlines:* 2/1 (fall), 11/1 (spring). *Application fee:* $100.

Degree Requirements 90 total credit hours; dissertation; written exam; defense of dissertation; residency.

CONTINUING EDUCATION PROGRAM

Contact Dr. M. Mauley, Program Director, School of Nursing, Columbia University, 630 West 168th Street, New York, NY 10032, 212-305-3414. *Fax:* 212-305-6937.

See full description on page 430.

DAEMEN COLLEGE
Nursing Department
Amherst, New York

Program • RN Baccalaureate

The College Independent comprehensive coed institution. Founded: 1947. *Primary accreditation:* regional. *Setting:* 37-acre suburban campus. *Total enrollment:* 1,938.

The Nursing Department Founded in 1979. *Nursing program faculty:* 15 (80% with doctorates). *Off-campus program sites:* Olean, Batavia, Jamestown.

▶ ***NOTEWORTHY***

Daemen College's BS in nursing program for RNs is ideal for registered nurses interested in personal development, career mobility, or attending graduate school. Daemen's upper-division BS nursing program offers full- or part-time study, liberal credit transfer policies, individualized attention, and tuition grants. For registered nurses these grants can underwrite up to 50% of tuition and fees. The grants are not based on financial need and are guaranteed through completion of the program. Daemen has accreditation from the National League for Nursing for its unique program for RNs. More information can be obtained by calling the Nursing Department at 716-839-8387.

Academic Facilities *Campus library:* 140,000 volumes (10,000 in health, 4,000 in nursing); 940 periodical subscriptions (250 health-care related). *Nursing school resources:* CAI, computer lab, nursing audiovisuals.

Student Life *Student services:* personal counseling, career counseling, institutionally sponsored work-study program, job placement, campus safety program, special assistance for disabled students. *Nursing student activities:* Nursing Honor Society.

Calendar Semesters.

NURSING STUDENT PROFILE

Undergraduate **Enrollment:** 400
Women: 96%; **Men:** 4%; **Minority:** 3%; **International:** 2%; **Part-time:** 90%

BACCALAUREATE PROGRAM

Contact Dr. Mary Lou Rusin, Professor and Chair, Nursing Department, Daemen College, 4380 Main Street, Amherst, NY 14226, 716-839-8387. *Fax:* 716-839-8516. *E-mail:* mrusin@daemen.edu

Expenses *Tuition:* $9950 full-time, $335 per credit hour part-time. *Full-time mandatory fees:* $70–$200. *Part-time mandatory fees:* $2–$68. *Room and board:* $5200. *Books and supplies per academic year:* $300.

Financial Aid Institutionally sponsored need-based grants/scholarships, institutionally sponsored non-need grants/scholarships, Federal Supplemental Educational Opportunity Grants, Federal Work-Study. 100% of undergraduate students in nursing programs received some form of financial aid in 1995–96.

RN Baccalaureate Program (BS)

Applying *Required:* minimum college GPA of 2.0, RN license, diploma or AD in nursing, high school transcript, transcript of college record. 56 prerequisite credits must be completed before admission to the nursing program. *Options:* Course work may be accelerated. *Application deadline:* rolling.

Degree Requirements 120 total credit hours, 45 in nursing.

DOMINICAN COLLEGE OF BLAUVELT
Division of Nursing
Orangeburg, New York

Programs • Generic Baccalaureate • RN Baccalaureate • Baccalaureate for Second Degree • LPN to Baccalaureate

The College Independent comprehensive coed institution. Founded: 1952. *Primary accreditation:* regional. *Setting:* 14-acre suburban campus. *Total enrollment:* 1,737.

The Division of Nursing Founded in 1973.

Academic Facilities *Campus library:* 103,000 volumes (5,650 in health); 670 periodical subscriptions (235 health-care related).

Calendar Semesters.

BACCALAUREATE PROGRAMS

Contact Director of Admissions, Division of Nursing, Dominican College of Blauvelt, 470 Western Highway, Orangeburg, NY 10962, 914-359-7800 Ext. 271. *Fax:* 914-359-2313.

Expenses *Tuition:* $9750 full-time, $325 per semester hour part-time. *Room and board:* $6000.

Financial Aid Institutionally sponsored need-based grants/scholarships, institutionally sponsored non-need grants/scholarships, Federal Nursing Student Loans, Federal Supplemental Educational Opportunity Grants, Federal Work-Study, New York State Tuition Assistance Program (TAP).

Generic Baccalaureate Program (BSN)

Applying *Required:* SAT I or ACT, English, math placement tests, minimum college GPA of 2.5, high school transcript, written essay.

Degree Requirements 123 total credit hours.

RN Baccalaureate Program (BSN)

Applying *Required:* English, math placement tests; NLN Mobility Profile II, minimum college GPA of 2.5, written essay.

Degree Requirements 123 total credit hours.

Baccalaureate for Second Degree Program (BSN)

Applying *Required:* English placement test, minimum college GPA of 2.5, written essay, transcript of college record.

Degree Requirements 123 total credit hours.

LPN to Baccalaureate Program (BSN)

Applying *Required:* English, math placement tests, minimum college GPA of 2.5, written essay. *Options:* Advanced standing available through credit by exam.

Degree Requirements 123 total credit hours.

See full description on page 438.

D'YOUVILLE COLLEGE
Division of Nursing
Buffalo, New York

Programs • Generic Baccalaureate • RN Baccalaureate • BSN to Master's • RN to Master's • Continuing Education

The College Independent comprehensive coed institution. Founded: 1908. *Primary accreditation:* regional. *Setting:* 7-acre urban campus. *Total enrollment:* 1,905.

The Division of Nursing Founded in 1942. *Nursing program faculty:* 20 (50% with doctorates).

Academic Facilities *Campus library:* 98,336 volumes (9,691 in health, 2,931 in nursing); 720 periodical subscriptions (1,228 health-care related). *Nursing school resources:* CAI, computer lab, nursing audiovisuals, interactive nursing skills videos, learning resource lab.

Student Life *Student services:* health clinic, personal counseling, career counseling, institutionally sponsored work-study program, job placement, campus safety program, special assistance for disabled students. *International student services:* counseling/support, ESL courses, Multicultural Student Office. *Nursing student activities:* Sigma Theta Tau, student nurses association.

Calendar Semesters.

NURSING STUDENT PROFILE

Undergraduate **Enrollment:** 229
Women: 86%; **Men:** 14%; **Minority:** 19%; **International:** 18%; **Part-time:** 36%
Graduate **Enrollment:** 171
Women: 97%; **Men:** 3%; **Minority:** 4%; **International:** 79%; **Part-time:** 87%

BACCALAUREATE PROGRAMS

Contact Mr. Ron Dannecker, Director of Admissions, D'Youville College, 320 Porter Avenue, Buffalo, NY 14201, 716-881-7600. *Fax:* 716-881-7790.

Expenses *Tuition:* $9510 full-time, ranges from $260 to $285 per credit part-time. *Full-time mandatory fees:* $340–$500. *Room and board:* $2370. *Books and supplies per academic year:* ranges from $600 to $700.

Financial Aid Institutionally sponsored need-based grants/scholarships, institutionally sponsored non-need grants/scholarships, Federal Nursing

Student Loans, Federal Pell Grants, Federal Supplemental Educational Opportunity Grants, Federal Work-Study, Federal Stafford Loans. 71% of undergraduate students in nursing programs received some form of financial aid in 1995–96. *Application deadline:* 4/15.

Generic Baccalaureate Program (BS)

Applying *Required:* SAT I, ACT, TOEFL for nonnative speakers of English, Skills Assessment Inventory, minimum high school GPA of 2.67, minimum college GPA of 2.5, 2 years of high school math, 3 years of high school science, high school chemistry, high school biology, high school transcript, transcript of college record, high school class rank: top 50%. *Options:* Advanced standing available through the following means: advanced placement exams, credit by exam. Course work may be accelerated. May apply for transfer of up to 65 total credits. *Application deadline:* rolling. *Application fee:* $25.

Degree Requirements 129 total credit hours, 48 in nursing.

RN Baccalaureate Program (BS)

Applying *Required:* TOEFL for nonnative speakers of English, minimum college GPA of 2.0, RN license, diploma or AD in nursing, 3 letters of recommendation, transcript of college record, minimum 1 year of work experience. *Options:* Advanced standing available through credit by exam. Course work may be accelerated. May apply for transfer of up to 65 total credits. *Application deadline:* rolling. *Application fee:* $25.

Degree Requirements 121 total credit hours, 40 in nursing.

MASTER'S PROGRAMS

Contact Dr. Carol Gutt, Director, Graduate Program in Nursing, Department of Nursing, D'Youville College, 320 Porter Avenue, Buffalo, NY 14201, 716-881-7783. *Fax:* 716-881-7760.

Areas of Study Clinical nurse specialist program in community health nursing.

Expenses *Tuition:* $5706 full-time, $317 per credit hour part-time. *Full-time mandatory fees:* $340–$500. *Room and board:* $2235. *Books and supplies per academic year:* ranges from $600 to $700.

Financial Aid Nurse traineeships, Federal Nursing Student Loans, institutionally sponsored need-based grants/scholarships, institutionally sponsored non-need-based grants/scholarships. *Application deadline:* 4/15.

BSN to Master's Program (MS)

Applying *Required:* bachelor's degree in nursing, minimum GPA of 3.0, RN license, statistics course, essay, interview, transcript of college record, computer course or equivalent. *Application deadline:* rolling. *Application fee:* $25.

Degree Requirements 39–42 total credit hours dependent upon track, 12–21 in nursing, 21–27 in theory/research, teaching, management, and addictions. Completion of publishable paper, service on a community board. Thesis required.

RN to Master's Program (MS)

Applying *Required:* minimum GPA of 2.5, RN license, 1 year of clinical experience, 3 letters of recommendation, transcript of college record, AD in nursing. *Application deadline:* rolling. *Application fee:* $20.

Degree Requirements 151–154 total credit hours dependent upon track, 43 in nursing, 108–111 in community addictions or management or teaching, theory/research. Completion of publishable paper, service on a community board, statistics, computer science. Thesis required.

CONTINUING EDUCATION PROGRAM

Contact Carol Coppola, Director, Continuing Education, D'Youville College, 320 Porter Avenue, Buffalo, NY 14201-1084, 716-881-7683. *Fax:* 716-881-7760.

ELMIRA COLLEGE
Nurse Education Program
Elmira, New York

Programs • Generic Baccalaureate • RN Baccalaureate • Accelerated RN Baccalaureate • Continuing Education

The College Independent 4-year coed college. Founded: 1855. *Primary accreditation:* regional. *Setting:* 42-acre small-town campus. *Total enrollment:* 1,104.

The Nurse Education Program Founded in 1972. *Nursing program faculty:* 5 (20% with doctorates).

▶ *NOTEWORTHY*

Many features distinguish the Elmira College nursing program from other nursing programs. Students in the Elmira College nursing program begin clinical experiences of 6 to 17 hours per week in the sophomore year. Students are admitted directly to the nursing program and do not have to qualify again. Clinical nursing experiences take place in a variety of community-based health-care agencies as well as in acute-care hospitals. Curriculum emphasis is on health maintenance within the community. Extracurricular activities and intercollegiate athletic participation are encouraged by the nursing faculty. A strong liberal arts component and a required community service experience ensure a well-rounded graduate.

Academic Facilities *Campus library:* 383,000 volumes (7,461 in health, 5,200 in nursing); 852 periodical subscriptions (72 health-care related). *Nursing school resources:* CAI, computer lab, nursing audiovisuals, interactive nursing skills videos, learning resource lab.

Student Life *Student services:* health clinic, personal counseling, career counseling, institutionally sponsored work-study program, job placement, campus safety program. *International student services:* counseling/support, special assistance for nonnative speakers of English, ESL courses. *Nursing student activities:* nursing club, student nurses association, Nursing Honor Society.

Calendar Modified 4-4-1.

NURSING STUDENT PROFILE

Undergraduate **Enrollment:** 175
Women: 90%; **Men:** 10%; **Minority:** 4%; **International:** 1%; **Part-time:** 52%

BACCALAUREATE PROGRAMS

Contact Mr. William Neal, Dean of Admissions, Elmira College, Elmira, NY 14901, 607-735-1724. *Fax:* 607-735-1718.

Expenses *Tuition:* $17,550 per academic year. *Full-time mandatory fees:* $400. *Room and board:* $5880. *Books and supplies per academic year:* $1000.

Financial Aid Institutionally sponsored need-based grants/scholarships, institutionally sponsored non-need grants/scholarships, Federal Pell Grants, Federal Perkins Loans, Federal Supplemental Educational Opportunity Grants, Federal Work-Study. 48% of undergraduate students in nursing programs received some form of financial aid in 1995–96. *Application deadline:* 3/1.

Generic Baccalaureate Program (BS)

Applying *Required:* SAT I, ACT, TOEFL for nonnative speakers of English, 3 years of high school math, 3 years of high school science, high school chemistry, high school biology, high school transcript, 2 letters of recommendation, written essay, transcript of college record. *Options:* Advanced standing available through the following means: advanced placement exams, credit by exam. Course work may be accelerated. May apply for transfer of up to 90 total credits. *Application deadline:* rolling. *Application fee:* $40.

Degree Requirements 120 total credit hours, 44 in nursing.

RN Baccalaureate Program (BS)

Applying *Required:* minimum college GPA of 2.0, interview, transcript of college record. *Options:* Advanced standing available through the following means: advanced placement exams, credit by exam. Course work may be accelerated. May apply for transfer of up to 90 total credits. *Application deadline:* rolling. *Application fee:* $40.

Degree Requirements 120 total credit hours, 44 in nursing.

Accelerated RN Baccalaureate Program (BS)

Applying *Required:* minimum college GPA of 2.0, RN license, diploma or AD in nursing, interview, transcript of college record. *Application deadline:* rolling. *Application fee:* $40.

Degree Requirements 120 total credit hours, 44 in nursing.

CONTINUING EDUCATION PROGRAM

Contact Dr. Anita B. Ogden, Director of Nurse Education and Professor, Nurse Education, Elmira College, Elmira, NY 14901, 607-735-1890. *Fax:* 607-735-1758. *E-mail:* aogden@elmira.edu

HARTWICK COLLEGE
Department of Nursing
Oneonta, New York

Programs • Generic Baccalaureate • RN Baccalaureate • Baccalaureate for Second Degree

The College Independent 4-year coed college. Founded: 1797. *Primary accreditation:* regional. *Setting:* 375-acre small-town campus. *Total enrollment:* 1,522.

The Department of Nursing Founded in 1943. *Nursing program faculty:* 13 (7% with doctorates). *Off-campus program sites:* New York City, Albany, Cooperstown.

Academic Facilities *Nursing school resources:* CAI, computer lab, nursing audiovisuals, interactive nursing skills videos, learning resource lab.

Student Life *Student services:* health clinic, personal counseling, career counseling, institutionally sponsored work-study program, job placement, campus safety program. *International student services:* counseling/support, special assistance for nonnative speakers of English. *Nursing student activities:* student nurses association.

Calendar 4-1-4.

NURSING STUDENT PROFILE

Undergraduate **Enrollment:** 165
Women: 94%; **Men:** 6%; **Minority:** 12%; **International:** 0%; **Part-time:** 19%

BACCALAUREATE PROGRAMS

Contact Dr. Dianne Miner, Chair, Bresee Hall, Department of Nursing, Hartwick College, Oneonta, NY 13820, 607-431-4780. *Fax:* 607-431-4850.

Expenses *Tuition:* $20,502 full-time, $2278 per course part-time. *Full-time mandatory fees:* $300. *Room and board:* $5310. *Room only:* $2660.

Generic Baccalaureate Program (BS)

Applying *Required:* ACT, minimum college GPA of 2.0, high school transcript, 2 letters of recommendation, written essay. *Application deadlines:* 2/15 (fall), 1/1 (spring). *Application fee:* $35.

Degree Requirements 40 course units, including 16 in nursing.

RN Baccalaureate Program (BS)

Applying *Required:* NLN Preadmission Examination-RN, RN license, high school transcript, 2 letters of recommendation, written essay, transcript of college record. *Application deadlines:* 5/30 (fall), 11/15 (spring). *Application fee:* $35.

Degree Requirements 40 course units, including 16 in nursing.

Baccalaureate for Second Degree Program (BS)

Applying *Required:* minimum high school GPA of 2.0, high school transcript, 2 letters of recommendation, transcript of college record. *Application deadline:* rolling. *Application fee:* $35.

Degree Requirements 18 total credit hours.

See full description on page 452.

HUNTER COLLEGE OF THE CITY UNIVERSITY OF NEW YORK
Hunter-Bellevue School of Nursing
New York, New York

Programs • Generic Baccalaureate • RN Baccalaureate • BSN to Master's • MS/MPH

The University State and locally supported comprehensive coed institution. Part of City University of New York System. Founded: 1870. *Primary accreditation:* regional. *Total enrollment:* 18,250.

The Hunter-Bellevue School of Nursing Founded in 1955. *Nursing program faculty:* 38 (66% with doctorates).

Academic Facilities *Campus library:* 73,000 volumes (36,000 in health, 3,800 in nursing); 2,327 periodical subscriptions (350 health-care related). *Nursing school resources:* CAI, computer lab, nursing audiovisuals, interactive nursing skills videos, learning resource lab, media production equipment, Internet connection.

Student Life *Student services:* child-care facilities, personal counseling, career counseling, job placement, campus safety program, special assistance for disabled students, emergency medical services, tutoring/study skills resource center. *International student services:* ESL courses, language lab. *Nursing student activities:* Sigma Theta Tau, student nurses association.

Calendar Semesters.

NURSING STUDENT PROFILE

Undergraduate **Enrollment:** 276
Women: 87%; **Men:** 13%; **Minority:** 47%; **Part-time:** 46%
Graduate **Enrollment:** 299
Women: 95%; **Men:** 5%; **Minority:** 40%; **Part-time:** 97%

BACCALAUREATE PROGRAMS

Contact Dr. Diane Rendon, Associate Professor and Director of Undergraduate Program, Hunter-Bellevue School of Nursing, Hunter College of the City University of New York, 425 East 25th Street, New York, NY 10010, 212-481-7596. *Fax:* 212-481-5078. *E-mail:* drendon@heijra.hunter.cuny.edu

Expenses *State resident tuition:* ranges from $2950 to $3200 full-time, ranges from $125 to $135 per credit part-time. *Nonresident tuition:* ranges from $6550 to $6800 full-time, ranges from $275 to $285 per credit part-time. *Full-time mandatory fees:* $57. *Part-time mandatory fees:* $41. *Room and board:* $8100–$11,700. *Room only:* $1890. *Books and supplies per academic year:* $500.

Financial Aid Institutionally sponsored need-based grants/scholarships, institutionally sponsored non-need grants/scholarships, Federal Supplemental Educational Opportunity Grants, Federal Work-Study. 50% of undergraduate students in nursing programs received some form of financial aid in 1995–96. *Application deadline:* 5/1.

Generic Baccalaureate Program (BS)

Applying *Required:* TOEFL for nonnative speakers of English, Hunter College Skills Assessment Test, minimum college GPA of 2.5, high school transcript, transcript of college record. 64 prerequisite credits must be completed before admission to the nursing program. *Options:* May apply for transfer of up to 95 total credits. *Application deadline:* 3/15. *Application fee:* $40.

Degree Requirements 128 total credit hours, 54 in nursing. 560 clinical hours.

RN Baccalaureate Program (BS)

Applying *Required:* Hunter College Skills Assessment Test, New York State Regents College exam for non-CUNY transfers with AAS in Nursing, minimum college GPA of 2.5, RN license, diploma or AD in nursing. 64 prerequisite credits must be completed before admission to the nursing program. *Options:* May apply for transfer of up to 24 total credits. *Application deadlines:* 3/15 (fall), 11/1 (spring). *Application fee:* $40.

Degree Requirements 128 total credit hours, 54 in nursing.

MASTER'S PROGRAMS

Contact Dr. Mary T. Ramshorn, Director of Graduate Program and Professor, Hunter-Bellevue School of Nursing, Hunter College of the City University of New York, 425 East 24th Street, New York, NY 10010, 212-481-4465. *Fax:* 212-481-5078. *E-mail:* mramshor@hejira.hunter.cuny.edu

Areas of Study Clinical nurse specialist programs in community health nursing, medical-surgical nursing, parent-child nursing, psychiatric–mental health nursing; nursing administration; nurse practitioner programs in child care/pediatrics, gerontology, advanced pediatric care.

Expenses *State resident tuition:* $4350 full-time, $185 per credit part-time. *Nonresident tuition:* $7600 full-time, $320 per credit part-time. *Full-time mandatory fees:* $13. *Room and board:* $8100–$11,700. *Room only:* $1890. *Books and supplies per academic year:* ranges from $400 to $600.

Financial Aid Nurse traineeships, graduate tuition waiver. 1% of master's level students in nursing programs received some form of financial aid in 1995-96. *Application deadline:* 5/1.

BSN to Master's Program (MS)

Applying *Required:* bachelor's degree in nursing, minimum GPA of 3.0, RN license, statistics course, professional liability/malpractice insurance, essay, 2 letters of recommendation, transcript of college record. *Application deadlines:* 12/1 (fall), 5/1 (spring). *Application fee:* $40.

Degree Requirements 42 total credit hours, 39–42 in nursing.

MS/MPH Program

Applying *Required:* GRE General Test, bachelor's degree in nursing, minimum GPA of 3.0, RN license, statistics course, professional liability/malpractice insurance, essay, 2 letters of recommendation, transcript of college record. *Application deadlines:* 12/1 (fall), 5/1 (spring). *Application fee:* $40.

Degree Requirements 57 total credit hours, 30 in nursing, 27 in community health education.

KEUKA COLLEGE
Division of Nursing
Keuka Park, New York

Programs • Generic Baccalaureate • RN Baccalaureate

The College Independent 4-year coed college, affiliated with American Baptist Churches in the U.S.A.. Founded: 1890. *Primary accreditation:* regional. *Setting:* 173-acre rural campus. *Total enrollment:* 921.

The Division of Nursing Founded in 1943. *Nursing program faculty:* 8 (25% with doctorates). *Off-campus program sites:* Elmira, Geneva.

Academic Facilities *Campus library:* 95,000 volumes (4,287 in health, 704 in nursing); 400 periodical subscriptions (55 health-care related). *Nursing school resources:* CAI, computer lab, nursing audiovisuals, interactive nursing skills videos, learning resource lab, observation laboratory.

Student Life *Student services:* health clinic, personal counseling, career counseling, institutionally sponsored work-study program, job placement, campus safety program, special assistance for disabled students. *Nursing student activities:* student nurses association, undergraduate research exchange.

Calendar Semesters.

NURSING STUDENT PROFILE

Undergraduate **Enrollment:** 81
Women: 95%; **Men:** 5%; **Minority:** 7%; **International:** 0%; **Part-time:** 31%

BACCALAUREATE PROGRAMS

Contact Dr. Margaret England, Chair, Division of Nursing, Keuka College, Keuka Park, NY 14478, 315-536-4411 Ext. 5273. *Fax:* 315-536-5216. *E-mail:* mengland@mail.keuka.edu

Expenses *Tuition:* $10,490 full-time, $360 per credit hour part-time. *Full-time mandatory fees:* $571–$656. *Room and board:* $5040. *Books and supplies per academic year:* $600.

Financial Aid Institutionally sponsored need-based grants/scholarships, institutionally sponsored non-need grants/scholarships, Federal Direct Loans, Federal Nursing Student Loans, Federal Pell Grants, Federal Perkins Loans, Federal Supplemental Educational Opportunity Grants, Federal Work-Study. 70% of undergraduate students in nursing programs received some form of financial aid in 1995–96. *Application deadline:* 3/1.

Generic Baccalaureate Program (BSN)

Applying *Required:* SAT I, ACT, minimum college GPA of 2.0, high school transcript, 2 letters of recommendation, transcript of college record. *Options:* May apply for transfer of up to 90 total credits. *Application deadline:* rolling. *Application fee:* $25.

Degree Requirements 122 total credit hours, 55 in nursing. 1 field period for every year at Keuka, senior field period must be in nursing.

RN Baccalaureate Program (BSN)

Applying *Required:* SAT I or ACT if high school diploma or equivalent is less than 5 years old, minimum college GPA of 2.0, RN license, interview, transcript of college record. *Options:* Advanced standing available through credit by exam. May apply for transfer of up to 90 total credits. *Application deadline:* rolling. *Application fee:* $25.

Degree Requirements 122 total credit hours, 55 in nursing. 1 field period for every year at Keuka, senior field period must be in nursing.

LEHMAN COLLEGE OF THE CITY UNIVERSITY OF NEW YORK
Department of Nursing
Bronx, New York

Programs • Generic Baccalaureate • Accelerated RN Baccalaureate • MS • Continuing Education

The University State and locally supported comprehensive coed institution. Part of City University of New York System. Founded: 1931. *Primary accreditation:* regional. *Setting:* 37-acre urban campus. *Total enrollment:* 9,599.

The Department of Nursing Founded in 1970. *Nursing program faculty:* 32 (47% with doctorates). *Off-campus program site:* New York City.

Academic Facilities *Campus library:* 600,000 volumes; 2,000 periodical subscriptions. *Nursing school resources:* CAI, computer lab, nursing audiovisuals, interactive nursing skills videos, learning resource lab, nursing laboratory.

Student Life *Student services:* health clinic, child-care facilities, personal counseling, career counseling, institutionally sponsored work-study program, campus safety program, special assistance for disabled students. *International student services:* counseling/support, special assistance for nonnative speakers of English, ESL courses. *Nursing student activities:* Sigma Theta Tau, student nurses association, National Student Nurses Association.

Calendar Semesters.

NURSING STUDENT PROFILE

Undergraduate **Enrollment:** 282
Women: 92%; **Men:** 8%; **Minority:** 34%
Graduate **Enrollment:** 116
Women: 91%; **Men:** 9%; **Minority:** 68%

BACCALAUREATE PROGRAMS

Contact Dr. Eulee Mead-Bennett, Director of Undergraduate Programs, Department of Nursing, Lehman College of the City University of New York, 250 Bedford Park Boulevard, West, Bronx, NY 10468, 718-960-8213. *Fax:* 718-960-8488.

Expenses *State resident tuition:* $3000 full-time, $125 per credit part-time. *Nonresident tuition:* $6600 full-time, $275 per credit part-time. *Full-time mandatory fees:* $35. *Books and supplies per academic year:* ranges from $500 to $600.

Financial Aid Federal Nursing Student Loans, Federal Perkins Loans, Federal Supplemental Educational Opportunity Grants, Federal Work-Study, New York State Tuition Assistance Program (TAP). 27% of undergraduate students in nursing programs received some form of financial aid in 1995–96.

Generic Baccalaureate Program (BS)

Applying *Required:* math, reading, and writing assessment tests, minimum college GPA of 2.75, high school transcript, interview, 3 letters of recommendation, transcript of college record. 20 prerequisite credits must be completed before admission to the nursing program. *Options:* Course work may be accelerated. May apply for transfer of up to 60 total credits. *Application deadline:* 7/1. *Application fee:* $35.

Degree Requirements 120 total credit hours, 75 in nursing.

Accelerated RN Baccalaureate Program (BS)

Applying *Required:* math, reading, and writing assessment tests, minimum college GPA of 2.75, RN license, diploma or AD in nursing, interview, 3 letters of recommendation, transcript of college record. 20 prerequisite credits must be completed before admission to the nursing program. *Application deadline:* 7/1. *Application fee:* $35.

Degree Requirements 120 total credit hours, 75 in nursing.

Lehman College of the City University of New York (continued)

MASTER'S PROGRAM

Contact Dr. Keville Fredrickson, Director, Graduate Program, Department of Nursing, Lehman College of the City University of New York, 250 Bedford Park Boulevard, West, Bronx, NY 10468, 718-960-8378. *Fax:* 718-960-8488.

Areas of Study Clinical nurse specialist programs in adult health nursing, gerontological nursing, pediatric nursing; nurse anesthesia; nursing administration; nursing education; nurse practitioner program in child care/pediatrics.

Expenses *State resident tuition:* $3330 full-time, $185 per credit part-time. *Nonresident tuition:* $5760 full-time, $320 per credit part-time. *Full-time mandatory fees:* $70.

Financial Aid Nurse traineeships, employment opportunities.

MS Program

Applying *Required:* GRE General Test, English proficiency exam, bachelor's degree in nursing, minimum GPA of 3.0, RN license, 1 year of clinical experience, professional liability/malpractice insurance, essay, interview, 3 letters of recommendation, transcript of college record. *Application deadline:* 3/1. *Application fee:* $35.

Degree Requirements 40 total credit hours, 30 in nursing, 10 in statistics and other specified areas. Project.

CONTINUING EDUCATION PROGRAM

Contact Dr. Jody Williams, Assistant Professor, Department of Nursing, Lehman College of the City University of New York, 250 Bedford Park Boulevard, West, Bronx, NY 10468, 718-960-8391. *Fax:* 718-960-8488.

LONG ISLAND UNIVERSITY, BROOKLYN CAMPUS

School of Nursing
Brooklyn, New York

Programs • Generic Baccalaureate • RN Baccalaureate • Accelerated MSN

The University Independent comprehensive coed institution. Part of Long Island University. Founded: 1926. *Primary accreditation:* regional. *Setting:* 10-acre urban campus. *Total enrollment:* 8,096.

The School of Nursing Founded in 1990. *Nursing program faculty:* 15 (33% with doctorates).

Academic Facilities *Campus library:* 235,118 volumes (10,850 in health, 800 in nursing); 2,205 periodical subscriptions (211 health-care related). *Nursing school resources:* CAI, computer lab, nursing audiovisuals, interactive nursing skills videos, learning resource lab.

Student Life *Student services:* health clinic, child-care facilities, personal counseling, career counseling, institutionally sponsored work-study program, job placement, campus safety program, special assistance for disabled students. *International student services:* counseling/support, special assistance for nonnative speakers of English, ESL courses. *Nursing student activities:* student nurses association.

Calendar Semesters.

NURSING STUDENT PROFILE

Undergraduate **Enrollment:** 618
Women: 93%; **Men:** 7%; **Minority:** 72%; **Part-time:** 25%

BACCALAUREATE PROGRAMS

Contact Ms. Letitia Galdamez, Director of Advisement, School of Nursing, Long Island University, Brooklyn Campus, 1 University Plaza, Brooklyn, NY 11201, 718-488-1512. *Fax:* 718-780-4019. *E-mail:* lgaldame@titan.liunet.edu

Expenses *Tuition:* $13,056 full-time, $408 per credit part-time. *Full-time mandatory fees:* $277–$497. *Part-time mandatory fees:* $147–$367. *Room and board:* $2040–$4500.

Financial Aid Federal Direct Loans, Federal Pell Grants, Federal Perkins Loans, Federal Work-Study. 100% of undergraduate students in nursing programs received some form of financial aid in 1995–96.

Generic Baccalaureate Program (BS)

Applying *Required:* TOEFL for nonnative speakers of English, Nelson-Denny Reading Exam, minimum college GPA of 2.5, high school transcript, interview, transcript of college record. *Options:* Advanced standing available through advanced placement exams. *Application deadlines:* 6/1 (fall), 12/1 (spring), 4/1 (summer). *Application fee:* $30.

Degree Requirements 128 total credit hours, 62 in nursing.

RN Baccalaureate Program (BS)

Applying *Required:* math and writing pretest, minimum college GPA of 2.5, RN license, diploma or AD in nursing, transcript of college record. *Options:* May apply for transfer of up to 29 total credits. *Application deadlines:* 6/1 (fall), 12/1 (spring), 4/1 (summer). *Application fee:* $30.

Degree Requirements 128 total credit hours, 59 in nursing. NLN Profile II for diploma students.

MASTER'S PROGRAM

Contact Dawn Kilts, Director, School of Nursing, Long Island University, Brooklyn Campus, 1 University Plaza, Brooklyn, NY 11201, 718-488-1059. *Fax:* 718-780-4019.

Areas of Study Nurse practitioner program in adult health.

Expenses *Tuition:* $15,372 full-time, $427 per credit part-time. *Full-time mandatory fees:* $277–$497. *Part-time mandatory fees:* $147–$367.

Financial Aid Graduate assistantships.

Accelerated MSN Program

Applying *Required:* bachelor's degree, minimum GPA of 3.0, RN license, 2 years of clinical experience, physical assessment course, interview, letter of recommendation, transcript of college record.

Degree Requirements 41 total credit hours, 38 in nursing, 3 in elective. Thesis required.

LONG ISLAND UNIVERSITY, C.W. POST CAMPUS

Department of Nursing
Brookville, New York

Programs • RN Baccalaureate • RN to Master's

The University Independent comprehensive coed institution. Part of Long Island University. Founded: 1954. *Primary accreditation:* regional. *Setting:* 305-acre small-town campus. *Total enrollment:* 8,060.

The Department of Nursing Founded in 1972. *Nursing program faculty:* 4 (75% with doctorates). *Off-campus program sites:* Southampton, Brentwood, Amityville.

Academic Facilities *Campus library:* 500,073 volumes (20,000 in nursing); 5,000 periodical subscriptions (300 health-care related). *Nursing school resources:* CAI, computer lab, nursing audiovisuals, learning resource lab.

Student Life *Student services:* health clinic, child-care facilities, personal counseling, career counseling, job placement, campus safety program. *International student services:* counseling/support, special assistance for nonnative speakers of English, ESL courses. *Nursing student activities:* student nurses association.

Calendar Semesters.

NURSING STUDENT PROFILE

Undergraduate **Enrollment:** 160
Women: 99%; **Men:** 1%; **Minority:** 5%; **Part-time:** 99%

BACCALAUREATE PROGRAM

Contact Dr. Theodora T. Grauer, Chairperson, Life Sciences Room 270, Department of Nursing, Long Island University, C. W. Post Campus, Brookville, NY 11548, 516-299-2320. *Fax:* 516-283-4081. *E-mail:* ttgrauer@hornet.liunet.edu

Expenses *Tuition:* $13,040 full-time, $408 per credit part-time. *Full-time mandatory fees:* $285+. *Part-time mandatory fees:* $52+. *Books and supplies per academic year:* ranges from $250 to $400.

Financial Aid Institutionally sponsored non-need grants/scholarships. *Application deadline:* 6/1.

RN Baccalaureate Program (BS)

Applying *Required:* TOEFL for nonnative speakers of English, minimum college GPA of 2.5, 3 years of high school math, 3 years of high school science, RN license, diploma or AD in nursing, transcript of college record, 1 year of clinical experience or passing grade on clinical performance exam. *Options:* May apply for transfer of up to 64 total credits. *Application deadline:* rolling. *Application fee:* $30.

Degree Requirements 128 total credit hours, 34 in nursing.

MASTER'S PROGRAM

Contact Dr. Theodora Grauer, Chairperson and Professor, Department of Nursing, Long Island University, C.W. Post Campus, Brookville, NY 11548, 516-299-2320. *Fax:* 516-299-2527. *E-mail:* ttgrauer@hornet.liunet.edu

Areas of Study Clinical nurse specialist program in adult health nursing; nurse practitioner program in family health.

Expenses *Tuition:* ranges from $7290 to $9315 full-time, $405 per credit part-time. *Part-time mandatory fees:* $142+.

Financial Aid Federal Direct Loans, employment opportunities, TAP (New York State Aid).

RN to Master's Program (MS)

Applying *Required:* GRE General Test, TOEFL for nonnative speakers of English, bachelor's degree in nursing, minimum GPA of 3.0, RN license, 2 years of clinical experience, professional liability/malpractice insurance, essay, interview, transcript of college record. *Application deadline:* rolling. *Application fee:* $30.

Degree Requirements 36–46 total credit hours dependent upon track, 36–46 in nursing. Research proposal.

MEDGAR EVERS COLLEGE OF THE CITY UNIVERSITY OF NEW YORK
Department of Nursing
Brooklyn, New York

Program • RN Baccalaureate

The University State and locally supported 4-year coed college. Part of City University of New York System. Founded: 1969. *Primary accreditation:* regional. *Setting:* 1-acre urban campus.

The Department of Nursing Founded in 1975.

Academic Facilities *Campus library:* 94,941 volumes (3,825 in health, 20,000 in nursing).

Calendar Semesters.

BACCALAUREATE PROGRAM

Contact Admissions Office, Department of Nursing, Medgar Evers College of the City University of New York, 1650 Bedford Avenue, Brooklyn, NY 11225, 718-270-6024. *Fax:* 718-270-6496.

RN Baccalaureate Program (BS)

Applying *Required:* reading, writing, and math proficiency exams, minimum college GPA of 2.5, RN license, diploma or AD in nursing, transcript of college record, health exams, immunizations. 64 prerequisite credits must be completed before admission to the nursing program. *Options:* Advanced standing available through credit by exam. *Application fee:* $40.

Degree Requirements 128 total credit hours, 64 in nursing.

MERCY COLLEGE
Department of Nursing
Dobbs Ferry, New York

Programs • RN Baccalaureate • MS

The College Independent comprehensive coed institution. Founded: 1951. *Primary accreditation:* regional. *Setting:* 20-acre small-town campus. *Total enrollment:* 6,792.

The Department of Nursing Founded in 1977. (80% with doctorates).

Academic Facilities *Campus library:* 293,000 volumes; 1,332 periodical subscriptions.

Student Life *Student services:* health clinic, career counseling, campus safety program. *Nursing student activities:* Sigma Theta Tau.

Calendar Semesters.

BACCALAUREATE PROGRAM

Contact Chairperson, Department of Nursing, Mercy College, 555 Broadway, Dobbs Ferry, NY 10522, 914-674-9331 Ext. 550. *Fax:* 914-674-9457.

Expenses *Tuition:* $9120 full-time, $285 per credit part-time. *Books and supplies per academic year:* $400.

RN Baccalaureate Program (BS)

Applying *Required:* minimum college GPA of 2.5, RN license, diploma or AD in nursing, transcript of college record. *Application fee:* $35.

MASTER'S PROGRAM

Contact Graduate Program Director, Department of Nursing, Mercy College, 555 Broadway, Dobbs Ferry, NY 10522, 914-674-9331 Ext. 550. *Fax:* 914-674-9457.

Areas of Study Clinical nurse specialist program in family health nursing.

Expenses *Tuition:* $350 per credit.

MS Program

Applying *Required:* GRE General Test or Miller Analogies Test, bachelor's degree in nursing, minimum GPA of 3.0, RN license, 1 year of clinical experience, physical assessment course, professional liability/malpractice insurance, interview, 2 letters of recommendation, transcript of college record. *Application fee:* $35.

See full description on page 482.

MOLLOY COLLEGE
Department of Nursing
Rockville Centre, New York

Programs • Generic Baccalaureate • RN Baccalaureate • Baccalaureate for Second Degree • International Nurse to Baccalaureate • MS • RN to Master's • Accelerated Master's for Nurses with Non-Nursing Degrees • Post-Master's • Continuing Education

The College Independent comprehensive coed institution. Founded: 1955. *Primary accreditation:* regional. *Setting:* 25-acre suburban campus. *Total enrollment:* 2,346.

The Department of Nursing Founded in 1957. *Nursing program faculty:* 87 (16% with doctorates).

▶ ***NOTEWORTHY***

Undergraduate programs in nursing are designed to prepare the nurse generalist for practice in a variety of health-care settings. Eligible students may pursue one of the following options: baccalaureate degree in nursing, registered nurse baccalaureate completion program, and dual degree for second degree students and registered nurse students. The Master of Science degree program combines academic, clinical, and research activities that educate graduate nurses for advanced clinical practice and role functions. Preparation as adult and pediatric nurse practitioner is offered in both the master's and post-master's programs. In addition, the post-master's program is available for role functions in education or administration.

Academic Facilities *Campus library:* 132,120 volumes (1,555 in health, 5,100 in nursing); 1,425 periodical subscriptions (290 health-care related). *Nursing school resources:* CAI, computer lab, nursing audiovisuals, interactive nursing skills videos, learning resource lab.

Student Life *Student services:* health clinic, child-care facilities, personal counseling, career counseling, institutionally sponsored work-study program, special assistance for disabled students. *International student services:*

Molloy College (continued)
counseling/support, ESL courses. *Nursing student activities:* Sigma Theta Tau, nursing club, student nurses association.

Calendar Semesters.

NURSING STUDENT PROFILE

Undergraduate **Enrollment:** 1020
Women: 94%; **Men:** 6%; **Minority:** 15%; **International:** 11%; **Part-time:** 34%

Graduate **Enrollment:** 214
Women: 97%; **Men:** 3%; **Minority:** 25%; **International:** 0%; **Part-time:** 95%

BACCALAUREATE PROGRAMS

Contact Mr. Wayne James, Director of Admissions, Department of Nursing, Molloy College, 1000 Hempstead Avenue, Rockville Centre, NY 11570, 516-678-5000 Ext. 233. *Fax:* 516-678-7295. *E-mail:* wayja01@molloy.edu

Expenses *Tuition:* $9600 full-time, $320 per credit part-time. *Full-time mandatory fees:* $579–$769. *Part-time mandatory fees:* $150–$300. *Books and supplies per academic year:* ranges from $700 to $900.

Financial Aid Institutionally sponsored need-based grants/scholarships, institutionally sponsored non-need grants/scholarships, Federal Nursing Student Loans, Federal Supplemental Educational Opportunity Grants, Federal Work-Study. 50% of undergraduate students in nursing programs received some form of financial aid in 1995–96. *Application deadline:* 4/15.

Generic Baccalaureate Program (BS)

Applying *Required:* SAT I, ACT, TOEFL for nonnative speakers of English, Nelson-Denny Reading Test, NLN Preadmission Examination, Engineering Diagnostic Test, minimum high school GPA of 3.0, minimum college GPA of 3.0, high school chemistry, high school biology, high school transcript, written essay, transcript of college record. *Options:* Advanced standing available through advanced placement exams. Course work may be accelerated. May apply for transfer of up to 98 total credits. *Application deadlines:* 5/15 (fall), 11/15 (spring). *Application fee:* $25.

Degree Requirements 129 total credit hours, 56 in nursing. Math screening, 47 core requirements, 24 related requirements, 2 electives.

RN Baccalaureate Program (BS)

Applying *Required:* TOEFL for nonnative speakers of English, Nelson-Denny Reading Test, minimum college GPA of 3.0, high school chemistry, high school biology, RN license, diploma or AD in nursing, high school transcript, written essay, transcript of college record. *Options:* Advanced standing available through the following means: advanced placement without credit, credit by exam. May apply for transfer of up to 98 total credits. *Application deadlines:* 5/15 (fall), 11/15 (spring). *Application fee:* $25.

Degree Requirements 129 total credit hours, 31 in nursing. Mathematics skills requirement.

Baccalaureate for Second Degree Program (BS)

Applying *Required:* TOEFL for nonnative speakers of English, Nelson-Denny Reading Test, minimum college GPA of 3.0, 3 years of high school math, 3 years of high school science, high school biology, high school transcript, interview, written essay, transcript of college record. *Options:* Course work may be accelerated. May apply for transfer of up to 98 total credits. *Application deadlines:* 5/15 (fall), 11/15 (spring). *Application fee:* $25.

Degree Requirements 129 total credit hours, 56 in nursing. Math screening.

International Nurse to Baccalaureate Program (BS)

Applying *Required:* SAT I, ACT, TOEFL for nonnative speakers of English, Nelson-Denny Reading Test, minimum college GPA of 3.0, high school biology, RN license, diploma or AD in nursing, high school transcript, written essay, transcript of college record. *Options:* Advanced standing available through the following means: advanced placement exams, credit by exam. Course work may be accelerated. May apply for transfer of up to 98 total credits. *Application deadlines:* 5/15 (fall), 11/15 (spring). *Application fee:* $25.

Degree Requirements 129 total credit hours, 56 in nursing. Math screening.

MASTER'S PROGRAMS

Contact Dr. Carol A. Clifford, RN, Director, Graduate Program, Department of Nursing, Molloy College, 1000 Hempstead Avenue, Rockville Centre, NY 11570, 516-256-2218. *Fax:* 516-678-9718. *E-mail:* clica01@molloy.edu

Areas of Study Clinical nurse specialist programs in adult health nursing, pediatric nursing; nursing administration; nursing education; nurse practitioner programs in adult health, child care/pediatrics.

Expenses *Tuition:* $6660 full-time, $370 per credit part-time. *Full-time mandatory fees:* $270.

Financial Aid Graduate assistantships, Federal Nursing Student Loans. 1% of master's level students in nursing programs received some form of financial aid in 1995-96. *Application deadline:* 4/15.

MS Program

Applying *Required:* TOEFL for nonnative speakers of English, bachelor's degree in nursing, minimum GPA of 3.0, RN license, 1 year of clinical experience, statistics course, interview, 3 letters of recommendation, transcript of college record, research course; physical assessment course and professional liability/malpractice insurance for nurse practitioner track. *Application deadlines:* 4/1 (fall), 11/1 (spring). *Application fee:* $60.

Degree Requirements 40–42 total credit hours dependent upon track, 35–37 in nursing. 202-585 clinical hours.

RN to Master's Program (MS)

Applying *Required:* TOEFL for nonnative speakers of English, Nelson-Denny Reading Test, Diagnostic Composition Test, minimum GPA of 3.3, RN license, 1 year of clinical experience, physical assessment course, statistics course, professional liability/malpractice insurance, essay, interview, 3 letters of recommendation, transcript of college record, BS in nursing earned concurrently with MS. *Application deadlines:* 4/1 (fall), 11/1 (spring). *Application fee:* $60.

Degree Requirements 160–162 total credit hours dependent upon track, 59–61 in nursing, 6–9 in mathematics, philosophy, and other specified areas.

Accelerated Master's for Nurses with Non-Nursing Degrees Program (MS)

Applying *Required:* TOEFL for nonnative speakers of English, Nelson-Denny Reading Test, Diagnostic Composition Test, bachelor's degree, minimum GPA of 3.3, RN license, 1 year of clinical experience, physical assessment course, statistics course, professional liability/malpractice insurance, essay, interview, 3 letters of recommendation, transcript of college record, BS in nursing earned concurrently with MS. *Application deadlines:* 4/1 (fall), 11/1 (spring). *Application fee:* $60.

Degree Requirements 169 total credit hours, 94 in nursing, 6–9 in mathematics, philosophy, and other specified areas. Thesis is optional.

Post-Master's Program

Applying *Required:* bachelor's degree in nursing, minimum GPA of 3.0, RN license, 1 year of clinical experience, physical assessment course, professional liability/malpractice insurance, essay, interview, 3 letters of recommendation, transcript of college record, nursing theory course for nursing management or nursing education; minimum 3.0 college GPA, malpractice insurance, 3 letters of recommendation, physical assessment course for nurse practitioner. *Application deadlines:* 4/1 (fall), 11/1 (spring). *Application fee:* $60.

Degree Requirements 15–20 total credit hours dependent upon track, 15–20 in nursing. 500 clinical hours for nurse practitioner track.

CONTINUING EDUCATION PROGRAM

Contact Mari Moriarty, RN, Coordinator, Continuing Education, Nursing, Department of Nursing, Molloy College, 1000 Hempstead Avenue, Rockville Centre, NY 11570, 516-678-5000 Ext. 260. *Fax:* 516-678-7295.

MOUNT SAINT MARY COLLEGE
Division of Nursing
Newburgh, New York

Programs • Generic Baccalaureate • Accelerated Baccalaureate • RN Baccalaureate • RN to Master's

The College Independent comprehensive coed institution. Founded: 1960. *Primary accreditation:* regional. *Setting:* 72-acre suburban campus. *Total enrollment:* 1,913.

The Division of Nursing Founded in 1967. *Nursing program faculty:* 10 (50% with doctorates).

▶ ***NOTEWORTHY***

Mount Saint Mary College's nursing program approaches nursing holistically with a focus on wellness and the traditional role of caring for the sick. The commitment to personal attention and the friendly atmosphere are especially strong in nursing. Academic courses provide students with the background and experience to succeed in caregiving and career advancement. Students study the liberal arts and sciences and complete 15 hours per week in one of 20 hospitals or clinics affiliated with the Mount. Students use some of the finest medical equipment and facilities available. Graduates are fully prepared to take the licensure exam for registered nurses. The recent passing rate of 94% earned Mount Saint Mary's College the second ranking among all nursing schools in New York State.

Academic Facilities *Campus library:* 110,561 volumes (4,385 in nursing); 660 periodical subscriptions (94 health-care related). *Nursing school resources:* CAI, computer lab, nursing audiovisuals, learning resource lab.

Student Life *Student services:* health clinic, personal counseling, career counseling, institutionally sponsored work-study program, job placement, campus safety program, special assistance for disabled students. *Nursing student activities:* Sigma Theta Tau, nursing club, student nurses association.

Calendar Semesters.

NURSING STUDENT PROFILE

Undergraduate **Enrollment:** 251
Women: 93%; **Men:** 7%; **Minority:** 14%; **International:** 1%; **Part-time:** 32%
Graduate **Enrollment:** 29
Women: 96%; **Men:** 4%; **Minority:** 4%; **International:** 0%; **Part-time:** 96%

BACCALAUREATE PROGRAMS

Contact Mr. J. Randall Ognibene, Director of Admissions, Division of Nursing, Mount Saint Mary College, 330 Powell Avenue, Newburgh, NY 12550, 914-561-0800. *Fax:* 914-562-6762.

Expenses *Tuition:* $9270 full-time, $309 per credit part-time. *Full-time mandatory fees:* $320. *Room and board:* $5000. *Books and supplies per academic year:* $600.

Financial Aid Institutionally sponsored need-based grants/scholarships, institutionally sponsored non-need grants/scholarships, Federal Nursing Student Loans, Federal Supplemental Educational Opportunity Grants, Federal Work-Study. *Application deadline:* 3/1.

Generic Baccalaureate Program (BSN)

Applying *Required:* SAT I, ACT, TOEFL for nonnative speakers of English, high school chemistry, high school biology, high school transcript, letter of recommendation, transcript of college record, optional essay, interview recommended. *Options:* Advanced standing available through the following means: advanced placement exams, advanced placement without credit, credit by exam. Course work may be accelerated. May apply for transfer of up to 90 total credits. *Application deadline:* rolling. *Application fee:* $20.

Degree Requirements 120 total credit hours, 46 in nursing. 39-credit Core Foundation requirement.

Accelerated Baccalaureate Program (BSN)

Applying *Required:* SAT I, TOEFL for nonnative speakers of English, high school chemistry, high school biology, high school transcript, letter of recommendation, transcript of college record. *Options:* Advanced standing available through the following means: advanced placement exams, advanced placement without credit, credit by exam. Course work may be accelerated. May apply for transfer of up to 90 total credits. *Application deadline:* rolling. *Application fee:* $20.

Degree Requirements 120 total credit hours, 46 in nursing. 39-credit Core Foundation requirement.

RN Baccalaureate Program (BSN)

Applying *Required:* SAT I, TOEFL for nonnative speakers of English, high school chemistry, high school biology, RN license, diploma or AD in nursing, 6 months of clinical work experience. *Options:* Advanced standing available through credit by exam. Course work may be accelerated. May apply for transfer of up to 90 total credits. *Application deadline:* rolling. *Application fee:* $20.

Degree Requirements 120 total credit hours, 46 in nursing. 39-credit Core Foundation requirement.

MASTER'S PROGRAM

Contact Sr. Leona Deboer, Graduate Nursing Program Coordinator and Professor, 330 Powell Avenue, Newburgh, NY 12550, 914-569-3138. *Fax:* 914-562-6762. *E-mail:* deboer@msmc.edu

Areas of Study Clinical nurse specialist program in adult health nursing.

Expenses *Tuition:* $7680 full-time, $320 per credit part-time. *Full-time mandatory fees:* $55. *Room and board:* $5000. *Books and supplies per academic year:* $600.

Financial Aid Graduate assistantships, Federal Direct Loans, employment opportunities, New York State TAP (Tuition Assistance Program), Sigma Theta Tau Grant. *Application deadline:* 3/1.

RN to Master's Program (MS)

Applying *Required:* GRE General Test, Miller Analogies Test, bachelor's degree in nursing, minimum GPA of 3.0, RN license, 1 year of clinical experience, physical assessment course, statistics course, professional liability/malpractice insurance, essay, interview, letter of recommendation, transcript of college record. *Application deadline:* rolling. *Application fee:* $20.

Degree Requirements 48 total credit hours, 48 in nursing. Cumulative research-based project.

NAZARETH COLLEGE OF ROCHESTER
Department of Nursing
Rochester, New York

Programs • RN Baccalaureate • RN to Master's

The College Independent comprehensive coed institution. Founded: 1924. *Primary accreditation:* regional. *Setting:* 75-acre suburban campus. *Total enrollment:* 2,802.

The Department of Nursing Founded in 1942. *Nursing program faculty:* 8 (44% with doctorates). *Off-campus program site:* Canandaigua.

Academic Facilities *Campus library:* 25,800 volumes (7,032 in health, 10,500 in nursing); 590 periodical subscriptions (109 health-care related). *Nursing school resources:* CAI, computer lab, nursing audiovisuals, learning resource lab.

Nazareth College of Rochester (continued)

Student Life *Student services:* health clinic, child-care facilities, personal counseling, career counseling, institutionally sponsored work-study program, job placement, campus safety program, special assistance for disabled students. *Nursing student activities:* Nursing Honor Society.

Calendar Semesters.

NURSING STUDENT PROFILE

Undergraduate **Enrollment:** 183
Women: 97%; **Men:** 3%; **Minority:** 2%; **International:** 0%; **Part-time:** 99%
Graduate **Enrollment:** 24
Women: 92%; **Men:** 8%; **Minority:** 0%; **International:** 0%; **Part-time:** 83%

BACCALAUREATE PROGRAM

Contact Dr. Margaret M. Andrews, Chairperson and Professor, Department of Nursing, Nazareth College of Rochester, 4245 East Avenue, Rochester, NY 14618-3790, 716-389-2710. *Fax:* 716-586-2452. *E-mail:* mmandrew@naz.edu

Expenses *Tuition:* $5963 full-time, $345 per credit part-time. *Full-time mandatory fees:* $262. *Part-time mandatory fees:* $60. *Room and board:* $1215. *Room only:* $1628.

Financial Aid Institutionally sponsored need-based grants/scholarships, institutionally sponsored non-need grants/scholarships, Federal Supplemental Educational Opportunity Grants, Federal Work-Study. *Application deadline:* 3/1.

RN Baccalaureate Program (BS)

Applying *Required:* TOEFL for nonnative speakers of English, minimum college GPA of 2.3, RN license, diploma or AD in nursing, written essay, transcript of college record. 60 prerequisite credits must be completed before admission to the nursing program. *Options:* Course work may be accelerated. May apply for transfer of up to 60 total credits. *Application deadline:* rolling. *Application fee:* $25.

Degree Requirements 120 total credit hours, 33 in nursing.

MASTER'S PROGRAM

Contact Patricia A. Hanson, Director, Gerontological Nurse Practitioner Program, Department of Nursing, Nazareth College of Rochester, 4245 East Avenue, Rochester, NY 14618-3790, 716-389-2711. *Fax:* 716-586-2452. *E-mail:* pahanson@naz.edu

Areas of Study Nurse practitioner program in gerontology.

Expenses *Tuition:* $9504 full-time, $396 per credit part-time. *Full-time mandatory fees:* $0.

Financial Aid Graduate assistantships.

RN to Master's Program (MS)

Applying *Required:* GRE General Test, Miller Analogies Test, bachelor's degree in nursing, bachelor's degree, RN license, physical assessment course, statistics course, essay, interview, 2 letters of recommendation, transcript of college record. *Application deadline:* rolling. *Application fee:* $45.

Degree Requirements 38 total credit hours.

NEW YORK UNIVERSITY
Division of Nursing
New York, New York

Programs • Generic Baccalaureate • RN Baccalaureate • Baccalaureate for Second Degree • Accelerated Baccalaureate for Second Degree • MA • MA/MSM • PhD • Continuing Education

The University Independent coed university. Founded: 1831. *Primary accreditation:* regional. *Setting:* 28-acre urban campus. *Total enrollment:* 35,825.

The Division of Nursing Founded in 1947. *Nursing program faculty:* 28 (85% with doctorates).

Academic Facilities *Campus library:* 3.2 million volumes (228,361 in health, 1,988 in nursing); 29,244 periodical subscriptions (3,049 health-care related). *Nursing school resources:* CAI, computer lab, nursing audiovisuals, interactive nursing skills videos, learning resource lab.

Student Life *Student services:* health clinic, child-care facilities, personal counseling, career counseling, institutionally sponsored work-study program, job placement, campus safety program, special assistance for disabled students. *International student services:* counseling/support, special assistance for nonnative speakers of English, ESL courses. *Nursing student activities:* Sigma Theta Tau, student nurses association.

Calendar Semesters.

NURSING STUDENT PROFILE

Undergraduate **Enrollment:** 480
Women: 97%; **Men:** 3%; **Minority:** 50%
Graduate **Enrollment:** 496
Women: 96%; **Men:** 4%; **Minority:** 43%; **Part-time:** 98%

BACCALAUREATE PROGRAMS

Contact Annette DeCoste, Recruitment Coordinator, 429 Shimkin Hall, School of Education, Division of Nursing, New York University, 50 West 4th Street, New York, NY 10012, 212-998-5317. *Fax:* 212-995-3143. *E-mail:* decoste@is.nyu.edu

Expenses *Tuition:* $20,756 full-time, $620 per credit part-time. *Room and board:* $7856. *Books and supplies per academic year:* $450.

Financial Aid Institutionally sponsored need-based grants/scholarships, institutionally sponsored non-need grants/scholarships, Federal Direct Loans, Federal Nursing Student Loans, Federal Pell Grants, Federal Perkins Loans, Federal Supplemental Educational Opportunity Grants, Federal Work-Study. 70% of undergraduate students in nursing programs received some form of financial aid in 1995–96. *Application deadline:* 4/1.

Generic Baccalaureate Program (BSN)

Applying *Required:* SAT I, TOEFL for nonnative speakers of English, minimum high school GPA of 2.8, 3 years of high school math, 3 years of high school science, high school biology, high school transcript, 2 letters of recommendation, written essay. *Options:* Advanced standing available through advanced placement exams. Course work may be accelerated. *Application deadlines:* 1/15 (fall), 12/1 (spring). *Application fee:* $45.

Degree Requirements 132 total credit hours, 45 in nursing.

RN Baccalaureate Program (BSN)

Applying *Required:* TOEFL for nonnative speakers of English, minimum college GPA of 2.8, RN license, diploma or AD in nursing, high school transcript, 2 letters of recommendation, written essay, transcript of college record. *Options:* Course work may be accelerated. May apply for transfer of up to 72 total credits. *Application deadline:* rolling. *Application fee:* $45.

Degree Requirements 132 total credit hours, 27 in nursing.

Baccalaureate for Second Degree Program (BSN)

Applying *Required:* TOEFL for nonnative speakers of English, minimum college GPA of 2.8, high school transcript, 2 letters of recommendation, written essay, transcript of college record, non-nursing baccalaureate degree. *Options:* Advanced standing available through advanced placement exams. Course work may be accelerated. May apply for transfer of up to 96 total credits. *Application deadline:* rolling. *Application fee:* $45.

Degree Requirements 132 total credit hours, 45 in nursing.

Accelerated Baccalaureate for Second Degree Program (BSN)

Applying *Required:* TOEFL for nonnative speakers of English, minimum college GPA of 3.0, high school transcript, interview, 2 letters of recommendation, written essay, transcript of college record, non-nursing baccalaureate degree, 2 references, 8 prerequisite courses. *Options:* May apply for transfer of up to 87 total credits. *Application deadline:* 2/1 (summer). *Application fee:* $45.

Degree Requirements 132 total credit hours, 45 in nursing.

MASTER'S PROGRAMS

Contact Christine Dunnery, Assistant Recruiter, 429 Shimkin Hall, School of Education, Division of Nursing, New York University, 50 West 4th Street, New York, NY 10012, 212-998-5336. *Fax:* 212-995-3143. *E-mail:* nursing.programs@nyu.edu

Areas of Study Clinical nurse specialist programs in adult health nursing, gerontological nursing, pediatric nursing, psychiatric–mental health nursing; nurse midwifery; nursing administration; nursing education; nurse practitioner programs in acute care, adult health, child care/pediatrics, gerontology, primary care, psychiatric–mental health.

Expenses *Tuition:* $630 per credit. *Room and board:* $8000–$9000. *Room only:* $5800–$8000. *Books and supplies per academic year:* ranges from $500 to $700.

Financial Aid Graduate assistantships, nurse traineeships, Federal Nursing Student Loans, institutionally sponsored loans, employment opportunities. 70% of master's level students in nursing programs received some form of financial aid in 1995-96. *Application deadline:* 3/1.

MA Program

Applying *Required:* TOEFL for nonnative speakers of English, bachelor's degree in nursing, minimum GPA of 3.0, RN license, statistics course, essay, 2 letters of recommendation, transcript of college record, resume. *Application deadlines:* 3/1 (fall), 12/1 (spring). *Application fee:* $40.

Degree Requirements 45–51 total credit hours dependent upon track, 33–42 in nursing, 9–15 in statistics and advanced sciences. English essay, final practicum.

MA/MSM Program

Applying *Required:* GRE General Test, TOEFL for nonnative speakers of English, bachelor's degree in nursing, minimum GPA of 3.0, RN license, statistics course, essay, 2 letters of recommendation, transcript of college record, resume. *Application deadlines:* 3/1 (fall), 12/1 (spring). *Application fee:* $40.

Degree Requirements 68 total credit hours, 38 in nursing, 30 in management. English essay, final practicum.

DOCTORAL PROGRAM

Contact Christina Dunnery, Assistant Recruiter, 429 Shimkin Hall, School of Education, Division of Nursing, New York University, 50 West 4th Street, New York, NY 10012, 212-998-5336. *Fax:* 212-995-3143. *E-mail:* nursing.programs@nyu.edu

Areas of Study Nursing research.

Expenses *Tuition:* $630 per credit. *Room and board:* $8000–$9000. *Room only:* $5800–$8000. *Books and supplies per academic year:* ranges from $200 to $700.

Financial Aid Graduate assistantships, nurse traineeships, fellowships, dissertation grants, grants, Federal Direct Loans, Federal Nursing Student Loans, opportunities for employment, institutionally sponsored need-based grants/scholarships, institutionally sponsored non-need-based grants/scholarships. *Application deadline:* 3/1.

PhD Program

Applying *Required:* GRE General Test (minimum combined score of 1000 on three tests), master's degree in nursing, master's degree, statistics course, 2 letters of recommendation, vitae, writing sample, competitive review by faculty committee, published work. *Application deadline:* 2/1. *Application fee:* $40.

Degree Requirements 54–60 total credit hours dependent upon track; 6 credits each in foundations and cognates, 18 credits in research, 24 credits in nursing; dissertation; oral exam; written exam; defense of dissertation; residency.

CONTINUING EDUCATION PROGRAM

Contact Ms. Laura Nagle, Continuing Education Coordinator, 429 Shimkin Hall, School of Education, Division of Nursing, New York University, 50 West 4th Street, New York, NY 10012, 212-998-5345. *Fax:* 212-995-4561. *E-mail:* nagle@is2.nyu.edu

See full description on page 484.

NIAGARA UNIVERSITY

College of Nursing
Niagara University, New York

Programs • Generic Baccalaureate • RN Baccalaureate • Accelerated Baccalaureate for Second Degree • Accelerated RN to Master's

The University Independent comprehensive coed institution. Founded: 1856. *Primary accreditation:* regional. *Setting:* 160-acre suburban campus. *Total enrollment:* 2,865.

The College of Nursing Founded in 1946. *Nursing program faculty:* 24 (17% with doctorates).

▶ ***NOTEWORTHY***

Niagara University has developed 2 new nursing programs for persons looking to change or enhance their careers. In fall 1995, Niagara began to offer an MS degree in nursing leading to certification as a family nurse practitioner. The 45-credit-hour program is designed to be completed full-time in a year plus 1 semester or part-time in 2 years plus 1 semester. Classes are offered in the fall, spring, and summer semesters. Applicants must have a BS in nursing and at least 1 year of experience as an RN. Persons who already have a non-nursing degree and want to enter the nursing profession can obtain a BS degree in nursing in 1 year through Niagara's accelerated program. Niagara University has been educating nurses for nearly 50 years in an atmosphere that fosters critical thinking, professionalism, and deep concern for the rights and dignity of the individual.

Academic Facilities *Campus library:* 301,000 volumes (9,743 in health); 1,500 periodical subscriptions (125 health-care related). *Nursing school resources:* CAI, computer lab, nursing audiovisuals, interactive nursing skills videos, learning resource lab.

Student Life *Student services:* health clinic, personal counseling, career counseling, institutionally sponsored work-study program, job placement, campus safety program, special assistance for disabled students. *International student services:* counseling/support, special assistance for nonnative speakers of English. *Nursing student activities:* Sigma Theta Tau, student nurses association.

Calendar Semesters.

NURSING STUDENT PROFILE

Undergraduate **Enrollment:** 253
Women: 87%; **Men:** 13%; **Minority:** 8%; **International:** 8%; **Part-time:** 36%
Graduate **Enrollment:** 28
Women: 100%; **Minority:** 4%; **International:** 7%; **Part-time:** 75%

BACCALAUREATE PROGRAMS

Contact Dr. Dolores A. Bower, RN, Dean, College of Nursing, Niagara University, PO Box 2203, Niagara University, NY 14109, 716-286-8312. *Fax:* 716-286-8308. *E-mail:* dab@niagara.edu

Expenses *Tuition:* $11,800 full-time, $356 per semester hour part-time. *Full-time mandatory fees:* $458. *Room and board:* $5388. *Books and supplies per academic year:* $700.

Financial Aid Institutionally sponsored need-based grants/scholarships, institutionally sponsored non-need grants/scholarships, Federal Nursing Student Loans, Federal Pell Grants, Federal Perkins Loans, Federal Supplemental Educational Opportunity Grants, Federal Work-Study. 89% of undergraduate students in nursing programs received some form of financial aid in 1995–96. *Application deadline:* 3/15.

Generic Baccalaureate Program (BS)

Applying *Required:* SAT I, ACT, TOEFL for nonnative speakers of English, minimum high school GPA of 3.3, minimum college GPA of 2.5, 3 years of high school math, 3 years of high school science, high school chemistry, high school biology, high school foreign language, high school transcript, letter of recommendation, written essay, transcript of college record. *Options:* Advanced standing available through advanced placement exams. Course work may be accelerated. May apply for transfer of up to 77 total credits. *Application deadline:* rolling. *Application fee:* $25.

Degree Requirements 123 total credit hours, 46 in nursing.

RN Baccalaureate Program (BS)

Applying *Required:* minimum college GPA of 2.5, RN license, diploma or AD in nursing, high school transcript, interview, transcript of college record. *Options:* Advanced standing available through credit by exam. May apply for transfer of up to 64 total credits. *Application deadline:* rolling. *Application fee:* $25.

Degree Requirements 122 total credit hours, 45 in nursing.

Accelerated Baccalaureate for Second Degree Program (BS)

Applying *Required:* TOEFL for nonnative speakers of English, minimum college GPA of 2.5, high school transcript, interview, transcript of college record, BS. 6 prerequisite credits must be completed before admission to the nursing program. *Options:* May apply for transfer of up to 68 total credits. *Application deadline:* rolling. *Application fee:* $25.

Degree Requirements 123 total credit hours, 46 in nursing.

Niagara University (continued)

MASTER'S PROGRAM

Contact Dr. Dianne Morrison-Beedy, Director of the Family Nurse Practitioner Program, College of Nursing, Graduate Division, Niagara University, PO Box 2203, Niagara University, NY 14109-2203, 716-286-8338. *Fax:* 716-286-8308. *E-mail:* dmb@niagara.edu

Areas of Study Nurse practitioner program in family health.

Expenses *Tuition:* $393 per credit hour. *Full-time mandatory fees:* $10. *Part-time mandatory fees:* $10. *Room and board:* $5138–$6330. *Books and supplies per academic year:* ranges from $300 to $2000.

Financial Aid Nurse traineeships, employment opportunities, TAP, graduate workstudy, Federal Family Education Loan Program. 25% of master's level students in nursing programs received some form of financial aid in 1995-96. *Application deadline:* 4/15.

MASTER'S FOR RN WITH BS DEGREE (MS)

Applying *Required:* GRE General Test, bachelor's degree in nursing, bachelor's degree, minimum GPA of 3.0, RN license, 1 year of clinical experience, physical assessment course, statistics course, professional liability/malpractice insurance, essay, interview, 2 letters of recommendation, transcript of college record, curriculum vitae, CPR Certificate. *Application deadline:* rolling.

Degree Requirements 45 total credit hours, 42 in nursing.

PACE UNIVERSITY

Lienhard School of Nursing
Westchester and New York, New York

Programs • Generic Baccalaureate • RN Baccalaureate • Baccalaureate for Second Degree • MS • Master's for Nurses with Non-Nursing Degrees • Accelerated Master's for Non-Nursing College Graduates • Post-Master's • Continuing Education

The University Independent coed university. Part of Pace University. Founded: 1906. *Primary accreditation:* regional. *Total enrollment:* 12,534.

The Lienhard School of Nursing Founded in 1973. *Nursing program faculty:* 30 (67% with doctorates).

Academic Facilities *Campus library:* 1.0 million volumes (16,200 in health, 3,000 in nursing); 4,000 periodical subscriptions (425 health-care related). *Nursing school resources:* CAI, computer lab, nursing audiovisuals, interactive nursing skills videos, learning resource lab.

Student Life *Student services:* health clinic, child-care facilities, personal counseling, career counseling, institutionally sponsored work-study program, job placement, campus safety program, special assistance for disabled students. *International student services:* counseling/support, special assistance for nonnative speakers of English, English language institute. *Nursing student activities:* Sigma Theta Tau, student nurses association.

Calendar Semesters.

NURSING STUDENT PROFILE

Undergraduate **Enrollment:** 650
Women: 93%; **Men:** 7%; **Minority:** 42%; **International:** 3%; **Part-time:** 49%
Graduate **Enrollment:** 335
Women: 91%; **Men:** 9%; **Minority:** 5%; **International:** 5%; **Part-time:** 94%

BACCALAUREATE PROGRAMS

Contact Office of Undergraduate Admission, Pace University, 861 Bedford Road, Pleasantville, NY 10570, 914-773-3746. *Fax:* 914-773-3851. *E-mail:* infoctr@nyo27.wan.pace.edu

Expenses *Tuition:* $12,710 full-time, $398 per credit part-time. *Full-time mandatory fees:* $320–$785. *Part-time mandatory fees:* $48–$107. *Room and board:* $5340. *Room only:* $3900–$4200. *Books and supplies per academic year:* $650.

Financial Aid Institutionally sponsored need-based grants/scholarships, institutionally sponsored non-need grants/scholarships, Federal Direct Loans, Federal Nursing Student Loans, Federal Pell Grants, Federal Perkins Loans, Federal Supplemental Educational Opportunity Grants, Federal Work-Study, institutionally sponsored payment plans. 54% of undergraduate students in nursing programs received some form of financial aid in 1995–96. *Application deadline:* 2/8.

GENERIC BACCALAUREATE PROGRAM (BS)

Applying *Required:* SAT I, ACT, TOEFL for nonnative speakers of English, minimum high school GPA of 2.5, minimum college GPA of 2.5, 4 years of high school math, 2 years of high school science, high school foreign language, written essay. *Options:* Advanced standing available through the following means: advanced placement exams, credit by exam. Course work may be accelerated. May apply for transfer of up to 96 total credits. *Application deadline:* rolling. *Application fee:* $35.

Degree Requirements 129 total credit hours, 63 in nursing. 66 credit hours of core requirements.

RN BACCALAUREATE PROGRAM (BS)

Applying *Required:* minimum college GPA of 2.5, RN license, diploma or AD in nursing, high school transcript, written essay, transcript of college record. 64 prerequisite credits must be completed before admission to the nursing program. *Options:* Advanced standing available through credit by exam. May apply for transfer of up to 68 total credits. *Application deadline:* rolling. *Application fee:* $35.

Degree Requirements 129 total credit hours, 63 in nursing. 66 credit hours of core requirements.

BACCALAUREATE FOR SECOND DEGREE PROGRAM (BSN)

Applying *Required:* GRE or Miller Analogies Test. *Options:* Advanced standing available through credit by exam. May apply for transfer of up to 96 total credits.

Degree Requirements 128 total credit hours, 50 in nursing.

MASTER'S PROGRAMS

Contact Office of Graduate Admission, Pace University, 1 Martine Avenue, White Plains, NY 10606, 914-422-4283. *Fax:* 914-422-4287.

Areas of Study Clinical nurse specialist programs in adult health nursing, psychiatric–mental health nursing; nurse practitioner programs in acute care, community health, family health, primary care.

Expenses *Tuition:* $475 per credit. *Full-time mandatory fees:* $48–$160+. *Room and board:* $5340. *Room only:* $3900–$4200.

Financial Aid Graduate assistantships, Federal Direct Loans, Federal Nursing Student Loans, employment opportunities, deferred payment plans.

MS PROGRAM

Applying *Required:* GRE General Test or Miller Analogies Test, TOEFL for nonnative speakers of English, bachelor's degree in nursing, RN license, 2 letters of recommendation, transcript of college record. *Application deadlines:* 7/31 (fall), 11/30 (spring), 4/30 (summer). *Application fee:* $60.

Degree Requirements 36–42 total credit hours dependent upon track. Special project.

MASTER'S FOR NURSES WITH NON-NURSING DEGREES PROGRAM (MS)

Applying *Required:* GRE General Test or Miller Analogies Test, TOEFL for nonnative speakers of English, bachelor's degree, RN license, essay, 2 letters of recommendation, transcript of college record. *Application deadlines:* 7/31 (fall), 11/30 (spring), 4/30 (summer). *Application fee:* $60.

ACCELERATED MASTER'S FOR NON-NURSING COLLEGE GRADUATES PROGRAM (MS)

Applying *Required:* GRE General Test or Miller Analogies Test, TOEFL for nonnative speakers of English, essay, 2 letters of recommendation, transcript of college record, BSN earned concurrently. *Application deadline:* 3/1 (summer). *Application fee:* $60.

Degree Requirements 30–33 total credit hours dependent upon track, 30–33 in nursing.

POST-MASTER'S PROGRAM

Applying *Required:* RN license, 1 year of clinical experience, essay, 2 letters of recommendation, transcript of college record. *Application deadlines:* 7/31 (fall), 11/30 (spring), 4/30 (summer). *Application fee:* $60.

Degree Requirements 18–27 total credit hours dependent upon track, 18–27 in nursing.

CONTINUING EDUCATION PROGRAM

Contact Dr. Geraldine Colombraro, Assistant Dean, Center for Continuing Education in Nursing and Health Care, Lienhard School of Nursing, Pace University, Bedford Road, Pleasantville, NY 10570, 914-773-3358. *Fax:* 914-773-3376.

See full description on page 490.

ROBERTS WESLEYAN COLLEGE

Division of Nursing
Rochester, New York

Programs • Generic Baccalaureate • RN Baccalaureate • Accelerated RN Baccalaureate • Continuing Education

The College Independent comprehensive coed institution, affiliated with Free Methodist Church of North America. Founded: 1866. *Primary accreditation:* regional. *Setting:* 75-acre suburban campus. *Total enrollment:* 1,267.

The Division of Nursing Founded in 1952. *Nursing program faculty:* 13 (15% with doctorates).

Academic Facilities *Campus library:* 99,857 volumes (5,537 in health, 4,200 in nursing); 730 periodical subscriptions (85 health-care related). *Nursing school resources:* CAI, computer lab, nursing audiovisuals, interactive nursing skills videos, learning resource lab.

Student Life *Student services:* health clinic, personal counseling, career counseling, institutionally sponsored work-study program, campus safety program, special assistance for disabled students. *International student services:* counseling/support, special assistance for nonnative speakers of English, ESL courses. *Nursing student activities:* nursing club, Nurses Christian Fellowship, Nursing Honor Society.

Calendar Semesters.

NURSING STUDENT PROFILE

Undergraduate **Enrollment:** 120
Women: 92%; **Men:** 8%; **Minority:** 6%; **International:** 2%; **Part-time:** 6%

BACCALAUREATE PROGRAMS

Contact Ms. Linda Kurtz, Director of Admissions, Roberts Wesleyan College, 2301 Westside Drive, Rochester, NY 14624-1997, 716-594-6400. *Fax:* 716-594-6371. *E-mail:* admissions@roberts.edu

Expenses *Tuition:* $11,412 per academic year. *Full-time mandatory fees:* $228. *Room and board:* $4056. *Room only:* $2766. *Books and supplies per academic year:* $520.

Financial Aid Institutionally sponsored need-based grants/scholarships, institutionally sponsored non-need grants/scholarships, Federal Nursing Student Loans, Federal Supplemental Educational Opportunity Grants, Federal Work-Study. *Application deadline:* 3/15.

Generic Baccalaureate Program (BS)

Applying *Required:* SAT I, ACT, TOEFL for nonnative speakers of English, high school chemistry, high school biology, high school transcript, letter of recommendation, written essay, transcript of college record. 30 prerequisite credits must be completed before admission to the nursing program. *Options:* May apply for transfer of up to 90 total credits. *Application deadline:* rolling. *Application fee:* $35.

Degree Requirements 125 total credit hours, 56 in nursing.

RN Baccalaureate Program (BS)

Applying *Required:* SAT I or ACT, TOEFL for nonnative speakers of English, minimum high school GPA of 2.5, minimum college GPA of 2.25, high school chemistry, high school biology, RN license, diploma or AD in nursing, high school foreign language, high school transcript, interview, letter of recommendation, written essay, transcript of college record, high school class rank: . *Application deadlines:* 2/1 (priority deadline for fall), rolling.

Degree Requirements 125 total credit hours, 56 in nursing.

Accelerated RN Baccalaureate Program (BS)

Applying *Required:* high school chemistry, high school biology, RN license, diploma or AD in nursing, letter of recommendation, written essay, transcript of college record, 2 years of work experience. 62 prerequisite credits must be completed before admission to the nursing program. *Options:* May apply for transfer of up to 90 total credits. *Application deadline:* rolling. *Application fee:* $35.

Degree Requirements 125 total credit hours, 56 in nursing.

CONTINUING EDUCATION PROGRAM

Contact Mrs. Sue Hodges, Director of Continuing Liberal Studies, Robert Wesleyan College, 2301 Westside Drive, Rochester, NY 14624-1997, 716-594-6481. *E-mail:* hodgess@roberts.edu

RUSSELL SAGE COLLEGE

Department of Nursing
Troy, New York

Programs • Generic Baccalaureate • RN Baccalaureate • Baccalaureate for Second Degree • MS • RN to Master's • Master's for Nurses with Non-Nursing Degrees • MS/MBA • Post-Master's

The College Independent 4-year women's college. Part of The Sage Colleges. Founded: 1916. *Primary accreditation:* regional. *Setting:* 8-acre urban campus. *Total enrollment:* 1,115.

The Department of Nursing Founded in 1934. *Nursing program faculty:* 18 (60% with doctorates).

Academic Facilities *Campus library:* 225,000 volumes (4,003 in health, 2,516 in nursing); 1,500 periodical subscriptions (400 health-care related). *Nursing school resources:* CAI, computer lab, nursing audiovisuals, interactive nursing skills videos.

Student Life *Student services:* health clinic, personal counseling, career counseling, institutionally sponsored work-study program, special assistance for disabled students. *International student services:* counseling/support. *Nursing student activities:* Sigma Theta Tau, nursing club, student nurses association.

Calendar Semesters.

NURSING STUDENT PROFILE

Undergraduate **Enrollment:** 252
Women: 96%; **Men:** 4%; **Minority:** 4%; **Part-time:** 30%
Graduate **Enrollment:** 270
Women: 98%; **Men:** 2%; **Minority:** 6%; **International:** 2%; **Part-time:** 77%

BACCALAUREATE PROGRAMS

Contact Dr. Lynne Golonka, Undergraduate Director, Department of Nursing, The Sage Colleges, Russell Sage College, Troy, NY 12180-4115, 518-270-2231. *Fax:* 518-270-2009. *E-mail:* golonl@sage.edu

Expenses *Tuition:* $13,400 full-time, $340 per credit hour part-time. *Full-time mandatory fees:* $270–$350. *Room and board:* $5100–$6900. *Room only:* $2770–$3710. *Books and supplies per academic year:* ranges from $300 to $500.

Financial Aid Institutionally sponsored need-based grants/scholarships, institutionally sponsored non-need grants/scholarships, Federal Supplemental Educational Opportunity Grants, Federal Work-Study. *Application deadline:* 3/15.

Generic Baccalaureate Program (BS)

Applying *Required:* SAT I, TOEFL for nonnative speakers of English, minimum high school GPA of 2.5, minimum college GPA of 2.5, high school chemistry, high school biology, high school transcript, interview, written essay, transcript of college record. 30 prerequisite credits must be completed before admission to the nursing program. *Options:* Course work may be accelerated. May apply for transfer of up to 75 total credits. *Application deadlines:* 5/1 (fall), 12/1 (spring). *Application fee:* $20.

Degree Requirements 120 total credit hours, 54 in nursing.

RN Baccalaureate Program (BS)

Applying *Required:* minimum high school GPA of 2.5, minimum college GPA of 2.5, high school chemistry, high school biology, RN license, diploma or AD in nursing, high school transcript, interview, transcript of college record. 58 prerequisite credits must be completed before admission to the nursing program. *Options:* Course work may be accelerated. May apply for transfer of up to 60 total credits. *Application deadline:* rolling. *Application fee:* $20.

Degree Requirements 120 total credit hours, 54 in nursing.

Baccalaureate for Second Degree Program (BS)

Applying *Required:* minimum college GPA of 2.5, high school chemistry, high school biology, high school transcript, interview, transcript of college record. 60 prerequisite credits must be completed before admission to the nursing program. *Options:* Course work may be accelerated. May apply for transfer of up to 75 total credits. *Application deadline:* rolling. *Application fee:* $20.

Degree Requirements 120 total credit hours, 54 in nursing.

Russell Sage College (continued)

MASTER'S PROGRAMS

Contact Dr. Ann Gothler, Director, Graduate Program in Nursing, Department of Nursing, The Sage Colleges, Russell Sage College, Troy, NY 12180-4115, 518-270-2384. *Fax:* 518-270-2009. *E-mail:* gothla@sage.edu

Areas of Study Clinical nurse specialist programs in community health nursing, medical-surgical nursing, psychiatric–mental health nursing; nursing administration; nursing education; nurse practitioner programs in acute care, adult health, family health, gerontology, psychiatric–mental health.

Expenses *Tuition:* $340 per credit hour. *Full-time mandatory fees:* $0. *Room and board:* $5080–$6000. *Room only:* $2770–$3210. *Books and supplies per academic year:* ranges from $350 to $700.

Financial Aid Graduate assistantships, nurse traineeships, Federal Nursing Student Loans, employment opportunities. *Application deadline:* 4/1.

MS Program

Applying *Required:* bachelor's degree in nursing, minimum GPA of 2.75, physical assessment course, statistics course, professional liability/malpractice insurance, essay, 2 letters of recommendation, transcript of college record, family nurse practitioner track requires RN license and 1 year of professional nursing experience. *Application deadline:* rolling. *Application fee:* $20.

Degree Requirements 42 total credit hours, 36–39 in nursing, 3–6 in other specified areas. Thesis or research project.

RN to Master's Program (MS)

Applying *Required:* minimum GPA of 2.5, RN license, interview, transcript of college record, minimum 3.2 GPA in nursing major after 15 credits. *Application deadline:* rolling. *Application fee:* $20.

Degree Requirements 120 total credit hours, 54 in nursing, 66 in biological science, chemistry, physics, nutrition, and other specified areas. Thesis or project.

Master's for Nurses with Non-Nursing Degrees Program (MS)

Applying *Required:* minimum GPA of 2.75, RN license, physical assessment course, statistics course, professional liability/malpractice insurance, essay, interview, 2 letters of recommendation, transcript of college record. *Application deadline:* rolling. *Application fee:* $20.

Degree Requirements 54–57 total credit hours dependent upon track, 48–53 in nursing, 3–6 in other specified areas. Thesis or research project.

MS/MBA Program

Applying *Required:* GMAT, minimum GPA of 2.75, RN license, physical assessment course, statistics course, professional liability/malpractice insurance, essay, interview, 2 letters of recommendation, transcript of college record. *Application deadline:* rolling. *Application fee:* $20.

Degree Requirements 66 total credit hours, 33 in nursing, 33 in business administration. Thesis or research project.

Post-Master's Program

Applying *Required:* RN license, 1 year of clinical experience, physical assessment course, statistics course, professional liability/malpractice insurance, essay, interview, transcript of college record. *Application deadline:* rolling. *Application fee:* $20.

Degree Requirements 12–24 total credit hours dependent upon track, 9–21 in nursing, 3–6 in pharmacology, pathophysiology.

ST. JOHN FISHER COLLEGE

Department of Nursing
Rochester, New York

Programs • Generic Baccalaureate • RN Baccalaureate • Baccalaureate for Second Degree • MS • Accelerated MS • RN to Master's • Continuing Education

The College Independent comprehensive coed institution, affiliated with Roman Catholic Church. Founded: 1948. *Primary accreditation:* regional. *Setting:* 125-acre suburban campus. *Total enrollment:* 2,045.

The Department of Nursing Founded in 1942. *Nursing program faculty:* 10 (50% with doctorates).

Academic Facilities *Campus library:* 160,000 volumes (4,200 in nursing); 950 periodical subscriptions (55 health-care related). *Nursing school resources:* CAI, computer lab, nursing audiovisuals, interactive nursing skills videos, learning resource lab.

Student Life *Student services:* health clinic, child-care facilities, personal counseling, career counseling, institutionally sponsored work-study program, job placement, campus safety program, special assistance for disabled students. *International student services:* counseling/support. *Nursing student activities:* Sigma Theta Tau, nursing club, student nurses association.

Calendar Semesters.

NURSING STUDENT PROFILE

Undergraduate **Enrollment:** 242
Women: 89%; **Men:** 11%; **Minority:** 11%; **International:** 0%; **Part-time:** 32%
Graduate **Enrollment:** 147
Women: 95%; **Men:** 5%; **Minority:** 3%; **International:** 0%; **Part-time:** 77%

BACCALAUREATE PROGRAMS

Contact Gerard Rooney, Dean of Enrollment Management, Admissions Office, St. John Fisher College, 3690 East Avenue, Rochester, NY 14618, 716-385-8064. *E-mail:* rooney@sjfc.edu

Expenses *Tuition:* $11,760 full-time, $295 per credit part-time. *Full-time mandatory fees:* $400. *Room and board:* $5580–$6140. *Room only:* $3950–$4340. *Books and supplies per academic year:* ranges from $300 to $500.

Financial Aid Institutionally sponsored need-based grants/scholarships, institutionally sponsored non-need grants/scholarships, Federal Supplemental Educational Opportunity Grants, Federal Work-Study. 75% of undergraduate students in nursing programs received some form of financial aid in 1995–96. *Application deadline:* 3/1.

Generic Baccalaureate Program (BS)

Applying *Required:* SAT I, ACT, TOEFL for nonnative speakers of English, minimum high school GPA of 3.0, minimum college GPA of 3.0, 3 years of high school math, 3 years of high school science, high school chemistry, high school biology, high school transcript, 2 letters of recommendation, written essay, transcript of college record. *Options:* Advanced standing available through the following means: advanced placement exams, credit by exam. Course work may be accelerated. *Application deadline:* rolling. *Application fee:* $25.

Degree Requirements 120 total credit hours, 52 in nursing. 68 credit hours of liberal arts/science.

RN Baccalaureate Program (BS)

Applying *Required:* TOEFL for nonnative speakers of English, minimum college GPA of 3.0, RN license, diploma or AD in nursing, 2 letters of recommendation, written essay, transcript of college record. 55 prerequisite credits must be completed before admission to the nursing program. *Options:* Advanced standing available through the following means: advanced placement exams, credit by exam. Course work may be accelerated. May apply for transfer of up to 90 total credits. *Application deadline:* rolling. *Application fee:* $25.

Degree Requirements 120 total credit hours, 52 in nursing. 68 credit hours of academic courses.

Baccalaureate for Second Degree Program (BS)

Applying *Required:* SAT I, ACT, TOEFL for nonnative speakers of English, minimum high school GPA of 3.0, minimum college GPA of 3.0, 3 years of high school math, 3 years of high school science, high school chemistry, high school biology, high school transcript, 2 letters of recommendation, written essay, transcript of college record. 55 prerequisite credits must be completed before admission to the nursing program. *Options:* Advanced standing available through the following means: advanced placement exams, credit by exam. Course work may be accelerated. *Application deadline:* rolling. *Application fee:* $25.

Degree Requirements 120 total credit hours, 52 in nursing. 68 credit hours of liberal arts/science.

MASTER'S PROGRAMS

Contact Dr. Kathleen Powers, Chair, Department of Nursing, St. John Fisher College, 3690 East Avenue, Rochester, NY 14618, 716-385-8241. *Fax:* 716-385-8466. *E-mail:* powers@sjfc.edu

Areas of Study Clinical nurse specialist program in managed care for high risk populations; nursing administration; nurse practitioner program in family health.

Expenses *Tuition:* $365 per credit. *Full-time mandatory fees:* $50–$150. *Books and supplies per academic year:* ranges from $100 to $300.

Financial Aid Nurse traineeships, employment opportunities, institutionally sponsored need-based grants/scholarships. 50% of master's level students in nursing programs received some form of financial aid in 1995-96.

MS Program

Applying *Required:* TOEFL for nonnative speakers of English, bachelor's degree in nursing, minimum GPA of 3.0, RN license, physical assessment course, statistics course, essay, 2 letters of recommendation, transcript of college record, nursing research course. *Application deadline:* rolling. *Application fee:* $30.

Degree Requirements 36 total credit hours, 30 in nursing, 6 in business administration. Project.

Accelerated MS Program

Applying *Required:* TOEFL for nonnative speakers of English, bachelor's degree in nursing, minimum GPA of 3.0, RN license, physical assessment course, statistics course, essay, 2 letters of recommendation, transcript of college record, nursing research course; students in final year of bachelor's degree in nursing may take graduate courses and apply them to this degree. *Application deadline:* rolling. *Application fee:* $30.

Degree Requirements 36 total credit hours, 30 in nursing, 6 in business administration. Project.

RN to Master's Program (MS)

Applying *Required:* TOEFL for nonnative speakers of English, bachelor's degree in nursing, minimum GPA of 3.0, RN license, physical assessment course, statistics course, professional liability/malpractice insurance, essay, 2 letters of recommendation, transcript of college record. *Application deadline:* rolling. *Application fee:* $30.

Degree Requirements 36 total credit hours, 30 in nursing, 6 in business administration. Project.

CONTINUING EDUCATION PROGRAM

Contact Greg Williams, Director, Continuing Education Office, St. John Fisher College, 3690 East Avenue, Rochester, NY 14618, 716-385-8317. *E-mail:* williams@sjfc.edu

ST. JOSEPH'S COLLEGE, NEW YORK

Nursing Department
Brooklyn, New York

Program • Generic Baccalaureate

The College Independent 4-year coed college. Founded: 1916. *Primary accreditation:* regional. *Total enrollment:* 1,216.

The Nursing Department Founded in 1987.

Academic Facilities *Campus library:* 336,505 volumes (1,900 in health, 2,300 in nursing); 923 periodical subscriptions (154 health-care related).

Calendar Semesters.

BACCALAUREATE PROGRAM

Contact Director, Nursing Department, St. Joseph's College, New York, 245 Clinton Avenue, Brooklyn, NY 11205-3688, 718-399-0068. *Fax:* 718-398-4936.

STATE UNIVERSITY OF NEW YORK AT BINGHAMTON

Decker School of Nursing
Binghamton, New York

Programs • Generic Baccalaureate • RN Baccalaureate • Accelerated RN Baccalaureate • Accelerated Baccalaureate for Second Degree • MS • Post-Master's • Continuing Education

The University State-supported coed university. Part of State University of New York System. Founded: 1946. *Primary accreditation:* regional. *Setting:* 606-acre suburban campus. *Total enrollment:* 11,952.

The Decker School of Nursing Founded in 1969. *Nursing program faculty:* 34 (39% with doctorates).

Academic Facilities *Campus library:* 1.5 million volumes; 8,800 periodical subscriptions. *Nursing school resources:* CAI, computer lab, nursing audiovisuals, interactive nursing skills videos, learning resource lab.

Student Life *Student services:* health clinic, child-care facilities, personal counseling, career counseling, institutionally sponsored work-study program, job placement, campus safety program, special assistance for disabled students. *International student services:* counseling/support, special assistance for nonnative speakers of English, ESL courses. *Nursing student activities:* Sigma Theta Tau, student nurses association.

Calendar Semesters.

NURSING STUDENT PROFILE

Undergraduate **Enrollment:** 294
Women: 95%; **Men:** 5%; **Minority:** 9%; **International:** 0%; **Part-time:** 12%
Graduate **Enrollment:** 133
Women: 92%; **Men:** 8%; **Minority:** 3%; **International:** 1%; **Part-time:** 66%

BACCALAUREATE PROGRAMS

Contact Ms. Marlene Payne, Coordinator, Undergraduate Program, Decker School of Nursing, State University of New York at Binghamton, PO Box 6000, Binghamton, NY 13902-6000, 607-777-4713. *Fax:* 607-777-4440. *E-mail:* mpayne@binghamton.edu

Expenses *State resident tuition:* $3400 full-time, $137 per credit hour part-time. *Nonresident tuition:* $4150 full-time, $346 per credit hour part-time. *Full-time mandatory fees:* $673. *Part-time mandatory fees:* $115–$587. *Room and board:* $3674–$6494. *Room only:* $2140–$4440.

Financial Aid Institutionally sponsored need-based grants/scholarships, institutionally sponsored non-need grants/scholarships, Federal Direct Loans, Federal Nursing Student Loans, Federal Pell Grants, Federal Supplemental Educational Opportunity Grants, Federal Work-Study. *Application deadline:* 3/1.

Generic Baccalaureate Program (BS)

Applying *Required:* SAT I, minimum high school GPA of 3.0, minimum college GPA of 2.7, 3 years of high school math, 3 years of high school science, high school chemistry, high school biology, high school transcript, 2 letters of recommendation, written essay, transcript of college record. 12 prerequisite credits must be completed before admission to the nursing program. *Options:* Course work may be accelerated. May apply for transfer of up to 76 total credits. *Application deadlines:* 12/1 (fall), 11/15 (spring). *Application fee:* $30.

Degree Requirements 128 total credit hours, 52 in nursing.

RN Baccalaureate Program (BS)

Applying *Required:* New York State Regents College exam, ACT PEP or NLN Mobility Profile II for diploma RNs, minimum college GPA of 2.7, RN license, diploma or AD in nursing, written essay, transcript of college record. 50 prerequisite credits must be completed before admission to the nursing program. *Options:* Course work may be accelerated. May apply for transfer of up to 84 total credits. *Application deadlines:* 12/1 (fall), 11/15 (spring). *Application fee:* $30.

Degree Requirements 128 total credit hours, 52 in nursing.

Accelerated RN Baccalaureate Program (BS)

Applying *Required:* minimum college GPA of 3.0, RN license, diploma or AD in nursing, interview, 2 letters of recommendation, written essay, transcript of college record. 70 prerequisite credits must be completed

State University of New York at Binghamton (continued)

before admission to the nursing program. *Options:* May apply for transfer of up to 84 total credits. *Application deadlines:* 12/1 (fall), 11/15 (spring). *Application fee:* $25.

Degree Requirements 128 total credit hours, 52 in nursing.

Accelerated Baccalaureate for Second Degree Program (BS)

Applying *Required:* minimum college GPA of 3.0, interview, 2 letters of recommendation, written essay, transcript of college record. 44 prerequisite credits must be completed before admission to the nursing program. *Options:* Course work may be accelerated. May apply for transfer of up to 76 total credits. *Application deadlines:* 12/1 (fall), 11/15 (spring). *Application fee:* $30.

Degree Requirements 128 total credit hours, 52 in nursing.

MASTER'S PROGRAMS

Contact Ms. Joyce Ferrario, Associate Dean and Coordinator, Graduate Program, Decker School of Nursing, State University of New York at Binghamton, PO Box 6000, Binghamton, NY 13902-6000, 607-777-4964. *Fax:* 607-777-4440.

Areas of Study Clinical nurse specialist programs in community health nursing, family health nursing, gerontological nursing; nursing administration; nursing education; nurse practitioner programs in community health, family health, gerontology, primary care.

Expenses *State resident tuition:* $5100 full-time, $213 per credit part-time. *Nonresident tuition:* $8416 full-time, $351 per credit part-time. *Full-time mandatory fees:* $2022. *Books and supplies per academic year:* ranges from $800 to $900.

Financial Aid Graduate assistantships, nurse traineeships, Federal Nursing Student Loans. 35% of master's level students in nursing programs received some form of financial aid in 1995-96. *Application deadline:* 3/31.

MS Program

Applying *Required:* GRE General Test, bachelor's degree in nursing, minimum GPA of 3.0, RN license, statistics course, essay, 2 letters of recommendation, transcript of college record. *Application deadline:* rolling. *Application fee:* $50.

Degree Requirements 48 total credit hours, 48 in nursing.

Post-Master's Program

Applying *Required:* minimum GPA of 3.0, RN license, statistics course, essay, 2 letters of recommendation, transcript of college record, MS in Nursing. *Application deadline:* rolling. *Application fee:* $50.

Degree Requirements 28–31 total credit hours dependent upon track, 28–31 in nursing.

CONTINUING EDUCATION PROGRAM

Contact Dean's Office, Decker School of Nursing, State University of New York at Binghamton, PO Box 6000, Binghamton, NY 13902-6000, 607-777-2311. *Fax:* 607-777-4440.

See full description on page 508.

STATE UNIVERSITY OF NEW YORK AT BUFFALO

School of Nursing
Buffalo, New York

Programs • Generic Baccalaureate • RN Baccalaureate • RN to Master's • Postbaccalaureate Doctorate • Continuing Education

The University State-supported coed university. Part of State University of New York System. Founded: 1846. *Primary accreditation:* regional. *Setting:* 1,350-acre suburban campus. *Total enrollment:* 24,493.

The School of Nursing Founded in 1936. *Nursing program faculty:* 53 (80% with doctorates).

Academic Facilities *Campus library:* 3.0 million volumes (250,000 in health, 25,000 in nursing); 15,000 periodical subscriptions (2,500 health-care related). *Nursing school resources:* CAI, computer lab, nursing audiovisuals, interactive nursing skills videos, learning resource lab, anesthesia simulator.

Student Life *Student services:* health clinic, child-care facilities, personal counseling, career counseling, institutionally sponsored work-study program, job placement, campus safety program, special assistance for disabled students. *International student services:* counseling/support, special assistance for nonnative speakers of English, ESL courses. *Nursing student activities:* Sigma Theta Tau, nursing club, student nurses association.

Calendar Semesters.

NURSING STUDENT PROFILE

Undergraduate **Enrollment:** 244
Women: 91%; **Men:** 9%; **Minority:** 18%; **International:** 2%; **Part-time:** 35%

Graduate **Enrollment:** 277
Women: 92%; **Men:** 8%; **Minority:** 10%; **International:** 2%; **Part-time:** 87%

BACCALAUREATE PROGRAMS

Contact Dr. William P. Harden, Assistant Dean, 1017 Kimball Tower, School of Nursing, State University of New York at Buffalo, Buffalo, NY 14214-3079, 716-829-2537. *Fax:* 716-829-2021. *E-mail:* wharden@nurse.buffalo.edu

Expenses *State resident tuition:* $3400 full-time, $137 per credit part-time. *Nonresident tuition:* $8300 full-time, $346 per credit part-time. *Full-time mandatory fees:* $759. *Part-time mandatory fees:* $27+. *Room and board:* $4365–$5985. *Room only:* $2645–$3745. *Books and supplies per academic year:* ranges from $400 to $500.

Financial Aid Institutionally sponsored need-based grants/scholarships, institutionally sponsored non-need grants/scholarships, Federal Nursing Student Loans, Federal Supplemental Educational Opportunity Grants, Federal Work-Study. 64% of undergraduate students in nursing programs received some form of financial aid in 1995–96. *Application deadline:* 1/15.

Generic Baccalaureate Program (BS)

Applying *Required:* SAT I, ACT, TOEFL for nonnative speakers of English, TSE for nonnative speakers of English, minimum high school GPA of 2.5, minimum college GPA of 2.9, high school chemistry, high school transcript, transcript of college record. 22 prerequisite credits must be completed before admission to the nursing program. *Options:* Advanced standing available through the following means: advanced placement exams, credit by exam. *Application deadline:* 3/15. *Application fee:* $25.

Degree Requirements 120 total credit hours, 56 in nursing.

RN Baccalaureate Program (BS)

Applying *Required:* TOEFL for nonnative speakers of English, TSE for nonnative speakers of English, high school chemistry, RN license, diploma or AD in nursing, transcript of college record. 22 prerequisite credits must be completed before admission to the nursing program. *Options:* Advanced standing available through the following means: advanced placement exams, credit by exam. Course work may be accelerated. *Application deadlines:* 3/15 (fall), 10/15 (spring). *Application fee:* $25.

Degree Requirements 120 total credit hours, 30 in nursing.

MASTER'S PROGRAM

Contact Dr. William P. Harden, Assistant Dean, 1017 Kimball Tower, School of Nursing, State University of New York at Buffalo, Buffalo, NY 14214-3079, 716-829-2537. *Fax:* 716-829-2021. *E-mail:* wharden@nurse.buffalo.edu

Areas of Study Clinical nurse specialist program in pediatric nursing; nurse anesthesia; nurse practitioner programs in adult health, child care/pediatrics, family health, school health, women's health.

Expenses *State resident tuition:* $5100 full-time, $213 per credit part-time. *Nonresident tuition:* $8416 full-time, $351 per credit part-time. *Full-time mandatory fees:* $512. *Part-time mandatory fees:* $52–$244. *Room and board:* $4365–$5985. *Room only:* $2645–$3745. *Books and supplies per academic year:* ranges from $400 to $500.

Financial Aid Graduate assistantships, nurse traineeships, Federal Nursing Student Loans. 31% of master's level students in nursing programs received some form of financial aid in 1995-96. *Application deadline:* 4/15.

RN to Master's Program (MS)

Applying *Required:* GRE General Test, TOEFL for nonnative speakers of English, bachelor's degree in nursing, minimum GPA of 3.0, RN license, 1 year of clinical experience, physical assessment course, statistics course, interview, 3 letters of recommendation, transcript of college record, minimum 1 year experience in projected specialty. *Application deadlines:* 4/15 (fall), 11/15 (spring). *Application fee:* $35.

Degree Requirements 36–45 total credit hours dependent upon track, 36–45 in nursing. Thesis, project, or comprehensive exam.

Distance learning Courses provided through computer-based media.

DOCTORAL PROGRAM

Contact Dr. William P. Harden, Assistant Dean, 1017 Kimball Tower, School of Nursing, State University of New York at Buffalo, Buffalo, NY 14214-3079, 716-829-2537. *Fax:* 716-829-2021. *E-mail:* wharden@nurse.buffalo.edu

Areas of Study Nursing administration, nursing research, clinical practice.

Expenses *State resident tuition:* $5100 full-time, $213 per credit part-time. *Nonresident tuition:* $8416 full-time, $351 per credit part-time. *Full-time mandatory fees:* $512. *Part-time mandatory fees:* $52–$244. *Room and board:* $4365–$5985. *Room only:* $2645–$3745. *Books and supplies per academic year:* ranges from $400 to $500.

Financial Aid Nurse traineeships, fellowships, dissertation grants. *Application deadline:* 4/15.

Postbaccalaureate Doctorate (DNS)

Applying *Required:* TOEFL for nonnative speakers of English, GRE General Test (minimum score of 500 on verbal section, 500 on quantitative section), 1 year of clinical experience, 1 year in proposed area of specialization, 1 scholarly paper, statistics course, interview, 3 letters of recommendation, vitae, writing sample, competitive review by faculty committee, BSN, minimum 3.25 GPA. *Application deadlines:* 3/15 (fall), 10/15 (spring). *Application fee:* $35.

Degree Requirements 75+ total credit hours dependent upon track; dissertation; written exam; defense of dissertation; residency.

CONTINUING EDUCATION PROGRAM

Contact Dr. Mary Finnick, Director of Continuing Education, 704 Kimball Tower, School of Nursing, State University of New York at Buffalo, Buffalo, NY 14214-3079, 716-829-3291. *Fax:* 716-829-2021.

STATE UNIVERSITY OF NEW YORK AT NEW PALTZ
Department of Nursing
New Paltz, New York

Programs • RN Baccalaureate • MS

The University State-supported comprehensive coed institution. Part of State University of New York System. Founded: 1828. *Primary accreditation:* regional. *Setting:* 216-acre rural campus. *Total enrollment:* 7,897.

The Department of Nursing Founded in 1982. *Nursing program faculty:* 9 (56% with doctorates). *Off-campus program sites:* Middletown, West Haverstraw, Poughkeepsie.

Academic Facilities *Campus library:* 398,000 volumes (10,699 in health, 9,072 in nursing); 1,510 periodical subscriptions (66 health-care related). *Nursing school resources:* CAI, computer lab, nursing audiovisuals, learning resource lab.

Student Life *Student services:* health clinic, child-care facilities, personal counseling, career counseling, institutionally sponsored work-study program, special assistance for disabled students. *International student services:* special assistance for nonnative speakers of English, ESL courses. *Nursing student activities:* nursing club.

Calendar Semesters.

NURSING STUDENT PROFILE

Undergraduate **Enrollment:** 205

Women: 96%; **Men:** 4%; **Minority:** 13%; **International:** 0%; **Part-time:** 92%

Graduate **Enrollment:** 25

Women: 97%; **Men:** 3%; **Minority:** 7%; **International:** 0%; **Part-time:** 45%

BACCALAUREATE PROGRAM

Contact Dr. Ide Katims, Acting Director, VLC 205, Department of Nursing, State University of New York at New Paltz, New Paltz, NY 12561, 914-257-2922. *Fax:* 914-257-2926.

Expenses *State resident tuition:* $3400 full-time, $137 per credit part-time. *Nonresident tuition:* $8300 full-time, $346 per credit part-time. *Full-time mandatory fees:* $176. *Part-time mandatory fees:* $11–$88.

Financial Aid Institutionally sponsored need-based grants/scholarships, Federal Supplemental Educational Opportunity Grants, Federal Work-Study. *Application deadline:* 4/1.

RN Baccalaureate Program (BS)

Applying *Required:* NLN Mobility Profile II, minimum college GPA of 2.5, RN license, diploma or AD in nursing, 3 letters of recommendation, written essay, transcript of college record, health exam, professional liability/malpractice insurance. 31 prerequisite credits must be completed before admission to the nursing program. *Options:* May apply for transfer of up to 42 total credits. *Application deadlines:* 6/1 (fall), 12/1 (spring). *Application fee:* $25.

Degree Requirements 120 total credit hours, 45 in nursing.

MASTER'S PROGRAM

Contact Dr. Ide Katims, Director, VLC 205, Department of Nursing, State University of New York at New Paltz, New Paltz, NY 12561, 914-257-2922. *Fax:* 914-257-2926. *E-mail:* katimsi@matrix.newpaltz.edu

Areas of Study Clinical nurse specialist programs in family health nursing, gerontological nursing.

Expenses *State resident tuition:* $5100 full-time, $213 per credit part-time. *Nonresident tuition:* $8416 full-time, $351 per credit part-time.

Financial Aid Nurse traineeships, institutionally sponsored non-need-based grants/scholarships. *Application deadline:* 4/1.

MS Program

Applying *Required:* GRE General Test, bachelor's degree in nursing, bachelor's degree, minimum GPA of 3.0, RN license, 1 year of clinical experience, physical assessment course, statistics course, professional liability/malpractice insurance, essay, interview, 3 letters of recommendation, transcript of college record, research course. *Application deadline:* rolling.

Degree Requirements 36 total credit hours.

Distance learning Courses provided through video.

STATE UNIVERSITY OF NEW YORK AT STONY BROOK
Health Sciences Center–School of Nursing
Stony Brook, New York

Programs • Generic Baccalaureate • RN Baccalaureate • Accelerated Baccalaureate for Second Degree • MS • RN to Master's • Accelerated RN to Master's • Post-Master's • Continuing Education

The University State-supported coed university. Part of State University of New York System. Founded: 1957. *Primary accreditation:* regional. *Setting:* 1,100-acre small-town campus. *Total enrollment:* 17,658.

The Health Sciences Center–School of Nursing Founded in 1970. *Nursing program faculty:* 55 (23% with doctorates).

Academic Facilities *Campus library:* 3,000 volumes (1,000 in health, 750 in nursing); 3,000 periodical subscriptions (1,800 health-care related). *Nursing school resources:* CAI, computer lab, nursing audiovisuals, interactive nursing skills videos, learning resource lab.

Student Life *Student services:* health clinic, child-care facilities, personal counseling, career counseling, institutionally sponsored work-study program, campus safety program, special assistance for disabled students. *International student services:* counseling/support, special assistance for nonnative speakers of English, ESL courses. *Nursing student activities:* Sigma Theta Tau, student nurses association.

Calendar Semesters.

NURSING STUDENT PROFILE

Undergraduate **Enrollment:** 205

Women: 93%; **Men:** 7%; **Minority:** 18%; **International:** 1%; **Part-time:** 50%

Graduate **Enrollment:** 541

Women: 98%; **Men:** 2%; **Minority:** 15%; **International:** 1%; **Part-time:** 99%

BACCALAUREATE PROGRAMS

Contact Ms. Joyce Lichter, Assistant to the Dean for Student Affairs, School of Nursing-Health Sciences Center, State University of New York at Stony Brook, Stony Brook, NY 11794-8240, 516-444-3200. *Fax:* 516-444-3136.

Expenses *State resident tuition:* $3400 full-time, $137 per credit part-time. *Nonresident tuition:* $7550 full-time, $314 per credit part-time. *Full-time mandatory fees:* $317. *Books and supplies per academic year:* $400.

Financial Aid Institutionally sponsored need-based grants/scholarships, institutionally sponsored non-need grants/scholarships, Federal Nursing

State University of New York at Stony Brook (continued)
Student Loans, Federal Supplemental Educational Opportunity Grants, Federal Work-Study. *Application deadline:* 3/1.

Generic Baccalaureate Program (BS)

Applying *Required:* SAT I, ACT, TOEFL for nonnative speakers of English, minimum high school GPA of 3.5, minimum college GPA of 2.5, 3 years of high school math, 3 years of high school science, 3 letters of recommendation, written essay, transcript of college record, CPR certification. 57 prerequisite credits must be completed before admission to the nursing program. *Application deadline:* 1/31. *Application fee:* $30.

Degree Requirements 128 total credit hours, 71 in nursing.

RN Baccalaureate Program (BS)

Applying *Required:* NLN Mobility Profile II, minimum college GPA of 2.5, RN license, diploma or AD in nursing, 3 letters of recommendation, written essay, transcript of college record, CPR certification. 57 prerequisite credits must be completed before admission to the nursing program. *Options:* Advanced standing available through credit by exam. *Application deadline:* 1/31. *Application fee:* $30.

Degree Requirements 128 total credit hours, 71 in nursing.

Accelerated Baccalaureate for Second Degree Program (BS)

Applying *Required:* minimum college GPA of 2.8, interview, 3 letters of recommendation, written essay, transcript of college record, bachelor's degree, CPR certification. *Application deadline:* 1/31. *Application fee:* $25.

Degree Requirements 69 total credit hours, 69 in nursing.

MASTER'S PROGRAMS

Contact Ms. Joyce Lichter, Assistant to the Dean for Student Affairs, School of Nursing-Health Sciences Center, State University of New York at Stony Brook, Stony Brook, NY 11794-8240, 516-444-3200. *Fax:* 516-444-3136.

Areas of Study Clinical nurse specialist programs in adult health nursing, critical care nursing, maternity-newborn nursing, medical-surgical nursing, pediatric nursing, perinatal nursing, psychiatric–mental health nursing, women's health nursing, midwifery; nurse midwifery; nurse practitioner programs in acute care, adult health, child care/pediatrics, neonatal health, psychiatric–mental health, women's health, midwifery.

Expenses *State resident tuition:* $5100 full-time, $213 per credit hour part-time. *Nonresident tuition:* $8416 full-time, $351 per credit hour part-time. *Full-time mandatory fees:* $104. *Part-time mandatory fees:* $6+. *Room only:* $3168–$4752.

Financial Aid Nurse traineeships, Federal Nursing Student Loans, tuition assistance program, Federal Work-Study. *Application deadline:* 4/1.

MS Program

Applying *Required:* minimum GPA of 3.0, RN license, physical assessment course, statistics course, essay, interview, 3 letters of recommendation, transcript of college record, CPR certification. *Application deadline:* 3/1. *Application fee:* $50.

Degree Requirements 45 total credit hours, 45 in nursing. 600 clinical hours.

Distance learning Courses provided on-line. Specific degree requirements include emphasis in midwifery track only.

RN to Master's Program (MS)

Applying *Required:* TOEFL for nonnative speakers of English, bachelor's degree in nursing, bachelor's degree, minimum GPA of 3.0, RN license, physical assessment course, statistics course, professional liability/malpractice insurance, essay, 3 letters of recommendation, transcript of college record. *Application deadline:* 3/1. *Application fee:* $50.

Degree Requirements 45 total credit hours, 45 in nursing. 600 clinical hours.

Distance learning Courses provided through computer-based media. Specific degree requirements include emphasis in midwifery track only.

Accelerated RN to Master's Program (MS)

Applying *Required:* TOEFL for nonnative speakers of English, minimum GPA of 3.0, RN license, physical assessment course, statistics course, transcript of college record, CPR certification, BS earned concurrently. *Application deadline:* 3/1. *Application fee:* $50.

Degree Requirements 45 total credit hours, 45 in nursing. 600 clinical hours.

Distance learning Courses provided on-line. Specific degree requirements include emphasis in midwifery track only.

Post-Master's Program

Applying *Required:* minimum GPA of 3.0, RN license, 1 year of clinical experience, physical assessment course, statistics course, professional liability/malpractice insurance, essay, 3 letters of recommendation, transcript of college record, master's degree in nursing. *Application deadline:* 3/1. *Application fee:* $50.

Degree Requirements 24 total credit hours, 18–24 in nursing. 600 clinical hours.

Distance learning Courses provided on-line. Specific degree requirements include emphasis in midwifery track only.

CONTINUING EDUCATION PROGRAM

Contact Mr. Gene Mundie, Director of Continuing Education, School of Nursing-Health Science Center, State University of New York at Stony Brook, Stony Brook, NY 11794-8240, 516-444-3289. *Fax:* 516-444-3136.

STATE UNIVERSITY OF NEW YORK COLLEGE AT BROCKPORT
Nursing Department
Brockport, New York

Programs • Generic Baccalaureate • RN Baccalaureate

The University State-supported comprehensive coed institution. Part of State University of New York System. Founded: 1867. *Primary accreditation:* regional. *Setting:* 591-acre small-town campus. *Total enrollment:* 9,047.

The Nursing Department Founded in 1978. *Nursing program faculty:* 21 (20% with doctorates). *Off-campus program site:* Alfred.

Academic Facilities *Campus library:* 413,000 volumes (22,222 in health, 1,574 in nursing); 95,100 periodical subscriptions (82 health-care related). *Nursing school resources:* CAI, computer lab, nursing audiovisuals, interactive nursing skills videos, learning resource lab.

Student Life *Student services:* health clinic, child-care facilities, personal counseling, career counseling, institutionally sponsored work-study program, job placement, campus safety program, special assistance for disabled students. *International student services:* counseling/support, ESL courses. *Nursing student activities:* nursing club, student nurses association, Nursing Honor Society.

Calendar Semesters.

NURSING STUDENT PROFILE

Undergraduate **Enrollment:** 165
Women: 89%; **Men:** 11%; **Minority:** 5%; **International:** 1%; **Part-time:** 24%

BACCALAUREATE PROGRAMS

Contact Dr. Kathryn Wood, Chairperson, Nursing Department, State University of New York College at Brockport, Brockport, NY 14420, 716-395-2355. *Fax:* 716-395-2160. *E-mail:* kwood@brockvma.cc.brockport.edu

Expenses *State resident tuition:* $2650 full-time, $105 per credit part-time. *Nonresident tuition:* $6550 full-time, $274 per credit part-time. *Room and board:* $4520. *Books and supplies per academic year:* $350.

Financial Aid Federal Pell Grants, Federal Stafford Loans, New York State Tuition Assistance Program (TAP). *Application deadline:* 2/15.

Generic Baccalaureate Program (BSN)

Applying *Required:* SAT I or ACT, minimum high school GPA of 2.3, minimum college GPA of 2.5, 3 years of high school math, 3 years of high school science, high school biology, high school foreign language, high school transcript, 3 letters of recommendation, transcript of college record. 33 prerequisite credits must be completed before admission to the nursing program. *Options:* Advanced standing available through the following means: advanced placement exams, credit by exam. May apply for transfer of up to 64–96 total credits. *Application deadlines:* 4/15 (fall), 12/15 (spring). *Application fee:* $50.

Degree Requirements 120 total credit hours, 52 in nursing.

RN Baccalaureate Program (BSN)

Applying *Required:* NLN Mobility Profile I and II, minimum college GPA of 2.5, 3 letters of recommendation, minimum 2.0 GPA in all prerequisites, New York RN license. 54 prerequisite credits must be completed before admission to the nursing program. *Options:* Advanced standing available through the following means: advanced placement exams, credit by exam. May apply for transfer of up to 65 total credits. *Application deadlines:* 1/15 (fall), 9/15 (spring).

Degree Requirements 120 total credit hours, 52 in nursing.

Distance learning Courses provided through on-line.

STATE UNIVERSITY OF NEW YORK COLLEGE AT PLATTSBURGH

Department of Nursing
Plattsburgh, New York

Programs • Generic Baccalaureate • RN Baccalaureate

The University State-supported comprehensive coed institution. Part of State University of New York System. Founded: 1889. *Primary accreditation:* regional. *Setting:* 265-acre small-town campus. *Total enrollment:* 5,590.

The Department of Nursing Founded in 1946. *Nursing program faculty:* 18 (17% with doctorates). *Off-campus program sites:* Glens Falls, Potsdam, Saranac Lake.

Academic Facilities *Campus library:* 300,900 volumes (19,430 in nursing); 1,438 periodical subscriptions (174 health-care related). *Nursing school resources:* CAI, computer lab, nursing audiovisuals, interactive nursing skills videos, nursing skills lab, virtual reality venipuncture simulator.

Student Life *Student services:* health clinic, child-care facilities, personal counseling, career counseling, institutionally sponsored work-study program, job placement, campus safety program, special assistance for disabled students. *International student services:* special assistance for non-native speakers of English. *Nursing student activities:* Sigma Theta Tau, student nurses association.

Calendar Semesters.

NURSING STUDENT PROFILE

Undergraduate **Enrollment:** 365

Women: 87%; **Men:** 13%; **Minority:** 6%; **International:** 5%; **Part-time:** 36%

BACCALAUREATE PROGRAMS

Contact Dr. Gretchen Crawford Beebe, Chairperson and Professor, Department of Nursing, State University of New York College at Plattsburgh, Plattsburgh, NY 12901, 518-564-3124. *Fax:* 518-564-3100. *E-mail:* beebegc@splava.cc.plattsburgh.edu

Expenses *State resident tuition:* $3400 full-time, $137 per credit hour part-time. *Nonresident tuition:* $8300 full-time, $346 per credit hour part-time. *Full-time mandatory fees:* $413. *Room and board:* $4326. *Books and supplies per academic year:* $600.

Financial Aid Institutionally sponsored need-based grants/scholarships, institutionally sponsored non-need grants/scholarships, Federal Direct Loans, Federal Nursing Student Loans, Federal Pell Grants, Federal Perkins Loans, Federal Supplemental Educational Opportunity Grants, Federal Work-Study, Federal Stafford Loans, New York State Tuition Assistance Program (TAP). *Application deadline:* 3/1.

Generic Baccalaureate Program (BS)

Applying *Required:* SAT I or ACT, TOEFL for nonnative speakers of English, minimum college GPA of 2.5, 3 years of high school math, 3 years of high school science, high school chemistry, high school biology, high school transcript, transcript of college record. *Options:* May apply for transfer of up to 89 total credits. *Application deadline:* rolling. *Application fee:* $25.

Degree Requirements 125 total credit hours, 54 in nursing.

RN Baccalaureate Program (BS)

Applying *Required:* minimum college GPA of 2.5, RN license, diploma or AD in nursing, transcript of college record. 60 prerequisite credits must be completed before admission to the nursing program. *Options:* Advanced standing available through credit by exam. May apply for transfer of up to 89 total credits. *Application deadline:* rolling. *Application fee:* $25.

Degree Requirements 125 total credit hours, 54 in nursing.

Distance learning Courses provided through video, audio, computer-based media. Specific degree requirements include residency, which can be met through teleteaching courses.

STATE UNIVERSITY OF NEW YORK HEALTH SCIENCE CENTER AT BROOKLYN

College of Nursing
Brooklyn, New York

Programs • Generic Baccalaureate • Master's

The University State-supported upper-level specialized coed institution. Part of State University of New York System. Founded: 1858. *Primary accreditation:* regional. *Total enrollment:* 1,604.

The College of Nursing Founded in 1967.

Academic Facilities *Campus library:* 241,969 volumes (241,969 in health); 1,301 periodical subscriptions (1,200 health-care related).

Calendar Semesters.

BACCALAUREATE PROGRAM

Contact Undergraduate Admission Office, College of Nursing, State University of New York Health Science Center at Brooklyn, 450 Clarkson Avenue, Box 60A, Brooklyn, NY 11203-2098, 718-270-2446.

MASTER'S PROGRAM

Contact Admissions Office, College of Nursing, State University of New York Health Science Center at Brooklyn, 450 Clarkson Avenue, Box 60A, Brooklyn, NY 11203, 718-270-2446.

STATE UNIVERSITY OF NEW YORK HEALTH SCIENCE CENTER AT SYRACUSE

College of Nursing
Syracuse, New York

Programs • RN Baccalaureate • RN to Master's • Post-Master's

The University State-supported specialized coed university. Part of State University of New York System. Founded: 1950. *Primary accreditation:* regional. *Setting:* 25-acre urban campus. *Total enrollment:* 1,130.

The College of Nursing Founded in 1986. *Nursing program faculty:* 7 (71% with doctorates).

Academic Facilities *Campus library:* 150,000 volumes (147,000 in health, 15,000 in nursing); 1,280 periodical subscriptions (1,254 health-care related).

Calendar Semesters.

BACCALAUREATE PROGRAM

Contact Chair, College of Nursing, State University of New York Health Science Center at Syracuse, 714 Irving Avenue, Syracuse, NY 13210, 315-464-4276. *Fax:* 315-464-5168.

Expenses *State resident tuition:* $3400 full-time, $137 per credit hour part-time. *Nonresident tuition:* $8300 full-time, $364 per credit hour part-time.

State University of New York Health Science Center at Syracuse (continued)

RN Baccalaureate Program (BS)

Applying *Required:* minimum college GPA of 2.0, RN license, diploma or AD in nursing, CPR certification. *Application deadline:* 2/1.

Degree Requirements 121–124 total credit hours dependent upon track, 58–61 in nursing.

MASTER'S PROGRAMS

Contact Chair, MSN Program, College of Nursing, State University of New York Health Science Center at Syracuse, 714 Irving Avenue, Syracuse, NY 13210, 315-464-4276. *Fax:* 315-464-5168.

Areas of Study Nurse practitioner programs in adult health, child care/pediatrics, family health.

Expenses *State resident tuition:* ranges from $5100 to $5500 full-time, $213 per credit hour part-time. *Nonresident tuition:* ranges from $5500 to $8461 full-time, $315 per credit hour part-time.

RN to Master's Program (MS)

Applying *Required:* bachelor's degree in nursing. *Application deadline:* 2/1.

Degree Requirements 40 total credit hours, 37 in nursing.

Post-Master's Program

Applying *Application deadline:* 2/1.

Degree Requirements 3 semesters of clinical/theory and pharmacy courses.

STATE UNIVERSITY OF NEW YORK INSTITUTE OF TECHNOLOGY AT UTICA/ROME

School of Nursing
Utica, New York

Programs • RN Baccalaureate • MSN

The University State-supported upper-level coed institution. Part of State University of New York System. Founded: 1966. *Primary accreditation:* regional. *Setting:* 800-acre suburban campus. *Total enrollment:* 2,578.

The School of Nursing Founded in 1966. *Nursing program faculty:* 11 (36% with doctorates). *Off-campus program site:* Albany.

Academic Facilities *Campus library:* 156,000 volumes (15,000 in nursing); 1,250 periodical subscriptions (335 health-care related). *Nursing school resources:* CAI, computer lab, nursing audiovisuals, interactive nursing skills videos, learning resource lab.

Student Life *Student services:* health clinic, personal counseling, career counseling, institutionally sponsored work-study program, job placement, campus safety program, special assistance for disabled students. *International student services:* counseling/support, special assistance for nonnative speakers of English. *Nursing student activities:* Sigma Theta Tau, nursing club, student nurses association.

Calendar Semesters.

NURSING STUDENT PROFILE

Undergraduate **Enrollment:** 398
Women: 92%; **Men:** 8%; **Minority:** 6%; **International:** 0%; **Part-time:** 77%
Graduate **Enrollment:** 78
Women: 96%; **Men:** 4%; **Minority:** 4%; **International:** 0%; **Part-time:** 76%

BACCALAUREATE PROGRAM

Contact Ms. Janet Owens, Staff Assistant, School of Nursing, State University of New York Institute of Technology at Utica/Rome, PO Box 3050, Utica, NY 13504-3050, 315-792-7295. *Fax:* 315-792-7555. *E-mail:* sieo@sunyit.edu

Expenses *State resident tuition:* $3400 full-time, $137 per credit hour part-time. *Nonresident tuition:* $8300 full-time, $346 per credit hour part-time. *Full-time mandatory fees:* $479. *Room and board:* $4630–$5670. *Room only:* $2630–$3470. *Books and supplies per academic year:* ranges from $200 to $500.

Financial Aid Institutionally sponsored need-based grants/scholarships, institutionally sponsored non-need grants/scholarships, Federal Direct Loans, Federal Nursing Student Loans, Federal Supplemental Educational Opportunity Grants, Federal Work-Study.

RN Baccalaureate Program (BS)

Applying *Required:* NLN Achievement Tests for diploma graduates, RN license, diploma or AD in nursing, transcript of college record, immunizations, 62 credits earned at another institution. 56 prerequisite credits must be completed before admission to the nursing program. *Options:* Course work may be accelerated. May apply for transfer of up to 64 total credits. *Application deadline:* rolling. *Application fee:* $25.

Degree Requirements 124 total credit hours, 62 in nursing.

MASTER'S PROGRAM

Contact Ms. Janet Owens, Staff Assistant, School of Nursing, State University of New York Institute of Technology at Utica/Rome, PO Box 3050, Utica, NY 13504-3050, 315-792-7295. *Fax:* 315-792-7555.

Areas of Study Nursing administration; nurse practitioner program in adult health.

Expenses *State resident tuition:* $5100 full-time, $213 per credit hour part-time. *Nonresident tuition:* $8416 full-time, $351 per credit hour part-time. *Full-time mandatory fees:* $379. *Room and board:* $4630–$5670. *Room only:* $2630–$3470. *Books and supplies per academic year:* ranges from $300 to $500.

Financial Aid Graduate assistantships, Federal Nursing Student Loans, employment opportunities, institutionally sponsored non-need-based grants/scholarships.

MSN Program

Applying *Required:* GRE General Test, bachelor's degree in nursing, minimum GPA of 3.0, RN license, 1 year of clinical experience, statistics course, essay, 3 letters of recommendation, transcript of college record, computer literacy, physical assessment course for nurse practitioner. *Application deadline:* rolling. *Application fee:* $35.

Degree Requirements 33–39 total credit hours dependent upon track, 24–33 in nursing, 6–9 in business, computer science, psychology, biology.

SYRACUSE UNIVERSITY

College of Nursing
Syracuse, New York

Programs • Baccalaureate for Second Degree • Accelerated Baccalaureate for Second Degree • MS • RN to Master's • MSN/MBA • Post-Master's

The University Independent coed university. Founded: 1870. *Primary accreditation:* regional. *Setting:* 200-acre urban campus. *Total enrollment:* 14,636.

The College of Nursing Founded in 1943. *Nursing program faculty:* 66 (93% with doctorates). *Off-campus program sites:* Elmira, Cortland, Binghamton.

Academic Facilities *Campus library:* 2.5 million volumes (26,000 in health, 7,000 in nursing); 10,568 periodical subscriptions (140 health-care related). *Nursing school resources:* CAI, computer lab, nursing audiovisuals, interactive nursing skills videos, learning resource lab.

Student Life *Student services:* health clinic, child-care facilities, personal counseling, career counseling, institutionally sponsored work-study program, job placement, campus safety program, special assistance for disabled students. *International student services:* counseling/support, special assistance for nonnative speakers of English, ESL courses. *Nursing student activities:* Sigma Theta Tau, nursing club, student nurses association, ALHANA (minority student group).

Calendar Semesters.

NURSING STUDENT PROFILE

Undergraduate **Enrollment:** 594
Women: 90%; **Men:** 10%; **Minority:** 17%; **International:** 1%; **Part-time:** 28%
Graduate **Enrollment:** 254
Women: 90%; **Men:** 10%; **Minority:** 7%; **International:** 4%; **Part-time:** 55%

BACCALAUREATE PROGRAMS

Contact Ms. Karen Gaughan, Director, Undergraduate Recruiting and Advising, College of Nursing, Syracuse University, 426 Ostrom Avenue,

Syracuse, NY 13244-3240, 315-443-2027. *Fax:* 315-443-9807. *E-mail:* kkgaugha@nur.syr.edu

Expenses *Tuition:* $16,710 per academic year. *Full-time mandatory fees:* $370. *Room and board:* $7220. *Room only:* $3920. *Books and supplies per academic year:* ranges from $500 to $800.

Financial Aid Institutionally sponsored need-based grants/scholarships, institutionally sponsored non-need grants/scholarships, Federal Direct Loans, Federal Nursing Student Loans, Federal Pell Grants, Federal Perkins Loans, Federal Supplemental Educational Opportunity Grants, Federal Work-Study. 57% of undergraduate students in nursing programs received some form of financial aid in 1995–96. *Application deadline:* 2/15.

Baccalaureate for Second Degree Program (BSN)

Applying *Required:* minimum college GPA of 2.8, transcript of college record, valid BA or BS from accredited institution. *Options:* Course work may be accelerated. May apply for transfer of up to 67 total credits. *Application deadlines:* 5/1 (fall), 12/1 (spring). *Application fee:* $40.

Degree Requirements 120 total credit hours, 53 in nursing.

Accelerated Baccalaureate for Second Degree Program (BSN)

Applying *Required:* SAT I or ACT, TOEFL for nonnative speakers of English, minimum college GPA of 2.5, 3 years of high school math, 3 years of high school science, high school chemistry, high school biology, high school foreign language, high school transcript, 3 letters of recommendation, written essay, high school class rank: top 40%. *Options:* Advanced standing available through advanced placement exams. Course work may be accelerated. May apply for transfer of up to 61 total credits. *Application deadline:* 2/1. *Application fee:* $40.

Degree Requirements 120 total credit hours, 59 in nursing.

MASTER'S PROGRAMS

Contact Ms. Janice M. Pedersen, Professional and Graduate Program Coordinator, College of Nursing, Syracuse University, 426 Ostrom Avenue, Syracuse, NY 13244-3240, 315-443-4272. *Fax:* 315-443-9807. *E-mail:* jmpeders@nursing.syr.edu

Areas of Study Clinical nurse specialist programs in adult health nursing, cardiovascular nursing, community health nursing, critical care nursing, family health nursing, gerontological nursing, maternity-newborn nursing, medical-surgical nursing, occupational health nursing, oncology nursing, parent-child nursing, pediatric nursing, perinatal nursing, psychiatric–mental health nursing, public health nursing, rehabilitation nursing, women's health nursing, school health; nursing administration; nursing education; nurse practitioner programs in child care/pediatrics, community health, family health, gerontology, occupational health, primary care, school health, women's health.

Expenses *Tuition:* $503 per credit hour. *Full-time mandatory fees:* $50. *Part-time mandatory fees:* $15. *Room and board:* $4725–$6145. *Room only:* $3540–$4960. *Books and supplies per academic year:* ranges from $600 to $1000.

Financial Aid Graduate assistantships, nurse traineeships, fellowships, Federal Nursing Student Loans, institutionally sponsored non-need-based grants/scholarships. 14% of master's level students in nursing programs received some form of financial aid in 1995-96. *Application deadline:* 1/30.

MS Program

Applying *Required:* GRE General Test, TOEFL for nonnative speakers of English, bachelor's degree in nursing, minimum GPA of 3.0, RN license, physical assessment course, statistics course, professional liability/malpractice insurance, essay, 3 letters of recommendation, transcript of college record. *Application deadline:* rolling. *Application fee:* $40.

Degree Requirements 45 total credit hours, 42 in nursing, 3 in related to specialty.

Distance learning Courses provided through correspondence, video, computer-based media, on-line. Specific degree requirements include 9-week on-campus residency over 3 years.

RN to Master's Program (MS)

Applying *Required:* GRE General Test, TOEFL for nonnative speakers of English, bachelor's degree in nursing, minimum GPA of 3.0, RN license, physical assessment course, statistics course, professional liability/malpractice insurance, essay, 3 letters of recommendation, transcript of college record. *Application deadline:* rolling. *Application fee:* $40.

Degree Requirements 45 total credit hours, 42 in nursing, 3 in related to specialty.

Distance learning Courses provided through correspondence, video, audio, computer-based media, on-line. Specific degree requirements include 9-week on-campus residency over 3 years.

MSN/MBA Program

Applying *Required:* GRE General Test or Miller Analogies Test, TOEFL for nonnative speakers of English, bachelor's degree in nursing, minimum GPA of 3.0, RN license, physical assessment course, statistics course, professional liability/malpractice insurance, essay, 3 letters of recommendation, transcript of college record. *Application deadlines:* 4/1 (summer), rolling. *Application fee:* $40.

Degree Requirements 78 total credit hours, 30 in nursing, 48 in management and other specified areas. 2 summer internships.

Distance learning Courses provided through correspondence, video, audio, computer-based media, on-line. Specific degree requirements include 9-week on-campus residency over 3 years.

Post-Master's Program

Applying *Required:* RN license, physical assessment course, professional liability/malpractice insurance, essay, transcript of college record, leadership experience. *Application deadline:* rolling. *Application fee:* $40.

Degree Requirements 13–15 total credit hours dependent upon track, 13–15 in nursing.

See full description on page 510.

TEACHERS COLLEGE, COLUMBIA UNIVERSITY
Department of Nursing Education
New York, New York

Programs • MA • Master of Education • Doctor of Education

The University Independent graduate specialized coed institution. Founded: 1887. *Primary accreditation:* regional. *Total enrollment:* 4,548.

The Department of Nursing Education Founded in 1899.

Academic Facilities *Campus library:* 5.5 million volumes; 63,403 periodical subscriptions.

Calendar Semesters.

MASTER'S PROGRAMS

Contact Coordinator, Department of Nursing Education, Teachers College, Columbia University, 525 West 120th Street, Box 150, New York, NY 10027, 212-678-3946. *Fax:* 212-678-4048.

Areas of Study Nursing education.

Expenses *Tuition:* $13,920 full-time, $580 per credit part-time.

Financial Aid Nurse traineeships.

MA Program

Applying *Required:* bachelor's degree in nursing, minimum GPA of 3.0, RN license, 1 year of clinical experience.

Master of Education Program (MED)

Applying *Required:* bachelor's degree in nursing, minimum GPA of 3.0, RN license, 1 year of clinical experience.

DOCTORAL PROGRAM

Contact Coordinator, Department of Nursing Education, Teachers College, Columbia University, 525 West 120th Street, Box 150, New York, NY 10027, 212-678-3421. *Fax:* 212-678-4004.

Expenses *Tuition:* $13,920 full-time, $580 per credit part-time.

Doctor of Education Program (EDD)

Applying *Required:* GRE General Test or Miller Analogies Test, TOEFL for nonnative speakers of English, master's degree in nursing, minimum 3.5 BSN GPA, RN licensure.

UNIVERSITY OF ROCHESTER
School of Nursing
Rochester, New York

Programs • Generic Baccalaureate • RN Baccalaureate • MS • RN to Master's • PhD • Postdoctoral

The University Independent coed university. Founded: 1850. *Primary accreditation:* regional. *Setting:* 534-acre suburban campus. *Total enrollment:* 8,120.

The School of Nursing Founded in 1923. *Nursing program faculty:* 233 (18% with doctorates).

Academic Facilities *Campus library:* 2.6 million volumes (233,900 in health); 10,500 periodical subscriptions (1,600 health-care related). *Nursing school resources:* CAI, computer lab, nursing audiovisuals, interactive nursing skills videos, learning resource lab.

Student Life *Student services:* health clinic, personal counseling, career counseling, institutionally sponsored work-study program, job placement, campus safety program, special assistance for disabled students, learning assistance center, academic advising. *International student services:* counseling/support, special assistance for nonnative speakers of English, ESL courses. *Nursing student activities:* Sigma Theta Tau, recruiter club, student nurses association.

Calendar Semesters.

NURSING STUDENT PROFILE

Undergraduate **Enrollment:** 240

Women: 87%; **Men:** 13%; **Minority:** 18%; **International:** 5%; **Part-time:** 35%

Graduate **Enrollment:** 266

Women: 94%; **Men:** 6%; **Minority:** 4%; **International:** 5%; **Part-time:** 61%

BACCALAUREATE PROGRAMS

Contact Dr. Mary Sue Jack, Assistant Dean of Student Affairs, School of Nursing, University of Rochester, 601 Elmwood Street, PO Box SON, Rochester, NY 14642, 716-275-2375. *Fax:* 716-473-1059.

Expenses *Tuition:* $19,630 full-time, $615 per credit hour part-time. *Full-time mandatory fees:* $435. *Room and board:* $5185–$6930. *Room only:* $4180. *Books and supplies per academic year:* $525.

Financial Aid Institutionally sponsored need-based grants/scholarships, Federal Nursing Student Loans, Federal Work-Study. 80% of undergraduate students in nursing programs received some form of financial aid in 1995–96. *Application deadline:* 3/31.

Generic Baccalaureate Program (BS)

Applying *Required:* SAT I or ACT, TOEFL for nonnative speakers of English, TSE for Professionals for nonnative speakers of English, minimum college GPA of 2.5, high school transcript, letter of recommendation, written essay, transcript of college record. 56 prerequisite credits must be completed before admission to the nursing program. *Options:* Advanced standing available through advanced placement exams. May apply for transfer of up to 64 total credits. *Application deadlines:* 1/15 (fall), 11/15 (spring). *Application fee:* $50.

Degree Requirements 128 total credit hours, 64 in nursing.

RN Baccalaureate Program (BS)

Applying *Required:* TOEFL for nonnative speakers of English, TSE for Professionals for nonnative speakers of English, minimum college GPA of 2.5, RN license, diploma or AD in nursing, letter of recommendation, written essay, transcript of college record. *Options:* Advanced standing available through advanced placement exams. May apply for transfer of up to 64–96 total credits. *Application deadline:* rolling. *Application fee:* $40.

Degree Requirements 128 total credit hours, 64 in nursing.

MASTER'S PROGRAMS

Contact Dr. Mary Sue Jack, Assistant Dean of Student Affairs, School of Nursing, University of Rochester, 601 Elmwood Street, PO Box SON, Rochester, NY 14642, 716-275-2375. *Fax:* 716-473-1059.

Areas of Study Clinical nurse specialist program in psychiatric–mental health nursing; nurse midwifery; nurse practitioner programs in acute care, adult health, child care/pediatrics, family health, gerontology, primary care, women's health.

Expenses *Tuition:* ranges from $11,070 to $13,530 full-time, $615 per credit hour part-time. *Full-time mandatory fees:* $435. *Room and board:* $5185–$6930. *Room only:* $4180. *Books and supplies per academic year:* $525.

Financial Aid Graduate assistantships, nurse traineeships, Federal Nursing Student Loans, institutionally sponsored loans, employment opportunities. 84% of master's level students in nursing programs received some form of financial aid in 1995-96. *Application deadline:* 6/1.

MS Program

Applying *Required:* Miller Analogies Test, TOEFL for nonnative speakers of English, GRE General Test (minimum combined score of 950 on quantitative and verbal sections), TSE for Professionals for nonnative speakers of English, bachelor's degree in nursing, minimum GPA of 3.0, RN license, physical assessment course, statistics course, essay, interview, 2 letters of recommendation, transcript of college record. *Application deadlines:* 2/15 (fall), 9/15 (spring). *Application fee:* $25.

Degree Requirements 36–49 total credit hours dependent upon track, 36–49 in nursing. Thesis or comprehensive exam.

RN to Master's Program (MS)

Applying *Required:* Miller Analogies Test, TOEFL for nonnative speakers of English, GRE General Test (minimum combined score of 950 on quantitative and verbal sections), TSE for Professionals for nonnative speakers of English, minimum GPA of 3.0, RN license, essay, interview, 2 letters of recommendation, transcript of college record. *Application deadlines:* 2/15 (fall), 9/15 (spring). *Application fee:* $40.

Degree Requirements 160 total credit hours, 96 in nursing, 64 in arts and sciences. Thesis or comprehensive exam.

DOCTORAL PROGRAM

Contact Dr. Madeline Schmitt, Director, PhD Program, School of Nursing, University of Rochester, 601 Elmwood Street, PO Box SON, Rochester, NY 14642, 716-275-2371. *Fax:* 716-473-1059. *E-mail:* mads@son.rochester.edu

Areas of Study Nursing research.

Expenses *Tuition:* ranges from $5535 to $7380 full-time, $615 per credit hour part-time. *Full-time mandatory fees:* $310. *Books and supplies per academic year:* $525.

Financial Aid Graduate assistantships, nurse traineeships, fellowships, dissertation grants, grants, opportunities for employment. *Application deadline:* 6/1.

PhD Program

Applying *Required:* GRE General Test, TOEFL for nonnative speakers of English, TSE for Professionals for nonnative speakers of English, master's degree in nursing, statistics course, interview, 3 letters of recommendation, vitae, writing sample, competitive review by faculty committee, 3.0 undergraduate GPA, 3.5 graduate GPA for approved courses. *Application deadline:* 2/1. *Application fee:* $25.

Degree Requirements 60 total credit hours; dissertation; written exam; defense of dissertation.

POSTDOCTORAL PROGRAM

Contact Dr. Madeline Schmitt, Director of the PhD Program, School of Nursing, University of Rochester, 601 Elmwood Street, PO Box SON, Rochester, NY 14642, 716-275-2371. *Fax:* 716-473-1059. *E-mail:* mads@son.rochester.edu

Areas of Study Stress and coping.

UNIVERSITY OF THE STATE OF NEW YORK, REGENTS COLLEGE
Nursing Program
Albany, New York

Programs • Generic Baccalaureate • Continuing Education

The University Independent 4-year coed college. Founded: 1970. *Primary accreditation:* regional. *Total enrollment:* 19,443.

The Nursing Program Founded in 1976. *Nursing program faculty:* 195 (30% with doctorates).

Academic Facilities *Nursing school resources:* nursing audiovisuals, on-line study groups.

Calendar Open enrollment.

NURSING STUDENT PROFILE

Undergraduate **Enrollment:** 11,310

Women: 82%; **Men:** 18%; **Minority:** 22%; **International:** 1%; **Part-time:** 100%

BACCALAUREATE PROGRAM

Contact Academic Adviser, Nursing Program, University of the State of New York, Regents College, 7 Columbia Circle, Albany, NY 12203, 518-464-8500. *Fax:* 518-465-8777. *E-mail:* rcinfo@cnsvax.albany.edu

Expenses *Tuition:* ranges from $595 to $1250 per academic year.

Financial Aid Institutionally sponsored need-based grants/scholarships, institutionally sponsored non-need grants/scholarships, The Chancellor's Scholarship.

Generic Baccalaureate Program (BSN)

Applying *Required:* admission open to students with specific health-care experience, determined by assessment. *Options:* Advanced standing available through credit by exam. Course work may be accelerated. *Application deadline:* rolling.

Degree Requirements 120 total credit hours, 48 in nursing.

Distance learning Courses provided through on-line.

CONTINUING EDUCATION PROGRAM

Contact Kathleen Santarcangelo, Program Coordinator, University of the State of New York, Regents College, 7 Columbia Circle, Albany, NY 12203, 518-464-8500. *E-mail:* rcinfo@cnsvax.albany.edu

See full description on page 560.

UTICA COLLEGE OF SYRACUSE UNIVERSITY
Department of Nursing
Utica, New York

Programs • Generic Baccalaureate • RN Baccalaureate

The University Independent 4-year coed college. Part of Syracuse University. Founded: 1946. *Primary accreditation:* regional. *Setting:* 132-acre suburban campus. *Total enrollment:* 1,762.

The Department of Nursing Founded in 1982.

Academic Facilities *Campus library:* 170,000 volumes (2,516 in health, 1,102 in nursing); 1,050 periodical subscriptions (116 health-care related).

Calendar Semesters.

BACCALAUREATE PROGRAMS

Contact Director, Office of Admissions, Utica College of Syracuse University, 1600 Burrstone Road, Utica, NY 13502-4892, 800-782-8884. *Fax:* 315-792-3292.

Expenses *Tuition:* $14,116 full-time, $471 per credit hour part-time. *Full-time mandatory fees:* $90. *Room and board:* $5272–$6186. *Room only:* $6186. *Books and supplies per academic year:* $500+.

Financial Aid Institutionally sponsored need-based grants/scholarships, institutionally sponsored non-need grants/scholarships, Federal Nursing Student Loans, Federal Pell Grants, Federal Perkins Loans, Federal Supplemental Educational Opportunity Grants, Federal Work-Study, Federal Stafford Loans, New York state aid. *Application deadline:* 3/15.

Generic Baccalaureate Program (BS)

Applying *Required:* TOEFL for nonnative speakers of English. *Options:* Advanced standing available through credit by exam. *Application deadline:* rolling. *Application fee:* $25.

Degree Requirements 128 total credit hours, 53 in nursing.

RN Baccalaureate Program (BS)

Applying *Required:* RN license, diploma or AD in nursing, high school transcript, transcript of college record. *Options:* Advanced standing available through credit by exam. *Application deadline:* rolling. *Application fee:* $25.

Degree Requirements 128 total credit hours, 53 in nursing.

WAGNER COLLEGE
Nursing Department
Staten Island, New York

Programs • Generic Baccalaureate • RN Baccalaureate • Baccalaureate for Second Degree • MS • Post-Master's • Continuing Education

The College Independent comprehensive coed institution. Founded: 1883. *Primary accreditation:* regional. *Setting:* 105-acre urban campus. *Total enrollment:* 1,919.

The Nursing Department Founded in 1943. *Nursing program faculty:* 12 (80% with doctorates).

Academic Facilities *Campus library:* 292,000 volumes (15,060 in health, 7,052 in nursing); 1,027 periodical subscriptions (160 health-care related). *Nursing school resources:* CAI, computer lab, nursing audiovisuals, learning resource lab.

Student Life *Student services:* health clinic, child-care facilities, personal counseling, career counseling, institutionally sponsored work-study program. *International student services:* counseling/support, ESL courses. *Nursing student activities:* Sigma Theta Tau, student nurses association.

Calendar Semesters.

NURSING STUDENT PROFILE

Undergraduate **Enrollment:** 203

Women: 75%; **Men:** 25%; **Minority:** 35%; **International:** 0%; **Part-time:** 25%

Graduate **Enrollment:** 116

Women: 90%; **Men:** 10%; **Minority:** 15%; **International:** 0%; **Part-time:** 80%

BACCALAUREATE PROGRAMS

Contact Dr. Mary Ann Kosiba, Chairperson, Nursing Department, Wagner College, 631 Howard Avenue, Staten Island, NY 10301, 718-390-3436. *Fax:* 718-390-3467.

Expenses *Tuition:* $15,300 full-time, $515 per credit part-time. *Full-time mandatory fees:* $50. *Room and board:* $2900.

Financial Aid Institutionally sponsored need-based grants/scholarships, institutionally sponsored non-need grants/scholarships, Federal Nursing Student Loans. *Application deadline:* 5/1.

Generic Baccalaureate Program (BS)

Applying *Required:* SAT I or ACT, minimum high school GPA of 2.7, minimum college GPA of 2.7, 3 years of high school math, 3 years of high school science, high school transcript, 3 letters of recommendation, written essay, transcript of college record, 2.7 GPA for internal/external transfers. *Options:* Advanced standing available through advanced placement exams. May apply for transfer of up to 98 total credits. *Application deadlines:* 5/1 (fall), 10/1 (spring). *Application fee:* $50.

Degree Requirements 128 total credit hours, 54 in nursing.

RN Baccalaureate Program (BS)

Applying *Required:* NLN Mobility Profile II, minimum college GPA of 2.7, RN license, diploma or AD in nursing, 3 letters of recommendation, written essay, transcript of college record. *Options:* May apply for transfer of up to 98 total credits. *Application deadlines:* 5/1 (fall), 10/1 (spring). *Application fee:* $50.

Degree Requirements 128 total credit hours, 54 in nursing.

Baccalaureate for Second Degree Program (BS)

Applying *Required:* NLN Mobility Profile II, minimum college GPA of 2.7, diploma or AD in nursing, 3 letters of recommendation, written essay, transcript of college record, nursing and science credits. *Options:* May apply for transfer of up to 98 total credits. *Application deadlines:* 5/1 (fall), 10/1 (spring). *Application fee:* $50.

Degree Requirements 128 total credit hours, 54 in nursing.

MASTER'S PROGRAMS

Contact Graduate Admissions, Nursing Department, Wagner College, 631 Howard Avenue, Staten Island, NY 10301, 718-390-3411. *Fax:* 718-390-3467.

Areas of Study Nursing administration; nursing education; nurse practitioner program in family health.

Expenses *Tuition:* $9360 full-time, $520 per credit part-time. *Full-time mandatory fees:* $0.

Financial Aid Graduate assistantships, nurse traineeships, Federal Nursing Student Loans, institutionally sponsored loans. *Application deadline:* 9/1.

Wagner College (continued)

MS Program

Applying *Required:* Miller Analogies Test may be required, bachelor's degree in nursing, minimum GPA of 2.7, RN license, statistics course, professional liability/malpractice insurance, interview, 3 letters of recommendation, transcript of college record, nursing research course, CPR certification. *Application deadline:* rolling. *Application fee:* $50.

Degree Requirements 43–45 total credit hours dependent upon track, 33–34 in nursing, 6–7 in instruction, evaluation, behavior management. 43 credit hours for family nurse practitioner thesis option or 45 for project option.

Post-Master's Program

Applying *Required:* 2 letters of recommendation, current curriculum vitae and resume, minimum 3.0 graduate GPA. *Application deadline:* rolling. *Application fee:* $50.

Degree Requirements 23 total credit hours, 23 in nursing.

CONTINUING EDUCATION PROGRAM

Contact Dr. Mary Ann Kosiba, Chairperson, Nursing Department, Wagner College, 631 Howard Avenue, Staten Island, NY 10301, 718-390-3436. *Fax:* 718-390-3467.

YORK COLLEGE OF THE CITY UNIVERSITY OF NEW YORK
Nursing Department
Jamaica, New York

Program • RN Baccalaureate

The University State and locally supported 4-year coed college. Part of City University of New York System. Founded: 1967. *Primary accreditation:* regional. *Setting:* 50-acre urban campus. *Total enrollment:* 6,111.

The Nursing Department Founded in 1985. *Nursing program faculty:* 5 (60% with doctorates).

Academic Facilities *Campus library:* 30,483 volumes (7,852 in health, 553 in nursing); 32,195 periodical subscriptions. *Nursing school resources:* CAI, computer lab, nursing audiovisuals, learning resource lab.

Calendar Semesters.

NURSING STUDENT PROFILE

Undergraduate **Enrollment:** 46
Women: 93%; **Men:** 7%; **Minority:** 93%; **Part-time:** 96%

BACCALAUREATE PROGRAM

Contact Dr. Pearl S. Bailey, Director, Nursing Program, Nursing Department, York College of the City University of New York, 94-20 Guy R. Brewer Boulevard, Jamaica, NY 11451, 718-262-2054. *Fax:* 718-262-2002.

Expenses *State resident tuition:* $3200 full-time, $135 part-time. *Nonresident tuition:* $6800 full-time, $285 part-time. *Full-time mandatory fees:* $5000–$7962. *Books and supplies per academic year:* ranges from $300 to $500.

Financial Aid Institutionally sponsored need-based grants/scholarships, institutionally sponsored non-need grants/scholarships, Federal Nursing Student Loans, Federal Work-Study.

RN Baccalaureate Program (BS)

Applying *Required:* CUNY assessment test, NLN Mobility Profile II, minimum college GPA of 2.5, RN license, transcript of college record, immunizations, professional liability/malpractice insurance. 60 prerequisite credits must be completed before admission to the nursing program. *Options:* Advanced standing available through credit by exam. Course work may be accelerated. May apply for transfer of up to 90 total credits. *Application deadline:* 4/1. *Application fee:* $40.

Degree Requirements 128 total credit hours, 48 in nursing. NLN Mobility Profile II exam, skills assessment test, pharmacology test.

NORTH CAROLINA

BARTON COLLEGE
School of Nursing
Wilson, North Carolina

Programs • Generic Baccalaureate • Accelerated RN Baccalaureate • Baccalaureate for Second Degree

The College Independent 4-year coed college, affiliated with Christian Church (Disciples of Christ). Founded: 1902. *Primary accreditation:* regional. *Setting:* 62-acre small-town campus. *Total enrollment:* 1,401.

The School of Nursing Founded in 1970. *Nursing program faculty:* 14 (14% with doctorates).

Academic Facilities *Campus library:* 160,993 volumes (4,915 in health); 981 periodical subscriptions (50 health-care related). *Nursing school resources:* CAI, computer lab, nursing audiovisuals, interactive nursing skills videos.

Student Life *Student services:* personal counseling, career counseling, institutionally sponsored work-study program, job placement, campus safety program, special assistance for disabled students. *International student services:* counseling/support, special assistance for nonnative speakers of English. *Nursing student activities:* Sigma Theta Tau, student nurses association.

Calendar Semesters.

NURSING STUDENT PROFILE

Undergraduate **Enrollment:** 96
Women: 90%; **Men:** 10%; **Minority:** 8%; **International:** 4%; **Part-time:** 0%

BACCALAUREATE PROGRAMS

Contact Dr. Pet Pruden, Dean, School of Nursing, Barton College, Wilson, NC 27893, 919-399-6400. *Fax:* 919-399-6416. *E-mail:* ppruden@e-mail.barton.edu

Expenses *Tuition:* $8342 full-time, $355 per credit hour part-time. *Full-time mandatory fees:* $642–$660. *Part-time mandatory fees:* $0–$20. *Room and board:* $4065–$4765. *Room only:* $2179–$2875. *Books and supplies per academic year:* ranges from $500 to $800.

Financial Aid Institutionally sponsored need-based grants/scholarships, institutionally sponsored non-need grants/scholarships, Federal Nursing Student Loans, Federal Pell Grants, Federal Perkins Loans, Federal Supplemental Educational Opportunity Grants, Federal Work-Study.

Generic Baccalaureate Program (BSN)

Applying *Required:* SAT I, minimum college GPA of 2.5, transcript of college record. 33 prerequisite credits must be completed before admission to the nursing program. *Options:* Advanced standing available through credit by exam. May apply for transfer of up to 64–83 total credits. *Application deadline:* 2/1. *Application fee:* $20.

Degree Requirements 128 total credit hours, 51 in nursing.

Accelerated RN Baccalaureate Program (BSN)

Applying *Required:* SAT I, NLN Mobility Profile II, minimum college GPA of 2.5, RN license, diploma or AD in nursing, transcript of college record. 9 prerequisite credits must be completed before admission to the nursing program. *Options:* Advanced standing available through the following means: advanced placement exams, credit by exam. Course work may be accelerated. May apply for transfer of up to 64–83 total credits. *Application deadline:* 2/1. *Application fee:* $20.

Degree Requirements 128 total credit hours, 51 in nursing.

Baccalaureate for Second Degree Program (BSN)

Applying *Required:* SAT I, transcript of college record. 9 prerequisite credits must be completed before admission to the nursing program. *Options:* Advanced standing available through the following means: advanced placement exams, advanced placement without credit, credit by exam. May apply for transfer of up to 64 total credits. *Application deadline:* 2/1. *Application fee:* $20.

Degree Requirements 128 total credit hours, 51 in nursing.

DUKE UNIVERSITY
School of Nursing
Durham, North Carolina

Programs • MSN • Post-Master's

The University Independent coed university, affiliated with United Methodist Church. Founded: 1838. *Primary accreditation:* regional. *Setting:* 8,500-acre suburban campus. *Total enrollment:* 11,512.

The School of Nursing Founded in 1930. *Nursing program faculty:* 18 (75% with doctorates). *Off-campus program site:* Fayetteville.

Academic Facilities *Campus library:* 4.3 million volumes (300,000 in health, 5,300 in nursing); 26,500 periodical subscriptions (4,600 health-care related). *Nursing school resources:* CAI, computer lab, nursing audiovisuals, clinical diagnostic lab.

Student Life *Student services:* health clinic, child-care facilities, personal counseling, career counseling, institutionally sponsored work-study program, job placement, campus safety program. *International student services:* counseling/support. *Nursing student activities:* Sigma Theta Tau.

Calendar Semesters.

NURSING STUDENT PROFILE

Graduate **Enrollment:** 225

Women: 93%; **Men:** 7%; **Minority:** 11%; **International:** 1%; **Part-time:** 80%

MASTER'S PROGRAMS

Contact Judy Carter, Admissions Officer and Financial Aid Specialist, Box 3322 Medical Center, Graduate School of Nursing, Duke University, Durham, NC 27710, 919-684-4248. *Fax:* 919-681-8899. *E-mail:* carte026@mc.duke.edu

Areas of Study Clinical nurse specialist programs in gerontological nursing, oncology nursing, pediatric nursing; nursing administration; nurse practitioner programs in adult health, child care/pediatrics, family health, gerontology, primary care, cardiovascular, adult oncology.

Expenses *Tuition:* $19,100 full-time, $531 per unit hour part-time. *Full-time mandatory fees:* $275–$860. *Room and board:* $8500. *Room only:* $4725. *Books and supplies per academic year:* ranges from $750 to $850.

Financial Aid Nurse traineeships, Federal Nursing Student Loans, employment opportunities, institutionally sponsored need-based grants/scholarships, institutionally sponsored non-need-based grants/scholarships. *Application deadline:* 6/1.

MSN Program

Applying *Required:* GRE General Test, Miller Analogies Test, TOEFL for nonnative speakers of English, Commission on Graduates of Foreign Nursing Schools exam for international students, bachelor's degree in nursing, minimum GPA of 3.0, RN license, physical assessment course, statistics course, professional liability/malpractice insurance, essay, interview, 3 letters of recommendation, transcript of college record. *Application deadlines:* 3/1 (fall), 11/1 (spring), 3/1 (summer). *Application fee:* $50.

Degree Requirements 39–45 total credit hours dependent upon track, 39–45 in nursing. Thesis, research utilization project, or non-thesis project.

Distance learning Courses provided through computer-based media, on-line. Specific degree requirements include one or two class meetings at Duke School of Nursing per semester for informatics minor of the Nursing Systems Administration degree.

Post-Master's Program

Applying *Required:* bachelor's degree in nursing, minimum GPA of 3.0, RN license, 1 year of clinical experience, physical assessment course, statistics course, professional liability/malpractice insurance, essay, interview, 2 letters of recommendation, transcript of college record, MSN. *Application deadlines:* 3/1 (fall), 11/1 (spring), 3/1 (summer). *Application fee:* $50.

Degree Requirements 12–30 total credit hours dependent upon track, 12–30 in nursing.

Distance learning Courses provided through computer-based media, on-line. Specific degree requirements include one or two campus visits per semester for nursing informatics.

See full description on page 444.

EAST CAROLINA UNIVERSITY
School of Nursing
Greenville, North Carolina

Programs • Generic Baccalaureate • Accelerated RN Baccalaureate • MSN

The University State-supported coed university. Part of University of North Carolina System. Founded: 1907. *Primary accreditation:* regional. *Setting:* 465-acre urban campus. *Total enrollment:* 16,339.

The School of Nursing Founded in 1960. *Nursing program faculty:* 58 (47% with doctorates). *Off-campus program sites:* Elizabeth City, Wilmington.

Academic Facilities *Campus library:* 1.1 million volumes; 6,895 periodical subscriptions (5,368 health-care related). *Nursing school resources:* CAI, computer lab, nursing audiovisuals, interactive nursing skills videos, learning resource lab, nursing clinical learning lab.

Student Life *Student services:* health clinic, personal counseling, career counseling, institutionally sponsored work-study program, job placement, campus safety program, special assistance for disabled students. *International student services:* counseling/support, special assistance for nonnative speakers of English, ESL courses. *Nursing student activities:* Sigma Theta Tau, student nurses association.

Calendar Semesters.

NURSING STUDENT PROFILE

Undergraduate **Enrollment:** 486

Women: 84%; **Men:** 16%; **Minority:** 12%; **Part-time:** 10%

Graduate **Enrollment:** 137

Women: 96%; **Men:** 4%; **Minority:** 23%; **Part-time:** 69%

BACCALAUREATE PROGRAMS

Contact Ms. Jeannie Yount, Director, Student Services, School of Nursing, East Carolina University, Greenville, NC 27858-4353, 919-328-6075. *Fax:* 919-328-4300.

Expenses *State resident tuition:* $874 full-time, $219 per semester part-time. *Nonresident tuition:* $8028 full-time, $2007 per semester part-time. *Full-time mandatory fees:* $893. *Part-time mandatory fees:* $455. *Room and board:* $3300–$5000. *Room only:* $1660–$3000. *Books and supplies per academic year:* ranges from $250 to $300.

Financial Aid Institutionally sponsored need-based grants/scholarships, institutionally sponsored non-need grants/scholarships, Federal Nursing Student Loans, Federal Pell Grants, Federal Perkins Loans, Federal Supplemental Educational Opportunity Grants, Federal Work-Study. *Application deadline:* 3/15.

Generic Baccalaureate Program (BSN)

Applying *Required:* SAT I or ACT, minimum college GPA of 2.2, 3 years of high school math, 3 years of high school science, high school transcript, transcript of college record. 41 prerequisite credits must be completed before admission to the nursing program. *Options:* Advanced standing available through credit by exam. Course work may be accelerated. May apply for transfer of up to 60 total credits. *Application deadlines:* 3/1 (fall), 6/1 (spring). *Application fee:* $35.

Degree Requirements 126 total credit hours, 62 in nursing.

Accelerated RN Baccalaureate Program (BSN)

Applying *Required:* minimum college GPA of 2.2, RN license, diploma or AD in nursing, interview, transcript of college record. 54 prerequisite credits must be completed before admission to the nursing program. *Options:* May apply for transfer of up to 60 total credits. *Application deadlines:* 3/1 (fall), 6/1 (spring). *Application fee:* $25.

Degree Requirements 126 total credit hours, 63 in nursing.

MASTER'S PROGRAM

Contact Dr. Therese Lawler, Associate Dean, School of Nursing, East Carolina University, Greenville, NC 27858-4353, 919-328-4302. *Fax:* 919-328-4300. *E-mail:* nulawler@ecuvm.cis.ecu.edu

East Carolina University (continued)

Areas of Study Clinical nurse specialist programs in adult health nursing, maternity-newborn nursing, medical-surgical nursing, pediatric nursing, psychiatric–mental health nursing; nurse midwifery; nursing administration; nurse practitioner program in primary care.

Expenses *State resident tuition:* $874 full-time, $219 per semester part-time. *Nonresident tuition:* $8028 full-time, $2007 per semester part-time. *Full-time mandatory fees:* $878. *Part-time mandatory fees:* $440. *Room and board:* $3300–$5000. *Room only:* $1660–$3000.

Financial Aid Graduate assistantships, nurse traineeships, Federal Nursing Student Loans. *Application deadline:* 3/15.

MSN Program

Applying *Required:* GRE General Test or Miller Analogies Test, bachelor's degree in nursing, bachelor's degree, minimum GPA of 2.5, RN license, 2 years of clinical experience, physical assessment course, statistics course, professional liability/malpractice insurance, essay, interview, 2 letters of recommendation, transcript of college record, research course. *Application deadlines:* 6/1 (fall), 10/15 (spring). *Application fee:* $40.

Degree Requirements 39–56 total credit hours dependent upon track. Thesis required.

GARDNER-WEBB UNIVERSITY
Davis School of Nursing
Statesville, North Carolina

Program • RN Baccalaureate

The University Independent Baptist comprehensive coed institution. Founded: 1905. *Primary accreditation:* regional. *Setting:* 200-acre small-town campus. *Total enrollment:* 2,511.

The Davis School of Nursing Founded in 1983. *Nursing program faculty:* 6 (50% with doctorates). *Off-campus program sites:* Forsyth, Charlotte, Boiling Springs.

Academic Facilities *Campus library:* 160,000 volumes (2,745 in nursing); 885 periodical subscriptions (102 health-care related). *Nursing school resources:* computer lab, nursing audiovisuals.

Student Life *Nursing student activities:* nursing club.

Calendar Semesters.

NURSING STUDENT PROFILE

Undergraduate **Enrollment:** 163
Women: 94%; **Men:** 6%; **Minority:** 10%; **International:** 0%; **Part-time:** 86%

BACCALAUREATE PROGRAM

Contact Ms. Wanda C. Stutts, Chair and Assistant Professor, Davis School of Nursing, Gardner-Webb University, Statesville Campus, PO Box 908, Statesville, NC 28687-0908, 704-872-3664. *Fax:* 704-878-2615.

Expenses *Tuition:* $5056 full-time, $158 per semester hour part-time. *Full-time mandatory fees:* $15.

Financial Aid Institutionally sponsored need-based grants/scholarships, institutionally sponsored non-need grants/scholarships, Federal Nursing Student Loans.

RN Baccalaureate Program (BSN)

Applying *Required:* minimum college GPA of 2.5, RN license, diploma or AD in nursing, 2 letters of recommendation, transcript of college record. 24 prerequisite credits must be completed before admission to the nursing program. *Options:* Advanced standing available through credit by exam. May apply for transfer of up to 64 total credits. *Application deadline:* rolling. *Application fee:* $15.

Degree Requirements 128 total credit hours, 30 in nursing.

LENOIR-RHYNE COLLEGE
Department of Nursing
Hickory, North Carolina

Programs • RN Baccalaureate • Accelerated RN Baccalaureate

The College Independent Lutheran comprehensive coed institution. Founded: 1891. *Primary accreditation:* regional. *Setting:* 100-acre small-town campus. *Total enrollment:* 1,555.

The Department of Nursing Founded in 1910. *Nursing program faculty:* 9 (35% with doctorates).

Academic Facilities *Campus library:* 130,000 volumes; 1,386 periodical subscriptions. *Nursing school resources:* CAI, computer lab, nursing audiovisuals, learning resource lab.

Student Life *Student services:* health clinic, personal counseling, career counseling, institutionally sponsored work-study program, job placement, campus safety program, special assistance for disabled students. *International student services:* counseling/support, special assistance for nonnative speakers of English, ESL courses. *Nursing student activities:* Sigma Theta Tau, student nurses association.

Calendar Semesters.

NURSING STUDENT PROFILE

Undergraduate **Enrollment:** 142
Women: 92%; **Men:** 8%; **Minority:** 6%; **International:** 0%; **Part-time:** 4%

BACCALAUREATE PROGRAMS

Contact Ms. Kaye Deal, Secretary, Department of Nursing, Lenoir-Rhyne College, PO Box 7292, Hickory, NC 28603, 704-328-7281. *Fax:* 704-328-7368.

Expenses *Tuition:* $10,980 full-time, $300 per credit hour part-time. *Full-time mandatory fees:* $436. *Room and board:* $4324. *Books and supplies per academic year:* $400.

Financial Aid Institutionally sponsored need-based grants/scholarships, institutionally sponsored non-need grants/scholarships, Federal Direct Loans, Federal Nursing Student Loans, Federal Pell Grants, Federal Perkins Loans, Federal Work-Study.

RN Baccalaureate Program (BS)

Applying *Required:* SAT I, 3 years of high school math, 1 year of high school science, high school chemistry, 2 letters of recommendation, written essay, transcript of college record. *Options:* Advanced standing available through the following means: advanced placement exams, credit by exam. Course work may be accelerated. May apply for transfer of up to 96 total credits. *Application deadline:* rolling. *Application fee:* $25.

Degree Requirements 128 total credit hours, 57 in nursing.

Accelerated RN Baccalaureate Program (BS)

Applying *Required:* minimum college GPA of 2.5, RN license, diploma or AD in nursing, letter of recommendation, transcript of college record. 56 prerequisite credits must be completed before admission to the nursing program. *Options:* Advanced standing available through the following means: advanced placement exams, credit by exam. Course work may be accelerated. May apply for transfer of up to 96 total credits. *Application deadline:* rolling. *Application fee:* $25.

Degree Requirements 128 total credit hours, 57 in nursing.

NORTH CAROLINA AGRICULTURAL AND TECHNICAL STATE UNIVERSITY
School of Nursing
Greensboro, North Carolina

Programs • Generic Baccalaureate • RN Baccalaureate

The University State-supported coed university. Part of University of North Carolina System. Founded: 1891. *Primary accreditation:* regional. *Setting:* 181-acre urban campus. *Total enrollment:* 7,840.

The School of Nursing Founded in 1953. *Nursing program faculty:* 27 (3% with doctorates). *Off-campus program site:* High Point.

Academic Facilities *Campus library:* 416,021 volumes (1,476 in health, 1,499 in nursing); 3,622 periodical subscriptions (223 health-care related). *Nursing school resources:* CAI, computer lab, nursing audiovisuals, interactive nursing skills videos, learning resource lab.

Student Life *Student services:* health clinic, personal counseling, career counseling, institutionally sponsored work-study program, job placement, campus safety program, special assistance for disabled students. *International student services:* counseling/support, special assistance for nonnative speakers of English. *Nursing student activities:* Sigma Theta Tau, nursing club, student nurses association.

Calendar Semesters.

NURSING STUDENT PROFILE

Undergraduate **Enrollment:** 361
Women: 89%; **Men:** 11%; **Minority:** 82%; **International:** 0%; **Part-time:** 5%

BACCALAUREATE PROGRAMS

Contact Dr. Janice Brewington, Interim Dean and Associate Professor, School of Nursing, North Carolina Agricultural and Technical State University, 1601 East Market Street, Greensboro, NC 27411, 910-334-7750. *Fax:* 910-334-7637. *E-mail:* brewingj@athena.ncat.edu

Expenses *State resident tuition:* $874 per academic year. *Nonresident tuition:* $4014 per academic year. *Full-time mandatory fees:* $344. *Part-time mandatory fees:* $15. *Room and board:* $3430. *Books and supplies per academic year:* $42.

Financial Aid Institutionally sponsored need-based grants/scholarships, institutionally sponsored non-need grants/scholarships, Federal Direct Loans, Federal Nursing Student Loans, Federal Pell Grants, Federal Perkins Loans, Federal Supplemental Educational Opportunity Grants, Federal Work-Study. 48% of undergraduate students in nursing programs received some form of financial aid in 1995–96. *Application deadline:* 3/15.

Generic Baccalaureate Program (BSN)

Applying *Required:* SAT I or ACT, minimum high school GPA of 3.0, high school transcript, transcript of college record. *Options:* May apply for transfer of up to 80 total credits. *Application deadlines:* 6/1 (fall), 12/1 (spring). *Application fee:* $25.

Degree Requirements 124 total credit hours, 62 in nursing.

RN Baccalaureate Program (BSN)

Applying *Required:* minimum college GPA of 2.6, RN license, diploma or AD in nursing, high school transcript, transcript of college record. *Options:* Advanced standing available through the following means: advanced placement exams, credit by exam. Course work may be accelerated. May apply for transfer of up to 80 total credits. *Application deadlines:* 6/1 (fall), 12/1 (spring). *Application fee:* $25.

Degree Requirements 124 total credit hours, 62 in nursing.

NORTH CAROLINA CENTRAL UNIVERSITY

Department of Nursing
Durham, North Carolina

Programs • Generic Baccalaureate • RN Baccalaureate • Accelerated RN Baccalaureate • Baccalaureate for Second Degree

The University State-supported comprehensive coed institution. Part of University of North Carolina System. Founded: 1910. *Primary accreditation:* regional. *Setting:* 103-acre urban campus. *Total enrollment:* 5,470.

The Department of Nursing Founded in 1948. *Nursing program faculty:* 13 (50% with doctorates). *Off-campus program sites:* Henderson, Sanford.

Academic Facilities *Campus library:* 600,000 volumes (12,000 in health, 3,854 in nursing); 3,197 periodical subscriptions. *Nursing school resources:* CAI, computer lab, nursing audiovisuals, learning resource lab, nursing skills lab.

Student Life *Student services:* health clinic, child-care facilities, personal counseling, career counseling, institutionally sponsored work-study program, job placement, campus safety program, special assistance for disabled students. *International student services:* counseling/support, ESL courses. *Nursing student activities:* student nurses association.

Calendar Semesters.

NURSING STUDENT PROFILE

Undergraduate **Enrollment:** 161
Women: 84%; **Men:** 16%; **Minority:** 75%; **International:** 3%; **Part-time:** 1%

BACCALAUREATE PROGRAMS

Contact Dr. W. Kaye McDonald, Chair, Department of Nursing, North Carolina Central University, PO Box 19798, Durham, NC 27707, 919-560-6431. *Fax:* 919-560-5343. *E-mail:* wmcdonal@wpo.nccu.edu

Expenses *State resident tuition:* $1789 full-time, $236 per credit hour part-time. *Nonresident tuition:* $4471 full-time, $1131 per credit hour part-time. *Full-time mandatory fees:* $48. *Room and board:* $1714. *Room only:* $820. *Books and supplies per academic year:* $1500.

Financial Aid Institutionally sponsored need-based grants/scholarships, institutionally sponsored non-need grants/scholarships, Federal Nursing Student Loans, Federal Supplemental Educational Opportunity Grants, Federal Work-Study. *Application deadline:* 4/1.

Generic Baccalaureate Program (BSN)

Applying *Required:* SAT I, ACT, minimum college GPA of 2.5, 3 years of high school math, 3 years of high school science, transcript of college record, high school transcript or GED certificate, immunizations. 49 prerequisite credits must be completed before admission to the nursing program. *Options:* Course work may be accelerated. May apply for transfer of up to 60 total credits. *Application deadline:* 2/1. *Application fee:* $35.

Degree Requirements 128 total credit hours, 62 in nursing.

RN Baccalaureate Program (BSN)

Applying *Required:* SAT I, ACT, minimum college GPA of 2.5, 3 years of high school math, 3 years of high school science, RN license, diploma or AD in nursing, transcript of college record, high school transcript or GED certificate, immunizations. 66 prerequisite credits must be completed before admission to the nursing program. *Options:* Advanced standing available through advanced placement exams. Course work may be accelerated. May apply for transfer of up to 60 total credits. *Application deadline:* 2/1. *Application fee:* $35.

Degree Requirements 128 total credit hours, 62 in nursing.

Accelerated RN Baccalaureate Program (BSN)

Applying *Required:* SAT I, ACT, minimum college GPA of 2.5, 3 years of high school math, 3 years of high school science, RN license, diploma or AD in nursing, transcript of college record, high school transcript or GED certificate, immunizations. *Options:* Course work may be accelerated. May apply for transfer of up to 60 total credits. *Application deadline:* 2/1. *Application fee:* $35.

Degree Requirements 128 total credit hours, 62 in nursing.

Baccalaureate for Second Degree Program (BSN)

Applying *Required:* SAT I, ACT, minimum college GPA of 2.5, 3 years of high school math, 3 years of high school science, high school transcript, transcript of college record, high school transcript or GED certificate, immunizations. 66 prerequisite credits must be completed before admission to the nursing program. *Options:* Advanced standing available through the following means: advanced placement exams, credit by exam. *Application deadline:* 2/1. *Application fee:* $35.

Degree Requirements 128 total credit hours, 62 in nursing.

QUEENS COLLEGE

Division of Nursing
Charlotte, North Carolina

Programs • Generic Baccalaureate • RN Baccalaureate

Queens College (continued)

The College Independent Presbyterian comprehensive coed institution. Founded: 1857. *Primary accreditation:* regional. *Setting:* 25-acre suburban campus. *Total enrollment:* 1,557.

The Division of Nursing Founded in 1980. *Nursing program faculty:* 7 (42% with doctorates).

Academic Facilities *Campus library:* 100,000 volumes (3,000 in health); 500 periodical subscriptions (50 health-care related). *Nursing school resources:* CAI, computer lab, nursing audiovisuals, interactive nursing skills videos, learning resource lab.

Student Life *Student services:* health clinic, personal counseling, career counseling, institutionally sponsored work-study program, job placement, campus safety program, special assistance for disabled students. *International student services:* counseling/support. *Nursing student activities:* Sigma Theta Tau, student nurses association.

Calendar Semesters.

NURSING STUDENT PROFILE

Undergraduate **Enrollment:** 60
Women: 90%; **Men:** 10%; **Minority:** 10%; **International:** 5%; **Part-time:** 25%

BACCALAUREATE PROGRAMS

Contact Dr. Joan S. McGill, Chair and Professor, Division of Nursing, Queens College, 1900 Selwyn Avenue, Charlotte, NC 28274, 704-337-2276. *Fax:* 704-337-2517. *E-mail:* jmcgill@aol.com

Expenses *Tuition:* $11,910 full-time, $215 per semester hour part-time. *Full-time mandatory fees:* $50–$100. *Part-time mandatory fees:* $50–$100. *Room and board:* $5380. *Room only:* $1525. *Books and supplies per academic year:* ranges from $50 to $300.

Financial Aid Institutionally sponsored need-based grants/scholarships, institutionally sponsored non-need grants/scholarships, Federal Direct Loans, Federal Pell Grants, Federal Perkins Loans, Federal Work-Study, North Carolina Nurse Scholars Program. 80% of undergraduate students in nursing programs received some form of financial aid in 1995–96. *Application deadline:* 2/1.

Generic Baccalaureate Program (BSN)

Applying *Required:* TOEFL for nonnative speakers of English, SAT, ACT, or CLEP, minimum college GPA of 2.5, high school foreign language, high school transcript, transcript of college record. 34 prerequisite credits must be completed before admission to the nursing program. *Options:* Advanced standing available through advanced placement exams. May apply for transfer of up to 60 total credits. *Application deadlines:* 8/1 (fall), 12/15 (spring). *Application fee:* $25.

Degree Requirements 120 total credit hours, 58 in nursing.

RN Baccalaureate Program (BSN)

Applying *Required:* NLN Mobility Profile II, minimum college GPA of 2.5, RN license, diploma or AD in nursing. *Options:* Advanced standing available through the following means: advanced placement exams, credit by exam. May apply for transfer of up to 60 total credits. *Application deadline:* 6/1. *Application fee:* $25.

Degree Requirements 120 total credit hours, 58 in nursing.

UNIVERSITY OF NORTH CAROLINA AT CHAPEL HILL

School of Nursing
Chapel Hill, North Carolina

Programs • Generic Baccalaureate • RN Baccalaureate • Baccalaureate for Second Degree • Master's for Nurses with Non-Nursing Degrees • Post-Master's • PhD • Postdoctoral • Continuing Education

The University State-supported coed university. Part of University of North Carolina System. Founded: 1789. *Primary accreditation:* regional. *Setting:* 789-acre suburban campus. *Total enrollment:* 24,439.

The School of Nursing Founded in 1951. *Nursing program faculty:* 98 (60% with doctorates). *Off-campus program sites:* Raleigh, Asheville.

Academic Facilities *Campus library:* 4.0 million volumes (290,000 in health); 44,000 periodical subscriptions (10,000 health-care related). *Nursing school resources:* CAI, computer lab, nursing audiovisuals, interactive nursing skills videos, learning resource lab.

Student Life *Student services:* health clinic, personal counseling, career counseling, institutionally sponsored work-study program, job placement, campus safety program, special assistance for disabled students. *International student services:* counseling/support, special assistance for nonnative speakers of English, ESL courses. *Nursing student activities:* Sigma Theta Tau, student nurses association.

Calendar Semesters.

NURSING STUDENT PROFILE

Undergraduate **Enrollment:** 321
Women: 91%; **Men:** 9%; **Minority:** 13%; **International:** 0%; **Part-time:** 0%
Graduate **Enrollment:** 230
Women: 93%; **Men:** 7%; **Minority:** 11%; **International:** 1%; **Part-time:** 65%

BACCALAUREATE PROGRAMS

Contact Dr. Carol Binzer, Director of Student Services, Carrington Hall, School of Nursing, University of North Carolina at Chapel Hill, College Box 7460, Chapel Hill, NC 27599, 919-966-4260. *Fax:* 919-966-3540. *E-mail:* cdbinzer@unc.edu

Expenses *State resident tuition:* $2162 per academic year. *Nonresident tuition:* $10,694 per academic year. *Full-time mandatory fees:* $1548. *Room and board:* $4500. *Books and supplies per academic year:* $600.

Financial Aid Institutionally sponsored need-based grants/scholarships, institutionally sponsored non-need grants/scholarships, Federal Nursing Student Loans, Federal Supplemental Educational Opportunity Grants, Federal Work-Study. 51% of undergraduate students in nursing programs received some form of financial aid in 1995–96. *Application deadline:* 3/1.

Generic Baccalaureate Program (BSN)

Applying *Required:* SAT I, TOEFL for nonnative speakers of English, 3 years of high school math, 2 years of high school science, high school biology, high school transcript, 2 letters of recommendation, written essay, transcript of college record. 67 prerequisite credits must be completed before admission to the nursing program. *Options:* May apply for transfer of up to 64 total credits. *Application deadline:* 1/15. *Application fee:* $55.

Degree Requirements 129 total credit hours, 62 in nursing.

RN Baccalaureate Program (BSN)

Applying *Required:* TOEFL for nonnative speakers of English, 3 years of high school math, 2 years of high school science, high school biology, RN license, diploma or AD in nursing, high school transcript, 2 letters of recommendation, written essay, transcript of college record, professional liability/malpractice insurance. 67 prerequisite credits must be completed before admission to the nursing program. *Options:* Course work may be accelerated. May apply for transfer of up to 64 total credits. *Application deadline:* 1/15. *Application fee:* $55.

Degree Requirements 129 total credit hours, 30 in nursing.

Baccalaureate for Second Degree Program (BSN)

Applying *Required:* TOEFL for nonnative speakers of English, 3 years of high school math, 2 years of high school science, high school biology, high school transcript, 2 letters of recommendation, written essay, transcript of college record. 60 prerequisite credits must be completed before admission to the nursing program. *Options:* May apply for transfer of up to 64 total credits.

Degree Requirements 122 total credit hours, 62 in nursing.

MASTER'S PROGRAMS

Contact Dr. Carol Binzer, Director of Student Services, Carrington Hall, School of Nursing, University of North Carolina at Chapel Hill, College Box 7460, Chapel Hill, NC 27599, 919-966-4260. *Fax:* 919-966-3540. *E-mail:* cdbinzer.uncson@mhs.unc.edu

Areas of Study Clinical nurse specialist programs in maternity-newborn nursing, pediatric nursing, psychiatric–mental health nursing, women's health nursing; nursing administration; nurse practitioner programs in adult health, child care/pediatrics, family health, primary care, psychiatric–mental health, women's health.

Expenses *State resident tuition:* $473. *Nonresident tuition:* $1540. *Full-time mandatory fees:* $380. *Part-time mandatory fees:* $300–$353. *Room and board:* $5852. *Books and supplies per academic year:* $700.

Financial Aid Graduate assistantships, nurse traineeships, Federal Nursing Student Loans, institutionally sponsored loans, employment opportunities. 29% of master's level students in nursing programs received some form of financial aid in 1995-96. *Application deadline:* 3/1.

Master's for Nurses with Non-Nursing Degrees Program (MSN)

Applying *Required:* GRE General Test, TOEFL for nonnative speakers of English, bachelor's degree in nursing, RN license, 1 year of clinical experience, physical assessment course, statistics course, professional liability/malpractice insurance, essay, interview, 3 letters of recommendation, transcript of college record, evaluation of coursework and bridge courses for non-BSN applicants. *Application deadlines:* 1/31 (fall), 10/15 (spring). *Application fee:* $55.

Degree Requirements 36–42 total credit hours dependent upon track, 36–42 in nursing. Thesis required.

Post-Master's Program

Applying *Required:* RN license, 1 year of clinical experience, physical assessment course, professional liability/malpractice insurance, essay, 2 letters of recommendation, transcript of college record, MSN degree. *Application deadlines:* 3/1, rolling.

Degree Requirements 18–24 total credit hours dependent upon track, 18–24 in nursing.

DOCTORAL PROGRAM

Contact Dr. Carol Binzer, Director of Student Services, Carrington Hall, School of Nursing, University of North Carolina at Chapel Hill, College Box 7460, Chapel Hill, NC 27599, 919-966-4260. *Fax:* 919-966-3540.

Areas of Study Nursing research.

Expenses *State resident tuition:* $473 per course. *Nonresident tuition:* $1540 per course. *Full-time mandatory fees:* $380. *Part-time mandatory fees:* $300–$353. *Room and board:* $5852. *Books and supplies per academic year:* $700.

Financial Aid Graduate assistantships, nurse traineeships, fellowships, dissertation grants, grants, institutionally sponsored loans, opportunities for employment. *Application deadline:* 3/1.

PhD Program

Applying *Required:* GRE General Test, TOEFL for nonnative speakers of English, master's degree in nursing, 1 year of clinical experience, 1 scholarly paper, statistics course, interview, 3 letters of recommendation, vitae, writing sample, competitive review by faculty committee, graduate-level nursing theory course. *Application deadlines:* 1/31 (fall), 10/15 (spring). *Application fee:* $55.

Degree Requirements 30 total credit hours; dissertation; oral exam; written exam; defense of dissertation; residency.

POSTDOCTORAL PROGRAM

Contact Dr. Merle Mishel, Professor, Carrington Hall, School of Nursing, College Box 7460, Chapel Hill, NC 27599, 919-966-5294. *Fax:* 919-966-7298. *E-mail:* mmishel.uncson@mhs.unc.edu

CONTINUING EDUCATION PROGRAM

Contact Laurice Ferris, Director of Continuing Education, Carrington Hall, School of Nursing, University of North Carolina at Chapel Hill, College Box 7460, Chapel Hill, NC 27599, 919-966-3638. *Fax:* 919-966-7298. *E-mail:* lferris.uncson@mhs.unc.edu

UNIVERSITY OF NORTH CAROLINA AT CHARLOTTE

College of Nursing and Health Professions
Charlotte, North Carolina

Programs • Generic Baccalaureate • RN Baccalaureate • BSN to Master's • MSN/MHA • Continuing Education

The University State-supported coed university. Part of University of North Carolina System. Founded: 1946. *Primary accreditation:* regional. *Setting:* 1,000-acre urban campus. *Total enrollment:* 15,895.

The College of Nursing and Health Professions Founded in 1965. *Nursing program faculty:* 38 (70% with doctorates). *Off-campus program site:* Asheville.

Academic Facilities *Campus library:* 415,446 volumes (28,338 in health, 2,152 in nursing); 12,664 periodical subscriptions (903 health-care related). *Nursing school resources:* CAI, computer lab, nursing audiovisuals, learning resource lab.

Student Life *Student services:* health clinic, personal counseling, career counseling, institutionally sponsored work-study program, job placement, campus safety program, special assistance for disabled students. *International student services:* counseling/support, special assistance for nonnative speakers of English, ESL courses. *Nursing student activities:* Sigma Theta Tau, student nurses association.

Calendar Semesters.

NURSING STUDENT PROFILE

Undergraduate **Enrollment:** 560
Women: 92%; **Men:** 8%; **Minority:** 15%; **International:** 0%; **Part-time:** 18%
Graduate **Enrollment:** 139
Women: 90%; **Men:** 10%; **Minority:** 6%; **International:** 1%; **Part-time:** 76%

BACCALAUREATE PROGRAMS

Contact Dr. Cynthia Beamon, Director of Student Affairs, College of Nursing and Health Professions, University of North Carolina at Charlotte, Charlotte, NC 28223, 704-547-4650. *Fax:* 704-547-3180.

Expenses *State resident tuition:* $1718 per academic year. *Nonresident tuition:* $8872 per academic year. *Full-time mandatory fees:* $52. *Room and board:* $1163–$1946. *Room only:* $835–$1151. *Books and supplies per academic year:* ranges from $800 to $1200.

Financial Aid Institutionally sponsored need-based grants/scholarships, institutionally sponsored non-need grants/scholarships, Federal Supplemental Educational Opportunity Grants, Federal Work-Study. *Application deadline:* 4/1.

Generic Baccalaureate Program (BSN)

Applying *Required:* SAT I or ACT, TOEFL or Michigan English Language Assessment Battery for nonnative speakers of English, minimum college GPA of 2.5, 3 years of high school math, 3 years of high school science, high school chemistry, high school biology, high school foreign language, high school transcript, transcript of college record. *Options:* May apply for transfer of up to 90 total credits. *Application deadline:* 1/15. *Application fee:* $25.

Degree Requirements 120 total credit hours, 56 in nursing.

RN Baccalaureate Program (BSN)

Applying *Required:* TOEFL or Michigan English Language Assessment Battery for nonnative speakers of English, minimum college GPA of 2.5, RN license, diploma or AD in nursing, transcript of college record. 41 prerequisite credits must be completed before admission to the nursing program. *Options:* Advanced standing available through credit by exam. May apply for transfer of up to 64 total credits. *Application deadline:* 9/30. *Application fee:* $25.

Degree Requirements 122 total credit hours, 66 in nursing.

MASTER'S PROGRAMS

Contact Dr. Cynthia Beamon, Director of Student Affairs, College of Nursing and Health Professions, University of North Carolina at Charlotte, Charlotte, NC 28223, 704-547-4684. *Fax:* 704-547-3180.

Areas of Study Clinical nurse specialist programs in adult health nursing, community health nursing, medical-surgical nursing, psychiatric–mental health nursing; nurse anesthesia; nursing education; nurse practitioner program in family health.

Expenses *State resident tuition:* $1718 full-time, $326 per semester part-time. *Nonresident tuition:* $8872 full-time, $2224 per semester part-time. *Full-time mandatory fees:* $0. *Room only:* $835–$1151. *Books and supplies per academic year:* ranges from $100 to $200.

Financial Aid Graduate assistantships, nurse traineeships, Federal Nursing Student Loans, institutionally sponsored loans, employment opportunities. *Application deadline:* 4/1.

BSN to Master's Program (MSN)

Applying *Required:* GRE General Test or Miller Analogies Test, bachelor's degree in nursing, minimum GPA of 3.0, RN license, statistics course, professional liability/malpractice insurance, essay, 3 letters of recommendation, transcript of college record, minimum of 1 year of critical-care experience with adults and certification in advanced cardiac life support for nurse anesthesia track. *Application deadlines:* 7/1 (fall), 11/15 (spring), 5/1 (summer). *Application fee:* $25.

Degree Requirements 38–70 total credit hours dependent upon track, 29–70 in nursing. Thesis or nursing project.

Distance learning Courses provided through video, audio.

University of North Carolina at Charlotte (continued)

MSN/MHA Program

Applying *Required:* GRE General Test, Miller Analogies Test, bachelor's degree in nursing, minimum GPA of 3.0, RN license, statistics course, professional liability/malpractice insurance, essay, letter of recommendation, transcript of college record. *Application deadlines:* 7/1 (fall), 11/15 (spring). *Application fee:* $35.

Degree Requirements 59 total credit hours, 23 in nursing, 36 in business administration. Thesis or nursing project.

CONTINUING EDUCATION PROGRAM

Contact Dr. Lienne Edwards, Director of Continuing Education, College of Nursing and Health Professions, University of North Carolina at Charlotte, Charlotte, NC 28223, 704-547-4672. *Fax:* 704-547-3180.

UNIVERSITY OF NORTH CAROLINA AT GREENSBORO

School of Nursing
Greensboro, North Carolina

Programs • Generic Baccalaureate • RN Baccalaureate • MSN

The University State-supported coed university. Part of University of North Carolina System. Founded: 1891. *Primary accreditation:* regional. *Setting:* 190-acre urban campus. *Total enrollment:* 12,644.

The School of Nursing Founded in 1966. *Nursing program faculty:* 40 (50% with doctorates). *Off-campus program site:* Hickory.

Academic Facilities *Campus library:* 148 periodical subscriptions. *Nursing school resources:* CAI, computer lab, nursing audiovisuals, interactive nursing skills videos, learning resource lab.

Student Life *Student services:* health clinic, child-care facilities, personal counseling, career counseling, institutionally sponsored work-study program, job placement, campus safety program, special assistance for disabled students. *International student services:* counseling/support, special assistance for nonnative speakers of English, ESL courses. *Nursing student activities:* Sigma Theta Tau, student nurses association, Black Nursing Student Association, Nursing Christian Fellowship.

Calendar Semesters.

NURSING STUDENT PROFILE

Undergraduate **Enrollment:** 756

Women: 92%; **Men:** 8%; **Minority:** 20%; **International:** 0%; **Part-time:** 29%

Graduate **Enrollment:** 261

Women: 93%; **Men:** 7%; **Minority:** 15%; **International:** 0%; **Part-time:** 38%

BACCALAUREATE PROGRAMS

Contact Dr. Virginia Karb, Associate Dean, School of Nursing, University of North Carolina at Greensboro, Greensboro, NC 27412, 910-334-5010 Ext. 567. *Fax:* 910-334-3628. *E-mail:* karbvb@florence.uncg.edu

Expenses *State resident tuition:* $1954 full-time, ranges from $81 to $161 per credit hour part-time. *Nonresident tuition:* $10,272 full-time, ranges from $428 to $1201 per credit hour part-time. *Full-time mandatory fees:* $585–$695. *Room and board:* $857–$1286. *Books and supplies per academic year:* $350.

Financial Aid Institutionally sponsored need-based grants/scholarships, institutionally sponsored non-need grants/scholarships, Federal Direct Loans, Federal Pell Grants, Federal Perkins Loans, Federal Supplemental Educational Opportunity Grants, Federal Work-Study. 47% of undergraduate students in nursing programs received some form of financial aid in 1995–96. *Application deadline:* 3/1.

Generic Baccalaureate Program (BSN)

Applying *Required:* SAT I or ACT, TOEFL for nonnative speakers of English, minimum college GPA of 2.0, 3 years of high school math, 3 years of high school science, high school biology, high school transcript, transcript of college record. 50 prerequisite credits must be completed before admission to the nursing program. *Options:* Advanced standing available through the following means: advanced placement exams, advanced placement without credit. *Application deadlines:* 8/1 (fall), 12/1 (spring). *Application fee:* $35.

Degree Requirements 122 total credit hours, 54 in nursing. Specified cognate courses.

RN Baccalaureate Program (BSN)

Applying *Required:* TOEFL for nonnative speakers of English, minimum college GPA of 2.0, RN license, diploma or AD in nursing, transcript of college record. *Options:* Advanced standing available through the following means: advanced placement exams, advanced placement without credit, credit by exam. *Application deadlines:* 8/1 (fall), 12/1 (spring). *Application fee:* $35.

Degree Requirements 122 total credit hours, 54–30 in nursing. Residency, university's liberal education requirements.

MASTER'S PROGRAM

Contact Eileen Kohlenberg, Director of Graduate Studies, School of Nursing, University of North Carolina at Greensboro, Greensboro, NC 27412-5001, 910-334-5010 Ext. 526. *Fax:* 910-334-3628. *E-mail:* kohlenbe@florence. uncg.edu

Areas of Study Nurse anesthesia; nursing administration; nursing education; nurse practitioner program in gerontology.

Expenses *State resident tuition:* $1955 full-time, $568 per semester part-time. *Nonresident tuition:* $10,273 full-time, $3687 per semester part-time. *Room and board:* $2100–$2400. *Room only:* $857–$1450. *Books and supplies per academic year:* ranges from $200 to $600.

Financial Aid Graduate assistantships, nurse traineeships, institutionally sponsored loans, employment opportunities, institutionally sponsored need-based grants/scholarships, institutionally sponsored non-need-based grants/scholarships. *Application deadline:* 3/1.

MSN Program

Applying *Required:* GRE General Test, Miller Analogies Test, bachelor's degree in nursing, minimum GPA of 3.0, RN license, 1 year of clinical experience, physical assessment course, statistics course, professional liability/malpractice insurance, 3 letters of recommendation, transcript of college record. *Application deadline:* rolling. *Application fee:* $35.

Degree Requirements 36–47 total credit hours dependent upon track, 33–47 in nursing. Thesis or advanced nursing project.

UNIVERSITY OF NORTH CAROLINA AT WILMINGTON

School of Nursing
Wilmington, North Carolina

Programs • Generic Baccalaureate • RN Baccalaureate

The University State-supported comprehensive coed institution. Part of University of North Carolina System. Founded: 1947. *Primary accreditation:* regional. *Setting:* 650-acre urban campus. *Total enrollment:* 8,601.

The School of Nursing Founded in 1985. *Nursing program faculty:* 16 (60% with doctorates). *Off-campus program site:* Jacksonville.

Academic Facilities *Campus library:* 403,748 volumes (14,509 in health, 1,913 in nursing); 5,044 periodical subscriptions (366 health-care related). *Nursing school resources:* CAI, computer lab, nursing audiovisuals, interactive nursing skills videos, learning resource lab.

Student Life *Student services:* health clinic, personal counseling, career counseling, institutionally sponsored work-study program, job placement, campus safety program, special assistance for disabled students. *International student services:* counseling/support. *Nursing student activities:* Sigma Theta Tau, nursing club, student nurses association.

Calendar Semesters.

NURSING STUDENT PROFILE

Undergraduate **Enrollment:** 160

Women: 90%; **Men:** 10%; **Minority:** 12%; **International:** 1%; **Part-time:** 0%

BACCALAUREATE PROGRAMS

Contact Ms. Peggy Segars, Executive Assistant, School of Nursing, University of North Carolina at Wilmington, 601 South College Road, Wilmington, NC 28403, 910-962-3784. *Fax:* 910-962-3723.

Expenses *State resident tuition:* $840 per academic year. *Nonresident tuition:* $7682 per academic year. *Full-time mandatory fees:* $824. *Room and board:* $3660–$4300. *Books and supplies per academic year:* ranges from $600 to $700.

Financial Aid Institutionally sponsored need-based grants/scholarships, Federal Direct Loans, Federal Nursing Student Loans, Federal Supplemental Educational Opportunity Grants, Federal Work-Study, North Carolina Student Incentive Grant Program, North Carolina Nurse Scholars Program.

Generic Baccalaureate Program (BS)

Applying *Required:* SAT I, ACT, TOEFL for nonnative speakers of English, English, math placement tests, minimum college GPA of 2.5, high school biology, high school transcript, written essay, transcript of college record. 70 prerequisite credits must be completed before admission to the nursing program. *Options:* Advanced standing available through the following means: advanced placement exams, credit by exam. May apply for transfer of up to 62–94 total credits. *Application deadline:* 12/1. *Application fee:* $25.

Degree Requirements 124 total credit hours, 54 in nursing.

Distance learning Courses provided through computer-based media.

RN Baccalaureate Program (BS)

Applying *Required:* SAT I, ACT, math placement, NLN Mobility Profile II, minimum college GPA of 2.5, RN license, diploma or AD in nursing, written essay, transcript of college record. *Options:* Advanced standing available through the following means: advanced placement exams, credit by exam. May apply for transfer of up to 62–94 total credits. *Application deadlines:* 12/1 (fall), 1/30 (summer). *Application fee:* $25.

Degree Requirements 124 total credit hours, 54 in nursing.

WESTERN CAROLINA UNIVERSITY

Department of Nursing
Cullowhee, North Carolina

Programs • Generic Baccalaureate • RN Baccalaureate

The University State-supported comprehensive coed institution. Part of University of North Carolina System. Founded: 1889. *Primary accreditation:* regional. *Setting:* 260-acre rural campus. *Total enrollment:* 6,651.

The Department of Nursing Founded in 1973. *Nursing program faculty:* 17 (30% with doctorates). *Off-campus program site:* Asheville.

Academic Facilities *Campus library:* 10,000 volumes in nursing; 70 health-care related periodical subscriptions. *Nursing school resources:* CAI, computer lab, nursing audiovisuals, interactive nursing skills videos, learning resource lab.

Student Life *Student services:* health clinic, personal counseling, career counseling, institutionally sponsored work-study program, job placement, campus safety program, special assistance for disabled students. *International student services:* counseling/support, special assistance for nonnative speakers of English, ESL courses. *Nursing student activities:* Sigma Theta Tau, student nurses association.

Calendar Semesters.

NURSING STUDENT PROFILE

Undergraduate **Enrollment:** 151
Women: 87%; **Men:** 13%; **Minority:** 2%; **Part-time:** 34%

BACCALAUREATE PROGRAMS

Contact Dr. Sharon Jacques, Acting Head, Department of Nursing, Western Carolina University, Cullowhee, NC 28723, 704-227-7467. *Fax:* 704-227-7446. *E-mail:* jacques@wpoff.wcu.edu

Expenses *State resident tuition:* $1732 full-time, $209 per course part-time. *Nonresident tuition:* $7682 full-time, $1064 per course part-time. *Room and board:* $2520–$2950. *Books and supplies per academic year:* ranges from $700 to $900.

Financial Aid Institutionally sponsored need-based grants/scholarships, institutionally sponsored non-need grants/scholarships, Federal Direct Loans, Federal Nursing Student Loans, Federal Pell Grants, Federal Perkins Loans, Federal Supplemental Educational Opportunity Grants, Federal Work-Study, state loan for nursing. *Application deadline:* 4/1.

Generic Baccalaureate Program (BSN)

Applying *Required:* SAT I, TOEFL for nonnative speakers of English, minimum college GPA of 2.25, 3 years of high school math, 3 years of high school science, written essay, transcript of college record. 60 prerequisite credits must be completed before admission to the nursing program. *Options:* Advanced standing available through credit by exam. May apply for transfer of up to 98 total credits. *Application deadline:* 2/15.

Degree Requirements 128 total credit hours, 53 in nursing. 22 credits in chemistry, psychology, anatomy and physiology, and microbiology.

RN Baccalaureate Program (BSN)

Applying *Required:* TOEFL for nonnative speakers of English, minimum college GPA of 2.25, RN license, diploma or AD in nursing, transcript of college record. 60 prerequisite credits must be completed before admission to the nursing program. *Options:* Advanced standing available through credit by exam. Course work may be accelerated. May apply for transfer of up to 98 total credits. *Application deadline:* rolling.

Degree Requirements 128 total credit hours, 53 in nursing.

WINSTON-SALEM STATE UNIVERSITY

Division of Nursing and Allied Health
Winston-Salem, North Carolina

Programs • Generic Baccalaureate • RN Baccalaureate • Baccalaureate for Second Degree • LPN to Baccalaureate

The University State-supported 4-year coed college. Part of University of North Carolina System. Founded: 1892. *Primary accreditation:* regional. *Setting:* 81-acre urban campus. *Total enrollment:* 2,863.

The Division of Nursing and Allied Health Founded in 1953.

Academic Facilities *Campus library:* 167,865 volumes (5,619 in nursing); 1,112 periodical subscriptions (890 health-care related).

Calendar Semesters.

BACCALAUREATE PROGRAMS

Contact University Admissions, Division of Nursing and Allied Health, Winston-Salem State University, 601 Martin Luther King, Jr. Drive, Winston-Salem, NC 27110, 919-750-2070.

Expenses *State resident tuition:* $648 full-time, $115 per 3 hours part-time. *Nonresident tuition:* $6742 full-time, $877 per 3 hours part-time. *Full-time mandatory fees:* $719.

Generic Baccalaureate Program (BSN)

Applying *Required:* SAT I, minimum college GPA of 2.6.

Degree Requirements 126 total credit hours.

RN Baccalaureate Program (BSN)

Applying *Required:* minimum college GPA of 2.0, RN license. *Options:* Course work may be accelerated.

Degree Requirements 126 total credit hours.

Baccalaureate for Second Degree Program (BSN)

Degree Requirements 126 total credit hours.

LPN to Baccalaureate Program (BSN)

Applying *Required:* SAT I, minimum college GPA of 2.6. *Options:* Course work may be accelerated.

Degree Requirements 126 total credit hours.

NORTH DAKOTA

DICKINSON STATE UNIVERSITY

Department of Nursing
Dickinson, North Dakota

Programs • RN Baccalaureate • LPN to Baccalaureate

Dickinson State University (continued)

The University State-supported 4-year coed college. Part of North Dakota University System. Founded: 1918. *Primary accreditation:* regional. *Setting:* 100-acre small-town campus. *Total enrollment:* 1,578.

The Department of Nursing Founded in 1967. *Nursing program faculty:* 14 (14% with doctorates).

Academic Facilities *Campus library:* 68,858 volumes (3,476 in health, 718 in nursing); 660 periodical subscriptions (90 health-care related). *Nursing school resources:* CAI, computer lab, nursing audiovisuals, learning resource lab.

Student Life *Student services:* health clinic, personal counseling, career counseling, institutionally sponsored work-study program, job placement. *International student services:* counseling/support. *Nursing student activities:* student nurses association.

Calendar Semesters.

NURSING STUDENT PROFILE

Undergraduate **Enrollment:** 126

Women: 93%; **Men:** 7%; **Minority:** 3%; **International:** 0%; **Part-time:** 26%

BACCALAUREATE PROGRAMS

Contact Dr. Sandra Affeldt, Chairperson, Department of Nursing, Dickinson State University, 291 Campus Drive, Dickinson, ND 58601-4896, 701-227-2172. *Fax:* 701-227-2006. *E-mail:* sandra_affeldt@dsu1.dsu1.nodak.edu

Expenses *State resident tuition:* $1970 full-time, $82 per credit hour part-time. *Nonresident tuition:* $2388 full-time, $199 per credit hour part-time. *Full-time mandatory fees:* $300–$450. *Part-time mandatory fees:* $300–$450. *Room and board:* $2302–$2840. *Room only:* $872–$1260. *Books and supplies per academic year:* ranges from $400 to $600.

Financial Aid Institutionally sponsored need-based grants/scholarships, institutionally sponsored non-need grants/scholarships, Federal Nursing Student Loans, Federal Pell Grants, Federal Perkins Loans, Federal Supplemental Educational Opportunity Grants, Federal Work-Study. *Application deadline:* 4/15.

RN Baccalaureate Program (BSN)

Applying *Required:* ACT, NCLEX-RN or NCLEX-PN exam, minimum college GPA of 2.5, 3 years of high school math, 3 years of high school science, high school chemistry, RN license, diploma or AD in nursing, high school transcript, 3 letters of recommendation, transcript of college record, immunizations, high school diploma or GED certificate. *Options:* Advanced standing available through credit by exam. Course work may be accelerated. *Application deadline:* 1/1. *Application fee:* $25.

Degree Requirements 130 total credit hours, 66 in nursing.

LPN to Baccalaureate Program (BSN)

Applying *Required:* ACT, TOEFL for nonnative speakers of English, NCLEX-RN or NCLEX-PN exam, minimum college GPA of 2.5, 3 years of high school math, 3 years of high school science, high school chemistry, RN license, diploma or AD in nursing, high school transcript, 3 letters of recommendation, transcript of college record, LPN license, proof of measles-rubella immunization, graduate of approved ASPN program, high school diploma or GED certificate. *Options:* Advanced standing available through credit by exam. *Application fee:* $25.

Degree Requirements 130 total credit hours.

JAMESTOWN COLLEGE
Department of Nursing
Jamestown, North Dakota

Programs • Generic Baccalaureate • RN Baccalaureate

The College Independent Presbyterian 4-year coed college. Founded: 1883. *Primary accreditation:* regional. *Setting:* 107-acre small-town campus. *Total enrollment:* 1,064.

The Department of Nursing Founded in 1950. *Nursing program faculty:* 8 (13% with doctorates). *Off-campus program site:* Fargo.

Academic Facilities *Campus library:* 117,620 volumes (990 in health, 983 in nursing); 490 periodical subscriptions (163 health-care related). *Nursing school resources:* CAI, computer lab, nursing audiovisuals, interactive nursing skills videos, learning resource lab.

Student Life *Student services:* personal counseling, career counseling, institutionally sponsored work-study program, job placement. *International student services:* counseling/support, special assistance for nonnative speakers of English, ESL courses. *Nursing student activities:* Sigma Theta Tau, student nurses association.

Calendar Semesters.

NURSING STUDENT PROFILE

Undergraduate **Enrollment:** 150

Women: 85%; **Men:** 15%; **Minority:** 1%; **International:** 1%; **Part-time:** 3%

BACCALAUREATE PROGRAMS

Contact Dr. Geneal E. Hall, Chairperson, Department of Nursing, Jamestown College, 6010 College Lane, Jamestown, ND 58405, 701-252-3467 Ext. 2497. *Fax:* 701-253-4318. *E-mail:* hall@acc.jc.edu

Expenses *Tuition:* $8420 full-time, $230 per semester credit part-time. *Full-time mandatory fees:* $500. *Part-time mandatory fees:* $250. *Room and board:* $3080. *Room only:* up to $1330. *Books and supplies per academic year:* ranges from $400 to $500.

Financial Aid Institutionally sponsored need-based grants/scholarships, institutionally sponsored non-need grants/scholarships, Federal Nursing Student Loans, Federal Supplemental Educational Opportunity Grants, Federal Work-Study. 73% of undergraduate students in nursing programs received some form of financial aid in 1995–96. *Application deadline:* 9/6.

Generic Baccalaureate Program (BA)

Applying *Required:* ACT, TOEFL for nonnative speakers of English, minimum college GPA of 2.5, high school transcript. 29 prerequisite credits must be completed before admission to the nursing program. *Options:* Advanced standing available through credit by exam. May apply for transfer of up to 64 total credits. *Application deadlines:* 8/15 (fall), 12/10 (spring). *Application fee:* $20.

Degree Requirements 128 total credit hours, 60 in nursing. English proficiency exam.

RN Baccalaureate Program (BA)

Applying *Required:* NLN Mobility Profile II, minimum college GPA of 2.5, RN license, diploma or AD in nursing, transcript of college record. 29 prerequisite credits must be completed before admission to the nursing program. *Options:* Course work may be accelerated. May apply for transfer of up to 64 total credits. *Application deadline:* 8/15. *Application fee:* $20.

Degree Requirements 128 total credit hours, 60 in nursing.

MEDCENTER ONE COLLEGE OF NURSING
Bismarck, North Dakota

Programs • Generic Baccalaureate • RN Baccalaureate • Accelerated LPN to Baccalaureate

The College Independent upper-level specialized primarily women's institution. Founded: 1988. *Primary accreditation:* regional. *Setting:* 15-acre small-town campus. *Total enrollment:* 83. Founded in 1988. *Nursing program faculty:* 13 (16% with doctorates).

Academic Facilities *Campus library:* 9,548 volumes (7,048 in health, 2,500 in nursing); 372 periodical subscriptions (350 health-care related). *Nursing school resources:* CAI, computer lab, nursing audiovisuals, interactive nursing skills videos, learning resource lab.

Student Life *Student services:* health clinic, personal counseling, career counseling, institutionally sponsored work-study program, job placement, campus safety program. *Nursing student activities:* student nurses association.

Calendar Semesters.

NURSING STUDENT PROFILE

Undergraduate **Enrollment:** 74

Women: 93%; **Men:** 7%; **Part-time:** 10%

BACCALAUREATE PROGRAMS

Contact Ms. Lisa F. Schauer, Registrar, Medcenter One College of Nursing, 512 North 7th Street, Bismarck, ND 58501, 701-323-6270. *Fax:* 701-323-6967.

Expenses *Tuition:* $2480 full-time, $103 per credit part-time. *Full-time mandatory fees:* $210. *Room only:* $780. *Books and supplies per academic year:* $500.

Financial Aid Institutionally sponsored need-based grants/scholarships, institutionally sponsored non-need grants/scholarships, Federal Nursing

Student Loans, Federal Pell Grants, Federal Perkins Loans, Federal Supplemental Educational Opportunity Grants, Federal Work-Study. 96% of undergraduate students in nursing programs received some form of financial aid in 1995–96. *Application deadline:* 5/1.

Generic Baccalaureate Program (BScN)

Applying *Required:* minimum college GPA of 2.5, interview, written essay, transcript of college record. 65 prerequisite credits must be completed before admission to the nursing program. *Options:* May apply for transfer of up to 101 total credits. *Application deadlines:* 3/26 (fall), 11/7 (spring), 4/1 (summer). *Application fee:* $40.

Degree Requirements 126 total credit hours.

RN Baccalaureate Program (BScN)

Applying *Required:* NLN Mobility Profile II, minimum college GPA of 2.5, RN license, diploma or AD in nursing, written essay, transcript of college record. *Options:* May apply for transfer of up to 101 total credits. *Application deadline:* rolling. *Application fee:* $40.

Degree Requirements 126 total credit hours.

Accelerated LPN to Baccalaureate Program (BSN)

Applying *Required:* NLN Mobility Profile I, minimum college GPA of 2.5, interview, written essay, transcript of college record, LPN license. *Options:* May apply for transfer of up to 101 total credits. *Application deadline:* rolling. *Application fee:* $40.

Degree Requirements 126 total credit hours.

MINOT STATE UNIVERSITY

College of Nursing
Minot, North Dakota

Programs • Generic Baccalaureate • Accelerated RN Baccalaureate • Accelerated LPN to Baccalaureate • Continuing Education

The University State-supported comprehensive coed institution. Part of North Dakota University System. Founded: 1913. *Primary accreditation:* regional. *Setting:* 103-acre small-town campus. *Total enrollment:* 3,761.

The College of Nursing Founded in 1969. *Nursing program faculty:* 12 (8% with doctorates).

Academic Facilities *Campus library:* 313,906 volumes (950 in health, 1,685 in nursing); 913 periodical subscriptions (46 health-care related). *Nursing school resources:* CAI, computer lab, nursing audiovisuals, interactive nursing skills videos, learning resource lab.

Student Life *Student services:* health clinic, personal counseling, career counseling, institutionally sponsored work-study program, job placement, special assistance for disabled students. *International student services:* counseling/support. *Nursing student activities:* student nurses association, Nursing Honor Society.

Calendar Semesters.

NURSING STUDENT PROFILE

Undergraduate **Enrollment:** 90

Women: 91%; **Men:** 9%; **Minority:** 3%; **International:** 0%; **Part-time:** 16%

BACCALAUREATE PROGRAMS

Contact Dr. Valeda C. Fabricius, Dean, College of Nursing, Minot State University, Minot, ND 58707, 701-858-3101. *Fax:* 701-858-4309. *E-mail:* fabriciu@warp6.cs.misu.nodak.edu

Expenses *State resident tuition:* $2720 full-time, $85 per credit part-time. *Nonresident tuition:* $6688 full-time, $209 per credit part-time. *Full-time mandatory fees:* $150. *Room and board:* $3155. *Room only:* $1311. *Books and supplies per academic year:* $600.

Financial Aid Institutionally sponsored need-based grants/scholarships, institutionally sponsored non-need grants/scholarships, Federal Nursing Student Loans, Federal Perkins Loans, Federal Supplemental Educational Opportunity Grants, Federal Work-Study. 87% of undergraduate students in nursing programs received some form of financial aid in 1995–96. *Application deadline:* 4/15.

Generic Baccalaureate Program (BSN)

Applying *Required:* minimum college GPA of 2.5, transcript of college record, minimum 2.0 GPA in each required supporting course. 50 prerequisite credits must be completed before admission to the nursing program. *Options:* Advanced standing available through the following means: advanced placement exams, credit by exam. Course work may be accelerated. May apply for transfer of up to 60 total credits. *Application deadline:* 10/15. *Application fee:* $25.

Degree Requirements 128 total credit hours, 64 in nursing.

Accelerated RN Baccalaureate Program (BSN)

Applying *Required:* minimum college GPA of 2.5, transcript of college record, minimum 2.0 GPA in each required supporting course. 50 prerequisite credits must be completed before admission to the nursing program. *Options:* Advanced standing available through the following means: advanced placement exams, credit by exam. May apply for transfer of up to 60 total credits. *Application deadline:* 10/15. *Application fee:* $25.

Degree Requirements 128 total credit hours, 64 in nursing.

Accelerated LPN to Baccalaureate Program (BSN)

Applying *Required:* minimum college GPA of 2.5, transcript of college record, minimum 2.0 GPA in each required supporting course. 50 prerequisite credits must be completed before admission to the nursing program. *Options:* Advanced standing available through the following means: advanced placement exams, credit by exam. May apply for transfer of up to 60 total credits. *Application deadline:* 10/15. *Application fee:* $25.

Degree Requirements 128 total credit hours, 64 in nursing.

CONTINUING EDUCATION PROGRAM

Contact Dr. Valeda C. Fabricius, Dean, College of Nursing, Minot State University, Minot, ND 58707, 701-858-3101. *Fax:* 701-858-4309. *E-mail:* fabriciu@warp6.cs.misu.nodak.edu

NORTH DAKOTA STATE UNIVERSITY

Tri-College University Nursing Consortium
Fargo, North Dakota

Program • Generic Baccalaureate

The University State-supported coed university. Part of North Dakota University System. Founded: 1890. *Primary accreditation:* regional. *Setting:* 2,100-acre urban campus. *Total enrollment:* 9,676.

The Tri-College University Nursing Consortium Founded in 1986. *Nursing program faculty:* 7 (14% with doctorates). *Off-campus program site:* Moorhead, MN.

Academic Facilities *Campus library:* 446,815 volumes (530 in health, 200 in nursing); 4,200 periodical subscriptions (94 health-care related). *Nursing school resources:* CAI, computer lab, nursing audiovisuals, learning resource lab.

Student Life *Student services:* health clinic, child-care facilities, personal counseling, career counseling, institutionally sponsored work-study program, job placement, campus safety program, special assistance for disabled students. *International student services:* counseling/support, ESL courses. *Nursing student activities:* Sigma Theta Tau, student nurses association.

Calendar Semesters.

NURSING STUDENT PROFILE

Undergraduate **Enrollment:** 51

Women: 88%; **Men:** 12%; **Minority:** 6%; **International:** 0%; **Part-time:** 4%

BACCALAUREATE PROGRAM

Contact Dr. Lois F. Nelson, Chair, Tri-College University Nursing Consortium, North Dakota State University, 136 Sudro, Fargo, ND 58105, 701-231-7395. *Fax:* 701-231-7606. *E-mail:* loinelso@plains.nodak.edu

Expenses *State resident tuition:* $2410 per academic year. *Nonresident tuition:* $5934 per academic year. *Full-time mandatory fees:* $480–$605. *Room and board:* $2806–$3018. *Books and supplies per academic year:* ranges from $150 to $550.

Financial Aid Institutionally sponsored need-based grants/scholarships, institutionally sponsored non-need grants/scholarships, Federal Nursing Student Loans, Federal Supplemental Educational Opportunity Grants, Federal Work-Study. *Application deadline:* 4/15.

North Dakota State University (continued)

Generic Baccalaureate Program (BS)

Applying *Required:* ACT, TOEFL for nonnative speakers of English, minimum college GPA of 2.5, 2 letters of recommendation, written essay, transcript of college record. 60 prerequisite credits must be completed before admission to the nursing program. *Options:* Advanced standing available through the following means: advanced placement exams, advanced placement without credit, credit by exam. *Application deadline:* 2/1.

Degree Requirements 122 total credit hours, 48 in nursing.

UNIVERSITY OF MARY

Division of Nursing
Bismarck, North Dakota

Programs • Generic Baccalaureate • RN Baccalaureate • Accelerated RN Baccalaureate • LPN to Baccalaureate • Master's

The University Independent Roman Catholic comprehensive coed institution. Founded: 1959. *Primary accreditation:* regional. *Setting:* 107-acre small-town campus. *Total enrollment:* 1,776.

Academic Facilities *Campus library:* 52,000 volumes; 515 periodical subscriptions (100 health-care related).

Student Life *Student services:* health clinic. *Nursing student activities:* Sigma Theta Tau.

Calendar Semesters.

BACCALAUREATE PROGRAMS

Contact Chairperson, Division of Nursing, University of Mary, 7500 University Drive, Bismarck, ND 58504, 701-255-7500 Ext. 470. *Fax:* 701-255-7687.

Expenses *Tuition:* $7230 full-time, $225 per credit part-time. *Full-time mandatory fees:* $100. *Room and board:* $2890–$3290. *Room only:* $1260–$1660.

Financial Aid Federal Nursing Student Loans, Federal Perkins Loans, Federal Supplemental Educational Opportunity Grants, Federal PLUS Loans, Federal Stafford Loans.

Generic Baccalaureate Program (BS)

Applying *Required:* SAT I or ACT, high school transcript, 3 letters of recommendation. *Application deadline:* rolling. *Application fee:* $15.

Degree Requirements 128 total credit hours.

RN Baccalaureate Program (BS)

Applying *Required:* RN license, diploma or AD in nursing, 3 letters of recommendation, transcript of college record. 30 prerequisite credits must be completed before admission to the nursing program. *Application deadline:* rolling. *Application fee:* $15.

Degree Requirements 128 total credit hours.

Accelerated RN Baccalaureate Program (BS)

Applying *Application deadline:* rolling. *Application fee:* $15.

LPN to Baccalaureate Program (BSN)

Applying *Required:* diploma or AD in nursing, transcript of college record, LPN license. *Application deadline:* rolling. *Application fee:* $15.

Degree Requirements 128 total credit hours.

MASTER'S PROGRAMS

Contact Chairperson, Division of Nursing, University of Mary, 7500 University Drive, Bismarck, ND 58504, 701-255-7500 Ext. 470. *Fax:* 701-255-7687.

UNIVERSITY OF NORTH DAKOTA

College of Nursing
Grand Forks, North Dakota

Programs • Generic Baccalaureate • RN Baccalaureate • MS

The University State-supported coed university. Part of North Dakota University System. Founded: 1883. *Primary accreditation:* regional. *Setting:* 570-acre small-town campus. *Total enrollment:* 11,512.

The College of Nursing Founded in 1947. *Nursing program faculty:* 60 (33% with doctorates). *Off-campus program sites:* Bemidji, Fargo, Jamestown.

Academic Facilities *Campus library:* 705,000 volumes (34,000 in health); 5,074 periodical subscriptions (1,074 health-care related). *Nursing school resources:* CAI, computer lab, nursing audiovisuals, interactive nursing skills videos, learning resource lab.

Student Life *Student services:* health clinic, child-care facilities, personal counseling, career counseling, institutionally sponsored work-study program, job placement, campus safety program, special assistance for disabled students. *International student services:* counseling/support, special assistance for nonnative speakers of English, ESL courses. *Nursing student activities:* Sigma Theta Tau, student nurses association.

Calendar Semesters.

NURSING STUDENT PROFILE

Undergraduate **Enrollment:** 301
Women: 84%; **Men:** 16%; **Minority:** 13%; **International:** 3%; **Part-time:** 15%
Graduate **Enrollment:** 150
Women: 92%; **Men:** 8%; **Minority:** 4%; **International:** 1%; **Part-time:** 70%

BACCALAUREATE PROGRAMS

Contact Ms. Sandra Benson, Director, Student Affairs, College of Nursing, University of North Dakota, Box 9025, Grand Forks, ND 58202, 701-777-4174. *Fax:* 701-777-4096. *E-mail:* sabenson@badlands.nodak.edu

Expenses *State resident tuition:* $2428 full-time, $88 per credit hour part-time. *Nonresident tuition:* ranges from $2956 to $5952 full-time, ranges from $98 to $235 per credit hour part-time. *Full-time mandatory fees:* $300. *Part-time mandatory fees:* $13+. *Room and board:* $2730. *Books and supplies per academic year:* ranges from $300 to $400.

Financial Aid Institutionally sponsored need-based grants/scholarships, institutionally sponsored non-need grants/scholarships, Federal Nursing Student Loans, Federal Perkins Loans, Federal Supplemental Educational Opportunity Grants, Federal Work-Study. *Application deadline:* 3/15.

Generic Baccalaureate Program (BS)

Applying *Required:* ACT, TOEFL for nonnative speakers of English, minimum high school GPA of 2.3, minimum college GPA of 2.5, high school transcript, transcript of college record. 24 prerequisite credits must be completed before admission to the nursing program. *Options:* May apply for transfer of up to 99 total credits. *Application deadlines:* 5/1 (fall), 5/1 (spring). *Application fee:* $20.

Degree Requirements 129 total credit hours, 61 in nursing.

RN Baccalaureate Program (BS)

Applying *Required:* TOEFL for nonnative speakers of English, minimum college GPA of 2.5, RN license, diploma or AD in nursing, transcript of college record. 24 prerequisite credits must be completed before admission to the nursing program. *Options:* May apply for transfer of up to 99 total credits. *Application deadlines:* 5/1 (fall), 5/1 (spring). *Application fee:* $20.

Degree Requirements 129 total credit hours, 61 in nursing.

MASTER'S PROGRAM

Contact Dr. Regina Monnig, Associate Dean and Director of Graduate Studies, College of Nursing, University of North Dakota, Box 9025, Grand Fork, ND 58202, 701-777-4552. *Fax:* 701-777-4096.

Areas of Study Clinical nurse specialist programs in adult health nursing, parent-child nursing, rural health nursing; nurse anesthesia; nurse practitioner program in family health.

Expenses *State resident tuition:* $2738 full-time, $97 per credit hour part-time. *Nonresident tuition:* ranges from $3302 to $6612 full-time, ranges from $120 to $258 per credit hour part-time. *Full-time mandatory fees:* $1000–$1500. *Part-time mandatory fees:* $42+. *Books and supplies per academic year:* ranges from $1000 to $2000.

Financial Aid Graduate assistantships, nurse traineeships, Federal Nursing Student Loans, institutionally sponsored loans, employment opportunities. *Application deadline:* 3/15.

MS Program

Applying *Required:* bachelor's degree in nursing, minimum GPA of 3.0, RN license, 1 year of clinical experience, statistics course, essay, interview, 3 letters of recommendation, transcript of college record, biochemistry for nurse anesthesia track. *Application deadlines:* 1/15 (family nurse practitioner or anesthesia track), rolling. *Application fee:* $20.

Degree Requirements 36–65 total credit hours dependent upon track, 18–45 in nursing, up to 18 in physiology, pharmacology, and other specified areas. Thesis or independent study.

Distance learning Courses provided through video, audio, computer-based media. Specific degree requirements include emphasis in rural health option only.

OHIO

ASHLAND UNIVERSITY
Department of Nursing
Ashland, Ohio

Program • RN Baccalaureate

The University Independent comprehensive coed institution, affiliated with Brethren Church. Founded: 1878. *Primary accreditation:* regional. *Setting:* 98-acre small-town campus. *Total enrollment:* 5,608.

The Department of Nursing Founded in 1981. *Nursing program faculty:* 3 (33% with doctorates). *Off-campus program sites:* Dover, Marion, Akron.

Academic Facilities *Campus library:* 300,000 volumes (5,000 in health, 2,000 in nursing); 1,000 periodical subscriptions (100 health-care related). *Nursing school resources:* CAI, computer lab, nursing audiovisuals, learning resource lab.

Student Life *Student services:* health clinic, child-care facilities, personal counseling, career counseling, institutionally sponsored work-study program, job placement, campus safety program, special assistance for disabled students. *International student services:* counseling/support, special assistance for nonnative speakers of English, ESL courses. *Nursing student activities:* Nursing Honor Society.

Calendar Semesters.

NURSING STUDENT PROFILE

Undergraduate **Enrollment:** 98

Women: 98%; **Men:** 2%; **Minority:** 5%; **International:** 0%; **Part-time:** 90%

BACCALAUREATE PROGRAM

Contact Dr. Ella Kick, Chair, School of Nursing, Ashland University, Ashland, OH 44805, 419-289-5244. *Fax:* 419-289-5989.

Expenses *Tuition:* $245 per credit hour. *Part-time mandatory fees:* $260. *Books and supplies per academic year:* ranges from $25 to $100.

Financial Aid Federal loans. 4% of undergraduate students in nursing programs received some form of financial aid in 1995–96. *Application deadline:* 7/15.

RN Baccalaureate Program (BSN)

Applying *Required:* minimum college GPA of 2.5, RN license, diploma or AD in nursing, transcript of college record. 31 prerequisite credits must be completed before admission to the nursing program. *Options:* Advanced standing available through credit by exam. Course work may be accelerated. May apply for transfer of up to 68 total credits. *Application deadlines:* 8/15 (fall), 1/1 (spring). *Application fee:* $15.

Degree Requirements 128 total credit hours, 30 in nursing.

BOWLING GREEN STATE UNIVERSITY
School of Nursing
Bowling Green, Ohio

Programs • Generic Baccalaureate • RN Baccalaureate

The University State-supported coed university. Founded: 1910. *Primary accreditation:* regional. *Setting:* 1,176-acre small-town campus. *Total enrollment:* 17,564.

The School of Nursing Founded in 1971. *Nursing program faculty:* 54 (31% with doctorates). *Off-campus program sites:* Huron, Lima, Archbald.

Academic Facilities *Campus library:* 1.7 million volumes; 6,034 periodical subscriptions. *Nursing school resources:* CAI, computer lab, nursing audiovisuals, learning resource lab.

Student Life *Student services:* health clinic, child-care facilities, personal counseling, career counseling, institutionally sponsored work-study program, job placement, campus safety program, special assistance for disabled students. *International student services:* counseling/support, special assistance for nonnative speakers of English, ESL courses. *Nursing student activities:* Sigma Theta Tau, nursing club, student nurses association.

Calendar Quarters.

NURSING STUDENT PROFILE

Undergraduate **Enrollment:** 274

Women: 94%; **Men:** 6%; **Minority:** 4%; **International:** 0%; **Part-time:** 44%

BACCALAUREATE PROGRAMS

Contact Ms. Gloria Pizana, Secretary, School of Nursing, Bowling Green State University, 102 Health Center, Bowling Green, OH 43403, 419-372-8760. *Fax:* 419-372-2897. *E-mail:* penriq@bgnet.bgsu.edu

Expenses *State resident tuition:* $3070 full-time, $197 per credit part-time. *Nonresident tuition:* $8512 full-time, $414 per credit part-time. *Full-time mandatory fees:* $190–$365. *Room and board:* $3956. *Room only:* $2068. *Books and supplies per academic year:* ranges from $1180 to $1290.

Financial Aid Institutionally sponsored need-based grants/scholarships, institutionally sponsored non-need grants/scholarships, Federal Direct Loans, Federal Nursing Student Loans, Federal Pell Grants, Federal Perkins Loans, Federal Supplemental Educational Opportunity Grants, Federal Work-Study. *Application deadline:* 4/1.

Generic Baccalaureate Program (BSN)

Applying *Required:* SAT I or ACT, TOEFL for nonnative speakers of English, minimum college GPA of 2.5, 3 years of high school math, 3 years of high school science, high school foreign language, high school transcript, transcript of college record. 24 prerequisite credits must be completed before admission to the nursing program. *Options:* Advanced standing available through the following means: advanced placement exams, credit by exam. *Application deadline:* 1/1. *Application fee:* $30.

Degree Requirements 123 total credit hours, 56 in nursing.

RN Baccalaureate Program (BSN)

Applying *Required:* NLN Mobility Profile II for diploma graduates, minimum college GPA of 2.5, RN license, diploma or AD in nursing, high school foreign language, high school transcript, transcript of college record, professional liability/malpractice insurance. 29 prerequisite credits must be completed before admission to the nursing program. *Options:* Advanced standing available through the following means: advanced placement exams, credit by exam. Course work may be accelerated. *Application deadline:* rolling. *Application fee:* $30.

Degree Requirements 123 total credit hours, 28 in nursing.

CAPITAL UNIVERSITY
School of Nursing
Columbus, Ohio

Programs • Generic Baccalaureate • RN Baccalaureate • MSN/MBA • MSN/JD • MSN/MDiv

The University Independent comprehensive coed institution, affiliated with Evangelical Lutheran Church in America. Founded: 1830. *Primary accreditation:* regional. *Setting:* 48-acre suburban campus. *Total enrollment:* 4,071.

The School of Nursing Founded in 1950. *Nursing program faculty:* 43 (53% with doctorates).

Capital University (continued)

▶ ***NOTEWORTHY***

Capital's nursing students gain experience in a number of health-care agencies, including Columbus Children's Hospital, Columbus City Health Department, Franklin County District Board of Health, Grant Medical Center, Heinzerling Memorial Foundation, Mt. Carmel Medical Center, Riverside Methodist Hospitals, St. Ann's Hospital, and Park Medical Center. Capital was selected as one of 40 colleges and universities in the United States as a Partner in Nursing Education by the U.S. Army. ROTC scholarship winners are awarded a $12,600 scholarship from the Army plus a room award and an additional scholarship from Capital.

Academic Facilities *Campus library:* 180,000 volumes (6,209 in health); 894 periodical subscriptions (82 health-care related). *Nursing school resources:* CAI, computer lab, nursing audiovisuals, learning resource lab.

Student Life *Student services:* health clinic, personal counseling, career counseling, institutionally sponsored work-study program, job placement. *International student services:* counseling/support, special assistance for nonnative speakers of English, ESL courses. *Nursing student activities:* Sigma Theta Tau, student nurses association.

Calendar Semesters.

NURSING STUDENT PROFILE

Undergraduate **Enrollment:** 368

Women: 90%; **Men:** 10%; **Minority:** 9%; **International:** 1%; **Part-time:** 23%

Graduate **Enrollment:** 48

Women: 95%; **Men:** 5%; **Minority:** 6%; **International:** 5%; **Part-time:** 56%

BACCALAUREATE PROGRAMS

Contact Ms. Beth Heiser, Director of Admission, Admission Office, Capital University, Columbus, OH 43209, 614-236-6101. *Fax:* 614-236-6820. *E-mail:* admissions@capital.edu

Expenses *Tuition:* $14,200 full-time, $474 per semester hour part-time. *Full-time mandatory fees:* $140–$560. *Room and board:* $4000. *Books and supplies per academic year:* $500.

Financial Aid Institutionally sponsored need-based grants/scholarships, institutionally sponsored non-need grants/scholarships, Federal Nursing Student Loans, Federal Pell Grants, Federal Perkins Loans, Federal Supplemental Educational Opportunity Grants, Federal Work-Study. 100% of undergraduate students in nursing programs received some form of financial aid in 1995–96. *Application deadline:* 2/15.

Generic Baccalaureate Program (BSN)

Applying *Required:* SAT I, ACT, TOEFL for nonnative speakers of English, minimum high school GPA of 2.5, minimum college GPA of 2.5, 3 years of high school math, 3 years of high school science, high school chemistry, high school biology, high school foreign language, high school transcript, transcript of college record. *Options:* Advanced standing available through the following means: advanced placement exams, advanced placement without credit, credit by exam. May apply for transfer of up to 104 total credits. *Application deadline:* rolling. *Application fee:* $15.

Degree Requirements 134 total credit hours, 68 in nursing.

RN Baccalaureate Program (BSN)

Applying *Required:* TOEFL for nonnative speakers of English, RN license, diploma or AD in nursing. *Options:* Advanced standing available through the following means: advanced placement exams, advanced placement without credit, credit by exam. Course work may be accelerated. May apply for transfer of up to 104 total credits. *Application deadline:* rolling. *Application fee:* $15.

Degree Requirements 134 total credit hours, 60 in nursing.

MASTER'S PROGRAMS

Contact Dr. Laurel Talabere, Associate Dean, Capital University, 2199 East Main Street, Columbus, OH 43209, 614-236-6378. *Fax:* 614-236-6157.

Areas of Study Clinical nurse specialist programs in community health nursing, family health nursing; nursing administration.

Expenses *Tuition:* $245 per semester hour. *Books and supplies per academic year:* $300.

Financial Aid Federal Direct Loans.

MSN/MBA Program

Applying *Required:* GRE General Test, TOEFL for nonnative speakers of English, bachelor's degree in nursing, minimum GPA of 3.0, RN license, 1 year of clinical experience, physical assessment course, statistics course, essay, transcript of college record, research course. *Application deadline:* rolling. *Application fee:* $25.

Degree Requirements 36 total credit hours, 27 in nursing, 9 in administration and ethics. Thesis required.

MSN/JD Program

Applying *Required:* GRE General Test, TOEFL for nonnative speakers of English, bachelor's degree in nursing, minimum GPA of 3.0, RN license, 1 year of clinical experience, physical assessment course, statistics course, essay, transcript of college record, research course. *Application deadline:* rolling. *Application fee:* $25.

Degree Requirements 36 total credit hours, 27 in nursing, 9 in administration and ethics. Thesis required.

MSN/MDiv Program

Applying *Required:* GRE General Test, TOEFL for nonnative speakers of English, bachelor's degree in nursing, minimum GPA of 3.0, RN license, 1 year of clinical experience, physical assessment course, statistics course, essay, transcript of college record, research course. *Application deadline:* rolling. *Application fee:* $25.

Degree Requirements 36 total credit hours, 27 in nursing, 9 in administration and ethics. Thesis required.

See full description on page 422.

CASE WESTERN RESERVE UNIVERSITY

The Frances Payne Bolton School of Nursing Cleveland, Ohio

Programs • Generic Baccalaureate • RN Baccalaureate • MSN • RN to Master's • Master's for Nurses with Non-Nursing Degrees • MSN/MBA • Post-Master's • PhD • ND • Continuing Education

The University Independent coed university. Founded: 1826. *Primary accreditation:* regional. *Setting:* 128-acre urban campus. *Total enrollment:* 9,747.

The Frances Payne Bolton School of Nursing Founded in 1898. *Nursing program faculty:* 91 (42% with doctorates).

Academic Facilities *Campus library:* 1.5 million volumes (139,537 in health, 22,000 in nursing); 6,000 periodical subscriptions (2,800 health-care related). *Nursing school resources:* CAI, computer lab, nursing audiovisuals, interactive nursing skills videos, learning resource lab.

Student Life *Student services:* health clinic, child-care facilities, personal counseling, career counseling, institutionally sponsored work-study program, job placement, campus safety program, special assistance for disabled students, minority scholars program. *International student services:* counseling/support, special assistance for nonnative speakers of English, ESL courses. *Nursing student activities:* Sigma Theta Tau, student nurses association.

Calendar Semesters.

NURSING STUDENT PROFILE

Undergraduate **Enrollment:** 251

Women: 90%; **Men:** 10%; **Minority:** 11%; **International:** 0%; **Part-time:** 10%

Graduate **Enrollment:** 428

Women: 89%; **Men:** 11%; **Minority:** 9%; **International:** 11%; **Part-time:** 35%

BACCALAUREATE PROGRAMS

Contact Ms. Regina Fraiya, Director of Student Services, Frances Payne Bolton School of Nursing, Case Western Reserve University, 10900 Euclid Avenue, Cleveland, OH 44106-4904, 800-825-2540 Ext. 2529. *Fax:* 216-368-2529. *E-mail:* emu4@po.cwru.edu

Expenses *Tuition:* $17,100 per academic year. *Full-time mandatory fees:* $287–$847. *Room and board:* $4700–$6290. *Room only:* $2870–$3860. *Books and supplies per academic year:* ranges from $300 to $700.

Financial Aid Institutionally sponsored need-based grants/scholarships, institutionally sponsored non-need grants/scholarships, Federal Direct

Loans, Federal Nursing Student Loans, Federal Perkins Loans, Federal Supplemental Educational Opportunity Grants, Federal Work-Study, Bolton Scholarship. 100% of undergraduate students in nursing programs received some form of financial aid in 1995–96. *Application deadline:* 3/1.

Generic Baccalaureate Program (BSN)

Applying *Required:* SAT I, ACT, TOEFL for nonnative speakers of English, minimum high school GPA of 3.0, minimum college GPA of 3.0, 3 years of high school math, 3 years of high school science, high school chemistry, high school biology, high school transcript, letter of recommendation, written essay, transcript of college record. *Options:* Advanced standing available through advanced placement exams. May apply for transfer of up to 60 total credits. *Application deadlines:* 2/1 (fall), 5/1 (summer).

Degree Requirements 122 total credit hours, 72 in nursing.

RN Baccalaureate Program (BSN)

Applying *Required:* TOEFL for nonnative speakers of English, minimum college GPA of 2.5, RN license, diploma or AD in nursing, transcript of college record. *Options:* May apply for transfer of up to 97 total credits. *Application deadlines:* 7/1 (fall), 11/1 (spring), 4/1 (summer).

Degree Requirements 122 total credit hours, 30 in nursing.

MASTER'S PROGRAMS

Contact Ms. Elaine Vincent, Assistant Director of Admission, Frances Payne Bolton School of Nursing, Case Western Reserve University, 10900 Euclid Avenue, Cleveland, OH 44106-4904, 216-368-2529. *Fax:* 216-368-3542. *E-mail:* emu4@po.cwru.edu

Areas of Study Clinical nurse specialist programs in community health nursing, critical care nursing, medical-surgical nursing, oncology nursing; nurse anesthesia; nurse midwifery; nursing administration; nursing education; nurse practitioner programs in acute care, adult health, child care/pediatrics, family health, gerontology, neonatal health, psychiatric–mental health, women's health.

Expenses *Tuition:* $17,100 full-time, $713 per semester hour part-time. *Full-time mandatory fees:* $30–$700. *Room and board:* $4940–$5980. *Room only:* $3110–$3550. *Books and supplies per academic year:* ranges from $500 to $600.

Financial Aid Graduate assistantships, nurse traineeships, Federal Nursing Student Loans, employment opportunities, institutionally sponsored need-based grants/scholarships. *Application deadline:* 3/1.

MSN Program

Applying *Required:* GRE General Test, Miller Analogies Test, TOEFL for nonnative speakers of English, bachelor's degree in nursing, minimum GPA of 3.0, RN license, physical assessment course, statistics course, professional liability/malpractice insurance, essay, 3 letters of recommendation, transcript of college record, national certification as nurse practitioner, midwife, or anesthetist for accelerated program. *Application deadlines:* 7/1 (fall), 11/1 (spring), 1/15 (nurse anesthesia program). *Application fee:* $75–175.

Degree Requirements 18–45 total credit hours dependent upon track, 18–40 in nursing, 18 in anthropology for MSN/MA in anthropology degree. Comprehensive exam in anthropology for MSN/MA in Anthropology degree.

RN to Master's Program (MSN)

Applying *Required:* GRE General Test, Miller Analogies Test, TOEFL for nonnative speakers of English, minimum GPA of 2.5, RN license, 1 year of clinical experience, physical assessment course, statistics course, professional liability/malpractice insurance, essay, 3 letters of recommendation, transcript of college record. *Application deadlines:* 7/1 (fall), 11/1 (spring), 4/1 (summer). *Application fee:* $75.

Degree Requirements 59 total credit hours, 59 in nursing. 19 credits of nursing courses to bridge from RN to MSN.

Master's for Nurses with Non-Nursing Degrees Program (MSN)

Applying *Required:* GRE General Test, Miller Analogies Test, TOEFL for nonnative speakers of English, bachelor's degree, minimum GPA of 3.0, RN license, statistics course, professional liability/malpractice insurance, essay, 3 letters of recommendation, transcript of college record, portfolio of experiences. *Application deadlines:* 7/1 (fall), 11/1 (spring), 4/1 (summer). *Application fee:* $175.

Degree Requirements 40 total credit hours, 40 in nursing.

MSN/MBA Program

Applying *Required:* TOEFL for nonnative speakers of English, GMAT, bachelor's degree in nursing, minimum GPA of 3.0, RN license, 2 years of clinical experience, professional liability/malpractice insurance, essay, 3 letters of recommendation, transcript of college record. *Application deadlines:* 5/1 (fall), 11/1 (spring), 3/1 (summer). *Application fee:* $75.

Degree Requirements 72 total credit hours, 27 in nursing, 45 in management.

Post-Master's Program

Applying *Required:* GRE General Test or Miller Analogies Test, minimum GPA of 3.0, RN license, statistics course, professional liability/malpractice insurance, essay, 3 letters of recommendation, transcript of college record. *Application deadlines:* 7/1 (fall), 11/1 (spring), 4/1 (summer). *Application fee:* $75.

Degree Requirements 21 total credit hours, 21 in nursing.

DOCTORAL PROGRAMS

Contact Dr. Beverly Roberts, PhD Coordinator, Frances Payne Bolton School of Nursing, Case Western Reserve University, 10900 Euclid Avenue, Cleveland, OH 44106-4904, 216-368-1200. *Fax:* 216-368-3542.

Areas of Study Nursing research.

Expenses *Tuition:* $17,100 full-time, $713 per semester hour part-time. *Full-time mandatory fees:* $10–$700. *Room and board:* $4940–$5980. *Room only:* $3110–$3550. *Books and supplies per academic year:* ranges from $500 to $700.

Financial Aid Grants, opportunities for employment. *Application deadline:* 3/1.

PhD Program

Applying *Required:* GRE General Test, TOEFL for nonnative speakers of English, statistics course, interview, 3 letters of recommendation, writing sample. *Application deadlines:* 3/1 (fall), 10/1 (spring), 2/1 (summer). *Application fee:* $25.

Degree Requirements 36 total credit hours; dissertation; oral exam; defense of dissertation; residency.

ND Program

Applying *Required:* GRE General Test, master's degree in nursing, statistics course, interview, 3 letters of recommendation, RN license, transcript of college record, national certification as nurse practitioner or advanced practice nurse, written essay, professional liability/malpractice insurance. *Application deadlines:* 6/1 (fall), 11/1 (spring), 3/1 (summer). *Application fee:* $75.

Degree Requirements 24 total credit hours; 24 hours in nursing; thesis.

Postbaccalaureate Doctorate (ND)

Applying *Required:* GRE General Test, statistics course, interview, 3 letters of recommendation, BSN, transcript of college record, written essay, professional liability/malpractice insurance. *Application deadline:* 6/1. *Application fee:* $75.

Degree Requirements thesis.

Doctorate for Nurses with Non-Nursing Degrees (ND)

Applying *Required:* GRE General Test, TOEFL for nonnative speakers of English, statistics course, interview, 3 letters of recommendation, BA/BS in non-nursing field, minimum 2.8 GPA, transcript of college record, written essay, professional liability/malpractice insurance. *Application deadline:* 6/1. *Application fee:* $75.

Degree Requirements 124 total credit hours; 121 hours in nursing, 3 hours in advanced statistics; residency; thesis.

CONTINUING EDUCATION PROGRAM

Contact Dr. Jeanne Novotny, Assistant Dean, Frances Payne Bolton School of Nursing, Case Western Reserve University, 10900 Euclid Avenue, Cleveland, OH 44106-4904, 216-368-2529. *Fax:* 216-368-3542.

See full description on page 424.

CEDARVILLE COLLEGE
Department of Nursing
Cedarville, Ohio

Programs • Generic Baccalaureate • RN Baccalaureate • LPN to Baccalaureate

The College Independent Baptist 4-year coed college. Founded: 1887. *Primary accreditation:* regional. *Setting:* 105-acre rural campus. *Total enrollment:* 2,454.

The Department of Nursing Founded in 1981. *Nursing program faculty:* 14 (36% with doctorates).

Academic Facilities *Campus library:* 150,000 volumes (10,000 in health, 2,300 in nursing); 1,050 periodical subscriptions (50 health-care related). *Nursing school resources:* CAI, interactive nursing skills videos.

Calendar Quarters.

BACCALAUREATE PROGRAMS

Contact Director of Admissions, Admissions, Cedarville College, PO Box 601, Cedarville, OH 45314, 513-766-7700. *Fax:* 513-766-2760. *E-mail:* admiss@cedarville.edu

Financial Aid Institutionally sponsored need-based grants/scholarships, institutionally sponsored non-need grants/scholarships, Federal Pell Grants, Federal Perkins Loans, Federal Supplemental Educational Opportunity Grants, Federal Work-Study, Federal Family Education Loan Program (FFELP), Ohio state grants. *Application deadline:* 2/15.

Generic Baccalaureate Program (BSN)

Applying *Required:* SAT I or ACT, minimum high school GPA of 2.5, high school transcript, letter of recommendation, written essay, high school class rank: , CPR certification. *Options:* Advanced standing available through credit by exam. *Application deadline:* rolling. *Application fee:* $30.

Degree Requirements 208–227 total credit hours dependent upon track, 98 in nursing. 227 hours required for cross-cultural nursing emphasis.

RN Baccalaureate Program (BSN)

Applying *Required:* SAT I or ACT, minimum high school GPA of 2.5, minimum college GPA of 2.5, RN license, diploma or AD in nursing, high school transcript, letter of recommendation, written essay, high school class rank: . *Application deadline:* rolling. *Application fee:* $30.

Degree Requirements 208 total credit hours, 98 in nursing.

LPN to Baccalaureate Program (BSN)

Applying *Required:* SAT I, TOEFL for nonnative speakers of English, minimum high school GPA of 2.5, minimum college GPA of 2.5, diploma or AD in nursing, high school transcript, letter of recommendation, written essay, high school class rank: , LPN license. *Application deadline:* rolling. *Application fee:* $30.

Degree Requirements 208 total credit hours, 98 in nursing.

CLEVELAND STATE UNIVERSITY
Department of Nursing
Cleveland, Ohio

Programs • Generic Baccalaureate • RN Baccalaureate • Continuing Education

The University State-supported coed university. Founded: 1964. *Primary accreditation:* regional. *Setting:* 70-acre urban campus. *Total enrollment:* 15,671.

The Department of Nursing Founded in 1975. *Nursing program faculty:* 10 (50% with doctorates).

Academic Facilities *Campus library:* 856,978 volumes (13,859 in health, 14,411 in nursing); 4,000 periodical subscriptions (148 health-care related). *Nursing school resources:* CAI, computer lab, nursing audiovisuals, interactive nursing skills videos, learning resource lab.

Student Life *Student services:* health clinic, child-care facilities, personal counseling, career counseling, institutionally sponsored work-study program, job placement, campus safety program, special assistance for disabled students. *International student services:* counseling/support, special assistance for nonnative speakers of English, ESL courses. *Nursing student activities:* Sigma Theta Tau, student nurses association.

Calendar Quarters.

NURSING STUDENT PROFILE

Undergraduate **Enrollment:** 218
Women: 83%; **Men:** 17%; **Minority:** 11%; **Part-time:** 12%

BACCALAUREATE PROGRAMS

Contact Mrs. Jule Monnens, Recruiter and Adviser, Rhodes Tower 915, Department of Nursing, Cleveland State University, 1860 East 22nd Street, Cleveland, OH 44115, 216-687-3810. *Fax:* 216-687-3556. *E-mail:* j.monnens@popmail.csuohio.edu

Expenses *State resident tuition:* $3333 full-time, $93 per quarter hour part-time. *Nonresident tuition:* $6665 full-time, $186 per quarter hour part-time. *Full-time mandatory fees:* $77. *Part-time mandatory fees:* $22–$55. *Room and board:* $4176. *Room only:* $2760. *Books and supplies per academic year:* $690.

Financial Aid Institutionally sponsored need-based grants/scholarships, institutionally sponsored non-need grants/scholarships.

Generic Baccalaureate Program (BSN)

Applying *Required:* SAT I or ACT, Michigan English Language Assessment Battery for nonnative speakers of English, minimum college GPA of 2.0, high school transcript, written essay, transcript of college record. 99 prerequisite credits must be completed before admission to the nursing program. *Options:* May apply for transfer of up to 99 total credits. *Application deadline:* 3/1. *Application fee:* $25.

Degree Requirements 209 total credit hours, 101 in nursing.

RN Baccalaureate Program (BSN)

Applying *Required:* Michigan English Language Assessment Battery for nonnative speakers of English, minimum college GPA of 2.0, RN license, diploma or AD in nursing, high school transcript, written essay, transcript of college record. 47 prerequisite credits must be completed before admission to the nursing program. *Options:* Advanced standing available through advanced placement without credit. *Application deadline:* 3/1.

Degree Requirements 195 total credit hours, 46 in nursing.

CONTINUING EDUCATION PROGRAM

Contact Vida Svarcas, Director, Nursing and Health Science Continuing Education, Euclid Building 103, Division of Continuing Education, Cleveland State University, 1824 East 24th Street, Cleveland, OH 44115, 216-687-4843. *Fax:* 216-687-9399.

COLLEGE OF MOUNT ST. JOSEPH
Department of Nursing
Cincinnati, Ohio

Programs • Generic Baccalaureate • RN Baccalaureate

The College Independent Roman Catholic comprehensive coed institution. Founded: 1920. *Primary accreditation:* regional. *Setting:* 75-acre suburban campus. *Total enrollment:* 2,349.

The Department of Nursing Founded in 1926. *Nursing program faculty:* 20 (21% with doctorates).

Academic Facilities *Campus library:* 91,875 volumes (2,800 in nursing); 768 periodical subscriptions (108 health-care related). *Nursing school resources:* CAI, computer lab, nursing audiovisuals, interactive nursing skills videos, learning resource lab.

Student Life *Student services:* health clinic, child-care facilities, personal counseling, career counseling, institutionally sponsored work-study program, job placement, campus safety program, special assistance for disabled students. *International student services:* counseling/support, special assistance for nonnative speakers of English, ESL courses. *Nursing* *student activities:* student nurses association, Nursing Honor Society, Ohio Student Nurses Association, National Student Nurses Association.

Calendar Semesters.

NURSING STUDENT PROFILE

Undergraduate **Enrollment:** 171

Women: 94%; **Men:** 6%; **Minority:** 10%; **International:** 1%; **Part-time:** 17%

BACCALAUREATE PROGRAMS

Contact Dr. Ignatius Perkins, Chair, Department of Nursing, College of Mount St. Joseph, 5701 Delhi Road, Cincinnati, OH 45233-1670, 513-244-4511. *Fax:* 513-244-4222. *E-mail:* ignatius_perkins@mail.msj.edu

Expenses *Tuition:* $11,300 full-time, $290 per credit hour part-time. *Full-time mandatory fees:* $420–$1230. *Room and board:* $4650–$6570. *Room only:* $2600–$4220. *Books and supplies per academic year:* ranges from $400 to $600.

Financial Aid Institutionally sponsored need-based grants/scholarships, institutionally sponsored non-need grants/scholarships, Federal Direct Loans, Federal Nursing Student Loans, Federal Pell Grants, Federal Perkins Loans, Federal Work-Study, health care organization-sponsored scholarships, endowed scholarships. 60% of undergraduate students in nursing programs received some form of financial aid in 1995–96. *Application deadline:* 4/15.

Generic Baccalaureate Program (BSN)

Applying *Required:* SAT I, ACT, TOEFL for nonnative speakers of English, minimum high school GPA of 2.25, minimum college GPA of 2.5, 2 years of high school math, 2 years of high school science, high school chemistry, high school foreign language, high school transcript, interview, transcript of college record. 28 prerequisite credits must be completed before admission to the nursing program. *Options:* Advanced standing available through the following means: advanced placement exams, credit by exam. Course work may be accelerated. May apply for transfer of up to 101 total credits. *Application deadlines:* 8/15 (fall), 12/1 (spring). *Application fee:* $100.

Degree Requirements 128 total credit hours, 53 in nursing. Religious studies, sociology, humanities, natural sciences.

RN Baccalaureate Program (BSN)

Applying *Required:* NLN Mobility Profile II, minimum college GPA of 2.5, RN license, diploma or AD in nursing, high school transcript, interview, transcript of college record, validation of prior learning through articulation agreements. 28 prerequisite credits must be completed before admission to the nursing program. *Options:* Advanced standing available through the following means: advanced placement exams, credit by exam. Course work may be accelerated. May apply for transfer of up to 101 total credits. *Application deadlines:* 8/1 (fall), 12/1 (spring). *Application fee:* $25.

Degree Requirements 128 total credit hours, 53 in nursing. Religious studies, sociology, humanities, natural sciences.

FRANCISCAN UNIVERSITY OF STEUBENVILLE
Department of Nursing
Steubenville, Ohio

Programs • Generic Baccalaureate • RN Baccalaureate

The University Independent Roman Catholic comprehensive coed institution. Founded: 1946. *Primary accreditation:* regional. *Setting:* 100-acre suburban campus. *Total enrollment:* 1,964.

The Department of Nursing Founded in 1979. *Nursing program faculty:* 12 (16% with doctorates).

Academic Facilities *Nursing school resources:* CAI, computer lab, nursing audiovisuals, learning resource lab.

Calendar Semesters.

NURSING STUDENT PROFILE

Undergraduate **Enrollment:** 156

Women: 89%; **Men:** 11%; **Minority:** 1%; **International:** 1%; **Part-time:** 15%

BACCALAUREATE PROGRAMS

Contact Ms. Carolyn Miller, Chairperson, Department of Nursing, Franciscan University of Steubenville, Steubenville, OH 43952, 614-283-6324. *Fax:* 614-283-6472.

Expenses *Tuition:* $8880 full-time, $370 per credit hour part-time. *Full-time mandatory fees:* $100–$200. *Room and board:* $4500. *Books and supplies per academic year:* ranges from $200 to $500.

Financial Aid Institutionally sponsored need-based grants/scholarships, institutionally sponsored non-need grants/scholarships, Federal Direct Loans, Federal Nursing Student Loans, Federal Supplemental Educational Opportunity Grants, Federal Work-Study. *Application deadline:* 3/1.

Generic Baccalaureate Program (BSN)

Applying *Required:* SAT I or ACT, minimum high school GPA of 2.5, minimum college GPA of 2.5, 3 years of high school math, 3 years of high school science, high school chemistry, high school biology, high school transcript, transcript of college record, high school class rank: top 33%, immunizations, health exam. *Options:* Advanced standing available through the following means: advanced placement exams, credit by exam. *Application deadline:* 5/30. *Application fee:* $20.

Degree Requirements 126 total credit hours, 57 in nursing.

RN Baccalaureate Program (BSN)

Applying *Required:* ACT PEP, minimum college GPA of 2.5, RN license, diploma or AD in nursing, high school transcript, transcript of college record, professional liability/malpractice insurance, immunizations, health exam. *Options:* Advanced standing available through the following means: advanced placement exams, credit by exam. *Application deadline:* rolling. *Application fee:* $20.

Degree Requirements 126 total credit hours, 57 in nursing.

FRANKLIN UNIVERSITY
Nursing Program
Columbus, Ohio

Program • RN Baccalaureate

The University Independent comprehensive coed institution. Founded: 1902. *Primary accreditation:* regional. *Setting:* 14-acre urban campus. *Total enrollment:* 4,073.

The Nursing Program Founded in 1981.

Academic Facilities *Campus library:* 200,000 volumes; 1,200 periodical subscriptions. *Nursing school resources:* nursing audiovisuals.

Student Life *Student services:* career counseling, campus safety program. *Nursing student activities:* student nurses association.

Calendar Trimesters.

BACCALAUREATE PROGRAM

Contact Dr. Louise J. Gallaway, Chairperson, Nursing Program, Franklin University, 201 South Grant Avenue, Columbus, OH 43215, 614-341-6318. *Fax:* 614-228-8478.

Expenses *Tuition:* ranges from $161 to $214 per credit hour. *Books and supplies per academic year:* $500.

Financial Aid *Application deadline:* 5/30.

RN Baccalaureate Program (BSN)

Applying *Required:* TOEFL for nonnative speakers of English, RN license, diploma or AD in nursing, high school transcript, interview, transcript of college record. *Options:* Advanced standing available through credit by exam. *Application deadline:* rolling.

Degree Requirements 130 total credit hours, 66 in nursing.

KENT STATE UNIVERSITY
School of Nursing
Kent, Ohio

Programs • Generic Baccalaureate • RN Baccalaureate • Accelerated RN Baccalaureate • Baccalaureate for Second Degree • LPN to Baccalaureate • MSN • MSN/MBA • MSN/MPA • Post-Master's

The University State-supported coed university. Part of Kent State University System. Founded: 1910. *Primary accreditation:* regional. *Setting:* 1,200-acre small-town campus. *Total enrollment:* 20,972.

The School of Nursing Founded in 1967. *Nursing program faculty:* 75 (77% with doctorates).

Academic Facilities *Campus library:* 1.5 million volumes.

Student Life *Student services:* health clinic, personal counseling, career counseling, job placement. *Nursing student activities:* Students for Professional Nursing, Ohio Nursing Students Association, Graduate Nurse Student Organization.

NURSING STUDENT PROFILE

Undergraduate **Enrollment:** 1000
Graduate **Enrollment:** 150
Part-time: 65%

BACCALAUREATE PROGRAMS

Contact Assistant Dean, Undergraduate and Student Affairs, School of Nursing, Kent State University, PO Box 5190, Kent, OH 44242-0001, 216-672-7930. *Fax:* 216-672-2433.

Expenses *State resident tuition:* $4288 full-time, $195 per credit part-time. *Full-time mandatory fees:* $735. *Room and board:* $200.

GENERIC BACCALAUREATE PROGRAM (BSN)

Applying *Required:* SAT I, ACT, minimum college GPA of 2.5. *Application fee:* $25.

RN BACCALAUREATE PROGRAM (BSN)

Applying *Required:* SAT I or ACT, minimum college GPA of 2.5, high school transcript. *Application fee:* $25.

ACCELERATED RN BACCALAUREATE PROGRAM (BSN)

Applying *Required:* SAT I or ACT, minimum college GPA of 2.5, high school transcript. *Application fee:* $25.

BACCALAUREATE FOR SECOND DEGREE PROGRAM (BSN)

Applying *Required:* SAT I or ACT, minimum college GPA of 2.5, high school transcript. *Application fee:* $25.

LPN TO BACCALAUREATE PROGRAM (BSN)

Applying *Required:* SAT I or ACT, minimum college GPA of 2.5, high school transcript. *Application fee:* $25.

MASTER'S PROGRAMS

Contact Assistant Dean, Undergraduate and Student Affairs, School of Nursing, Kent State University, PO Box 5190, Kent, OH 44242-0001, 216-672-7930. *Fax:* 216-672-2433.

Areas of Study Clinical nurse specialist programs in adult health nursing, gerontological nursing, parent-child nursing, psychiatric–mental health nursing; nursing administration; nursing education; nurse practitioner program in clinical nursing.

Expenses *State resident tuition:* $4568 full-time, $208 per credit part-time.

MSN PROGRAM

Applying *Required:* GRE General Test, Miller Analogies Test, bachelor's degree in nursing, minimum GPA of 3.0, RN license, essay, interview, 3 letters of recommendation, transcript of college record. *Application fee:* $25.

MSN/MBA PROGRAM

MSN/MPA PROGRAM

POST-MASTER'S PROGRAM

See full description on page 468.

LOURDES COLLEGE
Department of Nursing
Sylvania, Ohio

Programs • Generic Baccalaureate • RN Baccalaureate • Accelerated RN Baccalaureate • Continuing Education

The College Independent Roman Catholic 4-year coed college. Founded: 1958. *Primary accreditation:* regional. *Setting:* 90-acre suburban campus. *Total enrollment:* 1,589.

The Department of Nursing Founded in 1986. *Nursing program faculty:* 18 (6% with doctorates).

Academic Facilities *Campus library:* 64,000 volumes (300 in health, 475 in nursing); 375 periodical subscriptions (80 health-care related). *Nursing school resources:* CAI, computer lab, nursing audiovisuals, interactive nursing skills videos, learning resource lab.

Student Life *Student services:* personal counseling, career counseling, job placement, campus safety program, special assistance for disabled students. *International student services:* counseling/support. *Nursing student activities:* student nurses association, Nursing Honor Society.

Calendar Semesters.

NURSING STUDENT PROFILE

Undergraduate **Enrollment:** 454
Women: 92%; **Men:** 8%; **Minority:** 2%; **International:** 0%; **Part-time:** 75%

BACCALAUREATE PROGRAMS

Contact Ms. Catherine Kleiner, Recruiter and Adviser, Department of Nursing, Lourdes College, 6832 Convent Boulevard, Sylvania, OH 43560, 419-885-3211 Ext. 278.

Expenses *Tuition:* $250 per credit hour. *Full-time mandatory fees:* $10–$300.

Financial Aid Institutionally sponsored need-based grants/scholarships, Federal Nursing Student Loans, Federal Supplemental Educational Opportunity Grants, Federal Work-Study. *Application deadline:* 8/15.

GENERIC BACCALAUREATE PROGRAM (BSN)

Applying *Required:* SAT I or ACT, TOEFL for nonnative speakers of English, minimum college GPA of 2.5, high school chemistry, high school biology, high school transcript, letter of recommendation, written essay, transcript of college record. 63 prerequisite credits must be completed before admission to the nursing program. *Options:* May apply for transfer of up to 96 total credits. *Application deadline:* 1/15.

Degree Requirements 128 total credit hours, 59 in nursing.

RN BACCALAUREATE PROGRAM (BSN)

Applying *Required:* minimum college GPA of 2.5, RN license, diploma or AD in nursing. 63 prerequisite credits must be completed before admission to the nursing program. *Options:* Course work may be accelerated. May apply for transfer of up to 96 total credits. *Application deadlines:* 1/15 (fall), 10/15 (summer).

Degree Requirements 128 total credit hours, 59 in nursing.

ACCELERATED RN BACCALAUREATE PROGRAM (BSN)

Applying *Required:* minimum college GPA of 2.5, RN license, diploma or AD in nursing. *Options:* May apply for transfer of up to 96 total credits. *Application deadline:* 10/15 (summer).

Degree Requirements 128 total credit hours, 59 in nursing.

CONTINUING EDUCATION PROGRAM

Contact Dr. Janet Robinson, Administrative Coordinator for Nursing Continuing Education, Department of Nursing, Lourdes College, 6832 Convent Boulevard, Sylvania, OH 43560, 419-885-3211. *Fax:* 419-882-3786.

MALONE COLLEGE
Department of Nursing
Canton, Ohio

Programs • Generic Baccalaureate • RN Baccalaureate • LPN to Baccalaureate

The College Independent comprehensive coed institution, affiliated with Evangelical Friends Church–Eastern Region. Founded: 1892. *Primary accreditation:* regional. *Setting:* 78-acre suburban campus. *Total enrollment:* 1,979.

The Department of Nursing Founded in 1987. *Nursing program faculty:* 18 (11% with doctorates).

Academic Facilities *Campus library:* 137,856 volumes (400 in health, 2,500 in nursing); 1,538 periodical subscriptions (100 health-care related). *Nursing school resources:* CAI, computer lab, nursing audiovisuals, interactive nursing skills videos, learning resource lab.

Student Life *Student services:* health clinic, personal counseling, career counseling, institutionally sponsored work-study program, job placement, special assistance for disabled students. *International student services:* counseling/support, multicultural services. *Nursing student activities:* student nurses association, Malone Nurses Christian Fellowship and Malone College Honor Society of Nursing.

Calendar Trimesters.

NURSING STUDENT PROFILE

Undergraduate **Enrollment:** 183
Women: 93%; **Men:** 7%; **Minority:** 5%; **International:** 0%

BACCALAUREATE PROGRAMS

Contact Mr. Lee Sommers, Dean of Admissions, Malone College, 515 25th Street, NW, Canton, OH 44709, 330-471-8145. *Fax:* 330-454-6977.

Expenses *Tuition:* $10,620 full-time, $265 per credit hour part-time. *Full-time mandatory fees:* $540. *Room and board:* $4300. *Books and supplies per academic year:* ranges from $400 to $600.

Financial Aid Institutionally sponsored need-based grants/scholarships, institutionally sponsored non-need grants/scholarships, Federal Supplemental Educational Opportunity Grants, Federal Work-Study. *Application deadline:* 3/1.

Generic Baccalaureate Program (BSN)

Applying *Required:* ACT, minimum high school GPA of 2.5, 3 years of high school math, 3 years of high school science, high school chemistry, high school transcript, 3 letters of recommendation, written essay, transcript of college record. *Application deadlines:* 7/1 (fall), 11/5 (spring). *Application fee:* $20.

Degree Requirements 124 total credit hours, 60 in nursing.

RN Baccalaureate Program (BSN)

Applying *Required:* minimum college GPA of 2.0, RN license, diploma or AD in nursing, 3 letters of recommendation, transcript of college record, biological chemistry, human anatomy and physiology, minimum 2.25 GPA in nursing. 60 prerequisite credits must be completed before admission to the nursing program. *Options:* May apply for transfer of up to 82 total credits. *Application deadline:* rolling. *Application fee:* $25.

Degree Requirements 124 total credit hours, 37 in nursing. 6 hours theology/Bible literature.

LPN to Baccalaureate Program (BSN)

Applying *Required:* high school transcript, interview, letter of recommendation, transcript of college record, LPN license. *Options:* Advanced standing available through the following means: advanced placement without credit, credit by exam. *Application deadline:* rolling. *Application fee:* $20.

Degree Requirements 124 total credit hours, 60 in nursing. 12 credits received by college transfer credit or by Mobility exam.

MEDICAL COLLEGE OF OHIO
School of Nursing
Toledo, Ohio

Programs • MSN • Post-Master's • Continuing Education

The College State-supported graduate specialized coed institution. Founded: 1964. *Primary accreditation:* regional. *Total enrollment:* 1,048.

The School of Nursing Founded in 1971. *Nursing program faculty:* 54 (31% with doctorates). *Off-campus program sites:* Huron, Lima, Archbold.

Academic Facilities *Campus library:* 115,800 volumes (1,998 in nursing); 1,055 periodical subscriptions (1,055 health-care related). *Nursing school resources:* CAI, computer lab, nursing audiovisuals, learning resource lab.

Student Life *Student services:* health clinic, child-care facilities, personal counseling, career counseling, institutionally sponsored work-study program, job placement, campus safety program, special assistance for disabled students. *International student services:* counseling/support, special assistance for nonnative speakers of English, ESL courses. *Nursing student activities:* Sigma Theta Tau, student nurses association.

Calendar Semesters.

NURSING STUDENT PROFILE

Graduate **Enrollment:** 178
Women: 97%; **Men:** 3%; **Minority:** 3%; **International:** 0%; **Part-time:** 93%

MASTER'S PROGRAMS

Contact Dr. Ruth R. Alteneder, Associate Dean, Graduate Program, School of Nursing, Medical College of Ohio, PO Box 10008, Toledo, OH 43699-0008, 419-381-5860. *Fax:* 419-381-3022. *E-mail:* alteneder@cutter.mco.edu

Areas of Study Clinical nurse specialist programs in adult health nursing, parent-child nursing, psychiatric–mental health nursing; nursing education; nurse practitioner program in family health.

Expenses *State resident tuition:* $2640 full-time, $109 per credit hour part-time. *Nonresident tuition:* $4628 full-time, $193 per credit hour part-time. *Full-time mandatory fees:* $160–$228. *Books and supplies per academic year:* ranges from $500 to $750.

Financial Aid Nurse traineeships, employment opportunities, institutionally sponsored non-need-based grants/scholarships. *Application deadline:* 3/31.

MSN Program

Applying *Required:* GRE General Test, bachelor's degree in nursing, minimum GPA of 3.0, RN license, 1 year of clinical experience, physical assessment course, statistics course, professional liability/malpractice insurance, essay, 3 letters of recommendation, transcript of college record, computer literacy. *Application deadlines:* 3/31 (fall), 12/31 (spring), 8/31 (winter). *Application fee:* $30.

Degree Requirements 51–54 total credit hours dependent upon track, 51–54 in nursing.

Post-Master's Program

Applying *Required:* minimum GPA of 3.0, RN license, 1 year of clinical experience, physical assessment course, statistics course, professional liability/malpractice insurance, essay, 3 letters of recommendation, transcript of college record, MSN. *Application deadline:* 3/31. *Application fee:* $30.

Degree Requirements 39 total credit hours, 39 in nursing.

CONTINUING EDUCATION PROGRAM

Contact Dr. Diane Smolen, Director, Continuing Nursing Education, School of Nursing, Medical College of Ohio, PO Box 10008, Toledo, OH 43699-0008, 419-381-4237. *Fax:* 419-381-5881. *E-mail:* smolen@cutter.mco.edu

MIAMI UNIVERSITY
Department of Nursing
Oxford, Ohio

Program • RN Baccalaureate

The University State-related coed university. Part of Miami University System. Founded: 1809. *Primary accreditation:* regional. *Setting:* 1,900-acre small-town campus. *Total enrollment:* 15,601.

The Department of Nursing Founded in 1976. *Nursing program faculty:* 5 (60% with doctorates). *Off-campus program sites:* Hamilton, Middletown.

Academic Facilities *Campus library:* 1.4 million volumes (29,000 in nursing); 6,815 periodical subscriptions (852 health-care related). *Nursing*

Miami University (continued)

school resources: CAI, computer lab, nursing audiovisuals, interactive nursing skills videos, learning resource lab.

Student Life *Student services:* health clinic, child-care facilities, personal counseling, career counseling, special assistance for disabled students. *International student services:* counseling/support. *Nursing student activities:* Nursing Honor Society.

Calendar Semesters.

NURSING STUDENT PROFILE

Undergraduate **Enrollment:** 120

Women: 96%; **Men:** 4%; **Minority:** 10%; **International:** 0%; **Part-time:** 75%

BACCALAUREATE PROGRAM

Contact Dr. Eugenia M. Mills, Chair and Director, 113 Kreger Hall, Department of Nursing, Miami University, Oxford, OH 45056, 513-785-3282. *Fax:* 513-785-3284. *E-mail:* millsem@muohio.edu

Expenses *State resident tuition:* $2000 full-time, $145 per credit hour part-time. *Nonresident tuition:* $4715 full-time, $372 per credit hour part-time. *Full-time mandatory fees:* $255. *Room and board:* $2105. *Room only:* $975. *Books and supplies per academic year:* ranges from $100 to $150.

Financial Aid Institutionally sponsored need-based grants/scholarships, institutionally sponsored non-need grants/scholarships, Federal Nursing Student Loans, Federal Supplemental Educational Opportunity Grants. 3% of undergraduate students in nursing programs received some form of financial aid in 1995–96. *Application deadline:* 2/15.

RN Baccalaureate Program (BSN)

Applying *Required:* minimum college GPA of 2.5, RN license, diploma or AD in nursing, transcript of college record. *Options:* May apply for transfer of up to 64 total credits. *Application deadline:* rolling. *Application fee:* $25.

Degree Requirements 128 total credit hours, 34 in nursing.

THE OHIO STATE UNIVERSITY
College of Nursing
Columbus, Ohio

Programs • Generic Baccalaureate • RN Baccalaureate • MS/MBA • MS/MHA • PhD

The University State-supported coed university. Founded: 1870. *Primary accreditation:* regional. *Setting:* 3,303-acre urban campus. *Total enrollment:* 48,676.

The College of Nursing Founded in 1914. *Nursing program faculty:* 58 (57% with doctorates).

► ***NOTEWORTHY***

The Ohio State University offers the BSN in a 4-year, NLN-accredited undergraduate program. The graduate nursing program is ranked among the top in the country. The master's degree curriculum prepares students for advanced practice nursing (clinical nurse specialist, nurse practitioner, certified nurse/midwife) with the choice of several specialties, including adult health and illness; community health; parent-child: neonatal, pediatric, women's health, nurse midwifery; and psychiatric/mental health. The MS/MBA and MS/MHA are also available. Electives are offered in diverse areas, including administration and education. The PhD program prepares nurses to conduct research that contributes to the development of nursing science and can improve the practice of professional nursing. It includes a nursing science major, a cognate minor, a dissertation, and a research residency requirement of 3 quarters.

Academic Facilities *Campus library:* 4.8 million volumes (175,000 in health); 32,000 periodical subscriptions (6,000 health-care related). *Nursing school resources:* CAI, computer lab, nursing audiovisuals, interactive nursing skills videos, learning resource lab.

Student Life *Student services:* health clinic, child-care facilities, personal counseling, career counseling, institutionally sponsored work-study program, job placement, campus safety program, special assistance for disabled students. *International student services:* counseling/support, special assistance for nonnative speakers of English, ESL courses. *Nursing student activities:* Sigma Theta Tau, student nurses association, Alpha Tau Delta, Chi Eta Phi.

Calendar Quarters.

NURSING STUDENT PROFILE

Undergraduate **Enrollment:** 463

Women: 87%; **Men:** 13%; **Minority:** 12%; **International:** 1%; **Part-time:** 19%

Graduate **Enrollment:** 160

Women: 95%; **Men:** 5%; **Minority:** 8%; **International:** 1%; **Part-time:** 70%

BACCALAUREATE PROGRAMS

Contact Dr. Susan Missler, Academic Counselor, College of Nursing, The Ohio State University, 1585 Neil Avenue, Columbus, OH 43210-1289, 614-292-4041. *Fax:* 614-292-4535. *E-mail:* missler.1@osu.edu

Expenses *State resident tuition:* $3468 per academic year. *Nonresident tuition:* $10,335 per academic year. *Full-time mandatory fees:* $350–$500. *Room and board:* $4400. *Room only:* $3000. *Books and supplies per academic year:* ranges from $500 to $700.

Financial Aid Institutionally sponsored need-based grants/scholarships, institutionally sponsored non-need grants/scholarships, Federal Direct Loans, Federal Nursing Student Loans, Federal Pell Grants, Federal Perkins Loans, Federal Supplemental Educational Opportunity Grants, Federal Work-Study. 70% of undergraduate students in nursing programs received some form of financial aid in 1995–96. *Application deadline:* 3/1.

Generic Baccalaureate Program (BSN)

Applying *Required:* SAT I, ACT, TOEFL for nonnative speakers of English, minimum college GPA of 2.0, 3 years of high school math, 3 years of high school science, high school chemistry, high school biology, high school foreign language, high school transcript, transcript of college record. 45 prerequisite credits must be completed before admission to the nursing program. *Options:* Advanced standing available through the following means: advanced placement exams, advanced placement without credit, credit by exam. May apply for transfer of up to 150 total credits. *Application deadline:* 4/1. *Application fee:* $30.

Degree Requirements 196 total credit hours, 88 in nursing.

RN Baccalaureate Program (BSN)

Applying *Required:* TOEFL for nonnative speakers of English, minimum college GPA of 2.0, 3 years of high school math, 3 years of high school science, RN license, diploma or AD in nursing, written essay, transcript of college record. 45 prerequisite credits must be completed before admission to the nursing program. *Options:* Advanced standing available through the following means: advanced placement exams, advanced placement without credit, credit by exam. Course work may be accelerated. May apply for transfer of up to 150 total credits. *Application deadline:* 4/1. *Application fee:* $30.

Degree Requirements 196 total credit hours, 88 in nursing.

MASTER'S PROGRAMS

Contact Ms. Katherine Frazier, Administrative Secretary, College of Nursing, The Ohio State University, 1585 Neil Avenue, Columbus, OH 43210-1289, 614-292-8962. *Fax:* 614-292-4948. *E-mail:* frazier.7@osu.edu

Areas of Study Clinical nurse specialist programs in adult health nursing, community health nursing, maternity-newborn nursing, parent-child nursing, pediatric nursing, perinatal nursing, psychiatric–mental health nursing, women's health nursing; nurse midwifery; nurse practitioner programs in adult health, child care/pediatrics, neonatal health, psychiatric–mental health, women's health.

Expenses *State resident tuition:* $4941 full-time, $165 per credit hour part-time. *Nonresident tuition:* $12,831 full-time, $428 per credit hour part-time. *Full-time mandatory fees:* $350–$500. *Room and board:* $4400. *Room only:* $3000. *Books and supplies per academic year:* ranges from $200 to $1000.

Financial Aid Graduate assistantships, nurse traineeships, fellowships, Federal Direct Loans, Federal Nursing Student Loans, institutionally sponsored loans, employment opportunities. 24% of master's level students in nursing programs received some form of financial aid in 1995-96. *Application deadline:* 3/1.

MS/MBA Program

Applying *Required:* GRE General Test, TOEFL for nonnative speakers of English, bachelor's degree in nursing, minimum GPA of 3.0, RN license, physical assessment course, statistics course, professional liability/

malpractice insurance, essay, 3 letters of recommendation, transcript of college record. *Application deadlines:* 5/1 (fall), 2/1 (spring), 5/1 (winter, 11/1; summer). *Application fee:* $30.

Degree Requirements 52–60 total credit hours dependent upon track.

MS/MHA Program

Applying *Required:* GRE General Test, Miller Analogies Test, TOEFL for nonnative speakers of English, bachelor's degree in nursing, minimum GPA of 3.0, RN license, physical assessment course, statistics course, professional liability/malpractice insurance, essay, 3 letters of recommendation, transcript of college record. *Application deadlines:* 5/1 (fall), 2/1 (spring), 5/1 (winter 11/01, summer). *Application fee:* $30.

Degree Requirements 52–56 total credit hours dependent upon track.

DOCTORAL PROGRAM

Contact Dr. Mary Ellen Wewers, Associate Professor, College of Nursing, The Ohio State University, 1585 Neil Avenue, Columbus, OH 43210-1289, 614-292-8962. *Fax:* 614-292-4948. *E-mail:* wewers.1@osu.edu

Areas of Study Nursing research.

Expenses *State resident tuition:* $4941 full-time, $165 per credit hour part-time. *Nonresident tuition:* $12,831 full-time, $428 per credit hour part-time. *Full-time mandatory fees:* $75–$500. *Room and board:* $4400. *Room only:* $3000. *Books and supplies per academic year:* ranges from $200 to $1000.

Financial Aid Graduate assistantships, nurse traineeships, fellowships, dissertation grants, grants, Federal Direct Loans, institutionally sponsored loans, opportunities for employment. *Application deadline:* 3/1.

PhD Program

Applying *Required:* GRE General Test, TOEFL for nonnative speakers of English, master's degree in nursing, statistics course, 3 letters of recommendation, vitae, writing sample, competitive review by faculty committee. *Application deadline:* 1/15. *Application fee:* $30.

Degree Requirements 90 total credit hours; dissertation; oral exam; written exam; defense of dissertation; residency.

OHIO UNIVERSITY
School of Nursing
Athens, Ohio

Program • RN Baccalaureate

The University State-supported coed university. Part of Ohio University System. Founded: 1804. *Primary accreditation:* regional. *Setting:* 1,700-acre small-town campus. *Total enrollment:* 19,143.

The School of Nursing Founded in 1975. *Nursing program faculty:* 9 (78% with doctorates).

Academic Facilities *Campus library:* 1.3 million volumes; 10,935 periodical subscriptions.

Calendar Quarters.

BACCALAUREATE PROGRAM

Contact Dr. Kathleen Rose-Grippa, Director and Professor, McCracken Hall 312, School of Nursing, Ohio University, Athens, OH 45701, 614-593-4494. *Fax:* 614-593-0286.

Expenses *State resident tuition:* $4080 full-time, $125 per hour part-time. *Nonresident tuition:* $8574 full-time, $274 per hour part-time. *Full-time mandatory fees:* $377. *Room and board:* $3363–$5610. *Room only:* $1818–$2706.

Financial Aid Institutionally sponsored need-based grants/scholarships, Federal Direct Loans, Federal Pell Grants, Federal Perkins Loans, Federal Supplemental Educational Opportunity Grants, Federal Work-Study, Ohio state aid. *Application deadline:* 3/15.

RN Baccalaureate Program (BSN)

Applying *Required:* TOEFL for nonnative speakers of English, RN license, diploma or AD in nursing, transcript of college record, immunizations, CPR certification. *Options:* Advanced standing available through the following means: advanced placement exams, credit by exam. *Application fee:* $30.

OTTERBEIN COLLEGE
Nursing Program
Westerville, Ohio

Programs • Generic Baccalaureate • RN Baccalaureate • LPN to Baccalaureate • MSN • Continuing Education

The College Independent United Methodist comprehensive coed institution. Founded: 1847. *Primary accreditation:* regional. *Setting:* 140-acre suburban campus. *Total enrollment:* 2,478.

The Nursing Program Founded in 1979. *Nursing program faculty:* 33 (28% with doctorates).

Academic Facilities *Nursing school resources:* CAI, computer lab, nursing audiovisuals, learning resource lab.

Student Life *Student services:* health clinic, personal counseling, career counseling, institutionally sponsored work-study program, job placement, campus safety program. *International student services:* counseling/support, ESL courses. *Nursing student activities:* Sigma Theta Tau, student nurses association.

Calendar Quarters.

NURSING STUDENT PROFILE

Undergraduate **Enrollment:** 365
Women: 94%; **Men:** 6%; **Minority:** 11%; **International:** 0%; **Part-time:** 50%
Graduate **Enrollment:** 65
Women: 100%; **Minority:** 2%; **International:** 0%; **Part-time:** 98%

BACCALAUREATE PROGRAMS

Contact Dr. Judy M. Strayer, Chairperson, Nursing Program, Otterbein College, Westerville, OH 43081, 614-823-1614. *Fax:* 614-823-3131.

Expenses *Full-time mandatory fees:* $130. *Room and board:* $4569. *Books and supplies per academic year:* ranges from $150 to $200.

Financial Aid Institutionally sponsored need-based grants/scholarships, institutionally sponsored non-need grants/scholarships, Federal Direct Loans, Federal Nursing Student Loans, Federal Perkins Loans, Federal Supplemental Educational Opportunity Grants, Federal Work-Study. *Application deadline:* 4/1.

Generic Baccalaureate Program (BSN)

Applying *Required:* ACT, minimum college GPA of 2.5, high school transcript, transcript of college record. *Options:* Advanced standing available through the following means: advanced placement exams, credit by exam. May apply for transfer of up to 60 total credits. *Application deadline:* rolling. *Application fee:* $35.

Degree Requirements 138 total credit hours, 57 in nursing.

RN Baccalaureate Program (BSN)

Applying *Required:* minimum college GPA of 2.5, RN license, diploma or AD in nursing, high school transcript, transcript of college record. *Options:* Advanced standing available through the following means: advanced placement exams, credit by exam. Course work may be accelerated. May apply for transfer of up to 60 total credits. *Application deadline:* rolling. *Application fee:* $35.

Degree Requirements 138 total credit hours, 57 in nursing.

LPN to Baccalaureate Program (BSN)

Applying *Required:* NLN Achievement Tests in nutrition, pharmacology, fundamentals, and child-bearing, minimum college GPA of 2.5, high school transcript, interview, transcript of college record, graduate of LPN program, LPN license, 6 months experience. *Options:* Advanced standing available through the following means: advanced placement exams, credit by exam. Course work may be accelerated. May apply for transfer of up to 60 total credits. *Application deadline:* rolling. *Application fee:* $35.

Degree Requirements 138 total credit hours, 57 in nursing.

Otterbein College (continued)

MASTER'S PROGRAM

Contact Eda Mikolaj, Coordinator, Graduate Studies, Nursing Department, Otterbein College, 155 West Main Street, Westerville, OH 43081, 614-823-1614. *Fax:* 614-823-3131.

Areas of Study Clinical nurse specialist program in adult health nursing; nursing administration.

Expenses *Tuition:* $13,611 full-time, $190 per credit hour part-time. *Full-time mandatory fees:* $25. *Part-time mandatory fees:* $25. *Books and supplies per academic year:* $300.

Financial Aid Nurse traineeships, Federal Direct Loans, Federal Nursing Student Loans, employment opportunities.

MSN Program

Applying *Required:* GRE General Test. *Application deadline:* rolling.

CONTINUING EDUCATION PROGRAM

Contact Dr. John Kengla, Director, Department of Continuing Studies, Otterbein College, Westerville, OH 43081, 614-823-1356.

UNIVERSITY OF AKRON

College of Nursing
Akron, Ohio

Programs • Generic Baccalaureate • RN Baccalaureate • LPN to Baccalaureate • MSN • RN to Master's • Continuing Education

The University State-supported coed university. Founded: 1870. *Primary accreditation:* regional. *Setting:* 170-acre urban campus. *Total enrollment:* 25,098.

The College of Nursing Founded in 1967. *Nursing program faculty:* 55 (45% with doctorates). *Off-campus program site:* Lorain.

▶ ***NOTEWORTHY***

The BSN program was recently named a national Center for Nursing Excellence by the Army Nurse Corps for 4-year Army ROTC scholarship recipients. An outreach RN/BSN program will be offered at Lorain County Community College beginning in the summer of 1997. The graduate program is moving toward increased post-master's options, such as acute-care and adult nurse practitioner programs, in response to nursing workforce needs. The Center for Nursing is currently addressing the health-care needs of medically underserved populations in the Akron metropolitan area through a multidisciplinary approach utilizing advanced practice nurses and resident physicians.

Academic Facilities *Campus library:* 865,448 volumes (10,602 in health, 12,375 in nursing); 5,375 periodical subscriptions (574 health-care related). *Nursing school resources:* CAI, computer lab, nursing audiovisuals, interactive nursing skills videos, learning resource lab.

Student Life *Student services:* health clinic, child-care facilities, personal counseling, career counseling, institutionally sponsored work-study program, job placement, campus safety program, special assistance for disabled students. *International student services:* counseling/support, special assistance for nonnative speakers of English, ESL courses. *Nursing student activities:* Sigma Theta Tau, nursing club, student nurses association.

Calendar Semesters.

NURSING STUDENT PROFILE

Undergraduate **Enrollment:** 565
Women: 88%; **Men:** 12%; **Minority:** 11%; **International:** 0%; **Part-time:** 5%

Graduate **Enrollment:** 300
Women: 97%; **Men:** 3%; **Minority:** 1%; **International:** 0%; **Part-time:** 80%

BACCALAUREATE PROGRAMS

Contact Dr. Phyllis Fitzgerald, Assistant Dean for Student Affairs, College of Nursing, University of Akron, 209 Carroll Street, Akron, OH 44325-3701, 216-972-5103. *Fax:* 216-972-5737. *E-mail:* pfitzgerald@uakron.edu

Expenses *State resident tuition:* $3510 full-time, $135 per credit hour part-time. *Nonresident tuition:* $8017 full-time, $308 per credit hour part-time. *Full-time mandatory fees:* $65–$210. *Room and board:* $4240. *Books and supplies per academic year:* ranges from $500 to $1000.

Financial Aid Institutionally sponsored need-based grants/scholarships, institutionally sponsored non-need grants/scholarships, Federal Nursing Student Loans, Federal Supplemental Educational Opportunity Grants, Federal Work-Study. *Application deadline:* 5/31.

Generic Baccalaureate Program (BSN)

Applying *Required:* TOEFL for nonnative speakers of English, minimum college GPA of 2.5, 3 years of high school math, 3 years of high school science, high school chemistry, high school biology, high school transcript, transcript of college record, minimum 2.0 GPA in prerequisite college courses. 34 prerequisite credits must be completed before admission to the nursing program. *Options:* Advanced standing available through credit by exam. May apply for transfer of up to 67 total credits. *Application deadline:* 3/1. *Application fee:* $25.

Degree Requirements 134 total credit hours, 67 in nursing.

RN Baccalaureate Program (BSN)

Applying *Required:* TOEFL for nonnative speakers of English, minimum college GPA of 2.5, RN license, diploma or AD in nursing, transcript of college record. 34 prerequisite credits must be completed before admission to the nursing program. *Options:* Advanced standing available through credit by exam. Course work may be accelerated. May apply for transfer of up to 67 total credits. *Application deadline:* 3/1. *Application fee:* $25.

Degree Requirements 134 total credit hours, 32 in nursing.

LPN to Baccalaureate Program (BSN)

Applying *Required:* TOEFL for nonnative speakers of English, NLN Mobility Profile I, skills competency testing, minimum college GPA of 2.5, 3 letters of recommendation, written essay, transcript of college record, LPN license. 34 prerequisite credits must be completed before admission to the nursing program. *Options:* Advanced standing available through the following means: advanced placement exams, credit by exam. Course work may be accelerated. May apply for transfer of up to 67 total credits. *Application deadlines:* 3/1 (fall), 5/1 (summer). *Application fee:* $25.

Degree Requirements 134 total credit hours, 67 in nursing.

MASTER'S PROGRAMS

Contact Dr. Linda Linc, Interim Associate Dean, Graduate Program, College of Nursing, University of Akron, 209 Carroll Street, Akron, OH 44325-3701, 216-972-7555. *Fax:* 216-972-5737.

Areas of Study Clinical nurse specialist programs in adult health nursing, gerontological nursing, pediatric nursing, psychiatric–mental health nursing; nurse anesthesia; nursing administration; nursing education; nurse practitioner programs in acute care, child care/pediatrics, primary care.

Expenses *State resident tuition:* $159 per credit. *Nonresident tuition:* $302 per credit. *Full-time mandatory fees:* $20–$200. *Room and board:* $4062. *Books and supplies per academic year:* ranges from $300 to $600.

Financial Aid Graduate assistantships, nurse traineeships, fellowships, institutionally sponsored need-based grants/scholarships. *Application deadline:* 2/1.

MSN Program

Applying *Required:* GRE General Test or Miller Analogies Test, bachelor's degree in nursing, minimum GPA of 3.0, RN license, physical assessment course, statistics course, professional liability/malpractice insurance, essay, interview, 3 letters of recommendation, transcript of college record, minimum of 1 year of clinical experience in critical care for nurse anesthesia program. *Application deadline:* rolling. *Application fee:* $25.

Degree Requirements 36–44 total credit hours dependent upon track, 36–44 in nursing.

RN to Master's Program (MSN)

Applying *Required:* GRE General Test or Miller Analogies Test, minimum GPA of 3.0, RN license, physical assessment course, statistics course, professional liability/malpractice insurance, essay, interview, 3 letters of recommendation, transcript of college record. *Application deadline:* rolling. *Application fee:* $25.

Degree Requirements 170 total credit hours, 57 in nursing.

CONTINUING EDUCATION PROGRAM

Contact Mrs. Barbara Smith, Secretary for Continuing Education, College of Nursing, University of Akron, 209 Carroll Street, Akron, OH 44325-3701, 216-972-7554. *Fax:* 216-972-5737.

See full description on page 516.

UNIVERSITY OF CINCINNATI
College of Nursing and Health
Cincinnati, Ohio

Programs • Generic Baccalaureate • RN Baccalaureate • MSN • Accelerated MSN • MSN/MBA • PhD • Continuing Education

The University State-supported coed university. Part of University of Cincinnati System. Founded: 1819. *Primary accreditation:* regional. *Setting:* 137-acre urban campus. *Total enrollment:* 18,373.

The College of Nursing and Health Founded in 1889. *Nursing program faculty:* 95 (51% with doctorates).

Academic Facilities *Campus library:* 2.1 million volumes (221,630 in health, 21,306 in nursing); 19,431 periodical subscriptions (2,384 health-care related). *Nursing school resources:* CAI, computer lab, nursing audiovisuals, interactive nursing skills videos, learning resource lab.

Student Life *Student services:* health clinic, child-care facilities, personal counseling, career counseling, institutionally sponsored work-study program, campus safety program, special assistance for disabled students. *International student services:* counseling/support, ESL courses. *Nursing student activities:* Sigma Theta Tau, student nurses association.

Calendar Quarters.

NURSING STUDENT PROFILE

Undergraduate **Enrollment:** 675
Women: 91%; **Men:** 9%; **Minority:** 12%; **International:** 1%; **Part-time:** 35%

Graduate **Enrollment:** 271
Women: 94%; **Men:** 6%; **Minority:** 8%; **International:** 1%; **Part-time:** 52%

BACCALAUREATE PROGRAMS

Contact Dr. Donna Lauver, Program Coordinator, College of Nursing and Health, University of Cincinnati, PO Box 210038, Cincinnati, OH 45221-0038, 513-558-3600. *Fax:* 513-558-7523. *E-mail:* donna.lauver@uc.edu

Expenses *State resident tuition:* $4152 full-time, $115 per quarter credit part-time. *Nonresident tuition:* $10,464 full-time, $290 per quarter credit part-time. *Full-time mandatory fees:* $687–$1446. *Part-time mandatory fees:* $90–$849. *Books and supplies per academic year:* ranges from $660 to $1000.

Financial Aid Institutionally sponsored need-based grants/scholarships, institutionally sponsored non-need grants/scholarships, Federal Nursing Student Loans, Federal Pell Grants, Federal Perkins Loans, Federal Supplemental Educational Opportunity Grants, Federal Work-Study. *Application deadline:* 7/1.

Generic Baccalaureate Program (BSN)

Applying *Required:* SAT I, ACT, TOEFL for nonnative speakers of English, minimum college GPA of 2.5, high school math, high school chemistry, high school biology, high school foreign language, high school transcript, transcript of college record, high school class rank: top 33%. 48 prerequisite credits must be completed before admission to the nursing program. *Options:* Advanced standing available through the following means: advanced placement exams, credit by exam. May apply for transfer of up to 83 total credits. *Application deadline:* rolling. *Application fee:* $30.

Degree Requirements 189 total credit hours, 100 in nursing.

RN Baccalaureate Program (BSN)

Applying *Required:* TOEFL for nonnative speakers of English, NLN Mobility Profile II, RN license, diploma or AD in nursing, high school transcript, transcript of college record. *Options:* Advanced standing available through the following means: advanced placement exams, credit by exam. Course work may be accelerated. May apply for transfer of up to 79 total credits. *Application deadlines:* 7/15 (fall), 1/10 (spring), 10/1 (summer; 4/25, winter). *Application fee:* $30.

Degree Requirements 189 total credit hours, 100 in nursing.

Distance learning Courses provided through interactive television.

MASTER'S PROGRAMS

Contact Thomas West, Program Coordinator, College of Nursing and Health, University of Cincinnati, PO Box 210038, Cincinnati, OH 45221-0038, 513-558-3600. *Fax:* 513-558-7523. *E-mail:* tom.west@uc.edu

Areas of Study Clinical nurse specialist programs in adult health nursing, community health nursing, critical care nursing, occupational health nursing, pediatric nursing, perinatal nursing, psychiatric–mental health nursing, genetics nursing; nurse anesthesia; nurse midwifery; nursing administration; nurse practitioner programs in child care/pediatrics, family health, neonatal health.

Expenses *State resident tuition:* $5445 full-time, $182 per quarter credit part-time. *Nonresident tuition:* $10,383 full-time, $347 per quarter credit part-time. *Full-time mandatory fees:* $687–$1446. *Part-time mandatory fees:* $90–$849. *Room and board:* $5049–$5253. *Room only:* $383–$534. *Books and supplies per academic year:* ranges from $500 to $1000.

Financial Aid Graduate assistantships, nurse traineeships, fellowships, Federal Nursing Student Loans, institutionally sponsored non-need-based grants/scholarships. *Application deadline:* 9/1.

MSN Program

Applying *Required:* GRE General Test, TOEFL for nonnative speakers of English, bachelor's degree in nursing, minimum GPA of 3.0, RN license, 1 year of clinical experience, physical assessment course, statistics course, essay, interview, 3 letters of recommendation, transcript of college record. *Application deadline:* rolling. *Application fee:* $30.

Degree Requirements 60–82 total credit hours dependent upon track, 51–79 in nursing, up to 9 in varies with major. Project.

Distance learning Courses provided through interactive television. Specific degree requirements include selected courses.

Accelerated MSN Program

Applying *Required:* GRE General Test, TOEFL for nonnative speakers of English, minimum GPA of 3.0, essay, interview, 3 letters of recommendation, transcript of college record. *Application deadline:* rolling. *Application fee:* $30.

Degree Requirements 60–82 total credit hours dependent upon track, up to 9 in varies with major. Project.

Distance learning Courses provided through interactive television. Specific degree requirements include selected courses.

MSN/MBA Program

Applying *Required:* GRE General Test, TOEFL for nonnative speakers of English, bachelor's degree in nursing, minimum GPA of 3.0, RN license, 1 year of clinical experience, statistics course, essay, interview, 3 letters of recommendation, transcript of college record. *Application deadline:* rolling. *Application fee:* $30.

Degree Requirements 93 total credit hours, 49 in nursing, 44 in business and other specified areas. Project.

Distance learning Courses provided through interactive television. Specific degree requirements include selected courses.

DOCTORAL PROGRAM

Contact Tom West, Program Coordinator, School of Nursing and Health, University of Cincinnati, PO Box 210038, Cincinnati, OH 45221-0038, 513-558-3600. *Fax:* 513-558-7523.

Areas of Study Nursing research.

Expenses *State resident tuition:* $5445 full-time, $182 per quarter credit part-time. *Nonresident tuition:* $10,383 full-time, $347 per quarter credit part-time. *Full-time mandatory fees:* $687–$1446. *Part-time mandatory fees:* $90–$849. *Room and board:* $5049–$5253. *Room only:* $383–$534. *Books and supplies per academic year:* ranges from $600 to $1000.

Financial Aid Graduate assistantships, nurse traineeships, fellowships, dissertation grants, Federal Direct Loans, institutionally sponsored non-need-based grants/scholarships. *Application deadline:* 7/1.

PhD Program

Applying *Required:* GRE General Test, 1 year of clinical experience, statistics course, interview, 3 letters of recommendation, vitae, writing sample, competitive review by faculty committee, BSN or MSN. *Application deadline:* rolling. *Application fee:* $30.

Degree Requirements 135 total credit hours; dissertation; written exam; defense of dissertation; residency.

CONTINUING EDUCATION PROGRAM

Contact Ms. Anita Finkelman, Director, Continuing Education, College of Nursing and Health, University of Cincinnati, PO Box 210038, Cincinnati, OH 45221-0038, 513-558-5311. *Fax:* 513-558-7523. *E-mail:* anita.finkelman@uc.edu

See full description on page 526.

UNIVERSITY OF TOLEDO
Nursing Department
Toledo, Ohio

Programs • Generic Baccalaureate • RN Baccalaureate

The University State-supported coed university. Founded: 1872. *Primary accreditation:* regional. *Setting:* 305-acre suburban campus. *Total enrollment:* 21,991.

The Nursing Department Founded in 1971. *Nursing program faculty:* 54 (31% with doctorates). *Off-campus program sites:* Huron, Lima, Archbold.

Academic Facilities *Campus library:* 888,471 volumes; 4,736 periodical subscriptions. *Nursing school resources:* CAI, computer lab, nursing audiovisuals, learning resource lab.

Student Life *Student services:* health clinic, child-care facilities, personal counseling, career counseling, institutionally sponsored work-study program, job placement, campus safety program, special assistance for disabled students. *International student services:* counseling/support, special assistance for nonnative speakers of English, ESL courses. *Nursing student activities:* Sigma Theta Tau, student nurses association.

Calendar Quarters.

NURSING STUDENT PROFILE

Undergraduate **Enrollment:** 148

Women: 86%; **Men:** 14%; **Minority:** 13%; **International:** 1%; **Part-time:** 20%

BACCALAUREATE PROGRAMS

Contact Ms. Patricia Hoover, Coordinator of Nursing Advisement, College of Arts and Sciences, University of Toledo, 2801 West Bancroft, Toledo, OH 43606, 419-537-2673. *Fax:* 419-537-2157.

Expenses *State resident tuition:* $3588 full-time, $100 per credit part-time. *Nonresident tuition:* $8598 full-time, $239 per credit part-time. *Full-time mandatory fees:* $190–$300.

Financial Aid Institutionally sponsored need-based grants/scholarships, institutionally sponsored non-need grants/scholarships, Federal Direct Loans, Federal Nursing Student Loans, Federal Pell Grants, Federal Perkins Loans, Federal Supplemental Educational Opportunity Grants, Federal Work-Study. *Application deadline:* 4/1.

Generic Baccalaureate Program (BSN)

Applying *Required:* SAT I, ACT, TOEFL for nonnative speakers of English, minimum college GPA of 2.5, 3 years of high school math, 3 years of high school science, high school foreign language, high school transcript, transcript of college record. 46 prerequisite credits must be completed before admission to the nursing program. *Options:* Advanced standing available through the following means: advanced placement exams, credit by exam. May apply for transfer of up to 90 total credits. *Application deadline:* 1/1. *Application fee:* $30.

Degree Requirements 186 total credit hours, 84 in nursing.

RN Baccalaureate Program (BSN)

Applying *Required:* NLN Mobility Profile II for diploma graduates, minimum college GPA of 2.5, RN license, diploma or AD in nursing, high school foreign language, high school transcript, transcript of college record, professional liability/malpractice insurance. 46 prerequisite credits must be completed before admission to the nursing program. *Options:* Advanced standing available through the following means: advanced placement exams, credit by exam. Course work may be accelerated. May apply for transfer of up to 90 total credits. *Application deadline:* rolling. *Application fee:* $30.

Degree Requirements 186 total credit hours, 40 in nursing.

URSULINE COLLEGE
Division of Nursing
Pepper Pike, Ohio

Programs • Generic Baccalaureate • Accelerated RN Baccalaureate • Accelerated Baccalaureate for Second Degree • Continuing Education

The College Independent Roman Catholic comprehensive primarily women's institution. Founded: 1871. *Primary accreditation:* regional. *Setting:* 112-acre suburban campus. *Total enrollment:* 1,312.

The Division of Nursing Founded in 1975. *Nursing program faculty:* 34 (33% with doctorates).

▶ *NOTEWORTHY*

Ursuline College's nursing program prepares graduates for the future—for practice in the community, homes, and internationally recognized medical centers. Ursuline's curriculum focuses on the person, student, and patient/client. Small classes and clinical groups, plus a core curriculum based on how women learn best, help make this possible. Closely supervised by faculty members, students work with all age groups, from infants to the elderly; in a variety of urban and suburban settings, from hospitals to clinics to hospice; and in all specialties, including critical care, maternity, pediatrics, mental health, and community health. Combining courses in the liberal arts and professional subject matters provides a broad foundation and enables students to have experiences in direct patient care, teaching, leadership/management, and research. A special capstone course in a clinical specialty facilitates transition from senior to graduate.

Academic Facilities *Campus library:* 110,000 volumes (12,000 in health, 4,000 in nursing); 600 periodical subscriptions (190 health-care related). *Nursing school resources:* CAI, computer lab, nursing audiovisuals, interactive nursing skills videos.

Student Life *Student services:* health clinic, personal counseling, career counseling, institutionally sponsored work-study program, job placement, campus safety program, special assistance for disabled students. *International student services:* counseling/support. *Nursing student activities:* Sigma Theta Tau, student nurses association.

Calendar Semesters.

NURSING STUDENT PROFILE

Undergraduate **Enrollment:** 467

Women: 97%; **Men:** 3%; **Minority:** 18%; **International:** 1%; **Part-time:** 40%

BACCALAUREATE PROGRAMS

Contact Mr. Dennis Giacomino, Director of Admissions, Ursuline College, 2550 Lander Road, Pepper Pike, OH 44124-4398, 216-449-4203.

Expenses *Tuition:* $11,648 full-time, $364 per credit hour part-time. *Full-time mandatory fees:* $50–$820. *Room and board:* $4330. *Books and supplies per academic year:* ranges from $500 to $600.

Financial Aid Institutionally sponsored need-based grants/scholarships, institutionally sponsored non-need grants/scholarships, Federal Perkins Loans, Federal Supplemental Educational Opportunity Grants, Federal Work-Study, Federal Family Education Loan Program (FFELP). *Application deadline:* 3/1.

Generic Baccalaureate Program (BSN)

Applying *Required:* SAT I, ACT, minimum high school GPA of 2.5, minimum college GPA of 2.5, 1 year of high school math, 2 years of high school science, high school chemistry, high school biology, high school transcript, letter of recommendation, written essay, transcript of college record. *Options:* May apply for transfer of up to 64 total credits. *Application deadline:* rolling. *Application fee:* $25.

Degree Requirements 129 total credit hours, 58 in nursing.

Accelerated RN Baccalaureate Program (BSN)

Applying *Required:* SAT I, ACT, minimum high school GPA of 2.5, minimum college GPA of 2.5, 1 year of high school math, 2 years of high school science, high school chemistry, high school biology, RN license, high school transcript, letter of recommendation, written essay, transcript of college record. *Options:* May apply for transfer of up to 64 total credits. *Application fee:* $25.

Degree Requirements 129 total credit hours, 58 in nursing.

Accelerated Baccalaureate for Second Degree Program (BSN)

Applying *Required:* SAT I, TOEFL for nonnative speakers of English, minimum high school GPA of 2.5, minimum college GPA of 2.5, 1 year of high school math, 2 years of high school science, high school chemistry, high school biology, high school transcript, letter of recommendation, written essay, transcript of college record, baccalaureate degree. *Options:* May apply for transfer of up to 64 total credits. *Application fee:* $25.

Degree Requirements 58 total credit hours in nursing. Some core requirements.

CONTINUING EDUCATION PROGRAM

Contact Dr. Carole F. Cashion, Dean and Strawbridge Professor of Nursing, Division of Nursing, Ursuline College, 2550 Lander Road, Pepper Pike, OH 44124-4398, 216-646-8166. *Fax:* 216-449-4267.

WALSH UNIVERSITY
Baccalaureate Nursing Department
North Canton, Ohio

Program • RN Baccalaureate

The University Independent Roman Catholic comprehensive coed institution. Founded: 1958. *Primary accreditation:* regional. *Setting:* 58-acre small-town campus. *Total enrollment:* 1,485.

The Baccalaureate Nursing Department Founded in 1984.

Calendar Semesters.

BACCALAUREATE PROGRAM

Contact Chair, Baccalaureate Nursing Department, Walsh University, 2020 Easton Street, NW, North Canton, OH 44720, 216-490-7208. *Fax:* 216-490-7206.

Expenses *Tuition:* $10,200 per academic year. *Room and board:* $4760.

RN Baccalaureate Program (BSN)

Applying *Required:* RN license, diploma or AD in nursing, transcript of college record. 30 prerequisite credits must be completed before admission to the nursing program. *Application fee:* $15.

WRIGHT STATE UNIVERSITY
College of Nursing and Health
Dayton, Ohio

Programs • Generic Baccalaureate • RN Baccalaureate • MS • Master's for Nurses with Non-Nursing Degrees • MS/MBA

The University State-supported coed university. Founded: 1964. *Primary accreditation:* regional. *Setting:* 557-acre suburban campus. *Total enrollment:* 16,488.

The College of Nursing and Health Founded in 1973. *Nursing program faculty:* 36 (41% with doctorates). *Off-campus program site:* Celina.

Academic Facilities *Campus library:* 627,978 volumes (105,948 in health, 10,439 in nursing); 5,215 periodical subscriptions (1,113 health-care related). *Nursing school resources:* CAI, computer lab, nursing audiovisuals, interactive nursing skills videos, learning resource lab.

Student Life *Student services:* health clinic, child-care facilities, personal counseling, career counseling, institutionally sponsored work-study program, job placement, campus safety program, special assistance for disabled students. *International student services:* counseling/support, ESL courses. *Nursing student activities:* Sigma Theta Tau, student nurses association.

Calendar Quarters.

NURSING STUDENT PROFILE

Undergraduate **Enrollment:** 540

Women: 86%; **Men:** 14%; **Minority:** 10%; **International:** 1%; **Part-time:** 36%

Graduate **Enrollment:** 275

Women: 96%; **Men:** 4%; **Minority:** 7%; **International:** 1%; **Part-time:** 80%

BACCALAUREATE PROGRAMS

Contact Ms. Theresa Haghnazarian, Director, Student and Alumni Affairs, 401 Allyn Hall, Wright State University-Miami Valley College of Nursing and Health, Dayton, OH 45435, 937-775-3132. *Fax:* 937-775-4571.

Expenses *State resident tuition:* $3600 full-time, $112 per credit hour part-time. *Nonresident tuition:* $7200 full-time, $224 per credit hour part-time. *Full-time mandatory fees:* $110–$650. *Room and board:* $4500. *Books and supplies per academic year:* ranges from $300 to $800.

Financial Aid Institutionally sponsored need-based grants/scholarships, institutionally sponsored non-need grants/scholarships, Federal Direct Loans, Federal Nursing Student Loans, Federal Pell Grants, Federal Perkins Loans, Federal Supplemental Educational Opportunity Grants, Federal Work-Study, state scholarships and grants. 77% of undergraduate students in nursing programs received some form of financial aid in 1995–96. *Application deadline:* 3/31.

Generic Baccalaureate Program (BSN)

Applying *Required:* SAT I, ACT, TOEFL for nonnative speakers of English, minimum college GPA of 2.5, 3 years of high school math, 3 years of high school science, high school foreign language, high school transcript, transcript of college record. 48 prerequisite credits must be completed before admission to the nursing program. *Options:* Advanced standing available through credit by exam. Course work may be accelerated. May apply for transfer of up to 147 total credits. *Application deadlines:* 6/15 (fall), 12/15 (spring). *Application fee:* $30.

Degree Requirements 192 total credit hours, 88 in nursing.

RN Baccalaureate Program (BSN)

Applying *Required:* minimum college GPA of 2.5, 3 years of high school math, 3 years of high school science, RN license, diploma or AD in nursing, high school foreign language, transcript of college record. 48 prerequisite credits must be completed before admission to the nursing program. *Options:* Advanced standing available through credit by exam. Course work may be accelerated. May apply for transfer of up to 147 total credits. *Application deadline:* 8/1. *Application fee:* $30.

Degree Requirements 192 total credit hours.

MASTER'S PROGRAMS

Contact Ms. Theresa Haghnazarian, Director, Student and Alumni Affairs, 401 Allyn Hall, Wright State University-Miami Valley College of Nursing and Health, Dayton, OH 45435, 937-775-3132. *Fax:* 937-775-4571.

Areas of Study Clinical nurse specialist programs in adult health nursing, community health nursing, pediatric nursing; nursing administration; nursing education; nurse practitioner program in family health.

Expenses *State resident tuition:* $4551 full-time, $143 per credit hour part-time. *Nonresident tuition:* $8151 full-time, $255 per credit hour part-time. *Full-time mandatory fees:* $100–$500. *Room and board:* $4500. *Books and supplies per academic year:* ranges from $300 to $800.

Financial Aid Graduate assistantships, nurse traineeships, fellowships, Federal Direct Loans, Federal Nursing Student Loans, employment opportunities. 29% of master's level students in nursing programs received some form of financial aid in 1995-96. *Application deadline:* 3/31.

MS Program

Applying *Required:* GRE General Test, bachelor's degree in nursing, minimum GPA of 2.7, RN license, physical assessment course, statistics course, professional liability/malpractice insurance, essay, interview, 2 letters of recommendation, transcript of college record, special application and minimum 3.0 college GPA for family nurse practitioner track. *Application deadlines:* 3/1 (family nurse practitioner track), rolling. *Application fee:* $25.

Degree Requirements 48–64 total credit hours dependent upon track, 45–64 in nursing. Thesis required.

Master's for Nurses with Non-Nursing Degrees Program (MS)

Applying *Required:* GRE General Test, minimum GPA of 3.0, RN license, physical assessment course, statistics course, professional liability/malpractice insurance, essay, transcript of college record, baccalaureate degree in a specific academic discipline. *Application deadline:* rolling. *Application fee:* $25.

Degree Requirements 61–78 total credit hours dependent upon track, 53–70 in nursing, 8 in elementary statistics and other specified areas. Thesis required.

MS/MBA Program

Applying *Required:* GRE General Test, GMAT, bachelor's degree in nursing, minimum GPA of 2.7, RN license, physical assessment course, statistics course, professional liability/malpractice insurance, essay, transcript of college record. *Application deadline:* rolling. *Application fee:* $25.

Degree Requirements 78–93 total credit hours dependent upon track, 45–50 in nursing, 33 in business administration. Thesis required.

See full description on page 574.

XAVIER UNIVERSITY
Department of Nursing
Cincinnati, Ohio

Programs • Generic Baccalaureate • RN Baccalaureate • BSN to Master's

The University Independent Roman Catholic comprehensive coed institution. Founded: 1831. *Primary accreditation:* regional. *Setting:* 100-acre suburban campus. *Total enrollment:* 6,127.

The Department of Nursing Founded in 1978. *Nursing program faculty:* 12 (40% with doctorates).

Academic Facilities *Campus library:* 350,000 volumes (8,360 in health, 1,160 in nursing); 1,500 periodical subscriptions (100 health-care related). *Nursing school resources:* CAI, computer lab, nursing audiovisuals, interactive nursing skills videos, learning resource lab.

Student Life *Student services:* health clinic, personal counseling, career counseling, institutionally sponsored work-study program, job placement, campus safety program, special assistance for disabled students. *International student services:* counseling/support, ESL courses. *Nursing student activities:* nursing club, student nurses association, Nursing Honor Society.

Calendar Semesters.

NURSING STUDENT PROFILE

Undergraduate **Enrollment:** 155
Women: 94%; **Men:** 6%; **Minority:** 9%; **Part-time:** 39%
Graduate **Enrollment:** 12
Women: 100%; **Minority:** 8%; **Part-time:** 100%

BACCALAUREATE PROGRAMS

Contact Ms. Marilyn Gomez, Coordinator of Nursing Student Services, Department of Nursing, Xavier University, 3800 Victory Parkway, Cincinnati, OH 45207-7351, 513-745-4392. *Fax:* 513-745-1087. *E-mail:* gomez@admin.xu.edu

Expenses *Tuition:* $12,950 full-time, $315 per semester credit part-time. *Full-time mandatory fees:* $13–$63. *Room and board:* $4640–$5850. *Room only:* $2220–$3290. *Books and supplies per academic year:* ranges from $400 to $750.

Financial Aid Institutionally sponsored need-based grants/scholarships, institutionally sponsored non-need grants/scholarships, Federal Direct Loans, Federal Nursing Student Loans, Federal Perkins Loans, Federal Supplemental Educational Opportunity Grants, Federal Work-Study. 52% of undergraduate students in nursing programs received some form of financial aid in 1995–96. *Application deadline:* 2/15.

Generic Baccalaureate Program (BSN)

Applying *Required:* SAT I, ACT, TOEFL for nonnative speakers of English, minimum high school GPA of 2.4, minimum college GPA of 2.5, 3 years of high school math, 3 years of high school science, high school chemistry, high school foreign language, high school transcript, written essay, transcript of college record. *Options:* Advanced standing available through the following means: advanced placement exams, advanced placement without credit. *Application deadline:* rolling. *Application fee:* $25.

Degree Requirements 132 total credit hours, 62 in nursing.

RN Baccalaureate Program (BSN)

Applying *Required:* minimum college GPA of 2.0, high school chemistry, RN license, diploma or AD in nursing, high school transcript, transcript of college record. *Options:* Advanced standing available through the following means: advanced placement exams, advanced placement without credit, credit by exam. *Application deadlines:* 8/1 (fall), 11/1 (spring). *Application fee:* $25.

Degree Requirements 120 total credit hours, 45 in nursing.

MASTER'S PROGRAM

Contact Ms. Marilyn Gomez, Coordinator of Nursing Student Services, Department of Nursing, Xavier University, 3800 Victory Parkway, Cincinnati, OH 45207-7351, 513-745-4392. *Fax:* 513-745-1087. *E-mail:* gomez@admin.xu.edu

Areas of Study Nursing administration.

Expenses *Tuition:* $357 per semester credit. *Part-time mandatory fees:* $13.

Financial Aid Graduate assistantships, Federal Direct Loans, institutionally sponsored need-based grants/scholarships. 25% of master's level students in nursing programs received some form of financial aid in 1995-96. *Application deadline:* 7/1.

BSN to Master's Program (MSN)

Applying *Required:* Miller Analogies Test, bachelor's degree in nursing, minimum GPA of 2.8, RN license, physical assessment course, statistics course, letter of recommendation, transcript of college record. *Application deadline:* rolling.

Degree Requirements 36 total credit hours, 33 in nursing. Graduate project.

YOUNGSTOWN STATE UNIVERSITY
College of Health and Human Services, Department of Nursing
Youngstown, Ohio

Programs • Generic Baccalaureate • RN Baccalaureate

The University State-supported comprehensive coed institution. Founded: 1908. *Primary accreditation:* regional. *Setting:* 127-acre urban campus. *Total enrollment:* 13,273.

The College of Health and Human Services, Department of Nursing Founded in 1967. *Nursing program faculty:* 24 (27% with doctorates).

Academic Facilities *Campus library:* 554,270 volumes (6,358 in health); 3,363 periodical subscriptions (313 health-care related). *Nursing school resources:* CAI, computer lab, nursing audiovisuals, interactive nursing skills videos, learning resource lab.

Student Life *Student services:* health clinic, personal counseling, career counseling, institutionally sponsored work-study program, job placement, campus safety program, special assistance for disabled students. *International student services:* counseling/support. *Nursing student activities:* Sigma Theta Tau, student nurses association.

Calendar Quarters.

NURSING STUDENT PROFILE

Undergraduate **Enrollment:** 271
Women: 90%; **Men:** 10%; **Minority:** 5%; **International:** 0%; **Part-time:** 22%

BACCALAUREATE PROGRAMS

Contact Ms. Michelle White, Academic Adviser, Dean's Office, College of Health and Human Services, Youngstown State University, 1 University Plaza, Youngstown, OH 44555, 330-742-1768. *Fax:* 330-742-2309. *E-mail:* amcast07@ysub.ysu.edu

Expenses *State resident tuition:* $3366 full-time, $90 per credit hour part-time. *Nonresident tuition:* ranges from $4986 to $7002 full-time, ranges from $45 to $101 per credit hour part-time. *Full-time mandatory fees:* $180. *Room and board:* $4200. *Books and supplies per academic year:* $630.

Financial Aid Institutionally sponsored need-based grants/scholarships, institutionally sponsored non-need grants/scholarships, Federal Supplemental Educational Opportunity Grants, Federal Work-Study. *Application deadline:* 7/1.

Generic Baccalaureate Program (BSN)

Applying *Required:* ACT, minimum college GPA of 2.0, 3 years of high school math, high school chemistry, high school transcript, transcript of college record, minimum 2.5 GPA in pre-nursing courses. *Options:* Advanced standing available through credit by exam. *Application deadline:* 9/1 (winter). *Application fee:* $20.

Degree Requirements 211 total credit hours, 116 in nursing.

RN Baccalaureate Program (BSN)

Applying *Required:* ACT, minimum college GPA of 2.0, 3 years of high school math, high school chemistry, RN license, diploma or AD in nursing, high school transcript, transcript of college record, CPR certification, minimum 2.5 GPA in prerequisite courses. 52 prerequisite credits must be completed before admission to the nursing program. *Options:* Course work may be accelerated. *Application deadline:* 3/15. *Application fee:* $20.

Degree Requirements 190 total credit hours, 97 in nursing.

OKLAHOMA

EAST CENTRAL UNIVERSITY
Department of Nursing
Ada, Oklahoma

Programs • Generic Baccalaureate • RN Baccalaureate

The University State-supported comprehensive coed institution. Part of Oklahoma State Regents for Higher Education. Founded: 1909. *Primary accreditation:* regional. *Setting:* 140-acre small-town campus. *Total enrollment:* 4,378.

The Department of Nursing Founded in 1974. *Nursing program faculty:* 11 (33% with doctorates). *Off-campus program site:* Ardmore.

Academic Facilities *Campus library:* 2,108 volumes (917 in nursing); 803 periodical subscriptions (91 health-care related). *Nursing school resources:* CAI, computer lab, nursing audiovisuals, interactive nursing skills videos, learning resource lab.

Student Life *Student services:* health clinic, child-care facilities, personal counseling, career counseling, institutionally sponsored work-study program, job placement, campus safety program, special assistance for disabled students. *International student services:* counseling/support. *Nursing student activities:* nursing club, student nurses association.

Calendar Semesters.

NURSING STUDENT PROFILE

Undergraduate **Enrollment:** 320
Women: 80%; **Men:** 20%; **Minority:** 20%; **International:** 0%; **Part-time:** 25%

BACCALAUREATE PROGRAMS

Contact Dr. Elizabeth Schmelling, Chair, Department of Nursing, East Central University, Ada, OK 74820, 405-332-8000 Ext. 434. *Fax:* 405-332-1623. *E-mail:* eschmlng@mailclerk.ecok.edu

Expenses *State resident tuition:* $1696 full-time, $644 per semester part-time. *Nonresident tuition:* ranges from $1832 to $2296 full-time, $132 per credit part-time. *Full-time mandatory fees:* $40–$55. *Room and board:* $2296. *Books and supplies per academic year:* ranges from $400 to $700.

Financial Aid Institutionally sponsored need-based grants/scholarships, institutionally sponsored non-need grants/scholarships, Federal Direct Loans, Federal Nursing Student Loans, Federal Perkins Loans, Federal Supplemental Educational Opportunity Grants, Federal Work-Study.

Generic Baccalaureate Program (BS)

Applying *Required:* SAT I or ACT, TOEFL for nonnative speakers of English, minimum college GPA of 2.5, 3 years of high school math, high school science, high school chemistry, high school biology, high school foreign language, high school transcript, transcript of college record, high school diploma or GED certificate, immunizations. *Options:* Advanced standing available through the following means: advanced placement exams, credit by exam. May apply for transfer of up to 60 total credits. *Application deadline:* 9/1.

Degree Requirements 124 total credit hours.

RN Baccalaureate Program (BS)

Applying *Required:* SAT I or ACT, TOEFL for nonnative speakers of English, minimum college GPA of 2.5, 3 years of high school math, high school science, high school chemistry, high school biology, RN license, diploma or AD in nursing, high school foreign language, high school transcript, 2 letters of recommendation, transcript of college record, immunizations. *Options:* Advanced standing available through the following means: advanced placement exams, credit by exam. May apply for transfer of up to 60 total credits. *Application deadlines:* 9/1, rolling.

Degree Requirements 127 total credit hours.

LANGSTON UNIVERSITY
School of Nursing
Langston, Oklahoma

Program • Generic Baccalaureate

The University State-supported comprehensive coed institution. Part of Oklahoma State Regents for Higher Education. Founded: 1897. *Primary accreditation:* regional. *Setting:* 40-acre rural campus. *Total enrollment:* 4,200.

The School of Nursing Founded in 1978.

Calendar Semesters.

BACCALAUREATE PROGRAM

Contact Secretary, 302 University Women Building, School of Nursing, Langston University, Langston, OK 73050, 405-466-3411. *Fax:* 405-466-2915.

NORTHEASTERN STATE UNIVERSITY
Department of Nursing
Tahlequah, Oklahoma

Program • RN Baccalaureate

The University State-supported comprehensive coed institution. Part of Oklahoma State Regents for Higher Education. Founded: 1846. *Primary accreditation:* regional. *Setting:* 160-acre small-town campus. *Total enrollment:* 9,273.

The Department of Nursing Founded in 1982. *Nursing program faculty:* 5 (20% with doctorates). *Off-campus program site:* Muskogee.

Academic Facilities *Campus library:* 300,000 volumes (5,200 in health, 2,351 in nursing); 3,400 periodical subscriptions (91 health-care related). *Nursing school resources:* computer lab, nursing audiovisuals, Internet.

Student Life *Student services:* health clinic, personal counseling, career counseling, institutionally sponsored work-study program, job placement, campus safety program, multicultural services, veteran's services, center for tribal studies. *International student services:* counseling/support, special assistance for nonnative speakers of English, literacy center. *Nursing student activities:* Sigma Theta Tau, student nurses association.

Calendar Semesters.

NURSING STUDENT PROFILE

Undergraduate **Enrollment:** 24
Women: 88%; **Men:** 12%; **Minority:** 38%; **International:** 0%; **Part-time:** 92%

BACCALAUREATE PROGRAM

Contact Dr. Joyce A. Van Nostrand, Department Head, Department of Nursing, Northeastern State University, Tahlequah, OK 74464-2399, 918-458-2087. *Fax:* 918-458-2325. *E-mail:* vannostr@cherokee.nsuok.edu

Expenses *State resident tuition:* $1336 full-time, $56 per credit hour part-time. *Nonresident tuition:* $3292 full-time, $137 per credit hour part-time. *Full-time mandatory fees:* $80–$100. *Room and board:* $1896–$3800. *Room only:* $1084–$1740. *Books and supplies per academic year:* ranges from $150 to $350.

Financial Aid Institutionally sponsored need-based grants/scholarships, institutionally sponsored non-need grants/scholarships, Federal Direct Loans, Federal Perkins Loans, Federal Supplemental Educational Opportunity Grants, Federal Work-Study, scholarship for a progressing junior. 17% of undergraduate students in nursing programs received some form of financial aid in 1995–96. *Application deadline:* 7/1.

RN Baccalaureate Program (BSN)

Applying *Required:* ACT, ACT PEP for diploma RNs, minimum college GPA of 2.0, RN license, diploma or AD in nursing, 3 letters of recommendation, transcript of college record, CPR certification, Purified Protein Derivative Test, immunizations, professional liability/malpractice insurance. 78 prerequisite credits must be completed before admission to the nursing program. *Options:* May apply for transfer of up to 64 total credits. *Application deadline:* 1/1.

Degree Requirements 124 total credit hours, 32 in nursing. Program completion within 5 years of start of first clinical nursing course.

NORTHWESTERN OKLAHOMA STATE UNIVERSITY
School of Nursing
Alva, Oklahoma

Programs • Generic Baccalaureate • RN Baccalaureate

The University State-supported comprehensive coed institution. Part of Oklahoma State Regents for Higher Education. Founded: 1897. *Primary accreditation:* regional. *Setting:* 70-acre small-town campus. *Total enrollment:* 1,861.

The School of Nursing Founded in 1981. *Nursing program faculty:* 7. *Off-campus program site:* Enid.

Academic Facilities *Campus library:* 118,000 volumes (700 in health, 350 in nursing); 1,500 periodical subscriptions (60 health-care related). *Nursing school resources:* CAI, computer lab, nursing audiovisuals.

Student Life *Student services:* health clinic, personal counseling, career counseling, institutionally sponsored work-study program, job placement, special assistance for disabled students. *International student services:* counseling/support. *Nursing student activities:* student nurses association.

Calendar Semesters.

NURSING STUDENT PROFILE

Undergraduate **Enrollment:** 61
Women: 86%; **Men:** 14%; **Minority:** 1%; **International:** 0%; **Part-time:** 23%

BACCALAUREATE PROGRAMS

Contact Mrs. Doris Ferguson, Dean, School of Nursing, Northwestern Oklahoma State University, 709 Oklahoma Boulevard, Alva, OK 73717-9898, 405-327-8489. *Fax:* 405-327-1881. *E-mail:* dlfergus@ranger1.nwalva.edu

Expenses *State resident tuition:* $6555 full-time, ranges from $53 to $67 per credit hour part-time. *Nonresident tuition:* $16,277 full-time, ranges from $135 to $162 per credit hour part-time. *Full-time mandatory fees:* $30. *Books and supplies per academic year:* ranges from $250 to $300.

Financial Aid Institutionally sponsored need-based grants/scholarships, institutionally sponsored non-need grants/scholarships, Federal Nursing Student Loans, Federal Pell Grants. *Application deadline:* 7/1.

Generic Baccalaureate Program (BSN)

Applying *Required:* ACT, TOEFL for nonnative speakers of English, minimum college GPA of 2.5, 3 years of high school math, 3 years of high school science, high school chemistry, high school biology, RN license, high school transcript, interview, 3 letters of recommendation, transcript of college record, health exam. 30 prerequisite credits must be completed before admission to the nursing program. *Application deadline:* 4/1. *Application fee:* $15.

Degree Requirements 124 total credit hours, 61 in nursing.

RN Baccalaureate Program (BSN)

Applying *Required:* ACT, TOEFL for nonnative speakers of English, minimum college GPA of 2.5, RN license, diploma or AD in nursing, 3 letters of recommendation, transcript of college record, health exam. *Options:* Advanced standing available through credit by exam. May apply for transfer of up to 56 total credits. *Application deadline:* 8/16.

Degree Requirements 124 total credit hours, 61 in nursing.

OKLAHOMA BAPTIST UNIVERSITY
School of Nursing
Shawnee, Oklahoma

Programs • Generic Baccalaureate • RN Baccalaureate

The University Independent Southern Baptist comprehensive coed institution. Founded: 1910. *Primary accreditation:* regional. *Setting:* 125-acre small-town campus. *Total enrollment:* 2,322.

The School of Nursing Founded in 1952.

Academic Facilities *Campus library:* 120,000 volumes; 750 periodical subscriptions.

Calendar Semesters.

BACCALAUREATE PROGRAMS

Contact Dean, School of Nursing, Oklahoma Baptist University, 500 West University, Shawnee, OK 74801, 405-275-2850. *Fax:* 405-878-2069.

Expenses *Tuition:* $6500 full-time, $200 per credit hour part-time.

Financial Aid Institutionally sponsored need-based grants/scholarships, institutionally sponsored non-need grants/scholarships, Federal Pell Grants, Federal Perkins Loans, Federal Supplemental Educational Opportunity Grants, Federal Work-Study, Federal PLUS Loans, Federal Stafford Loans, state aid. *Application deadline:* 3/1.

Generic Baccalaureate Program (BSN)

Applying *Required:* SAT I or ACT, high school transcript, interview, 2 letters of recommendation, written essay. *Application fee:* $25.

Degree Requirements 132–134 total credit hours dependent upon track, 65 in nursing.

RN Baccalaureate Program (BSN)

Applying *Required:* minimum college GPA of 2.0, RN license, diploma or AD in nursing, high school transcript, interview, 2 letters of recommendation, written essay, transcript of college record. *Application deadline:* rolling. *Application fee:* $25.

Degree Requirements 65 total credit hours in nursing.

OKLAHOMA CITY UNIVERSITY
Kramer School of Nursing
Oklahoma City, Oklahoma

Programs • Generic Baccalaureate • RN Baccalaureate

The University Independent United Methodist comprehensive coed institution. Founded: 1904. *Primary accreditation:* regional. *Setting:* 65-acre suburban campus. *Total enrollment:* 4,660.

The Kramer School of Nursing Founded in 1981. *Nursing program faculty:* 10 (10% with doctorates).

Academic Facilities *Campus library:* 640,067 volumes (519 in health, 398 in nursing); 600 periodical subscriptions (60 health-care related). *Nursing school resources:* CAI, computer lab, nursing audiovisuals, learning resource lab.

Student Life *Student services:* health clinic, personal counseling, career counseling, institutionally sponsored work-study program, job placement, special assistance for disabled students. *International student services:* counseling/support, special assistance for nonnative speakers of English, ESL courses. *Nursing student activities:* student nurses association, OCU Nursing Honor Society, Blue Key Organization.

Calendar Semesters.

NURSING STUDENT PROFILE

Undergraduate **Enrollment:** 90
Women: 93%; **Men:** 7%; **Minority:** 34%; **International:** 5%; **Part-time:** 3%

BACCALAUREATE PROGRAMS

Contact Ms. Janey Wheeler, Student Services Coordinator, Kramer School of Nursing, Oklahoma City University, 2501 North Blackwelder, Box 96B, Oklahoma City, OK 73106, 405-521-5900. *Fax:* 405-521-5914. *E-mail:* jwheeler@frodo.okcu.edu

Expenses *Tuition:* $4025 full-time, $270 per hour part-time. *Full-time mandatory fees:* $200–$400. *Room and board:* $3500. *Books and supplies per academic year:* ranges from $500 to $700.

Financial Aid Institutionally sponsored need-based grants/scholarships, institutionally sponsored non-need grants/scholarships, Federal Direct Loans, Federal Nursing Student Loans, Federal Pell Grants, Federal Perkins Loans, Federal Supplemental Educational Opportunity Grants, Federal Work-Study. *Application deadline:* 3/1.

Generic Baccalaureate Program (BSN)

Applying *Required:* ACT, TOEFL for nonnative speakers of English, minimum college GPA of 2.5, 3 years of high school math, 3 years of high school science, high school chemistry, high school biology, high school transcript, interview, 2 letters of recommendation, written essay, transcript of college record. 25 prerequisite credits must be completed before admission to the nursing program. *Options:* Advanced standing available through advanced placement exams. May apply for transfer of up to 90 total credits. *Application deadlines:* 3/1 (fall), 11/1 (spring). *Application fee:* $20.

Degree Requirements 124 total credit hours, 62 in nursing.

RN Baccalaureate Program (BSN)

Applying *Required:* minimum college GPA of 2.5, RN license, diploma or AD in nursing, 2 letters of recommendation, transcript of college record. 38 prerequisite credits must be completed before admission to the nursing program. *Options:* May apply for transfer of up to 90 total credits. *Application deadline:* rolling. *Application fee:* $20.

Degree Requirements 124 total credit hours, 62 in nursing.

ORAL ROBERTS UNIVERSITY
Anna Vaughn School of Nursing
Tulsa, Oklahoma

Program • Generic Baccalaureate

The University Independent interdenominational coed university. Founded: 1963. *Primary accreditation:* regional. *Setting:* 500-acre urban campus. *Total enrollment:* 3,682.

The Anna Vaughn School of Nursing Founded in 1975. *Nursing program faculty:* 7 (14% with doctorates).

Academic Facilities *Campus library:* 697,045 volumes (79,981 in health, 1,941 in nursing); 1,737 periodical subscriptions (169 health-care related).

Student Life *Student services:* health clinic, career counseling. *Nursing student activities:* Sigma Theta Tau.

Calendar Semesters.

BACCALAUREATE PROGRAM

Contact Dr. Kenda Jezek, Dean, Anna Vaughn School of Nursing, Oral Roberts University, 7777 South Lewis Avenue, Tulsa, OK 74171, 918-495-6198. *Fax:* 918-495-6033.

Expenses *Tuition:* $9392 full-time, $398 per credit part-time.

Financial Aid Institutionally sponsored need-based grants/scholarships, institutionally sponsored non-need grants/scholarships, Federal Pell Grants, Federal Perkins Loans, Federal Supplemental Educational Opportunity Grants, Federal Work-Study, Federal PLUS Loans, Federal Stafford Loans, state aid. *Application deadline:* 3/31.

Generic Baccalaureate Program (BSN)

Applying *Required:* SAT I or ACT, TOEFL for nonnative speakers of English, minimum college GPA of 2.6, high school chemistry, high school biology, high school transcript, letter of recommendation, transcript of college record. *Options:* Advanced standing available through the following means: advanced placement exams, credit by exam. *Application deadline:* rolling.

Degree Requirements 130 total credit hours, 48 in nursing.

SOUTHERN NAZARENE UNIVERSITY
School of Nursing
Bethany, Oklahoma

Programs • Generic Baccalaureate • RN Baccalaureate • LPN to Baccalaureate

The University Independent Nazarene comprehensive coed institution. Founded: 1899. *Primary accreditation:* regional. *Setting:* 40-acre suburban campus. *Total enrollment:* 1,834.

The School of Nursing Founded in 1980. *Nursing program faculty:* 5 (20% with doctorates).

Academic Facilities *Campus library:* 168,247 volumes (1,737 in nursing); 602 periodical subscriptions (48 health-care related). *Nursing school resources:* CAI, computer lab, nursing audiovisuals, learning resource lab.

Student Life *Student services:* health clinic, personal counseling, career counseling, institutionally sponsored work-study program, job placement, special assistance for disabled students. *International student services:* counseling/support, special assistance for nonnative speakers of English. *Nursing student activities:* nursing club, student nurses association, honor society.

Calendar Semesters.

NURSING STUDENT PROFILE

Undergraduate **Enrollment:** 100
Women: 94%; **Men:** 6%; **Minority:** 9%; **International:** 0%; **Part-time:** 17%

BACCALAUREATE PROGRAMS

Contact Donna J. Eckhart, Chair and Professor, School of Nursing, Southern Nazarene University, 6729 Northwest 39th Expressway, Bethany, OK 73008, 405-491-6365. *Fax:* 405-491-6355.

Expenses *Tuition:* $7332 full-time, $241 per credit hour part-time. *Full-time mandatory fees:* $348–$518. *Room and board:* $2006. *Room only:* $1896. *Books and supplies per academic year:* $600.

Financial Aid Institutionally sponsored need-based grants/scholarships, institutionally sponsored non-need grants/scholarships, Federal Nursing Student Loans, Federal Pell Grants, Federal Perkins Loans, Federal Supplemental Educational Opportunity Grants, Federal Work-Study. 75% of undergraduate students in nursing programs received some form of financial aid in 1995–96. *Application deadline:* 3/1.

Generic Baccalaureate Program (BS)

Applying *Required:* SAT I, ACT, TOEFL for nonnative speakers of English, minimum college GPA of 2.5, high school transcript, interview, 3 letters of recommendation, written essay, transcript of college record. 38 prerequisite credits must be completed before admission to the nursing program. *Options:* Advanced standing available through the following means: advanced placement exams, credit by exam. May apply for transfer of up to 64 total credits. *Application deadline:* 3/1. *Application fee:* $25.

Degree Requirements 125 total credit hours, 56 in nursing.

RN Baccalaureate Program (BS)

Applying *Required:* SAT I, ACT, NLN Mobility Profile II, minimum college GPA of 2.5, RN license, diploma or AD in nursing, interview, transcript of college record. 38 prerequisite credits must be completed before admission to the nursing program. *Options:* Advanced standing available through the following means: advanced placement exams, credit by exam. May apply for transfer of up to 64 total credits. *Application deadline:* 3/1. *Application fee:* $25.

Degree Requirements 125 total credit hours, 56 in nursing.

LPN to Baccalaureate Program (BS)

Applying *Required:* SAT I, ACT, school-based challenge exams, minimum college GPA of 2.5, high school transcript, interview, 3 letters of recommendation, written essay, transcript of college record, LPN license, LPN transcript. 38 prerequisite credits must be completed before admission to the nursing program. *Options:* Advanced standing available through the following means: advanced placement exams, credit by exam. May apply for transfer of up to 64 total credits. *Application deadline:* 3/1. *Application fee:* $25.

Degree Requirements 125 total credit hours, 56 in nursing.

SOUTHWESTERN OKLAHOMA STATE UNIVERSITY
Division of Nursing
Weatherford, Oklahoma

Programs • Generic Baccalaureate • RN Baccalaureate

The University State-supported comprehensive coed institution. Part of Southwestern Oklahoma State University. Founded: 1901. *Primary accreditation:* regional. *Setting:* 73-acre small-town campus. *Total enrollment:* 4,623.

The Division of Nursing Founded in 1976. *Nursing program faculty:* 9.

Southwestern Oklahoma State University (continued)

Academic Facilities *Campus library:* 244,923 volumes (16,369 in health, 625 in nursing); 1,519 periodical subscriptions (296 health-care related). *Nursing school resources:* computer lab, nursing audiovisuals, interactive nursing skills videos, learning resource lab.

Student Life *Student services:* health clinic, child-care facilities, career counseling, institutionally sponsored work-study program. *Nursing student activities:* student nurses association.

Calendar Semesters.

NURSING STUDENT PROFILE

Undergraduate **Enrollment:** 80

Women: 92%; **Men:** 8%; **International:** 0%

BACCALAUREATE PROGRAMS

Contact Dr. Patricia Meyer, Chair, Division of Nursing, Southwestern Oklahoma State University, 100 Campus Drive, Weatherford, OK 73096-3098, 405-772-3261. *Fax:* 405-774-3795.

Expenses *State resident tuition:* $1688 per academic year. *Nonresident tuition:* $4219 per academic year. *Full-time mandatory fees:* $9. *Room and board:* $1992–$2560.

Financial Aid Institutionally sponsored long-term loans, Federal Nursing Student Loans, Federal Supplemental Educational Opportunity Grants, Federal Work-Study.

Generic Baccalaureate Program (BSN)

Applying *Required:* SAT I, ACT, TOEFL for nonnative speakers of English, minimum college GPA of 2.25, interview, 3 letters of recommendation, transcript of college record. 69 prerequisite credits must be completed before admission to the nursing program. *Options:* Advanced standing available through credit by exam. May apply for transfer of up to 64 total credits. *Application deadline:* 2/1.

Degree Requirements 124–125 total credit hours dependent upon track, 53 in nursing.

RN Baccalaureate Program (BSN)

Applying *Required:* minimum college GPA of 2.25, RN license, diploma or AD in nursing, high school transcript, interview, 3 letters of recommendation, transcript of college record. *Options:* Advanced standing available through the following means: advanced placement exams, credit by exam. Course work may be accelerated. May apply for transfer of up to 64 total credits. *Application deadline:* 3/1 (summer).

Degree Requirements 124–129 total credit hours dependent upon track, 53 in nursing.

UNIVERSITY OF CENTRAL OKLAHOMA

Department of Nursing
Edmond, Oklahoma

Programs • Generic Baccalaureate • RN Baccalaureate • LPN to Baccalaureate

The University State-supported comprehensive coed institution. Part of Oklahoma State Regents for Higher Education. Founded: 1890. *Primary accreditation:* regional. *Setting:* 200-acre suburban campus. *Total enrollment:* 15,334.

The Department of Nursing Founded in 1968. *Nursing program faculty:* 14 (14% with doctorates).

Academic Facilities *Campus library:* 850,000 volumes; 3,000 periodical subscriptions. *Nursing school resources:* CAI, computer lab, nursing audiovisuals, interactive nursing skills videos, learning resource lab.

Student Life *Student services:* health clinic, child-care facilities, personal counseling, career counseling, institutionally sponsored work-study program, job placement, campus safety program, special assistance for disabled students. *International student services:* counseling/support, special assistance for nonnative speakers of English. *Nursing student activities:* Sigma Theta Tau, student nurses association.

Calendar Semesters.

NURSING STUDENT PROFILE

Undergraduate **Enrollment:** 185

Women: 93%; **Men:** 7%; **Minority:** 10%; **International:** 2%; **Part-time:** 0%

BACCALAUREATE PROGRAMS

Contact Dr. Patricia LaGrow, Chairperson, Department of Nursing, University of Central Oklahoma, 100 North University Drive, Edmond, OK 73034-5209, 405-341-2980 Ext. 5000. *Fax:* 405-330-3824.

Expenses *State resident tuition:* $1400 per academic year. *Nonresident tuition:* $3352 per academic year. *Full-time mandatory fees:* $600–$650. *Room and board:* $2100–$3200. *Books and supplies per academic year:* ranges from $550 to $600.

Financial Aid Institutionally sponsored need-based grants/scholarships, institutionally sponsored non-need grants/scholarships, Federal Nursing Student Loans, Federal Work-Study.

Generic Baccalaureate Program (BSN)

Applying *Required:* SAT I, ACT, TOEFL for nonnative speakers of English, minimum college GPA of 2.75, 3 years of high school math, high school chemistry, high school biology, high school transcript, 3 letters of recommendation, written essay, transcript of college record. 64 prerequisite credits must be completed before admission to the nursing program. *Options:* May apply for transfer of up to 60 total credits. *Application deadline:* 1/15.

Degree Requirements 124 total credit hours, 48–56 in nursing.

RN Baccalaureate Program (BSN)

Applying *Required:* SAT I, ACT, TOEFL for nonnative speakers of English, 3 years of high school math, high school chemistry, high school biology, RN license, diploma or AD in nursing, high school transcript, 3 letters of recommendation, transcript of college record. 64 prerequisite credits must be completed before admission to the nursing program. *Options:* Course work may be accelerated. May apply for transfer of up to 60 total credits. *Application deadlines:* 1/15 (fall), 10/15 (spring).

Degree Requirements 124 total credit hours, 48–56 in nursing.

LPN to Baccalaureate Program (BSN)

Applying *Required:* SAT I, ACT, TOEFL for nonnative speakers of English, minimum college GPA of 2.75, high school math, high school chemistry, high school biology, 3 letters of recommendation, transcript of college record, LPN license. 64 prerequisite credits must be completed before admission to the nursing program. *Options:* Course work may be accelerated. May apply for transfer of up to 60 total credits. *Application deadlines:* 1/15 (fall), 10/15 (spring).

Degree Requirements 124 total credit hours, 48–56 in nursing.

UNIVERSITY OF OKLAHOMA HEALTH SCIENCES CENTER

College of Nursing
Oklahoma City, Oklahoma

Programs • Generic Baccalaureate • RN Baccalaureate • LPN to Baccalaureate • MS • Master's for Nurses with Non-Nursing Degrees • Continuing Education

The University State-supported upper-level coed institution. Part of University of Oklahoma. Founded: 1890. *Primary accreditation:* regional. *Setting:* 200-acre urban campus. *Total enrollment:* 2,960.

The College of Nursing Founded in 1911. *Nursing program faculty:* 52 (48% with doctorates). *Off-campus program sites:* Tulsa, Claremore.

Academic Facilities *Campus library:* 212,965 volumes (181,020 in health, 31,945 in nursing); 2,500 periodical subscriptions (2,500 health-care related). *Nursing school resources:* CAI, computer lab, nursing audiovisuals, interactive nursing skills videos, learning resource lab.

Student Life *Student services:* health clinic, child-care facilities, personal counseling, career counseling, institutionally sponsored work-study program, campus safety program, special assistance for disabled students.

International student services: counseling/support. *Nursing student activities:* Sigma Theta Tau, nursing club, student nurses association.

Calendar Semesters.

NURSING STUDENT PROFILE

Undergraduate **Enrollment:** 293

Women: 84%; **Men:** 16%; **Minority:** 23%; **International:** 0%; **Part-time:** 24%

Graduate **Enrollment:** 215

Women: 98%; **Men:** 2%; **Minority:** 11%; **International:** 0%; **Part-time:** 80%

BACCALAUREATE PROGRAMS

Contact Dr. Patricia Dolphin, Assistant Dean for Public and Support Services, College of Nursing, University of Oklahoma, PO Box 26901, Oklahoma City, OK 73190, 405-271-2125. *Fax:* 405-271-3443.

Expenses *State resident tuition:* $3700 full-time, $1850 per academic year part-time. *Nonresident tuition:* $5846 full-time, $2923 per academic year part-time. *Full-time mandatory fees:* $125–$300. *Part-time mandatory fees:* $100–$275. *Books and supplies per academic year:* ranges from $650 to $1500.

Financial Aid Institutionally sponsored need-based grants/scholarships, institutionally sponsored non-need grants/scholarships, Federal Nursing Student Loans, Federal Supplemental Educational Opportunity Grants, Federal Work-Study. 69% of undergraduate students in nursing programs received some form of financial aid in 1995–96. *Application deadline:* 3/1.

Generic Baccalaureate Program (BSN)

Applying *Required:* TOEFL for nonnative speakers of English, minimum college GPA of 2.5, written essay, transcript of college record. 67 prerequisite credits must be completed before admission to the nursing program. *Options:* May apply for transfer of up to 67 total credits. *Application deadline:* 1/15. *Application fee:* $50.

Degree Requirements 127 total credit hours, 60 in nursing.

RN Baccalaureate Program (BSN)

Applying *Required:* TOEFL for nonnative speakers of English, NLN Mobility Profile II, minimum college GPA of 2.5, RN license, diploma or AD in nursing, written essay, transcript of college record. 67 prerequisite credits must be completed before admission to the nursing program. *Options:* Advanced standing available through the following means: advanced placement exams, advanced placement without credit. Course work may be accelerated. May apply for transfer of up to 67 total credits. *Application deadline:* 1/15. *Application fee:* $50.

Degree Requirements 127 total credit hours, 60 in nursing.

LPN to Baccalaureate Program (BSN)

Applying *Required:* TOEFL for nonnative speakers of English, NLN Mobility Profile II, minimum college GPA of 2.5, written essay, transcript of college record, LPN license. 67 prerequisite credits must be completed before admission to the nursing program. *Options:* Advanced standing available through the following means: advanced placement exams, advanced placement without credit. Course work may be accelerated. May apply for transfer of up to 67 total credits. *Application deadline:* 1/15. *Application fee:* $50.

Degree Requirements 127 total credit hours, 60 in nursing.

MASTER'S PROGRAMS

Contact Dr. Patricia Dolphin, Assistant Dean for Public and Support Services, College of Nursing, University of Oklahoma, PO Box 26901, Oklahoma City, OK 73190, 405-271-2125. *Fax:* 405-271-3443.

Areas of Study Clinical nurse specialist programs in community health nursing, family health nursing, gerontological nursing, maternity-newborn nursing, medical-surgical nursing, pediatric nursing, psychiatric–mental health nursing; nursing administration; nursing education; nurse practitioner programs in child care/pediatrics, family health.

Expenses *State resident tuition:* $1604 full-time, $882 per academic year part-time. *Nonresident tuition:* $4486 full-time, $2582 per academic year part-time. *Full-time mandatory fees:* $140–$400. *Part-time mandatory fees:* $100–$300. *Books and supplies per academic year:* ranges from $650 to $1500.

Financial Aid Graduate assistantships, nurse traineeships, Federal Nursing Student Loans, employment opportunities. 26% of master's level students in nursing programs received some form of financial aid in 1995-96. *Application deadline:* 3/1.

MS Program

Applying *Required:* bachelor's degree in nursing, minimum GPA of 3.0, RN license, 2 years of clinical experience, statistics course, professional liability/malpractice insurance, 3 letters of recommendation, transcript of college record. *Application deadlines:* 6/1 (fall), 11/1 (spring), 4/1 (summer). *Application fee:* $50.

Degree Requirements 45 total credit hours, 35–39 in nursing, 6–10 in other specified areas. Thesis or comprehensive exam.

Master's for Nurses with Non-Nursing Degrees Program (MS)

Applying *Required:* TOEFL for nonnative speakers of English, bachelor's degree, minimum GPA of 3.0, RN license, 2 years of clinical experience, statistics course, professional liability/malpractice insurance, 3 letters of recommendation, transcript of college record. *Application deadlines:* 6/1 (fall), 11/1 (spring), 4/1 (summer). *Application fee:* $50.

Degree Requirements 59 total credit hours, 49–53 in nursing, 6–10 in other specified areas. Thesis or comprehensive exam.

CONTINUING EDUCATION PROGRAM

Contact Dr. Patricia Dolphin, Assistant Dean for Public and Support Services, College of Nursing, University of Oklahoma, PO Box 26901, Oklahoma City, OK 73190, 405-271-2125. *Fax:* 405-271-3443. *E-mail:* patricia-dolphin@uokhsc.edu

UNIVERSITY OF TULSA
School of Nursing
Tulsa, Oklahoma

Programs • Generic Baccalaureate • RN Baccalaureate

The University Independent coed university, affiliated with Presbyterian Church. Founded: 1894. *Primary accreditation:* regional. *Setting:* 100-acre urban campus. *Total enrollment:* 4,386.

The School of Nursing Founded in 1968. *Nursing program faculty:* 13 (30% with doctorates).

Academic Facilities *Campus library:* 632,145 volumes (4,300 in nursing); 2,700 periodical subscriptions (118 health-care related). *Nursing school resources:* CAI, computer lab, nursing audiovisuals, interactive nursing skills videos, learning resource lab.

Student Life *Student services:* health clinic, child-care facilities, personal counseling, career counseling, institutionally sponsored work-study program, job placement, campus safety program, special assistance for disabled students. *International student services:* counseling/support, special assistance for nonnative speakers of English, ESL courses. *Nursing student activities:* Sigma Theta Tau, student nurses association.

Calendar Semesters.

NURSING STUDENT PROFILE

Undergraduate **Enrollment:** 109

Women: 95%; **Men:** 5%; **Minority:** 18%; **Part-time:** 3%

BACCALAUREATE PROGRAMS

Contact Dr. Susan Gaston, Director, School of Nursing, University of Tulsa, 600 South College Avenue, Tulsa, OK 74104-3189, 918-631-3116. *Fax:* 918-631-2068. *E-mail:* gastonsk@centum.utulsa.edu

Expenses *Tuition:* $12,850 full-time, $460 per credit hour part-time. *Full-time mandatory fees:* $18–$60. *Room and board:* $3920–$5450. *Room only:* $2160–$3250. *Books and supplies per academic year:* ranges from $800 to $1200.

Financial Aid Institutionally sponsored need-based grants/scholarships, institutionally sponsored non-need grants/scholarships, Federal Direct Loans, Federal Perkins Loans, Federal Work-Study. *Application deadline:* 2/1.

Generic Baccalaureate Program (BSN)

Applying *Required:* SAT I or ACT, minimum college GPA of 2.5, high school transcript, written essay, transcript of college record. 17 prerequisite credits must be completed before admission to the nursing program. *Options:* Course work may be accelerated. May apply for transfer of up to 62 total credits. *Application deadline:* rolling. *Application fee:* $25.

Degree Requirements 124 total credit hours, 61 in nursing.

RN Baccalaureate Program (BSN)

Applying *Required:* minimum college GPA of 2.5, RN license, diploma or AD in nursing, high school transcript, written essay, transcript of college record. 17 prerequisite credits must be completed before admission to

University of Tulsa (continued)

the nursing program. *Options:* Advanced standing available through advanced placement exams. Course work may be accelerated. May apply for transfer of up to 62 total credits. *Application deadline:* rolling. *Application fee:* $25.

Degree Requirements 124 total credit hours, 61 in nursing.

OREGON

LINFIELD COLLEGE

Linfield-Good Samaritan School of Nursing
Portland, Oregon

Programs • Generic Baccalaureate • RN Baccalaureate • Continuing Education

The College Independent American Baptist 4-year coed college. Founded: 1849. *Primary accreditation:* regional. *Setting:* 110-acre small-town campus. *Total enrollment:* 1,588.

The Linfield-Good Samaritan School of Nursing Founded in 1983. *Nursing program faculty:* 20 (30% with doctorates).

Academic Facilities *Campus library:* 145,772 volumes (7,028 in health, 1,368 in nursing); 1,309 periodical subscriptions (325 health-care related). *Nursing school resources:* CAI, computer lab, nursing audiovisuals, interactive nursing skills videos, learning resource lab.

Student Life *Student services:* health clinic, personal counseling, career counseling, institutionally sponsored work-study program, job placement, campus safety program, special assistance for disabled students, tutoring, writing lab. *Nursing student activities:* Sigma Theta Tau, nursing club, student nurses association.

Calendar Semesters.

NURSING STUDENT PROFILE

Undergraduate **Enrollment:** 322

Women: 92%; **Men:** 8%; **Minority:** 11%; **International:** 1%; **Part-time:** 4%

BACCALAUREATE PROGRAMS

Contact Ms. Barbara Kuzio, Director, Enrollment Services, Linfield College-Portland Campus, 2215 Northwest Northrup Street, Portland, OR 97210, 503-413-8481. *Fax:* 503-413-6283. *E-mail:* bkuzio@linfield.edu

Expenses *Tuition:* $14,976 full-time, $468 per credit part-time. *Full-time mandatory fees:* $110–$338. *Room only:* $1816. *Books and supplies per academic year:* ranges from $400 to $800.

Financial Aid Institutionally sponsored need-based grants/scholarships, institutionally sponsored non-need grants/scholarships, Federal Nursing Student Loans, Federal Perkins Loans, Federal Supplemental Educational Opportunity Grants, Federal Work-Study, state need grants. 99% of undergraduate students in nursing programs received some form of financial aid in 1995–96. *Application deadline:* 8/30.

Generic Baccalaureate Program (BSN)

Applying *Required:* SAT I, ACT, TOEFL for nonnative speakers of English, minimum college GPA of 2.5, 3 years of high school math, 3 years of high school science, high school transcript, 2 letters of recommendation, written essay, transcript of college record. *Options:* May apply for transfer of up to 69 total credits. *Application deadlines:* 2/15 (fall), 3/1 (transfers). *Application fee:* $40.

Degree Requirements 133 total credit hours, 57 in nursing. Computer proficiency.

RN Baccalaureate Program (BSN)

Applying *Required:* NLN Mobility Profile II, minimum college GPA of 2.5, RN license, diploma or AD in nursing, 2 letters of recommendation, written essay, transcript of college record. *Options:* May apply for transfer of up to 65 total credits. *Application fee:* $40.

Degree Requirements 133 total credit hours, 57 in nursing. 30 semester credits must be completed at Linfield College.

CONTINUING EDUCATION PROGRAM

Contact Dr. Pamela Harris, Dean, School of Nursing, Linfield College, 2255 Northwest Northrup Street, Portland, OR 97210, 503-413-7163. *Fax:* 503-413-6846.

OREGON HEALTH SCIENCES UNIVERSITY

School of Nursing
Portland, Oregon

Programs • Generic Baccalaureate • RN Baccalaureate • MS/MN • RN to Master's • MS/MN/MPH • Post-Master's • PhD • Postdoctoral

The University State-related upper-level specialized coed institution. Part of Oregon State System of Higher Education. Founded: 1974. *Primary accreditation:* regional. *Setting:* 116-acre urban campus. *Total enrollment:* 1,771.

The School of Nursing Founded in 1926. *Nursing program faculty:* 173. *Off-campus program sites:* La Grande, Klamath Falls, Ashland.

Academic Facilities *Campus library:* 226,919 volumes (219,253 in health, 7,666 in nursing); 2,357 periodical subscriptions (2,357 health-care related). *Nursing school resources:* CAI, computer lab, nursing audiovisuals, interactive nursing skills videos, learning resource lab.

Student Life *Student services:* health clinic, child-care facilities, personal counseling, institutionally sponsored work-study program, campus safety program, special assistance for disabled students. *Nursing student activities:* Sigma Theta Tau, student nurses association.

Calendar Quarters.

NURSING STUDENT PROFILE

Undergraduate **Enrollment:** 490

Women: 87%; **Men:** 13%; **Minority:** 8%; **International:** 1%; **Part-time:** 31%

Graduate **Enrollment:** 245

Women: 92%; **Men:** 8%; **Minority:** 8%; **International:** 4%; **Part-time:** 38%

BACCALAUREATE PROGRAMS

Contact Office of Recruitment, Oregon Health Sciences University, 3181 Sam Jackson Park Road, Portland, OR 97201-3098, 503-494-7725. *Fax:* 503-494-4350. *E-mail:* proginfo@ohsu.edu

Expenses *State resident tuition:* ranges from $4428 to $6832 full-time, ranges from $190 to $315 per credit part-time. *Nonresident tuition:* ranges from $11,320 to $13,036 full-time, ranges from $190 to $315 per credit part-time. *Full-time mandatory fees:* $858.

Financial Aid Institutionally sponsored need-based grants/scholarships, Federal Nursing Student Loans, Federal Supplemental Educational Opportunity Grants, Federal Work-Study. *Application deadline:* 3/1.

Generic Baccalaureate Program (BS)

Applying *Required:* SAT I, minimum college GPA of 2.5, high school transcript, written essay, transcript of college record, computer skills. 91 prerequisite credits must be completed before admission to the nursing program. *Application deadline:* 2/15. *Application fee:* $40.

Degree Requirements 186 total credit hours, 95 in nursing.

RN Baccalaureate Program (BS)

Applying *Required:* SAT I, RN license, diploma or AD in nursing, high school transcript, transcript of college record. *Options:* May apply for transfer of up to 108 total credits. *Application deadline:* 2/15. *Application fee:* $40.

Degree Requirements 186 total credit hours, 93 in nursing.

MASTER'S PROGRAMS

Contact Office of Recruitment, Oregon Health Sciences University, 3181 Sam Jackson Park Road, Portland, OR 97201-3098, 503-494-7725. *Fax:* 503-494-4350. *E-mail:* proginfo@ohsu.edu

Areas of Study Clinical nurse specialist programs in adult health nursing, community health nursing, gerontological nursing, medical-surgical nursing, pediatric nursing, psychiatric–mental health nursing, public health nursing, women's health nursing; nurse midwifery; nurse practitioner programs in adult health, child care/pediatrics, family health, primary care, psychiatric–mental health, women's health.

Expenses *State resident tuition:* ranges from $4448 to $6832 full-time, ranges from $190 to $315 per credit part-time. *Nonresident tuition:* ranges from $11,320 to $13,036 full-time, ranges from $190 to $315 per credit part-time. *Full-time mandatory fees:* $1491.

Financial Aid Graduate assistantships, nurse traineeships, Federal Nursing Student Loans, institutionally sponsored loans, employment opportunities. *Application deadline:* 3/1.

MS/MN Program

Applying *Required:* GRE General Test, bachelor's degree in nursing, minimum GPA of 3.0, RN license, 1 year of clinical experience, physical assessment course, statistics course, essay, 3 letters of recommendation, transcript of college record. *Application deadline:* 1/15. *Application fee:* $40.

Degree Requirements 45 total credit hours, 39–42 in nursing. Research project (MS), additional clinical experience (MN).

RN to Master's Program (MS/MN)

Applying *Required:* GRE General Test, minimum GPA of 3.0, RN license, 1 year of clinical experience, physical assessment course, statistics course, essay, 3 letters of recommendation, transcript of college record. *Application deadline:* 1/15.

Degree Requirements 229–244 total credit hours dependent upon track, 130–135 in nursing. Research project (MS), additional clinical experience (MN).

MS/MN/MPH Program

Applying *Required:* GRE General Test, bachelor's degree in nursing, minimum GPA of 3.0, RN license, 1 year of clinical experience, physical assessment course, statistics course, essay, 3 letters of recommendation, transcript of college record. *Application deadline:* 1/15. *Application fee:* $40.

Degree Requirements 45 total credit hours, 39–42 in nursing, 3–6 in public health. Research project (MS), additional clinical experience (MN).

Post-Master's Program

Applying *Required:* minimum GPA of 3.0, RN license, essay, 3 letters of recommendation, transcript of college record. *Application deadline:* 1/15. *Application fee:* $40.

Degree Requirements 40–50 total credit hours dependent upon track, 40–50 in nursing.

DOCTORAL PROGRAM

Contact Office of Recruitment, Oregon Health Sciences University, 3181 Sam Jackson Park Road, Portland, OR 97201-3098, 503-494-7725. *Fax:* 503-494-4350. *E-mail:* proginfo@ohsu.edu

Areas of Study Nursing research, gerontology, families in health, illness and transition.

Expenses *State resident tuition:* $190 per credit. *Nonresident tuition:* $315 per credit. *Full-time mandatory fees:* $1491.

Financial Aid Graduate assistantships, fellowships, institutionally sponsored loans, opportunities for employment. *Application deadline:* 1/15.

PhD Program

Applying *Required:* GRE General Test, master's degree in nursing, 1 scholarly paper, statistics course, interview, 3 letters of recommendation, vitae, writing sample, competitive review by faculty committee, minimum 3.5 graduate GPA. *Application deadline:* 1/15. *Application fee:* $45.

Degree Requirements 90 total credit hours; dissertation; oral exam; written exam; defense of dissertation.

POSTDOCTORAL PROGRAM

Contact Ms. Virginia Tildern, Associate Dean of Research, Development, and Utilization, School of Nursing, Oregon Health Sciences University, 3181 Southwest Sam Jackson Park Road, Portland, OR 97201, 503-494-3857. *E-mail:* tildernu@ohsu.edu

Areas of Study Gerontological nursing; families in health, illness, and transition.

UNIVERSITY OF PORTLAND
School of Nursing
Portland, Oregon

Programs • Generic Baccalaureate • RN Baccalaureate • BSN to Master's • RN to Master's

The University Independent Roman Catholic comprehensive coed institution. Founded: 1901. *Primary accreditation:* regional. *Setting:* 95-acre suburban campus. *Total enrollment:* 2,331.

The School of Nursing Founded in 1934. *Nursing program faculty:* 34 (53% with doctorates).

Academic Facilities *Campus library:* 350,000 volumes (3,950 in health, 1,000 in nursing); 5,784 periodical subscriptions (141 health-care related). *Nursing school resources:* CAI, computer lab, nursing audiovisuals, interactive nursing skills videos, learning resource lab.

Student Life *Student services:* health clinic, personal counseling, career counseling, institutionally sponsored work-study program, job placement, campus safety program, special assistance for disabled students, adult student programs. *International student services:* counseling/support, special assistance for nonnative speakers of English, ESL courses. *Nursing student activities:* student nurses association, School of Nursing honor society.

Calendar Semesters.

NURSING STUDENT PROFILE

Undergraduate
Women: 89%; **Men:** 11%; **Minority:** 4%; **International:** 1%; **Part-time:** 9%
Graduate **Enrollment:** 69
Women: 99%; **Men:** 1%; **Minority:** 3%; **International:** 38%; **Part-time:** 7%

BACCALAUREATE PROGRAMS

Contact Mr. Daniel Reilly, Director, Admissions Office, School of Nursing, University of Portland, 5000 North Willamette Boulevard, Portland, OR 97203-5798, 503-283-7147. *Fax:* 503-283-7399.

Expenses *Tuition:* $14,300 full-time, $455 per semester credit hour part-time. *Full-time mandatory fees:* $40–$110. *Room and board:* $4380–$4610. *Books and supplies per academic year:* ranges from $250 to $500.

Financial Aid Institutionally sponsored need-based grants/scholarships, institutionally sponsored non-need grants/scholarships, Federal Nursing Student Loans, Federal Supplemental Educational Opportunity Grants, Federal Work-Study. *Application deadline:* 3/15.

Generic Baccalaureate Program (BSN)

Applying *Required:* SAT I or ACT, College Board Achievements, TOEFL for nonnative speakers of English, high school chemistry, high school transcript, written essay. 63 prerequisite credits must be completed before admission to the nursing program. *Application deadline:* 2/15. *Application fee:* $40.

Degree Requirements 130 total credit hours, 72 in nursing.

RN Baccalaureate Program (BSN)

Applying *Required:* NLN Mobility Profile Exams, minimum college GPA of 2.5, RN license. 55 prerequisite credits must be completed before admission to the nursing program. *Application deadline:* rolling. *Application fee:* $40.

Degree Requirements 130 total credit hours, 69 in nursing.

MASTER'S PROGRAMS

Contact Dr. Karl Wetzel, Dean, Graduate School, School of Nursing, University of Portland, 5000 North Willamette Boulevard, Portland, OR 97203-5798, 503-283-7107. *Fax:* 503-283-7399. *E-mail:* wetzel@uofport.edu

Areas of Study Clinical nurse specialist program in community health nursing; nurse practitioner program in adult health.

Expenses *Tuition:* $295 per summer semester hours. *Full-time mandatory fees:* $40–$110. *Room only:* $1750.

Financial Aid Federal Nursing Student Loans. 13% of master's level students in nursing programs received some form of financial aid in 1995-96. *Application deadline:* 3/15.

BSN to Master's Program (MS)

Applying *Required:* GRE General Test, bachelor's degree in nursing, minimum GPA of 2.5, RN license, 1 year of clinical experience, statistics

University of Portland (continued)

course, essay, 3 letters of recommendation, transcript of college record, minimum 3.0 GPA in nursing major. *Application deadline:* 12/31 (summer). *Application fee:* $30.

Degree Requirements 39 total credit hours, 36 in nursing, 3 in advanced physiology.

RN to Master's Program (MS)

Applying *Required:* GRE General Test, NLN Mobility Profile II, minimum GPA of 3.0, RN license, 1 year of clinical experience, statistics course, transcript of college record. *Application deadline:* rolling. *Application fee:* $40.

Degree Requirements 169 total credit hours, 160 in nursing, 9 in advanced physiology, theology, philosophy.

PENNSYLVANIA

ALLEGHENY UNIVERSITY OF THE HEALTH SCIENCES
School of Nursing
Philadelphia, Pennsylvania

Programs • RN Baccalaureate • MSN • RN to Master's • Continuing Education

The University Independent coed university. Founded: 1848. *Primary accreditation:* regional. *Total enrollment:* 1,736.

The School of Nursing Founded in 1977. *Nursing program faculty:* 15 (74% with doctorates). *Off-campus program site:* Bethlehem.

Academic Facilities *Campus library:* 90,000 volumes (69,500 in health, 15,500 in nursing); 1,300 periodical subscriptions (1,270 health-care related). *Nursing school resources:* CAI, computer lab, nursing audiovisuals, learning resource lab.

Student Life *Student services:* health clinic, personal counseling, institutionally sponsored work-study program, job placement, campus safety program. *International student services:* counseling/support, special assistance for nonnative speakers of English. *Nursing student activities:* Sigma Theta Tau, nursing club.

Calendar Semesters.

NURSING STUDENT PROFILE

Undergraduate **Enrollment:** 308
Women: 92%; **Men:** 8%; **Minority:** 24%; **Part-time:** 93%
Graduate **Enrollment:** 115
Women: 94%; **Men:** 6%; **Minority:** 3%; **Part-time:** 60%

BACCALAUREATE PROGRAM

Contact Ms. Margaret Lacey, RN, Director, BSN Program, Allegheny University of the Health Sciences, Broad and Vine Street MS 501, Philadelphia, PA 19102-1192, 215-762-7149. *E-mail:* laceym@allegheny.edu

Expenses *Tuition:* $9520 full-time, $415 per credit part-time. *Full-time mandatory fees:* $30.

Financial Aid Institutionally sponsored need-based grants/scholarships, Federal Nursing Student Loans, Federal Pell Grants, Federal Perkins Loans, Federal Supplemental Educational Opportunity Grants, Federal Work-Study. *Application deadline:* 8/1.

RN Baccalaureate Program (BSN)

Applying *Required:* RN license, diploma or AD in nursing, written essay, transcript of college record. 60 prerequisite credits must be completed before admission to the nursing program. *Options:* Course work may be accelerated. May apply for transfer of up to 90 total credits. *Application deadline:* rolling. *Application fee:* $30.

Degree Requirements 121 total credit hours, 61 in nursing.

MASTER'S PROGRAMS

Contact Dr. Marylou McHugh, RN, Associate Dean for Academic Affairs, School of Nursing, MS 501, Broad and Vine, Philadelphia, PA 19102-1192, 215-762-4946. *Fax:* 215-762-1259. *E-mail:* mchughm@allegheny.edu

Areas of Study Nurse anesthesia; nurse practitioner programs in acute care, child care/pediatrics, family health, women's health.

Expenses *Tuition:* $10,530 full-time, $585 per credit part-time. *Full-time mandatory fees:* $30. *Room and board:* $8550. *Books and supplies per academic year:* $650.

Financial Aid Nurse traineeships, institutionally sponsored loans, Perkins loans.

MSN Program

Applying *Required:* GRE General Test (minimum combined score of 1500 on three tests) or Miller Analogies Test, bachelor's degree in nursing, minimum GPA of 3.0, RN license, physical assessment course, statistics course, professional liability/malpractice insurance, interview, 2 letters of recommendation, transcript of college record. *Application deadline:* 4/1. *Application fee:* $50.

Degree Requirements 48–60 total credit hours dependent upon track, 48–60 in nursing.

RN to Master's Program (MSN)

Applying *Required:* GRE General Test (minimum combined score of 1500 on three tests) or Miller Analogies Test, bachelor's degree in nursing, minimum GPA of 3.0, RN license, 1 year of clinical experience, physical assessment course, statistics course, professional liability/malpractice insurance, interview, 2 letters of recommendation, transcript of college record. *Application deadline:* 4/1. *Application fee:* $50.

Degree Requirements 48–60 total credit hours dependent upon track, 48–60 in nursing.

CONTINUING EDUCATION PROGRAM

Contact Alice Stein, Associate Dean for Continuing Education, Allegheny University of the Health Sciences, Broad and Vine Streets, Philadelphia, PA 19102-1192. *E-mail:* steina@allegheny.edu

See full description on page 416.

ALLENTOWN COLLEGE OF ST. FRANCIS DE SALES
Department of Nursing and Health
Center Valley, Pennsylvania

Programs • Generic Baccalaureate • RN Baccalaureate • Baccalaureate for Second Degree • LPN to Baccalaureate • BSN to Master's • RN to Master's

The College Independent Roman Catholic comprehensive coed institution. Founded: 1962. *Primary accreditation:* regional. *Setting:* 300-acre suburban campus. *Total enrollment:* 2,220.

The Department of Nursing and Health Founded in 1975. *Nursing program faculty:* 12 (42% with doctorates).

Academic Facilities *Campus library:* 150,000 volumes; 900 periodical subscriptions (100 health-care related). *Nursing school resources:* CAI, computer lab, nursing audiovisuals, learning resource lab.

Student Life *Student services:* health clinic, personal counseling, career counseling, institutionally sponsored work-study program, job placement, campus safety program, special assistance for disabled students.

International student services: counseling/support. *Nursing student activities:* Sigma Theta Tau, student nurses association.

Calendar Semesters.

NURSING STUDENT PROFILE

Undergraduate **Enrollment:** 130
Women: 93%; **Men:** 7%; **Minority:** 4%; **International:** 0%; **Part-time:** 9%
Graduate **Enrollment:** 70
Women: 98%; **Men:** 2%; **Minority:** 0%; **International:** 0%; **Part-time:** 100%

BACCALAUREATE PROGRAMS

Contact Dr. Karen Moore Schaefer, Chair, Department of Nursing and Health, Allentown College of St. Francis de Sales, 2755 Station Avenue, Center Valley, PA 18034, 610-282-1100 Ext. 1271. *Fax:* 610-282-2254.

Expenses *Tuition:* $5495 full-time, $365 per credit part-time. *Full-time mandatory fees:* $750–$820. *Room and board:* $5050. *Books and supplies per academic year:* ranges from $400 to $600.

Financial Aid Institutionally sponsored need-based grants/scholarships, institutionally sponsored non-need grants/scholarships, Federal Direct Loans, Federal Nursing Student Loans, Federal Perkins Loans, Federal Supplemental Educational Opportunity Grants, Federal Work-Study. *Application deadline:* 5/1.

Generic Baccalaureate Program (BSN)

Applying *Required:* SAT I, ACT, TOEFL for nonnative speakers of English, minimum college GPA of 2.0, 3 years of high school math, 3 years of high school science, high school chemistry, high school biology, high school transcript, 3 letters of recommendation. *Options:* Course work may be accelerated. May apply for transfer of up to 60 total credits. *Application deadlines:* 6/1 (fall), 12/1 (spring). *Application fee:* $25.

Degree Requirements 132 total credit hours, 46 in nursing.

RN Baccalaureate Program (BSN)

Applying *Required:* TOEFL for nonnative speakers of English, minimum college GPA of 2.0, RN license, diploma or AD in nursing, high school transcript, interview, 2 letters of recommendation, written essay, transcript of college record, professional liability/malpractice insurance. *Options:* Advanced standing available through the following means: advanced placement exams, credit by exam. Course work may be accelerated. May apply for transfer of up to 60 total credits. *Application deadline:* rolling. *Application fee:* $35.

Degree Requirements 132 total credit hours, 26 in nursing.

Baccalaureate for Second Degree Program (BSN)

Applying *Required:* TOEFL for nonnative speakers of English, minimum college GPA of 2.0, high school transcript, interview, 2 letters of recommendation, written essay, transcript of college record. *Options:* Advanced standing available through credit by exam. Course work may be accelerated. *Application deadline:* rolling. *Application fee:* $35.

Degree Requirements 46 total credit hours in nursing.

LPN to Baccalaureate Program (BSN)

Applying *Required:* SAT I, ACT, TOEFL for nonnative speakers of English, minimum college GPA of 2.0, 3 years of high school math, 3 years of high school science, high school chemistry, high school biology, high school transcript, 2 letters of recommendation. *Options:* Advanced standing available through advanced placement exams. Course work may be accelerated. May apply for transfer of up to 60 total credits. *Application deadline:* rolling. *Application fee:* $25.

Degree Requirements 132 total credit hours, 46 in nursing.

MASTER'S PROGRAMS

Contact Dr. Karen Moore Schaefer, Chair, Department of Nursing and Health, Allentown College of St. Francis de Sales, 2755 Station Avenue, Center Valley, PA 18034, 610-282-1100 Ext. 1271. *Fax:* 610-282-2254.

Areas of Study Clinical nurse specialist programs in community health nursing, adult health in acute care; nursing administration.

Expenses *Tuition:* $6480 full-time, ranges from $360 to $385 per credit part-time. *Books and supplies per academic year:* ranges from $150 to $200.

Financial Aid Graduate assistantships, employment opportunities.

BSN to Master's Program (MSN)

Applying *Required:* GRE General Test, Miller Analogies Test, bachelor's degree in nursing, minimum GPA of 3.0, RN license, 1 year of clinical experience, physical assessment course, statistics course, professional liability/malpractice insurance, essay, interview, 3 letters of recommendation, transcript of college record. *Application deadline:* rolling. *Application fee:* $35.

Degree Requirements 39–48 total credit hours dependent upon track, 24–33 in nursing, 6–24 in electives for regular track; 24 hours in specific business administration courses for nursing administration track.

RN to Master's Program (MSN)

Applying *Required:* GRE General Test, Miller Analogies Test, TOEFL for nonnative speakers of English, minimum GPA of 3.0, RN license, essay, interview, 3 letters of recommendation. *Application deadline:* rolling. *Application fee:* $35.

BLOOMSBURG UNIVERSITY OF PENNSYLVANIA

Department of Nursing
Bloomsburg, Pennsylvania

Programs • Generic Baccalaureate • RN Baccalaureate • Baccalaureate for Second Degree • MSN

The University State-supported comprehensive coed institution. Part of Pennsylvania State System of Higher Education. Founded: 1839. *Primary accreditation:* regional. *Setting:* 192-acre small-town campus. *Total enrollment:* 7,312.

The Department of Nursing Founded in 1975. *Nursing program faculty:* 23 (40% with doctorates).

Academic Facilities *Campus library:* 352,290 volumes (11,949 in health); 1,500 periodical subscriptions (79 health-care related). *Nursing school resources:* CAI, computer lab, nursing audiovisuals, interactive nursing skills videos, learning resource lab, CINAHL.

Student Life *Student services:* health clinic, child-care facilities, personal counseling, career counseling, institutionally sponsored work-study program, campus safety program, special assistance for disabled students. *International student services:* counseling/support, special assistance for nonnative speakers of English, ESL courses. *Nursing student activities:* Sigma Theta Tau, student nurses association, Phi Kappa Phi.

Calendar Semesters.

NURSING STUDENT PROFILE

Undergraduate **Enrollment:** 285
Women: 83%; **Men:** 17%; **Part-time:** 10%
Graduate **Enrollment:** 30
Women: 97%; **Men:** 3%; **Part-time:** 94%

BACCALAUREATE PROGRAMS

Contact Dr. Christine Alichnie, Chairperson, Department of Nursing, Bloomsburg University of Pennsylvania, MCHS 3109, Bloomsburg, PA 17815, 717-389-4600. *Fax:* 717-389-3894. *E-mail:* husky.alich@bloomu.edu

Expenses *State resident tuition:* $3368 full-time, $140 per credit part-time. *Nonresident tuition:* $8566 full-time, $357 per credit part-time. *Full-time mandatory fees:* $688. *Room and board:* $2812–$3100. *Room only:* $1576–$1822. *Books and supplies per academic year:* $340.

Financial Aid Institutionally sponsored need-based grants/scholarships, institutionally sponsored non-need grants/scholarships, Federal Nursing Student Loans, Federal Supplemental Educational Opportunity Grants, Federal Work-Study. *Application deadline:* 3/15.

Generic Baccalaureate Program (BSN)

Applying *Required:* SAT I, minimum high school GPA of 3.0, 4 years of high school math, high school science, high school chemistry, high school transcript, high school class rank: top 25%. *Options:* Advanced standing available through the following means: advanced placement exams, credit by exam. *Application deadline:* 12/1. *Application fee:* $25.

Degree Requirements 128 total credit hours, 58 in nursing.

RN Baccalaureate Program (BSN)

Applying *Required:* minimum high school GPA of 3.0, minimum college GPA of 2.5, 4 years of high school math, 2 years of high school science, high school chemistry, RN license, diploma or AD in nursing, high school transcript, transcript of college record, high school class rank: top 25%.

Bloomsburg University of Pennsylvania (continued)

Options: Advanced standing available through the following means: advanced placement exams, credit by exam. May apply for transfer of up to 64 total credits. *Application deadline:* rolling. *Application fee:* $25.

Degree Requirements 128 total credit hours, 58 in nursing.

Baccalaureate for Second Degree Program (BSN)

Applying *Required:* SAT I, minimum college GPA of 2.5, high school transcript, transcript of college record, high school class rank: top 25%. *Options:* Advanced standing available through credit by exam. *Application deadline:* rolling. *Application fee:* $25.

Degree Requirements 128 total credit hours, 58 in nursing.

MASTER'S PROGRAM

Contact Dr. Sharon Haymaker, Coordinator of Graduate Program, Department of Nursing, Bloomsburg University of Pennsylvania, MCHS 3115, Bloomsburg, PA 17815, 717-389-4419. *Fax:* 717-389-4602. *E-mail:* haymaker@planetx.bloomu.edu

Areas of Study Clinical nurse specialist programs in adult health nursing, community health nursing; nurse practitioner program in adult health.

Expenses *State resident tuition:* $3368 full-time, $167 per credit part-time. *Nonresident tuition:* $6054 full-time, $336 per credit part-time. *Full-time mandatory fees:* $556. *Room and board:* $1096–$1504. *Room only:* $1162–$1792. *Books and supplies per academic year:* ranges from $200 to $400.

Financial Aid Graduate assistantships, nurse traineeships, Federal Nursing Student Loans, employment opportunities, institutionally sponsored non-need-based grants/scholarships. *Application deadline:* 3/15.

MSN Program

Applying *Required:* GRE General Test (minimum combined score of 1200 on three tests), bachelor's degree in nursing, minimum GPA of 3.0, RN license, 1 year of clinical experience, physical assessment course, statistics course, professional liability/malpractice insurance, essay, interview, 3 letters of recommendation, transcript of college record, resume. *Application deadline:* rolling. *Application fee:* $25.

Degree Requirements 39–42 total credit hours dependent upon track, 39 in nursing.

CALIFORNIA UNIVERSITY OF PENNSYLVANIA
Department of Nursing
California, Pennsylvania

Program • RN Baccalaureate

The University State-supported comprehensive coed institution. Part of Pennsylvania State System of Higher Education. Founded: 1852. *Primary accreditation:* regional. *Setting:* 148-acre small-town campus. *Total enrollment:* 6,015.

The Department of Nursing Founded in 1983. *Nursing program faculty:* 4 (50% with doctorates).

Academic Facilities *Campus library:* 354,210 volumes (3,664 in health, 1,941 in nursing); 1,470 periodical subscriptions (80 health-care related). *Nursing school resources:* CAI, computer lab, nursing audiovisuals.

Student Life *Student services:* health clinic, child-care facilities, personal counseling, career counseling, institutionally sponsored work-study program, job placement, campus safety program, special assistance for disabled students. *International student services:* counseling/support, special assistance for nonnative speakers of English, ESL courses. *Nursing student activities:* Nursing Honor Society.

Calendar Semesters.

NURSING STUDENT PROFILE

Undergraduate **Enrollment:** 112
Women: 98%; **Men:** 2%; **Minority:** 1%; **Part-time:** 88%

BACCALAUREATE PROGRAM

Contact Dr. Margaret Marcinek, Chairperson, Department of Nursing, California University of Pennsylvania, 250 University Avenue, Box 60, California, PA 15419-1394, 412-938-5739. *Fax:* 412-938-5832. *E-mail:* marcinek@cup.edu

Expenses *State resident tuition:* $3368 full-time, $140 per credit part-time. *Nonresident tuition:* $8566 full-time, $357 per credit part-time. *Full-time mandatory fees:* $936. *Part-time mandatory fees:* $244–$626. *Room and board:* $3500–$4508. *Room only:* $1604–$2512. *Books and supplies per academic year:* ranges from $150 to $300.

Financial Aid Institutionally sponsored need-based grants/scholarships, Federal Supplemental Educational Opportunity Grants, Federal Work-Study. 4% of undergraduate students in nursing programs received some form of financial aid in 1995–96. *Application deadline:* 4/1.

RN Baccalaureate Program (BSN)

Applying *Required:* NLN Mobility Profile II, RN license, diploma or AD in nursing, 2 letters of recommendation, written essay, transcript of college record. 67 prerequisite credits must be completed before admission to the nursing program. *Options:* Advanced standing available through the following means: advanced placement exams, credit by exam. May apply for transfer of up to 65 total credits. *Application deadline:* rolling. *Application fee:* $25.

Degree Requirements 128 total credit hours, 63 in nursing.

CARLOW COLLEGE
Division of Nursing
Pittsburgh, Pennsylvania

Programs • Generic Baccalaureate • RN Baccalaureate • Accelerated RN Baccalaureate • RN to Master's

The College Independent Roman Catholic comprehensive primarily women's institution. Founded: 1929. *Primary accreditation:* regional. *Setting:* 13-acre urban campus. *Total enrollment:* 2,058.

The Division of Nursing Founded in 1948. *Nursing program faculty:* 40 (40% with doctorates). *Off-campus program sites:* Beaver, Greensburg, Cranberry.

Academic Facilities *Campus library:* 111,336 volumes (13,360 in health, 5,567 in nursing); 200 periodical subscriptions (95 health-care related). *Nursing school resources:* CAI, nursing audiovisuals, learning resource lab.

Student Life *Student services:* child-care facilities, personal counseling, career counseling, institutionally sponsored work-study program, job placement, campus safety program. *Nursing student activities:* Sigma Theta Tau, nursing club, student nurses association.

Calendar Semesters.

NURSING STUDENT PROFILE

Undergraduate **Enrollment:** 600
Women: 89%; **Men:** 11%; **Minority:** 10%; **International:** 1%; **Part-time:** 2%

Graduate **Enrollment:** 127
Women: 90%; **Men:** 10%; **Minority:** 10%; **International:** 0%; **Part-time:** 0%

BACCALAUREATE PROGRAMS

Contact Ms. Carole Descak, Director of Admissions, Division of Nursing, Carlow College, 3333 Fifth Avenue, Pittsburgh, PA 15213, 412-578-6059.

Expenses *Tuition:* $11,064 full-time, $351 per credit part-time. *Full-time mandatory fees:* $400–$500. *Room and board:* $4434. *Books and supplies per academic year:* ranges from $300 to $375.

Financial Aid Institutionally sponsored need-based grants/scholarships, institutionally sponsored non-need grants/scholarships, Federal Nursing Student Loans, Federal Supplemental Educational Opportunity Grants, Federal Work-Study. *Application deadline:* 5/1.

Generic Baccalaureate Program (BSN)

Applying *Required:* SAT I, 3 years of high school math, 3 years of high school science, high school biology, high school transcript, interview, 3 letters of recommendation, transcript of college record. *Options:* May apply for transfer of up to 54 total credits. *Application deadline:* rolling. *Application fee:* $20.

Degree Requirements 125 total credit hours, 48 in nursing.

RN Baccalaureate Program (BSN)

Applying *Required:* RN license, diploma or AD in nursing, 1 year of nursing experience. *Options:* May apply for transfer of up to 54 total credits. *Application deadline:* rolling. *Application fee:* $15.

Degree Requirements 125 total credit hours, 53 in nursing.

Accelerated RN Baccalaureate Program (BSN)

Applying *Required:* RN license, diploma or AD in nursing, transcript of college record, 2 years of recent nursing experience. 30 prerequisite credits must be completed before admission to the nursing program. *Options:* May apply for transfer of up to 54 total credits. *Application deadline:* rolling. *Application fee:* $15.

Degree Requirements 125 total credit hours, 53 in nursing.

MASTER'S PROGRAM

Contact Tracey Kniess, Graduate Nursing Admissions Office, Division of Nursing, Carlow College, 3333 Fifth Avenue, Pittsburgh, PA 15213, 412-578-6711. *Fax:* 412-578-6321. *E-mail:* kniess@carlow.edu

Areas of Study Clinical nurse specialist program in case management; nurse practitioner programs in gerontology, family home health.

Expenses *Tuition:* $2094 full-time, $349 per credit part-time. *Full-time mandatory fees:* $200–$250. *Books and supplies per academic year:* ranges from $250 to $300.

Financial Aid Graduate assistantships, institutionally sponsored loans, institutionally sponsored need-based grants/scholarships, institutionally sponsored non-need-based grants/scholarships. 50% of master's level students in nursing programs received some form of financial aid in 1995-96. *Application deadline:* 8/1.

RN to Master's Program (MSN)

Applying *Required:* GRE General Test, bachelor's degree in nursing, minimum GPA of 3.0, RN license, 1 year of clinical experience, statistics course, professional liability/malpractice insurance, essay, interview, letter of recommendation, transcript of college record. *Application deadline:* rolling. *Application fee:* $35.

Degree Requirements 55 total credit hours. May take a project option. Thesis required.

Distance learning Courses provided through video.

CEDAR CREST COLLEGE
Nursing Department
Allentown, Pennsylvania

Programs • Generic Baccalaureate • RN Baccalaureate • MSN

The College Independent 4-year primarily women's college, affiliated with United Church of Christ. Founded: 1867. *Primary accreditation:* regional. *Setting:* 84-acre suburban campus. *Total enrollment:* 1,329.

The Nursing Department Founded in 1974. *Nursing program faculty:* 11 (45% with doctorates). *Off-campus program site:* Bethlehem.

▶ ***NOTEWORTHY***

Cedar Crest College offers undergraduate and master's degree programs in nursing. (Majors in nursing, allied health, and the sciences account for 45% of the College's total student enrollment.) The undergraduate nursing program includes clinical experiences at more than a dozen top-rated health-care facilities within 10 miles of the College, including Pennsylvania's largest teaching hospital. The MSN program provides nursing professionals with resources to expand their roles in an evolving health-care system geared toward advanced practice nursing. The program is led by a doctorally prepared faculty, including nurse practitioners with expertise in family and women's health.

Academic Facilities *Campus library:* 126,068 volumes (3,400 in health, 2,200 in nursing); 522 periodical subscriptions (84 health-care related). *Nursing school resources:* CAI, computer lab, nursing audiovisuals, learning resource lab.

Student Life *Student services:* health clinic, personal counseling, career counseling, institutionally sponsored work-study program, job placement, campus safety program, special assistance for disabled students. *International student services:* counseling/support, ESL courses. *Nursing student activities:* Sigma Theta Tau, student nurses association.

Calendar Semesters.

NURSING STUDENT PROFILE

Undergraduate **Enrollment:** 228

Women: 95%; **Men:** 5%; **Minority:** 3%; **International:** 1%; **Part-time:** 54%

Graduate **Enrollment:** 16

Women: 94%; **Men:** 6%; **Minority:** 6%; **International:** 0%; **Part-time:** 100%

BACCALAUREATE PROGRAMS

Contact Judith A. Neyhart, Vice President for Enrollment Management, Cedar Crest College, 100 College Drive, Allentown, PA 18104-6196, 610-740-3780. *Fax:* 610-606-4647. *E-mail:* ccc.udmis@cedarcrest.edu

Expenses *Tuition:* $15,210 full-time, $433 per credit hour part-time. *Full-time mandatory fees:* $300–$350. *Part-time mandatory fees:* $200–$250. *Room and board:* $4678–$5525. *Room only:* $2666–$2980. *Books and supplies per academic year:* ranges from $600 to $750.

Financial Aid Institutionally sponsored need-based grants/scholarships, institutionally sponsored non-need grants/scholarships, Federal Nursing Student Loans, Federal Supplemental Educational Opportunity Grants, Federal Work-Study. 59% of undergraduate students in nursing programs received some form of financial aid in 1995–96. *Application deadline:* 5/1.

Generic Baccalaureate Program (BS)

Applying *Required:* SAT I, TOEFL for nonnative speakers of English, 3 years of high school math, 3 years of high school science, high school chemistry, high school biology, high school transcript, interview. *Options:* Advanced standing available through the following means: advanced placement exams, credit by exam. May apply for transfer of up to 90 total credits. *Application deadline:* rolling. *Application fee:* $30.

Degree Requirements 122 total credit hours, 53 in nursing.

RN Baccalaureate Program (BS)

Applying *Required:* RN license, diploma or AD in nursing, high school transcript, interview, transcript of college record. *Options:* May apply for transfer of up to 90 total credits. *Application deadline:* rolling. *Application fee:* $30.

Degree Requirements 122 total credit hours, 53 in nursing.

MASTER'S PROGRAM

Contact Nancy Hollinger, Director of Lifelong Learning, Cedar Crest College, 100 College Drive, Allentown, PA 18104-6196, 610-740-3770. *Fax:* 610-740-3786.

Areas of Study Clinical nurse specialist programs in adult health nursing, gerontological nursing, women's health nursing; nursing administration.

Expenses *Tuition:* $7830 full-time, $435 per credit part-time. *Full-time mandatory fees:* $50–$250. *Part-time mandatory fees:* $10–$150. *Books and supplies per academic year:* ranges from $100 to $225.

Financial Aid Graduate assistantships.

MSN Program

Applying *Required:* GRE General Test, Miller Analogies Test, TOEFL for nonnative speakers of English, bachelor's degree in nursing, minimum GPA of 3.0, RN license, 1 year of clinical experience, physical assessment course, statistics course, professional liability/malpractice insurance, essay, interview, 3 letters of recommendation, transcript of college record. *Application deadline:* rolling. *Application fee:* $40.

Degree Requirements 37 total credit hours, 34 in nursing, 3 in advanced pathophysiology.

CLARION UNIVERSITY OF PENNSYLVANIA
School of Nursing
Oil City, Pennsylvania

Programs • RN Baccalaureate • Master's • Continuing Education

The University State-supported comprehensive coed institution. Part of Pennsylvania State System of Higher Education. Founded: 1867. *Primary accreditation:* regional. *Setting:* 100-acre rural campus. *Total enrollment:* 5,860.

The School of Nursing Founded in 1982. *Nursing program faculty:* 9 (55% with doctorates). *Off-campus program site:* Pittsburgh.

Academic Facilities *Campus library:* 30,000 volumes (3,000 in health, 4,200 in nursing); 500 periodical subscriptions (308 health-care related). *Nursing school resources:* CAI, computer lab, nursing audiovisuals, learning resource lab, in-house and Internet on-line indices.

Clarion University of Pennsylvania (continued)

Student Life *Student services:* child-care facilities, personal counseling, career counseling, job placement, campus safety program, special assistance for disabled students. *Nursing student activities:* Sigma Theta Tau, nursing club.

Calendar Semesters.

NURSING STUDENT PROFILE

Undergraduate **Enrollment:** 156
Women: 87%; **Men:** 13%; **Minority:** 7%; **International:** 0%; **Part-time:** 84%
Graduate **Enrollment:** 44
Women: 93%; **Men:** 7%; **Minority:** 5%; **International:** 0%; **Part-time:** 95%

BACCALAUREATE PROGRAM

Contact Dr. T. Audean Duespohl, Dean, School of Nursing, Clarion University of Pennsylvania, 1801 West First Street, Oil City, PA 16301, 814-677-6107. *Fax:* 814-676-0251. *E-mail:* duespohl@vaxb.clarion.edu

Expenses *State resident tuition:* $3368 full-time, $140 per credit part-time. *Nonresident tuition:* $8566 full-time, $357 per credit part-time. *Full-time mandatory fees:* $309. *Books and supplies per academic year:* $340.

Financial Aid Institutionally sponsored need-based grants/scholarships, institutionally sponsored non-need grants/scholarships, Federal Direct Loans, Federal Pell Grants, Federal Work-Study. *Application deadline:* 5/1.

RN Baccalaureate Program (BSN)

Applying *Required:* NLN Comprehensive Achievement Test (for those not meeting direct articulation requirements), minimum college GPA of 2.5, RN license, diploma or AD in nursing, 2 letters of recommendation, transcript of college record. *Options:* May apply for transfer of up to 65 total credits. *Application deadlines:* 6/1 (fall), 10/1 (spring). *Application fee:* $25.

Degree Requirements 128 total credit hours, 63 in nursing.

MASTER'S PROGRAM

Contact Dr. Joyce White, Coordinator, MSN Family Nurse Practitioner Program, Strain Behavioral Science Building, Slippery Rock University, Slippery Rock, PA 16057-1326, 412-738-2323. *Fax:* 412-738-2881.

Areas of Study Nurse practitioner program in family health.

CONTINUING EDUCATION PROGRAM

Contact Dr. T. A. Duespohl, Dean of Nursing, Clarion University of Pennsylvania, Vemango Campus, Oil City, PA 16301, 814-677-6107. *Fax:* 814-676-0251. *E-mail:* duespohl@vaxb.clarion.edu

COLLEGE MISERICORDIA

Nursing Department
Dallas, Pennsylvania

Programs • Generic Baccalaureate • Accelerated RN Baccalaureate • Baccalaureate for Second Degree • MSN • Accelerated MSN • RN to Master's • MSN/MOM

The College Independent Roman Catholic comprehensive coed institution. Founded: 1924. *Primary accreditation:* regional. *Setting:* 100-acre small-town campus. *Total enrollment:* 1,779.

The Nursing Department Founded in 1950. *Nursing program faculty:* 15 (40% with doctorates).

Academic Facilities *Campus library:* 67,495 volumes (3,700 in health, 5,550 in nursing); 727 periodical subscriptions (169 health-care related). *Nursing school resources:* CAI, computer lab, nursing audiovisuals, interactive nursing skills videos, learning resource lab.

Student Life *Student services:* health clinic, personal counseling, career counseling, institutionally sponsored work-study program, job placement, campus safety program, special assistance for disabled students. *International student services:* counseling/support. *Nursing student activities:* Sigma Theta Tau, student nurses association.

Calendar Semesters.

NURSING STUDENT PROFILE

Undergraduate **Enrollment:** 220
Women: 85%; **Men:** 15%; **Minority:** 1%; **International:** 0%; **Part-time:** 25%
Graduate **Enrollment:** 60
Women: 97%; **Men:** 3%; **Minority:** 2%; **International:** 0%; **Part-time:** 30%

BACCALAUREATE PROGRAMS

Contact Ms. Jane Dessoye, Executive Director, Admissions and Financial Aid, College Misericordia, 301 Lake Street, Dallas, PA 18612, 717-674-6460. *Fax:* 717-675-2441.

Expenses *Tuition:* $11,620 full-time, $280 per credit part-time. *Full-time mandatory fees:* $570–$650. *Part-time mandatory fees:* $3+. *Room and board:* $6066–$6566. *Room only:* $3240. *Books and supplies per academic year:* $500.

Financial Aid Institutionally sponsored need-based grants/scholarships, institutionally sponsored non-need grants/scholarships, Federal Nursing Student Loans, Federal Pell Grants, Federal Perkins Loans, Federal Supplemental Educational Opportunity Grants, Federal Work-Study. *Application deadline:* 3/1.

Generic Baccalaureate Program (BSN)

Applying *Required:* SAT I, ACT, minimum high school GPA of 2.5, 3 years of high school math, 3 years of high school science, high school chemistry, high school transcript, 2 letters of recommendation, written essay. *Options:* Advanced standing available through the following means: advanced placement exams, advanced placement without credit, credit by exam. Course work may be accelerated. May apply for transfer of up to 90 total credits. *Application deadline:* rolling. *Application fee:* $20.

Degree Requirements 129 total credit hours, 49 in nursing.

Accelerated RN Baccalaureate Program (BSN)

Applying *Required:* minimum high school GPA of 2.5, minimum college GPA of 2.5, high school chemistry, RN license, diploma or AD in nursing, high school transcript, 2 letters of recommendation, written essay, transcript of college record. *Options:* Advanced standing available through the following means: advanced placement exams, advanced placement without credit, credit by exam. Course work may be accelerated. May apply for transfer of up to 90 total credits. *Application deadline:* rolling. *Application fee:* $20.

Degree Requirements 130 total credit hours, 52 in nursing.

Baccalaureate for Second Degree Program (BSN)

Applying *Required:* minimum college GPA of 2.5, 2 letters of recommendation, written essay, transcript of college record. 20 prerequisite credits must be completed before admission to the nursing program. *Options:* Advanced standing available through the following means: advanced placement exams, advanced placement without credit, credit by exam. Course work may be accelerated. May apply for transfer of up to 90 total credits. *Application deadline:* rolling. *Application fee:* $20.

Degree Requirements 126 total credit hours, 49 in nursing.

MASTER'S PROGRAMS

Contact Dr. Helen J. Streubert, Chairperson and Professor, Nursing Department, College Misericordia, 301 Lake Street, Dallas, PA 18612, 717-674-6474. *Fax:* 717-674-8902. *E-mail:* hstreube@miseri.edu

Areas of Study Clinical nurse specialist programs in adult health nursing, community health nursing, parent-child nursing; nursing administration; nursing education; nurse practitioner program in family health.

Expenses *Tuition:* $7020 full-time, $390 per credit part-time. *Full-time mandatory fees:* $20–$50. *Books and supplies per academic year:* $500.

Financial Aid Graduate assistantships, nurse traineeships, Federal Stafford Loans. 42% of master's level students in nursing programs received some form of financial aid in 1995-96.

MSN Program

Applying *Required:* GRE General Test, Miller Analogies Test, bachelor's degree in nursing, minimum GPA of 2.5, RN license, physical assessment course, statistics course, essay, 3 letters of recommendation, transcript of college record, family nurse practitioner requires 1 year clinical experience, professional liability/malpractice insurance. *Application deadline:* rolling. *Application fee:* $20.

Degree Requirements 40–45 total credit hours dependent upon track, 34–45 in nursing, up to 6 in education/organizational management.

Accelerated MSN Program

Applying *Required:* GRE General Test, Miller Analogies Test, bachelor's degree in nursing, minimum GPA, RN license, physical assessment course, statistics course, professional liability/malpractice insurance, essay, 3 letters of recommendation, transcript of college record. *Application deadline:* rolling. *Application fee:* $20.

Degree Requirements 40–45 total credit hours dependent upon track, 34–45 in nursing.

RN to Master's Program (MSN)

Applying *Required:* GRE General Test, Miller Analogies Test, minimum GPA of 2.7, RN license, physical assessment course, statistics course, essay, 3 letters of recommendation, transcript of college record. *Application deadline:* rolling. *Application fee:* $20.

Degree Requirements 40 total credit hours, 36–40 in nursing, 6 in education/organizational management.

MSN/MOM Program

Applying *Required:* GRE General Test, Miller Analogies Test, bachelor's degree in nursing, minimum GPA of 2.5, RN license, physical assessment course, statistics course, essay, 3 letters of recommendation, transcript of college record. *Application deadline:* rolling. *Application fee:* $20.

Degree Requirements 67 total credit hours, 40 in nursing, 37 in organizational management.

DUQUESNE UNIVERSITY
School of Nursing
Pittsburgh, Pennsylvania

Programs • Generic Baccalaureate • RN Baccalaureate • Baccalaureate for Second Degree • BSN to Master's • MSN/MBA • Post-Master's • PhD • Continuing Education

The University Independent Roman Catholic coed university. Founded: 1878. *Primary accreditation:* regional. *Setting:* 40-acre urban campus. *Total enrollment:* 9,285.

The School of Nursing Founded in 1935. *Nursing program faculty:* 21 (48% with doctorates).

▶ *NOTEWORTHY*

Students in Duquesne University's undergraduate and master's degree programs enjoy the benefits of studying in Pittsburgh's world-class health-care facilities. The PhD program emphasizes faculty strengths in a variety of research areas and is offered on a part-time basis for students who cannot make the commitment to full-time study. Supporting the research efforts of faculty members and students is a Center for Nursing Research in partnership with Allegheny General Hospital. The School is an affiliate of the WHO Collaborating Center at George Mason University through the activities of the Center for International Nursing.

Academic Facilities *Campus library:* 473,576 volumes (43,787 in health, 1,560 in nursing); 5,759 periodical subscriptions (340 health-care related). *Nursing school resources:* CAI, computer lab, nursing audiovisuals, learning resource lab.

Student Life *Student services:* health clinic, child-care facilities, personal counseling, career counseling, institutionally sponsored work-study program, job placement, campus safety program, special assistance for disabled students, health education programs. *International student services:* counseling/support, special assistance for nonnative speakers of English, ESL courses. *Nursing student activities:* Sigma Theta Tau, student nurses association, Alpha Tau Delta, Chi Eta Phi.

Calendar Semesters.

NURSING STUDENT PROFILE

Undergraduate **Enrollment:** 320
Women: 85%; **Men:** 15%; **Minority:** 10%; **International:** 1%; **Part-time:** 18%
Graduate **Enrollment:** 161
Women: 98%; **Men:** 2%; **Minority:** 0%; **International:** 1%; **Part-time:** 95%

BACCALAUREATE PROGRAMS

Contact University Admissions Office, Administration Building, Duquesne University, Pittsburgh, PA 15282, 412-396-6220. *Fax:* 412-396-5644. *E-mail:* schaefer@duq2.cc.duq.edu

Expenses *Tuition:* $6210 full-time, $419 per credit part-time. *Part-time mandatory fees:* $35+. *Room and board:* $5803.

Financial Aid Institutionally sponsored need-based grants/scholarships, institutionally sponsored non-need grants/scholarships, Federal Nursing Student Loans, Federal Supplemental Educational Opportunity Grants, Federal Work-Study, endowment scholarships. *Application deadline:* 5/1.

Generic Baccalaureate Program (BSN)

Applying *Required:* SAT I, ACT, TOEFL for nonnative speakers of English, minimum high school GPA of 2.5, minimum college GPA of 2.5, 3 years of high school math, 3 years of high school science, high school chemistry, high school biology, high school transcript, letter of recommendation, written essay, transcript of college record, high school class rank: top 40%, must demonstrate exemplary personal conduct. *Options:* Advanced standing available through the following means: advanced placement exams, credit by exam. May apply for transfer of up to 60 total credits. *Application deadline:* rolling. *Application fee:* $45.

Degree Requirements 125 total credit hours, 75 in nursing.

RN Baccalaureate Program (BSN)

Applying *Required:* RN license, diploma or AD in nursing, high school transcript, interview, written essay, transcript of college record, 2.5 QPA from previous nursing school. *Options:* Advanced standing available through the following means: advanced placement exams, credit by exam. Course work may be accelerated. May apply for transfer of up to 60 total credits. *Application deadline:* rolling. *Application fee:* $45.

Degree Requirements 125 total credit hours, 75 in nursing.

Baccalaureate for Second Degree Program (BSN)

Applying *Required:* TOEFL for nonnative speakers of English, minimum college GPA of 2.5, high school transcript, interview, written essay, transcript of college record. 62 prerequisite credits must be completed before admission to the nursing program. *Options:* Advanced standing available through the following means: advanced placement exams, credit by exam. Course work may be accelerated. May apply for transfer of up to 62 total credits. *Application deadline:* rolling. *Application fee:* $45.

Degree Requirements 125 total credit hours, 75 in nursing.

MASTER'S PROGRAMS

Contact Dr. Jeri Milstead, Chair, MSN Program, 604 College Hall, School of Nursing, Duquesne University, 600 Forbes Avenue, Pittsburgh, PA 15282, 412-396-4865. *Fax:* 412-396-6346. *E-mail:* milstead@duq3.cc.duq.edu

Areas of Study Clinical nurse specialist program in gerontological nursing; nursing administration; nursing education; nurse practitioner program in family health.

Expenses *Tuition:* $7884 full-time, $438 per credit part-time. *Full-time mandatory fees:* $35–$473.

Financial Aid Graduate assistantships, nurse traineeships, institutionally sponsored loans. *Application deadline:* 5/31.

BSN to Master's Program (MSN)

Applying *Required:* Miller Analogies Test, TOEFL for nonnative speakers of English, bachelor's degree in nursing, minimum GPA of 2.75, RN license, 1 year of clinical experience, physical assessment course, statistics course, professional liability/malpractice insurance, essay, 2 letters of recommendation, transcript of college record, computer literacy. *Application deadlines:* 8/1 (fall), 12/1 (spring). *Application fee:* $40.

Degree Requirements 42–50 total credit hours dependent upon track, 42–50 in nursing.

Duquesne University (continued)

MSN/MBA Program

Applying *Required:* GRE General Test, bachelor's degree in nursing, minimum GPA of 2.75, RN license, 1 year of clinical experience, statistics course, professional liability/malpractice insurance, essay, 2 letters of recommendation, transcript of college record, computer literacy. *Application deadlines:* 8/1 (fall), 12/1 (spring). *Application fee:* $40.

Degree Requirements 74 total credit hours, 43 in nursing.

Post-Master's Program

Applying *Required:* bachelor's degree in nursing, RN license, professional liability/malpractice insurance, essay, letter of recommendation, transcript of college record, master's in nursing. *Application deadlines:* 8/1 (fall), 12/1 (spring). *Application fee:* $40.

Degree Requirements 24–34 total credit hours dependent upon track, 24–34 in nursing.

DOCTORAL PROGRAM

Contact Dr. Mary deChesnay, Dean of Nursing and Chair of PhD Program, 631 College Hall, School of Nursing, Duquesne University, 600 Forbes Avenue, Pittsburgh, PA 15282, 412-396-6553. *Fax:* 412-396-5974. *E-mail:* dechesna@duq2.cc.duq.edu

Areas of Study Nursing administration, nursing education, nursing research.

Expenses *Tuition:* $7884 full-time, $438 per credit part-time. *Full-time mandatory fees:* $35+.

Financial Aid Graduate assistantships, nurse traineeships. *Application deadline:* 5/1.

PhD Program

Applying *Required:* GRE General Test, TOEFL for nonnative speakers of English, master's degree in nursing, statistics course, interview, 3 letters of recommendation, vitae, writing sample, competitive review by faculty committee. *Application deadline:* 4/1. *Application fee:* $45.

Degree Requirements 57 total credit hours; dissertation; defense of dissertation; residency; comprehensive exam, qualifying exam.

CONTINUING EDUCATION PROGRAM

Contact Dr. Mary deChesnay, Dean of Nursing and Chair of PhD Program, 631 College Hall, School of Nursing, Duquesne University, 600 Forbes Avenue, Pittsburgh, PA 15282, 412-396-6553. *Fax:* 412-396-5974. *E-mail:* dechesna@duq2.cc.duq.edu

EASTERN COLLEGE

Department of Nursing
St. Davids, Pennsylvania

Program • RN Baccalaureate

The College Independent American Baptist comprehensive coed institution. Founded: 1932. *Primary accreditation:* regional. *Setting:* 107-acre small-town campus. *Total enrollment:* 2,155.

The Department of Nursing Founded in 1983. *Nursing program faculty:* 6 (33% with doctorates).

▶ ***NOTEWORTHY***

Eastern, an innovative Christian college of the arts and sciences, offers an NLN-accredited upper-division BSN degree for registered nurses. Courses are scheduled to accommodate the part-time working nurse. Students may attend part-time and full-time and participate in all campus activities. A Christian world view, emphasizing a holistic, caring approach to multicultural groups, serves as a foundation for all nursing courses. Eastern also offers a 1-year prenursing course of study that prepares students for admission into an affiliated diploma nursing program, after which students may return to Eastern to complete the BSN.

Academic Facilities *Campus library:* 128,878 volumes (5,000 in health); 1,170 periodical subscriptions (100 health-care related). *Nursing school resources:* computer lab, nursing audiovisuals, learning resource lab.

Student Life *Student services:* health clinic, personal counseling, career counseling, institutionally sponsored work-study program, job placement, special assistance for disabled students. *International student services:* counseling/support, special assistance for nonnative speakers of English. *Nursing student activities:* Nursing Honor Society.

Calendar Semesters.

NURSING STUDENT PROFILE

Undergraduate **Enrollment:** 136

Women: 91%; **Men:** 9%; **Minority:** 6%; **International:** 1%; **Part-time:** 98%

BACCALAUREATE PROGRAM

Contact Mr. Mark Seymour, Executive Director of Enrollment Management, Admissions Office, Eastern College, 10 Fairview Drive, St. Davids, PA 19087-3696, 610-341-5967. *Fax:* 610-341-1723. *E-mail:* admis@eastern.edu

Expenses *Tuition:* $9366 full-time, $295 per hour part-time. *Full-time mandatory fees:* $0. *Part-time mandatory fees:* $0. *Room and board:* $5230. *Room only:* $2510. *Books and supplies per academic year:* $450.

Financial Aid Federal Pell Grants, Federal Perkins Loans, Federal Supplemental Educational Opportunity Grants, Federal Work-Study, Federal Stafford Loans. *Application deadline:* 4/1.

RN Baccalaureate Program (BSN)

Applying *Required:* TOEFL for nonnative speakers of English, diploma or AD in nursing, high school transcript, interview, 2 letters of recommendation, transcript of college record, RN license or passage of NCLEX-RN exam. *Options:* May apply for transfer of up to 93 total credits. *Application deadline:* rolling. *Application fee:* $25.

Degree Requirements 127 total credit hours, 27 in nursing.

EAST STROUDSBURG UNIVERSITY OF PENNSYLVANIA

Department of Nursing
East Stroudsburg, Pennsylvania

Programs • Generic Baccalaureate • RN Baccalaureate • LPN to Baccalaureate

The University State-supported comprehensive coed institution. Part of Pennsylvania State System of Higher Education. Founded: 1893. *Primary accreditation:* regional. *Setting:* 183-acre small-town campus. *Total enrollment:* 5,491.

The Department of Nursing Founded in 1973. *Nursing program faculty:* 9 (44% with doctorates).

Academic Facilities *Campus library:* 411,084 volumes (18,800 in health, 1,570 in nursing); 2,145 periodical subscriptions (196 health-care related). *Nursing school resources:* CAI, computer lab, nursing audiovisuals, interactive nursing skills videos, learning resource lab.

Student Life *Student services:* health clinic, child-care facilities, personal counseling, career counseling, institutionally sponsored work-study program, job placement, campus safety program, special assistance for disabled students. *International student services:* counseling/support, special assistance for nonnative speakers of English, ESL courses. *Nursing student activities:* Sigma Theta Tau, student nurses association.

Calendar Semesters.

NURSING STUDENT PROFILE

Undergraduate **Enrollment:** 99

Women: 89%; **Men:** 11%; **Minority:** 7%; **International:** 1%; **Part-time:** 31%

BACCALAUREATE PROGRAMS

Contact Dr. Mark Kilker, Chairperson and Director, Department of Nursing, East Stroudsburg University of Pennsylvania, 200 Prospect Street, East Stroudsburg, PA 18301-2999, 717-422-3568. *Fax:* 717-422-3848. *E-mail:* mkilker@esu.edu

Expenses *State resident tuition:* $3368 full-time, $140 per credit part-time. *Nonresident tuition:* $8566 full-time, $357 per credit part-time. *Full-time*

mandatory fees: $827–$842. *Part-time mandatory fees:* $35+. *Room and board:* $3578–$3876. *Room only:* $2200–$2450. *Books and supplies per academic year:* ranges from $250 to $350.

Financial Aid Institutionally sponsored need-based grants/scholarships, institutionally sponsored non-need grants/scholarships, Federal Direct Loans, Federal Perkins Loans, Federal Supplemental Educational Opportunity Grants, Federal Work-Study. *Application deadline:* 3/1.

Generic Baccalaureate Program (BS)

Applying *Required:* SAT I, TOEFL for nonnative speakers of English, high school transcript, high school class rank: top 30%, 4 years of high school English, 2 years of laboratory science, 3 years of social studies, and 2 years of math, including 1 year of algebra. *Options:* Advanced standing available through the following means: advanced placement exams, credit by exam. *Application deadlines:* 3/1 (fall), 12/6 (spring). *Application fee:* $25.

Degree Requirements 128 total credit hours, 63 in nursing.

RN Baccalaureate Program (BS)

Applying *Required:* minimum college GPA of 2.5, RN license, diploma or AD in nursing, high school transcript, transcript of college record. *Options:* Advanced standing available through the following means: advanced placement exams, credit by exam. Course work may be accelerated. *Application deadlines:* 3/1 (fall), 12/6 (spring). *Application fee:* $25.

Degree Requirements 128 total credit hours, 63 in nursing.

LPN to Baccalaureate Program (BS)

Applying *Required:* minimum college GPA of 2.5, high school transcript, transcript of college record, LPN license, LPN transcripts. *Options:* Course work may be accelerated. *Application deadlines:* 3/1 (fall), 12/6 (spring). *Application fee:* $25.

Degree Requirements 128 total credit hours, 63 in nursing.

EDINBORO UNIVERSITY OF PENNSYLVANIA

Department of Nursing
Edinboro, Pennsylvania

Programs • Generic Baccalaureate • RN Baccalaureate • Baccalaureate for Second Degree • BSN to Master's

The University State-supported comprehensive coed institution. Part of Pennsylvania State System of Higher Education. Founded: 1857. *Primary accreditation:* regional. *Setting:* 585-acre small-town campus. *Total enrollment:* 7,477.

The Department of Nursing Founded in 1970. *Nursing program faculty:* 19 (32% with doctorates). *Off-campus program sites:* Erie, Meadville.

Academic Facilities *Campus library:* 400,000 volumes; 1,680 periodical subscriptions (105 health-care related). *Nursing school resources:* CAI, computer lab, nursing audiovisuals, learning resource lab.

Student Life *Student services:* health clinic, child-care facilities, personal counseling, career counseling, institutionally sponsored work-study program, campus safety program, special assistance for disabled students. *International student services:* counseling/support, special assistance for nonnative speakers of English. *Nursing student activities:* Sigma Theta Tau, student nurses association.

Calendar Semesters.

NURSING STUDENT PROFILE

Undergraduate **Enrollment:** 300
Women: 95%; **Men:** 5%; **Minority:** 1%; **International:** 1%; **Part-time:** 0%
Graduate **Enrollment:** 45
Women: 90%; **Men:** 10%; **Minority:** 0%; **International:** 0%; **Part-time:** 90%

BACCALAUREATE PROGRAMS

Contact Admissions Office, Department of Nursing, Edinboro University of Pennsylvania, Edinboro, PA 16444, 814-732-2761. *Fax:* 814-732-2420.

Expenses *State resident tuition:* $3224 full-time, $134 per credit part-time. *Nonresident tuition:* $8198 full-time, $342 per credit part-time. *Full-time mandatory fees:* $64–$120. *Room and board:* $2397–$4794. *Room only:* $1452–$2904. *Books and supplies per academic year:* ranges from $300 to $600.

Financial Aid Institutionally sponsored need-based grants/scholarships, Federal Direct Loans, Federal Nursing Student Loans, Federal Pell Grants, Federal Supplemental Educational Opportunity Grants, Federal Work-Study. *Application deadline:* 5/1.

Generic Baccalaureate Program (BSN)

Applying *Required:* SAT I, ACT, minimum college GPA of 2.5, high school chemistry, high school transcript, transcript of college record, high school class rank: top 40%. 32 prerequisite credits must be completed before admission to the nursing program. *Application deadline:* rolling. *Application fee:* $25.

Degree Requirements 128 total credit hours, 51 in nursing.

RN Baccalaureate Program (BSN)

Applying *Required:* minimum college GPA of 2.5, RN license, diploma or AD in nursing, high school transcript, transcript of college record. *Options:* Advanced standing available through advanced placement exams. *Application deadline:* rolling. *Application fee:* $25.

Degree Requirements 128 total credit hours, 51 in nursing.

Baccalaureate for Second Degree Program (BSN)

Applying *Required:* minimum college GPA of 2.5, interview, transcript of college record. *Application deadline:* 7/1. *Application fee:* $25.

Degree Requirements 51 total credit hours, 44 in nursing. 4 credits of anatomy and physiology, 3 credits of nutrition.

MASTER'S PROGRAM

Contact Dr. Judy Schilling, Department of Nursing, Edinboro University of Pennsylvania, 138 Centennial Hall, Edinboro, PA 16444, 814-732-4669. *Fax:* 814-732-2422.

Areas of Study Nurse practitioner program in family health.

Expenses *State resident tuition:* $3224 full-time, $179 per credit part-time. *Nonresident tuition:* $5794 full-time, $322 per credit part-time. *Full-time mandatory fees:* $378. *Part-time mandatory fees:* $42. *Books and supplies per academic year:* ranges from $200 to $300.

BSN to Master's Program (MSN)

Applying *Required:* GRE General Test or Miller Analogies Test, TOEFL for nonnative speakers of English, bachelor's degree in nursing, minimum GPA of 3.0, RN license, 1 year of clinical experience, statistics course, professional liability/malpractice insurance, interview, 3 letters of recommendation, transcript of college record. *Application deadline:* rolling. *Application fee:* $25.

Degree Requirements 45 total credit hours, 38 in nursing, 7 in pathophysiology and statistics. 500-hour internship with preceptor. Thesis required.

GANNON UNIVERSITY

Villa Maria School of Nursing
Erie, Pennsylvania

Programs • Generic Baccalaureate • RN Baccalaureate • MSN • MSN/MBA

The University Independent Roman Catholic comprehensive coed institution. Founded: 1925. *Primary accreditation:* regional. *Setting:* 13-acre urban campus. *Total enrollment:* 3,528.

The Villa Maria School of Nursing Founded in 1952. *Nursing program faculty:* 31 (12% with doctorates).

Academic Facilities *Campus library:* 245,000 volumes; 1,100 periodical subscriptions (150 health-care related). *Nursing school resources:* CAI, computer lab, nursing audiovisuals, interactive nursing skills videos, learning resource lab.

Student Life *Student services:* health clinic, personal counseling, career counseling, institutionally sponsored work-study program, job placement, campus safety program, special assistance for disabled students.

Gannon University (continued)
International student services: counseling/support, special assistance for nonnative speakers of English, ESL courses. *Nursing student activities:* Sigma Theta Tau, nursing club.

Calendar Semesters.

NURSING STUDENT PROFILE

Undergraduate **Enrollment:** 300
Women: 88%; **Men:** 12%; **Minority:** 4%; **International:** 1%; **Part-time:** 1%
Graduate **Enrollment:** 76
Women: 91%; **Men:** 9%; **Minority:** 3%; **International:** 0%; **Part-time:** 66%

BACCALAUREATE PROGRAMS

Contact Ms. Patricia Marshall, Director, Baccalaureate Program, Villa Maria School of Nursing, Gannon University, University Square, Erie, PA 16541, 814-871-5470. *Fax:* 814-871-5662.

Expenses *Tuition:* $10,870 full-time, $345 per credit hour part-time. *Full-time mandatory fees:* $125. *Room and board:* $2000. *Room only:* $1170. *Books and supplies per academic year:* $300.

Financial Aid Institutionally sponsored need-based grants/scholarships, institutionally sponsored non-need grants/scholarships, Federal Direct Loans, Federal Nursing Student Loans, Federal Perkins Loans, Federal Supplemental Educational Opportunity Grants. 67% of undergraduate students in nursing programs received some form of financial aid in 1995–96. *Application deadline:* 3/1.

Generic Baccalaureate Program (BSN)

Applying *Required:* SAT I or ACT, SAT II Writing Test, TOEFL for nonnative speakers of English, minimum high school GPA of 2.0, 2 years of high school math, 2 years of high school science, high school chemistry, high school biology, high school transcript, letter of recommendation, high school class rank: top 40%. *Options:* May apply for transfer of up to 45 total credits. *Application deadline:* rolling. *Application fee:* $25.

Degree Requirements 128 total credit hours, 52 in nursing.

RN Baccalaureate Program (BSN)

Applying *Required:* TOEFL for nonnative speakers of English, minimum college GPA of 2.5, RN license, diploma or AD in nursing, 3 letters of recommendation, transcript of college record. *Options:* Advanced standing available through the following means: advanced placement exams, credit by exam. May apply for transfer of up to 45 total credits. *Application deadline:* rolling. *Application fee:* $25.

Degree Requirements 128 total credit hours, 22 in nursing.

MASTER'S PROGRAMS

Contact Dr. Beverly J. Bartlett, MSN Program Director, Academic Center, Department of Nursing, Gannon University, University Square, Erie, PA 16541, 814-871-5463. *Fax:* 814-871-5662.

Areas of Study Clinical nurse specialist program in medical-surgical nursing; nurse anesthesia; nursing administration; nurse practitioner program in family health.

Expenses *Tuition:* $7560 full-time, $420 per credit hour part-time. *Books and supplies per academic year:* $200.

Financial Aid Nurse traineeships, Federal Nursing Student Loans, employment opportunities. 66% of master's level students in nursing programs received some form of financial aid in 1995-96. *Application deadline:* 3/1.

MSN Program

Applying *Required:* GRE General Test, Miller Analogies Test, bachelor's degree in nursing, minimum GPA of 3.0, RN license, 1 year of clinical experience, statistics course, 3 letters of recommendation, transcript of college record, advanced cardiac life support certification, experience as critical-care RN, written essay, interview, 4 letters of recommendation, 3 years clinical experience for nurse anesthesia track. *Application deadlines:* 8/15 (fall), 1/2 (spring). *Application fee:* $25.

Degree Requirements 42–48 total credit hours dependent upon track, 18–24 in nursing, 21–24 in research, anesthesia, physiology, finance. Thesis required.

MSN/MBA Program

Applying *Required:* GMAT, bachelor's degree in nursing, minimum GPA of 3.0, RN license, 1 year of clinical experience, statistics course, 3 letters of recommendation, transcript of college record. *Application deadlines:* 8/15 (fall), 1/2 (spring). *Application fee:* $25.

Degree Requirements 69 total credit hours, 18 in nursing, 51 in research, business. Thesis required.

See full description on page 448.

GWYNEDD-MERCY COLLEGE
Division of Nursing
Gwynedd Valley, Pennsylvania

Programs • RN Baccalaureate • MSN • Accelerated RN to Master's • Continuing Education

The College Independent Roman Catholic comprehensive coed institution. Founded: 1948. *Primary accreditation:* regional. *Setting:* 170-acre suburban campus. *Total enrollment:* 1,816.

The Division of Nursing Founded in 1968. *Nursing program faculty:* 21 (52% with doctorates).

▶ *NOTEWORTHY*

Gwynedd-Mercy College Division of Nursing is NLN accredited and widely recognized as the pioneer in clinic-based nursing education. The College has been teaching and graduating ASNs and BSNs since 1959. The students are in the health-care environment from day one, learning firsthand in hospitals, clinics, and nursing homes. With a pass rate of 95% on the national registry, it helps to have Gwynedd on a résumé. Along with the exposure to real-world nursing, there is Gwynedd's long-standing reputation for liberal arts excellence coupled with the financial assistance its students need. Gwynedd-Mercy College was ranked number 2 in the north region as a "best value college" by *U.S. News & World Report* in September 1996.

Academic Facilities *Campus library:* 95,000 volumes; 789 periodical subscriptions. *Nursing school resources:* CAI, computer lab, nursing audiovisuals, interactive nursing skills videos, learning resource lab.

Student Life *Student services:* child-care facilities, personal counseling, career counseling, institutionally sponsored work-study program, job placement. *International student services:* counseling/support, special assistance for nonnative speakers of English, ESL courses. *Nursing student activities:* Sigma Theta Tau, student nurses association.

Calendar Semesters.

NURSING STUDENT PROFILE

Undergraduate **Enrollment:** 313
Women: 90%; **Men:** 10%; **Minority:** 6%; **International:** 4%; **Part-time:** 60%
Graduate **Enrollment:** 100
Women: 97%; **Men:** 3%; **Minority:** 9%; **International:** 0%; **Part-time:** 80%

BACCALAUREATE PROGRAM

Contact Betsy Black, Assistant Chair of Undergraduate Nursing, Nursing Division, Gwynedd-Mercy College, Sumneytown Pike, Gwynedd Valley, PA 19437-0901, 215-641-5501 Ext. 5532. *Fax:* 215-641-5564.

Expenses *Tuition:* $12,670 full-time, $315 per credit part-time. *Full-time mandatory fees:* $15. *Room and board:* $5800.

Financial Aid Institutionally sponsored need-based grants/scholarships, Federal Direct Loans, Federal Nursing Student Loans, Federal Work-Study. 81% of undergraduate students in nursing programs received some form of financial aid in 1995–96. *Application deadline:* 4/30.

RN Baccalaureate Program (BSN)

Applying *Required:* SAT I, TOEFL for nonnative speakers of English, RN license, diploma or AD in nursing. 64 prerequisite credits must be completed before admission to the nursing program. *Options:* Advanced standing available through the following means: advanced placement exams, advanced placement without credit, credit by exam. May apply for transfer of up to 32 total credits. *Application deadline:* rolling. *Application fee:* $35.

Degree Requirements 129 total credit hours, 65 in nursing.

MASTER'S PROGRAMS

Contact Dr. Mary Dressler, Interim Dean, Nursing Division, Gwynedd-Mercy College, Sumneytown Pike, Gwynedd Valley, PA 19437-0901, 215-646-7300 Ext. 695. *Fax:* 215-641-5564.

Areas of Study Clinical nurse specialist programs in gerontological nursing, oncology nursing, pediatric nursing; nurse practitioner programs in adult health, child care/pediatrics.

Expenses *Tuition:* $7920 full-time, $340 per credit part-time. *Full-time mandatory fees:* $50.

Financial Aid Nurse traineeships. 20% of master's level students in nursing programs received some form of financial aid in 1995-96. *Application deadline:* 9/1.

MSN Program

Applying *Required:* Miller Analogies Test, minimum GPA of 3.0, RN license, 2 years of clinical experience, physical assessment course, statistics course, professional liability/malpractice insurance, interview, letter of recommendation, transcript of college record, BSN or NLN Comprehensive Nursing Achievement Test. *Application deadlines:* 7/15 (fall), 11/15 (spring). *Application fee:* $25.

Degree Requirements 39–46 total credit hours dependent upon track, 33–36 in nursing, 6–10 in biology, business, education, pharmacology, sociology. Thesis required.

Accelerated RN to Master's Program (MSN)

Applying *Required:* Miller Analogies Test, TOEFL for nonnative speakers of English, minimum GPA of 3.0, RN license, 1 year of clinical experience, physical assessment course, statistics course, professional liability/malpractice insurance, interview, 2 letters of recommendation, transcript of college record, BSN or NLN Comprehensive Achievement Test for baccalaureate students. *Application deadlines:* 7/15 (fall), 11/15 (spring). *Application fee:* $25.

Degree Requirements 39–46 total credit hours dependent upon track, 33 in nursing, 6 in business education, sociology. 4 credits in biology, 3 credits in pharmacology, 46 credits in practitioner program. Thesis required.

CONTINUING EDUCATION PROGRAM

Contact Ms. Ann Marie Vreeland, Coordinator of Continuing Education, Nursing Division, Gwynedd-Mercy College, Sumneytown Pike, Gwynedd Valley, PA 19437-0901, 215-646-7300 Ext. 553.

HOLY FAMILY COLLEGE
Division of Nursing
Philadelphia, Pennsylvania

Programs • Generic Baccalaureate • Accelerated RN Baccalaureate • Baccalaureate for Second Degree • Master's for Nurses with Non-Nursing Degrees • Master's for Non-Nursing College Graduates

The College Independent Roman Catholic comprehensive coed institution. Founded: 1954. *Primary accreditation:* regional. *Setting:* 47-acre suburban campus. *Total enrollment:* 2,760.

The Division of Nursing Founded in 1971. *Nursing program faculty:* 49 (12% with doctorates). *Off-campus program site:* Newtown.

Academic Facilities *Campus library:* 106,709 volumes (8,000 in health, 7,500 in nursing); 596 periodical subscriptions (100 health-care related). *Nursing school resources:* CAI, computer lab, nursing audiovisuals, interactive nursing skills videos, learning resource lab.

Student Life *Student services:* health clinic, personal counseling, career counseling, institutionally sponsored work-study program, campus safety program, special assistance for disabled students. *International student services:* counseling/support, special assistance for nonnative speakers of English. *Nursing student activities:* Sigma Theta Tau, nursing club, student nurses association.

Calendar Semesters.

NURSING STUDENT PROFILE	
Undergraduate	**Enrollment:** 600
Women: 88%; **Men:** 12%; **Minority:** 5%; **International:** 3%; **Part-time:** 37%	

BACCALAUREATE PROGRAMS

Contact Mrs. Liz Nagler, Acting Director of Admissions, Division of Nursing, Holy Family College, Grant and Frankford Avenues, Philadelphia, PA 19114-2094, 215-637-3050. *Fax:* 215-632-8067.

Expenses *Tuition:* $5120 full-time, $225 per credit hour part-time. *Full-time mandatory fees:* $600.

Financial Aid Institutionally sponsored need-based grants/scholarships, institutionally sponsored non-need grants/scholarships, Federal Nursing Student Loans, Federal Pell Grants, Federal Perkins Loans, Federal Supplemental Educational Opportunity Grants, Federal Work-Study. 70% of undergraduate students in nursing programs received some form of financial aid in 1995–96. *Application deadline:* 2/15.

Generic Baccalaureate Program (BSN)

Applying *Required:* SAT I or ACT, TOEFL for nonnative speakers of English, minimum college GPA of 2.5, high school chemistry, high school biology, high school foreign language, high school transcript, letter of recommendation, written essay, transcript of college record. *Options:* Advanced standing available through advanced placement exams. Course work may be accelerated. May apply for transfer of up to 60 total credits. *Application deadline:* rolling. *Application fee:* $25.

Degree Requirements 134 total credit hours, 62 in nursing.

Accelerated RN Baccalaureate Program (BSN)

Applying *Required:* SAT I or ACT, TOEFL for nonnative speakers of English, minimum college GPA of 2.5, high school chemistry, high school biology, high school foreign language, high school transcript, letter of recommendation, written essay. *Options:* Advanced standing available through advanced placement exams. May apply for transfer of up to 60 total credits. *Application deadline:* rolling. *Application fee:* $25.

Degree Requirements 134 total credit hours, 62 in nursing.

Baccalaureate for Second Degree Program (BSN)

Applying *Required:* TOEFL for nonnative speakers of English, minimum college GPA of 2.5, high school chemistry, high school biology, letter of recommendation, written essay, transcript of college record. *Options:* Advanced standing available through advanced placement exams. Course work may be accelerated. May apply for transfer of up to 60 total credits. *Application deadline:* rolling. *Application fee:* $25.

Degree Requirements 134 total credit hours, 62 in nursing.

MASTER'S PROGRAMS

Contact Graduate Studies Office, Holy Family College, Grant and Frankford Avenues, Philadelphia, PA 19114-2094.

Areas of Study Clinical nurse specialist program in community health nursing.

Expenses *Tuition:* $5310 full-time, $295 per credit part-time. *Full-time mandatory fees:* $130. *Books and supplies per academic year:* ranges from $300 to $500.

Financial Aid Graduate assistantships, Federal Direct Loans.

Master's for Nurses with Non-Nursing Degrees Program (MSN)

Applying *Required:* GRE General Test (minimum combined score of 1200 on three tests), Miller Analogies Test, TOEFL for nonnative speakers of English, bachelor's degree, minimum GPA of 2.5, RN license, 2 letters of recommendation, transcript of college record, coursework in nursing community health, nursing leadership management, and research. *Application deadline:* rolling. *Application fee:* $25.

Degree Requirements 39 total credit hours, 33–39 in nursing.

Master's for Non-Nursing College Graduates Program (MSN)

Applying *Required:* GRE General Test (minimum combined score of 1200 on three tests), Miller Analogies Test, TOEFL for nonnative speakers of

Holy Family College (continued)
English, bachelor's degree, minimum GPA of 2.5, RN license, 2 letters of recommendation, transcript of college record. *Application deadline:* rolling. *Application fee:* $25.

Degree Requirements 39 total credit hours, 33–39 in nursing.

See full description on page 456.

IMMACULATA COLLEGE
Nursing Department
Immaculata, Pennsylvania

Program • RN Baccalaureate

The College Independent Roman Catholic comprehensive primarily women's institution. Founded: 1920. *Primary accreditation:* regional. *Setting:* 400-acre suburban campus. *Total enrollment:* 2,053.

The Nursing Department Founded in 1984. *Nursing program faculty:* 6 (50% with doctorates).

Academic Facilities *Campus library:* 138,327 volumes (500 in health, 1,500 in nursing); 714 periodical subscriptions (84 health-care related). *Nursing school resources:* CAI, computer lab, nursing audiovisuals.

Student Life *Student services:* health clinic, personal counseling, career counseling, institutionally sponsored work-study program, campus safety program, special assistance for disabled students. *International student services:* counseling/support, special assistance for nonnative speakers of English. *Nursing student activities:* nursing club.

Calendar Semesters.

NURSING STUDENT PROFILE

Undergraduate **Enrollment:** 108
Women: 98%; **Men:** 2%; **Minority:** 5%; **International:** 1%; **Part-time:** 80%

BACCALAUREATE PROGRAM

Contact Ms. Janis Bates, Director, Continuing Education, Loyola Hall, Immaculata College, 1145 King Road, Immaculata, PA 19345, 610-647-4400.

Expenses *Tuition:* $11,400 full-time, $235 per credit part-time. *Full-time mandatory fees:* $180. *Room and board:* $5855. *Room only:* $3120. *Books and supplies per academic year:* ranges from $250 to $300.

RN Baccalaureate Program (BSN)

Applying *Required:* SAT I, RN license, diploma or AD in nursing, 3 letters of recommendation, verification of employment. 60 prerequisite credits must be completed before admission to the nursing program. *Options:* May apply for transfer of up to 66 total credits. *Application deadline:* rolling.

Degree Requirements 126 total credit hours, 54 in nursing. 27 upper division nursing credits.

INDIANA UNIVERSITY OF PENNSYLVANIA
Department of Nursing and Allied Health Professions
Indiana, Pennsylvania

Programs • Generic Baccalaureate • RN Baccalaureate • MSN

The University State-supported coed university. Part of Pennsylvania State System of Higher Education. Founded: 1875. *Primary accreditation:* regional. *Setting:* 342-acre small-town campus. *Total enrollment:* 13,879.

The Department of Nursing and Allied Health Professions Founded in 1968. *Nursing program faculty:* 25 (32% with doctorates).

Academic Facilities *Campus library:* 751,709 volumes (2,363 in health, 3,395 in nursing); 4,500 periodical subscriptions (225 health-care related). *Nursing school resources:* CAI, computer lab, nursing audiovisuals, interactive nursing skills videos, learning resource lab.

Student Life *Student services:* health clinic, child-care facilities, personal counseling, career counseling, institutionally sponsored work-study program, job placement, campus safety program, special assistance for disabled students. *International student services:* counseling/support, special assistance for nonnative speakers of English, ESL courses. *Nursing student activities:* Sigma Theta Tau, student nurses association, Alpha Tau Delta, Nursing Mentorship Program.

Calendar Semesters.

NURSING STUDENT PROFILE

Undergraduate **Enrollment:** 335
Women: 85%; **Men:** 15%; **Minority:** 10%; **International:** 5%; **Part-time:** 5%
Graduate **Enrollment:** 41
Women: 97%; **Men:** 3%; **Minority:** 1%; **International:** 2%; **Part-time:** 75%

BACCALAUREATE PROGRAMS

Contact Mr. Bill Nunn, Dean of Admissions, Room 216, Pratt Hall, Indiana University of Pennsylvania, Indiana, PA 15705, 412-357-2230. *Fax:* 412-357-6213. *E-mail:* billnunn@grove.iup.edu

Expenses *State resident tuition:* $3368 full-time, $140 per credit hour part-time. *Nonresident tuition:* $8566 full-time, $357 per credit hour part-time. *Full-time mandatory fees:* $500. *Room and board:* $3136. *Room only:* $1822. *Books and supplies per academic year:* ranges from $400 to $500.

Financial Aid Institutionally sponsored need-based grants/scholarships, institutionally sponsored non-need grants/scholarships, Federal Nursing Student Loans, Federal Perkins Loans, Federal Supplemental Educational Opportunity Grants, Federal Work-Study. *Application deadline:* 5/1.

Generic Baccalaureate Program (BSN)

Applying *Required:* SAT I, 2 years of high school math, 2 years of high school science, high school transcript, high school class rank: top 20%. *Options:* Advanced standing available through the following means: advanced placement exams, credit by exam. Course work may be accelerated. May apply for transfer of up to 60 total credits. *Application deadline:* rolling. *Application fee:* $30.

Degree Requirements 127 total credit hours, 53 in nursing. 55 credits in liberal studies.

RN Baccalaureate Program (BSN)

Applying *Required:* SAT I, TOEFL for nonnative speakers of English, high school math, high school science, RN license, diploma or AD in nursing, high school transcript, transcript of college record. *Options:* Advanced standing available through the following means: advanced placement exams, credit by exam. Course work may be accelerated. May apply for transfer of up to 60 total credits. *Application deadline:* rolling. *Application fee:* $30.

Degree Requirements 124 total credit hours, 50 in nursing. 55 credits in liberal studies.

MASTER'S PROGRAM

Contact Dr. David Lynch, Dean, Graduate School, Room 129, Stright Hall, Indiana University of Pennsylvania, Indiana, PA 15705, 412-357-2222. *Fax:* 412-357-7518. *E-mail:* dmlynch@grove.iup.edu

Areas of Study Nursing administration; nursing education.

Expenses *State resident tuition:* $3368 full-time, $187 per credit hour part-time. *Nonresident tuition:* $6054 full-time, $336 per credit hour part-time. *Full-time mandatory fees:* $608. *Part-time mandatory fees:* $206. *Books and supplies per academic year:* $150.

Financial Aid Graduate assistantships, nurse traineeships, employment opportunities. *Application deadline:* 5/1.

MSN Program

Applying *Required:* bachelor's degree in nursing, minimum GPA of 3.0, RN license, 2 years of clinical experience, physical assessment course, statistics course, professional liability/malpractice insurance, essay, 2 letters of recommendation, transcript of college record. *Application deadlines:* 8/15 (fall), 1/15 (spring), 5/15 (summer). *Application fee:* $20.

Degree Requirements 45 total credit hours, 39 in nursing, 6 in statistics and other specified areas.

KUTZTOWN UNIVERSITY OF PENNSYLVANIA
Department of Nursing
Kutztown, Pennsylvania

Program • RN Baccalaureate

The University State-supported comprehensive coed institution. Part of Pennsylvania State System of Higher Education. Founded: 1866. *Primary accreditation:* regional. *Setting:* 325-acre small-town campus. *Total enrollment:* 7,811.

The Department of Nursing Founded in 1977. *Nursing program faculty:* 5. *Off-campus program sites:* Allentown, Reading, Pottstown.

Academic Facilities *Campus library:* 350,000 volumes (33,000 in health, 12,000 in nursing). *Nursing school resources:* computer lab, nursing audiovisuals, interactive nursing skills videos.

Student Life *Student services:* health clinic, child-care facilities, personal counseling, career counseling, institutionally sponsored work-study program, job placement, campus safety program, special assistance for disabled students. *International student services:* counseling/support, special assistance for nonnative speakers of English, ESL courses. *Nursing student activities:* Sigma Theta Tau, nursing club, student nurses association.

Calendar Semesters.

NURSING STUDENT PROFILE

Undergraduate **Enrollment:** 140
Women: 97%; **Men:** 3%; **Minority:** 5%; **International:** 0%; **Part-time:** 98%

BACCALAUREATE PROGRAM

Contact Ms. Vera Brancato, Chairperson, Beekey Building, Room 219, Department of Nursing, Kutztown University, Kutztown, PA 19530, 610-683-4330. *Fax:* 610-683-1327. *E-mail:* brancato@kutztown.edu

Expenses *Tuition:* $3332 full-time, $144 per semester hour part-time. *Full-time mandatory fees:* $382–$492. *Room and board:* $3250. *Room only:* $2000. *Books and supplies per academic year:* ranges from $450 to $550.

Financial Aid Institutionally sponsored need-based grants/scholarships, institutionally sponsored non-need grants/scholarships, Federal Nursing Student Loans, Federal Supplemental Educational Opportunity Grants, Federal Work-Study. *Application deadline:* 3/15.

RN Baccalaureate Program (BSN)

Applying *Required:* RN license, diploma or AD in nursing, high school transcript, transcript of college record, CPR certification. *Options:* Advanced standing available through credit by exam. May apply for transfer of up to 64 total credits. *Application deadline:* rolling. *Application fee:* $25.

Degree Requirements 128 total credit hours, 51 in nursing.

LA ROCHE COLLEGE
Division of Nursing
Pittsburgh, Pennsylvania

Programs • RN Baccalaureate • MSN • RN to Master's • Continuing Education

The College Independent comprehensive coed institution, affiliated with Roman Catholic Church. Founded: 1963. *Primary accreditation:* regional. *Setting:* 80-acre suburban campus. *Total enrollment:* 1,630.

The Division of Nursing Founded in 1981. *Nursing program faculty:* 8 (50% with doctorates). *Off-campus program site:* Meadville.

Academic Facilities *Campus library:* 69,000 volumes; 604 periodical subscriptions. *Nursing school resources:* computer lab, nursing audiovisuals, learning resource lab.

Student Life *Student services:* health clinic, career counseling, institutionally sponsored work-study program. *International student services:* counseling/support, ESL courses. *Nursing student activities:* Sigma Theta Tau.

Calendar Semesters.

NURSING STUDENT PROFILE

Undergraduate **Enrollment:** 158
Women: 95%; **Men:** 5%; **Minority:** 1%; **Part-time:** 90%
Graduate **Enrollment:** 92
Women: 95%; **Men:** 5%; **Minority:** 2%; **Part-time:** 92%

BACCALAUREATE PROGRAM

Contact Ms. Yvonne Hennigan, Manager of Nursing Student Enrollment, Division of Nursing, La Roche College, 9000 Babcock Boulevard, Pittsburgh, PA 15237, 412-367-9257. *Fax:* 412-367-9277.

Expenses *Tuition:* $389 per credit. *Full-time mandatory fees:* $20–$65. *Books and supplies per academic year:* ranges from $50 to $200.

Financial Aid Institutionally sponsored need-based grants/scholarships, institutionally sponsored non-need grants/scholarships, Federal Pell Grants, Federal Perkins Loans, Federal Supplemental Educational Opportunity Grants, Federal Work-Study, Federal Stafford Loans, PHEAA State Grant. *Application deadline:* 5/1.

RN Baccalaureate Program (BSN)

Applying *Required:* TOEFL for nonnative speakers of English, NLN Mobility Profile II, direct articulation, PA articulation model, minimum college GPA of 2.5, RN license, diploma or AD in nursing, 2 letters of recommendation, transcript of college record. *Options:* Advanced standing available through credit by exam. May apply for transfer of up to 60–90 total credits. *Application deadline:* rolling. *Application fee:* $25.

Degree Requirements 120 total credit hours, 57 in nursing.

MASTER'S PROGRAMS

Contact Ms. Yvonne Hennigan, Manager of Nursing Student Enrollment, Division of Nursing, La Roche College, 9000 Babcock Boulevard, Pittsburgh, PA 15237, 412-367-9257. *Fax:* 412-367-9368.

Areas of Study Clinical nurse specialist programs in community health nursing, critical care nursing, gerontological nursing; nursing administration; nurse practitioner program in family health.

Expenses *Tuition:* $396 per credit. *Full-time mandatory fees:* $0. *Books and supplies per academic year:* ranges from $60 to $300.

Financial Aid Graduate assistantships, Federal Stafford Loans. *Application deadline:* 5/1.

MSN Program

Applying *Required:* GRE General Test, TOEFL for nonnative speakers of English, bachelor's degree in nursing, minimum GPA of 3.0, RN license, statistics course, professional liability/malpractice insurance, essay, interview, 2 letters of recommendation, transcript of college record, biomedical ethics course, 3 years nursing management experience for management track, 2 years experience for nurse practitioner track, 1 year critical care experience for critical care nursing track. *Application deadlines:* 12/31 (nurse practitioner), rolling. *Application fee:* $25.

Degree Requirements 39 total credit hours, 24–39 in nursing, 15 in management. Thesis or research project.

RN to Master's Program (MSN)

Applying *Required:* GRE General Test, TOEFL for nonnative speakers of English, minimum GPA of 3.0, RN license, statistics course, professional liability/malpractice insurance, essay, interview, 2 letters of recommendation, transcript of college record, biomedical ethics course, 3 years of nursing management experience for management track, 1 year of critical care for critical care nursing track. *Application deadline:* rolling. *Application fee:* $25.

Degree Requirements 150 total credit hours, 63 in nursing, 52 in undergraduate liberal arts.

CONTINUING EDUCATION PROGRAM

Contact Dr. Kathleen Sullivan, Nursing Chair, Division of Nursing, LaRoche College, 9000 Babcock Boulevard, Pittsburgh, PA 15237, 412-397-9300 Ext. 199. *Fax:* 412-367-9368.

LA SALLE UNIVERSITY
School of Nursing
Philadelphia, Pennsylvania

Programs • Generic Baccalaureate • RN Baccalaureate • MSN • RN to Master's

The University Independent Roman Catholic comprehensive coed institution. Founded: 1863. *Primary accreditation:* regional. *Setting:* 100-acre urban campus. *Total enrollment:* 5,449.

The School of Nursing Founded in 1980. *Nursing program faculty:* 19 (63% with doctorates). *Off-campus program site:* Newtown.

▶ *NOTEWORTHY*

La Salle University's School of Nursing is a national leader in preparing nurses to work in a reformed health-care system. With an emphasis on community health, public health, primary prevention/health promotion, and acute and chronic illness care, La Salle's undergraduate and graduate degree programs are perfectly positioned for the expanding role of nurses as primary-care practitioners. La Salle's location in Philadelphia—one of the leading health-care centers in the nation—provides opportunities for a variety of clinical experiences. In addition to formal ties with 7 health-care institutions, the School of Nursing operates 2 nurse-managed primary health-care facilities.

Academic Facilities *Campus library:* 320,000 volumes (7,932 in nursing); 1,571 periodical subscriptions (215 health-care related). *Nursing school resources:* CAI, computer lab, nursing audiovisuals, interactive nursing skills videos, learning resource lab.

Student Life *Student services:* health clinic, child-care facilities, personal counseling, career counseling, institutionally sponsored work-study program, job placement, campus safety program, special assistance for disabled students. *International student services:* counseling/support, special assistance for nonnative speakers of English, ESL courses. *Nursing student activities:* Sigma Theta Tau, student nurses association.

Calendar Semesters.

NURSING STUDENT PROFILE

Undergraduate **Enrollment:** 438
Women: 89%; **Men:** 11%; **Minority:** 21%; **Part-time:** 68%
Graduate **Enrollment:** 211
Women: 92%; **Men:** 8%; **Minority:** 9%; **Part-time:** 61%

BACCALAUREATE PROGRAMS

Contact Dr. Eileen Giardino, Interim Director, BSN Program, School of Nursing, La Salle University, Philadelphia, PA 19141-1199, 215-951-1430. *Fax:* 215-951-1896. *E-mail:* giardino@lasalle.edu

Expenses *Tuition:* $6885 full-time, $485 per credit hour part-time. *Full-time mandatory fees:* $165–$200. *Room only:* $3290–$3990. *Books and supplies per academic year:* ranges from $350 to $450.

Financial Aid Institutionally sponsored need-based grants/scholarships, institutionally sponsored non-need grants/scholarships, Federal Direct Loans, Federal Perkins Loans, Federal Supplemental Educational Opportunity Grants, Federal Work-Study. 38% of undergraduate students in nursing programs received some form of financial aid in 1995–96. *Application deadline:* 2/15.

Generic Baccalaureate Program (BSN)

Applying *Required:* SAT I or ACT, TOEFL or SAT II writing test for nonnative speakers of English, minimum high school GPA of 2.75, 3 years of high school math, 3 years of high school science, high school chemistry, high school biology, high school foreign language, high school transcript, letter of recommendation, written essay, transcript of college record, high school class rank: top 50%. *Options:* Advanced standing available through advanced placement exams. May apply for transfer of up to 70 total credits. *Application deadline:* rolling. *Application fee:* $30.

Degree Requirements 120 total credit hours, 50 in nursing.

RN Baccalaureate Program (BSN)

Applying *Required:* writing and math admissions test, RN license, diploma or AD in nursing, transcript of college record. 24 prerequisite credits must be completed before admission to the nursing program. *Options:* Advanced standing available through the following means: advanced placement exams, credit by exam. Course work may be accelerated. May apply for transfer of up to 70 total credits. *Application deadline:* rolling. *Application fee:* $30.

Degree Requirements 120 total credit hours, 50 in nursing.

MASTER'S PROGRAMS

Contact Dr. Zane Wolf, Director, MSN Program, School of Nursing, La Salle University, Philadelphia, PA 19141-1199, 215-951-1432. *Fax:* 215-951-1896. *E-mail:* wolf@lasalle.edu

Areas of Study Clinical nurse specialist programs in adult health nursing, community health nursing; nursing administration; nurse practitioner program in adult primary care.

Expenses *Tuition:* $415 per credit. *Full-time mandatory fees:* $0. *Books and supplies per academic year:* $500.

Financial Aid Graduate assistantships, nurse traineeships. 18% of master's level students in nursing programs received some form of financial aid in 1995-96. *Application deadline:* 7/1.

MSN Program

Applying *Required:* GRE General Test or Miller Analogies Test, bachelor's degree in nursing, minimum GPA of 3.0, RN license, 3 years of clinical experience, statistics course, professional liability/malpractice insurance, essay, 2 letters of recommendation, transcript of college record. *Application deadline:* rolling. *Application fee:* $30.

Degree Requirements 41 total credit hours, 35 in nursing.

RN to Master's Program (MSN)

Applying *Required:* GRE General Test or Miller Analogies Test, minimum GPA of 3.0, RN license, 1 year of clinical experience, statistics course, professional liability/malpractice insurance, essay, 2 letters of recommendation, transcript of college record, BSN earned concurrently. *Application deadline:* rolling. *Application fee:* $30.

Degree Requirements 152 total credit hours, 82 in nursing.

See full description on page 470.

LYCOMING COLLEGE
Department of Nursing
Williamsport, Pennsylvania

Programs • Generic Baccalaureate • RN Baccalaureate • Baccalaureate for Second Degree

The College Independent United Methodist 4-year coed college. Founded: 1812. *Primary accreditation:* regional. *Setting:* 35-acre small-town campus. *Total enrollment:* 1,469.

The Department of Nursing Founded in 1981.

Academic Facilities *Campus library:* 160,000 volumes (7,300 in health, 300 in nursing); 1,000 periodical subscriptions. *Nursing school resources:* computer lab.

Calendar Semesters.

BACCALAUREATE PROGRAMS

Contact Chairperson and Associate Professor, Department of Nursing, Lycoming College, 700 College Place, Williamsport, PA 17701, 717-321-4224. *Fax:* 717-321-4090.

Expenses *Tuition:* $15,400 full-time, $1925 per unit course part-time. *Room and board:* $4500. *Room only:* $2350.

Financial Aid Institutionally sponsored need-based grants/scholarships, Federal Direct Loans, Federal Pell Grants, Federal Perkins Loans, Federal Supplemental Educational Opportunity Grants, Federal Work-Study, Federal PLUS Loans, state grants. *Application deadline:* 4/1.

Generic Baccalaureate Program (BSN)

Applying *Required:* SAT I or ACT, TOEFL for nonnative speakers of English, minimum college GPA of 2.5, high school transcript, 2 letters of recommendation, transcript of college record. *Application deadline:* rolling. *Application fee:* $25.

Degree Requirements 128 total credit hours.

RN Baccalaureate Program (BSN)

Applying *Required:* SAT I, minimum college GPA of 2.5. *Options:* May apply for transfer of up to 64–96 total credits. *Application deadline:* rolling. *Application fee:* $25.

Degree Requirements 128 total credit hours.

Baccalaureate for Second Degree Program (BSN)

Applying *Required:* minimum college GPA of 2.5. *Options:* May apply for transfer of up to 64–96 total credits. *Application deadline:* rolling. *Application fee:* $25.

Degree Requirements 128 total credit hours.

MANSFIELD UNIVERSITY OF PENNSYLVANIA

Robert Packer Department of Health Sciences
Mansfield, Pennsylvania

Programs • Generic Baccalaureate • RN Baccalaureate

The University State-supported comprehensive coed institution. Part of Pennsylvania State System of Higher Education. Founded: 1857. *Primary accreditation:* regional. *Setting:* 205-acre small-town campus. *Total enrollment:* 2,954.

The Robert Packer Department of Health Sciences Founded in 1987. *Nursing program faculty:* 15 (20% with doctorates). *Off-campus program site:* Sayre.

Academic Facilities *Campus library:* 244,000 volumes (11,000 in health, 2,200 in nursing); 1,200 periodical subscriptions (525 health-care related). *Nursing school resources:* CAI, computer lab, nursing audiovisuals, learning resource lab.

Student Life *Student services:* health clinic, personal counseling, career counseling, institutionally sponsored work-study program, job placement, campus safety program, special assistance for disabled students. *International student services:* counseling/support, ESL courses. *Nursing student activities:* nursing club.

Calendar Semesters.

NURSING STUDENT PROFILE

Undergraduate **Enrollment:** 154
Women: 88%; **Men:** 12%; **Minority:** 6%; **International:** 1%; **Part-time:** 9%

BACCALAUREATE PROGRAMS

Contact Admissions Office, Robert Packer Department of Health Sciences, Mansfield University of Pennsylvania, Mansfield, PA 16933, 717-662-4243. *Fax:* 717-662-4121. *E-mail:* admissns@mnsfld.edu

Expenses *State resident tuition:* $3368 full-time, $187 per credit part-time. *Nonresident tuition:* $8566 full-time, $336 per credit part-time. *Full-time mandatory fees:* $846. *Part-time mandatory fees:* $49–$225. *Room and board:* $3586–$3612. *Books and supplies per academic year:* $450.

Financial Aid Institutionally sponsored need-based grants/scholarships, institutionally sponsored non-need grants/scholarships, Federal Pell Grants, Federal Perkins Loans, Federal Supplemental Educational Opportunity Grants, Federal Work-Study, Federal PLUS Loans, Federal Stafford Loans. 75% of undergraduate students in nursing programs received some form of financial aid in 1995–96. *Application deadline:* 4/15.

Generic Baccalaureate Program (BSN)

Applying *Required:* SAT I, ACT, minimum high school GPA of 2.5, minimum college GPA of 2.5, 2 years of high school math, high school chemistry, high school biology, high school transcript, high school class rank: top 40%. *Application deadline:* rolling. *Application fee:* $25.

Degree Requirements 131 total credit hours, 61 in nursing.

RN Baccalaureate Program (BSN)

Applying *Required:* NLN Mobility Profile II, RN license, diploma or AD in nursing, transcript of college record. *Options:* May apply for transfer of up to 100 total credits. *Application deadline:* rolling. *Application fee:* $25.

Degree Requirements 131 total credit hours, 61 in nursing.

MARYWOOD COLLEGE

Department of Nursing
Scranton, Pennsylvania

Programs • Generic Baccalaureate • RN Baccalaureate • LPN to Baccalaureate • Continuing Education

The College Independent Roman Catholic comprehensive coed institution. Founded: 1915. *Primary accreditation:* regional. *Setting:* 115-acre suburban campus. *Total enrollment:* 2,958.

The Department of Nursing Founded in 1976. *Nursing program faculty:* 6 (50% with doctorates).

Academic Facilities *Campus library:* 180,709 volumes (5,343 in health, 1,089 in nursing); 1,114 periodical subscriptions (136 health-care related). *Nursing school resources:* CAI, computer lab, nursing audiovisuals, interactive nursing skills videos, learning resource lab.

Student Life *Student services:* health clinic, child-care facilities, personal counseling, career counseling, institutionally sponsored work-study program, job placement, campus safety program, special assistance for disabled students. *International student services:* counseling/support, special assistance for nonnative speakers of English, ESL courses. *Nursing student activities:* Sigma Theta Tau, nursing club, student nurses association.

Calendar Semesters.

NURSING STUDENT PROFILE

Undergraduate **Enrollment:** 110
Women: 94%; **Men:** 6%; **Minority:** 3%; **International:** 0%; **Part-time:** 30%

BACCALAUREATE PROGRAMS

Contact Dr. Mary Alice Golden, Chairperson, Department of Nursing, Marywood College, 2300 Adams Avenue, Scranton, PA 18509, 717-348-6275. *Fax:* 717-348-1817.

Expenses *Tuition:* ranges from $9000 to $10,000 full-time, $385 per credit part-time. *Full-time mandatory fees:* $75–$175. *Room and board:* $4110–$4800. *Room only:* $2400. *Books and supplies per academic year:* ranges from $600 to $800.

Financial Aid Institutionally sponsored need-based grants/scholarships, institutionally sponsored non-need grants/scholarships, Federal Nursing Student Loans, Federal Supplemental Educational Opportunity Grants, Federal Work-Study. 95% of undergraduate students in nursing programs received some form of financial aid in 1995–96. *Application deadline:* 2/15.

Generic Baccalaureate Program (BSN)

Applying *Required:* SAT I or ACT, TOEFL for nonnative speakers of English, high school chemistry, high school biology, high school transcript, letter of recommendation, transcript of college record. *Options:* May apply for transfer of up to 68 total credits. *Application deadline:* rolling. *Application fee:* $20.

Degree Requirements 136 total credit hours, 55 in nursing.

RN Baccalaureate Program (BSN)

Applying *Required:* SAT I or ACT, TOEFL for nonnative speakers of English, high school chemistry, high school biology, RN license, high school transcript, letter of recommendation, transcript of college record. *Options:* May apply for transfer of up to 68 total credits. *Application deadline:* rolling. *Application fee:* $20.

Degree Requirements 136 total credit hours, 135 in nursing.

LPN to Baccalaureate Program (BSN)

Applying *Required:* SAT I or ACT, TOEFL for nonnative speakers of English, high school chemistry, high school biology, high school transcript, letter of recommendation, transcript of college record. *Options:* May apply for transfer of up to 68 total credits. *Application deadline:* rolling. *Application fee:* $20.

Degree Requirements 136 total credit hours, 55 in nursing.

CONTINUING EDUCATION PROGRAM

Contact Dr. Edna Wilson, Dean, Continuing Education, Department of Nursing, Marywood College, 2300 Adams Avenue, Scranton, PA 18509, 717-348-6237. *Fax:* 717-343-5030.

See full description on page 476.

MESSIAH COLLEGE

Department of Nursing
Grantham, Pennsylvania

Programs • Generic Baccalaureate • RN Baccalaureate • Baccalaureate for Second Degree

The College Independent 4-year coed college, affiliated with Brethren in Christ Church. Founded: 1909. *Primary accreditation:* regional. *Setting:* 360-acre small-town campus. *Total enrollment:* 2,428.

The Department of Nursing Founded in 1980. *Nursing program faculty:* 12 (50% with doctorates).

Academic Facilities *Campus library:* 180,000 volumes; 1,000 periodical subscriptions. *Nursing school resources:* CAI, computer lab, nursing audiovisuals, interactive nursing skills videos, learning resource lab.

Student Life *Student services:* health clinic, personal counseling, career counseling, institutionally sponsored work-study program, job placement, campus safety program, special assistance for disabled students. *International student services:* counseling/support. *Nursing student activities:* Sigma Theta Tau, student nurses association, Nurses Christian Fellowship.

Calendar Semesters.

NURSING STUDENT PROFILE

Undergraduate **Enrollment:** 240
Women: 94%; **Men:** 6%; **Minority:** 3%; **International:** 0%; **Part-time:** 1%

BACCALAUREATE PROGRAMS

Contact Dr. Sandra L. Jamison, Chairperson, Department of Nursing, Messiah College, Grantham, PA 17027, 717-691-6029. *Fax:* 717-691-6046. *E-mail:* nursing@mcis.messiah.edu

Expenses *Tuition:* $5435 per academic year. *Full-time mandatory fees:* $205. *Room and board:* $2255–$2640. *Room only:* $1220–$1340. *Books and supplies per academic year:* ranges from $450 to $475.

Financial Aid Institutionally sponsored need-based grants/scholarships, institutionally sponsored non-need grants/scholarships, Federal Direct Loans, Federal Nursing Student Loans, Federal Perkins Loans, Federal Supplemental Educational Opportunity Grants, Federal Work-Study. *Application deadline:* 4/1.

Generic Baccalaureate Program (BSN)

Applying *Required:* SAT I, ACT, high school transcript, 2 letters of recommendation, written essay, high school class rank: top 33%. 21 prerequisite credits must be completed before admission to the nursing program. *Options:* Advanced standing available through advanced placement exams. May apply for transfer of up to 96 total credits. *Application deadline:* rolling. *Application fee:* $20.

Degree Requirements 126 total credit hours, 47 in nursing. English proficiency exam.

RN Baccalaureate Program (BSN)

Applying *Required:* minimum college GPA of 2.5, RN license, diploma or AD in nursing, interview, 2 letters of recommendation, written essay, transcript of college record, 1 year of experience as RN. 21 prerequisite credits must be completed before admission to the nursing program. *Options:* Advanced standing available through advanced placement exams. Course work may be accelerated. May apply for transfer of up to 96 total credits. *Application deadline:* rolling. *Application fee:* $20.

Degree Requirements 126 total credit hours, 47 in nursing. English proficiency exam.

Baccalaureate for Second Degree Program (BSN)

Applying *Required:* minimum college GPA of 2.5, interview, 2 letters of recommendation, written essay, transcript of college record. 57 prerequisite credits must be completed before admission to the nursing program. *Options:* Advanced standing available through advanced placement exams. Course work may be accelerated. May apply for transfer of up to 96 total credits. *Application deadline:* rolling. *Application fee:* $20.

Degree Requirements 126 total credit hours, 47 in nursing. English proficiency exam.

MILLERSVILLE UNIVERSITY OF PENNSYLVANIA

Department of Nursing
Millersville, Pennsylvania

Programs • RN Baccalaureate • BSN to Master's

The University State-supported comprehensive coed institution. Part of Pennsylvania State System of Higher Education. Founded: 1855. *Primary accreditation:* regional. *Setting:* 245-acre small-town campus. *Total enrollment:* 7,510.

The Department of Nursing Founded in 1979. *Nursing program faculty:* 7 (71% with doctorates). *Off-campus program site:* Lancaster.

Academic Facilities *Campus library:* 370,000 volumes; 2,000 periodical subscriptions (82 health-care related). *Nursing school resources:* CAI, computer lab, nursing audiovisuals, interactive nursing skills videos, learning resource lab.

Student Life *Student services:* health clinic, personal counseling, career counseling, institutionally sponsored work-study program, job placement, campus safety program, special assistance for disabled students. *International student services:* counseling/support, special assistance for nonnative speakers of English, ESL courses. *Nursing student activities:* Sigma Theta Tau, nursing club.

Calendar Semesters.

NURSING STUDENT PROFILE

Undergraduate **Enrollment:** 161
Women: 89%; **Men:** 11%; **Minority:** 3%; **International:** 0%; **Part-time:** 84%
Graduate **Enrollment:** 28
Women: 93%; **Men:** 7%; **Minority:** 0%; **International:** 0%; **Part-time:** 100%

BACCALAUREATE PROGRAM

Contact Dr. Carol Y. Phillips, Chairperson, Department of Nursing, Millersville University of Pennsylvania, Millersville, PA 17551-0302, 717-872-3410. *Fax:* 717-872-3985. *E-mail:* cphillip@marauder.millersv.edu

Expenses *State resident tuition:* $3368 full-time, $140 per credit part-time. *Nonresident tuition:* $8566 full-time, $357 per credit part-time. *Full-time mandatory fees:* $900. *Room and board:* $4300. *Room only:* $2420. *Books and supplies per academic year:* ranges from $600 to $800.

Financial Aid Institutionally sponsored need-based grants/scholarships, institutionally sponsored non-need grants/scholarships, Federal Nursing Student Loans, Federal Supplemental Educational Opportunity Grants, Federal Work-Study. 75% of undergraduate students in nursing programs received some form of financial aid in 1995–96. *Application deadline:* 5/1.

RN Baccalaureate Program (BSN)

Applying *Required:* NLN Mobility Profile II, RN license, diploma or AD in nursing, high school transcript, fulfillment of articulation model. 60 prerequisite credits must be completed before admission to the nursing program. *Options:* Advanced standing available through the following means: advanced placement exams, credit by exam. Course work may be accelerated. May apply for transfer of up to 84 total credits. *Application deadline:* rolling. *Application fee:* $25.

Degree Requirements 125 total credit hours, 63 in nursing.

MASTER'S PROGRAM

Contact Dr. Ruth E. Davis, RNC, CRNP, Graduate Program Coordinator and Assistant Professor, Department of Nursing, Millersville University, PO Box 1002, Millersville, PA 17551-0302, 717-871-2183. *Fax:* 717-872-3985. *E-mail:* rdavis@marauder.millersv.edu

Areas of Study Nurse practitioner program in family health.

Expenses *State resident tuition:* $187 per credit. *Nonresident tuition:* $336 per credit. *Part-time mandatory fees:* $38. *Books and supplies per academic year:* ranges from $600 to $800.

Financial Aid Graduate assistantships, employment opportunities. 64% of master's level students in nursing programs received some form of financial aid in 1995-96.

BSN to Master's Program (MSN)

Applying *Required:* GRE General Test, bachelor's degree in nursing, minimum GPA of 3.0, RN license, 1 year of clinical experience, physical assessment course, statistics course, professional liability/malpractice insurance, essay, interview, 3 letters of recommendation, transcript of college record. *Application deadline:* 3/31.

Degree Requirements 42 total credit hours, 42 in nursing.

NEUMANN COLLEGE

Division of Nursing and Health Sciences
Aston, Pennsylvania

Programs • Generic Baccalaureate • Accelerated RN Baccalaureate • BSN to Master's

The College Independent Roman Catholic comprehensive coed institution. Founded: 1965. *Primary accreditation:* regional. *Setting:* 14-acre small-town campus. *Total enrollment:* 1,214.

The Division of Nursing and Health Sciences Founded in 1965. *Nursing program faculty:* 14 (35% with doctorates).

Academic Facilities *Campus library:* 84,000 volumes (6,000 in health, 5,000 in nursing); 700 periodical subscriptions (140 health-care related). *Nursing school resources:* CAI, computer lab, nursing audiovisuals, interactive nursing skills videos, learning resource lab.

Student Life *Student services:* health clinic, personal counseling, career counseling, institutionally sponsored work-study program, campus safety program. *International student services:* counseling/support. *Nursing student activities:* Sigma Theta Tau, nursing club, student nurses association.

Calendar Semesters.

NURSING STUDENT PROFILE

Undergraduate **Enrollment:** 450
Women: 80%; **Men:** 20%; **Minority:** 6%; **International:** 1%; **Part-time:** 47%

Graduate **Enrollment:** 12
Women: 100%; **Minority:** 2%; **International:** 0%; **Part-time:** 100%

BACCALAUREATE PROGRAMS

Contact Mr. Mark Osborn, Director of Admissions, Division of Nursing and Health Sciences, Neumann College, Concord Road, Aston, PA 19014, 610-558-5616. *Fax:* 610-459-1370. *E-mail:* mosborn@smtpgate.neumann.edu

Expenses *Tuition:* $13,100 full-time, $470 per credit part-time. *Full-time mandatory fees:* $220. *Books and supplies per academic year:* ranges from $200 to $400.

Financial Aid Institutionally sponsored need-based grants/scholarships, institutionally sponsored non-need grants/scholarships, Federal Nursing Student Loans, Federal Supplemental Educational Opportunity Grants, Federal Work-Study. 56% of undergraduate students in nursing programs received some form of financial aid in 1995–96.

Generic Baccalaureate Program (BS)

Applying *Required:* SAT I, ACT, TOEFL for nonnative speakers of English, minimum high school GPA of 2.0, minimum college GPA of 2.5, 2 years of high school math, 2 years of high school science, high school foreign language, high school transcript, interview, letter of recommendation, written essay, transcript of college record. *Options:* May apply for transfer of up to 90 total credits. *Application deadline:* 8/15. *Application fee:* $25.

Degree Requirements 126 total credit hours, 42 in nursing.

Accelerated RN Baccalaureate Program (BS)

Applying *Required:* minimum college GPA of 2.5, RN license, diploma or AD in nursing, interview, written essay, transcript of college record. 63 prerequisite credits must be completed before admission to the nursing program. *Options:* Course work may be accelerated. May apply for transfer of up to 90 total credits. *Application deadline:* rolling. *Application fee:* $25.

Degree Requirements 126 total credit hours, 30 in nursing.

MASTER'S PROGRAM

Contact Dr. Jill B. Derstine, Chair, Division of Nursing and Health Sciences, Neumann College, 1 Neumann Drive, Aston, PA 19014, 610-558-5560. *Fax:* 610-459-1370. *E-mail:* jderstin@smtpgate.neumann.edu

Areas of Study Clinical nurse specialist programs in gerontological nursing, rehabilitation nursing.

Expenses *Tuition:* $485 per credit. *Part-time mandatory fees:* $50. *Books and supplies per academic year:* ranges from $100 to $300.

BSN to Master's Program (MSN)

Applying *Required:* GRE General Test or Miller Analogies Test, TOEFL for nonnative speakers of English, bachelor's degree in nursing, RN license, physical assessment course, statistics course, interview, 3 letters of recommendation, transcript of college record, nursing research, basic computer course. *Application deadline:* rolling. *Application fee:* $50.

Degree Requirements 39 total credit hours, 39 in nursing.

PENNSYLVANIA STATE UNIVERSITY, UNIVERSITY PARK CAMPUS

School of Nursing
University Park, Pennsylvania

Programs • Generic Baccalaureate • RN Baccalaureate • MS • Post-Master's • Continuing Education

The University State-related coed university. Part of Pennsylvania State University. Founded: 1855. *Primary accreditation:* regional. *Setting:* 5,160-acre small-town campus. *Total enrollment:* 39,646.

The School of Nursing Founded in 1964. *Nursing program faculty:* 72 (32% with doctorates). *Off-campus program sites:* Hershey, Harrisburg, Shenango.

Academic Facilities *Campus library:* 2.5 million volumes (240,000 in health); 29,000 periodical subscriptions (3,000 health-care related). *Nursing school resources:* CAI, computer lab, nursing audiovisuals, interactive nursing skills videos, learning resource lab.

Student Life *Student services:* health clinic, child-care facilities, personal counseling, career counseling, institutionally sponsored work-study program, job placement, campus safety program, special assistance for disabled students. *International student services:* counseling/support, special assistance for nonnative speakers of English, ESL courses. *Nursing student activities:* Sigma Theta Tau, nursing club, student nurses association.

Calendar Semesters.

NURSING STUDENT PROFILE

Undergraduate **Enrollment:** 660
Women: 85%; **Men:** 15%; **Minority:** 4%; **International:** 0%; **Part-time:** 49%

Graduate **Enrollment:** 60
Women: 98%; **Men:** 2%; **Minority:** 1%; **International:** 1%; **Part-time:** 80%

BACCALAUREATE PROGRAMS

Contact Ms. Susan Youtz, Assistant Director of Undergraduate Program, 201 Health and Human Development, East, School of Nursing, Pennsylvania State University, University Park, PA 16802, 814-863-0245. *Fax:* 814-865-3779. *E-mail:* scy1@psu.edu

Expenses *State resident tuition:* $5434 full-time, $227 per credit part-time. *Nonresident tuition:* $11,774 full-time, $491 per credit part-time. *Full-time mandatory fees:* $95. *Part-time mandatory fees:* $95. *Room and board:* $1880–$2220. *Room only:* $1820. *Books and supplies per academic year:* $700.

Financial Aid Institutionally sponsored need-based grants/scholarships, Federal Nursing Student Loans, Federal Work-Study. *Application deadline:* 2/15.

Generic Baccalaureate Program (BS)

Applying *Required:* SAT I, TOEFL for nonnative speakers of English, minimum college GPA of 3.0, 3 years of high school math, 3 years of high school science, high school chemistry, high school biology, high school foreign language, high school transcript, transcript of college record. 55 prerequisite credits must be completed before admission to the nursing program. *Options:* Advanced standing available through the following means: advanced placement exams, credit by exam. *Application deadline:* 2/15. *Application fee:* $35.

Degree Requirements 130 total credit hours, 63 in nursing.

RN Baccalaureate Program (BS)

Applying *Required:* SAT I, TOEFL for nonnative speakers of English, RN license, diploma or AD in nursing, transcript of college record. 55 prerequisite credits must be completed before admission to the nursing program. *Application deadline:* rolling. *Application fee:* $35.

Degree Requirements 130 total credit hours, 63 in nursing.

Pennsylvania State University, University Park Campus (continued)

MASTER'S PROGRAMS

Contact Dr. Freida Holt, Interim Associate Director for Graduate Programs, 203 Health and Human Development, East, School of Nursing, Pennsylvania State University, University Park, PA 16802, 814-863-2211. *Fax:* 814-865-3779. *E-mail:* fmh1@psu.edu

Areas of Study Clinical nurse specialist programs in adult health nursing, community health nursing; nursing administration; nursing education; nurse practitioner programs in family health, neonatal health.

Expenses *State resident tuition:* $6078 full-time, $256 per credit part-time. *Nonresident tuition:* $12,516 full-time, $256 per credit part-time. *Full-time mandatory fees:* $95. *Part-time mandatory fees:* $95. *Room only:* $2200–$2530. *Books and supplies per academic year:* ranges from $200 to $400.

Financial Aid Graduate assistantships, nurse traineeships. 33% of master's level students in nursing programs received some form of financial aid in 1995-96. *Application deadline:* 3/1.

MS Program

Applying *Required:* GRE General Test, TOEFL for nonnative speakers of English, bachelor's degree in nursing, minimum GPA of 3.0, RN license, statistics course, professional liability/malpractice insurance, essay, 2 letters of recommendation, transcript of college record. *Application deadline:* 3/1. *Application fee:* $40.

Degree Requirements 39 total credit hours, 27 in nursing. Scholarly paper or thesis.

Post-Master's Program

Applying *Required:* bachelor's degree in nursing, minimum GPA of 3.0, RN license, statistics course, professional liability/malpractice insurance, essay, 2 letters of recommendation, transcript of college record. *Application deadline:* 3/1.

Degree Requirements 39 total credit hours, 39 in nursing.

Distance learning Courses provided through video.

CONTINUING EDUCATION PROGRAM

Contact Dr. Sally I. Wangsness, Associate Director for Commonwealth Educational System Programs, 201 Health and Human Development, East, School of Nursing, Pennsylvania State University, University Park, PA 16802, 814-863-0245. *Fax:* 814-865-3779. *E-mail:* siw2@psu.edu

SAINT FRANCIS COLLEGE
Department of Nursing
Loretto, Pennsylvania

Programs • Generic Baccalaureate • RN Baccalaureate

The College Independent Roman Catholic comprehensive coed institution. Founded: 1847. *Primary accreditation:* regional. *Setting:* 600-acre rural campus. *Total enrollment:* 1,886.

The Department of Nursing Founded in 1980. *Nursing program faculty:* 11 (9% with doctorates).

Academic Facilities *Campus library:* 179,325 volumes (2,520 in health); 792 periodical subscriptions (110 health-care related). *Nursing school resources:* CAI, computer lab, nursing audiovisuals, learning resource lab.

Student Life *Student services:* health clinic, personal counseling, career counseling, institutionally sponsored work-study program, job placement. *International student services:* counseling/support. *Nursing student activities:* student nurses association.

Calendar Semesters.

NURSING STUDENT PROFILE

Undergraduate **Enrollment:** 124
Women: 80%; **Men:** 20%; **Minority:** 2%; **International:** 1%; **Part-time:** 8%

BACCALAUREATE PROGRAMS

Contact Dr. Jean M. Samii, Chairperson and Professor, Department of Nursing, Saint Francis College, Loretto, PA 15940-0060, 814-472-3184. *Fax:* 814-472-3154.

Expenses *Full-time mandatory fees:* $475. *Room and board:* $5330–$5660. *Room only:* $2670. *Books and supplies per academic year:* $500.

Financial Aid Institutionally sponsored need-based grants/scholarships, institutionally sponsored non-need grants/scholarships, Federal Direct Loans, Federal Nursing Student Loans, Federal Supplemental Educational Opportunity Grants, Federal Work-Study. 58% of undergraduate students in nursing programs received some form of financial aid in 1995–96. *Application deadline:* 5/1.

Generic Baccalaureate Program (BSN)

Applying *Required:* SAT I or ACT, TOEFL for nonnative speakers of English, minimum high school GPA of 3.0, minimum college GPA of 2.5, 2 years of high school math, 2 years of high school science, high school chemistry, high school biology, high school transcript, interview, 2 letters of recommendation, transcript of college record, high school class rank: top 40%. *Options:* May apply for transfer of up to 64 total credits. *Application deadline:* rolling. *Application fee:* $30.

Degree Requirements 138 total credit hours, 62 in nursing.

RN Baccalaureate Program (BSN)

Applying *Required:* TOEFL for nonnative speakers of English, minimum college GPA of 2.5, RN license, diploma or AD in nursing, interview, letter of recommendation, written essay, transcript of college record. *Options:* May apply for transfer of up to 64 total credits. *Application deadline:* rolling. *Application fee:* $30.

Degree Requirements 138 total credit hours, 62 in nursing.

SLIPPERY ROCK UNIVERSITY OF PENNSYLVANIA
Department of Nursing
Slippery Rock, Pennsylvania

Programs • RN Baccalaureate • Baccalaureate for Second Degree • BSN to Master's • Post-Master's

The University State-supported comprehensive coed institution. Part of Pennsylvania State System of Higher Education. Founded: 1889. *Primary accreditation:* regional. *Setting:* 611-acre rural campus. *Total enrollment:* 7,493.

The Department of Nursing Founded in 1974. *Nursing program faculty:* 7 (50% with doctorates). *Off-campus program site:* Mars.

Academic Facilities *Campus library:* 419,480 volumes (19,604 in health, 1,396 in nursing); 1,723 periodical subscriptions (165 health-care related). *Nursing school resources:* CAI, computer lab, nursing audiovisuals, interactive nursing skills videos, microfilm/microfiche and a statewide network for accessing journals.

Student Life *Student services:* health clinic, child-care facilities, personal counseling, career counseling, institutionally sponsored work-study program, job placement, campus safety program, special assistance for disabled students. *International student services:* counseling/support. *Nursing student activities:* Sigma Theta Tau.

Calendar Semesters.

NURSING STUDENT PROFILE

Undergraduate **Enrollment:** 134
Women: 91%; **Men:** 9%; **Minority:** 0%; **International:** 0%; **Part-time:** 96%
Graduate **Enrollment:** 56
Women: 90%; **Men:** 10%; **Minority:** 14%; **International:** 0%; **Part-time:** 90%

BACCALAUREATE PROGRAMS

Contact Ms. Carla Hradisky, Associate Director, Admissions, 104 Maltby Building, Department of Nursing, Slippery Rock University of Pennsylvania, Slippery Rock, PA 16057, 412-738-2112. *Fax:* 412-738-2913.

Expenses *State resident tuition:* $3368 full-time, $140 per semester credit part-time. *Nonresident tuition:* $8566 full-time, $357 per semester credit part-time. *Full-time mandatory fees:* $801. *Part-time mandatory fees:* $71+. *Room and board:* $3552. *Books and supplies per academic year:* ranges from $300 to $600.

Financial Aid Federal Nursing Student Loans, Federal Work-Study. *Application deadline:* 5/1.

RN Baccalaureate Program (BSN)

Applying *Required:* RN license, diploma or AD in nursing, interview, transcript of college record. 35 prerequisite credits must be completed before admission to the nursing program. *Options:* Advanced standing available through credit by exam. May apply for transfer of up to 67 total credits. *Application deadline:* rolling.

Degree Requirements 128 total credit hours, 63 in nursing.

Baccalaureate for Second Degree Program (BSN)

Applying *Required:* RN license, diploma or AD in nursing, interview, transcript of college record. *Options:* Advanced standing available through credit by exam. May apply for transfer of up to 67 total credits. *Application deadline:* rolling.

MASTER'S PROGRAMS

Contact Dr. Joyce White, Director and Coordinator, 119 Behavioral Science Building, Department of Nursing, Slippery Rock University, Slippery Rock, PA 16057, 412-738-2323. *Fax:* 412-738-2881.

Areas of Study Nurse practitioner program in family health.

Expenses *State resident tuition:* $3368 full-time, $187 per credit part-time. *Nonresident tuition:* $6054 full-time, $336 per credit part-time. *Full-time mandatory fees:* $775. *Part-time mandatory fees:* $119–$666. *Room only:* $1860–$2410. *Books and supplies per academic year:* ranges from $300 to $500.

Financial Aid Graduate assistantships, Federal Direct Loans, Federal Nursing Student Loans, employment opportunities. 14% of master's level students in nursing programs received some form of financial aid in 1995-96. *Application deadline:* 4/1.

BSN to Master's Program (MSN)

Applying *Required:* GRE General Test, bachelor's degree in nursing, bachelor's degree, minimum GPA of 2.7, RN license, 1 year of clinical experience, statistics course, professional liability/malpractice insurance, essay, interview, 3 letters of recommendation, transcript of college record. *Application deadlines:* 7/1 (fall), 11/1 (spring).

Degree Requirements 45 total credit hours, 45 in nursing. Thesis or project.

Post-Master's Program

Applying *Required:* bachelor's degree in nursing, bachelor's degree, minimum GPA of 2.7, RN license, 1 year of clinical experience, statistics course, professional liability/malpractice insurance, essay, interview, 3 letters of recommendation, transcript of college record, MSN. *Application deadlines:* 7/1 (fall), 11/1 (spring).

Degree Requirements 45 total credit hours, 45 in nursing.

TEMPLE UNIVERSITY
College of Allied Health Professions, Department of Nursing Philadelphia, Pennsylvania

Programs • Generic Baccalaureate • RN Baccalaureate • MSN

The University State-related coed university. Founded: 1884. *Primary accreditation:* regional. *Setting:* 76-acre urban campus. *Total enrollment:* 26,477.

The College of Allied Health Professions, Department of Nursing Founded in 1969. *Nursing program faculty:* 35 (43% with doctorates).

Academic Facilities *Campus library:* 2.0 million volumes (100,000 in health, 1,500 in nursing); 16,000 periodical subscriptions (1,200 health-care related). *Nursing school resources:* CAI, computer lab, nursing audiovisuals, interactive nursing skills videos, learning resource lab.

Student Life *Student services:* health clinic, child-care facilities, personal counseling, career counseling, institutionally sponsored work-study program, job placement, campus safety program, special assistance for disabled students. *International student services:* counseling/support, special assistance for nonnative speakers of English, ESL courses. *Nursing student activities:* Sigma Theta Tau, student nurses association.

Calendar Semesters.

NURSING STUDENT PROFILE

Undergraduate **Enrollment:** 321
Women: 90%; **Men:** 10%; **Minority:** 34%; **International:** 0%; **Part-time:** 57%
Graduate **Enrollment:** 149
Women: 89%; **Men:** 11%; **Minority:** 38%; **International:** 8%; **Part-time:** 96%

BACCALAUREATE PROGRAMS

Contact Dr. Catherine A. Bevil, Chair and Professor, Department of Nursing, College of Allied Health Professions, Temple University, 3307 North Broad Street, Philadelphia, PA 19140, 215-707-1598. *Fax:* 215-707-1599.

Expenses *State resident tuition:* $6786 full-time, $236 per credit part-time. *Nonresident tuition:* $12,010 full-time, $353 per credit part-time. *Full-time mandatory fees:* $320. *Room and board:* $5200. *Books and supplies per academic year:* $300.

Financial Aid Institutionally sponsored need-based grants/scholarships, Federal Nursing Student Loans, Federal Work-Study. *Application deadline:* 5/1.

Generic Baccalaureate Program (BSN)

Applying *Required:* SAT I or ACT, TOEFL for nonnative speakers of English, minimum college GPA of 2.5, 3 years of high school math, 3 years of high school science, high school foreign language, high school transcript, written essay, transcript of college record. 55 prerequisite credits must be completed before admission to the nursing program. *Options:* May apply for transfer of up to 64 total credits. *Application deadline:* 1/31. *Application fee:* $20.

Degree Requirements 122 total credit hours, 67 in nursing.

RN Baccalaureate Program (BSN)

Applying *Required:* SAT I or ACT, TOEFL for nonnative speakers of English, minimum college GPA of 2.5, RN license, diploma or AD in nursing, high school foreign language, high school transcript, written essay, transcript of college record. 55 prerequisite credits must be completed before admission to the nursing program. *Options:* Advanced standing available through credit by exam. May apply for transfer of up to 64 total credits. *Application deadline:* rolling. *Application fee:* $20.

Degree Requirements 122 total credit hours, 67 in nursing.

MASTER'S PROGRAM

Contact Dr. Jean H. Woods, Acting Director of Graduate Studies in Nursing, Department of Nursing, College of Allied Health Professions, Temple University, 3307 North Broad Street, Philadelphia, PA 19140, 215-707-4626. *Fax:* 215-707-1599.

Areas of Study Clinical nurse specialist programs in adult health nursing, gerontological nursing, maternity-newborn nursing, psychiatric–mental health nursing; nurse practitioner program in adult health primary care.

Expenses *State resident tuition:* $287 per credit. *Nonresident tuition:* $400 per credit. *Full-time mandatory fees:* $92. *Books and supplies per academic year:* ranges from $150 to $300.

Financial Aid Graduate assistantships. *Application deadline:* 5/1.

MSN Program

Applying *Required:* GRE General Test, TOEFL for nonnative speakers of English, bachelor's degree in nursing, minimum GPA of 3.0, RN license, 1 year of clinical experience, physical assessment course, statistics course, interview, 2 letters of recommendation, transcript of college record. *Application deadlines:* 2/15 (nurse practitioner track), rolling. *Application fee:* $35.

Degree Requirements 36 total credit hours, 24 in nursing. Thesis or research project.

THIEL COLLEGE
Nursing Department
Greenville, Pennsylvania

Programs • Generic Baccalaureate • Baccalaureate for Second Degree
The College Independent 4-year coed college, affiliated with Evangelical Lutheran Church in America. Founded: 1866. *Primary accreditation:* regional. *Setting:* 135-acre rural campus. *Total enrollment:* 1,008.
The Nursing Department Founded in 1983. *Nursing program faculty:* 9 (20% with doctorates).
Academic Facilities *Campus library:* 135,000 volumes (5,400 in health, 1,300 in nursing); 925 periodical subscriptions (75 health-care related). *Nursing school resources:* CAI, computer lab, nursing audiovisuals, learning resource lab.
Student Life *Student services:* health clinic, personal counseling, career counseling, institutionally sponsored work-study program, job placement, campus safety program, special assistance for disabled students. *International student services:* counseling/support, special assistance for nonnative speakers of English, ESL courses. *Nursing student activities:* Sigma Theta Tau, student nurses association.
Calendar Semesters.

NURSING STUDENT PROFILE

Undergraduate **Enrollment:** 63
Women: 78%; **Men:** 22%; **Minority:** 1%; **International:** 1%; **Part-time:** 6%

BACCALAUREATE PROGRAMS

Contact Dr. Evelyn E. Ramming, Director and Chairperson, Nursing Department, Thiel College, 75 College Avenue, Greenville, PA 16125, 412-589-2053. *Fax:* 412-589-2021.
Expenses *Tuition:* $12,420 full-time, $394 per credit hour part-time. *Full-time mandatory fees:* $30–$85. *Room and board:* $5090. *Books and supplies per academic year:* ranges from $30 to $500.
Financial Aid Institutionally sponsored need-based grants/scholarships, institutionally sponsored non-need grants/scholarships, Federal Nursing Student Loans, Federal Supplemental Educational Opportunity Grants, Federal Work-Study. 94% of undergraduate students in nursing programs received some form of financial aid in 1995–96. *Application deadline:* 5/1.

Generic Baccalaureate Program (BSN)

Applying *Required:* TOEFL for nonnative speakers of English, minimum high school GPA of 2.0, minimum college GPA of 2.5, 3 years of high school math, 3 years of high school science, high school chemistry, high school biology, high school transcript, interview, transcript of college record. 30 prerequisite credits must be completed before admission to the nursing program. *Options:* May apply for transfer of up to 90 total credits. *Application deadlines:* 7/1 (fall), 11/1 (spring). *Application fee:* $25.
Degree Requirements 124 total credit hours, 45 in nursing. English competency exam.

Baccalaureate for Second Degree Program (BSN)

Applying *Required:* TOEFL for nonnative speakers of English, minimum high school GPA of 2.0, minimum college GPA of 2.5, 3 years of high school math, 3 years of high school science, high school chemistry, high school biology, high school transcript, interview, transcript of college record. 30 prerequisite credits must be completed before admission to the nursing program. *Options:* May apply for transfer of up to 90 total credits. *Application deadlines:* 7/1 (fall), 11/1 (spring). *Application fee:* $25.
Degree Requirements 124 total credit hours, 49 in nursing. English competency exam.

See full description on page 514.

THOMAS JEFFERSON UNIVERSITY
Department of Nursing
Philadelphia, Pennsylvania

Programs • Generic Baccalaureate • RN Baccalaureate • MSN • Accelerated MSN • Accelerated Master's for Non-Nursing College Graduates
The University Independent upper-level coed institution. Founded: 1824. *Primary accreditation:* regional. *Setting:* 13-acre urban campus. *Total enrollment:* 1,533.
The Department of Nursing Founded in 1970. *Nursing program faculty:* 22 (55% with doctorates).

▶ *NOTEWORTHY*

Thomas Jefferson University's Department of Nursing is a national leader in preparing baccalaureate and master's nursing students for the challenges of an ever-changing health-care environment. New programs include an accelerated option for MSN for second degree students and a post-master's family nurse practitioner option. Program emphases include primary care, disease prevention/health promotion, acute and chronic illness, and community and public health nursing. Students have interdisciplinary learning experiences and take advantage of a broad spectrum of available clinical experiences, ranging from the prestigious Jefferson Health System and its preferred affiliates to more than 80 other hospitals, ambulatory sites, and community agencies. The Department also maintains a Women's Center for Health Promotion to advance the health of the surrounding community, as well as student learning and faculty practice opportunities. The Department participates in an international exchange program, and the Learning Resource Center remains on the cutting edge of nursing informatics and educational technology. The diverse student body can elect full-or part-time study and convenient day or evening hours.

Academic Facilities *Campus library:* 169,000 volumes (146,000 in health, 4,700 in nursing); 2,500 periodical subscriptions (2,100 health-care related). *Nursing school resources:* CAI, computer lab, nursing audiovisuals, interactive nursing skills videos, learning resource lab.
Student Life *Student services:* health clinic, child-care facilities, personal counseling, career counseling, institutionally sponsored work-study program, job placement, campus safety program, special assistance for disabled students. *International student services:* counseling/support, special assistance for nonnative speakers of English, ESL courses. *Nursing student activities:* Sigma Theta Tau, recruiter club, student nurses association.
Calendar Semesters.

NURSING STUDENT PROFILE

Undergraduate **Enrollment:** 324
Women: 85%; **Men:** 15%; **Minority:** 29%; **International:** 1%; **Part-time:** 35%
Graduate **Enrollment:** 90
Women: 97%; **Men:** 3%; **Minority:** 10%; **International:** 2%; **Part-time:** 83%

BACCALAUREATE PROGRAMS

Contact Dr. Pamela G. Watson, Chair and Professor, Department of Nursing, Thomas Jefferson University, 130 South 9th Street, Suite 1251, Philadelphia, PA 19107, 215-955-8390. *Fax:* 215-923-1468. *E-mail:* watsonp@jeflin.tju.edu
Expenses *Tuition:* $14,920 full-time, $520 per credit part-time. *Full-time mandatory fees:* $50–$200. *Room and board:* $5805–$8550. *Room only:* $2205–$4950. *Books and supplies per academic year:* $1250.
Financial Aid Institutionally sponsored need-based grants/scholarships, institutionally sponsored non-need grants/scholarships, Federal Direct Loans, Federal Nursing Student Loans, Federal Pell Grants, Federal Perkins Loans, Federal Supplemental Educational Opportunity Grants, Federal Work-Study. 69% of undergraduate students in nursing programs received some form of financial aid in 1995–96. *Application deadline:* 5/1.

Generic Baccalaureate Program (BSN)

Applying *Required:* TOEFL for nonnative speakers of English, minimum college GPA of 2.5, high school transcript, 2 letters of recommendation, written essay, transcript of college record, lower-division college transcript. *Options:* Advanced standing available through the following means: advanced placement exams, credit by exam. May apply for transfer of up to 99 total credits. *Application deadline:* rolling. *Application fee:* $40.
Degree Requirements 123 total credit hours, 64 in nursing.

RN Baccalaureate Program (BSN)

Applying *Required:* TOEFL for nonnative speakers of English, minimum college GPA of 2.5, RN license, diploma or AD in nursing, high school transcript, 2 letters of recommendation, written essay, transcript of college record, lower-division college transcript. 59 prerequisite credits must be completed before admission to the nursing program. *Options:* Advanced standing available through the following means: advanced placement exams, credit by exam. Course work may be accelerated. May apply for transfer of up to 99 total credits. *Application deadline:* rolling. *Application fee:* $40.
Degree Requirements 122 total credit hours, 63 in nursing.

MASTER'S PROGRAMS

Contact Dr. Nancy Youngblood, Interim Director, Master's Degree Program in Nursing, Department of Nursing, Thomas Jefferson University, 130 South 9th Street, Suite 1200, Philadelphia, PA 19107, 215-955-7937. *Fax:* 215-923-1468.

Areas of Study Clinical nurse specialist programs in adult health nursing, community health nursing, critical care nursing, medical-surgical nursing, public health nursing, rehabilitation nursing; nurse practitioner program in family health.

Expenses *Tuition:* $17,250 full-time, $597 per credit part-time. *Full-time mandatory fees:* up to $1203. *Part-time mandatory fees:* up to $1203. *Room and board:* $5805–$8550. *Room only:* $2205–$4950. *Books and supplies per academic year:* $600.

Financial Aid Nurse traineeships, fellowships, Federal Nursing Student Loans, institutionally sponsored loans, institutionally sponsored non-need-based grants/scholarships. 22% of master's level students in nursing programs received some form of financial aid in 1995-96. *Application deadline:* 5/1.

MSN Program

Applying *Required:* GRE General Test, Miller Analogies Test, bachelor's degree in nursing, minimum GPA of 3.0, RN license, physical assessment course, statistics course, professional liability/malpractice insurance, essay, interview, 3 letters of recommendation, transcript of college record. *Application deadline:* rolling. *Application fee:* $50.

Degree Requirements 39–48 total credit hours dependent upon track, 30–39 in nursing, 9 in other specified areas.

Accelerated MSN Program

Applying *Required:* GRE General Test, Miller Analogies Test, bachelor's degree in nursing, minimum GPA of 3.0, RN license, physical assessment course, statistics course, professional liability/malpractice insurance, essay, interview, 3 letters of recommendation, transcript of college record. *Application deadline:* rolling. *Application fee:* $50.

Degree Requirements 39–48 total credit hours dependent upon track, 30–39 in nursing, 9 in other specified areas. Completion of advanced placement RN program.

Accelerated Master's for Non-Nursing College Graduates Program (MSN)

Applying *Required:* GRE General Test or Miller Analogies Test, bachelor's degree, minimum GPA of 3.0, essay, 2 letters of recommendation, transcript of college record, BA or BS in non-nursing related discipline. *Application deadline:* rolling. *Application fee:* $50.

Degree Requirements 92 total credit hours, 92 in nursing.

UNIVERSITY OF PENNSYLVANIA
School of Nursing
Philadelphia, Pennsylvania

Programs • Generic Baccalaureate • Accelerated RN Baccalaureate • Accelerated Baccalaureate for Second Degree • BSN to Master's • MSN • Master's for Non-Nursing College Graduates • MSN/MBA • Post-Master's • PhD • PhD/MBA • Postdoctoral • Continuing Education

The University Independent coed university. Founded: 1740. *Primary accreditation:* regional. *Setting:* 260-acre urban campus. *Total enrollment:* 22,148.

The School of Nursing Founded in 1935. *Nursing program faculty:* 46 (100% with doctorates).

Academic Facilities *Campus library:* 4.2 million volumes (175,980 in health, 175,980 in nursing); 33,384 periodical subscriptions (2,788 health-care related). *Nursing school resources:* CAI, computer lab, nursing audiovisuals, interactive nursing skills videos, learning resource lab, TV production studio, online data base including Medline and nursing data bases, World Wide Web, Internet.

Student Life *Student services:* health clinic, child-care facilities, personal counseling, career counseling, institutionally sponsored work-study program, job placement, campus safety program, special assistance for disabled students, Department of Academic Support, writing center. *International student services:* counseling/support, special assistance for nonnative speakers of English, ESL courses. *Nursing student activities:* Sigma Theta Tau, student nurses association, nursing student forum, graduate student organization, doctoral student organization.

Calendar Semesters.

NURSING STUDENT PROFILE

Undergraduate **Enrollment:** 466
Women: 96%; **Men:** 4%; **Minority:** 16%; **International:** 3%; **Part-time:** 8%
Graduate **Enrollment:** 423
Women: 97%; **Men:** 3%; **Minority:** 12%; **International:** 5%; **Part-time:** 70%

BACCALAUREATE PROGRAMS

Contact Ms. Marian Matez, Assistant Dean for Undergraduate Admissions, Nursing Education Building, School of Nursing, University of Pennsylvania, Philadelphia, PA 19104-6096, 215-898-4271. *Fax:* 215-573-8439. *E-mail:* matez@pobox.upenn.edu

Expenses *Tuition:* $18,964 full-time, $2423 per course unit part-time. *Full-time mandatory fees:* $2386. *Room and board:* $7330. *Books and supplies per academic year:* $1760.

Financial Aid Institutionally sponsored need-based grants/scholarships, institutionally sponsored non-need grants/scholarships, Federal Direct Loans, Federal Nursing Student Loans, Federal Pell Grants, Federal Perkins Loans, Federal Supplemental Educational Opportunity Grants, Federal Work-Study. 85% of undergraduate students in nursing programs received some form of financial aid in 1995–96. *Application deadline:* 3/31.

Generic Baccalaureate Program (BSN)

Applying *Required:* SAT I or ACT, TOEFL for nonnative speakers of English, SAT II in writing, science, and applicant's choice (ACT can be substituted for both the SAT I and SAT II), minimum high school GPA of 3.0, 3 years of high school math, 4 years of high school science, high school chemistry, high school biology, high school foreign language, high school transcript, interview, 3 letters of recommendation, written essay, high school class rank: top 10%. *Options:* Advanced standing available through the following means: advanced placement exams, advanced placement without credit. Course work may be accelerated. May apply for transfer of up to 24 total credits. *Application deadline:* 1/1. *Application fee:* $55.

Degree Requirements 120 total credit hours, 84 in nursing.

Accelerated RN Baccalaureate Program (BSN)

Applying *Required:* SAT I, ACT, TOEFL for nonnative speakers of English, SAT II in writing, science, and applicant's choice (ACT can be substituted for both the SAT I and SAT II), minimum college GPA of 3.0, RN license, diploma or AD in nursing, high school transcript, interview, 3 letters of recommendation, written essay, transcript of college record. 24 prerequisite credits must be completed before admission to the nursing program. *Options:* Advanced standing available through the following means: advanced placement exams, advanced placement without credit, credit by exam. Course work may be accelerated. *Application deadlines:* 4/1 (fall), 10/15 (spring). *Application fee:* $55.

Degree Requirements 120 total credit hours, 84 in nursing. 20 course units must be completed at the University of Pennsylvania.

Accelerated Baccalaureate for Second Degree Program (BSN)

Applying *Required:* SAT I or ACT, TOEFL for nonnative speakers of English, minimum college GPA of 3.0, high school transcript, interview, 3 letters of recommendation, written essay, transcript of college record. *Options:* Advanced standing available through credit by exam. Course work may be accelerated. *Application deadlines:* 4/1 (fall), 10/15 (spring). *Application fee:* $55.

Degree Requirements 120 total credit hours, 84 in nursing. 20 course units must be completed at the University of Pennsylvania.

MASTER'S PROGRAMS

Contact Ms. Susan K. Ogle, Associate Director of Admissions and Student Affairs, Nursing Education Building, School of Nursing, University of Pennsylvania, Philadelphia, PA 19104-6096, 215-898-3301. *Fax:* 215-573-8439. *E-mail:* sogle@pobox.upenn.edu

Areas of Study Clinical nurse specialist programs in oncology nursing, perinatal nursing, psychiatric–mental health nursing; nurse midwifery; nursing administration; nurse practitioner programs in acute care, adult

University of Pennsylvania (continued)

health, child care/pediatrics, community health, family health, gerontology, neonatal health, occupational health, primary care, women's health, adult critical care, pediatric critical care, perinatal care, adult and pediatric oncology, home care.

Expenses *Tuition:* $19,226 full-time, $2581 per course unit part-time. *Full-time mandatory fees:* $1464. *Part-time mandatory fees:* $555. *Room and board:* $8168. *Books and supplies per academic year:* $3442.

Financial Aid Graduate assistantships, nurse traineeships, fellowships, Federal Direct Loans, Federal Nursing Student Loans, institutionally sponsored loans, institutionally sponsored need-based grants/scholarships, institutionally sponsored non-need-based grants/scholarships. 85% of master's level students in nursing programs received some form of financial aid in 1995-96. *Application deadline:* 3/31.

BSN to Master's Program (MSN)

Applying *Required:* GRE General Test, TOEFL for nonnative speakers of English, bachelor's degree in nursing, minimum GPA of 3.0, RN license, physical assessment course, statistics course, essay, interview, 3 letters of recommendation, transcript of college record, willingness to travel to transmission center. *Application deadline:* 2/15. *Application fee:* $55.

Degree Requirements 48 total credit hours.

Distance learning Courses provided through correspondence, video, audio, computer-based media, on-line, interactive real time audiovisual transmission.

MSN Program

Applying *Required:* GRE General Test, TOEFL for nonnative speakers of English, bachelor's degree in nursing, minimum GPA of 3.0, RN license, physical assessment course, statistics course, essay, interview, 3 letters of recommendation, transcript of college record. *Application deadline:* 2/15. *Application fee:* $55.

Degree Requirements 36–48 total credit hours dependent upon track.

Master's for Non-Nursing College Graduates Program (MSN)

Applying *Required:* GRE General Test, TOEFL for nonnative speakers of English, bachelor's degree, minimum GPA of 3.0, essay, interview, 3 letters of recommendation, transcript of college record, BSN degree earned concurrently. *Application deadline:* 12/1. *Application fee:* $55.

MSN/MBA Program

Applying *Required:* GRE General Test, TOEFL for nonnative speakers of English, GMAT, bachelor's degree in nursing, minimum GPA of 3.0, RN license, physical assessment course, statistics course, essay, interview, 3 letters of recommendation, transcript of college record, summer preterm study in accounting, statistics, and economics. *Application deadline:* 2/15. *Application fee:* $55.

Degree Requirements 69 total credit hours, 30 in nursing, 39 in health-care management, small business planning, and consultation.

Post-Master's Program

Applying *Required:* GRE General Test, TOEFL for nonnative speakers of English, bachelor's degree in nursing, RN license, physical assessment course, statistics course, essay, interview, 3 letters of recommendation, transcript of college record, MSN. *Application deadline:* 2/15. *Application fee:* $55.

DOCTORAL PROGRAMS

Contact Dr. Anne Keane, Interim Associate Dean and Director of Graduate Studies, Nursing Education Building, School of Nursing, University of Pennsylvania, Philadelphia, PA 19104-6096, 215-898-4150. *Fax:* 215-573-6659. *E-mail:* akeane@pobox.upenn.edu

Areas of Study Nursing administration, nursing education, nursing research, clinical practice, nursing policy.

Expenses *Tuition:* $20,644 full-time, $2769 per course unit part-time. *Full-time mandatory fees:* $1464. *Room and board:* $8168. *Books and supplies per academic year:* $3442.

Financial Aid Graduate assistantships, fellowships, Federal Direct Loans, institutionally sponsored loans, opportunities for employment, institutionally sponsored non-need-based grants/scholarships. *Application deadline:* 3/31.

PhD Program

Applying *Required:* GRE General Test, TOEFL for nonnative speakers of English, statistics course, interview, 3 letters of recommendation, competitive review by faculty committee, BSN or MSN. *Application deadline:* 1/1. *Application fee:* $55.

Degree Requirements 42–63 total credit hours dependent upon track; dissertation; oral exam; written exam; defense of dissertation.

PhD/MBA Program

Applying *Required:* GRE General Test, TOEFL for nonnative speakers of English, GMAT, statistics course, interview, 3 letters of recommendation, competitive review by faculty committee, BSN or MSN. *Application deadline:* 1/1. *Application fee:* $55.

Degree Requirements dissertation; oral exam; written exam; defense of dissertation.

POSTDOCTORAL PROGRAM

Contact Dr. Anne Keane, Interim Associate Dean and Director of Graduate Studies, Nursing Education Building, School of Nursing, University of Pennsylvania, Philadelphia, PA 19104-6096, 215-898-4150. *Fax:* 215-573-6659. *E-mail:* akeane@pobox.upenn.edu

Areas of Study Nursing research training, psychosocial oncology, historical research and writing.

CONTINUING EDUCATION PROGRAM

Contact Ms. Kathleen Burke, Coordinator, Center for Continuing Nursing Education, Nursing Education Building, School of Nursing, University of Pennsylvania, Philadelphia, PA 19104-6096, 215-898-4522. *Fax:* 215-898-6320. *E-mail:* burkekg@pobox.upenn.edu

See full description on page 548.

UNIVERSITY OF PITTSBURGH
School of Nursing
Pittsburgh, Pennsylvania

Programs • Generic Baccalaureate • Accelerated RN Baccalaureate • Baccalaureate for Second Degree • MSN • RN to Master's • Master's for Second Degree • PhD • Postdoctoral • Continuing Education

The University State-related coed university. Part of University of Pittsburgh System. Founded: 1787. *Primary accreditation:* regional. *Setting:* 132-acre urban campus. *Total enrollment:* 26,083.

The School of Nursing Founded in 1939. *Nursing program faculty:* 80 (58% with doctorates). *Off-campus program sites:* Bradford, Johnstown.

Academic Facilities *Campus library:* 3.4 million volumes (369,995 in health, 20,000 in nursing); 24,964 periodical subscriptions (2,558 health-care related). *Nursing school resources:* CAI, computer lab, nursing audiovisuals, interactive nursing skills videos, learning resource lab, clinical lab.

Student Life *Student services:* health clinic, child-care facilities, personal counseling, career counseling, institutionally sponsored work-study program, job placement, campus safety program, special assistance for disabled students, learning skills center. *International student services:* ESL courses, Office of International Services. *Nursing student activities:* Sigma Theta Tau, student nurses association.

Calendar Semesters.

NURSING STUDENT PROFILE

Undergraduate **Enrollment:** 527
Women: 86%; **Men:** 14%; **Minority:** 7%; **International:** 1%; **Part-time:** 30%
Graduate **Enrollment:** 349
Women: 93%; **Men:** 7%; **Minority:** 7%; **International:** 1%; **Part-time:** 66%

BACCALAUREATE PROGRAMS

Contact Ms. Cherie Remley, Director of Student Affairs, School of Nursing, University of Pittsburgh, 3500 Victoria Street, Pittsburgh, PA 15261, 412-624-2407. *Fax:* 412-624-2401. *E-mail:* nursao+@pitt.edu

Expenses *State resident tuition:* $6968 full-time, $238 per credit part-time. *Nonresident tuition:* $15,048 full-time, $500 per credit part-time. *Full-time*

mandatory fees: $262. *Part-time mandatory fees:* $75. *Room and board:* $2870–$4882. *Room only:* $2130–$3470. *Books and supplies per academic year:* ranges from $350 to $550.

Financial Aid Institutionally sponsored need-based grants/scholarships, institutionally sponsored non-need grants/scholarships, Federal Nursing Student Loans, Federal Supplemental Educational Opportunity Grants, Federal Work-Study. *Application deadline:* 4/1.

Generic Baccalaureate Program (BSN)

Applying *Required:* SAT I, TOEFL for nonnative speakers of English, 3 years of high school math, 3 years of high school science, high school chemistry, high school transcript, high school class rank: top 30%. *Application deadline:* rolling. *Application fee:* $35.

Degree Requirements 127 total credit hours, 82 in nursing.

Accelerated RN Baccalaureate Program (BSN)

Applying *Required:* TOEFL for nonnative speakers of English, ACT PEP or articulation agreement, RN license, diploma or AD in nursing, transcript of college record. 50 prerequisite credits must be completed before admission to the nursing program. *Options:* May apply for transfer of up to 90 total credits. *Application deadline:* rolling. *Application fee:* $35.

Degree Requirements 120 total credit hours, 64 in nursing.

Baccalaureate for Second Degree Program (BSN)

Applying *Required:* TOEFL for nonnative speakers of English, interview, written essay, transcript of college record, bachelor's degree or 90 credits toward degree in another field. 29 prerequisite credits must be completed before admission to the nursing program. *Options:* May apply for transfer of up to 63 total credits. *Application deadline:* 12/1 (summer). *Application fee:* $35.

Degree Requirements 127 total credit hours, 62 in nursing. Must attend full-time for 4 consecutive terms.

MASTER'S PROGRAMS

Contact Ms. Cherie Remley, Director of Student Affairs, School of Nursing, University of Pittsburgh, 3500 Victoria Street, Pittsburgh, PA 15261, 412-624-2407. *Fax:* 412-624-2401. *E-mail:* nursao+@pitt.edu

Areas of Study Nurse anesthesia; nursing administration; nursing education; nurse practitioner programs in acute care, child care/pediatrics, family health, primary care, women's health, psychiatric primary care.

Expenses *State resident tuition:* $8654 full-time, $358 per credit part-time. *Nonresident tuition:* $17,658 full-time, $729 per credit part-time. *Full-time mandatory fees:* $232. *Part-time mandatory fees:* $68. *Room and board:* $2870–$4882. *Room only:* $2130–$3470. *Books and supplies per academic year:* ranges from $350 to $550.

Financial Aid Graduate assistantships, nurse traineeships, Federal Nursing Student Loans, institutionally sponsored need-based grants/scholarships. *Application deadline:* 6/1.

MSN Program

Applying *Required:* GRE General Test or Miller Analogies Test, TOEFL for nonnative speakers of English, bachelor's degree in nursing, minimum GPA of 3.0, RN license, 1 year of clinical experience, statistics course, professional liability/malpractice insurance, essay, interview, 3 letters of recommendation, transcript of college record. *Application deadline:* rolling. *Application fee:* $35–40.

Degree Requirements 48–52 total credit hours dependent upon track, 36–42 in nursing.

RN to Master's Program (MSN)

Applying *Required:* GRE General Test or Miller Analogies Test, RN license, 1 year of clinical experience, statistics course, professional liability/malpractice insurance, essay, interview, 3 letters of recommendation, transcript of college record, students earn BSN upon completion of 30 credits. *Application deadline:* rolling. *Application fee:* $35.

Degree Requirements 168–172 total credit hours dependent upon track, 66–76 in nursing.

Master's for Second Degree Program (MSN)

Applying *Required:* RN license, 1 year of clinical experience, professional liability/malpractice insurance, essay, interview, letter of recommendation, transcript of college record, MSN. *Application deadline:* rolling. *Application fee:* $35–40.

Degree Requirements 30+ total credit hours dependent upon track, 30+ in nursing.

DOCTORAL PROGRAM

Contact Ms. Cherie Remley, Director of Student Affairs, School of Nursing, University of Pittsburgh, 3500 Victoria Street, Pittsburgh, PA 15261, 412-624-2407. *Fax:* 412-624-2401. *E-mail:* nursao+@pitt.edu

Areas of Study Nursing research.

Expenses *State resident tuition:* ranges from $4327 to $12,981 full-time, $358 per credit part-time. *Nonresident tuition:* ranges from $4327 to $12,981 full-time, $729 per credit part-time. *Full-time mandatory fees:* $232. *Part-time mandatory fees:* $68. *Room and board:* $2870–$4882. *Room only:* $2130–$3470.

Financial Aid Graduate assistantships, fellowships, Federal Nursing Student Loans, institutionally sponsored need-based grants/scholarships, institutionally sponsored non-need-based grants/scholarships, in-state tuition rates for full-time out-of-state students. *Application deadline:* 6/1.

PhD Program

Applying *Required:* GRE General Test, TOEFL for nonnative speakers of English, statistics course, interview, 3 letters of recommendation, vitae, competitive review by faculty committee, match between applicant's area of research interest and that of available faculty, appropriate master's degree for the intended research area. *Application deadlines:* 4/1 (fall), 10/1 (spring). *Application fee:* $30.

Degree Requirements 60 total credit hours; dissertation; oral exam; written exam; defense of dissertation; residency; 12 credits in other specified areas taken outside of the School of Nursing.

POSTDOCTORAL PROGRAM

Contact Dr. Leslie Hoffman, Department Chair, Acute and Tertiary Care, School of Nursing, University of Pittsburgh, 3500 Victoria Street, Pittsburgh, PA 15261, 412-624-4722. *Fax:* 412-624-2401. *E-mail:* nursao+@pitt.edu

Areas of Study Individualized study.

CONTINUING EDUCATION PROGRAM

Contact Joeta D'Este, Nurse Educator, 517 Nese-Barkan Building, School of Nursing, University of Pittsburgh, Pittsburgh, PA 15213, 412-647-8236. *E-mail:* nursao+@pitt.edu

See full description on page 550.

UNIVERSITY OF SCRANTON
Department of Nursing
Scranton, Pennsylvania

Programs • Generic Baccalaureate • RN Baccalaureate • BSN to Master's

The University Independent Roman Catholic (Jesuit) comprehensive coed institution. Founded: 1888. *Primary accreditation:* regional. *Setting:* 50-acre urban campus. *Total enrollment:* 4,931.

The Department of Nursing Founded in 1981. *Nursing program faculty:* 13 (84% with doctorates).

Academic Facilities *Campus library:* 310,710 volumes (5,735 in nursing); 2,059 periodical subscriptions (105 health-care related). *Nursing school resources:* CAI, computer lab, nursing audiovisuals, interactive nursing skills videos, learning resource lab.

Student Life *Student services:* health clinic, personal counseling, career counseling, institutionally sponsored work-study program, job placement, campus safety program, special assistance for disabled students. *International student services:* counseling/support, special assistance for

University of Scranton (continued)

nonnative speakers of English, ESL courses. *Nursing student activities:* Sigma Theta Tau, student nurses association.

Calendar Semesters.

NURSING STUDENT PROFILE

Undergraduate **Enrollment:** 187
Women: 94%; **Men:** 6%; **Minority:** 2%; **International:** 1%; **Part-time:** 4%
Graduate **Enrollment:** 26
Women: 100%; **Minority:** 0%; **International:** 0%; **Part-time:** 68%

BACCALAUREATE PROGRAMS

Contact Rev. Bernard L. McIlhenny, Dean of Admissions, Department of Admissions, University of Scranton, 800 Linden Street, Scranton, PA 18510-4699, 717-941-7540. *Fax:* 717-941-6369.

Expenses *Tuition:* $14,800 full-time, $415 per credit part-time. *Full-time mandatory fees:* $870+. *Room and board:* $4843. *Room only:* $3512–$3622. *Books and supplies per academic year:* ranges from $200 to $400.

Financial Aid Institutionally sponsored need-based grants/scholarships, institutionally sponsored non-need grants/scholarships, Federal Direct Loans, Federal Pell Grants, Federal Perkins Loans, Federal Supplemental Educational Opportunity Grants, Federal Work-Study. *Application deadline:* 2/15.

Generic Baccalaureate Program (BSN)

Applying *Required:* SAT I, TOEFL for nonnative speakers of English, minimum college GPA of 2.5, 3 years of high school math, 3 years of high school science, high school chemistry, high school biology, high school foreign language, high school transcript, 2 letters of recommendation, transcript of college record. *Options:* Advanced standing available through advanced placement exams. May apply for transfer of up to 74 total credits. *Application deadlines:* 3/1 (fall), 12/1 (spring). *Application fee:* $30.

Degree Requirements 137 total credit hours, 57 in nursing.

RN Baccalaureate Program (BSN)

Applying *Required:* RN license, diploma or AD in nursing, high school transcript, 3 letters of recommendation, transcript of college record, nursing school transcript, 2-3 letters of recommendation. *Options:* Advanced standing available through credit by exam. May apply for transfer of up to 74 total credits. *Application deadlines:* 12/1, rolling. *Application fee:* $30.

Degree Requirements 133 total credit hours, 57 in nursing.

MASTER'S PROGRAM

Contact Dr. Mary Jane Hanson, Director, Graduate Nursing Program, Department of Nursing, University of Scranton, Scranton, PA 18510, 717-941-4060. *Fax:* 717-941-4201.

Areas of Study Nurse practitioner program in family health.

Expenses *Tuition:* $9545 full-time, $415 per credit part-time. *Full-time mandatory fees:* $220.

Financial Aid Graduate assistantships, nurse traineeships. 77% of master's level students in nursing programs received some form of financial aid in 1995-96.

BSN to Master's Program (MS)

Applying *Required:* GRE General Test, bachelor's degree in nursing, minimum GPA of 3.0, RN license, 1 year of clinical experience, physical assessment course, statistics course, professional liability/malpractice insurance, essay, interview, 3 letters of recommendation, transcript of college record. *Application deadline:* 3/1. *Application fee:* $35.

Degree Requirements 46 total credit hours, 41 in nursing, 5 in elective.

VILLANOVA UNIVERSITY

College of Nursing
Villanova, Pennsylvania

Programs • Generic Baccalaureate • Accelerated RN Baccalaureate • Baccalaureate for Second Degree • MSN • Continuing Education

The University Independent Roman Catholic comprehensive coed institution. Founded: 1842. *Primary accreditation:* regional. *Setting:* 222-acre suburban campus. *Total enrollment:* 10,514.

The College of Nursing Founded in 1953. *Nursing program faculty:* 45 (70% with doctorates). *Off-campus program site:* York.

Academic Facilities *Campus library:* 925,000 volumes (19,000 in health, 3,550 in nursing); 5,050 periodical subscriptions (250 health-care related). *Nursing school resources:* CAI, computer lab, nursing audiovisuals, interactive nursing skills videos, learning resource lab.

Student Life *Student services:* health clinic, personal counseling, career counseling, institutionally sponsored work-study program, campus safety program, special assistance for disabled students, campus ministry. *International student services:* counseling/support, special assistance for nonnative speakers of English, ESL courses. *Nursing student activities:* Sigma Theta Tau, nursing club, student nurses association.

Calendar Semesters.

NURSING STUDENT PROFILE

Undergraduate **Enrollment:** 424
Women: 96%; **Men:** 4%; **Minority:** 9%; **International:** 2%; **Part-time:** 11%
Graduate **Enrollment:** 150
Women: 97%; **Men:** 3%; **Minority:** 4%; **International:** 2%; **Part-time:** 92%

BACCALAUREATE PROGRAMS

Contact Dr. Andrea Hollingsworth, Director, Undergraduate Program, College of Nursing, Villanova University, Villanova, PA 19085-1690, 610-519-4900. *Fax:* 610-519-7997.

Expenses *Tuition:* $18,360 full-time, $425 per credit part-time. *Full-time mandatory fees:* $260. *Room and board:* $6260–$8260. *Room only:* $3290–$4810. *Books and supplies per academic year:* ranges from $100 to $300.

Financial Aid Institutionally sponsored need-based grants/scholarships, institutionally sponsored non-need grants/scholarships, Federal Direct Loans, Federal Nursing Student Loans, Federal Pell Grants, Federal Perkins Loans, Federal Supplemental Educational Opportunity Grants, Federal Work-Study. 84% of undergraduate students in nursing programs received some form of financial aid in 1995–96. *Application deadline:* 2/15.

Generic Baccalaureate Program (BSN)

Applying *Required:* SAT I or ACT, TOEFL for nonnative speakers of English, minimum high school GPA of 3.0, 3 years of high school math, 3 years of high school science, high school chemistry, high school biology, high school foreign language, high school transcript, letter of recommendation, written essay, transcript of college record. *Options:* Course work may be accelerated. May apply for transfer of up to 67 total credits. *Application deadline:* 1/15. *Application fee:* $45.

Degree Requirements 133 total credit hours, 69 in nursing.

Accelerated RN Baccalaureate Program (BSN)

Applying *Required:* TOEFL for nonnative speakers of English, minimum college GPA of 2.5, RN license, diploma or AD in nursing, transcript of college record. *Options:* Advanced standing available through credit by exam. May apply for transfer of up to 90 total credits. *Application deadlines:* 4/15 (fall), 11/15 (spring). *Application fee:* $45.

Degree Requirements 133 total credit hours, 24 in nursing.

Baccalaureate for Second Degree Program (BSN)

Applying *Required:* SAT I, TOEFL for nonnative speakers of English, minimum high school GPA of 3.0, minimum college GPA of 2.5, 3 years of high school math, 3 years of high school science, high school chemistry, high school biology, transcript of college record. *Options:* Course work may be accelerated. May apply for transfer of up to 67 total credits. *Application deadlines:* 4/15 (fall), 11/15 (spring). *Application fee:* $45.

Degree Requirements 133 total credit hours, 69 in nursing.

MASTER'S PROGRAM

Contact Dr. Claire Manfredi, Director, Graduate Program, College of Nursing, Villanova University, Villanova, PA 19085-1690, 610-519-4934. *Fax:* 610-519-7997. *E-mail:* cmanfredi@email.vill.edu

Areas of Study Nurse anesthesia; nursing administration; nursing education; nurse practitioner program in adult health.

Expenses *Tuition:* $410 per credit. *Full-time mandatory fees:* $60. *Books and supplies per academic year:* ranges from $200 to $400.

Financial Aid Graduate assistantships, nurse traineeships, Federal Nursing Student Loans, institutionally sponsored need-based grants/scholarships. 10% of master's level students in nursing programs received some form of financial aid in 1995-96. *Application deadline:* 4/1.

MSN Program

Applying *Required:* GRE General Test or Miller Analogies Test, TOEFL for nonnative speakers of English, GRE General Test (minimum score of 450

on verbal section), bachelor's degree in nursing, minimum GPA of 3.0, RN license, 1 year of clinical experience, physical assessment course, statistics course, essay, interview, 3 letters of recommendation, transcript of college record. *Application deadlines:* 7/1 (summer), rolling. *Application fee:* $25.

Degree Requirements 45 total credit hours, 33–39 in nursing, up to 6 in higher education, financial management, organization.

CONTINUING EDUCATION PROGRAM

Contact Dr. Lynore DeSilets, Director, Continuing Education, College of Nursing, Villanova University, Villanova, PA 19085-1690, 610-519-4931. *Fax:* 610-519-7997.

See full description on page 566.

WAYNESBURG COLLEGE
Department of Nursing
Waynesburg, Pennsylvania

Programs • Generic Baccalaureate • LPN to Baccalaureate • Continuing Education

The College Independent comprehensive coed institution, affiliated with Presbyterian Church (U.S.A.). Founded: 1849. *Primary accreditation:* regional. *Setting:* 30-acre small-town campus. *Total enrollment:* 1,292.

The Department of Nursing Founded in 1983. *Nursing program faculty:* 10 (30% with doctorates).

Academic Facilities *Campus library:* 90,958 volumes (2,960 in health, 1,902 in nursing); 579 periodical subscriptions (82 health-care related). *Nursing school resources:* CAI, computer lab, nursing audiovisuals, learning resource lab, clinical skills lab.

Student Life *Student services:* health clinic, personal counseling, career counseling, institutionally sponsored work-study program, job placement, campus safety program, special assistance for disabled students. *International student services:* counseling/support. *Nursing student activities:* Sigma Theta Tau, student nurses association.

Calendar Semesters.

NURSING STUDENT PROFILE

Undergraduate **Enrollment:** 186
Women: 89%; **Men:** 11%; **Minority:** 1%; **International:** 0%; **Part-time:** 1%

BACCALAUREATE PROGRAMS

Contact Ms. Robin Moore, Dean of Admissions, Miller Hall, Department of Nursing, Waynesburg College, Waynesburg, PA 15370, 412-627-8191 Ext. 333. *Fax:* 412-627-6416. *E-mail:* rlmoore@waynesburg.edu

Expenses *Tuition:* $9800 per academic year. *Full-time mandatory fees:* $300–$350. *Room and board:* $2010. *Room only:* $2040. *Books and supplies per academic year:* ranges from $300 to $600.

Financial Aid Institutionally sponsored need-based grants/scholarships, institutionally sponsored non-need grants/scholarships, Federal Nursing Student Loans, Federal Perkins Loans, Federal Supplemental Educational Opportunity Grants, Federal Work-Study, institutionally sponsored short-term loans. 88% of undergraduate students in nursing programs received some form of financial aid in 1995–96. *Application deadline:* 3/15.

Generic Baccalaureate Program (BSN)

Applying *Required:* minimum high school GPA of 2.0, minimum college GPA of 2.5, 2 years of high school math, 2 years of high school science, high school chemistry, high school biology, high school transcript, interview, transcript of college record. 24 prerequisite credits must be completed before admission to the nursing program. *Options:* Advanced standing available through the following means: advanced placement exams, credit by exam. May apply for transfer of up to 63 total credits. *Application deadline:* rolling. *Application fee:* $15.

Degree Requirements 126 total credit hours, 63 in nursing.

LPN to Baccalaureate Program (BSN)

Applying *Required:* minimum high school GPA of 2.0, minimum college GPA of 2.5, 2 years of high school math, 2 years of high school science, high school chemistry, high school biology, high school transcript, interview, transcript of college record, LPN diploma. 24 prerequisite credits must be completed before admission to the nursing program. *Options:* Course work may be accelerated. May apply for transfer of up to 63 total credits. *Application deadline:* rolling. *Application fee:* $15.

Degree Requirements 126 total credit hours, 63 in nursing.

CONTINUING EDUCATION PROGRAM

Contact Dr. Joan Clites, Director and Chair, Department of Nursing, Waynesburg College, Waynesburg, PA 15370-1222, 412-852-3356. *Fax:* 412-627-6416. *E-mail:* jclites@wayncsburg.edu

WEST CHESTER UNIVERSITY OF PENNSYLVANIA
Department of Nursing
West Chester, Pennsylvania

Programs • Generic Baccalaureate • RN Baccalaureate • BSN to Master's

The University State-supported comprehensive coed institution. Part of Pennsylvania State System of Higher Education. Founded: 1871. *Primary accreditation:* regional. *Setting:* 547-acre small-town campus. *Total enrollment:* 11,055.

The Department of Nursing Founded in 1975. *Nursing program faculty:* 17 (24% with doctorates).

NURSING STUDENT PROFILE

Undergraduate **Enrollment:** 190
Women: 90%; **Men:** 10%
Graduate **Enrollment:** 38
Women: 95%; **Men:** 5%

BACCALAUREATE PROGRAMS

Contact Ms. Kathy Hein, Assistant Director of Admissions, Messikomer Building, Department of Nursing, West Chester University of Pennsylvania, 100 West Rosedale Avenue, West Chester, PA 19383, 610-436-3411.

Expenses *State resident tuition:* $3224 full-time, $134 per credit part-time. *Nonresident tuition:* $8198 full-time, $342 per credit part-time.

Generic Baccalaureate Program (BSN)

Applying *Required:* SAT I, TOEFL for nonnative speakers of English, 2 years of high school math, 2 years of high school science, high school transcript, written essay. *Application deadline:* rolling. *Application fee:* $25.

Degree Requirements 130 total credit hours, 50 in nursing.

RN Baccalaureate Program (BSN)

Applying *Required:* SAT I, TOEFL for nonnative speakers of English, RN license, diploma or AD in nursing. *Options:* Advanced standing available through credit by exam. *Application deadline:* rolling. *Application fee:* $25.

Degree Requirements 130 total credit hours, 50 in nursing.

MASTER'S PROGRAM

Contact Dr. Janet S. Hickman, Graduate Program Coordinator, Department of Nursing, West Chester University of Pennsylvania, 100 South Church Street, West Chester, PA 19383, 610-436-2258.

Areas of Study Clinical nurse specialist program in community health nursing; nursing administration; nursing education.

Expenses *State resident tuition:* $3224 full-time, $179 per credit part-time. *Nonresident tuition:* $5794 full-time, $322 per credit part-time.

BSN to Master's Program (MSN)

Applying *Required:* GRE General Test or Miller Analogies Test, bachelor's degree in nursing, minimum GPA of 2.5, RN license, 2 years of clinical experience, physical assessment course, statistics course, 3 letters of recommendation, transcript of college record. *Application deadlines:* 4/15 (fall), 10/15 (spring).

Degree Requirements 39 total credit hours, 36 in nursing, 3 in epidemiology. Thesis or other relative electives.

WIDENER UNIVERSITY
School of Nursing
Chester, Pennsylvania

Programs • Generic Baccalaureate • RN Baccalaureate • MSN • RN to Master's • Post-Master's • DNSc

The University Independent comprehensive coed institution. Founded: 1821. *Primary accreditation:* regional. *Setting:* 115-acre suburban campus. *Total enrollment:* 8,630.

The School of Nursing Founded in 1968. *Nursing program faculty:* 29 (72% with doctorates). *Off-campus program site:* Harrisburg.

Academic Facilities *Campus library:* 767,747 volumes (144,327 in health, 10,468 in nursing); 4,348 periodical subscriptions (245 health-care related). *Nursing school resources:* CAI, computer lab, nursing audiovisuals, interactive nursing skills videos, learning resource lab.

Student Life *Student services:* health clinic, child-care facilities, personal counseling, career counseling, institutionally sponsored work-study program, job placement, campus safety program. *International student services:* counseling/support. *Nursing student activities:* Sigma Theta Tau, student nurses association.

Calendar Semesters.

NURSING STUDENT PROFILE

Undergraduate **Enrollment:** 527
Women: 88%; **Men:** 12%; **Minority:** 21%; **International:** 3%; **Part-time:** 44%
Graduate **Enrollment:** 224
Women: 96%; **Men:** 4%; **Minority:** 3%; **International:** 1%; **Part-time:** 97%

BACCALAUREATE PROGRAMS

Contact Dr. Jane Brennan, Acting Assistant Dean for Undergraduate Studies, School of Nursing, Widener University, One University Place, Chester, PA 19013, 610-499-4210. *Fax:* 610-499-4216.

Expenses *Tuition:* $13,900 full-time, $463 per credit part-time. *Full-time mandatory fees:* $20. *Room and board:* $5910–$6730. *Books and supplies per academic year:* ranges from $225 to $400.

Financial Aid Institutionally sponsored need-based grants/scholarships, institutionally sponsored non-need grants/scholarships, Federal Pell Grants, Federal Perkins Loans, Federal Supplemental Educational Opportunity Grants, Federal Work-Study. 81% of undergraduate students in nursing programs received some form of financial aid in 1995–96. *Application deadline:* 4/1.

Generic Baccalaureate Program (BSN)

Applying *Required:* SAT I, TOEFL for nonnative speakers of English, high school chemistry, high school biology, high school transcript, 2 letters of recommendation, written essay. *Options:* Advanced standing available through credit by exam. May apply for transfer of up to 60 total credits. *Application deadline:* rolling. *Application fee:* $25.

Degree Requirements 122 total credit hours, 64 in nursing.

RN Baccalaureate Program (BSN)

Applying *Required:* TOEFL for nonnative speakers of English, minimum college GPA of 2.0, RN license, diploma or AD in nursing, interview, transcript of college record. *Options:* Advanced standing available through credit by exam. Course work may be accelerated. May apply for transfer of up to 90 total credits. *Application deadline:* rolling.

Degree Requirements 122 total credit hours, 34 in nursing.

MASTER'S PROGRAMS

Contact Dr. Mary Walker, Assistant Dean for Graduate Studies, School of Nursing, Widener University, One University Place, Chester, PA 19013, 610-499-4208. *Fax:* 610-499-4216. *E-mail:* mary.b.walker@widener.edu

Areas of Study Clinical nurse specialist programs in adult health nursing, community health nursing, critical care nursing; nurse practitioner program in family health.

Expenses *Tuition:* $7110 full-time, $395 per credit part-time. *Books and supplies per academic year:* ranges from $475 to $550.

Financial Aid Nurse traineeships, employment opportunities. *Application deadline:* 4/1.

MSN Program

Applying *Required:* GRE General Test, bachelor's degree in nursing, minimum GPA of 3.0, RN license, 1 year of clinical experience, statistics course, professional liability/malpractice insurance, essay, interview, 2 letters of recommendation, transcript of college record. *Application deadlines:* 7/15 (fall), 11/15 (spring), 3/15 (summer). *Application fee:* $25.

Degree Requirements 38–44 total credit hours dependent upon track, 32–38 in nursing.

RN to Master's Program (MSN)

Applying *Required:* GRE General Test, minimum GPA of 3.0, RN license, 1 year of clinical experience, statistics course, professional liability/malpractice insurance, essay, interview, 2 letters of recommendation, transcript of college record. *Application deadlines:* 7/15 (fall), 11/15 (spring), 3/15 (summer). *Application fee:* $25.

Degree Requirements 38–44 total credit hours dependent upon track, 32–38 in nursing.

Post-Master's Program

Applying *Required:* RN license, 1 year of clinical experience, professional liability/malpractice insurance, interview, 2 letters of recommendation, transcript of college record. *Application deadlines:* 7/15 (fall), 11/15 (spring), 3/15 (summer). *Application fee:* $25.

Degree Requirements 15 total credit hours, 15 in nursing.

DOCTORAL PROGRAM

Contact Dr. Mary Walker, Assistant Dean for Graduate Studies, School of Nursing, Widener University, One University Place, Chester, PA 19013, 610-499-4208. *Fax:* 610-499-4216. *E-mail:* mary.b.walker@widener.edu

Areas of Study Nursing education.

Expenses *Tuition:* $7560 full-time, $420 per credit part-time. *Books and supplies per academic year:* ranges from $500 to $600.

Financial Aid Nurse traineeships.

DNSc Program

Applying *Required:* GRE General Test (minimum combined score of 1500 on three tests), master's degree in nursing, year of clinical experience, statistics course, interview, 2 letters of recommendation, vitae, writing sample, competitive review by faculty committee, graduate course in nursing theories and conceptual models. *Application deadlines:* 11/15 (spring), 3/15 (summer). *Application fee:* $25.

Degree Requirements 63 total credit hours; 15 credits dissertation research; dissertation; oral exam; written exam; defense of dissertation.

See full description on page 572.

WILKES UNIVERSITY
Department of Nursing
Wilkes-Barre, Pennsylvania

Programs • Generic Baccalaureate • RN Baccalaureate • MS

The University Independent comprehensive coed institution. Founded: 1933. *Primary accreditation:* regional. *Setting:* 25-acre urban campus. *Total enrollment:* 2,600.

The Department of Nursing Founded in 1972. *Nursing program faculty:* 11 (55% with doctorates).

Academic Facilities *Campus library:* 213,462 volumes (13,450 in health, 12,210 in nursing); 1,084 periodical subscriptions (70 health-care related). *Nursing school resources:* CAI, computer lab, nursing audiovisuals, interactive nursing skills videos, learning resource lab.

Student Life *Student services:* health clinic, personal counseling, career counseling, institutionally sponsored work-study program, job placement, campus safety program, special assistance for disabled students. *International student services:* counseling/support, special assistance for

nonnative speakers of English. *Nursing student activities:* Sigma Theta Tau, nursing club, student nurses association.

Calendar Semesters.

NURSING STUDENT PROFILE

Undergraduate **Enrollment:** 230
Women: 90%; **Men:** 10%; **Minority:** 1%; **Part-time:** 40%
Graduate **Enrollment:** 31
Women: 100%; **Part-time:** 95%

BACCALAUREATE PROGRAMS

Contact Dr. Ann M. Kolanowski, Chairperson and Professor, Department of Nursing, Wilkes University, 109 South Franklin Street, Wilkes-Barre, PA 18766, 717-831-4074. *Fax:* 717-831-7807. *E-mail:* akolano@wilkes1.wilkes.edu

Expenses *Tuition:* $12,586 full-time, $359 per credit part-time. *Full-time mandatory fees:* $580. *Room and board:* $5540–$6158. *Room only:* $3440–$3890. *Books and supplies per academic year:* ranges from $100 to $200.

Financial Aid Institutionally sponsored need-based grants/scholarships, institutionally sponsored non-need grants/scholarships, Federal Nursing Student Loans, Federal Pell Grants, Federal Perkins Loans, Federal Supplemental Educational Opportunity Grants, Federal Work-Study. 24% of undergraduate students in nursing programs received some form of financial aid in 1995–96. *Application deadline:* 3/1.

Generic Baccalaureate Program (BS)

Applying *Required:* SAT I or ACT, minimum college GPA of 2.0, 3 years of high school math, 3 years of high school science, high school chemistry, high school biology, high school foreign language, high school transcript, written essay. *Options:* Advanced standing available through advanced placement exams. *Application deadline:* rolling. *Application fee:* $30.

Degree Requirements 129 total credit hours, 55 in nursing.

RN Baccalaureate Program (BS)

Applying *Required:* minimum college GPA of 2.0, RN license, diploma or AD in nursing, transcript of college record. *Options:* Advanced standing available through advanced placement exams. Course work may be accelerated. *Application deadline:* rolling. *Application fee:* $30.

Degree Requirements 129 total credit hours, 55 in nursing.

MASTER'S PROGRAM

Contact Dr. Mary Ann Saueraker, Associate Professor, Department of Nursing, Wilkes University, 109 South Franklin Street, Wilkes-Barre, PA 18766, 717-831-4076. *Fax:* 717-831-7807.

Areas of Study Clinical nurse specialist program in gerontological nursing; nurse anesthesia.

Expenses *Tuition:* $437 per credit. *Books and supplies per academic year:* ranges from $100 to $300.

Financial Aid Graduate assistantships, nurse traineeships. 35% of master's level students in nursing programs received some form of financial aid in 1995-96. *Application deadline:* 3/1.

MS Program

Applying *Required:* GRE General Test, Miller Analogies Test, bachelor's degree in nursing, minimum GPA of 3.0, RN license, 1 year of clinical experience, physical assessment course, statistics course, professional liability/malpractice insurance, essay, 3 letters of recommendation, transcript of college record. *Application deadline:* rolling. *Application fee:* $30.

Degree Requirements 36 total credit hours, 24–27 in nursing, 9–12 in statistics and other specified areas. 1 year of critical care experience for anesthesia program.

YORK COLLEGE OF PENNSYLVANIA

Department of Nursing
York, Pennsylvania

Programs • Generic Baccalaureate • RN Baccalaureate • LPN to Baccalaureate

The College Independent comprehensive coed institution. Founded: 1787. *Primary accreditation:* regional and Accrediting Commission for the Independent Colleges and Schools of the Career College Association. *Setting:* 80-acre suburban campus. *Total enrollment:* 5,054.

The Department of Nursing Founded in 1977. *Nursing program faculty:* 15 (67% with doctorates). *Off-campus program sites:* Harrisburg, Chambersburg, Camp Hill.

Academic Facilities *Campus library:* 128,827 volumes (12,079 in health, 881 in nursing); 1,261 periodical subscriptions (250 health-care related). *Nursing school resources:* CAI, computer lab, nursing audiovisuals, learning resource lab, CD-ROM.

Student Life *Student services:* health clinic, personal counseling, career counseling, institutionally sponsored work-study program, job placement, campus safety program, special assistance for disabled students. *International student services:* counseling/support, special assistance for nonnative speakers of English. *Nursing student activities:* Sigma Theta Tau, student nurses association.

Calendar Semesters.

NURSING STUDENT PROFILE

Undergraduate **Enrollment:** 453
Women: 89%; **Men:** 11%; **Minority:** 2%; **International:** 1%; **Part-time:** 27%

BACCALAUREATE PROGRAMS

Contact Ms. Nancy Spataro, Office of Admissions, Department of Nursing, York College of Pennsylvania, York, PA 17405-7199, 717-846-7788 Ext. 1368. *Fax:* 717-849-1607.

Expenses *Tuition:* $5525 full-time, $207 per credit hour part-time. *Full-time mandatory fees:* $672. *Room and board:* $4490. *Room only:* $2000. *Books and supplies per academic year:* $400.

Financial Aid Institutionally sponsored need-based grants/scholarships, institutionally sponsored non-need grants/scholarships, Federal Direct Loans, Federal Nursing Student Loans, Federal Perkins Loans, Federal Supplemental Educational Opportunity Grants, Federal Work-Study. 60% of undergraduate students in nursing programs received some form of financial aid in 1995–96. *Application deadline:* 5/1.

Generic Baccalaureate Program (BS)

Applying *Required:* SAT I or ACT, TOEFL for nonnative speakers of English, minimum high school GPA of 2.5, 3 years of high school math, 3 years of high school science, high school chemistry, high school biology, high school transcript, 2 letters of recommendation, written essay, transcript of college record, high school class rank: top 40%. 27 prerequisite credits must be completed before admission to the nursing program. *Options:* Advanced standing available through the following means: advanced placement exams, credit by exam. May apply for transfer of up to 102 total credits. *Application deadline:* rolling. *Application fee:* $20.

Degree Requirements 132 total credit hours, 54 in nursing.

RN Baccalaureate Program (BS)

Applying *Required:* minimum college GPA of 2.8, RN license, diploma or AD in nursing, transcript of college record. 27 prerequisite credits must be completed before admission to the nursing program. *Options:* Advanced standing available through the following means: advanced placement exams, advanced placement without credit, credit by exam. May apply for transfer of up to 102 total credits. *Application deadline:* rolling. *Application fee:* $20.

Degree Requirements 128 total credit hours, 54 in nursing.

Distance learning Courses provided through video, audio.

LPN to Baccalaureate Program (BS)

Applying *Required:* minimum college GPA of 2.8, LPN license, LPN school transcript. 27 prerequisite credits must be completed before admission to the nursing program. *Options:* Advanced standing available through the following means: advanced placement exams, advanced placement without credit, credit by exam. May apply for transfer of up to 102 total credits. *Application deadline:* rolling. *Application fee:* $20.

Degree Requirements 128 total credit hours, 54 in nursing.

PUERTO RICO

INTER AMERICAN UNIVERSITY OF PUERTO RICO, METROPOLITAN CAMPUS

Carmen Torres de Tiburcio School of Nursing
San Juan, Puerto Rico

Programs • Generic Baccalaureate • Continuing Education

The University Independent comprehensive coed institution. Part of Inter American University of Puerto Rico. Founded: 1960. *Primary accreditation:* regional. *Total enrollment:* 13,910.

The Carmen Torres de Tiburcio School of Nursing Founded in 1976. *Nursing program faculty:* 15 (14% with doctorates).

Academic Facilities *Campus library:* 120,389 volumes (13,538 in nursing); 24,862 periodical subscriptions (239 health-care related). *Nursing school resources:* nursing audiovisuals, learning resource lab.

Student Life *Student services:* career counseling, institutionally sponsored work-study program, job placement, special assistance for disabled students. *Nursing student activities:* student nurses association.

Calendar Semesters, Special trimester program in English for non-Spanish-speaking students.

NURSING STUDENT PROFILE

Undergraduate **Enrollment:** 315
Women: 81%; **Men:** 19%; **Minority:** 96%; **International:** 1%; **Part-time:** 10%

BACCALAUREATE PROGRAM

Contact Dr. Gloria E. Ortiz, Director, Carmen Torres de Tiburcio School of Nursing, Inter American University of Puerto Rico, Metropolitan Campus, PO Box 191293, San Juan, PR 00919-1293, 787-763-3066. *Fax:* 787-250-1242. *E-mail:* angtorr@ns.inter.edu

Expenses *Tuition:* ranges from $3040 to $3230 full-time, $95 per credit hour part-time. *Full-time mandatory fees:* $602. *Room and board:* $1600–$3000. *Room only:* $1250–$2400. *Books and supplies per academic year:* ranges from $800 to $1000.

Financial Aid Institutionally sponsored need-based grants/scholarships, Federal Nursing Student Loans, Federal Supplemental Educational Opportunity Grants, Federal Work-Study. *Application deadline:* 4/29.

Generic Baccalaureate Program (BSN)

Applying *Required:* 3 College Board Achievements, minimum high school GPA of 2.0, high school transcript, transcript of college record. *Options:* Advanced standing available through the following means: advanced placement exams, credit by exam. *Application deadlines:* 5/15 (fall), 11/15 (spring), 4/15 (summer). *Application fee:* $15.

Degree Requirements 129 total credit hours, 71 in nursing.

CONTINUING EDUCATION PROGRAM

Contact Dr. Gloria E. Ortiz, Director, Carmen Torres de Tiburcio School of Nursing, Inter American University of Puerto Rico, Metropolitan Campus, PO Box 191293, San Juan, PR 00919-1293, 787-763-3066. *Fax:* 787-250-1242.

PONTIFICAL CATHOLIC UNIVERSITY OF PUERTO RICO

Department of Nursing
Ponce, Puerto Rico

Programs • Generic Baccalaureate • MSN

The University Independent Roman Catholic comprehensive coed institution. Founded: 1948. *Primary accreditation:* regional. *Setting:* 120-acre urban campus. *Total enrollment:* 11,786.

The Department of Nursing Founded in 1956. *Nursing program faculty:* 31 (23% with doctorates).

Calendar Semesters.

NURSING STUDENT PROFILE

Undergraduate **Enrollment:** 603
Women: 95%; **Men:** 5%
Graduate **Enrollment:** 63
Women: 99%; **Men:** 1%

BACCALAUREATE PROGRAM

Contact Carmen Madera, Chair, Department of Nursing, Pontifical Catholic University of Puerto Rico, Avenue Las Americas, Station 6, Ponce, PR 00732, 787-841-2000 Ext. 259. *Fax:* 787-840-4295.

Expenses *Tuition:* $2280 full-time, $95 per credit part-time.

Generic Baccalaureate Program (BSN)

Applying *Required:* College Board Entrance Examination, minimum high school GPA of 2.5, high school transcript, interview. *Application deadlines:* 6/1 (fall), 11/1 (spring). *Application fee:* $20.

Degree Requirements 143 total credit hours, 69 in nursing.

MASTER'S PROGRAM

Contact Ms. Lourdes Maldonado, Chair, Department of Nursing, Pontifical Catholic University of Puerto Rico, Avenue Las Americas, Station 6, Ponce, PR 00732, 787-841-2000 Ext. 259.

Areas of Study Clinical nurse specialist programs in medical-surgical nursing, psychiatric–mental health nursing; nursing administration; nursing education.

Expenses *Tuition:* $2340 full-time, $130 per credit part-time.

MSN Program

Applying *Required:* GRE General Test, bachelor's degree in nursing, minimum GPA of 2.75, RN license, 2 years of clinical experience, statistics course, essay, interview, transcript of college record. *Application deadline:* 6/1. *Application fee:* $20.

Degree Requirements 46 total credit hours, 10–12 in electives.

UNIVERSIDAD METROPOLITANA

Department of Nursing
San Juan, Puerto Rico

Programs • Generic Baccalaureate • RN Baccalaureate

The Institution Independent comprehensive coed institution. Part of Ana G. Méndez University System. Founded: 1980. *Primary accreditation:* regional. *Total enrollment:* 3,200.

The Department of Nursing Founded in 1981. *Nursing program faculty:* 36.

Academic Facilities *Campus library:* 55,070 volumes (3,401 in health, 814 in nursing); 437 periodical subscriptions (66 health-care related).

Calendar Semesters.

NURSING STUDENT PROFILE

Undergraduate **Enrollment:** 280
Women: 84%; **Men:** 16%

BACCALAUREATE PROGRAMS

Contact Mrs. Carmen Bigas, Director of Admissions, Department of Nursing, Universidad Metropolitana, PO Box 21150, San Juan, PR 00928-1150, 787-766-1717.

Expenses *Tuition:* $2640 full-time, $110 per credit part-time.

Generic Baccalaureate Program (BSN)

Applying *Required:* College Board Achievements, minimum high school GPA of 2.0, high school biology, high school transcript, interview. *Application deadline:* rolling. *Application fee:* $15.

Degree Requirements 125 total credit hours, 32 in nursing.

RN Baccalaureate Program (BSN)

Applying *Required:* College Board Achievements, RN license, diploma or AD in nursing, high school transcript, interview, transcript of college record. *Options:* Advanced standing available through advanced placement exams. *Application deadline:* rolling. *Application fee:* $15.

Degree Requirements 125 total credit hours, 32 in nursing.

UNIVERSITY OF PUERTO RICO, HUMACAO UNIVERSITY COLLEGE
Nursing Department
Humacao, Puerto Rico

Program • Generic Baccalaureate

The University Commonwealth-supported 4-year coed college. Part of University of Puerto Rico System. Founded: 1962. *Primary accreditation:* regional. *Setting:* 62-acre suburban campus. *Total enrollment:* 4,228.

BACCALAUREATE PROGRAM

Contact Director, Nursing Department, University of Puerto Rico, Humacao University College, Humacao, PR 00791, 787-852-2525 Ext. 9346.

UNIVERSITY OF PUERTO RICO, MAYAGÜEZ CAMPUS
Nursing Department
Mayagüez, Puerto Rico

Programs • Generic Baccalaureate • Continuing Education

The University Commonwealth-supported coed university. Part of University of Puerto Rico System. Founded: 1911. *Primary accreditation:* regional. *Setting:* 315-acre urban campus. *Total enrollment:* 11,123.

The Nursing Department Founded in 1963. *Nursing program faculty:* 23 (13% with doctorates).

Academic Facilities *Campus library:* 939,809 volumes; 2,188 periodical subscriptions (68 health-care related). *Nursing school resources:* computer lab, nursing audiovisuals, learning resource lab.

Student Life *Student services:* health clinic, personal counseling, career counseling, institutionally sponsored work-study program, job placement, campus safety program, special assistance for disabled students. *International student services:* counseling/support. *Nursing student activities:* Sigma Theta Tau, student nurses association.

Calendar Semesters.

NURSING STUDENT PROFILE

Undergraduate **Enrollment:** 261
Women: 78%; **Men:** 22%; **International:** 0%; **Part-time:** 3%

BACCALAUREATE PROGRAM

Contact Dr. Hayden Ri¾s, Director, Nursing Department, University of Puerto Rico, Mayaguez Campus, PO Box 5000, College Station, Mayaguez, PR 00681-5000, 787-265-3842. *Fax:* 787-832-3875.

Expenses *State resident tuition:* $1500 full-time, $30 per credit part-time. *Full-time mandatory fees:* $70.

Financial Aid Institutionally sponsored long-term loans, Federal Nursing Student Loans, Federal Work-Study.

GENERIC BACCALAUREATE PROGRAM (BS)

Applying *Required:* SAT I, high school transcript. *Options:* May apply for transfer of up to 72 total credits. *Application deadline:* 12/18. *Application fee:* $15.

Degree Requirements 144 total credit hours, 57 in nursing.

CONTINUING EDUCATION PROGRAM

Contact Dr. Hayden Rios, Director, Nursing Department, University of Puerto Rico, Mayaguez Campus, PO Box 5000, College Station, Mayaguez, PR 00681-5000, 787-265-3842. *Fax:* 787-265-1225.

UNIVERSITY OF PUERTO RICO, MEDICAL SCIENCES CAMPUS
School of Nursing
San Juan, Puerto Rico

Programs • Generic Baccalaureate • Accelerated RN Baccalaureate • MSN • Continuing Education

The University Commonwealth-supported coed university. Part of University of Puerto Rico System. Founded: 1950. *Primary accreditation:* regional. *Setting:* 11-acre urban campus. *Total enrollment:* 2,881.

The School of Nursing Founded in 1941. *Nursing program faculty:* 31 (23% with doctorates).

Academic Facilities *Campus library:* 137,244 volumes (2,000 in health, 2,070 in nursing); 1,517 periodical subscriptions (1,517 health-care related). *Nursing school resources:* computer lab, nursing audiovisuals, interactive nursing skills videos, learning resource lab.

Calendar Semesters.

NURSING STUDENT PROFILE

Undergraduate **Enrollment:** 339
Women: 75%; **Men:** 25%; **Minority:** 100%; **Part-time:** 25%
Graduate **Enrollment:** 143
Women: 95%; **Men:** 5%; **Minority:** 100%; **Part-time:** 29%

BACCALAUREATE PROGRAMS

Contact Ms. Irma Rosa Ortiz de Pérez, Director, BSN Department, School of Nursing, University of Puerto Rico Medical Sciences Campus, PO Box 365067, San Juan, PR 00936-5067, 787-759-3644. *Fax:* 787-767-7070.

Expenses *State resident tuition:* $1100 per academic year. *Nonresident tuition:* $2400 per academic year. *Full-time mandatory fees:* $400. *Room and board:* $3000. *Room only:* $2000. *Books and supplies per academic year:* $400.

Financial Aid Institutionally sponsored need-based grants/scholarships, Federal Direct Loans, Federal Nursing Student Loans, Federal Pell Grants, Federal Perkins Loans, Federal Supplemental Educational Opportunity Grants, Federal Work-Study, legislative, institutional scholarships. *Application deadline:* 4/30.

GENERIC BACCALAUREATE PROGRAM (BSN)

Applying *Required:* SAT I, minimum high school GPA of 2.0, minimum college GPA of 2.0, interview, transcript of college record. 36 prerequisite credits must be completed before admission to the nursing program. *Options:* Course work may be accelerated. May apply for transfer of up to 72 total credits. *Application deadline:* 2/15. *Application fee:* $25.

Degree Requirements 131 total credit hours, 55 in nursing. Hepatitis B vaccine, other immunizations, and physical exam.

ACCELERATED RN BACCALAUREATE PROGRAM (BSN)

Applying *Required:* SAT I, minimum high school GPA of 2.0, minimum college GPA of 2.0, RN license, diploma or AD in nursing, interview, transcript of college record. *Options:* May apply for transfer of up to 72 total credits. *Application deadline:* 2/15. *Application fee:* $25.

Degree Requirements 131 total credit hours, 55 in nursing.

MASTER'S PROGRAM

Contact Dr. Martha Rivero, Director, MSN Department, School of Nursing, University of Puerto Rico Medical Sciences Campus, PO Box 365067, San Juan, PR 00936-5067, 787-758-2525 Ext. 3105. *Fax:* 787-767-7070.

Areas of Study Clinical nurse specialist program in critical care nursing; nurse anesthesia; nursing administration; nursing education.

Expenses *State resident tuition:* $2049 per academic year. *Full-time mandatory fees:* $555. *Room and board:* $3000. *Room only:* $2000. *Books and supplies per academic year:* $500.

Financial Aid Graduate assistantships, nurse traineeships, Federal Nursing Student Loans, employment opportunities. *Application deadline:* 2/15.

University of Puerto Rico, Medical Sciences Campus (continued)

MSN Program

Applying *Required:* GRE General Test, bachelor's degree in nursing, RN license, 2 years of clinical experience, physical assessment course, statistics course, interview, transcript of college record, curriculum vitae. *Application deadline:* 3/16. *Application fee:* $25.

Degree Requirements 48–56 total credit hours dependent upon track, 48–56 in nursing. Thesis required.

CONTINUING EDUCATION PROGRAM

Contact Ms. Maribel Rodriguez, Coordinator, School of Nursing, University of Puerto Rico Medical Sciences Campus, PO Box 365067, San Juan, PR 00936-5067, 787-758-2525 Ext. 3104. *Fax:* 787-767-7070.

UNIVERSITY OF THE SACRED HEART

Nursing Program
Santurce, Puerto Rico

Programs • Generic Baccalaureate • Accelerated RN Baccalaureate • Continuing Education

The University Independent Roman Catholic comprehensive coed institution. Founded: 1935. *Primary accreditation:* regional. *Setting:* 33-acre urban campus. *Total enrollment:* 5,199.

The Nursing Program Founded in 1972. *Nursing program faculty:* 5 (20% with doctorates).

Academic Facilities *Nursing school resources:* computer lab, nursing audiovisuals, learning resource lab.

Student Life *Student services:* health clinic, personal counseling, career counseling, institutionally sponsored work-study program, job placement, campus safety program, special assistance for disabled students. *International student services:* special assistance for nonnative speakers of English, ESL courses. *Nursing student activities:* Sigma Theta Tau, recruiter club, student nurses association.

Calendar Semesters.

NURSING STUDENT PROFILE

Undergraduate **Enrollment:** 120

Women: 80%; **Men:** 20%; **Minority:** 100%; **International:** 0%; **Part-time:** 10%

BACCALAUREATE PROGRAMS

Contact Dr. Amelia E. Yordan, Director, Nursing Program, University of the Sacred Heart, PO Box 12383, Loiza Station, Santurce, PR 00914-0383, 787-728-1515 Ext. 2427. *Fax:* 787-727-1250.

Expenses *Tuition:* $115 per credit. *Full-time mandatory fees:* $175. *Room and board:* $1000. *Books and supplies per academic year:* $200.

Financial Aid Institutionally sponsored need-based grants/scholarships, Federal Direct Loans, Federal Pell Grants, Federal Perkins Loans, Federal Supplemental Educational Opportunity Grants, Federal Work-Study. 95% of undergraduate students in nursing programs received some form of financial aid in 1995–96. *Application deadline:* 6/1.

Generic Baccalaureate Program (BSN)

Applying *Required:* College Board Entrance Examination, minimum high school GPA of 2.5, high school transcript, interview, 2 letters of recommendation, transcript of college record. 38 prerequisite credits must be completed before admission to the nursing program. *Options:* Advanced standing available through advanced placement exams. Course work may be accelerated. May apply for transfer of up to 68 total credits. *Application deadlines:* 8/1 (fall), 12/1 (spring). *Application fee:* $15.

Degree Requirements 138 total credit hours, 57 in nursing.

Accelerated RN Baccalaureate Program (BSN)

Applying *Required:* College Board Entrance Examination, minimum high school GPA of 2.5, diploma or AD in nursing, high school transcript, interview, 2 letters of recommendation, transcript of college record. *Options:* Advanced standing available through credit by exam. May apply for transfer of up to 29 total credits. *Application deadlines:* 8/1 (fall), 12/1 (spring). *Application fee:* $15.

Degree Requirements 138 total credit hours, 57 in nursing.

CONTINUING EDUCATION PROGRAM

Contact Dr. Amelia E. Yordan, Director, Nursing Program, University of the Sacred Heart, PO Box 12383, Loiza Station, Santurce, PR 00914-0383, 787-728-1515 Ext. 2427. *Fax:* 787-727-1250.

RHODE ISLAND

RHODE ISLAND COLLEGE

Department of Nursing
Providence, Rhode Island

Programs • Generic Baccalaureate • RN Baccalaureate

The College State-supported comprehensive coed institution. Founded: 1854. *Primary accreditation:* regional. *Setting:* 125-acre urban campus. *Total enrollment:* 9,900.

The Department of Nursing Founded in 1970. *Nursing program faculty:* 28.

Academic Facilities *Campus library:* 378,000 volumes (2,802 in health, 8,783 in nursing); 1,500 periodical subscriptions (69 health-care related).

Calendar Semesters.

BACCALAUREATE PROGRAMS

Contact Acting Director, Admissions Office, Rhode Island College, 600 Mt. Pleasant Avenue, Providence, RI 02908, 401-456-8234. *Fax:* 401-456-8379.

Financial Aid Institutionally sponsored need-based grants/scholarships, institutionally sponsored non-need grants/scholarships, Federal Nursing Student Loans, Federal Perkins Loans, Federal Supplemental Educational Opportunity Grants, Federal Work-Study, Federal PLUS Loans, Federal Stafford Loans, state aid. *Application deadline:* 3/1.

Generic Baccalaureate Program (BS)

Applying *Required:* SAT I, TOEFL for nonnative speakers of English, 3 years of high school math, high school foreign language, high school transcript, letter of recommendation. *Application deadlines:* 6/1 (transfer), rolling. *Application fee:* $25.

Degree Requirements 120 total credit hours, 55–57 in nursing.

RN Baccalaureate Program (BS)

Applying *Required:* SAT I, TOEFL for nonnative speakers of English, RN license, diploma or AD in nursing, high school transcript, transcript of college record. 8 prerequisite credits must be completed before admission to the nursing program. *Application deadlines:* 6/1 (transfer), rolling. *Application fee:* $25.

Degree Requirements 120 total credit hours, 55–57 in nursing.

SALVE REGINA UNIVERSITY

Department of Nursing
Newport, Rhode Island

Programs • Generic Baccalaureate • RN Baccalaureate

The University Independent Roman Catholic comprehensive coed institution. Founded: 1934. *Primary accreditation:* regional. *Setting:* 100-acre suburban campus. *Total enrollment:* 1,943.

The Department of Nursing Founded in 1948. *Nursing program faculty:* 11 (36% with doctorates).

▶ ***NOTEWORTHY***

The Salve Regina nursing curriculum involves a 4-year clinical component based on a liberal arts foundation, blending professional and classroom preparation for the BSN. Applicants accepted by the University who wish to major in nursing must also be accepted by the nursing committee on admission. An early licensure option is offered to those meeting the eligibility criteria. Students who choose this option may take a state licensure examination after completing at least 2 years of study. Clinicals, held throughout Rhode Island and southern Massachusetts, are small in size, allowing for extensive interaction with faculty and hospital staff members.

Academic Facilities *Campus library:* 109,572 volumes (5,388 in health, 746 in nursing); 787 periodical subscriptions (101 health-care related). *Nursing school resources:* CAI, computer lab, nursing audiovisuals, learning resource lab.

Student Life *Student services:* health clinic, personal counseling, career counseling, institutionally sponsored work-study program, job placement, campus safety program, special assistance for disabled students. *International student services:* counseling/support, special assistance for nonnative speakers of English, ESL courses. *Nursing student activities:* nursing club, student nurses association.

Calendar Semesters.

NURSING STUDENT PROFILE

Undergraduate **Enrollment:** 124
Women: 93%; **Men:** 7%; **Minority:** 7%; **International:** 0%; **Part-time:** 13%

BACCALAUREATE PROGRAMS

Contact Ms. Laura E. McPhie, Dean of Enrollment Services/Admissions, Admissions Office, Salve Regina University, 100 Ochre Point Avenue, Newport, RI 02840-4192, 401-847-6650 Ext. 2908. *Fax:* 401-848-2823. *E-mail:* sruadmis@salve3.salve.edu

Expenses *Tuition:* $14,990 full-time, $500 per credit part-time. *Full-time mandatory fees:* $300. *Part-time mandatory fees:* $170. *Room and board:* $6900. *Books and supplies per academic year:* $500.

Financial Aid Institutionally sponsored need-based grants/scholarships, institutionally sponsored non-need grants/scholarships, Federal Nursing Student Loans, Federal Pell Grants, Federal Perkins Loans, Federal Supplemental Educational Opportunity Grants, Federal Work-Study. 81% of undergraduate students in nursing programs received some form of financial aid in 1995–96. *Application deadline:* 3/1.

Generic Baccalaureate Program (BSN)

Applying *Required:* SAT I or ACT, 3 years of high school math, high school chemistry, high school biology, high school foreign language, high school transcript, 2 letters of recommendation, written essay, transcript of college record. *Options:* Advanced standing available through the following means: advanced placement exams, credit by exam. Course work may be accelerated. May apply for transfer of up to 92 total credits. *Application deadline:* rolling. *Application fee:* $25.

Degree Requirements 128 total credit hours, 65 in nursing.

RN Baccalaureate Program (BSN)

Applying *Required:* RN license, diploma or AD in nursing, high school transcript, 2 letters of recommendation, written essay, transcript of college record. 60 prerequisite credits must be completed before admission to the nursing program. *Options:* Advanced standing available through the following means: advanced placement exams, credit by exam. Course work may be accelerated. May apply for transfer of up to 92 total credits. *Application deadline:* rolling. *Application fee:* $25.

Degree Requirements 128 total credit hours, 33 in nursing.

UNIVERSITY OF RHODE ISLAND

College of Nursing
Kingston, Rhode Island

Programs • Generic Baccalaureate • RN Baccalaureate • MS • PhD

The University State-supported coed university. Part of Rhode Island State System of Higher Education. Founded: 1892. *Primary accreditation:* regional. *Setting:* 1,200-acre small-town campus. *Total enrollment:* 13,698.

The College of Nursing Founded in 1945. *Nursing program faculty:* 33 (50% with doctorates).

Academic Facilities *Nursing school resources:* CAI, computer lab, nursing audiovisuals, interactive nursing skills videos, learning resource lab.

Student Life *Student services:* health clinic, personal counseling, career counseling, campus safety program, special assistance for disabled students. *International student services:* counseling/support, ESL courses. *Nursing student activities:* Sigma Theta Tau, student nurses association.

Calendar Semesters.

NURSING STUDENT PROFILE

Undergraduate **Enrollment:** 477
Women: 88%; **Men:** 12%; **Minority:** 12%; **International:** 1%; **Part-time:** 10%
Graduate **Enrollment:** 125
Women: 92%; **Men:** 8%; **Minority:** 8%; **International:** 4%; **Part-time:** 75%

BACCALAUREATE PROGRAMS

Contact Ms. Ruth Waldman, Assistant Dean, White Hall, College of Nursing, University of Rhode Island, Kingston, RI 02881, 401-792-2766. *Fax:* 401-792-2061.

Expenses *State resident tuition:* $4817 full-time, $131 per credit part-time. *Nonresident tuition:* $12,509 full-time, $452 per credit part-time. *Full-time mandatory fees:* $1250. *Room and board:* $5500–$6000. *Books and supplies per academic year:* ranges from $400 to $600.

Financial Aid Institutionally sponsored need-based grants/scholarships, Federal Direct Loans, Federal Nursing Student Loans, Federal Perkins Loans, Federal Supplemental Educational Opportunity Grants, Federal Work-Study. 73% of undergraduate students in nursing programs received some form of financial aid in 1995–96. *Application deadline:* 3/1.

Generic Baccalaureate Program (BS)

Applying *Required:* SAT I, 3 years of high school math, 2 years of high school science, high school foreign language, high school transcript, high school class rank: top 40%. *Options:* Advanced standing available through advanced placement exams. May apply for transfer of up to 64 total credits. *Application deadlines:* 3/1 (fall), 11/1 (spring). *Application fee:* $30–45.

Degree Requirements 125 total credit hours, 60 in nursing.

RN Baccalaureate Program (BS)

Applying *Required:* minimum college GPA of 2.4, RN license, diploma or AD in nursing, transcript of college record. *Options:* Advanced standing available through the following means: advanced placement exams, credit by exam. May apply for transfer of up to 64 total credits. *Application deadlines:* 3/1 (fall), 11/1 (spring). *Application fee:* $30–45.

Degree Requirements 120 total credit hours, 45 in nursing.

MASTER'S PROGRAM

Contact Dr. Donna Schwartz-Barcott, Director of Graduate Programs, White Hall, College of Nursing, University of Rhode Island, Kingston, RI 02881, 401-874-2766. *Fax:* 401-874-2061.

Areas of Study Clinical nurse specialist programs in critical care nursing, gerontological nursing, maternity-newborn nursing, psychiatric–mental health nursing; nurse midwifery; nursing administration; nursing education; nurse practitioner program in family health.

Expenses *State resident tuition:* $4799 full-time, $184 per credit part-time. *Nonresident tuition:* $10,593 full-time, $506 per credit part-time. *Full-time mandatory fees:* $1400.

Financial Aid Graduate assistantships, Federal Direct Loans, employment opportunities. 12% of master's level students in nursing programs received some form of financial aid in 1995-96.

MS Program

Applying *Required:* GRE General Test or Miller Analogies Test, bachelor's degree in nursing, minimum GPA of 3.0, RN license, 1 year of clinical experience, statistics course, essay, 3 letters of recommendation, transcript of college record, 2 years of clinical experience for primary health care. *Application deadlines:* 4/15 (fall), 11/15 (spring). *Application fee:* $30–45.

Degree Requirements 40–45 total credit hours dependent upon track.

Distance learning Courses provided through video, computer-based media.

DOCTORAL PROGRAM

Contact Dr. Donna Schwartz-Barcott, Director of Graduate Programs, White Hall, College of Nursing, University of Rhode Island, Kingston, RI 02881, 401-874-2766. *Fax:* 401-874-2061.

Areas of Study Nursing research, nursing theory.

Expenses *State resident tuition:* $4799 full-time, $184 per credit part-time. *Nonresident tuition:* $10,593 full-time, $506 per credit part-time. *Full-time mandatory fees:* $1400.

Financial Aid Graduate assistantships, opportunities for employment.

University of Rhode Island (continued)

PhD Program

Applying *Required:* GRE General Test, master's degree in nursing, 2 scholarly papers, statistics course, 3 letters of recommendation, statement of purpose and goals. *Application deadlines:* 7/15 (fall), 11/15 (spring). *Application fee:* $30.

Degree Requirements 61 total credit hours; dissertation; oral exam; written exam; defense of dissertation.

Distance learning Courses provided through video, computer-based media.

SOUTH CAROLINA

CLEMSON UNIVERSITY

School of Nursing, College of Health, Education, and Human Development
Clemson, South Carolina

Programs • Generic Baccalaureate • Accelerated RN Baccalaureate • MS • Continuing Education

The University State-supported coed university. Founded: 1889. *Primary accreditation:* regional. *Setting:* 1,400-acre small-town campus. *Total enrollment:* 15,434.

The School of Nursing, College of Health, Education, and Human Development Founded in 1965. *Nursing program faculty:* 35 (65% with doctorates). *Off-campus program site:* Greenville.

Academic Facilities *Campus library:* 797,997 volumes (29,800 in health, 50,900 in nursing); 6,831 periodical subscriptions (877 health-care related). *Nursing school resources:* CAI, computer lab, nursing audiovisuals, interactive nursing skills videos, learning resource lab, telecampus.

Student Life *Student services:* health clinic, personal counseling, career counseling, institutionally sponsored work-study program, job placement, campus safety program, special assistance for disabled students. *International student services:* counseling/support, special assistance for nonnative speakers of English. *Nursing student activities:* Sigma Theta Tau, student nurses association.

Calendar Semesters.

NURSING STUDENT PROFILE

Undergraduate **Enrollment:** 479
Women: 94%; **Men:** 6%; **Minority:** 12%; **International:** 0%; **Part-time:** 8%

Graduate **Enrollment:** 98
Women: 94%; **Men:** 6%; **Minority:** 5%; **International:** 1%; **Part-time:** 50%

BACCALAUREATE PROGRAMS

Contact Ms. Beth Hearn, Director of Student Services, 309 Edwards Hall, Clemson University, Box 341704, Clemson, SC 29634-1704, 803-656-5495. *Fax:* 803-656-5488. *E-mail:* mary2@clemson.edu

Expenses *State resident tuition:* $2880 full-time, $120 per hour part-time. *Nonresident tuition:* $8126 full-time, $340 per hour part-time. *Full-time mandatory fees:* $140. *Room and board:* $2940–$3974. *Room only:* $1450–$2200. *Books and supplies per academic year:* $450.

Financial Aid Institutionally sponsored need-based grants/scholarships, institutionally sponsored non-need grants/scholarships, Federal Perkins Loans, Federal Supplemental Educational Opportunity Grants, Federal Work-Study, Federal PLUS Loans, Federal Stafford Loans. 12% of undergraduate students in nursing programs received some form of financial aid in 1995–96. *Application deadline:* 4/1.

Generic Baccalaureate Program (BS)

Applying *Required:* SAT I, ACT, TOEFL for nonnative speakers of English, 3 years of high school math, 3 years of high school science, high school chemistry, high school biology, high school foreign language, high school transcript, written essay, transcript of college record. *Options:* Advanced standing available through advanced placement exams. May apply for transfer of up to 105 total credits. *Application deadline:* rolling. *Application fee:* $35.

Degree Requirements 137 total credit hours, 64 in nursing.

Accelerated RN Baccalaureate Program (BS)

Applying *Required:* minimum college GPA of 2.5, RN license, diploma or AD in nursing, interview, transcript of college record. 79 prerequisite credits must be completed before admission to the nursing program. *Options:* Advanced standing available through credit by exam. Course work may be accelerated. May apply for transfer of up to 105 total credits. *Application deadline:* rolling. *Application fee:* $35.

Degree Requirements 137 total credit hours, 64 in nursing.

MASTER'S PROGRAM

Contact Ms. Beth Hearn, Director of Student Services, 309 Edwards Hall, Clemson University, Box 341704, Clemson, SC 29634-1704, 803-656-5495. *Fax:* 803-656-5488. *E-mail:* mary2@clemson.edu

Areas of Study Clinical nurse specialist programs in adult health nursing, gerontological nursing, maternity-newborn nursing, pediatric nursing; nursing administration; nursing education; nurse practitioner program in family health.

Expenses *State resident tuition:* $2922 full-time, $120 per hour part-time. *Nonresident tuition:* $5844 full-time, $240 per hour part-time. *Full-time mandatory fees:* $95. *Room and board:* $2940–$3974. *Room only:* $1450–$2200. *Books and supplies per academic year:* $500.

Financial Aid Graduate assistantships, nurse traineeships, Federal Nursing Student Loans, employment opportunities. 19% of master's level students in nursing programs received some form of financial aid in 1995-96. *Application deadline:* 3/1.

MS Program

Applying *Required:* TOEFL for nonnative speakers of English, GRE General Test (minimum score of 500 on each of three parts recommended), bachelor's degree in nursing, minimum GPA of 3.0, RN license, 1 year of clinical experience, physical assessment course, statistics course, professional liability/malpractice insurance, essay, 2 letters of recommendation, transcript of college record. *Application deadlines:* 7/15 (fall), 12/1 (spring). *Application fee:* $30.

Degree Requirements 35–45 total credit hours dependent upon track, 35–45 in nursing. Thesis or project.

CONTINUING EDUCATION PROGRAM

Contact Ms. Olivia Shanahan, Director of Continuing Education, Clemson University, PO Box 341711, Clemson, SC 29634-1711, 803-656-3078. *Fax:* 803-656-5488. *E-mail:* olivia@clemson.edu

LANDER UNIVERSITY

School of Nursing
Greenwood, South Carolina

Programs • Generic Baccalaureate • RN Baccalaureate • Baccalaureate for Second Degree

The University State-supported comprehensive coed institution. Part of South Carolina Commission on Higher Education. Founded: 1872. *Primary accreditation:* regional. *Setting:* 100-acre small-town campus. *Total enrollment:* 2,780.

The School of Nursing Founded in 1957. *Nursing program faculty:* 10 (30% with doctorates).

Academic Facilities *Campus library:* 247,972 volumes (5,570 in health); 935 periodical subscriptions (68 health-care related). *Nursing school resources:* CAI, computer lab, nursing audiovisuals.

Student Life *Student services:* health clinic, personal counseling, career counseling, job placement, campus safety program. *Nursing student activities:* Sigma Theta Tau, nursing club, student nurses association.

Calendar Semesters.

NURSING STUDENT PROFILE

Undergraduate **Enrollment:** 220
Women: 87%; **Men:** 13%; **Minority:** 17%; **International:** 1%; **Part-time:** 14%

BACCALAUREATE PROGRAMS

Contact Dr. Barbara T. Freese, Dean and Professor, School of Nursing, Lander University, Greenwood, SC 29649-2099, 864-388-8337. *Fax:* 864-388-8890.

Expenses *State resident tuition:* $3550 full-time, $142 per credit hour part-time. *Nonresident tuition:* $5382 full-time, $217 per credit hour part-time. *Full-time mandatory fees:* $80–$200. *Room and board:* $2800–$3200. *Books and supplies per academic year:* ranges from $200 to $500.

Financial Aid Institutionally sponsored need-based grants/scholarships, institutionally sponsored non-need grants/scholarships, Federal Pell

Grants, Federal Perkins Loans, Federal Supplemental Educational Opportunity Grants, Federal Work-Study. *Application deadline:* 4/15.

Generic Baccalaureate Program (BSN)

Applying *Required:* SAT I or ACT, minimum college GPA of 2.5, 3 years of high school math, high school foreign language, high school transcript, transcript of college record, 2 years of high school lab science. 30 prerequisite credits must be completed before admission to the nursing program. *Options:* Advanced standing available through credit by exam. Course work may be accelerated. May apply for transfer of up to 64 total credits. *Application deadline:* 8/4. *Application fee:* $15.

Degree Requirements 126 total credit hours, 56 in nursing.

RN Baccalaureate Program (BSN)

Applying *Required:* minimum college GPA of 2.5, 3 years of high school math, RN license, diploma or AD in nursing, high school foreign language, transcript of college record, 1 year of clinical experience, 2 years of high school lab science. 30 prerequisite credits must be completed before admission to the nursing program. *Options:* Advanced standing available through credit by exam. May apply for transfer of up to 64 total credits. *Application deadline:* rolling. *Application fee:* $15.

Degree Requirements 126 total credit hours, 56 in nursing.

Baccalaureate for Second Degree Program (BSN)

Applying *Required:* minimum college GPA of 2.5, 3 years of high school math, high school foreign language, transcript of college record, 2 years of high school lab science. *Options:* Advanced standing available through credit by exam. *Application deadline:* rolling. *Application fee:* $15.

Degree Requirements 126 total credit hours, 56 in nursing.

MEDICAL UNIVERSITY OF SOUTH CAROLINA
College of Nursing
Charleston, South Carolina

Programs • Generic Baccalaureate • RN Baccalaureate • LPN to Baccalaureate • MSN • RN to Master's • Master's for Nurses with Non-Nursing Degrees • Post-Master's • PhD • Continuing Education

The University State-supported upper-level coed institution. Founded: 1824. *Primary accreditation:* regional. *Setting:* 55-acre urban campus. *Total enrollment:* 2,209.

The College of Nursing Founded in 1883. *Nursing program faculty:* 70 (90% with doctorates). *Off-campus program site:* Florence.

Academic Facilities *Campus library:* 210,000 volumes; 2,900 periodical subscriptions (2,800 health-care related). *Nursing school resources:* computer lab, nursing audiovisuals, interactive nursing skills videos, learning resource lab.

Student Life *Student services:* health clinic, child-care facilities, personal counseling, career counseling, institutionally sponsored work-study program, job placement, campus safety program, special assistance for disabled students, wellness center. *International student services:* counseling/support. *Nursing student activities:* Sigma Theta Tau, student nurses association.

Calendar Semesters.

NURSING STUDENT PROFILE

Undergraduate **Enrollment:** 264
Women: 80%; **Men:** 20%; **Minority:** 16%; **Part-time:** 10%
Graduate **Enrollment:** 140
Women: 95%; **Men:** 5%; **Minority:** 10%; **International:** 10%; **Part-time:** 60%

BACCALAUREATE PROGRAMS

Contact Ms. Mardi Long, Director of Student Services, College of Nursing, Medical University of South Carolina, 171 Ashley Avenue, Charleston, SC 29425, 803-792-8515. *Fax:* 803-792-9258.

Expenses *State resident tuition:* $3202 full-time, $125 per semester hour part-time. *Nonresident tuition:* $9318 full-time, $352 per semester hour part-time. *Full-time mandatory fees:* $0–$100. *Part-time mandatory fees:* $0–$75. *Books and supplies per academic year:* ranges from $600 to $800.

Financial Aid Institutionally sponsored need-based grants/scholarships, institutionally sponsored non-need grants/scholarships, Federal Direct Loans, Federal Nursing Student Loans, Federal Pell Grants, Federal Perkins Loans, Federal Supplemental Educational Opportunity Grants, Federal Work-Study. 45% of undergraduate students in nursing programs received some form of financial aid in 1995–96.

Generic Baccalaureate Program (BSN)

Applying *Required:* SAT I, ACT, MAT for students age 23 and over, minimum college GPA of 2.5, written essay, transcript of college record. 60 prerequisite credits must be completed before admission to the nursing program. *Options:* Advanced standing available through the following means: advanced placement exams, credit by exam. May apply for transfer of up to 66 total credits. *Application deadlines:* 2/15 (fall), 9/15 (spring). *Application fee:* $50.

Degree Requirements 124 total credit hours, 64 in nursing.

RN Baccalaureate Program (BSN)

Applying *Required:* SAT I, ACT, MAT for students age 23 and over, minimum college GPA of 2.5, RN license, diploma or AD in nursing, written essay, transcript of college record. 60 prerequisite credits must be completed before admission to the nursing program. *Options:* Advanced standing available through the following means: advanced placement exams, credit by exam. Course work may be accelerated. May apply for transfer of up to 90 total credits. *Application deadlines:* 2/15 (fall), 9/15 (spring). *Application fee:* $50.

Degree Requirements 124 total credit hours, 34 in nursing.

LPN to Baccalaureate Program (BSN)

Applying *Required:* SAT I, ACT, MAT for students age 23 and over, minimum college GPA of 2.5, written essay, transcript of college record, LPN license. 60 prerequisite credits must be completed before admission to the nursing program. *Options:* Advanced standing available through the following means: advanced placement exams, credit by exam. Course work may be accelerated. May apply for transfer of up to 66 total credits. *Application deadlines:* 2/15 (fall), 9/15 (spring). *Application fee:* $50.

Degree Requirements 124 total credit hours, 64 in nursing.

MASTER'S PROGRAMS

Contact Ms. Mardi Long, Director of Student Services, College of Nursing, Medical University of South Carolina, 171 Ashley Avenue, Charleston, SC 29425, 803-792-8515. *Fax:* 803-792-9258.

Areas of Study Clinical nurse specialist programs in adult health nursing, critical care nursing, family health nursing, gerontological nursing, maternity-newborn nursing, parent-child nursing, perinatal nursing, psychiatric–mental health nursing, women's health nursing; nurse anesthesia; nurse midwifery; nursing administration; nurse practitioner programs in adult health, child care/pediatrics, family health, gerontology, neonatal health, psychiatric–mental health.

Expenses *State resident tuition:* $3014 full-time, $142 per semester hour part-time. *Nonresident tuition:* $3862 full-time, $187 per semester hour part-time. *Full-time mandatory fees:* $0–$100. *Part-time mandatory fees:* $0–$75. *Books and supplies per academic year:* ranges from $300 to $1000.

Financial Aid Graduate assistantships, nurse traineeships, fellowships, Federal Nursing Student Loans, institutionally sponsored loans, employment opportunities, institutionally sponsored need-based grants/scholarships, institutionally sponsored non-need-based grants/scholarships. 40% of master's level students in nursing programs received some form of financial aid in 1995-96.

MSN Program

Applying *Required:* GRE General Test (minimum combined score of 1000 on 2 sections), bachelor's degree in nursing, minimum GPA of 3.0, RN license, 2 years of clinical experience, physical assessment course, statistics course, professional liability/malpractice insurance, interview, 3 letters of recommendation, transcript of college record, computer literacy. *Application deadlines:* 2/15 (fall), 10/15 (spring), 2/15 (summer). *Application fee:* $50.

Degree Requirements 36–48 total credit hours dependent upon track, 36–48 in nursing. Scholarly project.

RN to Master's Program (MSN)

Applying *Required:* GRE General Test, minimum GPA of 3.0, RN license, 1 year of clinical experience, physical assessment course, statistics course,

Medical University of South Carolina (continued)
professional liability/malpractice insurance, interview, 3 letters of recommendation, transcript of college record, computer literacy, 60 semester hours prerequisite course work. *Application deadlines:* 2/15 (fall), 10/15 (spring), 2/15 (summer). *Application fee:* $50.

Degree Requirements 73 total credit hours, 73 in nursing. Scholarly project.

Master's for Nurses with Non-Nursing Degrees Program (MSN)

Applying *Required:* GRE General Test, minimum GPA of 3.0, RN license, 1 year of clinical experience, physical assessment course, statistics course, professional liability/malpractice insurance, interview, 3 letters of recommendation, transcript of college record, computer literacy. *Application deadlines:* 2/15 (fall), 10/15 (spring), 2/15 (summer). *Application fee:* $50.

Degree Requirements 73 total credit hours, 73 in nursing. Scholarly project.

Post-Master's Program

Applying *Required:* minimum GPA of 3.0, RN license, 2 years of clinical experience, physical assessment course, statistics course, professional liability/malpractice insurance, 3 letters of recommendation, transcript of college record. *Application deadlines:* 2/15 (fall), 10/15 (spring), 2/15 (summer). *Application fee:* $50.

Degree Requirements 36 total credit hours, 36 in nursing.

DOCTORAL PROGRAM

Contact Dr. Marie Lobo, Interim Director of Doctoral Studies, College of Nursing, Medical University of South Carolina, 171 Ashley Avenue, Charleston, SC 29425, 803-792-2819.

Areas of Study Individualized study.

Expenses *State resident tuition:* $3014 full-time, $142 per semester hour part-time. *Nonresident tuition:* $3862 full-time, $187 per semester hour part-time. *Full-time mandatory fees:* $0.

PhD Program

Applying *Required:* TOEFL for nonnative speakers of English, GRE General Test (minimum combined score of 1000 on verbal and quantitative sections), master's degree in nursing, 2 scholarly papers, interview, 3 letters of recommendation, vitae, writing sample, competitive review by faculty committee, application to University of South Carolina, Columbia. *Application deadline:* 4/1. *Application fee:* $35.

Degree Requirements 60 total credit hours; 27 core course credits, 3-credit research internship, 18 elective and cognate credits, 12-credit dissertation; dissertation; oral exam; written exam; defense of dissertation; residency.

CONTINUING EDUCATION PROGRAM

Contact Director of Continuing Education, College of Nursing, Medical University of South Carolina, 171 Ashley Avenue, Charleston, SC 29425, 803-792-8786. *Fax:* 803-792-2969.

SOUTH CAROLINA STATE UNIVERSITY

Department of Nursing
Orangeburg, South Carolina

Programs • Generic Baccalaureate • RN Baccalaureate

The University State-supported comprehensive coed institution. Part of South Carolina Commission on Higher Education. Founded: 1896. *Primary accreditation:* regional. *Setting:* 160-acre small-town campus. *Total enrollment:* 4,993.

The Department of Nursing Founded in 1988. *Nursing program faculty:* 6 (50% with doctorates).

Academic Facilities *Campus library:* 278,399 volumes (9,960 in health, 375 in nursing); 1,340 periodical subscriptions (66 health-care related). *Nursing school resources:* CAI, computer lab, nursing audiovisuals, learning resource lab.

Student Life *Student services:* health clinic, personal counseling, career counseling, institutionally sponsored work-study program, job placement, campus safety program, tutoring. *International student services:* counseling/support, special assistance for nonnative speakers of English. *Nursing student activities:* student nurses association, Chi Eta Phi nursing sorority.

Calendar Semesters.

NURSING STUDENT PROFILE

Undergraduate **Enrollment:** 27
Women: 93%; **Men:** 7%; **Minority:** 85%; **International:** 3%; **Part-time:** 22%

BACCALAUREATE PROGRAMS

Contact Mrs. Carrie James, Assistant Professor, Department of Nursing, South Carolina State University, 300 College Street, NE, PO Box 7158, Orangeburg, SC 29117-0001, 803-536-8608. *Fax:* 803-533-3628. *E-mail:* zf_cjames@floyd.scsu.edu

Expenses *State resident tuition:* $2250 full-time, $104 per semester hour part-time. *Nonresident tuition:* $5700 full-time, $208 per semester hour part-time. *Full-time mandatory fees:* $33–$150. *Room and board:* $2692–$2986. *Room only:* $1172–$1466. *Books and supplies per academic year:* ranges from $200 to $300.

Financial Aid Institutionally sponsored need-based grants/scholarships, institutionally sponsored non-need grants/scholarships, Federal Direct Loans, Federal Pell Grants, Federal Supplemental Educational Opportunity Grants, Federal Work-Study. 85% of undergraduate students in nursing programs received some form of financial aid in 1995–96. *Application deadline:* 7/15.

Generic Baccalaureate Program (BSN)

Applying *Required:* SAT I or ACT, minimum high school GPA of 2.5, minimum college GPA of 2.5, 3 years of high school math, 3 years of high school science, high school chemistry, high school biology, high school transcript, 2 letters of recommendation, transcript of college record. 49 prerequisite credits must be completed before admission to the nursing program. *Options:* Advanced standing available through the following means: advanced placement exams, credit by exam. Course work may be accelerated. May apply for transfer of up to 62 total credits. *Application deadlines:* 7/31 (fall), 11/30 (spring). *Application fee:* $35.

Degree Requirements 129 total credit hours, 64 in nursing. English proficiency exam.

RN Baccalaureate Program (BSN)

Applying *Required:* SAT I or ACT, minimum high school GPA of 2.5, minimum college GPA of 2.5, RN license, diploma or AD in nursing, high school transcript, letter of recommendation, transcript of college record. *Options:* Advanced standing available through advanced placement exams. Course work may be accelerated. May apply for transfer of up to 62 total credits. *Application deadlines:* 7/31 (fall), 11/30 (spring). *Application fee:* $35.

Degree Requirements 129 total credit hours, 64 in nursing. English proficiency exam.

UNIVERSITY OF SOUTH CAROLINA

College of Nursing
Columbia, South Carolina

Programs • Generic Baccalaureate • Accelerated RN Baccalaureate • MN • MS • MN/MPH • MS/MPH • Post-Master's • PhD

The University State-supported coed university. Part of University of South Carolina System. Founded: 1801. *Primary accreditation:* regional. *Setting:* 242-acre urban campus. *Total enrollment:* 26,346.

The College of Nursing Founded in 1957. *Nursing program faculty:* 43 (62% with doctorates).

Academic Facilities *Campus library:* 2.6 million volumes; 19,232 periodical subscriptions (2,108 health-care related). *Nursing school resources:* CAI, computer lab, nursing audiovisuals, interactive nursing skills videos, learning resource lab, clinical simulation lab.

Student Life *Student services:* health clinic, personal counseling, career counseling, institutionally sponsored work-study program, job placement, campus safety program, special assistance for disabled students. *International student services:* counseling/support, special assistance for

nonnative speakers of English, ESL courses. *Nursing student activities:* Sigma Theta Tau, recruiter club, nursing club, student nurses association.

Calendar Semesters.

NURSING STUDENT PROFILE

Undergraduate **Enrollment:** 695
Women: 90%; **Men:** 10%; **Minority:** 27%; **Part-time:** 26%
Graduate **Enrollment:** 228
Women: 96%; **Men:** 4%; **Minority:** 9%; **International:** 2%; **Part-time:** 78%

BACCALAUREATE PROGRAMS

Contact Mrs. Karen Waganer, Assistant Dean, College of Nursing, University of South Carolina, Columbia, SC 29208, 803-777-7412. *Fax:* 803-777-0616.

Expenses *State resident tuition:* $3788 full-time, $156 per credit hour part-time. *Nonresident tuition:* $9666 full-time, $386 per credit hour part-time. *Full-time mandatory fees:* $150–$170. *Room and board:* $3692. *Room only:* $1792–$2148. *Books and supplies per academic year:* ranges from $400 to $600.

Financial Aid Institutionally sponsored need-based grants/scholarships, institutionally sponsored non-need grants/scholarships, Federal Nursing Student Loans, Federal Supplemental Educational Opportunity Grants, Federal Work-Study. *Application deadline:* 4/15.

Generic Baccalaureate Program (BSN)

Applying *Required:* SAT I, TOEFL for nonnative speakers of English, minimum college GPA of 2.5, 3 years of high school math, 2 years of high school science, high school foreign language, high school transcript, transcript of college record. 23 prerequisite credits must be completed before admission to the nursing program. *Options:* Advanced standing available through the following means: advanced placement exams, credit by exam. Course work may be accelerated. May apply for transfer of up to 98 total credits. *Application deadlines:* 8/1 (fall), 12/1 (spring), 5/15 (summer). *Application fee:* $25.

Degree Requirements 128 total credit hours, 73 in nursing.

Accelerated RN Baccalaureate Program (BSN)

Applying *Required:* TOEFL for nonnative speakers of English, minimum college GPA of 2.5, RN license, diploma or AD in nursing, transcript of college record. 23 prerequisite credits must be completed before admission to the nursing program. *Options:* Advanced standing available through the following means: advanced placement exams, credit by exam. Course work may be accelerated. May apply for transfer of up to 98 total credits. *Application deadlines:* 8/1 (fall), 12/1 (spring), 5/15 (summer). *Application fee:* $25.

Degree Requirements 128 total credit hours, 73 in nursing.

MASTER'S PROGRAMS

Contact Ms. Becki Dangerfield, Student Services Specialist, College of Nursing, University of South Carolina, Columbia, SC 29208, 803-777-7412. *Fax:* 803-777-0616.

Areas of Study Clinical nurse specialist programs in community health nursing, psychiatric–mental health nursing; nursing administration; nurse practitioner programs in acute care, adult health, child care/pediatrics, family health, gerontology, psychiatric–mental health, women's health.

Expenses *State resident tuition:* $4176 full-time, $205 per semester hour part-time. *Nonresident tuition:* $8480 full-time, $415 per semester hour part-time. *Full-time mandatory fees:* $35.

Financial Aid Graduate assistantships, nurse traineeships, Federal Nursing Student Loans. *Application deadline:* 4/15.

MN Program

Applying *Required:* Miller Analogies Test, TOEFL for nonnative speakers of English, GRE General Test (minimum combined score of 1000 on verbal and quantitative sections), bachelor's degree in nursing, minimum GPA of 2.5, RN license, physical assessment course, essay, 2 letters of recommendation, transcript of college record, minimum 3.0 GPA in professional nursing courses. *Application deadlines:* 4/15 (fall), 10/15 (spring), 4/15 (summer). *Application fee:* $35.

Degree Requirements 36–45 total credit hours dependent upon track, 33–39 in nursing, 3–6 in statistics, epidemiology.

MS Program

Applying *Required:* Miller Analogies Test, TOEFL for nonnative speakers of English, GRE General Test (minimum combined score of 1000 on verbal and quantitative sections), bachelor's degree in nursing, minimum GPA of 2.5, RN license, physical assessment course, essay, 2 letters of recommendation, transcript of college record, minimum 3.0 GPA in professional nursing courses. *Application deadlines:* 4/15 (fall), 10/15 (spring), 4/15 (summer). *Application fee:* $35.

Degree Requirements 36–45 total credit hours dependent upon track, 33–42 in nursing, 3–6 in statistics, epidemiology. Thesis required.

MN/MPH Program

Applying *Required:* GRE General Test (minimum combined score of 1000 on verbal and quantitative sections), bachelor's degree in nursing, minimum GPA of 2.5, RN license, 2 letters of recommendation, transcript of college record, minimum 3.0 GPA in professional nursing courses. *Application deadlines:* 4/15 (fall), 10/15 (spring), 4/15 (summer). *Application fee:* $35.

Degree Requirements 51 total credit hours, 30 in nursing, 21 in public health.

MS/MPH Program

Applying *Required:* TOEFL for nonnative speakers of English, GRE General Test (minimum combined score of 1000 on verbal and quantitative sections), bachelor's degree in nursing, minimum GPA of 3.0, RN license, 2 letters of recommendation, transcript of college record, minimum 3.0 GPA in professional nursing courses. *Application deadlines:* 4/15 (fall), 10/15 (spring), 4/15 (summer). *Application fee:* $35.

Degree Requirements 54 total credit hours, 33 in nursing, 21 in public health. Thesis required.

Post-Master's Program

Applying *Required:* Miller Analogies Test, TOEFL for nonnative speakers of English, GRE General Test (minimum combined score of 1000 on verbal and quantitative sections), minimum GPA of 3.0, RN license, essay, letter of recommendation, transcript of college record. Master's in nursing. *Application deadlines:* 4/15 (fall), 10/15 (spring), 4/15 (summer). *Application fee:* $35.

Degree Requirements 21–27 total credit hours dependent upon track, 21–27 in nursing.

DOCTORAL PROGRAM

Contact Dr. Sue W. Young, Associate Dean, Academic Programs, College of Nursing, University of South Carolina, Columbia, SC 29208, 803-777-7113. *Fax:* 803-777-0616.

Areas of Study Individualized study.

Expenses *State resident tuition:* $4176 full-time, $205 per semester hour part-time. *Nonresident tuition:* $8480 full-time, $415 per semester hour part-time. *Full-time mandatory fees:* $35.

Financial Aid Graduate assistantships, nurse traineeships, fellowships, dissertation grants, grants, Federal Nursing Student Loans, opportunities for employment. *Application deadline:* 4/15.

PhD Program

Applying *Required:* TOEFL for nonnative speakers of English, GRE General Test (minimum combined score of 1000 on verbal and quantitative sections), master's degree in nursing, 2 scholarly papers, interview, 3 letters of recommendation, vitae, writing sample, competitive review by faculty committee. *Application deadline:* 2/1. *Application fee:* $35.

Degree Requirements 60 total credit hours; 27 core course credits, 3-credit research internship, 18 elective and cognate credits, 12-credit dissertation; dissertation; oral exam; written exam; defense of dissertation; residency.

UNIVERSITY OF SOUTH CAROLINA–AIKEN

School of Nursing
Aiken, South Carolina

Program • RN Baccalaureate

The University State-supported comprehensive coed institution. Part of University of South Carolina System. Founded: 1961. *Primary accreditation:* regional. *Setting:* 144-acre small-town campus. *Total enrollment:* 3,256.

The School of Nursing Founded in 1985. *Nursing program faculty:* 4 (100% with doctorates). *Off-campus program site:* Beaufort.

Academic Facilities *Campus library:* 120,444 volumes (5,302 in nursing); 967 periodical subscriptions (57 health-care related). *Nursing school*

University of South Carolina–Aiken (continued)
resources: CAI, computer lab, nursing audiovisuals, interactive nursing skills videos, learning resource lab.

Student Life *Student services:* child-care facilities, personal counseling, career counseling, institutionally sponsored work-study program, job placement, special assistance for disabled students. *Nursing student activities:* student nurses association, Nursing Honor Society.

Calendar Semesters.

NURSING STUDENT PROFILE

Undergraduate **Enrollment:** 107
Women: 95%; **Men:** 5%; **Minority:** 18%; **International:** 0%; **Part-time:** 70%

BACCALAUREATE PROGRAM

Contact Dr. Trudy G. Groves, BSN Program Director, School of Nursing, University of South Carolina-Aiken, 171 University Parkway, Aiken, SC 29801, 803-648-6851. *Fax:* 803-641-3362. *E-mail:* trudyg@aiken.sc.edu

Expenses *State resident tuition:* $2708 full-time, $119 per semester hour part-time. *Nonresident tuition:* $6770 full-time, $298 per semester hour part-time. *Full-time mandatory fees:* $70. *Books and supplies per academic year:* ranges from $200 to $400.

Financial Aid Institutionally sponsored need-based grants/scholarships, institutionally sponsored non-need grants/scholarships, Federal Nursing Student Loans. 75% of undergraduate students in nursing programs received some form of financial aid in 1995–96. *Application deadline:* 2/15.

RN Baccalaureate Program (BSN)

Applying *Required:* minimum college GPA of 2.0, RN license, diploma or AD in nursing, 2 letters of recommendation, transcript of college record. *Options:* Advanced standing available through the following means: advanced placement exams, credit by exam. Course work may be accelerated. May apply for transfer of up to 90 total credits. *Application deadlines:* 7/15 (fall), 11/15 (spring). *Application fee:* $25.

Degree Requirements 120 total credit hours, 36 in nursing.

UNIVERSITY OF SOUTH CAROLINA–SPARTANBURG
Mary Black School of Nursing
Spartanburg, South Carolina

Programs • Generic Baccalaureate • RN Baccalaureate

The University State-supported comprehensive coed institution. Part of University of South Carolina System. Founded: 1967. *Primary accreditation:* regional. *Setting:* 298-acre urban campus. *Total enrollment:* 3,420.

The Mary Black School of Nursing Founded in 1977. *Nursing program faculty:* 11 (55% with doctorates). *Off-campus program site:* Greenville.

Academic Facilities *Campus library:* 91,000 volumes (600 in health, 600 in nursing); 1,108 periodical subscriptions (107 health-care related). *Nursing school resources:* CAI, computer lab, nursing audiovisuals, interactive nursing skills videos, learning resource lab.

Student Life *Student services:* health clinic, child-care facilities, personal counseling, career counseling, institutionally sponsored work-study program, job placement, campus safety program, special assistance for disabled students. *International student services:* counseling/support, special assistance for nonnative speakers of English. *Nursing student activities:* Sigma Theta Tau, student nurses association.

Calendar Semesters.

NURSING STUDENT PROFILE

Undergraduate **Enrollment:** 108
Women: 94%; **Men:** 6%; **Minority:** 18%; **Part-time:** 24%

BACCALAUREATE PROGRAMS

Contact Dr. Jim Ferrell, Division Chair, Mary Black School of Nursing, University of South Carolina at Spartanburg, 800 University Way, Spartanburg, SC 29303, 864-503-5463. *Fax:* 864-503-5411.

Expenses *State resident tuition:* $2578 full-time, $113 per semester hour part-time. *Nonresident tuition:* $6446 full-time, $283 per semester hour part-time. *Full-time mandatory fees:* $25.

Financial Aid Institutionally sponsored need-based grants/scholarships, Federal Nursing Student Loans, Federal Pell Grants, Federal Supplemental Educational Opportunity Grants, Federal Work-Study. *Application deadline:* 7/1.

Generic Baccalaureate Program (BSN)

Applying *Required:* SAT I or ACT, TOEFL for nonnative speakers of English, minimum high school GPA of 2.0, minimum college GPA of 2.5, 3 years of high school math, 2 years of high school science, high school chemistry, high school biology, high school foreign language, high school transcript, transcript of college record, immunizations. 68 prerequisite credits must be completed before admission to the nursing program. *Options:* Advanced standing available through the following means: advanced placement exams, credit by exam. Course work may be accelerated. *Application deadline:* 3/1. *Application fee:* $25.

Degree Requirements 134 total credit hours, 69 in nursing.

RN Baccalaureate Program (BSN)

Applying *Required:* TOEFL for nonnative speakers of English, minimum college GPA of 2.5, RN license, diploma or AD in nursing, high school transcript, transcript of college record. *Options:* Course work may be accelerated. May apply for transfer of up to 104 total credits. *Application deadline:* 3/1. *Application fee:* $25.

Degree Requirements 134 total credit hours, 30 in nursing.

Distance learning Courses provided through closed circuit television.

SOUTH DAKOTA

AUGUSTANA COLLEGE
Department of Nursing
Sioux Falls, South Dakota

Programs • Generic Baccalaureate • RN Baccalaureate • Master's

The College Independent comprehensive coed institution, affiliated with Evangelical Lutheran Church in America. Founded: 1860. *Primary accreditation:* regional. *Setting:* 110-acre urban campus. *Total enrollment:* 1,778.

The Department of Nursing Founded in 1941. *Nursing program faculty:* 15 (60% with doctorates).

Academic Facilities *Campus library:* 228,000 volumes (4,875 in health, 711 in nursing); 922 periodical subscriptions (69 health-care related). *Nursing school resources:* CAI, computer lab, nursing audiovisuals, interactive nursing skills videos, learning resource lab.

Student Life *Student services:* health clinic, child-care facilities, personal counseling, career counseling, institutionally sponsored work-study program, job placement, campus safety program, special assistance for disabled students. *International student services:* counseling/support, special assistance for nonnative speakers of English. *Nursing student activities:* Sigma Theta Tau, student nurses association.

Calendar 4-1-4.

NURSING STUDENT PROFILE

Undergraduate **Enrollment:** 135
Women: 96%; **Men:** 4%; **Minority:** 1%; **International:** 2%; **Part-time:** 13%
Graduate **Enrollment:** 17
Women: 88%; **Men:** 12%; **Minority:** 0%; **International:** 0%; **Part-time:** 100%

BACCALAUREATE PROGRAMS

Contact Dr. Mary Brendtro, Chair, Department of Nursing, Augustana College, 2001 South Summit Avenue, Sioux Falls, SD 57197, 605-336-4721. *Fax:* 605-336-4723. *E-mail:* brendtro@inst.augie.edu

Expenses *Tuition:* $12,350 full-time, ranges from $200 to $366 per credit part-time. *Full-time mandatory fees:* $150. *Room and board:* $3701–$4532. *Room only:* $1788–$2512. *Books and supplies per academic year:* $500.

Financial Aid Institutionally sponsored need-based grants/scholarships, institutionally sponsored non-need grants/scholarships, Federal Nursing Student Loans, Federal Perkins Loans, Federal Supplemental Educational Opportunity Grants, Federal Work-Study, Federal Stafford loans. 95% of undergraduate students in nursing programs received some form of financial aid in 1995–96. *Application deadline:* 3/1.

Generic Baccalaureate Program (BA)

Applying *Required:* SAT I or ACT, TOEFL for nonnative speakers of English, minimum college GPA of 2.7, high school transcript, 2 letters of recommendation, written essay, transcript of college record, high school class rank: top 50%. 30 prerequisite credits must be completed before admission to the nursing program. *Options:* Advanced standing available through the following means: advanced placement exams, advanced placement without credit, credit by exam. May apply for transfer of up to 78 total credits. *Application deadline:* rolling. *Application fee:* $25.

Degree Requirements 130 total credit hours, 48 in nursing.

RN Baccalaureate Program (BA)

Applying *Required:* minimum college GPA of 2.7, RN license, diploma or AD in nursing, interview, 2 letters of recommendation, written essay, transcript of college record. 30 prerequisite credits must be completed before admission to the nursing program. *Options:* Advanced standing available through the following means: advanced placement exams, advanced placement without credit, credit by exam. May apply for transfer of up to 78 total credits. *Application deadline:* rolling. *Application fee:* $25.

Degree Requirements 130 total credit hours, 48 in nursing.

MASTER'S PROGRAMS

Contact Dr. Margot Nelson, Coordinator, Graduate Program, 2001 South Summit Avenue, Sioux Falls, SD 57197, 605-336-4729. *Fax:* 605-336-4723. *E-mail:* mnelson@inst.augie.edu

Areas of Study Clinical nurse specialist program in community health nursing.

Expenses *Tuition:* ranges from $2070 to $3870 per year. *Part-time mandatory fees:* $65–$185. *Books and supplies per academic year:* ranges from $270 to $1000.

Financial Aid Federal Direct Loans, employing institution support. 41% of master's level students in nursing programs received some form of financial aid in 1995-96. *Application deadline:* 5/1.

MOUNT MARTY COLLEGE

Nursing Program
Yankton, South Dakota

Programs • Generic Baccalaureate • RN Baccalaureate • LPN to Baccalaureate

The College Independent Roman Catholic comprehensive coed institution. Founded: 1936. *Primary accreditation:* regional. *Setting:* 80-acre small-town campus. *Total enrollment:* 915.

The Nursing Program Founded in 1962. *Nursing program faculty:* 10 (30% with doctorates).

Academic Facilities *Campus library:* 76,864 volumes; 420 periodical subscriptions. *Nursing school resources:* CAI, computer lab, nursing audiovisuals, interactive nursing skills videos, learning resource lab.

Student Life *Student services:* health clinic, child-care facilities, personal counseling, career counseling, institutionally sponsored work-study program, job placement, special assistance for disabled students. *International student services:* counseling/support, special assistance for nonnative speakers of English. *Nursing student activities:* nursing club, student nurses association.

Calendar Semesters.

NURSING STUDENT PROFILE

Undergraduate **Enrollment:** 83
Women: 87%; **Men:** 13%; **Minority:** 6%; **International:** 1%; **Part-time:** 0%

BACCALAUREATE PROGRAMS

Contact Admissions Department, Nursing Program, Mount Marty College, 1105 West 8th Street, Yankton, SD 57078-3724, 800-658-4552. *Fax:* 605-668-1357.

Expenses *Tuition:* $7998 per academic year. *Full-time mandatory fees:* $936. *Room and board:* $3733. *Books and supplies per academic year:* $200.

Financial Aid Institutionally sponsored need-based grants/scholarships, institutionally sponsored non-need grants/scholarships, Federal Nursing Student Loans, Federal Pell Grants, Federal Perkins Loans, Federal Supplemental Educational Opportunity Grants, Federal Work-Study, DHHS Scholarships for Disadvantaged Students. 86% of undergraduate students in nursing programs received some form of financial aid in 1995–96. *Application deadline:* 3/15.

Generic Baccalaureate Program (BS)

Applying *Required:* SAT I, ACT, TOEFL for nonnative speakers of English, minimum college GPA of 2.7, high school transcript, transcript of college record. 48 prerequisite credits must be completed before admission to the nursing program. *Options:* Advanced standing available through the following means: advanced placement exams, credit by exam. May apply for transfer of up to 96 total credits. *Application deadline:* 12/15.

Degree Requirements 128 total credit hours, 53 in nursing.

RN Baccalaureate Program (BS)

Applying *Required:* NLN Mobility Profile Exams, minimum college GPA of 2.7, RN license, diploma or AD in nursing, transcript of college record. 31 prerequisite credits must be completed before admission to the nursing program. *Options:* Advanced standing available through credit by exam. May apply for transfer of up to 96 total credits. *Application deadline:* 12/5.

Degree Requirements 128 total credit hours, 53 in nursing.

LPN to Baccalaureate Program (BS)

Applying *Required:* NLN Mobility Profile Exams, minimum college GPA of 2.7, transcript of college record, LPN license. *Options:* Advanced standing available through credit by exam. May apply for transfer of up to 96 total credits. *Application deadline:* 12/5.

Degree Requirements 128 total credit hours, 53 in nursing.

PRESENTATION COLLEGE

Department of Nursing
Aberdeen, South Dakota

Programs • Generic Baccalaureate • RN Baccalaureate

The College Independent Roman Catholic 4-year primarily women's college. Founded: 1951. *Primary accreditation:* regional. *Setting:* 100-acre small-town campus. *Total enrollment:* 369.

The Department of Nursing Founded in 1966. *Nursing program faculty:* 13.

Academic Facilities *Campus library:* 30,000 volumes (727 in health, 1,200 in nursing); 322 periodical subscriptions (108 health-care related). *Nursing school resources:* CAI, computer lab, nursing audiovisuals, learning resource lab, Internet.

Student Life *Student services:* personal counseling, career counseling, institutionally sponsored work-study program, job placement, campus safety program. *International student services:* counseling/support. *Nursing student activities:* nursing club, student nurses association, Nursing Honor Society.

Calendar Semesters.

NURSING STUDENT PROFILE

Undergraduate **Enrollment:** 91
Women: 94%; **Men:** 6%; **Minority:** 35%; **International:** 2%; **Part-time:** 18%

BACCALAUREATE PROGRAMS

Contact Mr. Thomas E. Stenvig, Chair, Department of Nursing, Presentation College, 1500 North Main Street, Aberdeen, SD 57401, 605-229-8472. *Fax:* 605-229-8489. *E-mail:* tstenvig@mail.pbvm.edu

Expenses *Tuition:* $6820 full-time, $215 per credit part-time. *Full-time mandatory fees:* $425–$850. *Part-time mandatory fees:* $425–$850. *Room and board:* $3046. *Books and supplies per academic year:* ranges from $500 to $1000.

Financial Aid Institutionally sponsored need-based grants/scholarships, institutionally sponsored non-need grants/scholarships, Federal Pell Grants, Federal Perkins Loans, Federal Work-Study, Indian Health Service Scholarships. 79% of undergraduate students in nursing programs received some form of financial aid in 1995–96. *Application deadline:* 4/1.

Generic Baccalaureate Program (BS)

Applying *Required:* SAT I, ACT, TOEFL for nonnative speakers of English, minimum high school GPA of 2.0, minimum college GPA of 2.0, high school chemistry, high school biology, high school transcript, transcript of college record. *Options:* May apply for transfer of up to 60 total credits. *Application deadline:* rolling. *Application fee:* $15.

Degree Requirements 122 total credit hours, 54 in nursing.

Presentation College (continued)

RN Baccalaureate Program (BS)

Applying *Required:* minimum college GPA of 2.0, diploma or AD in nursing, transcript of college record, RN license or pending passage of NCLEX. 60 prerequisite credits must be completed before admission to the nursing program. *Options:* Advanced standing available through advanced placement exams. May apply for transfer of up to 90 total credits. *Application deadline:* rolling. *Application fee:* $15.

Degree Requirements 130 total credit hours, 65 in nursing.

SOUTH DAKOTA STATE UNIVERSITY

College of Nursing
Brookings, South Dakota

Programs • Generic Baccalaureate • RN Baccalaureate • MS • Continuing Education

The University State-supported coed university. Founded: 1881. *Primary accreditation:* regional. *Setting:* 260-acre rural campus. *Total enrollment:* 8,840.

The College of Nursing Founded in 1935. *Nursing program faculty:* 80 (15% with doctorates). *Off-campus program sites:* Sioux Falls, Rapid City, Aberdeen.

Academic Facilities *Campus library:* 474,903 volumes (4,256 in health, 23,204 in nursing); 3,052 periodical subscriptions (202 health-care related). *Nursing school resources:* CAI, computer lab, nursing audiovisuals, learning resource lab.

Student Life *Student services:* health clinic, child-care facilities, personal counseling, career counseling, institutionally sponsored work-study program, job placement, campus safety program, special assistance for disabled students. *International student services:* counseling/support, special assistance for nonnative speakers of English, ESL courses. *Nursing student activities:* Sigma Theta Tau, recruiter club, student nurses association.

Calendar Semesters.

NURSING STUDENT PROFILE

Undergraduate **Enrollment:** 523
Women: 88%; **Men:** 12%; **Minority:** 24%; **International:** 1%; **Part-time:** 36%

Graduate **Enrollment:** 144
Women: 98%; **Men:** 2%; **Minority:** 2%; **International:** 0%; **Part-time:** 26%

BACCALAUREATE PROGRAMS

Contact Rosemary Chappell, Coordinator, Nursing Student Services, Nursing-Family/Consumer Science-Arts/Science Building, College of Nursing, South Dakota State University, Box 2275, Brookings, SD 57007-0098, 605-688-4106. *Fax:* 605-688-6119. *E-mail:* chappelr@ur.sdstate.edu

Expenses *State resident tuition:* $1696 full-time, $53 per credit hour part-time. *Nonresident tuition:* ranges from $3168 to $5376 full-time, ranges from $99 to $168 per credit hour part-time. *Full-time mandatory fees:* $1715+. *Room and board:* $2459–$3423. *Room only:* $1354–$1814. *Books and supplies per academic year:* $580.

Financial Aid Institutionally sponsored need-based grants/scholarships, institutionally sponsored non-need grants/scholarships, Federal Nursing Student Loans, Federal Perkins Loans, Federal Supplemental Educational Opportunity Grants, Federal Work-Study, state incentive grants. 50% of undergraduate students in nursing programs received some form of financial aid in 1995–96. *Application deadline:* 9/1.

Generic Baccalaureate Program (BS)

Applying *Required:* ACT, TOEFL for nonnative speakers of English, minimum college GPA of 2.5, 2 years of high school math, 3 years of high school science, high school transcript, transcript of college record, high school class rank: top 50%, 3 letters of recommendation for nursing students transferring from another institution. 32 prerequisite credits must be completed before admission to the nursing program. *Options:* Advanced standing available through the following means: advanced placement exams, credit by exam. May apply for transfer of up to 32–112 total credits. *Application deadline:* rolling. *Application fee:* $15.

Degree Requirements 136 total credit hours, 56 in nursing.

RN Baccalaureate Program (BS)

Applying *Required:* minimum college GPA of 2.5, RN license, diploma or AD in nursing, high school transcript, transcript of college record. 20 prerequisite credits must be completed before admission to the nursing program. *Options:* Advanced standing available through the following means: advanced placement exams, credit by exam. May apply for transfer of up to 32–112 total credits. *Application deadline:* rolling. *Application fee:* $15.

Degree Requirements 136 total credit hours, 56 in nursing.

MASTER'S PROGRAM

Contact Dr. Barbara Heater, Head, Graduate Nursing, Nursing-Family/Consumer Science-Arts and Science Building, College of Nursing, South Dakota State University, Box 2275, Brookings, SD 57007-0098, 605-688-4114. *Fax:* 605-688-6073. *E-mail:* heaterb@ur.sdstate.edu

Areas of Study Clinical nurse specialist programs in gerontological nursing, medical-surgical nursing, parent-child nursing; nursing administration; nursing education; nurse practitioner program in family health.

Expenses *State resident tuition:* $1435 full-time, $80 per semester hour part-time. *Nonresident tuition:* $4234 full-time, $235 per semester hour part-time. *Full-time mandatory fees:* $324. *Room and board:* $2965. *Room only:* $1345. *Books and supplies per academic year:* $580.

Financial Aid Graduate assistantships, nurse traineeships, fellowships, Federal Nursing Student Loans, institutionally sponsored loans, employment opportunities, institutionally sponsored need-based grants/scholarships, institutionally sponsored non-need-based grants/scholarships, Federal Stafford Loans, Federal Perkins Loans, State Incentive Grants, Federal Work-Study. 17% of master's level students in nursing programs received some form of financial aid in 1995-96. *Application deadline:* 3/15.

MS Program

Applying *Required:* bachelor's degree in nursing, minimum GPA of 3.0, RN license, 1 year of clinical experience, physical assessment course, statistics course, professional liability/malpractice insurance, essay, interview, 3 letters of recommendation, transcript of college record. *Application deadlines:* 1/15 (fall), 7/1 (spring). *Application fee:* $15.

Degree Requirements 40–54 total credit hours dependent upon track, 32–46 in nursing, 4 in pharmacotherapeutics. Thesis or project.

CONTINUING EDUCATION PROGRAM

Contact Ms. Alice Gehrke, Coordinator, Continuing Nursing Education, Nursing-Family/Consumer Science-Arts/Science Building, College of Nursing, South Dakota State University, Brookings, SD 57007-0098, 605-688-5745. *Fax:* 605-688-6119. *E-mail:* gehrkea@ur.sdstate.edu

TENNESSEE

AUSTIN PEAY STATE UNIVERSITY

School of Nursing
Clarksville, Tennessee

Programs • Generic Baccalaureate • Accelerated RN Baccalaureate

The University State-supported comprehensive coed institution. Part of State University and Community College System of Tennessee. Founded: 1927. *Primary accreditation:* regional. *Setting:* 200-acre suburban campus. *Total enrollment:* 7,556.

The School of Nursing Founded in 1972. *Nursing program faculty:* 19 (26% with doctorates).

▶ ***NOTEWORTHY***

This is a highly competitive nursing program in an expanding University and a growing community. Outstanding faculty members, including 40% who are certified advanced practice nurses and 26% who are doctorally prepared, each teach theory and clinical practice. The Lenora C. Reuther Chair of Excellence holder is a nationally recognized scholar. Students enjoy a reputation of excellence with employing agencies nationwide. Nontraditional students include international students, AMEDD students, and retired and former members of the military. Students' clinicals in a variety of community settings, including Nashville, prepare them to practice in any kind of health-care facility as beginning and future-oriented professional practitioners of nursing.

Academic Facilities *Nursing school resources:* computer lab, nursing audiovisuals, interactive nursing skills videos.

Student Life *Student services:* health clinic, child-care facilities, personal counseling, career counseling, institutionally sponsored work-study program, job placement, campus safety program, special assistance for disabled students, nontraditional student program. *International student services:* counseling/support, special assistance for nonnative speakers of English, ESL courses. *Nursing student activities:* Sigma Theta Tau, student nurses association.

Calendar Semesters.

NURSING STUDENT PROFILE

Undergraduate **Enrollment:** 157

Women: 75%; **Men:** 25%; **Minority:** 13%; **International:** 2%; **Part-time:** 0%

BACCALAUREATE PROGRAMS

Contact Dr. Wynella B. Badgett, Professor and Dean, School of Nursing, Austin Peay State University, PO Box 4658, Clarksville, TN 37044, 615-648-7710. *Fax:* 615-648-5998. *E-mail:* badgettw@apsu02.apsu.edu

Expenses *State resident tuition:* $1922 per academic year. *Nonresident tuition:* $4130 per academic year. *Full-time mandatory fees:* $84.

Financial Aid Institutionally sponsored need-based grants/scholarships, institutionally sponsored non-need grants/scholarships, Federal Nursing Student Loans, Federal Perkins Loans, Federal Work-Study.

GENERIC BACCALAUREATE PROGRAM (BSN)

Applying *Required:* ACT, TOEFL for nonnative speakers of English, ACT COMP, minimum high school GPA of 2.75, minimum college GPA of 2.8, 3 years of high school math, 3 years of high school science, high school foreign language, high school transcript, written essay, transcript of college record. 60 prerequisite credits must be completed before admission to the nursing program. *Options:* May apply for transfer of up to 60 total credits. *Application deadline:* 2/1. *Application fee:* $5.

Degree Requirements 137 total credit hours, 67 in nursing.

ACCELERATED RN BACCALAUREATE PROGRAM (BSN)

Applying *Required:* TOEFL for nonnative speakers of English, assessment test in math and English for students 21 or older, ACT COMP, minimum high school GPA of 2.75, minimum college GPA of 2.8, 3 years of high school math, 3 years of high school science, RN license, diploma or AD in nursing, high school foreign language, high school transcript, transcript of college record. 60 prerequisite credits must be completed before admission to the nursing program. *Options:* May apply for transfer of up to 60 total credits. *Application deadline:* 2/1.

Degree Requirements 137 total credit hours, 67 in nursing.

BELMONT UNIVERSITY
School of Nursing
Nashville, Tennessee

Programs • Generic Baccalaureate • Accelerated RN Baccalaureate • Baccalaureate for Second Degree

The University Independent Baptist comprehensive coed institution. Founded: 1951. *Primary accreditation:* regional. *Setting:* 34-acre urban campus. *Total enrollment:* 3,009.

The School of Nursing *Nursing program faculty:* 9 (44% with doctorates).

Academic Facilities *Campus library:* 157,000 volumes; 850 periodical subscriptions (100 health-care related).

Calendar Semesters.

BACCALAUREATE PROGRAMS

Contact Admission, Progression, Graduation Committee, School of Nursing, Belmont University, 1900 Belmont Boulevard, Nashville, TN 37212, 615-385-6436. *Fax:* 615-386-4563.

GENERIC BACCALAUREATE PROGRAM (BSN)

Applying *Required:* SAT I or ACT, TOEFL for nonnative speakers of English, minimum college GPA of 2.5, high school science, 4 years high school English. *Options:* Advanced standing available through the following means: advanced placement exams, credit by exam. *Application fee:* $25.

Degree Requirements 128 total credit hours, 63 in nursing.

ACCELERATED RN BACCALAUREATE PROGRAM (BSN)

Applying *Required:* SAT I or ACT, TOEFL for nonnative speakers of English, minimum high school GPA of 2.0, RN license, transcript of college record. *Options:* Advanced standing available through the following means: advanced placement exams, credit by exam. *Application deadline:* rolling. *Application fee:* $25.

Degree Requirements 128 total credit hours, 63 in nursing.

BACCALAUREATE FOR SECOND DEGREE PROGRAM (BSN)

Applying *Required:* SAT I or ACT, TOEFL for nonnative speakers of English, minimum high school GPA of 2.0, transcript of college record. 30 prerequisite credits must be completed before admission to the nursing program. *Options:* Advanced standing available through the following means: advanced placement exams, credit by exam. *Application deadline:* rolling. *Application fee:* $25.

Degree Requirements 128 total credit hours, 63 in nursing.

CARSON-NEWMAN COLLEGE
Division of Nursing
Jefferson City, Tennessee

Programs • Generic Baccalaureate • RN Baccalaureate

The College Independent Southern Baptist comprehensive coed institution. Founded: 1851. *Primary accreditation:* regional. *Setting:* 100-acre small-town campus. *Total enrollment:* 2,207.

The Division of Nursing Founded in 1982. *Nursing program faculty:* 10 (33% with doctorates).

Academic Facilities *Campus library:* 189,895 volumes (1,425 in health, 1,575 in nursing); 1,385 periodical subscriptions (67 health-care related). *Nursing school resources:* CAI, computer lab, interactive nursing skills videos, learning resource lab.

Student Life *Student services:* health clinic, child-care facilities, personal counseling, career counseling, institutionally sponsored work-study program, campus safety program, special assistance for disabled students, tutoring. *International student services:* counseling/support, ESL courses. *Nursing student activities:* student nurses association.

Calendar Semesters.

NURSING STUDENT PROFILE

Undergraduate **Enrollment:** 165

Women: 93%; **Men:** 7%; **Minority:** 2%; **International:** 1%; **Part-time:** 14%

BACCALAUREATE PROGRAMS

Contact Dr. Ann Harley, Dean, CNC Box 71883, Division of Nursing, Carson-Newman College, Jefferson City, TN 37760, 423-471-3425. *Fax:* 423-471-4574.

Expenses *Tuition:* $9480 full-time, $370 per hour part-time. *Full-time mandatory fees:* $500. *Part-time mandatory fees:* $276. *Room and board:* $2160. *Room only:* $1400. *Books and supplies per academic year:* ranges from $400 to $600.

Financial Aid Institutionally sponsored need-based grants/scholarships, institutionally sponsored non-need grants/scholarships, Federal Nursing Student Loans, Federal Work-Study. *Application deadline:* 4/1.

GENERIC BACCALAUREATE PROGRAM (BSN)

Applying *Required:* SAT I, ACT, TOEFL for nonnative speakers of English, minimum high school GPA of 2.0, minimum college GPA of 2.5, high school transcript, high school class rank: top 50%. 39 prerequisite credits must be completed before admission to the nursing program. *Application deadlines:* 9/1 (fall), 9/1 (spring). *Application fee:* $25.

Degree Requirements 129 total credit hours, 65 in nursing.

Carson-Newman College (continued)

RN Baccalaureate Program (BSN)

Applying *Required:* minimum college GPA of 2.5, RN license, diploma or AD in nursing, transcript of college record. 39 prerequisite credits must be completed before admission to the nursing program. *Application deadlines:* 9/1 (fall), 9/1 (spring). *Application fee:* $25.

Degree Requirements 129 total credit hours, 65 in nursing.

EAST TENNESSEE STATE UNIVERSITY

College of Nursing
Johnson City, Tennessee

Programs • Generic Baccalaureate • Accelerated RN Baccalaureate • LPN to Baccalaureate • MSN • Post-Master's

The University State-supported coed university. Part of State University and Community College System of Tennessee. Founded: 1911. *Primary accreditation:* regional. *Setting:* 366-acre small-town campus. *Total enrollment:* 11,718.

The College of Nursing Founded in 1954. *Nursing program faculty:* 51 (37% with doctorates). *Off-campus program sites:* Mountain City, Rogersville.

Academic Facilities *Nursing school resources:* CAI, computer lab, nursing audiovisuals, learning resource lab, nursing resource center.

Student Life *Student services:* health clinic, child-care facilities, personal counseling, career counseling, institutionally sponsored work-study program, job placement, campus safety program, special assistance for disabled students. *International student services:* counseling/support, special assistance for nonnative speakers of English, ESL courses. *Nursing student activities:* Sigma Theta Tau, student nurses association, Student Advisory Council.

Calendar Semesters.

NURSING STUDENT PROFILE

Undergraduate **Enrollment:** 280
Women: 87%; **Men:** 13%; **Minority:** 3%; **International:** 0%; **Part-time:** 17%

Graduate **Enrollment:** 56
Women: 93%; **Men:** 7%; **Minority:** 0%, **International:** 0%; **Part-time:** 46%

BACCALAUREATE PROGRAMS

Contact Ms. Gloria R. Gammell, Director, Career Counseling and Advisement, Office of Student Services, College of Nursing, East Tennessee State University, PO Box 70617, Johnson City, TN 37614-0617, 423-439-5880. *Fax:* 423-439-7477. *E-mail:* etsucon@nursserv.east-tenn-st.edu

Expenses *State resident tuition:* $1730 full-time, $77 per semester hour part-time. *Nonresident tuition:* $5860 full-time, $258 per semester hour part-time. *Full-time mandatory fees:* $20–$500. *Room only:* $690–$820. *Books and supplies per academic year:* ranges from $200 to $300.

Financial Aid Institutionally sponsored non-need grants/scholarships, Federal Perkins Loans, Federal Supplemental Educational Opportunity Grants, Federal Work-Study, scholarships for disadvantaged students, private scholarships and grants for nursing students. *Application deadline:* 7/1.

Generic Baccalaureate Program (BSN)

Applying *Required:* SAT I or ACT, TOEFL for nonnative speakers of English, minimum high school GPA of 2.3, minimum college GPA of 2.6, 3 years of high school math, 2 years of high school science, high school biology, high school foreign language, high school transcript, transcript of college record. 53 prerequisite credits must be completed before admission to the nursing program. *Options:* Advanced standing available through the following means: advanced placement exams, credit by exam. May apply for transfer of up to 61 total credits. *Application deadlines:* 2/1 (fall), 10/1 (spring). *Application fee:* $5.

Degree Requirements 137 total credit hours, 78 in nursing.

Accelerated RN Baccalaureate Program (BSN)

Applying *Required:* SAT I or ACT, TOEFL for nonnative speakers of English, minimum college GPA of 2.6, 3 years of high school math, 2 years of high school science, RN license, diploma or AD in nursing, high school foreign language, high school transcript, minimum 2.0 in each previous nursing course, Tennessee RN license. 60 prerequisite credits must be completed before admission to the nursing program. *Options:* Advanced standing available through the following means: advanced placement exams, advanced placement without credit, credit by exam. May apply for transfer of up to 83 total credits. *Application deadlines:* 2/1 (fall), 10/1 (spring). *Application fee:* $5.

Degree Requirements 137 total credit hours, 78 in nursing.

LPN to Baccalaureate Program (BSN)

Applying *Required:* SAT I or ACT, minimum high school GPA of 2.3, minimum college GPA of 2.6, 3 years of high school math, 2 years of high school science, high school foreign language, high school transcript, Tennessee LPN license, LPN transcript with a minimum GPA of 3.0. 53 prerequisite credits must be completed before admission to the nursing program. *Options:* Advanced standing available through advanced placement exams. May apply for transfer of up to 61 total credits. *Application deadlines:* 2/1 (fall), 10/1 (spring). *Application fee:* $5.

Degree Requirements 137 total credit hours, 78 in nursing.

MASTER'S PROGRAMS

Contact Dr. Patricia Smith, Associate Dean, Graduate Programs and Research, Office of Graduate Programs and Research, College of Nursing, East Tennessee State University, PO Box 70664, Johnson City, TN 37614-0664, 423-439-7472. *Fax:* 423-439-7477. *E-mail:* etsu@nursserv.east-tenn-st.edu

Areas of Study Nurse practitioner programs in adult health, family health.

Expenses *State resident tuition:* $2256 full-time, $113 per semester hour part-time. *Nonresident tuition:* $6386 full-time, $294 per semester hour part-time. *Full-time mandatory fees:* $50–$150. *Room only:* $700–$1000. *Books and supplies per academic year:* ranges from $600 to $800.

Financial Aid Graduate assistantships, nurse traineeships, Federal Nursing Student Loans, employment opportunities, National Health Service Corps Scholarships and Loans, privately funded scholarships. *Application deadline:* 7/1.

MSN Program

Applying *Required:* GRE General Test, TOEFL for nonnative speakers of English, bachelor's degree in nursing, minimum GPA of 3.0, RN license, physical assessment course, statistics course, professional liability/malpractice insurance, essay, 3 letters of recommendation, transcript of college record, research course. *Application deadline:* 1/15. *Application fee:* $5.

Degree Requirements 48 total credit hours, 48 in nursing.

Post-Master's Program

Applying *Required:* minimum GPA of 3.0, RN license, essay, 3 letters of recommendation, transcript of college record, master's degree in nursing. *Application deadline:* 1/15. *Application fee:* $5.

Degree Requirements 19 total credit hours, 19 in nursing.

MIDDLE TENNESSEE STATE UNIVERSITY

Department of Nursing
Murfreesboro, Tennessee

Programs • Generic Baccalaureate • RN Baccalaureate • Continuing Education

The University State-supported coed university. Part of State University and Community College System of Tennessee. Founded: 1911. *Primary accreditation:* regional. *Setting:* 500-acre urban campus. *Total enrollment:* 17,424.

The Department of Nursing Founded in 1987. *Nursing program faculty:* 21 (29% with doctorates).

Academic Facilities *Campus library:* 604,017 volumes (17,231 in health); 3,507 periodical subscriptions (82 health-care related). *Nursing school resources:* CAI, computer lab, nursing audiovisuals, interactive nursing skills videos, learning resource lab.

Student Life *Student services:* health clinic, child-care facilities, personal counseling, career counseling, institutionally sponsored work-study program, job placement, campus safety program, special assistance for

disabled students. *International student services:* counseling/support, special assistance for nonnative speakers of English, ESL courses. *Nursing student activities:* Sigma Theta Tau, nursing club, student nurses association.

Calendar Semesters.

NURSING STUDENT PROFILE

Undergraduate **Enrollment:** 827
Women: 89%; **Men:** 11%; **Minority:** 10%; **International:** 1%; **Part-time:** 5%

BACCALAUREATE PROGRAMS

Contact Dr. Judith H. Wakim, Chair and Professor, Department of Nursing, Middle Tennessee State University, Box 81, Murfreesboro, TN 37132, 615-898-2446. *Fax:* 615-898-5441. *E-mail:* jwakim@mtsu.edu

Expenses *State resident tuition:* $2022 full-time, $76 per semester hour part-time. *Nonresident tuition:* $6358 full-time, $266 per semester hour part-time. *Full-time mandatory fees:* $18–$20. *Room and board:* $2430. *Books and supplies per academic year:* ranges from $350 to $400.

Financial Aid Institutionally sponsored need-based grants/scholarships, institutionally sponsored non-need grants/scholarships, Federal Supplemental Educational Opportunity Grants, Federal Work-Study. *Application deadline:* 3/1.

Generic Baccalaureate Program (BSN)

Applying *Required:* ACT, score in 50th percentile or higher on American Psychological Association-Registered Nurse Entrance Exam, score in 90th percentile or higher on math computation test, minimum college GPA of 2.5, transcript of college record. 72 prerequisite credits must be completed before admission to the nursing program. *Options:* Advanced standing available through the following means: advanced placement exams, credit by exam. Course work may be accelerated. May apply for transfer of up to 109 total credits. *Application deadlines:* 2/1 (fall), 10/1 (spring). *Application fee:* $5.

Degree Requirements 142 total credit hours, 70 in nursing.

RN Baccalaureate Program (BSN)

Applying *Required:* ACT, minimum college GPA of 2.5, RN license, diploma or AD in nursing, transcript of college record. 64 prerequisite credits must be completed before admission to the nursing program. *Options:* Advanced standing available through the following means: advanced placement without credit, credit by exam. Course work may be accelerated. May apply for transfer of up to 94 total credits. *Application deadline:* rolling. *Application fee:* $5.

Degree Requirements 142 total credit hours, 48 in nursing.

CONTINUING EDUCATION PROGRAM

Contact Dr. Carmen Westwick, Chair of Excellence in Nursing, Department of Nursing, Middle Tennessee State University, Box 81, Murfreesboro, TN 37132, 615-898-5957.

SOUTHERN ADVENTIST UNIVERSITY
School of Nursing
Collegedale, Tennessee

Programs • RN Baccalaureate • Accelerated RN Baccalaureate

The University Independent Seventh-day Adventist 4-year coed college. Founded: 1892. *Primary accreditation:* regional. *Setting:* 1,000-acre small-town campus. *Total enrollment:* 1,591.

The School of Nursing Founded in 1957. *Nursing program faculty:* 22. *Off-campus program sites:* Orlando, Bradenton, Hudson.

Academic Facilities *Campus library:* 109 health-care related periodical subscriptions. *Nursing school resources:* CAI, computer lab, nursing audiovisuals, interactive nursing skills videos, learning resource lab.

Calendar Semesters.

NURSING STUDENT PROFILE

Undergraduate **Enrollment:** 369
Women: 78%; **Men:** 22%; **Minority:** 18%; **Part-time:** 57%

BACCALAUREATE PROGRAMS

Contact Ms. Linda Marlowe, Admissions and Progressions Coordinator, School of Nursing, Southern Adventist University, PO Box 370, Collegedale, TN 37315, 615-238-2941. *E-mail:* marlowe@southern.edu

Expenses *Tuition:* $9156 full-time, $389 part-time. *Full-time mandatory fees:* $403. *Part-time mandatory fees:* $13+. *Room and board:* $3782–$4000. *Room only:* $1620. *Books and supplies per academic year:* ranges from $548 to $650.

Financial Aid Federal Direct Loans, Federal Nursing Student Loans, Federal Pell Grants, Federal Perkins Loans, Federal Work-Study. 87% of undergraduate students in nursing programs received some form of financial aid in 1995–96. *Application deadline:* 3/15.

RN Baccalaureate Program (BS)

Applying *Required:* NLN Mobility Profile II, minimum high school GPA of 2.5, minimum college GPA of 2.5, RN license, diploma or AD in nursing, high school transcript, 3 letters of recommendation, transcript of college record, minimum 1 year work experience for every 5 years as RN. *Options:* May apply for transfer of up to 79 total credits. *Application deadline:* rolling. *Application fee:* $20.

Degree Requirements 124 total credit hours, 64 in nursing.

Accelerated RN Baccalaureate Program (BS)

Applying *Required:* NLN Mobility Profile II, minimum high school GPA of 2.5, minimum college GPA of 2.7, RN license, diploma or AD in nursing, high school transcript, 3 letters of recommendation, transcript of college record, minimum 1 year work experience for every 5 years as RN. *Options:* May apply for transfer of up to 72 total credits. *Application deadline:* rolling. *Application fee:* $20.

Degree Requirements 124 total credit hours, 64 in nursing.

TENNESSEE STATE UNIVERSITY
School of Nursing
Nashville, Tennessee

Programs • Generic Baccalaureate • Accelerated RN Baccalaureate • BSN to Master's

The University State-supported comprehensive coed institution. Part of State University and Community College System of Tennessee. Founded: 1912. *Primary accreditation:* regional. *Setting:* 450-acre urban campus. *Total enrollment:* 8,464.

The School of Nursing Founded in 1976. *Nursing program faculty:* 10 (50% with doctorates).

Academic Facilities *Campus library:* 355,000 volumes (50,000 in health, 25,000 in nursing); 1,300 periodical subscriptions (300 health-care related). *Nursing school resources:* CAI, computer lab, nursing audiovisuals, interactive nursing skills videos, learning resource lab.

Student Life *Student services:* health clinic, child-care facilities, personal counseling, career counseling, institutionally sponsored work-study program, job placement, campus safety program, special assistance for

Tennessee State University (continued)

disabled students. *International student services:* counseling/support, ESL courses. *Nursing student activities:* student nurses association, honor society.

Calendar Semesters.

NURSING STUDENT PROFILE

Undergraduate **Enrollment:** 150
Women: 60%; **Men:** 40%; **Minority:** 39%; **International:** 1%; **Part-time:** 10%
Graduate **Enrollment:** 30
Women: 97%; **Men:** 3%; **Minority:** 50%; **International:** 6%; **Part-time:** 80%

BACCALAUREATE PROGRAMS

Contact Dr. Barbara E. Brown, Director of BSN Program and Professor, School of Nursing, Tennessee State University, 3500 John A. Merritt Boulevard, PO Box 9590, Nashville, TN 37209-1561, 615-963-5273. *Fax:* 615-963-5049.

Expenses *State resident tuition:* $2000 full-time, $50 per hour part-time. *Nonresident tuition:* $6000 full-time, $200 per hour part-time. *Room and board:* $1360–$1560. *Room only:* $710–$910. *Books and supplies per academic year:* ranges from $300 to $450.

Financial Aid Institutionally sponsored need-based grants/scholarships, institutionally sponsored non-need grants/scholarships, Federal Nursing Student Loans, Federal Supplemental Educational Opportunity Grants, Federal Work-Study. 60% of undergraduate students in nursing programs received some form of financial aid in 1995–96. *Application deadline:* 3/1.

Generic Baccalaureate Program (BSN)

Applying *Required:* SAT I, ACT, minimum college GPA of 2.5, high school chemistry, transcript of college record. 58 prerequisite credits must be completed before admission to the nursing program. *Options:* May apply for transfer of up to 60 total credits. *Application deadlines:* 9/15 (spring), 2/15 (summer). *Application fee:* $5.

Degree Requirements 133 total credit hours, 53 in nursing.

Accelerated RN Baccalaureate Program (BSN)

Applying *Required:* minimum college GPA of 2.5, RN license, diploma or AD in nursing, transcript of college record. *Options:* May apply for transfer of up to 60 total credits. *Application deadline:* 2/15 (summer). *Application fee:* $5.

Degree Requirements 133 total credit hours, 53 in nursing.

MASTER'S PROGRAM

Contact Dr. Barbara E. Brown, MSN Program Director, School of Nursing, Tennessee State University, 3500 John A. Merritt Boulevard, Box 9590, Nashville, TN 37209-1561, 615-963-5261. *Fax:* 615-963-7614.

Areas of Study Nurse practitioner program in advanced family health.

Expenses *State resident tuition:* $2400 full-time, $50 per hour part-time. *Nonresident tuition:* $5600 full-time, $200 per hour part-time.

BSN to Master's Program (MSN)

Applying *Required:* GRE General Test or Miller Analogies Test, bachelor's degree in nursing, minimum GPA of 3.0, RN license, physical assessment course, statistics course, professional liability/malpractice insurance, essay, interview, 2 letters of recommendation, transcript of college record. *Application deadline:* 3/15. *Application fee:* $5.

Degree Requirements 38 total credit hours, 32 in nursing, 6 in elective. Thesis or project.

TENNESSEE TECHNOLOGICAL UNIVERSITY
School of Nursing
Cookeville, Tennessee

Programs • Generic Baccalaureate • RN Baccalaureate • Continuing Education

The University State-supported coed university. Part of State University and Community College System of Tennessee. Founded: 1915. *Primary accreditation:* regional. *Setting:* 235-acre small-town campus. *Total enrollment:* 8,166.

The School of Nursing Founded in 1980. *Nursing program faculty:* 11 (9% with doctorates).

Academic Facilities *Campus library:* 760,000 volumes; 3,000 periodical subscriptions. *Nursing school resources:* CAI, computer lab, nursing audiovisuals, interactive nursing skills videos, learning resource lab, CINAHL.

Student Life *Student services:* health clinic, child-care facilities, personal counseling, career counseling, institutionally sponsored work-study program, job placement, campus safety program, special assistance for disabled students. *International student services:* counseling/support, special assistance for nonnative speakers of English, ESL courses. *Nursing student activities:* Sigma Theta Tau, student nurses association.

Calendar Semesters.

NURSING STUDENT PROFILE

Undergraduate **Enrollment:** 124
Women: 92%; **Men:** 8%; **Minority:** 1%; **International:** 0%; **Part-time:** 24%

BACCALAUREATE PROGRAMS

Contact Ms. Susan Buchanan, Executive Aide, School of Nursing, Tennessee Technological University, Cookeville, TN 38505, 615-372-3203. *Fax:* 615-372-6244.

Expenses *State resident tuition:* $1840 full-time, $82 per hour part-time. *Nonresident tuition:* $6000 full-time, $181 per hour part-time. *Full-time mandatory fees:* $46. *Room and board:* $3360. *Room only:* $1600. *Books and supplies per academic year:* ranges from $450 to $500.

Financial Aid Institutionally sponsored need-based grants/scholarships, institutionally sponsored non-need grants/scholarships, Federal Work-Study. *Application deadline:* 5/1.

Generic Baccalaureate Program (BSN)

Applying *Required:* ACT, TOEFL for nonnative speakers of English, 3 years of high school math, 3 years of high school science, high school foreign language, high school transcript, transcript of college record, 1 unit of visual or performing arts. 66 prerequisite credits must be completed before admission to the nursing program. *Options:* May apply for transfer of up to 72 total credits. *Application deadline:* 2/1.

Degree Requirements 132 total credit hours, 60 in nursing.

RN Baccalaureate Program (BSN)

Applying *Required:* ACT, TOEFL for nonnative speakers of English, RN license, diploma or AD in nursing, transcript of college record. 39 prerequisite credits must be completed before admission to the nursing program. *Options:* May apply for transfer of up to 108 total credits. *Application deadlines:* 8/1 (fall), 12/15 (spring), 5/15 (summer).

Degree Requirements 132 total credit hours, 57 in nursing.

CONTINUING EDUCATION PROGRAM

Contact Ms. Gloria Russell, Continuing Education Coordinator and Associate Professor, School of Nursing, Tennessee Technological University, Cookeville, TN 38505, 615-372-3549. *Fax:* 615-372-6244.

UNION UNIVERSITY
School of Nursing
Jackson, Tennessee

Programs • Generic Baccalaureate • RN Baccalaureate • LPN to Baccalaureate

The University Independent Southern Baptist comprehensive coed institution. Founded: 1823. *Primary accreditation:* regional. *Setting:* 230-acre small-town campus. *Total enrollment:* 1,973.

The School of Nursing Founded in 1962. *Nursing program faculty:* 15 (13% with doctorates).

Academic Facilities *Campus library:* 91,250 volumes (4,050 in nursing); 1,080 periodical subscriptions (51 health-care related). *Nursing school resources:* CAI, computer lab, nursing audiovisuals, interactive nursing skills videos, learning resource lab.

Student Life *Student services:* health clinic, personal counseling, career counseling, job placement, campus safety program, special assistance for disabled students, wellness center. *International student services:* counseling/support. *Nursing student activities:* Sigma Theta Tau, student nurses association, Baptist Student Nurses Fellowship.

Calendar 4-1-4.

NURSING STUDENT PROFILE

Undergraduate **Enrollment:** 275
Women: 90%; **Men:** 10%; **Minority:** 13%; **International:** 1%; **Part-time:** 20%

BACCALAUREATE PROGRAMS

Contact Dr. Carla D. Sanderson, Dean, School of Nursing, Union University, 2447 Highway 45 Bypass, North, Jackson, TN 38305, 901-661-5200. *Fax:* 901-661-5175. *E-mail:* csanders@buster.uu.edu

Expenses *Tuition:* $6950 full-time, $290 per semester hour part-time. *Full-time mandatory fees:* $110–$300. *Room and board:* $2570. *Room only:* $1600. *Books and supplies per academic year:* ranges from $350 to $500.

Financial Aid Institutionally sponsored need-based grants/scholarships, institutionally sponsored non-need grants/scholarships, Federal Direct Loans, Federal Nursing Student Loans, Federal Perkins Loans, Federal Supplemental Educational Opportunity Grants, Federal Work-Study. 69% of undergraduate students in nursing programs received some form of financial aid in 1995–96. *Application deadline:* 5/15.

Generic Baccalaureate Program (BSN)

Applying *Required:* ACT, TOEFL for nonnative speakers of English, minimum college GPA of 2.5, high school transcript, interview, transcript of college record. 64 prerequisite credits must be completed before admission to the nursing program. *Options:* Advanced standing available through credit by exam. May apply for transfer of up to 102 total credits. *Application deadline:* rolling. *Application fee:* $25.

Degree Requirements 134 total credit hours, 67 in nursing.

RN Baccalaureate Program (BSN)

Applying *Required:* ACT, TOEFL for nonnative speakers of English, minimum college GPA of 2.0, RN license, diploma or AD in nursing, transcript of college record. 60 prerequisite credits must be completed before admission to the nursing program. *Options:* Advanced standing available through credit by exam. May apply for transfer of up to 102 total credits. *Application deadline:* rolling. *Application fee:* $25.

Degree Requirements 138 total credit hours, 30 in nursing.

LPN to Baccalaureate Program (BSN)

Applying *Required:* ACT, minimum college GPA of 2.0, transcript of college record. 60 prerequisite credits must be completed before admission to the nursing program. *Options:* Advanced standing available through credit by exam. May apply for transfer of up to 102 total credits. *Application deadline:* rolling. *Application fee:* $25.

Degree Requirements 138 total credit hours, 40 in nursing.

THE UNIVERSITY OF MEMPHIS
Loewenberg School of Nursing
Memphis, Tennessee

Programs • Generic Baccalaureate • RN Baccalaureate • Continuing Education

The University State-supported coed university. Part of State University and Community College System of Tennessee. Founded: 1912. *Primary accreditation:* regional. *Setting:* 1,100-acre urban campus. *Total enrollment:* 19,977.

The Loewenberg School of Nursing Founded in 1967. *Nursing program faculty:* 20 (50% with doctorates).

Academic Facilities *Campus library:* 1.0 million volumes; 9,300 periodical subscriptions. *Nursing school resources:* CAI, computer lab, nursing audiovisuals, interactive nursing skills videos, learning resource lab.

Student Life *Student services:* health clinic, child-care facilities, personal counseling, career counseling, institutionally sponsored work-study program, job placement, campus safety program, special assistance for disabled students. *International student services:* counseling/support, special assistance for nonnative speakers of English. *Nursing student activities:* Sigma Theta Tau, student nurses association.

Calendar Semesters.

NURSING STUDENT PROFILE

Undergraduate **Enrollment:** 260
Women: 81%; **Men:** 19%; **Minority:** 15%; **International:** 3%; **Part-time:** 39%

BACCALAUREATE PROGRAMS

Contact Ms. Sheila Hall, Assistant to the Dean, Loewenberg School of Nursing, University of Memphis, Memphis, TN 38152, 901-678-2003. *Fax:* 901-678-4906. *E-mail:* shall@cc.memphis.edu

Expenses *State resident tuition:* $2180 full-time, $96 per hour part-time. *Nonresident tuition:* $6516 full-time, $286 per hour part-time. *Full-time mandatory fees:* $215. *Part-time mandatory fees:* $65. *Room only:* $1480–$2730.

Financial Aid Institutionally sponsored need-based grants/scholarships, institutionally sponsored non-need grants/scholarships, Federal Nursing Student Loans, Federal Supplemental Educational Opportunity Grants, Federal Work-Study. *Application deadline:* 4/1.

Generic Baccalaureate Program (BSN)

Applying *Required:* SAT I, ACT, TOEFL for nonnative speakers of English, minimum college GPA of 2.5, minimum 2.4 GPA in prerequisite sciences. 38 prerequisite credits must be completed before admission to the nursing program. *Options:* Advanced standing available through credit by exam. Course work may be accelerated. May apply for transfer of up to 60 total credits. *Application deadlines:* 2/15 (fall), 10/1 (spring). *Application fee:* $5.

Degree Requirements 132 total credit hours, 63 in nursing.

RN Baccalaureate Program (BSN)

Applying *Required:* ACT, TOEFL for nonnative speakers of English, RN license, diploma or AD in nursing, recent or current clinical practice. 38 prerequisite credits must be completed before admission to the nursing program. *Options:* Course work may be accelerated. May apply for transfer of up to 60 total credits. *Application deadline:* rolling. *Application fee:* $5.

Degree Requirements 132 total credit hours, 31 in nursing.

CONTINUING EDUCATION PROGRAM

Contact Ms. Sheila Hall, Assistant to the Dean, Loewenberg School of Nursing, University of Memphis, Memphis, TN 38152, 901-678-2003. *Fax:* 901-678-4906.

UNIVERSITY OF TENNESSEE AT CHATTANOOGA
School of Nursing
Chattanooga, Tennessee

Programs • Generic Baccalaureate • RN Baccalaureate • Accelerated MSN • Continuing Education

The University State-supported comprehensive coed institution. Part of University of Tennessee System. Founded: 1886. *Primary accreditation:* regional. *Setting:* 101-acre urban campus. *Total enrollment:* 8,331.

The School of Nursing Founded in 1973. *Nursing program faculty:* 16 (40% with doctorates).

Academic Facilities *Nursing school resources:* CAI, computer lab, nursing audiovisuals, interactive nursing skills videos, learning resource lab, interactive teleconference facilities.

Student Life *Student services:* health clinic, child-care facilities, personal counseling, career counseling, institutionally sponsored work-study program, job placement, campus safety program, special assistance for disabled students. *International student services:* counseling/support. *Nursing student activities:* Sigma Theta Tau, nursing club, student nurses association.

Calendar Semesters.

NURSING STUDENT PROFILE

Undergraduate **Enrollment:** 190
Women: 85%; **Men:** 15%; **Minority:** 12%
Graduate **Enrollment:** 60
Women: 70%; **Men:** 30%; **Minority:** 15%; **Part-time:** 30%

BACCALAUREATE PROGRAMS

Contact Ms. Martha Butterfield, Undergraduate Coordinator, School of Nursing, University of Tennessee at Chattanooga, Chattanooga, TN 37403-2598, 423-755-4652. *E-mail:* martha-butterfield@utc.edu

Expenses *State resident tuition:* $1790 full-time, $68 per hour part-time. *Nonresident tuition:* $4336 full-time, $145 per hour part-time. *Full-time mandatory fees:* $274+. *Part-time mandatory fees:* $48+. *Room only:* $1500–$2350.

Financial Aid Institutionally sponsored need-based grants/scholarships, institutionally sponsored non-need grants/scholarships, Federal Direct Loans, Federal Nursing Student Loans, Federal Pell Grants, Federal Perkins Loans, Federal Supplemental Educational Opportunity Grants, Federal Work-Study. *Application deadline:* 2/1.

Generic Baccalaureate Program (BSN)

Applying *Required:* SAT I, ACT, minimum high school GPA of 2.0, minimum college GPA of 2.5, 3 years of high school math, 2 years of high school science, high school foreign language, high school transcript, interview, 2 letters of recommendation, transcript of college record. 45 prerequisite credits must be completed before admission to the nursing program. *Options:* Advanced standing available through the following means: advanced placement exams, credit by exam. Course work may be accelerated. *Application deadline:* rolling. *Application fee:* $25.

Degree Requirements 128 total credit hours.

RN Baccalaureate Program (BSN)

Applying *Required:* ACT PEP, minimum college GPA of 2.0, RN license, diploma or AD in nursing, high school transcript, transcript of college record, health exam, immunizations. *Options:* Advanced standing available through the following means: advanced placement exams, credit by exam. Course work may be accelerated. *Application deadline:* rolling. *Application fee:* $25.

Degree Requirements 128 total credit hours.

MASTER'S PROGRAM

Contact Dr. Maria Smith, Coordinator, Graduate Program, School of Nursing, University of Tennessee at Chattanooga, 615 McCallie Avenue, Chattanooga, TN 37403, 423-755-4646. *Fax:* 423-755-4668. *E-mail:* maria-smith@utc.edu

Areas of Study Clinical nurse specialist program in adult health nursing; nurse anesthesia; nursing administration; nursing education; nurse practitioner program in family health.

Expenses *State resident tuition:* $1026 full-time, $114 per hour part-time. *Nonresident tuition:* $1629 full-time, $181 per hour part-time. *Full-time mandatory fees:* $60+. *Part-time mandatory fees:* $48+.

Financial Aid Graduate assistantships, nurse traineeships, fellowships, Federal Direct Loans, Federal Nursing Student Loans.

Accelerated MSN Program

Applying *Required:* GRE General Test, bachelor's degree in nursing, minimum GPA of 3.0, RN license, 1 year of clinical experience, physical assessment course, statistics course, professional liability/malpractice insurance, essay, interview, 3 letters of recommendation, transcript of college record. *Application deadlines:* 4/1 (fall), 11/1 (anesthesia track). *Application fee:* $25.

Degree Requirements 40–52 total credit hours dependent upon track.

CONTINUING EDUCATION PROGRAM

Contact Dr. Pamela Holder, Director, School of Nursing, University of Tennessee at Chattanooga, 615 McCallie Avenue, Chattanooga, TN 37403-2598, 423-755-4750. *Fax:* 423-755-4668. *E-mail:* pam-holder@utc.edu

THE UNIVERSITY OF TENNESSEE AT MARTIN
Department of Nursing
Martin, Tennessee

Programs • Generic Baccalaureate • RN Baccalaureate

The University State-supported comprehensive coed institution. Part of University of Tennessee System. Founded: 1927. *Primary accreditation:* regional. *Setting:* 250-acre small-town campus. *Total enrollment:* 5,812.

The Department of Nursing Founded in 1989. *Nursing program faculty:* 18 (17% with doctorates). *Off-campus program site:* Jackson.

Academic Facilities *Campus library:* 250,000 volumes (9,500 in health, 1,350 in nursing); 1,500 periodical subscriptions (70 health-care related). *Nursing school resources:* CAI, computer lab, nursing audiovisuals, interactive nursing skills videos, learning resource lab.

Student Life *Student services:* health clinic, child-care facilities, personal counseling, career counseling, institutionally sponsored work-study program, job placement, campus safety program, special assistance for disabled students. *International student services:* counseling/support, special assistance for nonnative speakers of English, ESL courses. *Nursing student activities:* student nurses association, Nursing Honor Society.

Calendar Semesters.

NURSING STUDENT PROFILE

Undergraduate **Enrollment:** 138
Women: 97%; **Men:** 3%; **Minority:** 9%; **International:** 0%; **Part-time:** 28%

BACCALAUREATE PROGRAMS

Contact Dr. Victoria Seng, Chair and Associate Professor, Department of Nursing, University of Tennessee at Martin, Martin, TN 38238, 901-587-7131. *Fax:* 901-587-7841. *E-mail:* vseng@utm.edu

Expenses *State resident tuition:* $2014 full-time, $86 per semester hour part-time. *Nonresident tuition:* $6350 full-time, $267 per semester hour part-time. *Full-time mandatory fees:* $150–$250. *Part-time mandatory fees:* $150–$250. *Room only:* $1530. *Books and supplies per academic year:* ranges from $250 to $500.

Financial Aid Institutionally sponsored need-based grants/scholarships, institutionally sponsored non-need grants/scholarships, Federal Direct Loans, Federal Perkins Loans, Federal Work-Study. *Application deadline:* 3/1.

Generic Baccalaureate Program (BSN)

Applying *Required:* ACT, TOEFL for nonnative speakers of English, minimum high school GPA of 2.6, 3 years of high school math, 2 years of high school science, high school foreign language, high school transcript, transcript of college record, CPR certification, first aid certification, immunizations. 34 prerequisite credits must be completed before admission to the nursing program. *Options:* May apply for transfer of up to 105 total credits. *Application deadline:* 8/25. *Application fee:* $15.

Degree Requirements 136 total credit hours, 73 in nursing.

RN Baccalaureate Program (BSN)

Applying *Required:* minimum college GPA of 2.0, 3 years of high school math, 3 years of high school science, RN license, diploma or AD in nursing, high school foreign language, high school transcript, transcript of college record, CPR certification, first aid certification, immunizations. *Options:* Advanced standing available through the following means: advanced placement exams, credit by exam. May apply for transfer of up to 104 total credits. *Application deadline:* 8/25. *Application fee:* $15.

Degree Requirements 134 total credit hours, 58 in nursing.

Distance learning Courses provided through video.

UNIVERSITY OF TENNESSEE, KNOXVILLE

College of Nursing Knoxville, Tennessee

Programs • Generic Baccalaureate • Accelerated RN Baccalaureate • BSN to Master's • Master's for Non-Nursing College Graduates • PhD • Continuing Education

The University State-supported coed university. Part of University of Tennessee System. Founded: 1794. *Primary accreditation:* regional. *Setting:* 526-acre urban campus. *Total enrollment:* 25,704.

The College of Nursing Founded in 1971. *Nursing program faculty:* 41 (51% with doctorates).

Academic Facilities *Campus library:* 2.0 million volumes (40,818 in health, 3,412 in nursing); 6,168 periodical subscriptions (480 health-care related). *Nursing school resources:* computer lab, nursing audiovisuals, learning resource lab.

Student Life *Student services:* health clinic, personal counseling, campus safety program. *International student services:* counseling/support, referral to ESL courses sponsored by city. *Nursing student activities:* Sigma Theta Tau, student nurses association.

Calendar Semesters.

NURSING STUDENT PROFILE

Undergraduate **Enrollment:** 230

Women: 91%; **Men:** 9%; **Minority:** 7%; **International:** 2%; **Part-time:** 15%

Graduate **Enrollment:** 121

Women: 86%; **Men:** 14%; **Minority:** 4%; **International:** 4%; **Part-time:** 35%

BACCALAUREATE PROGRAMS

Contact Student Services Office, College of Nursing, University of Tennessee, Knoxville, 1200 Volunteer Boulevard, Knoxville, TN 37996-4180, 423-974-7606. *Fax:* 423-974-3569.

Expenses *State resident tuition:* $2060 full-time, $90 per credit hour part-time. *Nonresident tuition:* $6276 full-time, $264 per credit hour part-time. *Full-time mandatory fees:* $156. *Part-time mandatory fees:* $25+. *Room and board:* $3460–$4250. *Room only:* $1710–$2270.

Financial Aid Institutionally sponsored need-based grants/scholarships, institutionally sponsored non-need grants/scholarships, Federal Pell Grants, Federal Perkins Loans, Federal Supplemental Educational Opportunity Grants.

Generic Baccalaureate Program (BSN)

Applying *Required:* SAT I, ACT, TOEFL for nonnative speakers of English, minimum college GPA of 2.0, 3 years of high school math, 3 years of high school science, high school chemistry, high school biology, high school foreign language, transcript of college record, GED certificate or high school transcript. *Application deadline:* 1/15.

Degree Requirements 123 total credit hours, 59 in nursing. 60 of the 123 credits must be taken at a 4-year institution.

Accelerated RN Baccalaureate Program (BSN)

Applying *Required:* SAT I, ACT, TOEFL for nonnative speakers of English, minimum college GPA of 2.0, 3 years of high school math, 3 years of high school science, high school chemistry, high school biology, RN license, diploma or AD in nursing, high school foreign language, transcript of college record, GED certificate or high school transcript. *Options:* Advanced standing available through the following means: advanced placement exams, credit by exam. Course work may be accelerated. May apply for transfer of up to 64 total credits. *Application deadlines:* 3/1 (fall), 10/1 (spring), 4/1 (summer). *Application fee:* $25.

Degree Requirements 123 total credit hours, 59 in nursing. 60 of the 123 credits must be taken at a 4-year institution.

MASTER'S PROGRAMS

Contact Student Services Office, College of Nursing, University of Tennessee, Knoxville, 1200 Volunteer Boulevard, Knoxville, TN 37996-4180, 423-974-7606.

Areas of Study Clinical nurse specialist programs in adult health nursing, maternity-newborn nursing, pediatric nursing, psychiatric–mental health nursing, women's health nursing; nursing administration; nurse practitioner programs in child care/pediatrics, family health, neonatal health, primary care, women's health.

Expenses *State resident tuition:* $2464 full-time, $142 per credit hour part-time. *Nonresident tuition:* $6800 full-time, $378 per credit hour part-time. *Full-time mandatory fees:* $156. *Part-time mandatory fees:* $9+. *Room and board:* $3460–$4250. *Room only:* $1710–$2270. *Books and supplies per academic year:* ranges from $500 to $600.

Financial Aid Nurse traineeships, fellowships, institutionally sponsored need-based grants/scholarships, institutionally sponsored non-need-based grants/scholarships.

BSN to Master's Program (MSN)

Applying *Required:* GRE (minimum combined score of 1000 on verbal and math sections), bachelor's degree in nursing, minimum GPA of 3.0, RN license, 1 year of clinical experience, physical assessment course, essay, 3 letters of recommendation, transcript of college record. *Application deadlines:* 2/1 (fall), 10/15 (spring). *Application fee:* $25.

Degree Requirements 36 total credit hours, 33 in nursing, 3 in statistics. Additional clinical hours may be required for nurse practitioner concentrations.

Master's for Non-Nursing College Graduates Program (MSN)

Applying *Required:* TOEFL for nonnative speakers of English, GRE (minimum combined score of 1000 on verbal and math sections), bachelor's degree, minimum GPA of 3.0, essay, 3 letters of recommendation, transcript of college record. *Application deadline:* 2/1. *Application fee:* $25.

Degree Requirements 77 total credit hours, 74 in nursing, 3 in statistics.

DOCTORAL PROGRAM

Contact Student Services Office, College of Nursing, University of Tennessee, Knoxville, 1200 Volunteer Boulevard, Knoxville, TN 37996-4180, 423-974-7606.

Areas of Study Nursing administration, nursing education, nursing research, individualized cognate areas.

Expenses *State resident tuition:* $2464 full-time, $142 per credit hour part-time. *Nonresident tuition:* $6800 full-time, $378 per credit hour part-time. *Full-time mandatory fees:* $156. *Part-time mandatory fees:* $9+. *Room and board:* $3460–$4250. *Room only:* $1710–$2270. *Books and supplies per academic year:* ranges from $500 to $600.

Financial Aid Institutionally sponsored non-need-based grants/scholarships.

PhD Program

Applying *Required:* TOEFL for nonnative speakers of English, GRE General Test (minimum combined score of 1000 on verbal and quantitative sections), master's degree in nursing, interview, 3 letters of recommendation, competitive review by faculty committee, minimum 3.3 GPA. *Application deadline:* 2/15. *Application fee:* $25.

Degree Requirements 72 total credit hours; dissertation; written exam; defense of dissertation.

CONTINUING EDUCATION PROGRAM

Contact Maureen Nalle, Director, Continuing Education, College of Nursing, University of Tennessee, Knoxville, 1200 Volunteer Boulevard, Knoxville, TN 37996-4180, 423-974-4151.

UNIVERSITY OF TENNESSEE, MEMPHIS

College of Nursing
Memphis, Tennessee

Programs • MSN • Post-Master's • PhD • Continuing Education

The University State-supported upper-level coed institution. Part of University of Tennessee System. Founded: 1911. *Primary accreditation:* regional. *Setting:* 55-acre urban campus. *Total enrollment:* 2,080.

The College of Nursing Founded in 1949. *Nursing program faculty:* 35 (71% with doctorates). *Off-campus program sites:* Jackson, Knoxville.

Academic Facilities *Campus library:* 175,000 volumes; 1,550 periodical subscriptions (1,550 health-care related). *Nursing school resources:* CAI, computer lab, nursing audiovisuals, interactive nursing skills videos, learning resource lab.

Student Life *Student services:* health clinic, personal counseling, institutionally sponsored work-study program, campus safety program, special assistance for disabled students. *International student services:* counseling/support, special assistance for nonnative speakers of English. *Nursing student activities:* Sigma Theta Tau, student nurses association.

Calendar Semesters.

NURSING STUDENT PROFILE

Graduate **Enrollment:** 132
Women: 88%; **Men:** 12%; **Minority:** 23%; **Part-time:** 48%

MASTER'S PROGRAMS

Contact Mrs. Muriel Rice, Assistant Dean, Student Affairs, College of Nursing, University of Tennessee, Memphis, 877 Madison Avenue, Room 602, Memphis, TN 38163, 901-448-6125. *Fax:* 901-448-4121.

Areas of Study Clinical nurse specialist programs in critical care nursing, public health nursing; nurse anesthesia; nursing administration; nurse practitioner programs in child care/pediatrics, family health, gerontology, neonatal health, psychiatric–mental health.

Expenses *State resident tuition:* $3486 full-time, $194 per hour part-time. *Nonresident tuition:* $9584 full-time, $532 per hour part-time. *Full-time mandatory fees:* $726–$826. *Room and board:* $6460–$7800. *Books and supplies per academic year:* ranges from $1800 to $2000.

Financial Aid Nurse traineeships, institutionally sponsored loans. *Application deadline:* 2/15.

MSN Program

Applying *Required:* bachelor's degree in nursing, minimum GPA of 2.75, RN license, physical assessment course, essay, interview, 3 letters of recommendation, transcript of college record. *Application deadline:* 1/15. *Application fee:* $50.

Degree Requirements 33–35 total credit hours dependent upon track, 33–35 in nursing. Thesis required.

Distance learning Courses provided through interactive television.

Post-Master's Program

Applying *Required:* minimum GPA of 2.75, RN license, physical assessment course, essay, interview, 3 letters of recommendation, transcript of college record. *Application deadline:* 1/15. *Application fee:* $50.

Degree Requirements 15–25 total credit hours dependent upon track, 15–25 in nursing.

Distance learning Courses provided through interactive television.

DOCTORAL PROGRAM

Contact Dr. Donna Hathaway, Director of Nursing Research, College of Nursing, University of Tennessee, Memphis, 877 Madison Avenue, Room 641B, Memphis, TN 38163, 901-448-6135. *Fax:* 901-448-4121.

Areas of Study Nursing research.

Expenses *State resident tuition:* $3486 full-time, $194 per credit hour part-time. *Nonresident tuition:* $9584 full-time, $532 per credit hour part-time. *Full-time mandatory fees:* $711.

Financial Aid Stipends. *Application deadline:* 1/15.

PhD Program

Applying *Required:* GRE General Test (minimum combined score of 1500 on three tests), interview, 3 letters of recommendation, vitae, writing sample, competitive review by faculty committee. *Application deadline:* 1/15. *Application fee:* $50.

Degree Requirements 41+ total credit hours dependent upon track; 24 hours dissertation research; dissertation; oral exam; written exam; defense of dissertation.

CONTINUING EDUCATION PROGRAM

Contact Ms. Mary Goode, Staff Assistant, College of Nursing, University of Tennessee, Memphis, 877 Madison Avenue, Room 620, Memphis, TN 38163, 901-448-6100. *Fax:* 901-448-4121.

VANDERBILT UNIVERSITY

School of Nursing
Nashville, Tennessee

Programs • RN to Master's • Master's for Nurses with Non-Nursing Degrees • Master's for Non-Nursing College Graduates • Accelerated Master's for Non-Nursing College Graduates • MSN/MBA • Post-Master's • PhD

The University Independent coed university. Founded: 1873. *Primary accreditation:* regional. *Setting:* 330-acre urban campus. *Total enrollment:* 10,074.

The School of Nursing Founded in 1909. *Nursing program faculty:* 60.

Academic Facilities *Campus library:* 2.4 million volumes (189,389 in health); 17,009 periodical subscriptions (2,105 health-care related). *Nursing school resources:* CAI, computer lab, nursing audiovisuals, interactive nursing skills videos, learning resource lab.

Student Life *Student services:* health clinic, child-care facilities, personal counseling, career counseling, campus safety program, special assistance for disabled students. *International student services:* counseling/support, ESL courses. *Nursing student activities:* Sigma Theta Tau, student nurses association.

Calendar Trimesters.

NURSING STUDENT PROFILE

Graduate **Enrollment:** 468
Women: 87%; **Men:** 13%; **Minority:** 8%; **International:** 1%; **Part-time:** 18%

MASTER'S PROGRAMS

Contact Karen Lawrimore, Admissions Coordinator, 101 Godchaux Hall, School of Nursing, Vanderbilt University, Nashville, TN 37240, 615-322-3800. *Fax:* 615-343-0333. *E-mail:* karen.lawrimore@mcmail.vanderbilt.edu

Areas of Study Clinical nurse specialist program in parent-child nursing; nurse midwifery; nursing administration; nurse practitioner programs in acute care, adult health, family health, gerontology, neonatal health, occupational health, primary care, psychiatric–mental health, women's health.

Expenses *Tuition:* $22,458 full-time, $624 per credit hour part-time. *Full-time mandatory fees:* $1076. *Room and board:* $515–$715. *Books and supplies per academic year:* ranges from $1000 to $1500.

Financial Aid Federal Nursing Student Loans, institutionally sponsored loans, institutionally sponsored need-based grants/scholarships, institutionally sponsored non-need-based grants/scholarships. 98% of master's level students in nursing programs received some form of financial aid in 1995-96. *Application deadline:* 5/1.

RN to Master's Program (MSN)

Applying *Required:* TOEFL for nonnative speakers of English, GRE General Test (minimum combined score of 1000 on quantitative and verbal sections) or Miller Analogies Test (minimum score of 50), minimum GPA of 3.0, RN license, statistics course, interview, 3 letters of recommendation, transcript of college record, 72 semester hours of college courses including anatomy, human growth and development, microbiology, nutrition, and physiology. *Application deadline:* rolling. *Application fee:* $50.

Degree Requirements 88–99 total credit hours dependent upon track, 88 in nursing.

Master's for Nurses with Non-Nursing Degrees Program (MSN)

Applying *Required:* TOEFL for nonnative speakers of English, GRE General Test (minimum combined score of 1000 on quantitative and verbal sections) or Miller Analogies Test (minimum score of 50), minimum GPA of 3.0, RN license, statistics course, interview, 3 letters of recommendation, transcript of college record, 72 semester hours of college courses including anatomy, human growth and development, microbiology, nutrition, and physiology. *Application deadline:* rolling. *Application fee:* $50.

Degree Requirements 88–99 total credit hours dependent upon track, 88 in nursing.

Master's for Non-Nursing College Graduates Program (MSN)

Applying *Required:* TOEFL for nonnative speakers of English, GRE General Test (minimum combined score of 1000 on quantitative and verbal sections) or Miller Analogies Test (minimum score of 50), bachelor's degree, minimum GPA of 3.0, statistics course, interview, 3 letters of recommendation, transcript of college record, 72 semester hours of college courses including anatomy, human growth and development, microbiology, nutrition, and physiology. *Application deadline:* rolling. *Application fee:* $50.

Degree Requirements 88–99 total credit hours dependent upon track, 88 in nursing.

Accelerated Master's for Non-Nursing College Graduates Program (MSN)

Applying *Required:* TOEFL for nonnative speakers of English, GRE General Test (minimum combined score of 1000 on quantitative and verbal sections) or Miller Analogies Test (minimum score of 50), minimum GPA of 3.0, statistics course, interview, 3 letters of recommendation, transcript of college record, 72 semester hours including human anatomy and physiology, microbiology, nutrition, human growth and development. *Application deadline:* rolling. *Application fee:* $50.

Degree Requirements 88–99 total credit hours dependent upon track, 88 in nursing.

MSN/MBA Program

Applying *Required:* TOEFL for nonnative speakers of English, GMAT, bachelor's degree in nursing, minimum GPA of 3.0, statistics course, interview, 3 letters of recommendation, transcript of college record, 72 semester hours including human anatomy and physiology, microbiology, and life span development. *Application deadline:* rolling. *Application fee:* $100.

Degree Requirements 70 total credit hours, 39 in nursing, 31 in financial management, marketing, economics, and accounting. 5 semesters of full-time enrollment including one full-time summer semester.

Post-Master's Program

Applying *Required:* TOEFL for nonnative speakers of English, GRE General Test (minimum combined score of 1000 on quantitative and verbal sections) or Miller Analogies Test (minimum score of 50), minimum GPA of 3.0, RN license, interview, 3 letters of recommendation, transcript of college record, MSN from NLN accredited school. *Application deadline:* rolling. *Application fee:* $50.

Degree Requirements 21–24 total credit hours dependent upon track, 21–24 in nursing.

DOCTORAL PROGRAM

Contact Dr. Gail Ingersoll, Associate Dean for Research and Director of the Graduate Program, Godchaux Hall, School of Nursing, Vanderbilt University, Nashville, TN 37240, 615-343-4173. *Fax:* 615-343-7711. *E-mail:* gail.ingersoll@mcmail.vanderbilt.edu

Areas of Study Nursing research.

Expenses *Tuition:* $14,940 full-time, $830 per credit hour part-time. *Full-time mandatory fees:* $919–$959. *Books and supplies per academic year:* $300.

Financial Aid Graduate assistantships, fellowships, dissertation grants, opportunities for employment. *Application deadline:* 1/15.

PhD Program

Applying *Required:* GRE General Test, TOEFL for nonnative speakers of English, master's degree in nursing, statistics course, interview, 3 letters of recommendation, competitive review by faculty committee. *Application deadline:* 1/15. *Application fee:* $40.

Degree Requirements 72 total credit hours; dissertation; oral exam; written exam; defense of dissertation.

See full description on page 564.

TEXAS

ABILENE CHRISTIAN UNIVERSITY

Abilene Intercollegiate School of Nursing
Abilene, Texas

Programs • Generic Baccalaureate • RN Baccalaureate • MSN

The University Independent comprehensive coed institution, affiliated with Church of Christ. Founded: 1906. *Primary accreditation:* regional. *Setting:* 208-acre urban campus. *Total enrollment:* 4,436.

The Abilene Intercollegiate School of Nursing Founded in 1979. *Nursing program faculty:* 15 (40% with doctorates).

Academic Facilities *Campus library:* 564,813 volumes; 2,157 periodical subscriptions.

Calendar Semesters.

BACCALAUREATE PROGRAMS

Contact Academic Adviser, Abilene Intercollegiate School of Nursing, Abilene Christian University, 2149 Hickory Street, Abilene, TX 79601, 915-672-2441.

Expenses *Tuition:* $9100 full-time, $260 per credit hour part-time.

Financial Aid Federal Pell Grants, Federal Perkins Loans, Federal Supplemental Educational Opportunity Grants, Federal Work-Study, Federal PLUS Loans, Federal Stafford Loans, state grants, College Access Loan. *Application deadline:* 3/1.

Generic Baccalaureate Program (BSN)

Applying *Required:* SAT I or ACT, minimum college GPA of 2.5, high school transcript, 2 letters of recommendation, immunizations, health exam, CPR certification. *Application deadline:* 2/15. *Application fee:* $25.

Degree Requirements 135 total credit hours, 62 in nursing.

RN Baccalaureate Program (BSN)

Applying *Required:* high school transcript, transcript of college record, immunizations, health exam, CPR certification. *Application deadline:* 2/15. *Application fee:* $25.

Degree Requirements 135 total credit hours, 62 in nursing.

MASTER'S PROGRAM

Areas of Study Nursing administration.

MSN Program

Applying *Required:* GRE General Test or Miller Analogies Test, TOEFL for nonnative speakers of English, bachelor's degree in nursing, 1 year of clinical experience, statistics course, 3 letters of recommendation, transcript of college record. *Application deadlines:* 3/1 (fall), 10/15 (spring), 3/1 (summer).

Degree Requirements 39–42 total credit hours dependent upon track, 27–30 in nursing, 12 in support courses. Thesis or professional paper.

ANGELO STATE UNIVERSITY
Department of Nursing
San Angelo, Texas

Programs • RN Baccalaureate • RN to Master's

The University State-supported comprehensive coed institution. Part of Texas State University System. Founded: 1928. *Primary accreditation:* regional. *Setting:* 268-acre urban campus. *Total enrollment:* 6,103.

The Department of Nursing Founded in 1968. *Nursing program faculty:* 24 (8% with doctorates).

Academic Facilities *Nursing school resources:* computer lab, nursing audiovisuals, interactive nursing skills videos, learning resource lab.

Student Life *Student services:* health clinic, personal counseling, career counseling, institutionally sponsored work-study program, job placement, campus safety program, special assistance for disabled students. *Nursing student activities:* Sigma Theta Tau, student nurses association.

Calendar Semesters.

NURSING STUDENT PROFILE

Undergraduate **Enrollment:** 308
Women: 92%; **Men:** 8%; **Minority:** 5%; **International:** 0%; **Part-time:** 53%
Graduate **Enrollment:** 25
Women: 100%

BACCALAUREATE PROGRAM

Contact Dr. Leslie Mayrand, Head, Department of Nursing, Angelo University, PO Box 10902, San Angelo, TX 76909, 915-942-2224. *Fax:* 915-962-2236.

Expenses *State resident tuition:* $768 full-time, $32 per credit hour part-time. *Nonresident tuition:* $4104 full-time, $171 per credit hour part-time. *Full-time mandatory fees:* $92–$675. *Room and board:* $3500–$4048. *Room only:* $2096+.

Financial Aid Institutionally sponsored need-based grants/scholarships, institutionally sponsored non-need grants/scholarships.

RN Baccalaureate Program (BSN)

Applying *Required:* SAT I or ACT, minimum college GPA of 2.5, RN license, diploma or AD in nursing. 60 prerequisite credits must be completed before admission to the nursing program. *Options:* May apply for transfer of up to 90 total credits. *Application deadlines:* 8/15 (fall), 11/15 (spring).

Degree Requirements 133 total credit hours, 34 in nursing.

MASTER'S PROGRAM

Contact Mildred Roberson, Graduate Adviser, MSN Program, Department of Nursing, Angelo University, PO Box 10902, San Angelo, TX 76909, 915-942-2224. *Fax:* 915-942-2236.

Areas of Study Clinical nurse specialist programs in medical-surgical nursing, parent-child nursing.

Expenses *State resident tuition:* $320 full-time, $32 per semester credit hour part-time. *Nonresident tuition:* $1710 full-time, $171 per semester credit hour part-time. *Full-time mandatory fees:* $92–$675.

RN to Master's Program (MSN)

Applying *Required:* GRE General Test, Miller Analogies Test, physical assessment course, statistics course. *Application deadline:* 2/1.

Degree Requirements 47 total credit hours, 29 in nursing, 18 in required core courses. Thesis required.

BAYLOR UNIVERSITY
School of Nursing
Dallas, Texas

Programs • Generic Baccalaureate • RN Baccalaureate • Baccalaureate for Second Degree • MSN

The University Independent Baptist coed university. Founded: 1845. *Primary accreditation:* regional. *Setting:* 432-acre urban campus. *Total enrollment:* 12,202.

The School of Nursing Founded in 1950. *Nursing program faculty:* 30 (52% with doctorates).

Academic Facilities *Campus library:* 6,000 volumes (1,000 in health, 5,000 in nursing); 106 periodical subscriptions (106 health-care related). *Nursing school resources:* CAI, computer lab, nursing audiovisuals, interactive nursing skills videos, learning resource lab, physical assessment lab.

Student Life *Student services:* health clinic, personal counseling, career counseling, institutionally sponsored work-study program, campus safety program. *Nursing student activities:* Sigma Theta Tau, nursing club, student nurses association.

Calendar Semesters.

NURSING STUDENT PROFILE

Undergraduate **Enrollment:** 250
Women: 93%; **Men:** 7%; **Minority:** 17%; **International:** 2%; **Part-time:** 0%
Graduate **Enrollment:** 30
Women: 100%; **Minority:** 7%; **International:** 7%; **Part-time:** 100%

BACCALAUREATE PROGRAMS

Contact Dr. Carole Hanks, Director, Pre-Nursing Program, School of Nursing, Baylor University, PO Box 97333, Waco, TX 76798, 817-755-1821. *Fax:* 214-820-4770. *E-mail:* carole_hanks@baylor.edu

Expenses *Tuition:* $8640 full-time, $288 per credit hour part-time. *Full-time mandatory fees:* $640–$1150. *Room only:* $1700. *Books and supplies per academic year:* ranges from $400 to $700.

Financial Aid Institutionally sponsored need-based grants/scholarships, institutionally sponsored non-need grants/scholarships, Federal Nursing Student Loans, Federal Work-Study. 60% of undergraduate students in nursing programs received some form of financial aid in 1995–96. *Application deadline:* 7/1.

Generic Baccalaureate Program (BSN)

Applying *Required:* SAT I, ACT, TOEFL for nonnative speakers of English, minimum college GPA of 2.7, 3 letters of recommendation, transcript of college record, completion of nursing prerequisite courses. 63 prerequisite credits must be completed before admission to the nursing program. *Options:* May apply for transfer of up to 68 total credits. *Application deadlines:* 1/15 (fall), 8/15 (spring).

Degree Requirements 128 total credit hours, 65 in nursing.

RN Baccalaureate Program (BSN)

Applying *Required:* TOEFL for nonnative speakers of English, NLN Mobility Profile II for advanced placement, minimum college GPA of 2.7, RN license, diploma or AD in nursing, 3 letters of recommendation, transcript of college record. 63 prerequisite credits must be completed before admission to the nursing program. *Options:* Advanced standing available through the following means: advanced placement exams, credit by exam. Course work may be accelerated. May apply for transfer of up to 68 total credits. *Application deadlines:* 1/15 (fall), 8/15 (spring).

Degree Requirements 128 total credit hours, 65 in nursing.

Baccalaureate for Second Degree Program (BSN)

Applying *Required:* TOEFL for nonnative speakers of English, minimum college GPA of 2.7, 3 letters of recommendation, transcript of college record. 63 prerequisite credits must be completed before admission to the nursing program. *Options:* May apply for transfer of up to 68 total credits. *Application deadlines:* 1/15 (fall), 8/15 (spring).

Degree Requirements 128 total credit hours, 65 in nursing.

MASTER'S PROGRAM

Contact Dr. Pauline Johnson, Director, Graduate Program, School of Nursing, Baylor University, 3700 Worth Street, Dallas, TX 75246, 214-820-3361. *Fax:* 214-820-4770. *E-mail:* pauline_johnson@baylor.edu

Expenses *Tuition:* $5040 full-time, $280 per credit hour part-time. *Full-time mandatory fees:* $23–$320. *Room only:* $1700. *Books and supplies per academic year:* $300.

Financial Aid Graduate assistantships, institutionally sponsored loans. 90% of master's level students in nursing programs received some form of financial aid in 1995-96. *Application deadline:* 7/1.

MSN Program

Applying *Required:* GRE General Test, TOEFL for nonnative speakers of English, bachelor's degree in nursing, minimum GPA of 2.7, RN license,

1 year of clinical experience, statistics course, 3 letters of recommendation, transcript of college record, minimum 3.0 college GPA in nursing. *Application deadline:* 7/1.

Degree Requirements 40 total credit hours, 34 in nursing. Thesis or project.

HARDIN-SIMMONS UNIVERSITY
Abilene Intercollegiate School of Nursing
Abilene, Texas

Programs • Generic Baccalaureate • RN Baccalaureate • BSN to Master's

The University Independent Baptist comprehensive coed institution. Founded: 1891. *Primary accreditation:* regional. *Setting:* 40-acre urban campus. *Total enrollment:* 2,374.

The Abilene Intercollegiate School of Nursing Founded in 1979.

Academic Facilities *Campus library:* 195,000 volumes; 1,000 periodical subscriptions.

Calendar Semesters.

BACCALAUREATE PROGRAMS

Contact Academic Adviser, Abilene Intercollegiate School of Nursing, Hardin-Simmons University, 2149 Hickory Street, Abilene, TX 79601, 915-672-2441.

Expenses *Tuition:* ranges from $4140 to $4230 full-time, ranges from $230 to $235 per credit hour part-time. *Full-time mandatory fees:* $240.

Financial Aid Institutionally sponsored need-based grants/scholarships, institutionally sponsored non-need grants/scholarships, Federal Direct Loans, Federal Perkins Loans, Federal Supplemental Educational Opportunity Grants, Federal Work-Study, state grants and loans.

Generic Baccalaureate Program (BSN)

Applying *Required:* SAT I or ACT, TOEFL for nonnative speakers of English, 3 years of high school math, 3 years of high school science, high school chemistry, high school biology, high school transcript, 2 letters of recommendation. *Application fee:* $25.

Degree Requirements 130 total credit hours, 62 in nursing.

RN Baccalaureate Program (BSN)

Applying *Required:* SAT I or ACT, minimum college GPA of 2.5, RN license, diploma or AD in nursing, high school transcript, 2 letters of recommendation, transcript of college record, immunizations, health exam. *Application fee:* $25.

Degree Requirements 130 total credit hours, 62 in nursing.

MASTER'S PROGRAM

Areas of Study Nurse practitioner program in family health.

Expenses *Tuition:* $4320 full-time, $240 per semester hour part-time. *Full-time mandatory fees:* $240.

Financial Aid Institutionally sponsored need-based grants/scholarships, institutionally sponsored non-need-based grants/scholarships.

BSN to Master's Program (MSN)

Applying *Required:* GRE General Test, Miller Analogies Test, bachelor's degree in nursing, minimum GPA of 2.7, RN license, 1 year of clinical experience, statistics course, 3 letters of recommendation. *Application fee:* $25.

Degree Requirements 39–42 total credit hours dependent upon track, 39–42 in nursing. Thesis or professional paper, comprehensive exam.

HOUSTON BAPTIST UNIVERSITY
College of Nursing
Houston, Texas

Programs • Generic Baccalaureate • RN Baccalaureate • BSN to Master's

The University Independent Baptist comprehensive coed institution. Founded: 1960. *Primary accreditation:* regional. *Setting:* 158-acre urban campus. *Total enrollment:* 2,142.

The College of Nursing Founded in 1967. *Nursing program faculty:* 19.

Student Life *Student services:* health clinic, personal counseling, career counseling, institutionally sponsored work-study program, special assistance for disabled students. *International student services:* institute for English. *Nursing student activities:* Sigma Theta Tau, student nurses association.

Calendar Quarters.

NURSING STUDENT PROFILE

Undergraduate **Enrollment:** 145

Women: 85%; **Men:** 15%; **Minority:** 45%; **Part-time:** 0%

BACCALAUREATE PROGRAMS

Contact Dr. Nancy Yuill, Dean, College of Nursing, Houston Baptist University, 7502 Fondren Street, Houston, TX 77074, 281-649-3420. *Fax:* 281-649-3489.

Expenses *Tuition:* $7800 full-time, $260 per semester hour part-time. *Full-time mandatory fees:* $400.

Generic Baccalaureate Program (BSN)

Applying *Required:* written essay, transcript of college record, high school transcript or GED certificate. *Options:* Advanced standing available through credit by exam. *Application deadline:* rolling. *Application fee:* $25.

Degree Requirements 132 total credit hours, 54 in nursing.

RN Baccalaureate Program (BSN)

Applying *Required:* minimum college GPA of 2.5, RN license, diploma or AD in nursing, written essay, transcript of college record. *Application deadline:* rolling. *Application fee:* $25.

Degree Requirements 132 total credit hours, 54 in nursing.

MASTER'S PROGRAM

Contact Dr. Brenda Binder, Director, MSN Program, College of Nursing, Houston Baptist University, Houston, TX 77074, 281-649-2385. *Fax:* 281-649-3489.

Areas of Study Nurse practitioner program in family health.

Expenses *Tuition:* ranges from $3900 to $4550 full-time, $325 per semester hour part-time.

Financial Aid Institutionally sponsored loans.

BSN to Master's Program (MSN)

Applying *Required:* GRE General Test (minimum combined score of 900 on three tests), bachelor's degree in nursing, minimum GPA of 2.5. *Application deadline:* 2/15. *Application fee:* $25.

Degree Requirements 47 total credit hours, 47 in nursing.

INCARNATE WORD COLLEGE
Department of Nursing
San Antonio, Texas

Programs • Generic Baccalaureate • RN Baccalaureate • MSN • MSN/MBA • Continuing Education

The College Independent Roman Catholic comprehensive coed institution. Founded: 1881. *Primary accreditation:* regional. *Setting:* 54-acre urban campus. *Total enrollment:* 3,076.

The Department of Nursing Founded in 1935. *Nursing program faculty:* 32 (47% with doctorates).

Academic Facilities *Campus library:* 15,046 volumes (5,245 in nursing); 191 periodical subscriptions (177 health-care related). *Nursing school*

Incarnate Word College (continued)

resources: CAI, computer lab, nursing audiovisuals, interactive nursing skills videos, learning resource lab, OPAC, CINAHL, CORAL on-line catalogs.

Student Life *Student services:* health clinic, personal counseling, career counseling, institutionally sponsored work-study program, job placement, campus safety program, special assistance for disabled students. *International student services:* counseling/support, special assistance for nonnative speakers of English, ESL courses. *Nursing student activities:* student nurses association, Nursing Honor Society.

Calendar Semesters.

NURSING STUDENT PROFILE

Undergraduate **Enrollment:** 254
Women: 84%; **Men:** 16%; **Minority:** 61%; **Part-time:** 1%
Graduate **Enrollment:** 146
Women: 92%; **Men:** 8%; **Minority:** 40%; **Part-time:** 76%

BACCALAUREATE PROGRAMS

Contact Dr. Brenda S. Jackson, Director, Department of Nursing, University of the Incarnate Word, 4301 Broadway, San Antonio, TX 78209, 210-829-6029. *Fax:* 210-829-3174. *E-mail:* jackson@universe.uiwtx.edu

Expenses *Tuition:* $10,060 full-time, $310 per semester hour part-time. *Full-time mandatory fees:* $200–$320. *Room and board:* $1930–$3780. *Books and supplies per academic year:* $300.

Financial Aid Institutionally sponsored need-based grants/scholarships, institutionally sponsored non-need grants/scholarships, Federal Nursing Student Loans, Federal Perkins Loans, Federal Supplemental Educational Opportunity Grants, Federal Work-Study. 80% of undergraduate students in nursing programs received some form of financial aid in 1995–96. *Application deadline:* 4/1.

Generic Baccalaureate Program (BSN)

Applying *Required:* SAT I, ACT, TOEFL for nonnative speakers of English, minimum college GPA of 2.5. 42 prerequisite credits must be completed before admission to the nursing program. *Options:* May apply for transfer of up to 56 total credits. *Application deadlines:* 10/1 (fall), 3/1 (spring). *Application fee:* $20.

Degree Requirements 135 total credit hours, 56 in nursing.

RN Baccalaureate Program (BSN)

Applying *Required:* TOEFL for nonnative speakers of English, minimum college GPA of 2.5, RN license, diploma or AD in nursing, transcript of college record. 42 prerequisite credits must be completed before admission to the nursing program. *Options:* Advanced standing available through credit by exam. Course work may be accelerated. May apply for transfer of up to 56 total credits. *Application deadlines:* 10/1 (fall), 3/1 (spring). *Application fee:* $20.

Degree Requirements 135 total credit hours, 56 in nursing.

MASTER'S PROGRAMS

Contact Dr. Brenda S. Jackson, Director, MSN Program, Department of Nursing, University of the Incarnate Word, 4301 Broadway, San Antonio, TX 78209, 210-829-6029. *Fax:* 210-829-3174.

Areas of Study Clinical nurse specialist program in adult health nursing.

Expenses *Tuition:* $330 per semester hour. *Full-time mandatory fees:* $165–$200. *Room and board:* $1930–$3780. *Books and supplies per academic year:* $300.

Financial Aid Nurse traineeships, employment opportunities. *Application deadline:* 4/1.

MSN Program

Applying *Required:* GRE General Test (minimum combined score of 1200 on three tests), Miller Analogies Test, TOEFL for nonnative speakers of English, bachelor's degree in nursing, minimum GPA of 2.5, RN license, 1 year of clinical experience, physical assessment course, statistics course, 3 letters of recommendation, transcript of college record. *Application deadline:* rolling. *Application fee:* $20.

Degree Requirements 45 total credit hours, 30–39 in nursing, 6 in education, management. Thesis or comprehensive exam.

MSN/MBA Program

Applying *Required:* GRE General Test (minimum combined score of 1200 on three tests), Miller Analogies Test, GMAT, bachelor's degree in nursing, RN license, physical assessment course, statistics course, professional liability/malpractice insurance, 3 letters of recommendation, transcript of college record. *Application deadline:* rolling. *Application fee:* $20.

Degree Requirements 66 total credit hours, 30 in nursing, 3 in education. Thesis or comprehensive exam in nursing, Capstone practicum as nurse executive.

CONTINUING EDUCATION PROGRAM

Contact Ms. Jennifer Cook, Coordinator of Continuing Education, Department of Nursing, University of the Incarnate Word, 4301 Broadway, San Antonio, TX 78209, 210-829-6029. *Fax:* 210-829-3174.

LAMAR UNIVERSITY–BEAUMONT
Department of Nursing
Beaumont, Texas

Programs • Generic Baccalaureate • RN Baccalaureate

The University State-supported coed university. Part of Texas State University System. Founded: 1923. *Primary accreditation:* regional. *Setting:* 200-acre urban campus. *Total enrollment:* 8,356.

The Department of Nursing Founded in 1974. *Nursing program faculty:* 28.

Calendar Semesters.

BACCALAUREATE PROGRAMS

Contact Department of Nursing, Lamar University-Beaumont, Student Advising Center, PO Box 10081, Beaumont, TX 77710, 409-880-8868. *Fax:* 409-880-1865.

Expenses *State resident tuition:* $960 full-time, $192 per six semester hours part-time. *Nonresident tuition:* $5328 full-time, $246 per hour part-time. *Full-time mandatory fees:* $846. *Part-time mandatory fees:* $486. *Books and supplies per academic year:* $554.

Financial Aid Institutionally sponsored long-term loans, institutionally sponsored non-need grants/scholarships, Federal Pell Grants, Federal Perkins Loans, Federal Supplemental Educational Opportunity Grants, Federal Work-Study, Federal PLUS Loans, Federal Stafford Loans, state grants. *Application deadline:* 4/1.

Generic Baccalaureate Program (BSN)

Applying *Required:* SAT I or ACT, Texas Academic Skills Program test, minimum college GPA of 2.0, high school math, high school chemistry, high school biology. 38 prerequisite credits must be completed before admission to the nursing program. *Options:* Advanced standing available through the following means: advanced placement exams, credit by exam. *Application deadline:* rolling.

Degree Requirements 143 total credit hours, 70 in nursing.

RN Baccalaureate Program (BSN)

Applying *Required:* Texas Academic Skills Program test, minimum college GPA of 2.0, high school transcript, transcript of college record. *Options:* Advanced standing available through the following means: advanced placement exams, credit by exam. *Application deadline:* rolling.

Degree Requirements 142 total credit hours, 71 in nursing.

MCMURRY UNIVERSITY
Abilene Intercollegiate School of Nursing
Abilene, Texas

Programs • Generic Baccalaureate • RN Baccalaureate

The University Independent United Methodist 4-year coed college. Founded: 1923. *Primary accreditation:* regional. *Setting:* 41-acre urban campus. *Total enrollment:* 1,457.

The Abilene Intercollegiate School of Nursing Founded in 1979.

Academic Facilities *Campus library:* 142,019 volumes. *Nursing school resources:* computer lab.

Calendar Semesters.

BACCALAUREATE PROGRAMS

Contact Academic Adviser, Abilene Intercollegiate School of Nursing, McMurry University, 2149 Hickory Street, Abilene, TX 79601, 915-672-2441.

Expenses *Tuition:* $7200 full-time, ranges from $235 to $240 per semester hour part-time. *Full-time mandatory fees:* $750. *Room and board:* $3770. *Books and supplies per academic year:* $444.

Financial Aid Institutionally sponsored need-based grants/scholarships, institutionally sponsored non-need grants/scholarships, Federal Perkins Loans, Federal Supplemental Educational Opportunity Grants, Federal Work-Study, Federal PLUS Loans, Federal Stafford Loans. *Application deadline:* 3/15.

Generic Baccalaureate Program (BSN)

Applying *Required:* SAT I or ACT, TOEFL for nonnative speakers of English, minimum college GPA of 2.5, 3 years of high school math, 3 years of high school science, high school chemistry, high school biology, high school transcript, interview, 2 letters of recommendation. *Options:* Advanced standing available through the following means: advanced placement exams, credit by exam. *Application fee:* $20.

RN Baccalaureate Program (BSN)

Applying *Required:* NLN Mobility Profile II, high school transcript, transcript of college record. *Options:* Advanced standing available through credit by exam. *Application fee:* $20.

MIDWESTERN STATE UNIVERSITY
Nursing Program
Wichita Falls, Texas

Programs • Generic Baccalaureate • RN Baccalaureate • Master's • Continuing Education

The University State-supported comprehensive coed institution. Founded: 1922. *Primary accreditation:* regional. *Setting:* 172-acre small-town campus. *Total enrollment:* 5,833.

The Nursing Program Founded in 1986. *Nursing program faculty:* 14 (21% with doctorates).

Academic Facilities *Campus library:* 500,000 volumes (200 in health, 775 in nursing); 700 periodical subscriptions (70 health-care related). *Nursing school resources:* CAI, computer lab, nursing audiovisuals, learning resource lab.

Student Life *Student services:* health clinic, personal counseling, career counseling, institutionally sponsored work-study program, job placement, campus safety program, special assistance for disabled students. *International student services:* counseling/support, ESL courses. *Nursing student activities:* Sigma Theta Tau, student nurses association.

Calendar Semesters.

NURSING STUDENT PROFILE

Undergraduate **Enrollment:** 470
Women: 84%; **Men:** 16%; **Minority:** 23%; **Part-time:** 1%
Graduate **Enrollment:** 34
Women: 91%; **Men:** 9%; **Minority:** 47%; **International:** 0%; **Part-time:** 100%

BACCALAUREATE PROGRAMS

Contact Ms. Catherine Rudy, BSN Admissions Coordinator, Midwestern State University, 3410 Taft Boulevard, Wichita Falls, TX 76308, 817-689-4595. *Fax:* 817-689-4513.

Expenses *State resident tuition:* $1244 full-time, $322 per semester part-time. *Nonresident tuition:* $4676 full-time, $1180 per semester part-time. *Full-time mandatory fees:* $436–$600. *Room and board:* $3266–$3366. *Books and supplies per academic year:* ranges from $250 to $500.

Financial Aid Institutionally sponsored need-based grants/scholarships, institutionally sponsored non-need grants/scholarships, Federal Pell Grants, Federal Supplemental Educational Opportunity Grants, Federal Work-Study. 56% of undergraduate students in nursing programs received some form of financial aid in 1995–96. *Application deadline:* 4/15.

Generic Baccalaureate Program (BSN)

Applying *Required:* SAT I, ACT, TOEFL for nonnative speakers of English, minimum college GPA of 2.5, high school transcript, 3 letters of recommendation, transcript of college record. 45 prerequisite credits must be completed before admission to the nursing program. *Options:* May apply for transfer of up to 66–84 total credits. *Application deadlines:* 8/7 (fall), 12/15 (spring).

Degree Requirements 140 total credit hours, 59 in nursing.

RN Baccalaureate Program (BSN)

Applying *Required:* NLN Mobility Profile II, minimum college GPA of 2.5, RN license, diploma or AD in nursing, transcript of college record. *Options:* Advanced standing available through credit by exam. May apply for transfer of up to 60 total credits. *Application deadlines:* 8/7 (fall), 12/15 (spring).

Degree Requirements 139 total credit hours, 30 in nursing.

MASTER'S PROGRAMS

Contact Catherine Rudy, Nursing Programs Admission and Certification Assistant, Midwestern State University, 3410 Taft Boulevard, Wichita Falls, TX 76308. *Fax:* 817-689-4513.

Areas of Study Nursing education; nurse practitioner program in family health.

Expenses *State resident tuition:* $2066 full-time, ranges from $32 to $186 per semester credit hour part-time. *Nonresident tuition:* $9864 full-time, ranges from $237 to $288 per semester credit hour part-time. *Full-time mandatory fees:* $61. *Part-time mandatory fees:* $61. *Room and board:* $3366–$3470. *Books and supplies per academic year:* $750.

Financial Aid Graduate assistantships, institutionally sponsored need-based grants/scholarships, institutionally sponsored non-need-based grants/scholarships. 12% of master's level students in nursing programs received some form of financial aid in 1995-96.

CONTINUING EDUCATION PROGRAM

Contact Ms. Billye R. Goss, Director, Continuing Education, Midwestern State University, 3410 Taft Boulevard, Wichita Falls, TX 76308, 817-689-4726.

PRAIRIE VIEW A&M UNIVERSITY
College of Nursing
Houston, Texas

Programs • Generic Baccalaureate • RN Baccalaureate

The University State-supported comprehensive coed institution. Part of Texas A&M University System. Founded: 1878. *Primary accreditation:* regional. *Setting:* 1,440-acre small-town campus. *Total enrollment:* 5,999.

The College of Nursing Founded in 1918. *Nursing program faculty:* 29.

Academic Facilities *Campus library:* 243,860 volumes; 1,717 periodical subscriptions. *Nursing school resources:* CAI, computer lab, nursing audiovisuals, interactive nursing skills videos, learning resource lab.

Student Life *Student services:* health clinic, personal counseling, career counseling, campus safety program. *International student services:* counseling/support, international student club. *Nursing student activities:* Sigma Theta Tau, student nurses association, Male Student Club.

Calendar Semesters.

NURSING STUDENT PROFILE

Undergraduate **Enrollment:** 279
Women: 88%; **Men:** 12%; **Minority:** 90%; **International:** 0%; **Part-time:** 28%

BACCALAUREATE PROGRAMS

Contact Dr. Lillian Bernard, Associate Dean, College of Nursing, Prairie View A&M University, 6436 Fannin Street, Houston, TX 77030, 713-797-7000.

Expenses *State resident tuition:* $806 full-time, $245 per course part-time. *Nonresident tuition:* $2808 full-time, $791 per course part-time. *Full-time mandatory fees:* $15. *Books and supplies per academic year:* $500.

Financial Aid Institutionally sponsored need-based grants/scholarships, Federal Nursing Student Loans, Federal Supplemental Educational Opportunity Grants. *Application deadline:* 3/1.

Prairie View A&M University (continued)

Generic Baccalaureate Program (BS)

Applying *Required:* ACT, Nursing Entrance Test, minimum high school GPA of 2.0. 61 prerequisite credits must be completed before admission to the nursing program. *Options:* May apply for transfer of up to 62 total credits. *Application deadlines:* 3/1 (fall), 10/1 (spring). *Application fee:* $10.

Degree Requirements 131 total credit hours, 70 in nursing.

RN Baccalaureate Program (BS)

Applying *Required:* minimum college GPA of 2.5, RN license, diploma or AD in nursing, interview, transcript of college record. 61 prerequisite credits must be completed before admission to the nursing program. *Options:* Course work may be accelerated. May apply for transfer of up to 61 total credits. *Application deadlines:* 9/1 (fall), 1/5 (spring). *Application fee:* $10.

Degree Requirements 131 total credit hours, 70 in nursing.

SOUTHWESTERN ADVENTIST COLLEGE

Department of Nursing
Keene, Texas

Program • RN Baccalaureate

The College Independent Seventh-day Adventist comprehensive coed institution. Founded: 1894. *Primary accreditation:* regional. *Setting:* 150-acre rural campus. *Total enrollment:* 1,001.

The Department of Nursing Founded in 1985. *Nursing program faculty:* 11 (18% with doctorates).

Academic Facilities *Campus library:* 101,050 volumes (3,107 in nursing); 468 periodical subscriptions (41 health-care related). *Nursing school resources:* CAI, computer lab, nursing audiovisuals, interactive nursing skills videos.

Student Life *Student services:* health clinic, personal counseling, career counseling. *International student services:* counseling/support, ESL courses. *Nursing student activities:* student nurses association.

Calendar Semesters.

NURSING STUDENT PROFILE

Undergraduate **Enrollment:** 45

Women: 80%; **Men:** 20%; **Minority:** 5%; **International:** 2%; **Part-time:** 11%

BACCALAUREATE PROGRAM

Contact Dr. Catherine Turner, Chair, Department of Nursing, Southwestern Adventist University, Keene, TX 76059, 817-645-3921 Ext. 236. *Fax:* 817-556-4744. *E-mail:* turnerc@swau.edu

Expenses *Tuition:* $6000 full-time, $333 per credit part-time. *Full-time mandatory fees:* $290–$342. *Room and board:* $3812. *Books and supplies per academic year:* $500.

Financial Aid Institutionally sponsored need-based grants/scholarships, institutionally sponsored non-need grants/scholarships, Federal Perkins Loans, Federal Supplemental Educational Opportunity Grants, Federal Work-Study. *Application deadline:* 3/15.

RN Baccalaureate Program (BS)

Applying *Required:* minimum high school GPA of 3.25, minimum college GPA of 2.5, 2 years of high school math, 2 years of high school science, high school chemistry, high school biology, RN license, diploma or AD in nursing, high school transcript, interview, 3 letters of recommendation, transcript of college record. *Application deadline:* 7/1.

Degree Requirements 60 total credit hours, 33 in nursing.

STEPHEN F. AUSTIN STATE UNIVERSITY

Division of Nursing
Nacogdoches, Texas

Programs • Generic Baccalaureate • RN Baccalaureate

The University State-supported comprehensive coed institution. Part of Texas Higher Education Coordinating Board. Founded: 1923. *Primary accreditation:* regional. *Setting:* 400-acre small-town campus. *Total enrollment:* 11,758.

The Division of Nursing Founded in 1978. *Nursing program faculty:* 12.

Academic Facilities *Campus library:* 601,441 volumes; 3,200 periodical subscriptions.

Calendar Semesters.

BACCALAUREATE PROGRAMS

Contact Division of Nursing, Stephen F. Austin State University, Nacogdoches, TX 75962, 409-568-3604. *Fax:* 409-568-1635.

Expenses *State resident tuition:* ranges from $960 to $1088 full-time, ranges from $32 to $100 per semester hour part-time. *Nonresident tuition:* ranges from $6660 to $7548 full-time, $222 per semester hour part-time. *Part-time mandatory fees:* $36+. *Room and board:* $3504–$3992.

Financial Aid Federal Pell Grants, Federal Perkins Loans, Federal Supplemental Educational Opportunity Grants, Federal Work-Study, Federal Stafford Loans, state aid. *Application deadline:* 4/15.

Generic Baccalaureate Program (BSN)

Applying *Required:* SAT I or ACT, minimum college GPA of 2.5, high school transcript, transcript of college record, high school class rank: . *Options:* Advanced standing available through credit by exam.

Degree Requirements 130 total credit hours, 48 in nursing. Comprehensive final.

RN Baccalaureate Program (BSN)

Applying *Required:* minimum college GPA of 2.5, RN license, diploma or AD in nursing, transcript of college record. *Options:* Advanced standing available through credit by exam. May apply for transfer of up to 66 total credits. *Application deadline:* rolling.

Degree Requirements 130 total credit hours, 48 in nursing. Comprehensive final.

TEXAS A&M UNIVERSITY–CORPUS CHRISTI

Department of Nursing and Health Science
Corpus Christi, Texas

Programs • Generic Baccalaureate • RN Baccalaureate • Master's

The University State-supported comprehensive coed institution. Part of Texas A&M University System. Founded: 1947. *Primary accreditation:* regional. *Setting:* 240-acre suburban campus. *Total enrollment:* 5,545.

The Department of Nursing and Health Science Founded in 1974.

Academic Facilities *Campus library:* 321,134 volumes (4,895 in health, 2,022 in nursing); 1,582 periodical subscriptions (116 health-care related).

Calendar Semesters.

NURSING STUDENT PROFILE

Undergraduate **Enrollment:** 200

Women: 80%; **Men:** 20%

BACCALAUREATE PROGRAMS

Contact Dr. Mary Jane Hamilton, Undergraduate Coordinator, Department of Nursing and Health Science, Texas A&M University-Corpus Christi, 6300 Ocean Drive, Corpus Christi, TX 78412, 512-994-5797. *Fax:* 512-994-2484. *E-mail:* hamilton@falcon@tarmucc.edu

Expenses *State resident tuition:* $1858 full-time, $217 per credit part-time. *Nonresident tuition:* $6994 full-time, $343 per credit part-time.

Generic Baccalaureate Program (BSN)

Applying *Required:* TOEFL for nonnative speakers of English.

Degree Requirements 134 total credit hours, 62 in nursing.

RN Baccalaureate Program (BSN)

Degree Requirements 128+ total credit hours dependent upon track, 62 in nursing.

MASTER'S PROGRAMS

Contact Graduate Coordinator, Department of Nursing and Health Science, Texas A&M University-Corpus Christi, 6300 Ocean Drive, Corpus Christi, TX 78412, 512-994-2712. *Fax:* 512-994-2484.

See full description on page 512.

TEXAS CHRISTIAN UNIVERSITY
Harris College of Nursing
Fort Worth, Texas

Programs • Generic Baccalaureate • RN Baccalaureate • Continuing Education

The University Independent coed university, affiliated with Christian Church (Disciples of Christ). Founded: 1873. *Primary accreditation:* regional. *Setting:* 237-acre suburban campus. *Total enrollment:* 7,050.

The Harris College of Nursing Founded in 1946. *Nursing program faculty:* 26 (61% with doctorates).

Academic Facilities *Campus library:* 1.2 million volumes (16,505 in health, 3,063 in nursing); 3,900 periodical subscriptions (180 health-care related). *Nursing school resources:* CAI, computer lab, nursing audiovisuals, interactive nursing skills videos, learning resource lab.

Student Life *Student services:* health clinic, personal counseling, career counseling, institutionally sponsored work-study program, job placement, campus safety program, special assistance for disabled students. *International student services:* counseling/support. *Nursing student activities:* Sigma Theta Tau, student nurses association.

Calendar Semesters.

NURSING STUDENT PROFILE

Undergraduate **Enrollment:** 353
Women: 90%; **Men:** 10%; **Minority:** 20%; **International:** 7%; **Part-time:** 6%

BACCALAUREATE PROGRAMS

Contact Laura Thielke, Assistant to the Dean, Harris College of Nursing, Texas Christian University, 2800 West Bowie, TCU Box 298620, Fort Worth, TX 76129, 817-921-7497. *Fax:* 817-191-7704. *E-mail:* l.thielke@tcu.edu

Expenses *Tuition:* $9700 full-time, $314 per semester hour part-time. *Full-time mandatory fees:* $585–$843. *Room and board:* $3500. *Books and supplies per academic year:* ranges from $650 to $1000.

Financial Aid Institutionally sponsored need-based grants/scholarships, institutionally sponsored non-need grants/scholarships, Federal Direct Loans, Federal Nursing Student Loans, Federal Perkins Loans, Federal Supplemental Educational Opportunity Grants, Federal Work-Study. 50% of undergraduate students in nursing programs received some form of financial aid in 1995–96. *Application deadline:* 5/1.

Generic Baccalaureate Program (BSN)

Applying *Required:* SAT I or ACT, TOEFL for nonnative speakers of English, 3 years of high school math, 3 years of high school science, high school transcript, interview, written essay, transcript of college record. 40 prerequisite credits must be completed before admission to the nursing program. *Options:* Advanced standing available through the following means: advanced placement exams, credit by exam. May apply for transfer of up to 66 total credits. *Application deadlines:* 2/15 (fall), 12/1 (spring). *Application fee:* $30.

Degree Requirements 125 total credit hours, 57 in nursing.

RN Baccalaureate Program (BSN)

Applying *Required:* TOEFL for nonnative speakers of English, minimum college GPA of 2.25, RN license, diploma or AD in nursing, interview, written essay, transcript of college record, portfolio evaluation for credit. 40 prerequisite credits must be completed before admission to the nursing program. *Options:* Advanced standing available through credit by exam. May apply for transfer of up to 66 total credits. *Application deadlines:* 2/15 (fall), 12/1 (spring). *Application fee:* $30.

Degree Requirements 125 total credit hours, 57 in nursing.

CONTINUING EDUCATION PROGRAM

Contact Faculty Relations Committee, Harris College of Nursing, Texas Christian University, 2800 West Bowie, PO Box 32899, Fort Worth, TX 76129, 817-921-7652. *Fax:* 817-921-7704.

TEXAS TECH UNIVERSITY HEALTH SCIENCES CENTER
School of Nursing
Lubbock, Texas

Programs • Generic Baccalaureate • RN Baccalaureate • RN to Master's • MSN/MBA • Post-Master's • Continuing Education

The University State-supported graduate specialized coed institution. Founded: 1969. *Primary accreditation:* specialized. *Total enrollment:* 1,276.

The School of Nursing Founded in 1981. *Nursing program faculty:* 40 (32% with doctorates). *Off-campus program sites:* Odessa, Tyler.

▶ ***NOTEWORTHY***

The School of Nursing has a distinctive background and guiding theme that frames faculty and student activities. Reintegration is the term originated at Tech to designate a return to the role nurses originally assumed—an integration of education, practice, scholarship, and service. This concept brings a dynamic, distinctive approach to the faculty role and the curricula of the undergraduate and graduate programs. The School of Nursing offers entry points in the undergraduate program for generic students and registered nurses. The graduate program, comprising both a master's program and a joint doctoral program with the University of Texas Health Science Center at San Antonio, has a variety of majors, including a family nurse practitioner program. The School of Nursing focuses on primary care and rural health.

Academic Facilities *Campus library:* 227,754 volumes (227,754 in health, 8,445 in nursing); 2,515 periodical subscriptions (2,515 health-care related). *Nursing school resources:* CAI, computer lab, nursing audiovisuals, interactive nursing skills videos, learning resource lab.

Student Life *Student services:* health clinic, personal counseling, career counseling, job placement, campus safety program, special assistance for disabled students. *International student services:* counseling/support, special assistance for nonnative speakers of English, ESL courses. *Nursing student activities:* Sigma Theta Tau, recruiter club, student nurses association.

Calendar Semesters.

NURSING STUDENT PROFILE

Undergraduate **Enrollment:** 411
Women: 88%; **Men:** 12%; **Minority:** 21%; **International:** 1%; **Part-time:** 22%
Graduate **Enrollment:** 76
Women: 92%; **Men:** 8%; **Minority:** 16%; **International:** 5%; **Part-time:** 85%

BACCALAUREATE PROGRAMS

Contact Ms. Kathryn Quilliam, Director of Student Affairs, School of Nursing, Texas Tech University Health Sciences Center, 3601 4th Street, Lubbock, TX 79430, 806-743-2737. *Fax:* 806-743-1622. *E-mail:* sonkqg@ttuhsc.edu

Expenses *State resident tuition:* $1560 full-time, $760 per academic year part-time. *Nonresident tuition:* $7500 full-time, $4150 per academic year part-time. *Full-time mandatory fees:* $1028–$1300. *Part-time mandatory fees:* $300–$600. *Room and board:* $3225–$3945. *Books and supplies per academic year:* ranges from $500 to $700.

Financial Aid Institutionally sponsored need-based grants/scholarships, institutionally sponsored non-need grants/scholarships, Federal Nursing Student Loans, Federal Pell Grants, Federal Supplemental Educational

Texas Tech University Health Sciences Center (continued)
Opportunity Grants. 36% of undergraduate students in nursing programs received some form of financial aid in 1995–96. *Application deadline:* 5/1.

Generic Baccalaureate Program (BSN)

Applying *Required:* SAT I, ACT, TOEFL for nonnative speakers of English, minimum high school GPA of 2.0, minimum college GPA of 2.0, RN license, diploma or AD in nursing, high school transcript, 2 letters of recommendation, written essay, transcript of college record. *Options:* Advanced standing available through the following means: advanced placement exams, credit by exam. Course work may be accelerated. May apply for transfer of up to 96 total credits. *Application deadlines:* 5/15 (fall), 10/15 (spring), 2/15 (summer). *Application fee:* $30.

Degree Requirements 126 total credit hours, 70 in nursing.

Distance learning Courses provided through video, computer-based media, on-line.

RN Baccalaureate Program (BSN)

Applying *Required:* TOEFL for nonnative speakers of English, minimum college GPA of 2.0, RN license, diploma or AD in nursing, 2 letters of recommendation, written essay, transcript of college record. *Options:* Advanced standing available through the following means: advanced placement exams, credit by exam. Course work may be accelerated. May apply for transfer of up to 96 total credits. *Application deadlines:* 5/15 (fall), 2/15 (summer). *Application fee:* $30.

Degree Requirements 126 total credit hours, 70 in nursing.

Distance learning Courses provided through video.

MASTER'S PROGRAMS

Contact Ms. Kathryn Quilliam, Director of Student Affairs, School of Nursing, Texas Tech University Health Sciences Center, 3601 4th Street, Lubbock, TX 79430, 806-743-2737. *Fax:* 806-743-1622. *E-mail:* sonkqg@ttuhsc.edu

Areas of Study Clinical nurse specialist programs in community health nursing, gerontological nursing; nursing administration; nursing education; nurse practitioner program in family health.

Expenses *State resident tuition:* $1460 full-time, $600 per academic year part-time. *Nonresident tuition:* $5300 full-time, $3500 per academic year part-time. *Full-time mandatory fees:* $700–$800. *Part-time mandatory fees:* $200–$400. *Room and board:* $3225–$3945. *Books and supplies per academic year:* ranges from $200 to $500.

Financial Aid Nurse traineeships, Federal Nursing Student Loans, institutionally sponsored loans, institutionally sponsored need-based grants/scholarships, institutionally sponsored non-need-based grants/scholarships, grants. 13% of master's level students in nursing programs received some form of financial aid in 1995-96. *Application deadline:* 5/1.

RN to Master's Program (MSN)

Applying *Required:* GRE General Test, Miller Analogies Test, TOEFL for nonnative speakers of English, bachelor's degree in nursing, minimum GPA of 3.0, RN license, 1 year of clinical experience, statistics course, essay, 3 letters of recommendation, transcript of college record. *Application deadlines:* 6/1 (fall), 10/1 (spring), 3/1 (summer). *Application fee:* $30.

Degree Requirements 36 total credit hours, 27 in nursing, 9 in physiology, statistics, computer science. Basic cardiac life support certification. Thesis required.

Distance learning Courses provided through video, computer-based media, on-line.

MSN/MBA Program

Applying *Required:* GRE General Test, Miller Analogies Test, GMAT, bachelor's degree in nursing, minimum GPA of 3.0, RN license, 1 year of clinical experience, statistics course, essay, 4 letters of recommendation, transcript of college record. *Application deadlines:* 6/1 (fall), 10/1 (spring), 3/1 (summer). *Application fee:* $30.

Degree Requirements 69 total credit hours, 30 in nursing, 39 in business, computer science, physiology, statistics. Thesis required.

Distance learning Courses provided through video, computer-based media, on-line.

Post-Master's Program

Applying *Required:* GRE General Test, Miller Analogies Test, minimum GPA of 3.0, RN license, 1 year of clinical experience, statistics course, essay, 3 letters of recommendation, transcript of college record, MSN. *Application deadlines:* 6/1 (fall), 10/1 (spring), 3/1 (summer). *Application fee:* $30.

Degree Requirements 18 total credit hours, 18 in nursing. Advanced cardiac life support certification.

Distance learning Courses provided through video, computer-based media, on-line.

CONTINUING EDUCATION PROGRAM

Contact Ms. Shelley Burson, Director of Continuing Nursing Education, School of Nursing, Texas Tech University Health Sciences Center, 3601 4th Street, Lubbock, TX 79430, 806-743-2734. *Fax:* 806-743-1622. *E-mail:* sonszb@ttuhsc.edu

TEXAS WOMAN'S UNIVERSITY
College of Nursing
Denton, Texas

Programs • Generic Baccalaureate • RN Baccalaureate • Baccalaureate for Second Degree • MS • PhD

The University State-supported primarily women's university. Founded: 1901. *Primary accreditation:* regional. *Setting:* 270-acre suburban campus. *Total enrollment:* 9,852.

The College of Nursing Founded in 1954. *Nursing program faculty:* 109 (41% with doctorates). *Off-campus program sites:* Dallas, Houston.

Academic Facilities *Campus library:* 776,747 volumes (51,503 in health, 26,463 in nursing); 3,072 periodical subscriptions (446 health-care related). *Nursing school resources:* CAI, computer lab, nursing audiovisuals, learning resource lab.

Student Life *Student services:* health clinic, child-care facilities, personal counseling, career counseling, institutionally sponsored work-study program, job placement, campus safety program, special assistance for disabled students. *Nursing student activities:* Sigma Theta Tau, student nurses association.

Calendar Semesters.

NURSING STUDENT PROFILE

Undergraduate **Enrollment:** 716
Women: 91%; **Men:** 9%; **Minority:** 25%; **International:** 1%; **Part-time:** 62%
Graduate **Enrollment:** 489
Women: 98%; **Men:** 2%; **Minority:** 17%; **International:** 1%; **Part-time:** 87%

BACCALAUREATE PROGRAMS

Contact Dr. Betty Adams, Assistant Dean, College of Nursing, Texas Woman's University, Texas Woman's University Station, PO Box 425498, Denton, TX 76204-5498, 817-898-2401. *Fax:* 817-898-2437.

Expenses *State resident tuition:* ranges from $792 to $1032 full-time, $32 per semester hour part-time. *Nonresident tuition:* ranges from $6089 to $7934 full-time, $246 per semester hour part-time. *Full-time mandatory fees:* $176–$784.

Financial Aid Institutionally sponsored need-based grants/scholarships, institutionally sponsored non-need grants/scholarships, Federal Nursing Student Loans, Federal Work-Study. 92% of undergraduate students in nursing programs received some form of financial aid in 1995–96. *Application deadline:* 4/1.

Generic Baccalaureate Program (BS)

Applying *Required:* SAT I, TOEFL for nonnative speakers of English, minimum college GPA of 3.0. 67 prerequisite credits must be completed before admission to the nursing program. *Options:* May apply for transfer of up to 72 total credits. *Application deadlines:* 2/1 (fall), 9/1 (spring). *Application fee:* $25.

Degree Requirements 129 total credit hours, 58 in nursing.

RN Baccalaureate Program (BS)

Applying *Required:* RN license, diploma or AD in nursing, transcript of college record. 67 prerequisite credits must be completed before admission to the nursing program. *Options:* Advanced standing available through the following means: advanced placement without credit, credit by exam. May apply for transfer of up to 72 total credits. *Application deadlines:* 7/15 (fall), 12/15 (spring). *Application fee:* $25.

Degree Requirements 124 total credit hours, 53 in nursing.

Baccalaureate for Second Degree Program (BS)

Applying *Required:* minimum college GPA of 3.0. 37 prerequisite credits must be completed before admission to the nursing program. *Application deadlines:* 2/1 (fall), 9/1 (spring). *Application fee:* $25.

Degree Requirements 99 total credit hours, 58 in nursing.

MASTER'S PROGRAM

Contact Dr. Rose Nieswiadomy, College of Nursing, Texas Woman's University, 1810 Inwood Road, Dallas, TX 75235-7299, 214-689-6554. *Fax:* 214-689-6539.

Areas of Study Clinical nurse specialist programs in adult health nursing, community health nursing, maternity-newborn nursing, pediatric nursing, psychiatric–mental health nursing; nurse practitioner programs in adult health, child care/pediatrics, family health, women's health.

Expenses *State resident tuition:* ranges from $988 to $1222 full-time, $52 per semester hour part-time. *Nonresident tuition:* ranges from $5054 to $6251 full-time, $266 per semester hour part-time. *Full-time mandatory fees:* $176–$636.

Financial Aid Graduate assistantships, nurse traineeships, Federal Nursing Student Loans, institutionally sponsored need-based grants/scholarships, institutionally sponsored non-need-based grants/scholarships. 6% of master's level students in nursing programs received some form of financial aid in 1995-96. *Application deadline:* 4/1.

MS Program

Applying *Required:* TOEFL for nonnative speakers of English, GRE General Test (minimum combined score of 750 on verbal and quantitative sections), bachelor's degree in nursing, minimum GPA of 3.0, RN license, 1 year of clinical experience, statistics course, professional liability/malpractice insurance, transcript of college record. *Application deadline:* rolling. *Application fee:* $25.

Degree Requirements 38–47 total credit hours dependent upon track, 35–44 in nursing, 3 in pathophysiology.

DOCTORAL PROGRAM

Contact Dr. Maisie Kashka, Associate Professor, College of Nursing, Texas Woman's University, Texas Woman's University Station, PO Box 425498, Denton, TX 76204-5498, 817-898-2401. *Fax:* 817-898-2437.

Areas of Study Nursing research, theory development.

Expenses *State resident tuition:* $1560 full-time, $52 per semester hour part-time. *Nonresident tuition:* $7980 full-time, $266 per semester hour part-time. *Full-time mandatory fees:* $176–$636.

Financial Aid Graduate assistantships, nurse traineeships, grants, institutionally sponsored loans, opportunities for employment, institutionally sponsored need-based grants/scholarships, institutionally sponsored non-need-based grants/scholarships. *Application deadline:* 4/1.

PhD Program

Applying *Required:* GRE General Test (minimum combined score of 1000 on verbal and quantitative sections), master's degree in nursing, statistics course, 2 letters of recommendation, graduate-level courses in research and theory, statement of research and professional goals, RN license. *Application deadline:* rolling. *Application fee:* $25.

Degree Requirements 60 total credit hours; 36 hours in major, 15 hours in electives, 9 hours in statistics; dissertation; written exam; defense of dissertation; residency; proficiency in two research tools (foreign languages, statistics, computer science).

UNIVERSITY OF MARY HARDIN-BAYLOR

Scott and White School of Nursing
Belton, Texas

Programs • Generic Baccalaureate • RN Baccalaureate

The University Independent Southern Baptist comprehensive coed institution. Founded: 1845. *Primary accreditation:* regional. *Setting:* 100-acre small-town campus. *Total enrollment:* 2,270.

The Scott and White School of Nursing Founded in 1968. *Nursing program faculty:* 13 (46% with doctorates).

Academic Facilities *Campus library:* 147,243 volumes (7,511 in health, 4,903 in nursing); 1,030 periodical subscriptions (138 health-care related). *Nursing school resources:* CAI, computer lab, nursing audiovisuals, interactive nursing skills videos, learning resource lab.

Student Life *Student services:* personal counseling, career counseling, institutionally sponsored work-study program, job placement, campus safety program, special assistance for disabled students. *International student services:* counseling/support, special assistance for nonnative speakers of English, ESL courses. *Nursing student activities:* student nurses association, Nu Sigma Lambda (Honor Society), Nurses Christian Fellowship.

Calendar Semesters.

NURSING STUDENT PROFILE

Undergraduate **Enrollment:** 150

Women: 87%; **Men:** 13%; **Minority:** 17%; **Part-time:** 18%

BACCALAUREATE PROGRAMS

Contact Dr. Grace Labaj, Associate Dean, Scott and White School of Nursing, University of Mary Hardin-Baylor, UMHB Box 8015, Belton, TX 76513, 817-939-4662. *Fax:* 817-939-4535.

Expenses *Tuition:* $6960 full-time, $224 per semester hour part-time. *Full-time mandatory fees:* $180.

Financial Aid Institutionally sponsored need-based grants/scholarships, institutionally sponsored non-need grants/scholarships, Federal Supplemental Educational Opportunity Grants, Federal Work-Study. *Application deadline:* 6/1.

Generic Baccalaureate Program (BSN)

Applying *Required:* SAT I, ACT, minimum college GPA of 2.75, high school transcript, transcript of college record. 58 prerequisite credits must be completed before admission to the nursing program. *Options:* May apply for transfer of up to 58 total credits. *Application deadlines:* 6/1 (fall), 10/15 (spring). *Application fee:* $35.

Degree Requirements 124 total credit hours, 63 in nursing.

RN Baccalaureate Program (BSN)

Applying *Required:* SAT I, ACT, minimum college GPA of 2.75, RN license, diploma or AD in nursing, high school transcript, transcript of college record. 58 prerequisite credits must be completed before admission to the nursing program. *Options:* Advanced standing available through advanced placement exams. May apply for transfer of up to 58 total credits. *Application deadlines:* 6/1 (fall), 10/15 (spring). *Application fee:* $35.

Degree Requirements 124 total credit hours, 63 in nursing.

UNIVERSITY OF TEXAS AT ARLINGTON

School of Nursing
Arlington, Texas

Programs • Generic Baccalaureate • RN Baccalaureate • MSN • Continuing Education

The University State-supported coed university. Part of University of Texas System. Founded: 1895. *Primary accreditation:* regional. *Setting:* 395-acre suburban campus. *Total enrollment:* 22,121.

The School of Nursing Founded in 1971. *Nursing program faculty:* 61 (61% with doctorates). *Off-campus program sites:* Paris, Waco, Sherman.

Academic Facilities *Campus library:* 913,745 volumes (35,500 in health, 23,000 in nursing); 2,706 periodical subscriptions (104 health-care related). *Nursing school resources:* CAI, computer lab, nursing audiovisuals, learning resource lab.

Student Life *Student services:* health clinic, personal counseling, career counseling, institutionally sponsored work-study program, job placement, campus safety program, special assistance for disabled students.

University of Texas at Arlington (continued)

International student services: counseling/support, special assistance for nonnative speakers of English, ESL courses. *Nursing student activities:* Sigma Theta Tau, student nurses association.

Calendar Semesters.

NURSING STUDENT PROFILE

Undergraduate **Enrollment:** 465
Women: 85%; **Men:** 15%; **Minority:** 24%; **International:** 4%; **Part-time:** 11%
Graduate **Enrollment:** 254
Women: 97%; **Men:** 3%; **Minority:** 11%; **International:** 0%; **Part-time:** 69%

BACCALAUREATE PROGRAMS

Contact Ms. Shannon Williams, Administrative Assistant for Student Affairs, School of Nursing, University of Texas at Arlington, Box 19407, Arlington, TX 76019-0407, 817-272-2776 Ext. 4797. *Fax:* 817-272-5006. *E-mail:* williams@uta.edu

Expenses *State resident tuition:* $2342 full-time, ranges from $39 to $237 per hour part-time. *Nonresident tuition:* $9190 full-time, ranges from $275 to $363 per hour part-time. *Full-time mandatory fees:* $238–$2600. *Room and board:* $1910–$2870. *Room only:* $1310–$1470. *Books and supplies per academic year:* ranges from $900 to $1250.

Financial Aid Institutionally sponsored need-based grants/scholarships, institutionally sponsored non-need grants/scholarships, Federal Work-Study. *Application deadline:* 3/31.

Generic Baccalaureate Program (BSN)

Applying *Required:* TOEFL for nonnative speakers of English, minimum college GPA of 2.0, transcript of college record. 60 prerequisite credits must be completed before admission to the nursing program. *Application deadlines:* 9/1 (fall), 2/15 (spring). *Application fee:* $25.

Degree Requirements 128 total credit hours, 62 in nursing.

RN Baccalaureate Program (BSN)

Applying *Required:* TOEFL for nonnative speakers of English, minimum college GPA of 2.0, RN license, diploma or AD in nursing, transcript of college record. 60 prerequisite credits must be completed before admission to the nursing program. *Options:* Course work may be accelerated. *Application deadlines:* 9/1 (fall), 2/15 (spring). *Application fee:* $25.

Degree Requirements 128 total credit hours, 62 in nursing.

Distance learning Courses provided through video.

MASTER'S PROGRAM

Contact Dr. Susan K. Grove, Assistant Dean and Director of Graduate Studies, School of Nursing, University of Texas at Arlington, Box 19407, Arlington, TX 76019-0407, 817-272-2776 Ext. 4794. *Fax:* 817-272-5006. *E-mail:* grove@uta.edu

Areas of Study Nursing administration; nursing education; nurse practitioner programs in acute care, adult health, child care/pediatrics, family health, gerontology, psychiatric–mental health.

Expenses *State resident tuition:* $1683 full-time, $93 per hour part-time. *Nonresident tuition:* $5219 full-time, ranges from $314 to $324 per hour part-time. *Books and supplies per academic year:* $1200.

Financial Aid Graduate assistantships, nurse traineeships, Federal Nursing Student Loans, institutionally sponsored loans.

MSN Program

Applying *Required:* GRE General Test (minimum combined score of 1000 on analytical and verbal sections), bachelor's degree in nursing, minimum GPA of 3.0, RN license, physical assessment course, statistics course, professional liability/malpractice insurance, essay, interview, 3 letters of recommendation, transcript of college record. *Application deadlines:* 6/23 (fall), 10/20 (spring), 3/29 (summer).

Degree Requirements 46 total credit hours, 40 in nursing, 6 in other specified areas.

CONTINUING EDUCATION PROGRAM

Contact Ms. Jean Ashwill, Director of Continuing Education, School of Nursing, University of Texas at Arlington, Box 19407, Arlington, TX 76019-0407, 817-272-2776. *Fax:* 817-272-5006.

UNIVERSITY OF TEXAS AT AUSTIN
School of Nursing
Austin, Texas

Programs • Generic Baccalaureate • RN Baccalaureate • MSN • Master's for Nurses with Non-Nursing Degrees • MSN/MBA • PhD

The University State-supported coed university. Part of University of Texas System. Founded: 1883. *Primary accreditation:* regional. *Setting:* 350-acre urban campus. *Total enrollment:* 47,905.

The School of Nursing Founded in 1890.

Academic Facilities *Campus library:* 6.5 million volumes.

Student Life *Student services:* health clinic, personal counseling, career counseling, job placement, campus safety program. *International student services:* ESL courses. *Nursing student activities:* Sigma Theta Tau.

Calendar Semesters.

BACCALAUREATE PROGRAMS

Contact Assistant Dean for Student Affairs, School of Nursing, University of Texas at Austin, 1700 Red River Street, Austin, TX 78701-1499, 512-471-7311 Ext. 204. *Fax:* 512-471-4910.

Expenses *State resident tuition:* $1488 full-time, ranges from $32 to $152 per semester hour part-time. *Nonresident tuition:* $5904 full-time, $246 per semester hour part-time.

Financial Aid Institutionally sponsored need-based grants/scholarships, institutionally sponsored non-need grants/scholarships, Federal Perkins Loans, Federal Supplemental Educational Opportunity Grants, Federal PLUS Loans, Federal Stafford Loans. *Application deadline:* 3/31.

Generic Baccalaureate Program (BSN)

Applying *Required:* SAT I or ACT, TOEFL for nonnative speakers of English, minimum college GPA of 2.5, 3 years of high school math, high school foreign language, high school transcript. 69 prerequisite credits must be completed before admission to the nursing program. *Options:* Advanced standing available through credit by exam. *Application deadlines:* 2/1 (fall), 10/1 (spring), 2/1 (summer). *Application fee:* $65.

Degree Requirements 139–140 total credit hours dependent upon track, 67 in nursing.

RN Baccalaureate Program (BSN)

Applying *Required:* SAT I or ACT, TOEFL for nonnative speakers of English, minimum college GPA of 2.5, 3 years of high school math, high school foreign language, high school transcript. *Options:* Advanced standing available through credit by exam. *Application deadlines:* 2/1 (fall), 10/1 (spring), 2/1 (summer). *Application fee:* $65.

Degree Requirements 139–140 total credit hours dependent upon track, 67 in nursing.

MASTER'S PROGRAMS

Contact Graduate Program, School of Nursing, University of Texas at Austin, 1700 Red River Street, Austin, TX 78701-1499, 512-471-7311. *Fax:* 512-471-4910.

Areas of Study Clinical nurse specialist programs in adult health nursing, community health nursing, parent-child nursing, psychiatric–mental health nursing.

Expenses *State resident tuition:* $1392 full-time, ranges from $64 to $184 per semester hour part-time. *Nonresident tuition:* $5004 full-time, $278 per semester hour part-time.

Financial Aid *Application deadline:* 3/31.

MSN Program

Applying *Required:* GRE General Test, bachelor's degree in nursing, minimum GPA of 3.0, letter of recommendation, transcript of college record. *Application deadlines:* 2/1 (fall), 10/1 (spring), 2/1 (summer). *Application fee:* $60.

Degree Requirements 39 total credit hours, 27 in nursing. Thesis is optional.

MASTER'S FOR NURSES WITH NON-NURSING DEGREES PROGRAM (MSN)

Applying *Required:* GRE General Test, minimum GPA of 3.0, RN license, letter of recommendation, transcript of college record. *Application deadlines:* 2/1 (fall), 10/1 (spring), 2/1 (summer).

Degree Requirements Thesis is optional.

MSN/MBA PROGRAM

Applying *Required:* GRE General Test, GMAT, bachelor's degree in nursing, statistics course. *Application deadlines:* 2/1 (fall), 10/1 (spring), 2/1 (summer).

Degree Requirements 72 total credit hours, 27 in nursing.

DOCTORAL PROGRAM

Contact Graduate and International Admissions Center, University of Texas at Austin, PO Box 7608, Austin, TX 78713-7608, 512-471-6500. *Fax:* 512-471-5003.

Areas of Study Advanced practice nursing.

Expenses *State resident tuition:* $1392 full-time, ranges from $64 to $184 per semester hour part-time. *Nonresident tuition:* $5004 full-time, $278 per semester hour part-time.

Financial Aid Grants. *Application deadline:* 3/31.

PHD PROGRAM

Applying *Required:* GRE General Test, master's degree in nursing, statistics course, 3 letters of recommendation, research placement examination, professional background review, professional liability/malpractice insurance, RN license. *Application deadlines:* 2/1 (fall), 10/1 (spring), 2/1 (summer).

Degree Requirements 64 total credit hours; dissertation.

UNIVERSITY OF TEXAS AT EL PASO

College of Nursing and Health Sciences El Paso, Texas

Programs • Generic Baccalaureate • Accelerated RN Baccalaureate • MSN • Post-Master's • Continuing Education

The University State-supported coed university. Part of University of Texas System. Founded: 1913. *Primary accreditation:* regional. *Setting:* 360-acre urban campus. *Total enrollment:* 16,275.

The College of Nursing and Health Sciences Founded in 1972. *Nursing program faculty:* 43 (40% with doctorates).

Academic Facilities *Campus library:* 930,925 volumes (93,092 in nursing). *Nursing school resources:* CAI, computer lab, nursing audiovisuals, interactive nursing skills videos, learning resource lab, clinical simulation lab.

Student Life *Student services:* health clinic, child-care facilities, personal counseling, career counseling, institutionally sponsored work-study program, job placement, special assistance for disabled students, tutoring. *International student services:* counseling/support, special assistance for nonnative speakers of English, ESL courses, work-study, tutoring. *Nursing student activities:* Sigma Theta Tau, student nurses association.

Calendar Semesters.

NURSING STUDENT PROFILE

Undergraduate **Enrollment:** 476
Women: 80%; **Men:** 20%; **Minority:** 65%; **International:** 1%; **Part-time:** 20%
Graduate **Enrollment:** 124
Women: 80%; **Men:** 20%; **Minority:** 45%; **International:** 1%; **Part-time:** 69%

BACCALAUREATE PROGRAMS

Contact Dr. Helen M. Castillo, Chair, Nursing Department, College of Nursing and Health Sciences, University of Texas at El Paso, 1101 North Campbell Street, El Paso, TX 79902, 915-747-8217. *Fax:* 915-747-7207. *E-mail:* hcastill@mail.utep.edu

Expenses *State resident tuition:* $1678 full-time, $461 per semester part-time. *Nonresident tuition:* $6814 full-time, $1745 per semester part-time. *Full-time mandatory fees:* $455–$512. *Part-time mandatory fees:* $114–$264.

Financial Aid Institutionally sponsored need-based grants/scholarships, institutionally sponsored non-need grants/scholarships, Federal Nursing Student Loans, Federal Supplemental Educational Opportunity Grants, Federal Work-Study.

GENERIC BACCALAUREATE PROGRAM (BSN)

Applying *Required:* SAT I, ACT, TOEFL for nonnative speakers of English, 3 years of high school math, 3 years of high school science, high school chemistry, high school biology, high school transcript, written essay. 68 prerequisite credits must be completed before admission to the nursing program. *Options:* Advanced standing available through the following means: advanced placement exams, credit by exam. Course work may be accelerated. May apply for transfer of up to 66 total credits. *Application deadlines:* 7/1 (fall), 11/1 (spring), 4/1 (summer). *Application fee:* $15.

Degree Requirements 136 total credit hours, 68 in nursing.

ACCELERATED RN BACCALAUREATE PROGRAM (BSN)

Applying *Required:* SAT I, ACT, TOEFL for nonnative speakers of English, 3 years of high school math, 3 years of high school science, high school chemistry, high school biology, RN license, diploma or AD in nursing, high school foreign language, high school transcript, transcript of college record. *Options:* Advanced standing available through advanced placement exams. Course work may be accelerated. May apply for transfer of up to 66 total credits. *Application deadlines:* 7/1 (fall), 11/1 (spring), 4/1 (summer). *Application fee:* $15.

Degree Requirements 136 total credit hours, 68 in nursing.

MASTER'S PROGRAMS

Contact Dr. Helen M. Castillo, Chair, Nursing Department, College of Nursing and Health Sciences, University of Texas at El Paso, 1101 North Campbell Street, El Paso, TX 79902, 915-747-8217. *Fax:* 915-747-7207. *E-mail:* hcastill@mail.utep.edu

Areas of Study Clinical nurse specialist programs in adult health nursing, parent-child nursing, psychiatric–mental health nursing, women's health nursing; nurse midwifery; nursing administration; nurse practitioner programs in adult health, child care/pediatrics, community health, family health, women's health.

Expenses *State resident tuition:* $1678 full-time, $461 per semester part-time. *Nonresident tuition:* $6814 full-time, $1745 per semester part-time.

Financial Aid Graduate assistantships, nurse traineeships, Federal Nursing Student Loans, employment opportunities.

MSN PROGRAM

Applying *Required:* GRE General Test, Miller Analogies Test, bachelor's degree in nursing, minimum GPA of 3.0, RN license, physical assessment course, statistics course, professional liability/malpractice insurance, interview, 2 letters of recommendation, transcript of college record. *Application deadlines:* 7/1 (fall), 11/15 (spring), 4/1 (summer). *Application fee:* $15.

Degree Requirements 36–41 total credit hours dependent upon track, 36–41 in nursing. Up to 54 credit hours in nursing for nurse practitioner specialties.

POST-MASTER'S PROGRAM

Applying *Required:* minimum GPA of 3.0, RN license, physical assessment course, statistics course, professional liability/malpractice insurance, interview, 2 letters of recommendation, transcript of college record. *Application deadline:* 7/1. *Application fee:* $15.

Degree Requirements Thesis is optional.

CONTINUING EDUCATION PROGRAM

Contact Ms. Lisa Hennessy, Continuing Education, College of Nursing and Health Sciences, University of Texas at El Paso, 1101 North Campbell street, El Paso, TX 79902, 915-747-7218. *Fax:* 915-747-7207.

UNIVERSITY OF TEXAS AT TYLER

Division of Nursing Tyler, Texas

Programs • Generic Baccalaureate • RN Baccalaureate • MSN • MSN/MBA • Post-Master's

The University State-supported upper-level coed institution. Part of University of Texas System. Founded: 1971. *Primary accreditation:* regional. *Setting:* 200-acre urban campus. *Total enrollment:* 3,789.

The Division of Nursing Founded in 1978.

Academic Facilities *Campus library:* 190,000 volumes; 1,300 periodical subscriptions. *Nursing school resources:* CAI, computer lab, nursing audiovisuals, interactive nursing skills videos, learning resource lab.

Calendar Semesters.

University of Texas at Tyler (continued)

BACCALAUREATE PROGRAMS

Contact Admissions Office, University of Texas at Tyler, Tyler, TX 75799, 903-566-7201.

Expenses *State resident tuition:* $1632 full-time, ranges from $32 to $156 per semester hour part-time. *Nonresident tuition:* $6768 full-time, $282 per semester hour part-time. *Books and supplies per academic year:* ranges from $50 to $125.

Financial Aid Institutionally sponsored need-based grants/scholarships, institutionally sponsored non-need grants/scholarships, Federal Direct Loans, Federal Nursing Student Loans, Federal Pell Grants, Federal Perkins Loans, Federal Work-Study, state aid. *Application deadline:* 7/1.

Generic Baccalaureate Program (BSN)

Applying *Required:* minimum college GPA of 2.75, high school chemistry, high school transcript, transcript of college record, CPR certification, immunizations. *Application deadlines:* 3/15 (fall), 10/15 (spring).

Degree Requirements 54 total credit hours in nursing.

RN Baccalaureate Program (BSN)

Applying *Required:* minimum college GPA of 2.75, RN license, diploma or AD in nursing, transcript of college record. *Application deadlines:* 3/15 (fall), 10/15 (spring).

Degree Requirements 54 total credit hours in nursing.

MASTER'S PROGRAMS

Contact Graduate Coordinator, Division of Nursing, University of Texas at Tyler, Tyler, TX 75799, 903-566-7320. *Fax:* 903-566-2513.

Areas of Study Nurse midwifery; nurse practitioner program in family health.

Expenses *State resident tuition:* $1224 full-time, ranges from $32 to $156 per semester hour part-time. *Nonresident tuition:* $5076 full-time, $282 per semester hour part-time.

MSN Program

Applying *Required:* GRE General Test (minimum combined score of 1000 on three tests) or Miller Analogies Test, bachelor's degree in nursing, minimum GPA of 3.0, RN license, 4 letters of recommendation.

Degree Requirements 38 total credit hours, 35 in nursing, 3 in management. Thesis or professional paper.

MSN/MBA Program

Applying *Required:* GRE General Test or Miller Analogies Test, TOEFL for nonnative speakers of English, GMAT, bachelor's degree in nursing, minimum GPA of 3.0, RN license, statistics course, 4 letters of recommendation, accounting course, computer science course. *Application deadlines:* 3/15 (fall), 10/15 (spring).

Degree Requirements 74 total credit hours, 29 in nursing, 45 in administration.

Post-Master's Program

Applying *Application deadlines:* 3/15 (fall), 10/15 (spring).

Degree Requirements 18 total credit hours, 18 in nursing.

UNIVERSITY OF TEXAS HEALTH SCIENCE CENTER AT SAN ANTONIO

School of Nursing
San Antonio, Texas

Programs • Generic Baccalaureate • Accelerated Baccalaureate • MSN • RN to Master's • BSN to Doctorate • Continuing Education

The University State-supported upper-level specialized coed institution. Part of University of Texas System. Founded: 1976. *Primary accreditation:* regional. *Setting:* 100-acre suburban campus. *Total enrollment:* 2,828.

The School of Nursing Founded in 1969. *Nursing program faculty:* 73 (66% with doctorates). *Off-campus program sites:* Brownsville, Lubbock, Corpus Christi.

Academic Facilities *Campus library:* 205,641 volumes (205,641 in health, 20,564 in nursing); 2,600 periodical subscriptions (150 health-care related). *Nursing school resources:* CAI, computer lab, nursing audiovisuals, interactive nursing skills videos, learning resource lab, electronic classroom.

Student Life *Student services:* health clinic, personal counseling, career counseling, campus safety program, special assistance for disabled students. *International student services:* counseling/support, International Nursing Student Alliance. *Nursing student activities:* Sigma Theta Tau, student nurses association, Latin American Nursing Student Association, Mary Mahoney Nursing Student Association.

Calendar Semesters.

NURSING STUDENT PROFILE

Undergraduate **Enrollment:** 500
Women: 80%; **Men:** 20%; **Minority:** 30%; **International:** 1%; **Part-time:** 5%

Graduate **Enrollment:** 200
Women: 92%; **Men:** 8%; **Minority:** 12%; **International:** 1%; **Part-time:** 80%

BACCALAUREATE PROGRAMS

Contact Ms. Mary Anne Lynch, Assistant to the Registrar, School of Nursing, University of Texas Health Science Center at San Antonio, 7703 Floyd Curl Drive, San Antonio, TX 78284-7702, 210-567-2670.

Expenses *State resident tuition:* $864 full-time, $32 per semester credit hour part-time. *Nonresident tuition:* $6642 full-time, $246 per semester credit hour part-time. *Full-time mandatory fees:* $220–$300. *Part-time mandatory fees:* $100–$200. *Books and supplies per academic year:* ranges from $1000 to $1500.

Financial Aid Institutionally sponsored need-based grants/scholarships, institutionally sponsored non-need grants/scholarships, Federal Nursing Student Loans, Federal Pell Grants, Federal Perkins Loans, Federal Supplemental Educational Opportunity Grants. 50% of undergraduate students in nursing programs received some form of financial aid in 1995–96. *Application deadline:* 6/1.

Generic Baccalaureate Program (BSN)

Applying *Required:* Texas Academic Skills Program test, minimum college GPA of 2.0, 3 letters of recommendation, transcript of college record, minimum 2.3 GPA in 60 hours of prerequisites, non-cognitive questionnaire. 60 prerequisite credits must be completed before admission to the nursing program. *Options:* Course work may be accelerated. May apply for transfer of up to 30 total credits. *Application deadlines:* 4/1 (fall), 10/1 (spring). *Application fee:* $20.

Degree Requirements 120 total credit hours, 54 in nursing.

Accelerated Baccalaureate Program (BSN)

Applying *Required:* Texas academic skills program test, minimum college GPA of 2.0, transcript of college record, prior experience in nursing as RN or LPN with one year clinical experience, minimum 2.3 GPA in 60 hours of prerequisites. 60 prerequisite credits must be completed before admission to the nursing program. *Options:* Advanced standing available through credit by exam. May apply for transfer of up to 0 total credits. *Application deadlines:* 4/1 (fall), 10/1 (spring). *Application fee:* $20.

Degree Requirements 120 total credit hours, 54 in nursing.

MASTER'S PROGRAMS

Contact Ms. Magda Young, Graduate Admissions, Office of Student Services, University of Texas Health Science Center at San Antonio, 7703 Floyd Curl Drive, San Antonio, TX 78284-7702, 210-567-2661. *Fax:* 210-567-2685.

Areas of Study Clinical nurse specialist program in adult health nursing; nursing administration; nursing education; nurse practitioner program in family health.

Expenses *State resident tuition:* $576 full-time, $32 per semester credit hour part-time. *Nonresident tuition:* $4428 full-time, $246 per semester credit hour part-time. *Full-time mandatory fees:* $250–$300. *Part-time mandatory fees:* $100–$200. *Books and supplies per academic year:* ranges from $450 to $1000.

Financial Aid Graduate assistantships, nurse traineeships, Federal Nursing Student Loans, employment opportunities. 20% of master's level students in nursing programs received some form of financial aid in 1995-96. *Application deadline:* 6/1.

MSN Program

Applying *Required:* Miller Analogies Test, GRE General Test (minimum combined score of 1000 on verbal and quantitative sections), bachelor's degree in nursing, minimum GPA of 3.0, RN license, statistics course, 4 letters of recommendation, transcript of college record, CPR certification, computer literacy, immunizations, clinical experience depending on track. *Application deadlines:* 4/1 (fall), 10/1 (spring). *Application fee:* $10.

Degree Requirements 36–53 total credit hours dependent upon track, 30–53 in nursing.

Distance learning Courses provided through video, audio.

RN to Master's Program (MSN)

Applying *Required:* Miller Analogies Test, GRE General Test (minimum combined score of 1000 on verbal and quantitative sections), minimum GPA of 3.0, RN license, statistics course, 4 letters of recommendation, transcript of college record, ADN or diploma in nursing, CPR certification, computer literacy, immunization records. *Application deadlines:* 4/1 (fall), 10/1 (spring). *Application fee:* $10.

Degree Requirements 108–161 total credit hours dependent upon track, 45–72 in nursing.

Distance learning Courses provided through video, audio.

DOCTORAL PROGRAM

Contact Ms. Magda Young, Graduate Admissions, Office of Student Services, University of Texas Health Science Center at San Antonio, 7703 Floyd Curl Drive, San Antonio, TX 78284-7702, 210-567-2661. *Fax:* 210-567-2685.

Areas of Study Nursing research, clinical practice.

Expenses *State resident tuition:* $576 full-time, $32 per semester credit hour part-time. *Nonresident tuition:* $4428 full-time, $246 per semester credit hour part-time. *Full-time mandatory fees:* $250–$300. *Part-time mandatory fees:* $100–$200. *Books and supplies per academic year:* ranges from $900 to $1500.

Financial Aid Graduate assistantships, nurse traineeships, grants, Federal Direct Loans, opportunities for employment. *Application deadline:* 6/1.

BSN to Doctorate Program (PhD)

Applying *Required:* GRE General Test (minimum combined score of 1000 on verbal and quantitative sections), statistics course, interview, 4 letters of recommendation, competitive review by faculty committee, BSN from an NLN-accredited school of nursing, current licensure as RN in Texas, minimum 3.0 GPA. *Application deadline:* 4/1. *Application fee:* $10.

Degree Requirements 80 total credit hours; 18 credit hours in theory/research/science, 14 in clinical practice, 13 in profession/socialization, 14 in support courses, 9 in electives, 12 in dissertation research; dissertation; oral exam; written exam; defense of dissertation.

Distance learning Courses provided through video, audio.

CONTINUING EDUCATION PROGRAM

Contact Ms. Deidre Fisher, Director, Continuing Education, School of Nursing, University of Texas Health Science Center at San Antonio, 7703 Floyd Curl Drive, San Antonio, TX 78284-7946, 210-567-5850. *Fax:* 210-567-5929. *E-mail:* fisherd@uthscasa.edu

UNIVERSITY OF TEXAS–HOUSTON HEALTH SCIENCE CENTER

School of Nursing
Houston, Texas

Programs • Generic Baccalaureate • Accelerated RN Baccalaureate • BSN to Master's • MSN/MPH • Post-Master's • DSN • Continuing Education

The University State-supported upper-level coed institution. Part of University of Texas System. Founded: 1943. *Primary accreditation:* regional. *Total enrollment:* 3,097.

The School of Nursing Founded in 1972. *Nursing program faculty:* 86 (52% with doctorates). *Off-campus program site:* Fort Sam Houston.

Academic Facilities *Campus library:* 254,968 volumes (247,490 in health, 7,478 in nursing); 4,642 periodical subscriptions (4,642 health-care related). *Nursing school resources:* CAI, computer lab, nursing audiovisuals, learning resource lab.

Student Life *Student services:* health clinic, child-care facilities, personal counseling, campus safety program, special assistance for disabled students. *International student services:* counseling/support. *Nursing student activities:* Sigma Theta Tau, student nurses association, student assembly organization.

Calendar Semesters.

NURSING STUDENT PROFILE

Undergraduate **Enrollment:** 172
Women: 88%; **Men:** 12%; **Minority:** 32%; **International:** 2%; **Part-time:** 28%
Graduate **Enrollment:** 450
Women: 79%; **Men:** 21%; **Minority:** 23%; **International:** 1%; **Part-time:** 54%

BACCALAUREATE PROGRAMS

Contact Ms. Eleanor Evans, Pre-Admissions Counselor, School of Nursing, University of Texas-Houston Health Science Center, 1100 Holcombe Boulevard, #6.100, Houston, TX 77030, 713-500-2104. *Fax:* 713-500-2107. *E-mail:* eevans@sonl.nur.uth.tmc.edu

Expenses *State resident tuition:* $1224 full-time, $612 per academic year part-time. *Nonresident tuition:* $8856 full-time, $4428 per academic year part-time. *Full-time mandatory fees:* $349. *Part-time mandatory fees:* $287. *Room and board:* $8240. *Books and supplies per academic year:* ranges from $200 to $500.

Financial Aid Institutionally sponsored need-based grants/scholarships, Federal Nursing Student Loans, Federal Supplemental Educational Opportunity Grants. 94% of undergraduate students in nursing programs received some form of financial aid in 1995–96. *Application deadline:* 5/1.

Generic Baccalaureate Program (BSN)

Applying *Required:* TOEFL for nonnative speakers of English, minimum college GPA of 2.75, interview, written essay, transcript of college record, 3.0 GPA in science courses. 60 prerequisite credits must be completed before admission to the nursing program. *Options:* Course work may be accelerated. May apply for transfer of up to 60 total credits. *Application deadlines:* 9/1 (fall), 11/1 (RN-BSN summer admission). *Application fee:* $10.

Degree Requirements 125 total credit hours, 65 in nursing.

Accelerated RN Baccalaureate Program (BSN)

Applying *Required:* TOEFL for nonnative speakers of English, minimum college GPA of 2.75, RN license, diploma or AD in nursing, interview, written essay, transcript of college record, 3.0 GPA in prerequisite science courses. 60 prerequisite credits must be completed before admission to the nursing program. *Options:* Course work may be accelerated. May apply for transfer of up to 60 total credits. *Application deadline:* 11/1 (summer only). *Application fee:* $10.

Degree Requirements 125 total credit hours, 65 in nursing.

MASTER'S PROGRAMS

Contact Ms. Eleanor Evans, Pre-Admissions Counselor, School of Nursing, University of Texas-Houston Health Science Center, 1100 Holcombe Boulevard, #6.100, Houston, TX 77030, 713-500-2104. *Fax:* 713-500-2107. *E-mail:* eevans@sonl.nur.uth.tmc.edu

Areas of Study Clinical nurse specialist programs in gerontological nursing, oncology nursing, perinatal nursing, psychiatric–mental health nursing, women's health nursing, neonatal nursing, emergency care nursing, acute care; nurse anesthesia; nursing administration; nursing education; nurse practitioner programs in acute care, adult health, child care/pediatrics, emergency care, family health, gerontology, neonatal health, psychiatric–mental health, women's health, oncology, perinatal care.

Expenses *State resident tuition:* $918 full-time, $612 per academic year part-time. *Nonresident tuition:* $6642 full-time, $4428 per academic year part-time. *Full-time mandatory fees:* $349. *Part-time mandatory fees:* $287. *Room and board:* $8240. *Books and supplies per academic year:* ranges from $200 to $500.

Financial Aid Graduate assistantships, nurse traineeships, Federal Nursing Student Loans, institutionally sponsored need-based grants/scholarships. 25% of master's level students in nursing programs received some form of financial aid in 1995-96. *Application deadline:* 5/1.

BSN to Master's Program (MSN)

Applying *Required:* GRE General Test, Miller Analogies Test, TOEFL for nonnative speakers of English, bachelor's degree in nursing, minimum GPA of 3.0, RN license, 1 year of clinical experience, statistics course,

University of Texas–Houston Health Science Center (continued)

professional liability/malpractice insurance, interview, 3 letters of recommendation, transcript of college record. *Application deadlines:* 5/1 (fall), 9/1 (spring), 1/1 (summer). *Application fee:* $50.

Degree Requirements 50 total credit hours, 50 in nursing. Thesis required.

Distance learning Courses provided through teleconference.

MSN/MPH Program

Applying *Required:* GRE General Test, Miller Analogies Test, TOEFL for nonnative speakers of English, bachelor's degree in nursing, minimum GPA of 3.0, RN license, 1 year of clinical experience, statistics course, professional liability/malpractice insurance, interview, 3 letters of recommendation, transcript of college record, must also apply to the School of Public Health. *Application deadlines:* 5/1 (fall), 9/1 (spring), 1/1 (summer). *Application fee:* $50.

Degree Requirements 61 total credit hours, 61 in nursing. Thesis required for dual degree. Thesis required.

Distance learning Courses provided through teleconference.

Post-Master's Program

Applying *Required:* minimum GPA of 3.0, RN license, professional liability/malpractice insurance, interview, 3 letters of recommendation, transcript of college record, MSN. *Application deadlines:* 5/1 (fall), 9/1 (spring), 1/1 (summer). *Application fee:* $50.

Degree Requirements 19–31 total credit hours dependent upon track, 19–31 in nursing.

Distance learning Courses provided through teleconference.

DOCTORAL PROGRAM

Contact Dr. Janet Meininger, Coordinator, DSN Program and Professor, School of Nursing, University of Texas-Houston Health Science Center, 1100 Holcombe Bouelvard, Room #5.518, Houston, TX 77030, 713-500-2124. *Fax:* 713-500-2142. *E-mail:* jmeining@sonl.nur.uth.tmc.edu

Areas of Study Nursing research, clinical practice.

Expenses *State resident tuition:* $918 full-time, $612 per academic year part-time. *Nonresident tuition:* $6642 full-time, $4428 per academic year part-time. *Full-time mandatory fees:* $239. *Books and supplies per academic year:* ranges from $200 to $500.

Financial Aid Graduate assistantships, nurse traineeships, Federal Nursing Student Loans. *Application deadline:* 5/1.

DSN Program

Applying *Required:* GRE General Test, TOEFL for nonnative speakers of English, master's degree in nursing, year of clinical experience, interview, letter of recommendation, vitae. *Application deadline:* 1/1. *Application fee:* $100.

Degree Requirements 65 total credit hours; dissertation; candidacy exam (comprised of written paper and oral exam).

CONTINUING EDUCATION PROGRAM

Contact Dr. Gwendolyn Sherwood, Coordinator of Continuing Education, School of Nursing, University of Texas-Houston Health Science Center, 1100 Holcombe Boulevard, #6.250, Houston, TX 77030, 713-500-2000. *Fax:* 713-500-2026. *E-mail:* ericks@son1.nur.uth.tmc.edu

UNIVERSITY OF TEXAS MEDICAL BRANCH AT GALVESTON

School of Nursing
Galveston, Texas

Programs • Generic Baccalaureate • RN Baccalaureate • MSN • Post-Master's • Continuing Education

The University State-supported upper-level coed institution. Part of University of Texas System. Founded: 1891. *Primary accreditation:* regional. *Setting:* 82-acre small-town campus. *Total enrollment:* 2,249.

The School of Nursing Founded in 1890. *Nursing program faculty:* 88 (62% with doctorates). *Off-campus program sites:* Baytown, Beaumont, Nacogdoches.

Academic Facilities *Campus library:* 241,364 volumes; 2,823 periodical subscriptions. *Nursing school resources:* CAI, computer lab, nursing audiovisuals, interactive nursing skills videos, learning resource lab.

Student Life *Student services:* health clinic, child-care facilities, personal counseling, career counseling, institutionally sponsored work-study program, job placement, campus safety program, special assistance for disabled students. *International student services:* counseling/support, special assistance for nonnative speakers of English, ESL courses. *Nursing student activities:* Sigma Theta Tau, student nurses association.

Calendar Semesters.

NURSING STUDENT PROFILE

Undergraduate **Enrollment:** 311
Women: 85%; **Men:** 15%; **Minority:** 31%; **International:** 0%; **Part-time:** 22%
Graduate **Enrollment:** 172
Women: 89%; **Men:** 11%; **Minority:** 9%; **International:** 0%; **Part-time:** 70%

BACCALAUREATE PROGRAMS

Contact Office of Student Affairs, School of Nursing, University of Texas Medical Branch at Galveston, 301 University Boulevard, Galveston, TX 77555-1029, 409-772-6111. *Fax:* 409-772-8282.

Expenses *State resident tuition:* $768 full-time, $32 per credit hour part-time. *Nonresident tuition:* $5904 full-time, $246 per credit part-time. *Full-time mandatory fees:* $442.

Financial Aid Institutionally sponsored need-based grants/scholarships, institutionally sponsored non-need grants/scholarships, Federal Nursing Student Loans, Federal Supplemental Educational Opportunity Grants, Federal Work-Study.

Generic Baccalaureate Program (BSN)

Applying *Required:* Nursing Entrance Test, minimum college GPA of 2.5, 3 letters of recommendation, written essay, transcript of college record, CPR certification. 60 prerequisite credits must be completed before admission to the nursing program. *Options:* May apply for transfer of up to 97 total credits. *Application deadline:* 3/1. *Application fee:* $10.

Degree Requirements 127 total credit hours, 67 in nursing.

RN Baccalaureate Program (BSN)

Applying *Required:* RN license, written essay, transcript of college record. 60 prerequisite credits must be completed before admission to the nursing program. *Options:* Advanced standing available through advanced placement exams. Course work may be accelerated. May apply for transfer of up to 97 total credits. *Application deadlines:* 3/1 (fall), 11/1 (spring). *Application fee:* $10.

Degree Requirements 127 total credit hours, 67 in nursing.

MASTER'S PROGRAMS

Contact Dr. Jeanette C. Hartshorn, Professor and Associate Dean for Academic Administration, School of Nursing, University of Texas Medical Branch at Galveston, 1100 Mechanic Street, Route J-29, Galveston, TX 77555-1029, 409-772-7311. *Fax:* 409-747-1519. *E-mail:* jhartsho@sonpo.utmb.edu

Areas of Study Nurse midwifery; nursing administration; nursing education; nurse practitioner programs in acute care, adult health, child care/pediatrics, family health, gerontology, neonatal health, women's health.

Expenses *State resident tuition:* $576 full-time, $32 per credit hour part-time. *Nonresident tuition:* $4428 full-time, $246 per credit hour part-time. *Full-time mandatory fees:* $393–$408. *Room and board:* $1745. *Room only:* $400. *Books and supplies per academic year:* ranges from $750 to $900.

Financial Aid Graduate assistantships, nurse traineeships, Federal Nursing Student Loans, employment opportunities. *Application deadline:* 4/1.

MSN Program

Applying *Required:* Miller Analogies Test, GRE General Test (minimum combined score of 1100 on verbal and qualitative sections), bachelor's degree in nursing, minimum GPA of 3.0, RN license, statistics course, professional liability/malpractice insurance, 3 letters of recommendation, transcript of college record. *Application deadlines:* 4/1 (fall), 10/1 (spring). *Application fee:* $25.

Degree Requirements 39–60 total credit hours dependent upon track, 36–60 in nursing.

Distance learning Courses provided through video, audio, computer-based media. Specific degree requirements include acceptance into an official off-site campus.

Post-Master's Program

Applying *Required:* minimum GPA of 3.0, statistics course, professional liability/malpractice insurance, transcript of college record, master's degree in nursing. *Application deadlines:* 4/1 (fall), 10/1 (spring). *Application fee:* $25.

Degree Requirements 33 total credit hours, 33 in nursing.

Distance learning Courses provided through video, audio, computer-based media. Specific degree requirements include acceptance into an official off-site campus.

CONTINUING EDUCATION PROGRAM

Contact Ms. Phyllis Waters, Director of Continuing Education, School of Nursing, University of Texas Medical Branch at Galveston, 1100 Mechanic Street, Route J-29, Galveston, TX 77555-1029, 409-772-4812.

UNIVERSITY OF TEXAS–PAN AMERICAN
Department of Nursing
Edinburg, Texas

Programs • Generic Baccalaureate • RN Baccalaureate • MSN

The University State-supported comprehensive coed institution. Part of University of Texas System. Founded: 1927. *Primary accreditation:* regional. *Setting:* 200-acre rural campus. *Total enrollment:* 13,360.

The Department of Nursing Founded in 1967. *Nursing program faculty:* 17.

Academic Facilities *Campus library:* 324,308 volumes (13,155 in health, 6,000 in nursing); 2,254 periodical subscriptions (239 health-care related).

Calendar Semesters.

BACCALAUREATE PROGRAMS

Contact Coordinator, BSN Program, School of Health Sciences, Department of Nursing, University of Texas-Pan American, 1201 West University Drive, Edinburg, TX 78539, 210-381-3491. *Fax:* 210-381-2384.

Expenses *State resident tuition:* $32 per credit hour. *Nonresident tuition:* $222 per credit hour.

Financial Aid Institutionally sponsored need-based grants/scholarships, institutionally sponsored non-need grants/scholarships, Federal Direct Loans, Federal Pell Grants, Federal Perkins Loans, Federal Supplemental Educational Opportunity Grants, Federal Work-Study, Federal Family Education Loan Program (FFELP). *Application deadline:* 4/15.

Generic Baccalaureate Program (BSN)

Applying *Required:* SAT I or ACT, TOEFL for nonnative speakers of English, Texas Academic Skills Program test, minimum college GPA of 2.5, high school math, high school science, high school foreign language, high school transcript, CPR certification, immunizations. 80 prerequisite credits must be completed before admission to the nursing program. *Application deadlines:* 2/1 (fall), 9/1 (spring), 2/1 (summer).

Degree Requirements 132 total credit hours.

RN Baccalaureate Program (BSN)

Applying *Required:* SAT I or ACT, minimum college GPA of 2.5, RN license, high school transcript, transcript of college record, CPR certification, immunizations. 100 prerequisite credits must be completed before admission to the nursing program. *Options:* Advanced standing available through credit by exam. *Application deadline:* 10/1.

Degree Requirements 132 total credit hours.

MASTER'S PROGRAM

Contact Dr. Barbara Tucker, MSN Coordinator, Health Sciences Building, Room 2.204, Department of Nursing, University of Texas-Pan American, 1201 West University Drive, Edinburg, TX 78539, 210-381-3495. *Fax:* 210-381-2384.

Areas of Study Clinical nurse specialist program in adult health nursing; nursing administration; nursing education.

MSN Program

Applying *Required:* GRE General Test or Miller Analogies Test, bachelor's degree in nursing, minimum GPA of 3.0, physical assessment course, statistics course, 3 letters of recommendation, immunization.

Degree Requirements 43 total credit hours, 43 in nursing. Thesis or project.

WEST TEXAS A&M UNIVERSITY
Division of Nursing
Canyon, Texas

Programs • Generic Baccalaureate • RN Baccalaureate • LPN to Baccalaureate • MSN

The University State-supported comprehensive coed institution. Part of Texas A&M University System. Founded: 1909. *Primary accreditation:* regional. *Setting:* 128-acre small-town campus. *Total enrollment:* 6,630.

The Division of Nursing Founded in 1974. *Nursing program faculty:* 25. *Off-campus program site:* Amarillo.

Academic Facilities *Campus library:* 1.0 million volumes (16,000 in health, 8,000 in nursing); 1,800 periodical subscriptions (64 health-care related). *Nursing school resources:* CAI, computer lab, nursing audiovisuals, interactive nursing skills videos, learning resource lab.

Student Life *Student services:* health clinic, child-care facilities, personal counseling, career counseling, institutionally sponsored work-study program, job placement, campus safety program, special assistance for disabled students. *International student services:* counseling/support, special assistance for nonnative speakers of English, ESL courses. *Nursing student activities:* Sigma Theta Tau, student nurses association.

Calendar Semesters.

NURSING STUDENT PROFILE

Undergraduate **Enrollment:** 480
Women: 78%; **Men:** 22%; **Minority:** 15%; **International:** 1%; **Part-time:** 27%
Graduate **Enrollment:** 96
Women: 93%; **Men:** 7%; **Minority:** 13%; **International:** 0%; **Part-time:** 84%

BACCALAUREATE PROGRAMS

Contact Dr. M. Joleen Walsh, Head, Division of Nursing, West Texas A&M University, 313A Old Main, Canyon, TX 79016-0001, 806-656-2630. *Fax:* 806-656-2632. *E-mail:* jwalsh@wtamu.edu

Expenses *State resident tuition:* $768 full-time, $120 per hour part-time. *Nonresident tuition:* $5904 full-time, $246 per hour part-time. *Full-time mandatory fees:* $433. *Room only:* $1308. *Books and supplies per academic year:* ranges from $200 to $300.

Financial Aid Institutionally sponsored need-based grants/scholarships, institutionally sponsored non-need grants/scholarships, Federal Direct Loans, Federal Perkins Loans, Federal Supplemental Educational Opportunity Grants, Federal Work-Study, state grants and loans. *Application deadline:* 5/1.

Generic Baccalaureate Program (BSN)

Applying *Required:* SAT I or ACT, NLN Admissions Test, minimum college GPA of 2.0, 4 years of high school math, 3 years of high school science, transcript of college record, high school class rank: top 50%, GED certificate or high school transcript. *Options:* May apply for transfer of up to 66 total credits. *Application deadlines:* 2/1 (fall), 10/1 (spring), 2/1 (summer). *Application fee:* $30.

Degree Requirements 130 total credit hours, 109 in nursing.

RN Baccalaureate Program (BSN)

Applying *Required:* SAT I or ACT, minimum college GPA of 2.0, 4 years of high school math, 3 years of high school science, RN license, diploma or AD in nursing, high school transcript, transcript of college record, high school class rank: top 50%. *Options:* Advanced standing available through the following means: advanced placement exams, credit by exam. Course work may be accelerated. *Application deadlines:* 2/1 (fall), 10/1 (spring), 2/1 (summer).

Degree Requirements 130 total credit hours, 40 in nursing.

LPN to Baccalaureate Program (BSN)

Applying *Required:* TOEFL for nonnative speakers of English, NLN Admissions Test, high school transcript, interview, 2 letters of recommendation, transcript of college record. 24 prerequisite credits must be completed before admission to the nursing program. *Options:* Advanced standing available through the following means: advanced placement exams, credit by exam. May apply for transfer of up to 60 total credits. *Application deadlines:* 2/1 (fall), 10/1 (spring), 2/1 (summer). *Application fee:* $30.

Degree Requirements 130 total credit hours, 105 in nursing.

West Texas A&M University (continued)

MASTER'S PROGRAM

Contact Dr. M. Joleen Walsh, Head, Division of Nursing, West Texas A&M University, 313A Old Main, Canyon, TX 79016-0001, 806-656-2630. *Fax:* 806-656-2632.

Areas of Study Nursing administration; nursing education; nurse practitioner program in family health.

Expenses *State resident tuition:* $444 full-time, $120 per credit part-time. *Nonresident tuition:* $3012 full-time, $246 per credit part-time. *Full-time mandatory fees:* $373. *Books and supplies per academic year:* ranges from $250 to $300.

Financial Aid Nurse traineeships, fellowships. *Application deadline:* 5/1.

MSN Program

Applying *Required:* GRE General Test, bachelor's degree in nursing, minimum GPA of 3.0, RN license, statistics course, professional liability/malpractice insurance, 2 letters of recommendation, transcript of college record. *Application deadline:* rolling.

Degree Requirements 38 total credit hours, 32 in nursing.

UTAH

BRIGHAM YOUNG UNIVERSITY
College of Nursing
Provo, Utah

Programs • Generic Baccalaureate • Accelerated RN Baccalaureate • MSN • MSN/MBA • MSN/MPA

The University Independent coed university, affiliated with Church of Jesus Christ of Latter-day Saints. Founded: 1875. *Primary accreditation:* regional. *Setting:* 638-acre suburban campus. *Total enrollment:* 30,465.

The College of Nursing Founded in 1952.

Academic Facilities *Campus library:* 3.3 million volumes (24,471 in health, 3,482 in nursing); 20,000 periodical subscriptions (131 health-care related). *Nursing school resources:* computer lab.

Calendar Semesters.

BACCALAUREATE PROGRAMS

Contact Advisement Center Director, 551 A SWKT, College of Nursing, Brigham Young University, PO Box 25531, Provo, UT 84602, 801-378-7211. *Fax:* 801-378-3198.

Expenses *Tuition:* ranges from $2530 to $3800 full-time, ranges from $130 to $195 per credit hour part-time.

Generic Baccalaureate Program (BS)

Applying *Required:* minimum college GPA of 3.0. *Application deadlines:* 2/15 (fall), 2/15 (spring), 10/1 (summer; 2/15 winter).

Accelerated RN Baccalaureate Program (BS)

Applying *Required:* minimum college GPA of 3.0. *Application deadlines:* 2/15 (fall), 2/15 (spring), 10/1 (summer; 2/15 winter).

MASTER'S PROGRAMS

Contact Graduate Program Secretary, 500 SWKT, College of Nursing, Brigham Young University, Provo, UT 84602, 801-378-4142. *Fax:* 801-378-3198.

Areas of Study Nursing administration; nurse practitioner program in family health.

Expenses *Tuition:* ranges from $2980 to $4470 full-time, ranges from $165 to $248 per credit hour part-time.

MSN Program

Applying *Required:* GRE General Test, bachelor's degree in nursing, minimum GPA of 3.0, RN license, statistics course, professional liability/malpractice insurance, essay, interview, 3 letters of recommendation, resume. *Application deadline:* 2/1.

Degree Requirements 42–48 total credit hours dependent upon track. Thesis required.

MSN/MBA Program

Applying *Required:* GRE General Test, bachelor's degree in nursing, minimum GPA of 3.0, RN license, statistics course, professional liability/malpractice insurance, essay, interview, 3 letters of recommendation, resume. *Application deadline:* 2/1.

MSN/MPA Program

Applying *Required:* GRE General Test, bachelor's degree in nursing, minimum GPA of 3.0, RN license, statistics course, professional liability/malpractice insurance, essay, interview, 3 letters of recommendation, resume. *Application deadline:* 2/1.

UNIVERSITY OF UTAH
College of Nursing
Salt Lake City, Utah

Programs • Generic Baccalaureate • RN Baccalaureate • MS • RN to Master's • Post-Master's • PhD • Postdoctoral • Continuing Education

The University State-supported coed university. Part of Utah System of Higher Education. Founded: 1850. *Primary accreditation:* regional. *Setting:* 1,500-acre urban campus. *Total enrollment:* 25,423.

The College of Nursing Founded in 1942. *Nursing program faculty:* 87 (47% with doctorates). *Off-campus program sites:* Cedar Park, St. George, Sandy.

Academic Facilities *Campus library:* 3.1 million volumes (45,937 in health, 1,755 in nursing); 16,531 periodical subscriptions (1,419 health-care related). *Nursing school resources:* CAI, computer lab, nursing audiovisuals, interactive nursing skills videos, learning resource lab.

Student Life *Student services:* health clinic, personal counseling, career counseling, institutionally sponsored work-study program, campus safety program, special assistance for disabled students. *International student services:* counseling/support, ESL courses. *Nursing student activities:* Sigma Theta Tau, student nurses association.

Calendar Quarters.

NURSING STUDENT PROFILE

Undergraduate **Enrollment:** 274
Women: 83%; **Men:** 17%; **Minority:** 5%; **International:** 1%; **Part-time:** 17%
Graduate **Enrollment:** 247
Women: 89%; **Men:** 11%; **Minority:** 2%; **International:** 4%; **Part-time:** 51%

BACCALAUREATE PROGRAMS

Contact Ms. Tillie Wilber, Academic Adviser, College of Nursing, University of Utah, 25 South Medical Drive, Salt Lake City, UT 84112, 801-581-3414. *Fax:* 801-581-4642. *E-mail:* twilber@nurfac.nurs.utah.edu

Expenses *State resident tuition:* $2112 per academic year. *Nonresident tuition:* $6456 per academic year. *Full-time mandatory fees:* $66. *Room and board:* $4555. *Books and supplies per academic year:* ranges from $500 to $700.

Financial Aid Institutionally sponsored need-based grants/scholarships, institutionally sponsored non-need grants/scholarships, Federal Nursing Student Loans, Federal Pell Grants, Federal Perkins Loans, Federal Supplemental Educational Opportunity Grants, Federal Work-Study. *Application deadline:* 2/1.

Generic Baccalaureate Program (BS)

Applying *Required:* ACT, TOEFL for nonnative speakers of English, TSE for nonnative speakers of English, minimum college GPA of 2.8, 3 letters of recommendation, written essay, transcript of college record, resume. 59 prerequisite credits must be completed before admission to the nursing program. *Options:* Advanced standing available through advanced placement exams. *Application deadlines:* 4/5 (fall), 9/10 (spring), 9/10 (winter).

Degree Requirements 183 total credit hours, 90 in nursing. Minimum 2.0 GPA in all nursing courses.

RN Baccalaureate Program (BS)

Applying *Required:* ACT, TOEFL for nonnative speakers of English, TSE for nonnative speakers of English, minimum college GPA of 3.0, RN license, diploma or AD in nursing, 3 letters of recommendation, written essay, transcript of college record, resume. 59 prerequisite credits must be completed before admission to the nursing program. *Options:* Advanced standing available through advanced placement exams. *Application deadline:* 3/1.

Degree Requirements 183 total credit hours, 45 in nursing.

MASTER'S PROGRAMS

Contact Ms. Joyce Rathbun, Academic Adviser, College of Nursing, University of Utah, 25 South Medical Drive, Salt Lake City, UT 84112, 801-581-3414. *Fax:* 801-581-4642. *E-mail:* jrathbun@nurfac.nurs.utah.edu

Areas of Study Clinical nurse specialist programs in adult health nursing, community health nursing, oncology nursing, pediatric nursing, psychiatric–mental health nursing, clinical informatics nursing; nurse midwifery; nursing administration; nursing education; nurse practitioner programs in acute care, adult health, child care/pediatrics, community health, family health, gerontology, neonatal health, occupational health, psychiatric–mental health, women's health.

Expenses *State resident tuition:* $2820 full-time, ranges from $55 to $59 per credit hour part-time. *Nonresident tuition:* $6651 full-time, ranges from $159 to $163 per credit hour part-time. *Full-time mandatory fees:* $50–$150. *Books and supplies per academic year:* ranges from $400 to $700.

Financial Aid Graduate assistantships, nurse traineeships, fellowships, Federal Nursing Student Loans. *Application deadline:* 7/1.

MS Program

Applying *Required:* GRE General Test, TOEFL for nonnative speakers of English, TSE for nonnative speakers of English, bachelor's degree in nursing, minimum GPA of 3.0, RN license, statistics course, professional liability/malpractice insurance, essay, 3 letters of recommendation, transcript of college record, immunizations. *Application deadline:* 4/1. *Application fee:* $30.

Degree Requirements 45–72 total credit hours dependent upon track, 45–72 in nursing. Thesis or project.

Distance learning Courses provided through video, audio. Specific degree requirements include emphasis in family nurse practitioner and community health tracks; core courses for all tracks available.

RN to Master's Program (MS)

Applying *Required:* GRE General Test, TOEFL for nonnative speakers of English, ACT, TSE for nonnative speakers of English, minimum GPA of 3.0, RN license, 2 years of clinical experience, essay, interview, 3 letters of recommendation, transcript of college record, resume. *Application deadline:* 4/1.

Degree Requirements 228 total credit hours, 135 in nursing. Thesis or project.

Distance learning Courses provided through Ed-Net interactive television. Specific degree requirements include emphasis in family nurse practitioner and community health tracks; core courses for all tracks available.

Post-Master's Program

Applying *Required:* GRE General Test, TOEFL for nonnative speakers of English, TSE for nonnative speakers of English, minimum GPA of 3.0, RN license, statistics course, professional liability/malpractice insurance, essay, 3 letters of recommendation, transcript of college record, immunizations, MS in nursing. *Application deadline:* 4/1. *Application fee:* $30.

DOCTORAL PROGRAM

Contact Dr. Imogene Rigdon, Associate Dean for Academic Affairs, College of Nursing, University of Utah, 25 South Medical Drive, Salt Lake City, UT 84112, 801-581-8480. *Fax:* 801-581-4642. *E-mail:* irigdon@nurfac.nurs.utah.edu

Areas of Study Nursing administration, nursing education, nursing research, clinical practice, information systems.

Expenses *State resident tuition:* $2820 full-time, ranges from $55 to $59 per credit hour part-time. *Nonresident tuition:* $6651 full-time, ranges from $159 to $163 per credit hour part-time. *Full-time mandatory fees:* $50–$75. *Books and supplies per academic year:* ranges from $400 to $700.

Financial Aid Graduate assistantships, fellowships, dissertation grants, opportunities for employment, institutionally sponsored need-based grants/scholarships, institutionally sponsored non-need-based grants/scholarships. *Application deadline:* 7/1.

PhD Program

Applying *Required:* GRE General Test, TOEFL for nonnative speakers of English, TSE for nonnative speakers of English, master's degree in nursing, interview, 3 letters of recommendation, vitae, writing sample, competitive review by faculty committee. *Application deadline:* 2/1. *Application fee:* $30.

Degree Requirements 60 total credit hours; dissertation; oral exam; defense of dissertation; residency; written exam or synthesis course.

POSTDOCTORAL PROGRAM

Contact Dr. Lillian Nail, Associate Dean for Research, College of Nursing, University of Utah, 25 South Medical Drive, Salt Lake City, UT 84112, 801-581-8271. *Fax:* 801-581-4642. *E-mail:* lillian@nurfac.nurs.utah.edu

Areas of Study Nursing interventions.

CONTINUING EDUCATION PROGRAM

Contact Lynn Hollister, Director of Community Service, College of Nursing, University of Utah, 25 South Medical Drive, Salt Lake City, UT 84112, 801-581-8756. *Fax:* 801-581-4642. *E-mail:* lhollist@nurfac.nurs.utah.edu

WEBER STATE UNIVERSITY
Nursing Program
Ogden, Utah

Program • RN Baccalaureate

The University State-supported comprehensive coed institution. Part of Utah System of Higher Education. Founded: 1889. *Primary accreditation:* regional. *Setting:* 422-acre urban campus. *Total enrollment:* 13,996.

The Nursing Program Founded in 1987. *Nursing program faculty:* 48 (10% with doctorates).

▶ ***NOTEWORTHY***

Through 50 departments and programs in 7 colleges, Weber State offers undergraduate liberal education in the arts, humanities, and natural and social sciences as well as vocational and professional programs in the allied health professions, business, education, applied sciences, and technology. The Nursing Program is located in the College of Health Professions. The baccalaureate nursing program is designed for graduates of associate degree and diploma programs. Recognizing that RN students bring a variety of knowledge and expertise to their academic pursuits, the faculty is committed to a flexible program based on individual student needs. The program prepares nurses for increased responsibilities and leadership within the health-care system.

Academic Facilities *Campus library:* 275,000 volumes (700 in health, 800 in nursing); 2,000 periodical subscriptions (120 health-care related). *Nursing school resources:* CAI, computer lab, nursing audiovisuals, interactive nursing skills videos, learning resource lab.

Student Life *Student services:* health clinic, personal counseling, career counseling, institutionally sponsored work-study program, job placement, campus safety program, special assistance for disabled students. *International student services:* counseling/support. *Nursing student activities:* Sigma Theta Tau, student nurses association.

Calendar Quarters.

NURSING STUDENT PROFILE

Undergraduate **Enrollment:** 272
Women: 89%; **Men:** 11%; **Minority:** 2%; **International:** 0%

BACCALAUREATE PROGRAM

Contact Mr. Robert Holt, Admission Counselor, Nursing Program, College of Health Professionals, Weber State University, 3750 Harrison Boulevard, Ogden, UT 84408-3914, 801-626-6128. *Fax:* 801-626-6397. *E-mail:* rholt@weber.edu

Expenses *State resident tuition:* $1863 full-time, $114 per credit hour part-time. *Nonresident tuition:* $5448 full-time, $318 per credit hour part-time. *Full-time mandatory fees:* $150. *Books and supplies per academic year:* $1750.

Financial Aid Institutionally sponsored need-based grants/scholarships, institutionally sponsored non-need grants/scholarships, Federal Nursing Student Loans, Federal Work-Study. *Application deadline:* 5/2.

Weber State University (continued)

RN Baccalaureate Program (BSN)

Applying *Required:* ACT, RN license, diploma or AD in nursing, 3 letters of recommendation, transcript of college record. *Options:* Advanced standing available through credit by exam. Course work may be accelerated. May apply for transfer of up to 132 total credits. *Application deadline:* 4/1. *Application fee:* $20.

Degree Requirements 183 total credit hours, 51 in nursing.

WESTMINSTER COLLEGE OF SALT LAKE CITY

St. Mark's Westminster School of Nursing
Salt Lake City, Utah

Programs • Generic Baccalaureate • Accelerated RN Baccalaureate • BSN to Master's

The College Independent comprehensive coed institution. Founded: 1875. *Primary accreditation:* regional. *Setting:* 27-acre urban campus. *Total enrollment:* 2,009.

The St. Mark's Westminster School of Nursing Founded in 1968. *Nursing program faculty:* 25 (20% with doctorates).

Academic Facilities *Campus library:* 87,738 volumes (3,700 in health); 419 periodical subscriptions (40 health-care related). *Nursing school resources:* CAI, computer lab, nursing audiovisuals, interactive nursing skills videos, learning resource lab.

Student Life *Student services:* personal counseling, career counseling, institutionally sponsored work-study program, job placement, campus safety program, special assistance for disabled students. *International student services:* counseling/support, special assistance for nonnative speakers of English, ESL courses. *Nursing student activities:* Sigma Theta Tau, nursing club, student nurses association.

Calendar Semesters.

NURSING STUDENT PROFILE

Undergraduate **Enrollment:** 215
Women: 91%; **Men:** 9%; **Minority:** 8%; **International:** 0%; **Part-time:** 17%
Graduate **Enrollment:** 29
Women: 97%; **Men:** 3%; **Minority:** 11%; **International:** 0%; **Part-time:** 7%

BACCALAUREATE PROGRAMS

Contact Dr. A. Gretchen McNeely, Dean, St. Mark's Westminster School of Nursing, Westminster College of Salt Lake City, 1840 South 1300, East, Salt Lake City, UT 84105, 801-488-4234. *Fax:* 801-466-6916. *E-mail:* g-mcneel@wcslc.edu

Expenses *Tuition:* $10,200 full-time, $340 per hour part-time. *Full-time mandatory fees:* $70–$105. *Part-time mandatory fees:* $15–$25. *Room and board:* $4358–$5328. *Books and supplies per academic year:* $600.

Financial Aid Institutionally sponsored need-based grants/scholarships, institutionally sponsored non-need grants/scholarships, Federal Direct Loans, Federal Perkins Loans, Federal Supplemental Educational Opportunity Grants, Federal Work-Study. 87% of undergraduate students in nursing programs received some form of financial aid in 1995–96.

Generic Baccalaureate Program (BSN)

Applying *Required:* SAT I or ACT, TOEFL or Michigan English Language Assessment Battery for nonnative speakers of English, minimum college GPA of 2.5, 3 letters of recommendation, written essay, transcript of college record, goals statement. 41 prerequisite credits must be completed before admission to the nursing program. *Options:* Advanced standing available through advanced placement exams. May apply for transfer of up to 88 total credits. *Application deadline:* 10/10.

Degree Requirements 124 total credit hours, 57 in nursing.

Accelerated RN Baccalaureate Program (BSN)

Applying *Required:* SAT I or ACT, TOEFL or Michigan English Language Assessment Battery for nonnative speakers of English, minimum college GPA of 2.5, RN license, diploma or AD in nursing, 3 letters of recommendation, written essay, transcript of college record, academic progression plan. 42 prerequisite credits must be completed before admission to the nursing program. *Options:* Advanced standing available through the following means: advanced placement exams, credit by exam. Course work may be accelerated. May apply for transfer of up to 88 total credits. *Application deadline:* rolling.

Degree Requirements 124 total credit hours, 28 in nursing. 36 credit hours in residence.

MASTER'S PROGRAM

Contact Nick McClure, Associate Director of Admissions, St. Mark's-Westminster School of Nursing, Westminster College of Salt Lake City, 1840 South 1300 East, Salt Lake City, UT 84105, 800-748-4753. *Fax:* 801-466-6916. *E-mail:* n-mcclur@wcslc.edu

Areas of Study Nurse practitioner program in family health.

Expenses *Tuition:* $382 per hour. *Part-time mandatory fees:* $86. *Room and board:* $4358–$5328. *Books and supplies per academic year:* ranges from $400 to $600.

Financial Aid Federal Direct Loans, institutionally sponsored loans, institutionally sponsored need-based grants/scholarships, institutionally sponsored non-need-based grants/scholarships. 41% of master's level students in nursing programs received some form of financial aid in 1995-96.

BSN to Master's Program (MSN)

Applying *Required:* bachelor's degree in nursing, minimum GPA of 3.0, RN license, 1 year of clinical experience, physical assessment course, statistics course, professional liability/malpractice insurance, essay, 3 letters of recommendation, transcript of college record, resume/vita. *Application deadline:* 3/15. *Application fee:* $25.

Degree Requirements 38 total credit hours, 34 in nursing.

VERMONT

NORWICH UNIVERSITY

Division of Nursing
Montpelier, Vermont

Program • RN Baccalaureate

The University Independent comprehensive coed institution. Founded: 1819. *Primary accreditation:* regional. *Setting:* 1,125-acre small-town campus. *Total enrollment:* 2,556.

The Division of Nursing Founded in 1961.

Academic Facilities *Campus library:* 230,000 volumes; 1,300 periodical subscriptions.

Calendar Semesters.

BACCALAUREATE PROGRAM

Contact Office of Admission, Division of Nursing, Norwich University, Vermont College, Montpelier, VT 05602.

Expenses *Tuition:* ranges from $14,000 to $15,000 full-time, $365 per credit hour part-time.

Financial Aid Institutionally sponsored need-based grants/scholarships, institutionally sponsored non-need grants/scholarships, Federal Perkins Loans, Federal Supplemental Educational Opportunity Grants, Federal Work-Study, Federal PLUS Loans, Federal Stafford Loans.

RN Baccalaureate Program (BSN)

Applying *Required:* SAT I or ACT, minimum college GPA of 2.0, 3 years of high school math, 3 years of high school science, RN license, diploma or AD in nursing, high school transcript, letter of recommendation, transcript of college record. *Options:* Advanced standing available through credit by exam. May apply for transfer of up to 76 total credits. *Application deadline:* rolling.

Degree Requirements 123 total credit hours, 65 in nursing.

UNIVERSITY OF VERMONT
School of Nursing
Burlington, Vermont

Programs • Generic Baccalaureate • RN Baccalaureate • MS • Master's for Nurses with Non-Nursing Degrees • Post-Master's

The University State-supported coed university. Founded: 1791. *Primary accreditation:* regional. *Setting:* 425-acre small-town campus. *Total enrollment:* 9,111.

The School of Nursing Founded in 1943. *Nursing program faculty:* 24.

▶ ***NOTEWORTHY***

The baccalaureate program at the University of Vermont is designed to address the needs of RNs as well as basic students. Assessment of prior learning is key to placement within the program. The master's program focuses on clinical specialization. Three tracks are offered: community health, adult health, and primary care. Students in the primary care track complete practitioner requirements for ANP or FNP certification. Students completing the adult or community health track are eligible for CNS certification. In addition to accepting students with a BSN, the RN with a non-nursing baccalaureate may apply. Part-time study and evening courses are available.

Academic Facilities *Campus library:* 1.1 million volumes (104,338 in health, 7,800 in nursing); 6,239 periodical subscriptions (1,300 health-care related). *Nursing school resources:* CAI, computer lab, nursing audiovisuals, interactive nursing skills videos, learning resource lab.

Student Life *Student services:* health clinic, child-care facilities, personal counseling, career counseling, institutionally sponsored work-study program, job placement, campus safety program, special assistance for disabled students, learning co-op. *International student services:* counseling/support, special assistance for nonnative speakers of English, learning co-op. *Nursing student activities:* Sigma Theta Tau, student nurses association.

Calendar Semesters.

NURSING STUDENT PROFILE

Undergraduate
Women: 93%; **Men:** 7%; **Minority:** 3%; **International:** 2%; **Part-time:** 10%
Graduate **Enrollment:** 42
Women: 98%; **Men:** 2%; **Part-time:** 50%

BACCALAUREATE PROGRAMS

Contact Dr. Carol Gilbert, Associate Dean, Rowell Building, Room 216, School of Nursing, University of Vermont, Burlington, VT 05405-0068, 802-656-3830. *Fax:* 802-656-8306. *E-mail:* ashansen@zoo.uvm.edu

Expenses *State resident tuition:* $6732 full-time, $281 per credit part-time. *Nonresident tuition:* $16,824 full-time, $701 per credit part-time.

Financial Aid *Application deadline:* 3/1.

Generic Baccalaureate Program (BSN)

Applying *Required:* SAT I or ACT, 3 years of high school math, 3 years of high school science, high school chemistry, high school biology. *Application deadlines:* 2/1 (fall), 11/1 (spring).

RN Baccalaureate Program (BSN)

Applying *Required:* SAT I or ACT, minimum college GPA of 2.5, 3 years of high school math, 3 years of high school science, high school chemistry, high school biology, RN license. *Application deadline:* 2/1.

MASTER'S PROGRAMS

Contact Dr. Carol Gilbert, Chairperson, Rowell Building, Room 216, School of Nursing, University of Vermont, Burlington, VT 05405-0068, 802-656-3830. *Fax:* 802-656-8306.

Areas of Study Clinical nurse specialist programs in adult health nursing, community health nursing; nurse practitioner program in primary care.

Expenses *State resident tuition:* $281 per credit. *Nonresident tuition:* $701 per credit.

MS Program

Applying *Required:* GRE General Test, bachelor's degree in nursing, minimum GPA of 3.0, RN license, statistics course, 3 letters of recommendation. *Application deadlines:* 4/1 (fall), 11/15 (spring). *Application fee:* $25.

Degree Requirements 42 total credit hours. Thesis, project, or comprehensive exam.

Master's for Nurses with Non-Nursing Degrees Program (MS)

Applying *Required:* GRE General Test, bachelor's degree, minimum GPA of 3.0, RN license, statistics course, 3 letters of recommendation. *Application deadlines:* 4/1 (fall), 11/15 (spring). *Application fee:* $25.

Degree Requirements 42 total credit hours. Thesis, project, or comprehensive exam.

Post-Master's Program

Applying *Required:* minimum GPA of 3.0, 3 letters of recommendation, master's degree in nursing. *Application deadline:* 4/1. *Application fee:* $30.

Degree Requirements 30 total credit hours. Project.

VIRGINIA

CHRISTOPHER NEWPORT UNIVERSITY
Department of Nursing
Newport News, Virginia

Programs • Generic Baccalaureate • RN Baccalaureate • BSN to Master's

The University State-supported comprehensive coed institution. Founded: 1961. *Primary accreditation:* regional. *Setting:* 113-acre suburban campus. *Total enrollment:* 4,558.

The Department of Nursing Founded in 1986. *Nursing program faculty:* 7 (43% with doctorates).

Academic Facilities *Campus library:* 305,000 volumes (1,000 in nursing); 1,381 periodical subscriptions (60 health-care related). *Nursing school resources:* CAI, computer lab, nursing audiovisuals, learning resource lab.

Student Life *Student services:* health clinic, personal counseling, career counseling, institutionally sponsored work-study program, job placement, campus safety program, special assistance for disabled students. *International student services:* counseling/support. *Nursing student activities:* nursing club, student nurses association, Nursing Honor Society.

Calendar Semesters.

NURSING STUDENT PROFILE

Undergraduate **Enrollment:** 240
Women: 97%; **Men:** 3%; **Minority:** 20%; **International:** 0%; **Part-time:** 70%
Graduate **Enrollment:** 12
Women: 92%; **Men:** 8%; **Minority:** 13%; **Part-time:** 92%

BACCALAUREATE PROGRAMS

Contact Ms. Suzanne Perini, Senior Secretary, Department of Nursing, Christopher Newport University, 50 Shoe Lane, Newport News, VA 23606-2998, 757-594-7252. *Fax:* 757-594-7862.

Expenses *State resident tuition:* $1529 full-time, $139 per credit part-time. *Nonresident tuition:* $3641 full-time, $331 per credit part-time. *Full-time mandatory fees:* $40. *Books and supplies per academic year:* $250.

Financial Aid Institutionally sponsored need-based grants/scholarships, institutionally sponsored non-need grants/scholarships, Federal Nursing Student Loans, Federal Supplemental Educational Opportunity Grants, Federal Work-Study, private foundation scholarships.

Generic Baccalaureate Program (BSN)

Applying *Required:* SAT I, minimum college GPA of 2.5, high school chemistry, high school transcript, transcript of college record, community service. 60 prerequisite credits must be completed before admission to the nursing program. *Options:* Advanced standing available through the following means: advanced placement exams, credit by exam. May apply for transfer of up to 92 total credits. *Application deadline:* rolling. *Application fee:* $20.

Degree Requirements 120 total credit hours, 61 in nursing.

RN Baccalaureate Program (BSN)

Applying *Required:* minimum college GPA of 2.5, RN license, diploma or AD in nursing, transcript of college record, community service. 60

Christopher Newport University (continued)
prerequisite credits must be completed before admission to the nursing program. *Options:* May apply for transfer of up to 92 total credits. *Application deadline:* rolling. *Application fee:* $20.

Degree Requirements 120 total credit hours, 29 in nursing.

MASTER'S PROGRAM

Contact Dr. Karin Polifko-Harris, Graduate Nursing Program Director, 50 Shoe Lane, Newport News, VA 23606, 757-594-7252. *Fax:* 757-594-7862.

Expenses *State resident tuition:* $139 per credit. *Nonresident tuition:* $331 per credit.

BSN to Master's Program (MSN)

Applying *Required:* GRE General Test, bachelor's degree in nursing, minimum GPA, RN license, 1 year of clinical experience, physical assessment course, statistics course, professional liability/malpractice insurance, 3 letters of recommendation, transcript of college record. *Application deadline:* rolling.

Degree Requirements 40 total credit hours, 28 in nursing, 12 in organization theory. Thesis required.

EASTERN MENNONITE UNIVERSITY
Nursing Department
Harrisonburg, Virginia

Programs • Generic Baccalaureate • RN Baccalaureate

The University Independent Mennonite comprehensive coed institution. Founded: 1917. *Primary accreditation:* regional. *Setting:* 92-acre small-town campus. *Total enrollment:* 1,182.

The Nursing Department Founded in 1967. *Nursing program faculty:* 9 (33% with doctorates).

Academic Facilities *Campus library:* 139,229 volumes (950 in health, 2,700 in nursing); 1,119 periodical subscriptions (54 health-care related). *Nursing school resources:* CAI, computer lab, nursing audiovisuals, interactive nursing skills videos.

Student Life *Student services:* health clinic, personal counseling, career counseling, institutionally sponsored work-study program, job placement. *International student services:* counseling/support, ESL courses. *Nursing student activities:* nursing club.

Calendar Semesters.

NURSING STUDENT PROFILE

Undergraduate **Enrollment:** 114
Women: 91%; **Men:** 9%; **Minority:** 4%; **International:** 0%; **Part-time:** 1%

BACCALAUREATE PROGRAMS

Contact Dr. Marie S. Morris, Head, Nursing Department, Eastern Mennonite College, 1200 Park Road, Harrisonburg, VA 22801, 540-432-4186. *Fax:* 540-432-4444.

Expenses *Tuition:* $11,130 full-time, $430 per semester hour part-time. *Full-time mandatory fees:* $30–$100. *Room and board:* $4200. *Books and supplies per academic year:* ranges from $132 to $818.

Financial Aid Institutionally sponsored need-based grants/scholarships, institutionally sponsored non-need grants/scholarships, Federal Direct Loans, Federal Nursing Student Loans, Federal Perkins Loans, Federal Supplemental Educational Opportunity Grants, Federal Work-Study. 100% of undergraduate students in nursing programs received some form of financial aid in 1995–96. *Application deadline:* 5/1.

Generic Baccalaureate Program (BSN)

Applying *Required:* SAT I or ACT, TOEFL for nonnative speakers of English, minimum high school GPA of 2.0, minimum college GPA of 2.0, high school chemistry, high school biology, high school transcript, 2 letters of recommendation, written essay, transcript of college record. 30 prerequisite credits must be completed before admission to the nursing program. *Options:* Course work may be accelerated. *Application deadline:* rolling. *Application fee:* $15.

Degree Requirements 128 total credit hours, 56 in nursing.

RN Baccalaureate Program (BS)

Applying *Required:* SAT I, ACT, TOEFL for nonnative speakers of English, minimum high school GPA of 2.0, minimum college GPA of 2.0, RN license, diploma or AD in nursing, high school transcript, 2 letters of recommendation, written essay, minimum college GPA of 2.4 for nursing courses at the junior level. 30 prerequisite credits must be completed before admission to the nursing program. *Options:* Advanced standing available through credit by exam. Course work may be accelerated. May apply for transfer of up to 65 total credits. *Application deadline:* rolling. *Application fee:* $15.

Degree Requirements 128 total credit hours, 56 in nursing.

GEORGE MASON UNIVERSITY
College of Nursing and Health Science
Fairfax, Virginia

Programs • Generic Baccalaureate • Accelerated RN Baccalaureate • LPN to Baccalaureate • Master's for Nurses with Non-Nursing Degrees • MSN/MBA • PhD

The University State-supported coed university. Founded: 1957. *Primary accreditation:* regional. *Setting:* 677-acre suburban campus. *Total enrollment:* 24,172.

The College of Nursing and Health Science Founded in 1993. *Nursing program faculty:* 68 (47% with doctorates).

Academic Facilities *Campus library:* 900,000 volumes (16,172 in nursing); 9,200 periodical subscriptions (200 health-care related).

Calendar Semesters.

BACCALAUREATE PROGRAMS

Contact Mrs. Rosemarie Brenkus, Coordinator, Student Academic Affairs, College of Nursing and Health Science, George Mason University, Mailstop 3C4, 4400 University Drive, Fairfax, VA 22030-4444, 703-993-1914. *Fax:* 703-993-1942. *E-mail:* rbrenkus@osfi.gmu.edu

Expenses *State resident tuition:* $4248 full-time, $177 per credit hour part-time. *Nonresident tuition:* $11,952 full-time, $498 per credit hour part-time.

Generic Baccalaureate Program (BSN)

Applying *Required:* SAT I or ACT, TOEFL for nonnative speakers of English, 2 years of high school math, high school foreign language, high school transcript, interview, written essay, transcript of college record, high school class rank: top 50%. *Application deadlines:* 2/1 (fall), 11/1 (spring), 3/15 (transfer students - fall admission). *Application fee:* $30.

Degree Requirements 120 total credit hours, 57–60 in nursing.

Accelerated RN Baccalaureate Program (BSN)

Applying *Required:* SAT I or ACT. *Application deadlines:* 2/1 (fall), 11/1 (spring), 3/15 (transfer students - fall admission). *Application fee:* $30.

Degree Requirements 120 total credit hours, 57–60 in nursing.

LPN to Baccalaureate Program (BSN)

Applying *Required:* SAT I or ACT. *Application deadlines:* 2/1 (fall), 11/1 (spring), 3/15 (transfer students - fall admission). *Application fee:* $30.

Degree Requirements 120 total credit hours, 57–60 in nursing.

MASTER'S PROGRAMS

Contact Associate Dean, Graduate Programs and Research, College of Nursing and Health Science, George Mason University, Mailstop 3C4, 4400 University Drive, Fairfax, VA 22030-4444, 703-993-1913. *Fax:* 703-993-1942.

Areas of Study Nursing administration; nurse practitioner programs in adult health, family health, gerontology, primary care.

Expenses *State resident tuition:* $4248 full-time, $177 per credit hour part-time. *Nonresident tuition:* $11,952 full-time, $498 per credit hour part-time.

Master's for Nurses with Non-Nursing Degrees Program (MSN)

Applying *Required:* GRE General Test, TOEFL for nonnative speakers of English, bachelor's degree, minimum GPA of 3.0, 1 year of clinical experience, statistics course, professional liability/malpractice insurance,

3 letters of recommendation, transcript of college record, undergraduate research course, immunizations. *Application deadlines:* 2/1 (fall), 11/1 (spring). *Application fee:* $30.

Degree Requirements 36–42 total credit hours dependent upon track.

MSN/MBA Program

Applying *Required:* TOEFL for nonnative speakers of English, GMAT, bachelor's degree in nursing, minimum GPA of 3.2, 1 year of clinical experience, statistics course, professional liability/malpractice insurance, 3 letters of recommendation, transcript of college record, calculus, immunizations. *Application deadlines:* 2/1 (fall), 11/1 (spring). *Application fee:* $30.

Degree Requirements 57 total credit hours.

DOCTORAL PROGRAM

Contact Associate Dean, Graduate Programs and Research, College of Nursing and Health Science, George Mason University, Mailstop 3C4, 4400 University Place, Fairfax, VA 22030-4444, 703-993-1947. *Fax:* 703-993-1942.

Expenses *State resident tuition:* $4248 full-time, $177 per credit hour part-time. *Nonresident tuition:* $11,952 full-time, $498 per credit hour part-time.

Financial Aid Grants.

PhD Program

Applying *Required:* Miller Analogies Test, TOEFL for nonnative speakers of English, master's degree, 1 year of clinical experience, interview, 3 letters of recommendation, writing sample, licensure to practice professional nursing. *Application deadline:* 2/1. *Application fee:* $30.

Degree Requirements dissertation; oral exam.

HAMPTON UNIVERSITY
School of Nursing
Hampton, Virginia

Programs • Generic Baccalaureate • RN Baccalaureate • LPN to Baccalaureate • MS

The University Independent comprehensive coed institution. Founded: 1868. *Primary accreditation:* regional. *Setting:* 210-acre urban campus. *Total enrollment:* 6,035.

The School of Nursing Founded in 1944.

Academic Facilities *Campus library:* 393,247 volumes (125 in nursing); 1,152 periodical subscriptions.

Calendar Semesters.

BACCALAUREATE PROGRAMS

Contact Chairperson, School of Nursing, Hampton University, Hampton, VA 23668, 804-727-5251. *Fax:* 804-874-9412.

Expenses *Tuition:* $12,826 full-time, $200 per credit hour part-time.

Financial Aid *Application deadline:* 3/31.

Generic Baccalaureate Program (BS)

Applying *Required:* SAT I or ACT, TOEFL for nonnative speakers of English, minimum high school GPA of 2.0, 3 years of high school math, high school chemistry, high school biology, high school foreign language, high school transcript. *Options:* Advanced standing available through the following means: advanced placement exams, credit by exam. *Application deadlines:* 6/1 (fall), 12/15 (spring). *Application fee:* $15.

Degree Requirements 130 total credit hours, 68 in nursing. Comprehensive exam.

RN Baccalaureate Program (BS)

Applying *Required:* minimum college GPA of 2.3, RN license, diploma or AD in nursing, transcript of college record. *Options:* Advanced standing available through credit by exam. *Application deadlines:* 6/1 (fall), 12/15 (spring). *Application fee:* $15.

Degree Requirements 130 total credit hours, 60 in nursing. Comprehensive exam.

LPN to Baccalaureate Program (BS)

Applying *Required:* diploma or AD in nursing, transcript of college record, LPN license. *Options:* Advanced standing available through credit by exam. *Application deadlines:* 6/1 (fall), 12/15 (spring). *Application fee:* $15.

Degree Requirements 130 total credit hours, 59 in nursing. Comprehensive exam.

MASTER'S PROGRAM

Contact Chairperson, Department of Graduate Nursing Education, School of Nursing, Hampton University, Hampton, VA 23668, 804-727-5780. *Fax:* 804-874-9412.

Areas of Study Clinical nurse specialist programs in adult health nursing, community health nursing, psychiatric–mental health nursing; nursing administration; nursing education; nurse practitioner programs in family health, gerontology.

Expenses *Tuition:* $12,826 full-time, $200 per credit part-time.

MS Program

Applying *Required:* GRE General Test, TOEFL for nonnative speakers of English, California psychological inventory, bachelor's degree in nursing, minimum GPA of 3.0, RN license, 1 year of clinical experience, physical assessment course, statistics course, interview, 2 letters of recommendation, transcript of college record.

Degree Requirements 47–50 total credit hours dependent upon track.

JAMES MADISON UNIVERSITY
Department of Nursing
Harrisonburg, Virginia

Programs • Generic Baccalaureate • RN Baccalaureate • Baccalaureate for Second Degree • LPN to Baccalaureate

The University State-supported comprehensive coed institution. Founded: 1908. *Primary accreditation:* regional. *Setting:* 472-acre small-town campus. *Total enrollment:* 11,927.

The Department of Nursing Founded in 1980. *Nursing program faculty:* 8 (37% with doctorates).

Academic Facilities *Campus library:* 567,577 volumes (67,716 in health, 12,054 in nursing); 2,298 periodical subscriptions (129 health-care related). *Nursing school resources:* CAI, computer lab, nursing audiovisuals, interactive nursing skills videos, learning resource lab.

Student Life *Student services:* health clinic, personal counseling, career counseling, institutionally sponsored work-study program, job placement, campus safety program, special assistance for disabled students. *International student services:* counseling/support, special assistance for nonnative speakers of English, ESL courses. *Nursing student activities:* nursing club, student nurses association.

Calendar Semesters.

NURSING STUDENT PROFILE

Undergraduate **Enrollment:** 212
Women: 97%; **Men:** 3%; **Minority:** 6%; **International:** 0%; **Part-time:** 1%

BACCALAUREATE PROGRAMS

Contact Dr. Vida S. Huber, Head, Harrison Annex, Office B8, Department of Nursing, James Madison University, Harrisonburg, VA 22807, 703-568-6314. *Fax:* 703-568-7896. *E-mail:* huberrs@jmu.edu

Expenses *State resident tuition:* $4104 full-time, $1701 per semester part-time. *Nonresident tuition:* $8580 full-time, $3355 per semester part-time. *Full-time mandatory fees:* $25. *Part-time mandatory fees:* $25. *Room and board:* $4666. *Books and supplies per academic year:* ranges from $400 to $700.

Financial Aid Institutionally sponsored need-based grants/scholarships, institutionally sponsored non-need grants/scholarships, Federal Direct Loans, Federal Nursing Student Loans, Federal Pell Grants, Federal Perkins Loans, Federal Supplemental Educational Opportunity Grants, Federal Work-Study. *Application deadline:* 1/15.

Generic Baccalaureate Program (BSN)

Applying *Required:* SAT I, minimum college GPA of 2.7, written essay, transcript of college record. 31 prerequisite credits must be completed before admission to the nursing program. *Options:* Advanced standing available through the following means: advanced placement exams,

James Madison University (continued)

advanced placement without credit, credit by exam. *Application deadlines:* 11/15 (fall), 11/1 (spring), 2/1 (transfer applicants). *Application fee:* $25.

Degree Requirements 120 total credit hours, 61 in nursing.

RN Baccalaureate Program (BSN)

Applying *Required:* SAT I, minimum college GPA of 2.7, RN license, diploma or AD in nursing, written essay, transcript of college record. 31 prerequisite credits must be completed before admission to the nursing program. *Options:* Advanced standing available through the following means: advanced placement exams, advanced placement without credit, credit by exam. Course work may be accelerated. *Application deadlines:* 1/15 (fall), 11/1 (spring), 2/1 (transfer applicants). *Application fee:* $25.

Degree Requirements 120 total credit hours, 61 in nursing.

Baccalaureate for Second Degree Program (BSN)

Applying *Required:* minimum college GPA of 2.7, written essay, transcript of college record. 31 prerequisite credits must be completed before admission to the nursing program. *Options:* Advanced standing available through the following means: advanced placement exams, advanced placement without credit, credit by exam. *Application deadlines:* 1/15 (fall), 11/1 (spring), 2/1 (transfer applicants). *Application fee:* $25.

Degree Requirements 61 total credit hours in nursing.

LPN to Baccalaureate Program (BSN)

Applying *Required:* SAT I, minimum college GPA of 2.7, written essay, transcript of college record. 31 prerequisite credits must be completed before admission to the nursing program. *Options:* Advanced standing available through the following means: advanced placement exams, advanced placement without credit, credit by exam. *Application deadlines:* 1/15 (fall), 11/1 (spring). *Application fee:* $25.

Degree Requirements 120 total credit hours, 61 in nursing.

LIBERTY UNIVERSITY

Department of Nursing
Lynchburg, Virginia

Programs • Generic Baccalaureate • RN Baccalaureate • LPN to Baccalaureate

The University Independent nondenominational comprehensive coed institution. Founded: 1971. *Primary accreditation:* regional and TRACS. *Setting:* 160-acre suburban campus. *Total enrollment:* 5,138.

The Department of Nursing Founded in 1987. *Nursing program faculty:* 10 (20% with doctorates).

Academic Facilities *Campus library:* 300,000 volumes (3,632 in health, 3,000 in nursing); 46 health-care related periodical subscriptions. *Nursing school resources:* CAI, computer lab, nursing audiovisuals, interactive nursing skills videos, learning resource lab.

Student Life *Student services:* health clinic, personal counseling, career counseling, institutionally sponsored work-study program, job placement, campus safety program, special assistance for disabled students. *International student services:* counseling/support, special assistance for nonnative speakers of English, ESL courses. *Nursing student activities:* nursing club, student nurses association.

Calendar Semesters.

NURSING STUDENT PROFILE

Undergraduate **Enrollment:** 333
Women: 85%; **Men:** 15%; **Minority:** 4%; **International:** 10%; **Part-time:** 6%

BACCALAUREATE PROGRAMS

Contact Dr. Dea Britt, Chair, Department of Nursing, 1971 University Boulevard, Lynchburg, VA 24502-2269, 804-582-2519. *Fax:* 804-582-2554.

Expenses *Tuition:* $7350 full-time, $245 per credit hour part-time. *Full-time mandatory fees:* $360–$400. *Room and board:* $4600. *Books and supplies per academic year:* ranges from $250 to $350.

Financial Aid Institutionally sponsored need-based grants/scholarships, institutionally sponsored non-need grants/scholarships, Federal Nursing Student Loans, Federal Supplemental Educational Opportunity Grants, Federal Work-Study. 80% of undergraduate students in nursing programs received some form of financial aid in 1995–96. *Application deadline:* 4/1.

Generic Baccalaureate Program (BSN)

Applying *Required:* SAT I, ACT, TOEFL for nonnative speakers of English, minimum college GPA of 2.75, 3 years of high school math, 3 years of high school science, high school chemistry, high school biology, high school transcript, 2 letters of recommendation, written essay, transcript of college record. 14 prerequisite credits must be completed before admission to the nursing program. *Options:* Advanced standing available through the following means: advanced placement exams, credit by exam. May apply for transfer of up to 20 total credits. *Application deadline:* 3/1. *Application fee:* $35.

Degree Requirements 126 total credit hours, 54 in nursing.

RN Baccalaureate Program (BS)

Applying *Required:* TOEFL for nonnative speakers of English, minimum college GPA of 2.5, RN license, diploma or AD in nursing, letter of recommendation, transcript of college record. *Options:* Course work may be accelerated. May apply for transfer of up to 31 total credits. *Application deadline:* rolling. *Application fee:* $35.

Degree Requirements 126 total credit hours, 23 in nursing.

LPN to Baccalaureate Program (BSN)

Applying *Required:* SAT I, TOEFL for nonnative speakers of English, minimum college GPA of 2.75, high school math, high school science, high school chemistry, high school biology, high school transcript, 2 letters of recommendation, transcript of college record, LPN license. 14 prerequisite credits must be completed before admission to the nursing program. *Options:* Advanced standing available through credit by exam. May apply for transfer of up to 8 total credits. *Application deadline:* 3/1. *Application fee:* $35.

Degree Requirements 126 total credit hours, 54 in nursing.

LYNCHBURG COLLEGE

Department of Nursing
Lynchburg, Virginia

Programs • Generic Baccalaureate • RN Baccalaureate • Baccalaureate for Second Degree

The College Independent comprehensive coed institution, affiliated with Christian Church (Disciples of Christ). Founded: 1903. *Primary accreditation:* regional. *Setting:* 214-acre suburban campus. *Total enrollment:* 1,963.

The Department of Nursing Founded in 1978. *Nursing program faculty:* 10 (50% with doctorates).

Academic Facilities *Campus library:* 20,535 volumes (6,388 in nursing); 758 periodical subscriptions (84 health-care related). *Nursing school resources:* CAI, computer lab, nursing audiovisuals, interactive nursing skills videos, learning resource lab.

Student Life *Student services:* health clinic, personal counseling, career counseling, institutionally sponsored work-study program, campus safety program. *International student services:* counseling/support. *Nursing student activities:* Sigma Theta Tau, student nurses association.

Calendar Semesters.

NURSING STUDENT PROFILE

Undergraduate **Enrollment:** 120
Women: 94%; **Men:** 6%; **Minority:** 26%; **International:** 1%; **Part-time:** 7%

BACCALAUREATE PROGRAMS

Contact Dr. Nancy I. Whitman, Chairperson, Department of Nursing, Lynchburg College, 1501 Lakeside Drive, Lynchburg, VA 24501-3199, 804-544-8324. *Fax:* 804-544-8499. *E-mail:* whitman@lynchburg.edu

Expenses *Tuition:* $7360 full-time, $245 per semester hour part-time. *Full-time mandatory fees:* $125. *Room and board:* $2200–$2500. *Books and supplies per academic year:* ranges from $400 to $500.

Financial Aid Institutionally sponsored need-based grants/scholarships, institutionally sponsored non-need grants/scholarships, Federal Direct Loans, Federal Pell Grants, Federal Perkins Loans, Federal Supplemental Educational Opportunity Grants, Federal Work-Study, Virginia Foundation for Independent Colleges (VFIC) scholarships, Virginia Tuition Assistant Grant (VTAG). 100% of undergraduate students in nursing programs received some form of financial aid in 1995–96. *Application deadline:* 4/1.

Generic Baccalaureate Program (BSN)

Applying *Required:* SAT I, ACT, 3 College Board Achievements, TOEFL for nonnative speakers of English, minimum high school GPA of 2.0, minimum college GPA of 2.0, 3 years of high school math, 3 years of high school science, high school chemistry, high school biology, high school foreign language, high school transcript, 2 letters of recommendation, written essay, transcript of college record, students 25 years of age or older enter through ACCESS admissions only, requirements vary slightly. 28 prerequisite credits must be completed before admission to the nursing program. *Options:* May apply for transfer of up to 60 total credits. *Application deadlines:* 4/1 (fall), 11/15 (spring), 4/15 (summer). *Application fee:* $30.

Degree Requirements 124 total credit hours, 73 in nursing.

RN Baccalaureate Program (BSN)

Applying *Required:* minimum college GPA of 2.0, RN license, diploma or AD in nursing, high school transcript, interview, written essay, transcript of college record. 28 prerequisite credits must be completed before admission to the nursing program. *Options:* Advanced standing available through credit by exam. Course work may be accelerated. May apply for transfer of up to 76 total credits. *Application deadline:* rolling. *Application fee:* $30.

Degree Requirements 124 total credit hours, 73 in nursing.

Baccalaureate for Second Degree Program (BSN)

Applying *Required:* minimum college GPA of 2.0, interview, 2 letters of recommendation, written essay, transcript of college record, students 25 years of age or older enter through ACCESS admissions only, requirements vary. 28 prerequisite credits must be completed before admission to the nursing program. *Options:* May apply for transfer of up to 76 total credits. *Application deadlines:* 8/15 (fall), 12/1 (spring), 5/1 (summer). *Application fee:* $30.

Degree Requirements 124 total credit hours, 73 in nursing.

MARYMOUNT UNIVERSITY
School of Nursing
Arlington, Virginia

Programs • RN Baccalaureate • MSN • RN to Master's

The University Independent comprehensive coed institution, affiliated with Roman Catholic Church. Founded: 1950. *Primary accreditation:* regional. *Setting:* 21-acre suburban campus. *Total enrollment:* 3,812.

The School of Nursing Founded in 1966. *Nursing program faculty:* 46 (31% with doctorates).

▶ ***NOTEWORTHY***

Marymount University is an independent, coeducational Catholic university in Arlington, Virginia, just minutes from Washington, D.C. Marymount offers a unique ladder program allowing students to complete the AAS in Nursing degree—becoming eligible to take state board exams and attain licensure as a registered nurse—and then progress directly to the BSN degree program. The School of Nursing also offers the BSN completion program for RNs, an accelerated program for individuals with a prior bachelor's degree, and the MSN degree. All programs are accredited by the National League for Nursing.

Academic Facilities *Campus library:* 8,127 volumes in health, 1,044 in nursing. *Nursing school resources:* CAI, computer lab, nursing audiovisuals, interactive nursing skills videos, learning resource lab.

Student Life *Student services:* health clinic, personal counseling, career counseling, special assistance for disabled students. *International student services:* counseling/support, special assistance for nonnative speakers of English. *Nursing student activities:* Sigma Theta Tau, student nurses association.

Calendar Semesters.

NURSING STUDENT PROFILE

Undergraduate **Enrollment:** 410
Women: 88%; **Men:** 12%
Graduate **Enrollment:** 87
Women: 91%; **Men:** 9%

BACCALAUREATE PROGRAM

Contact Office of Admissions, School of Nursing, Marymount University, Arlington, VA 22207-4299, 703-284-1500. *Fax:* 703-284-1693.

Expenses *Tuition:* $12,400 full-time, $400 per credit part-time. *Full-time mandatory fees:* $140–$315. *Room and board:* $5640.

RN Baccalaureate Program (BSN)

Applying *Required:* SAT II Writing Test, challenge exam for diploma graduates, NLN exam, minimum college GPA of 2.0, RN license, diploma or AD in nursing, high school transcript, 2 letters of recommendation, transcript of college record, CPR certification, immunizations. *Options:* Course work may be accelerated. *Application deadline:* rolling. *Application fee:* $30.

Degree Requirements 133 total credit hours, 66 in nursing.

MASTER'S PROGRAMS

Contact Office of Admissions, School of Nursing, Marymount University, Arlington, VA 22207-4299, 703-284-1500. *Fax:* 703-284-1693.

Areas of Study Nursing administration; nursing education; nurse practitioner programs in family health, primary care.

Expenses *Tuition:* $7740 full-time, $430 per credit part-time. *Full-time mandatory fees:* $0. *Room and board:* $5640.

MSN Program

Applying *Required:* bachelor's degree in nursing, minimum GPA of 3.0, RN license, statistics course, professional liability/malpractice insurance, interview, 2 letters of recommendation, transcript of college record, 2 years of clinical experience required for the primary care family nurse practitioner track. *Application deadline:* rolling. *Application fee:* $30.

Degree Requirements 36–40 total credit hours dependent upon track, 27–31 in nursing.

RN to Master's Program (MSN)

Applying *Required:* bachelor's degree in nursing, minimum GPA of 3.0, RN license, physical assessment course, statistics course, professional liability/malpractice insurance, interview, 2 letters of recommendation, transcript of college record, pathophysiology, community health, nursing leadership, nursing research, and upper division validation exam; 2 years of clinical experience for family nurse practitioner track. *Application deadline:* rolling. *Application fee:* $30.

Degree Requirements 36–40 total credit hours dependent upon track, 27–31 in nursing.

NORFOLK STATE UNIVERSITY
Department of Nursing
Norfolk, Virginia

Programs • Baccalaureate for Second Degree • LPN to Baccalaureate

The University State-supported comprehensive coed institution. Part of Commonwealth of Virginia Council of Higher Education. Founded: 1935. *Primary accreditation:* regional. *Setting:* 130-acre urban campus. *Total enrollment:* 8,667.

The Department of Nursing Founded in 1981.

Academic Facilities *Campus library:* 300,000 volumes (16,000 in health, 2,500 in nursing). *Nursing school resources:* computer lab.

Calendar Semesters.

Norfolk State University (continued)

BACCALAUREATE PROGRAMS

Contact Ms. Rebecca B. Rice, Head, Department of Nursing, Norfolk State University, 2401 Corprew Avenue, Norfolk, VA 23504, 804-683-9014. *Fax:* 804-683-8241.

Expenses *Books and supplies per academic year:* ranges from $500 to $600.

Financial Aid Institutionally sponsored need-based grants/scholarships, institutionally sponsored non-need grants/scholarships, Federal Direct Loans, Federal Nursing Student Loans, Federal Pell Grants, Federal Perkins Loans, Federal Supplemental Educational Opportunity Grants, Federal Work-Study, Federal PLUS Loans, Federal Stafford Loans, state aid.

Baccalaureate for Second Degree Program (BSN)

Applying *Required:* minimum college GPA of 2.5, transcript of college record, physical examination, CPR certification. *Options:* Advanced standing available through the following means: advanced placement exams, credit by exam. May apply for transfer of up to 90 total credits. *Application deadline:* 12/1. *Application fee:* $20.

Degree Requirements 133 total credit hours, 49 in nursing.

LPN to Baccalaureate Program (BSN)

Applying *Required:* SAT I or ACT, minimum college GPA of 2.5, high school transcript, transcript of college record, LPN license, physical examination, CPR certification. *Options:* Advanced standing available through the following means: advanced placement exams, credit by exam. *Application fee:* $20.

Degree Requirements 124 total credit hours, 61 in nursing.

OLD DOMINION UNIVERSITY
School of Nursing
Norfolk, Virginia

Programs • Generic Baccalaureate • RN Baccalaureate • MSN • Continuing Education

The University State-supported coed university. Founded: 1930. *Primary accreditation:* regional. *Setting:* 172-acre urban campus. *Total enrollment:* 17,113.

The School of Nursing Founded in 1963. *Nursing program faculty:* 22 (36% with doctorates).

Academic Facilities *Campus library:* 851,194 volumes (40,598 in health); 6,789 periodical subscriptions. *Nursing school resources:* CAI, computer lab, nursing audiovisuals, learning resource lab.

Student Life *Student services:* health clinic, personal counseling, career counseling, institutionally sponsored work-study program, job placement, campus safety program, special assistance for disabled students. *International student services:* counseling/support, special assistance for nonnative speakers of English. *Nursing student activities:* Sigma Theta Tau, student nurses association.

Calendar Semesters.

NURSING STUDENT PROFILE

Undergraduate **Enrollment:** 524
Women: 91%; **Men:** 9%; **Minority:** 20%; **International:** 1%; **Part-time:** 38%
Graduate **Enrollment:** 180
Women: 95%; **Men:** 5%; **Minority:** 3%; **International:** 0%; **Part-time:** 36%

BACCALAUREATE PROGRAMS

Contact Ms. Phyllis Barham, Chief Academic Adviser, 358 Technology Building, School of Nursing, Old Dominion University, Norfolk, VA 23529-0500, 804-683-5245. *Fax:* 804-683-5253. *E-mail:* pdb100f@giraffe.tech.odu.edu

Expenses *State resident tuition:* $4121 full-time, $134 per credit part-time. *Nonresident tuition:* $10,640 full-time, $346 per credit part-time. *Full-time mandatory fees:* $48. *Part-time mandatory fees:* $10. *Books and supplies per academic year:* ranges from $300 to $500.

Financial Aid Institutionally sponsored need-based grants/scholarships, institutionally sponsored non-need grants/scholarships, Federal Work-Study. *Application deadline:* 2/1.

Generic Baccalaureate Program (BSN)

Applying *Required:* SAT I, TOEFL for nonnative speakers of English, minimum college GPA of 2.0, transcript of college record. 22 prerequisite credits must be completed before admission to the nursing program. *Options:* May apply for transfer of up to 90 total credits. *Application deadline:* 2/1. *Application fee:* $30.

Degree Requirements 120–123 total credit hours dependent upon track, 66 in nursing. Exit writing exam, senior assessment exam.

RN Baccalaureate Program (BSN)

Applying *Required:* TOEFL for nonnative speakers of English, minimum college GPA of 2.0, RN license, diploma or AD in nursing, transcript of college record. 29 prerequisite credits must be completed before admission to the nursing program. *Application deadline:* 2/1. *Application fee:* $30.

Degree Requirements 120–123 total credit hours dependent upon track, 66 in nursing. Exit writing exam, senior assessment exam.

Distance learning Courses provided through video, audio.

MASTER'S PROGRAM

Contact Dr. Betty Alexy, Graduate Program Director, 359-C Technology Building, School of Nursing, Old Dominion University, Norfolk, VA 23529-0500, 804-683-5257. *Fax:* 804-683-5253. *E-mail:* bbal00f@giraffe.tech.odu.edu

Areas of Study Clinical nurse specialist programs in community health nursing, critical care nursing, perinatal nursing; nurse anesthesia; nursing administration; nurse practitioner programs in child care/pediatrics, family health, neonatal health.

Expenses *State resident tuition:* $171 per credit. *Nonresident tuition:* $453 per credit. *Part-time mandatory fees:* $10.

Financial Aid Graduate assistantships, nurse traineeships, Federal Nursing Student Loans. 50% of master's level students in nursing programs received some form of financial aid in 1995-96. *Application deadline:* 2/1.

MSN Program

Applying *Required:* GRE General Test or Miller Analogies Test, bachelor's degree in nursing, minimum GPA of 2.5, RN license, 1 year of clinical experience, physical assessment course, statistics course, essay, interview, 3 letters of recommendation, transcript of college record, minimum 3.0 GPA in nursing major. *Application deadline:* 2/1. *Application fee:* $30.

Degree Requirements 36–83 total credit hours dependent upon track, 36–83 in nursing. Comprehensive exam.

CONTINUING EDUCATION PROGRAM

Contact Ms. Shirley Glover, Assistant Dean, College of Health Sciences, 203 Health Sciences Building, College of Health Sciences, Old Dominion University, Norfolk, VA 23529-0500, 804-683-4256. *Fax:* 804-683-5674.

RADFORD UNIVERSITY
School of Nursing
Radford, Virginia

Programs • Generic Baccalaureate • RN Baccalaureate • MSN • Continuing Education

The University State-supported comprehensive coed institution. Founded: 1910. *Primary accreditation:* regional. *Setting:* 177-acre small-town campus. *Total enrollment:* 8,687.

The School of Nursing Founded in 1971. *Nursing program faculty:* 32 (45% with doctorates). *Off-campus program site:* Roanoke.

Academic Facilities *Campus library:* 243,023 volumes (7,212 in health, 954 in nursing); 2,406 periodical subscriptions (147 health-care related). *Nursing school resources:* CAI, computer lab, nursing audiovisuals, learning resource lab.

Student Life *Student services:* health clinic, personal counseling, career counseling, institutionally sponsored work-study program, campus safety program, special assistance for disabled students. *International student*

services: counseling/support, special assistance for nonnative speakers of English, ESL courses. *Nursing student activities:* Sigma Theta Tau, student nurses association.

Calendar Semesters.

NURSING STUDENT PROFILE

Undergraduate **Enrollment:** 172
Women: 93%; **Men:** 7%; **Minority:** 5%; **International:** 1%; **Part-time:** 8%
Graduate **Enrollment:** 40
Women: 90%; **Men:** 10%; **Minority:** 5%; **International:** 5%; **Part-time:** 50%

BACCALAUREATE PROGRAMS

Contact Dr. Janet Hardy Boettcher, Chair and Professor, School of Nursing, Radford University, Box 6964, Radford, VA 24142, 540-831-5415. *Fax:* 540-831-6299. *E-mail:* jboettch@runet.edu

Expenses *State resident tuition:* $3146 full-time, $132 per credit hour part-time. *Nonresident tuition:* $7720 full-time, $322 per credit hour part-time. *Full-time mandatory fees:* $0. *Room and board:* $4310–$4312. *Books and supplies per academic year:* $500.

Financial Aid Institutionally sponsored need-based grants/scholarships, institutionally sponsored non-need grants/scholarships, Federal Nursing Student Loans, Federal Supplemental Educational Opportunity Grants, Federal Work-Study. 64% of undergraduate students in nursing programs received some form of financial aid in 1995–96. *Application deadline:* 3/1.

Generic Baccalaureate Program (BS)

Applying *Required:* SAT I or ACT, SAT II Writing Test, TOEFL for nonnative speakers of English, 3 years of high school math, high school chemistry, high school biology, high school transcript. 30 prerequisite credits must be completed before admission to the nursing program. *Options:* Advanced standing available through the following means: advanced placement exams, credit by exam. May apply for transfer of up to 95 total credits. *Application deadline:* 12/15. *Application fee:* $15.

Degree Requirements 125 total credit hours, 60 in nursing.

RN Baccalaureate Program (BS)

Applying *Required:* SAT II Writing Test, TOEFL for nonnative speakers of English, RN license, diploma or AD in nursing, transcript of college record, nursing practice within last 5 years. 30 prerequisite credits must be completed before admission to the nursing program. *Options:* May apply for transfer of up to 95 total credits. *Application deadline:* rolling. *Application fee:* $15.

Degree Requirements 125 total credit hours, 60 in nursing.

Distance learning Courses provided through video, audio.

MASTER'S PROGRAM

Contact Dr. Karolyn Givens, Coordinator, Graduate Program, School of Nursing, Radford University, Box 6964, Radford, VA 24142, 540-831-5113. *Fax:* 540-831-6299. *E-mail:* kgivens@runet.edu

Areas of Study Clinical nurse specialist programs in adult health nursing, home health nursing; nurse practitioner program in family health.

Expenses *State resident tuition:* $3304 full-time, $138 per credit hour part-time. *Nonresident tuition:* $6488 full-time, $271 per credit hour part-time. *Full-time mandatory fees:* $0. *Room and board:* $4310–$4312. *Books and supplies per academic year:* ranges from $200 to $300.

Financial Aid Graduate assistantships, nurse traineeships, Federal Nursing Student Loans, employment opportunities, institutionally sponsored need-based grants/scholarships. 20% of master's level students in nursing programs received some form of financial aid in 1995-96. *Application deadline:* 3/1.

MSN Program

Applying *Required:* GRE General Test, Miller Analogies Test, TOEFL for nonnative speakers of English, bachelor's degree in nursing, minimum GPA of 3.0, RN license, 1 year of clinical experience, physical assessment course, statistics course, interview, 2 letters of recommendation, transcript of college record. *Application deadline:* rolling. *Application fee:* $15.

Degree Requirements 35 total credit hours, 32 in nursing, 3 in statistics. Comprehensive exam/directed study.

CONTINUING EDUCATION PROGRAM

Contact Janet Hardy Boettcher, Chair, Box 6964 RU Station, Radford, VA 24141, 540-831-5415. *Fax:* 540-831-6299. *E-mail:* jboettch@runet.edu

UNIVERSITY OF VIRGINIA
School of Nursing
Charlottesville, Virginia

Programs • Generic Baccalaureate • RN Baccalaureate • Baccalaureate for Second Degree • BSN to Master's • MSN • MSN/MBA • PhD • Continuing Education

The University State-supported coed university. Founded: 1819. *Primary accreditation:* regional. *Setting:* 1,094-acre suburban campus. *Total enrollment:* 18,055.

The School of Nursing Founded in 1901. *Nursing program faculty:* 58 (50% with doctorates).

Academic Facilities *Campus library:* 3.3 million volumes (169,796 in health); 44,349 periodical subscriptions (2,917 health-care related). *Nursing school resources:* CAI, computer lab, nursing audiovisuals, interactive nursing skills videos, learning resource lab.

Student Life *Student services:* health clinic, child-care facilities, personal counseling, career counseling, institutionally sponsored work-study program, job placement, campus safety program, special assistance for disabled students. *International student services:* counseling/support, special assistance for nonnative speakers of English. *Nursing student activities:* Sigma Theta Tau, student nurses association.

Calendar Semesters.

NURSING STUDENT PROFILE

Undergraduate **Enrollment:** 291
Women: 95%; **Men:** 5%; **Minority:** 17%; **International:** 1%; **Part-time:** 6%
Graduate **Enrollment:** 171
Women: 92%; **Men:** 8%; **Minority:** 9%; **International:** 2%; **Part-time:** 64%

BACCALAUREATE PROGRAMS

Contact Ms. Susan Kennel, Director of Undergraduate Student Services, McLeod Hall, School of Nursing, University of Virginia, Charlottesville, VA 22903-3395, 804-924-0068. *Fax:* 804-982-1809. *E-mail:* sek2q@virginia.edu

Expenses *State resident tuition:* $4652 per academic year. *Nonresident tuition:* $14,438 per academic year. *Full-time mandatory fees:* $38. *Room and board:* $2464–$4770. *Room only:* $1816–$2704. *Books and supplies per academic year:* ranges from $250 to $450.

Financial Aid Institutionally sponsored need-based grants/scholarships, institutionally sponsored non-need grants/scholarships, Federal Direct Loans, Federal Nursing Student Loans, Federal Pell Grants, Federal Perkins Loans, Federal Supplemental Educational Opportunity Grants, Federal Work-Study. 52% of undergraduate students in nursing programs received some form of financial aid in 1995–96. *Application deadline:* 4/1.

Generic Baccalaureate Program (BSN)

Applying *Required:* SAT I or ACT, 3 College Board Achievements, TOEFL for nonnative speakers of English, 4 years of high school math, high school chemistry, high school biology, high school foreign language, high school transcript, written essay. *Options:* Advanced standing available through the following means: advanced placement exams, advanced placement without credit. May apply for transfer of up to 66 total credits. *Application deadline:* 1/2. *Application fee:* $40.

Degree Requirements 120 total credit hours, 67 in nursing.

RN Baccalaureate Program (BSN)

Applying *Required:* SAT I, TOEFL for nonnative speakers of English, minimum college GPA of 2.0, RN license, diploma or AD in nursing, high school transcript, written essay, transcript of college record, human anatomy and physiology course. 52 prerequisite credits must be completed before admission to the nursing program. *Options:* May apply for transfer of up to 52 total credits. *Application deadline:* 3/1. *Application fee:* $40.

Degree Requirements 120 total credit hours, 68 in nursing.

Baccalaureate for Second Degree Program (BSN)

Applying *Required:* SAT I, TOEFL for nonnative speakers of English, GRE general test, minimum college GPA of 2.0, high school transcript, 3 letters of recommendation, written essay, transcript of college record, human anatomy and physiology course, statistics course. 59 prerequisite credits

University of Virginia (continued)

must be completed before admission to the nursing program. *Options:* May apply for transfer of up to 66 total credits. *Application deadline:* 3/1. *Application fee:* $40.

Degree Requirements 120 total credit hours, 61 in nursing.

MASTER'S PROGRAMS

Contact Dr. Gregg E. Newschwander, Assistant Dean for Student Affairs, McLeod Hall, School of Nursing, University of Virginia, Charlottesville, VA 22903-3395, 804-924-0067. *Fax:* 804-982-1809. *E-mail:* gen2z@virginia.edu

Areas of Study Clinical nurse specialist programs in adult health nursing, community health nursing, critical care nursing, psychiatric–mental health nursing, home health nursing; nurse practitioner programs in acute care, child care/pediatrics, family health, primary care, women's health.

Expenses *State resident tuition:* $4652 per academic year. *Nonresident tuition:* $14,438 per academic year. *Full-time mandatory fees:* $32. *Room and board:* $2464–$4770. *Room only:* $1816–$2704. *Books and supplies per academic year:* ranges from $300 to $650.

Financial Aid Graduate assistantships, nurse traineeships, fellowships, Federal Direct Loans, Federal Nursing Student Loans, institutionally sponsored loans, employment opportunities, institutionally sponsored need-based grants/scholarships, institutionally sponsored non-need-based grants/scholarships. 26% of master's level students in nursing programs received some form of financial aid in 1995-96. *Application deadline:* 4/1.

BSN to Master's Program (MSN)

Applying *Required:* GRE General Test, TOEFL for nonnative speakers of English, bachelor's degree in nursing, minimum GPA of 3.0, RN license, 1 year of clinical experience, physical assessment course, statistics course, essay, 3 letters of recommendation, transcript of college record. *Application deadlines:* 4/1 (fall), 3/1 (acute care nurse practitioner track, summer admission only). *Application fee:* $40.

Degree Requirements 47–57 total credit hours dependent upon track.

MSN Program

Applying *Required:* GRE General Test, TOEFL for nonnative speakers of English, bachelor's degree in nursing, minimum GPA of 3.0, RN license, physical assessment course, statistics course, essay, interview, 3 letters of recommendation, transcript of college record, managerial experience recommended. *Application deadlines:* 4/1 (fall), 12/1 (spring), 4/1 (summer). *Application fee:* $40.

Degree Requirements 42 total credit hours, 39 in nursing.

MSN/MBA Program

Applying *Required:* GRE General Test, TOEFL for nonnative speakers of English, GMAT, bachelor's degree in nursing, minimum GPA of 3.0, RN license, 2 years of clinical experience, physical assessment course, essay, letter of recommendation, transcript of college record. *Application deadlines:* 4/1 (fall), 12/1 (spring). *Application fee:* $120.

Degree Requirements 93 total credit hours, 24 in nursing, 69 in business.

DOCTORAL PROGRAM

Contact Dr. Gregg E. Newschwander, Assistant Dean for Student Affairs, McLeod Hall, School of Nursing, University of Virginia, Charlottesville, VA 22903-3395, 804-924-0067. *Fax:* 804-982-1809. *E-mail:* gen2z@virginia.edu

Areas of Study Nursing research.

Expenses *State resident tuition:* $4652 per academic year. *Nonresident tuition:* $14,438 per academic year. *Full-time mandatory fees:* $32. *Room and board:* $2464–$4770. *Room only:* $1816–$2704. *Books and supplies per academic year:* ranges from $300 to $650.

Financial Aid Graduate assistantships, fellowships, dissertation grants, grants, Federal Direct Loans, institutionally sponsored loans, opportunities for employment, institutionally sponsored need-based grants/scholarships, institutionally sponsored non-need-based grants/scholarships. *Application deadline:* 4/1.

PhD Program

Applying *Required:* GRE General Test, TOEFL for nonnative speakers of English, 1 scholarly paper, statistics course, interview, 3 letters of recommendation, vitae, writing sample, competitive review by faculty committee, BSN, minimum 3.0 GPA, current RN license. *Application deadline:* 4/1. *Application fee:* $40.

Degree Requirements 71 total credit hours; 18 credits in nursing, 23 credits in research, 18 credits in cognates/electives, 12 credits in dissertation research; dissertation; oral exam; written exam; defense of dissertation; residency.

CONTINUING EDUCATION PROGRAM

Contact Ms. Jane Fruchtnicht, Director, Health Sciences Center, University of Virginia, Box 147, Charlottesville, VA 22908, 804-924-2502.

See full description on page 562.

VIRGINIA COMMONWEALTH UNIVERSITY
School of Nursing
Richmond, Virginia

Programs • Generic Baccalaureate • RN Baccalaureate • Master's for Nurses with Non-Nursing Degrees • Accelerated Master's for Non-Nursing College Graduates • PhD

The University State-supported coed university. Founded: 1838. *Primary accreditation:* regional. *Setting:* 99-acre urban campus. *Total enrollment:* 21,349.

The School of Nursing Founded in 1893. *Nursing program faculty:* 38 (74% with doctorates). *Off-campus program sites:* Roanoke, Newport News.

Academic Facilities *Campus library:* 1.0 million volumes (277,218 in health, 4,857 in nursing); 8,400 periodical subscriptions (2,738 health-care related). *Nursing school resources:* CAI, computer lab, nursing audiovisuals, interactive nursing skills videos.

Student Life *Student services:* health clinic, personal counseling, career counseling, institutionally sponsored work-study program, job placement, campus safety program, special assistance for disabled students. *International student services:* counseling/support, ESL courses. *Nursing student activities:* Sigma Theta Tau, student nurses association.

Calendar Semesters.

NURSING STUDENT PROFILE

Undergraduate **Enrollment:** 366
Women: 92%; **Men:** 8%; **Minority:** 12%; **International:** 1%; **Part-time:** 55%
Graduate **Enrollment:** 207
Women: 95%; **Men:** 5%; **Minority:** 9%; **International:** 1%; **Part-time:** 51%

BACCALAUREATE PROGRAMS

Contact Ms. Susan Lipp, Director of Enrollment and Student Services, School of Nursing, Virginia Commonwealth University, PO Box 567, Richmond, VA 23298-0567, 804-828-5171. *Fax:* 804-828-7743. *E-mail:* slipp@gems.vcu.edu

Expenses *State resident tuition:* $1563 full-time, $130 per credit hour part-time. *Nonresident tuition:* $5525 full-time, $460 per credit hour part-time. *Full-time mandatory fees:* $893. *Room and board:* $3864–$5235. *Room only:* $2244–$3545.

Financial Aid Institutionally sponsored need-based grants/scholarships, institutionally sponsored non-need grants/scholarships, Federal Nursing Student Loans, Federal Work-Study. *Application deadline:* 3/1.

Generic Baccalaureate Program (BS)

Applying *Required:* SAT I, TOEFL for nonnative speakers of English, minimum college GPA of 2.5, high school transcript, 3 letters of recommendation, written essay, transcript of college record. 30 prerequisite credits must be completed before admission to the nursing program. *Application deadlines:* 12/15 (fall), 12/15 (summer). *Application fee:* $25.

Degree Requirements 127 total credit hours, 71 in nursing.

RN Baccalaureate Program (BS)

Applying *Required:* SAT I, TOEFL for nonnative speakers of English, minimum college GPA of 2.5, RN license, diploma or AD in nursing, high school transcript, 3 letters of recommendation, written essay, transcript of college record. 59 prerequisite credits must be completed before admission to the nursing program. *Application deadlines:* 2/1 (fall), 11/1 (summer). *Application fee:* $25.

Degree Requirements 124 total credit hours, 62 in nursing.

MASTER'S PROGRAMS

Contact Susan Lipp, Director of Enrollment and Student Services, School of Nursing, Virginia Commonwealth University, PO Box 567, Richmond, VA 23298-0567, 804-828-5171. *Fax:* 804-828-7743.

Areas of Study Clinical nurse specialist programs in adult health nursing, family health nursing, pediatric nursing, psychiatric–mental health nursing, women's health nursing, adult health immunocompetence nursing; nursing administration; nurse practitioner programs in acute care, adult health, child care/pediatrics, family health, women's health, adult health immunocompetence nursing.

Expenses *State resident tuition:* $1905 full-time, $212 per credit hour part-time. *Nonresident tuition:* $5525 full-time, $614 per credit hour part-time. *Full-time mandatory fees:* $893. *Room and board:* $3864–$5235. *Room only:* $2244–$3545.

Financial Aid Graduate assistantships, nurse traineeships. *Application deadline:* 3/1.

Master's for Nurses with Non-Nursing Degrees Program (MS)

Applying *Required:* GRE General Test, TOEFL for nonnative speakers of English, minimum GPA of 2.7, RN license, physical assessment course, statistics course, essay, interview, 3 letters of recommendation, transcript of college record. *Application deadline:* 2/1. *Application fee:* $25.

Degree Requirements 42–52 total credit hours dependent upon track, 42–52 in nursing. Culminating research experience.

Accelerated Master's for Non-Nursing College Graduates Program (MS)

Applying *Required:* GRE General Test, TOEFL for nonnative speakers of English, bachelor's degree, minimum GPA of 2.7, statistics course, essay, 3 letters of recommendation, transcript of college record. *Application deadline:* 2/1 (summer). *Application fee:* $25.

Degree Requirements 96–106 total credit hours dependent upon track, 96–106 in nursing. Culminating research experience.

DOCTORAL PROGRAM

Contact Susan Lipp, Director of Enrollment and Student Services, School of Nursing, Virginia Commonwealth University, PO Box 567, Richmond, VA 23298-0567, 804-828-5171. *Fax:* 804-828-7743.

Areas of Study Nursing administration, Human Health and Illness, Biology of Health and Illness.

Expenses *State resident tuition:* $1905 full-time, $212 per credit hour part-time. *Nonresident tuition:* $5525 full-time, $614 per credit hour part-time. *Full-time mandatory fees:* $893. *Room and board:* $3864–$5235. *Room only:* $2244–$3545.

PhD Program

Applying *Required:* GRE General Test, TOEFL for nonnative speakers of English, statistics course, interview, 3 letters of recommendation, vitae, competitive review by faculty committee, baccalaureate or master's degree in nursing. *Application deadline:* 4/1. *Application fee:* $25.

Degree Requirements 64–70 total credit hours dependent upon track; dissertation; written exam; defense of dissertation.

VIRGIN ISLANDS

UNIVERSITY OF THE VIRGIN ISLANDS
Division of Nursing
Charlotte Amalie, St. Thomas, Virgin Islands

Programs • Generic Baccalaureate • RN Baccalaureate

The University Territory-supported comprehensive coed institution. Founded: 1962. *Primary accreditation:* regional. *Setting:* 175-acre small-town campus. *Total enrollment:* 3,054.

The Division of Nursing Founded in 1981. *Nursing program faculty:* 6 (50% with doctorates).

Academic Facilities *Nursing school resources:* CAI, computer lab, nursing audiovisuals, interactive nursing skills videos.

Student Life *Student services:* health clinic, personal counseling, career counseling, institutionally sponsored work-study program. *Nursing student activities:* student nurses association.

Calendar Semesters.

NURSING STUDENT PROFILE

Undergraduate **Enrollment:** 74
Women: 98%; **Men:** 2%; **Minority:** 90%; **Part-time:** 50%

BACCALAUREATE PROGRAMS

Contact Admissions Office, Division of Nursing Education, University of the Virgin Islands, Charlotte Amalie, St. Thomas, VI 00802-9990, 809-776-9200. *E-mail:* judith.edwin@uvi.edu

Expenses *State resident tuition:* $2010 full-time, $67 per credit hour part-time. *Nonresident tuition:* $6030 full-time, $201 per credit hour part-time. *Full-time mandatory fees:* $320–$420. *Room and board:* $4510–$4850. *Books and supplies per academic year:* ranges from $650 to $750.

Financial Aid Institutionally sponsored need-based grants/scholarships, institutionally sponsored non-need grants/scholarships, Federal Direct Loans, Federal Supplemental Educational Opportunity Grants, Federal Work-Study. *Application deadline:* 4/15.

Generic Baccalaureate Program (BS)

Applying *Required:* SAT I, 2 years of high school math, 2 years of high school science, high school transcript, 2 letters of recommendation. *Options:* Advanced standing available through the following means: advanced placement exams, credit by exam. *Application deadlines:* 4/15 (fall), 11/15 (spring). *Application fee:* $20.

Degree Requirements 128 total credit hours, 63 in nursing. Computer literacy, English proficiency exams.

RN Baccalaureate Program (BS)

Applying *Required:* SAT I, 2 years of high school math, 2 years of high school science, 2 letters of recommendation, transcript of college record, RN license or equivalent. *Options:* Advanced standing available through the following means: advanced placement exams, credit by exam. *Application deadlines:* 4/15 (fall), 11/15 (spring). *Application fee:* $20.

Degree Requirements 128 total credit hours, 63 in nursing. Computer literacy, English proficiency exams.

WASHINGTON

EASTERN WASHINGTON UNIVERSITY
Intercollegiate Center for Nursing Education
Spokane, Washington

Programs • Generic Baccalaureate • RN Baccalaureate • BSN to Master's • Continuing Education

The University State-supported comprehensive coed institution. Part of Washington Higher Education Coordinating Board. Founded: 1882. *Primary accreditation:* regional. *Setting:* 335-acre small-town campus. *Total enrollment:* 8,078.

The Intercollegiate Center for Nursing Education Founded in 1968. *Nursing program faculty:* 65 (38% with doctorates). *Off-campus program sites:* Vancouver, Richland, Yakima.

Academic Facilities *Campus library:* 421,164 volumes (12,120 in nursing); 5,231 periodical subscriptions (1,000 health-care related). *Nursing school resources:* CAI, computer lab, nursing audiovisuals, interactive nursing skills videos, learning resource lab, interactive audiovisual telecommunication classrooms, TV production studio, multimedia classroom.

Student Life *Student services:* health clinic, child-care facilities, personal counseling, career counseling, institutionally sponsored work-study program, job placement, campus safety program, special assistance for disabled students, veteran's services, learning skills center. *International student services:* counseling/support, special assistance for nonnative speakers of English, ESL courses. *Nursing student activities:* Sigma Theta Tau, student nurses association, multicultural club, Nurses Christian Fellowship.

Calendar Semesters.

NURSING STUDENT PROFILE

Undergraduate **Enrollment:** 334
Women: 81%; **Men:** 19%; **Minority:** 10%; **International:** 2%; **Part-time:** 24%
Graduate **Enrollment:** 80
Women: 89%; **Men:** 11%; **Minority:** 0%; **International:** 3%; **Part-time:** 78%

BACCALAUREATE PROGRAMS

Contact Ms. Peggy Peterson, Nursing Recruiter/Adviser, Eastern Washington University, Mail Stop #140, Cheney, WA 99004, 509-359-6246. *Fax:* 509-359-6927.

Expenses *State resident tuition:* $3024 full-time, $151 per semester credit part-time. *Nonresident tuition:* $4264 full-time, $426 per semester credit part-time. *Full-time mandatory fees:* $664–$666. *Part-time mandatory fees:* $540–$542. *Books and supplies per academic year:* ranges from $710 to $935.

Financial Aid Institutionally sponsored need-based grants/scholarships, institutionally sponsored non-need grants/scholarships, Federal Direct Loans, Federal Nursing Student Loans, Federal Perkins Loans, Federal Supplemental Educational Opportunity Grants, Federal Work-Study. 80% of undergraduate students in nursing programs received some form of financial aid in 1995–96. *Application deadline:* 3/1.

Generic Baccalaureate Program (BSN)

Applying *Required:* SAT I, ACT, algebra clearance test, writing test, minimum college GPA of 2.5, 2 years of high school science, high school foreign language, high school transcript, written essay, transcript of college record, immunizations. 60 prerequisite credits must be completed before admission to the nursing program. *Options:* May apply for transfer of up to 60 total credits. *Application deadlines:* 2/15 (fall), 9/1 (spring). *Application fee:* $35.

Degree Requirements 120 total credit hours, 61 in nursing.

Distance learning Courses provided through two-way audiovisual microwave television.

RN Baccalaureate Program (BSN)

Applying *Required:* SAT I, ACT, minimum college GPA of 2.5, high school transcript, written essay, transcript of college record, immunizations. 60 prerequisite credits must be completed before admission to the nursing program. *Options:* Advanced standing available through credit by exam. May apply for transfer of up to 60 total credits. *Application deadline:* rolling. *Application fee:* $35.

Degree Requirements 120 total credit hours, 61 in nursing.

Distance learning Courses provided through two-way audiovisual microwave television.

MASTER'S PROGRAM

Contact Dr. Marian Sheafor, Associate Dean for Academic Affairs, Intercollegiate Center for Nursing Education, Eastern Washington University, 2917 West Fort George Wright Drive, Spokane, WA 99224-5291, 509-324-7335. *Fax:* 509-324-7336. *E-mail:* sheafor@wsu.edu

Areas of Study Clinical nurse specialist programs in adult health nursing, community health nursing, psychiatric–mental health nursing; nurse practitioner program in family health.

Expenses *State resident tuition:* $4748 full-time, $237 per semester credit part-time. *Nonresident tuition:* $5947 full-time, $595 per semester credit part-time. *Full-time mandatory fees:* $60–$100. *Books and supplies per academic year:* $700.

Financial Aid Graduate assistantships, nurse traineeships, fellowships, Federal Direct Loans, Federal Nursing Student Loans, institutionally sponsored loans, employment opportunities, institutionally sponsored need-based grants/scholarships, institutionally sponsored non-need-based grants/scholarships. 33% of master's level students in nursing programs received some form of financial aid in 1995-96. *Application deadline:* 2/15.

BSN to Master's Program (MN)

Applying *Required:* bachelor's degree in nursing, minimum GPA of 3.0, RN license, physical assessment course, statistics course, essay, 3 letters of recommendation, transcript of college record, CPR certification, immunizations, word processing skills; interview for family nurse practitioner track. *Application deadlines:* 3/15 (fall), 11/1 (spring). *Application fee:* $35.

Degree Requirements 39–45 total credit hours dependent upon track, 29–34 in nursing, 10–11 in courses supportive to major and interests. Other research clinical projects, thesis optional. Thesis required.

Distance learning Courses provided through two-way audiovisual microwave television.

CONTINUING EDUCATION PROGRAM

Contact Dr. Barbara Johnston, Assistant Dean for Continuing Education, Intercollegiate Center for Nursing Education, Eastern Washington University, 2917 West Fort George Wright Drive, Spokane, WA 99204-5291, 509-324-7356. *Fax:* 509-324-7836.

GONZAGA UNIVERSITY
Department of Nursing
Spokane, Washington

Programs • RN Baccalaureate • MSN • Post-Master's

The University Independent Roman Catholic comprehensive coed institution. Founded: 1887. *Primary accreditation:* regional. *Setting:* 94-acre urban campus. *Total enrollment:* 4,785.

The Department of Nursing Founded in 1978.

Calendar Semesters.

BACCALAUREATE PROGRAM

Contact Community Liaison, Department of Nursing, Gonzaga University, Spokane, WA 99258, 509-328-4220. *Fax:* 509-484-2818.

Expenses *Tuition:* $13,900 full-time, $425 per credit part-time.

Financial Aid Institutionally sponsored need-based grants/scholarships, institutionally sponsored non-need grants/scholarships, Federal Pell Grants, Federal Perkins Loans, Federal Supplemental Educational Opportunity Grants, Federal Work-Study, Federal PLUS Loans, Federal Stafford Loans. *Application deadline:* 2/1.

RN Baccalaureate Program (BSN)

Applying *Required:* SAT I or ACT, TOEFL for nonnative speakers of English, minimum college GPA of 2.0, RN license, diploma or AD in nursing, high school transcript, 3 letters of recommendation, transcript of college record. *Options:* Advanced standing available through the following means: advanced placement exams, credit by exam. May apply for transfer of up to 64 total credits. *Application deadline:* rolling. *Application fee:* $40.

Degree Requirements 128 total credit hours, 66 in nursing.

MASTER'S PROGRAMS

Areas of Study Nursing administration; nursing education; nurse practitioner program in family health.

Expenses *Tuition:* $385 per credit hour.

MSN Program

Applying *Required:* Miller Analogies Test, bachelor's degree in nursing, minimum GPA of 3.0, RN license, essay, 2 letters of recommendation, transcript of college record. *Application deadlines:* 4/1 (fall), 11/15 (spring), 4/1 (summer).

Degree Requirements 43 total credit hours, 43 in nursing.

Post-Master's Program

Applying *Required:* RN license, essay, 2 letters of recommendation, transcript of college record, master's degree in nursing. *Application deadlines:* 4/1 (fall), 11/15 (spring), 4/1 (summer).

Degree Requirements 25 total credit hours, 25 in nursing. Thesis required.

PACIFIC LUTHERAN UNIVERSITY
School of Nursing
Tacoma, Washington

Programs • Generic Baccalaureate • Accelerated RN Baccalaureate • LPN to Baccalaureate • MSN • Continuing Education

The University Independent comprehensive coed institution, affiliated with Evangelical Lutheran Church in America. Founded: 1890. *Primary accreditation:* regional. *Setting:* 126-acre suburban campus. *Total enrollment:* 3,579.

The School of Nursing Founded in 1959. *Nursing program faculty:* 27 (65% with doctorates).

Academic Facilities *Campus library:* 311,194 volumes (16,889 in nursing); 2,091 periodical subscriptions (120 health-care related). *Nursing school resources:* CAI, computer lab, nursing audiovisuals, interactive nursing skills videos, learning resource lab.

Student Life *Student services:* health clinic, child-care facilities, personal counseling, career counseling, institutionally sponsored work-study program, campus safety program, special assistance for disabled students. *International student services:* counseling/support, special assistance for nonnative speakers of English, ESL courses. *Nursing student activities:* Sigma Theta Tau, student nurses association.

Calendar 4-1-4.

NURSING STUDENT PROFILE

Undergraduate **Enrollment:** 260

Women: 90%; **Men:** 10%; **Minority:** 15%; **International:** 1%; **Part-time:** 4%

Graduate **Enrollment:** 65

Women: 90%; **Men:** 10%; **Minority:** 32%; **International:** 2%; **Part-time:** 55%

BACCALAUREATE PROGRAMS

Contact Ms. Audrey Masenhimer, Admissions Assistant, School of Nursing, Pacific Lutheran University, Tacoma, WA 98447-0003, 206-535-7677. *Fax:* 206-535-7590.

Expenses *Tuition:* $13,312 full-time, $455 per credit hour part-time. *Full-time mandatory fees:* $345–$375. *Room and board:* $4426. *Room only:* $2300. *Books and supplies per academic year:* ranges from $100 to $500.

Financial Aid Institutionally sponsored need-based grants/scholarships, institutionally sponsored non-need grants/scholarships, Federal Direct Loans, Federal Nursing Student Loans, Federal Supplemental Educational Opportunity Grants, Federal Work-Study. *Application deadline:* 3/1.

Generic Baccalaureate Program (BSN)

Applying *Required:* TOEFL for nonnative speakers of English, Speaking Proficiency English Assessment Kit for nonnative speakers of English, minimum high school GPA of 2.5, minimum college GPA of 2.5, 3 years of high school math, 2 years of high school science, high school foreign language, high school transcript, 2 letters of recommendation, written essay, transcript of college record. 16 prerequisite credits must be completed before admission to the nursing program. *Options:* May apply for transfer of up to 64 total credits. *Application deadlines:* 3/1 (fall), 3/1 (spring). *Application fee:* $35.

Degree Requirements 128 total credit hours, 57 in nursing.

Accelerated RN Baccalaureate Program (BSN)

Applying *Required:* TOEFL for nonnative speakers of English, Speaking Proficiency English Assessment Kit for nonnative speakers of English, minimum college GPA of 2.5, 3 years of high school math, 2 years of high school science, RN license, diploma or AD in nursing, high school foreign language, high school transcript, 2 letters of recommendation, written essay, transcript of college record. 64 prerequisite credits must be completed before admission to the nursing program. *Options:* May apply for transfer of up to 64 total credits. *Application deadline:* 12/1. *Application fee:* $35.

Degree Requirements 128 total credit hours, 51 in nursing.

LPN to Baccalaureate Program (BSN)

Applying *Required:* TOEFL for nonnative speakers of English, Speaking Proficiency English Assessment Kit for nonnative speakers of English, minimum college GPA of 2.5, 3 years of high school math, 2 years of high school science, high school foreign language, high school transcript, 2 letters of recommendation, written essay, transcript of college record, LPN license or military equivalent. 35 prerequisite credits must be completed before admission to the nursing program. *Options:* Advanced standing available through credit by exam. May apply for transfer of up to 64 total credits. *Application deadline:* 12/1. *Application fee:* $35.

Degree Requirements 128 total credit hours, 57 in nursing.

MASTER'S PROGRAM

Contact Dr. Cleo Pass, Associate Dean, Graduate Nursing Education, School of Nursing, Pacific Lutheran University, Tacoma, WA 98447-0003, 206-536-5002. *Fax:* 206-535-7590.

Areas of Study Clinical nurse specialist program in continuity of care nursing; nursing administration; nurse practitioner programs in family health, gerontology, women's health.

Expenses *Tuition:* $455 per credit hour. *Full-time mandatory fees:* $125–$175. *Room only:* $2240.

Financial Aid Graduate assistantships, nurse traineeships, Federal Direct Loans, Federal Nursing Student Loans, employment opportunities. *Application deadline:* 3/1.

MSN Program

Applying *Required:* GRE General Test, bachelor's degree in nursing, minimum GPA of 3.0, RN license, physical assessment course, statistics course, professional liability/malpractice insurance, essay, interview, 2 letters of recommendation, transcript of college record. *Application deadlines:* 3/1 (nurse practitioner track), rolling. *Application fee:* $35.

Degree Requirements 32–36 total credit hours dependent upon track, 32–36 in nursing. Thesis is optional.

CONTINUING EDUCATION PROGRAM

Contact Dr. Patsy Maloney, Director, Center for Continued Nursing Learning, School of Nursing, Pacific Lutheran University, Tacoma, WA 98447-0003, 206-535-7685. *Fax:* 206-535-7590.

SAINT MARTIN'S COLLEGE
Department of Nursing
Lacey, Washington

Programs • RN Baccalaureate • RN to Master's • Continuing Education

Saint Martin's College (continued)

The College Independent Roman Catholic comprehensive coed institution. Founded: 1895. *Primary accreditation:* regional. *Setting:* 380-acre suburban campus. *Total enrollment:* 923.

The Department of Nursing Founded in 1985. *Nursing program faculty:* 6 (60% with doctorates).

Academic Facilities *Campus library:* 85,621 volumes (2,400 in health, 1,500 in nursing); 794 periodical subscriptions (87 health-care related). *Nursing school resources:* CAI, computer lab, nursing audiovisuals, learning resource lab.

Student Life *Student services:* personal counseling, career counseling, institutionally sponsored work-study program, job placement, campus safety program, special assistance for disabled students. *International student services:* counseling/support, special assistance for nonnative speakers of English, ESL courses. *Nursing student activities:* nursing club, student nurses association.

Calendar Semesters.

NURSING STUDENT PROFILE

Undergraduate **Enrollment:** 40
Women: 98%; **Men:** 2%; **Minority:** 6%; **International:** 0%; **Part-time:** 90%
Graduate **Enrollment:** 30
Women: 98%; **Men:** 2%; **Minority:** 5%; **International:** 0%; **Part-time:** 70%

BACCALAUREATE PROGRAM

Contact Ms. Julia Miller, Associate Professor, Department of Nursing, Saint Martin's College, Lacey, WA 98503, 360-438-4376. *Fax:* 360-459-4124.

Expenses *Tuition:* $12,610 full-time, $420 per semester credit part-time. *Full-time mandatory fees:* $70–$240. *Room and board:* $4590–$5440. *Books and supplies per academic year:* ranges from $400 to $600.

Financial Aid Institutionally sponsored need-based grants/scholarships, institutionally sponsored non-need grants/scholarships, Federal Direct Loans, Federal Perkins Loans, Federal Supplemental Educational Opportunity Grants, Federal Work-Study. 40% of undergraduate students in nursing programs received some form of financial aid in 1995–96. *Application deadline:* 3/1.

RN Baccalaureate Program (BSN)

Applying *Required:* TOEFL for nonnative speakers of English, minimum high school GPA of 2.0, minimum college GPA of 2.0, RN license, diploma or AD in nursing, high school transcript, 2 letters of recommendation, written essay, transcript of college record. 12 prerequisite credits must be completed before admission to the nursing program. *Options:* Course work may be accelerated. May apply for transfer of up to 96 total credits. *Application deadlines:* 7/1 (fall), 11/1 (spring). *Application fee:* $25.

Degree Requirements 52 total credit hours, 31 in nursing.

MASTER'S PROGRAM

Contact Dr. Maura Egan, Director of MSN Program, Department of Nursing, St. Martin's College, Lacey, WA 98503-1297, 360-438-4376. *Fax:* 360-459-4124.

Areas of Study Nurse practitioner program in family health.

Expenses *Tuition:* $6300 full-time, $420 per semester credit part-time. *Full-time mandatory fees:* $25–$50. *Part-time mandatory fees:* $25–$50. *Room and board:* $5440. *Books and supplies per academic year:* ranges from $150 to $250.

Financial Aid Federal Direct Loans, institutionally sponsored loans, employment opportunities, institutionally sponsored need-based grants/scholarships, institutionally sponsored non-need-based grants/scholarships. 40% of master's level students in nursing programs received some form of financial aid in 1995-96. *Application deadline:* 3/1.

RN to Master's Program (MSN)

Applying *Required:* GRE General Test, bachelor's degree in nursing, minimum GPA of 2.0, RN license, 1 year of clinical experience, physical assessment course, statistics course, professional liability/malpractice insurance, essay, interview, 2 letters of recommendation, transcript of college record. *Application deadlines:* 7/1 (fall), 11/1 (spring). *Application fee:* $25.

Degree Requirements 30 total credit hours, 30 in nursing. Clinical project or thesis.

CONTINUING EDUCATION PROGRAM

Contact Dr. Maddy deGive, Professor, Continuing Education in Nursing, Saint Martin's College, Lacey, WA 98503, 360-438-4376. *Fax:* 360-459-4124. *E-mail:* mdegive@stmartin.edu

SEATTLE PACIFIC UNIVERSITY
School of Health Sciences
Seattle, Washington

Programs • Generic Baccalaureate • RN Baccalaureate • MSN • Post-Master's

The University Independent Free Methodist comprehensive coed institution. Founded: 1891. *Primary accreditation:* regional. *Setting:* 35-acre urban campus. *Total enrollment:* 3,437.

The School of Health Sciences Founded in 1952. *Nursing program faculty:* 16.

Academic Facilities *Campus library:* 200,000 volumes; 1,400 periodical subscriptions (175 health-care related).

Calendar Quarters.

BACCALAUREATE PROGRAMS

Contact Associate Dean, School of Health Sciences, Seattle Pacific University, 3307 3rd Avenue West, Seattle, WA 98119, 206-281-2233. *Fax:* 206-281-2767.

Expenses *Tuition:* $13,680 full-time, ranges from $218 to $382 per credit part-time.

Financial Aid Institutionally sponsored need-based grants/scholarships, institutionally sponsored non-need grants/scholarships, Federal Nursing Student Loans, Federal Perkins Loans, Federal Supplemental Educational Opportunity Grants, Federal Work-Study, Federal PLUS Loans, Federal Stafford Loans. *Application deadline:* 3/1.

Generic Baccalaureate Program (BS)

Applying *Required:* SAT I or ACT, TOEFL for nonnative speakers of English, minimum high school GPA of 2.0, minimum college GPA of 2.65, 2 years of high school math, 2 years of high school science, high school chemistry, high school transcript, 2 letters of recommendation, transcript of college record. 25 prerequisite credits must be completed before admission to the nursing program. *Application deadline:* rolling. *Application fee:* $35.

Degree Requirements 180 total credit hours, 75 in nursing. Last 15 credits must be taken at Seattle Pacific University.

RN Baccalaureate Program (BS)

Applying *Required:* RN license, diploma or AD in nursing, high school transcript, 2 letters of recommendation, transcript of college record. *Application deadline:* rolling. *Application fee:* $35.

Degree Requirements 180 total credit hours, 75 in nursing.

MASTER'S PROGRAMS

Contact Dr. Annalee R. Oakes, Director, Graduate Program, School of Health Sciences, Seattle Pacific University, 3307 3rd Avenue West, Seattle, WA 98119, 206-281-2608. *Fax:* 206-281-2767.

Areas of Study Nursing administration; nursing education; nurse practitioner programs in adult health, family health, gerontology.

Expenses *Tuition:* ranges from $275 to $300 per credit hour.

MSN Program

Applying *Required:* GRE General Test, bachelor's degree in nursing, minimum GPA of 3.0, RN license, statistics course, essay, 3 letters of recommendation, 3.50 GPA for nurse practitioner pathways. *Application deadline:* rolling. *Application fee:* $35.

Degree Requirements 45 total credit hours, 45 in nursing. 14 additional credits to complete nurse practitioner pathways. Thesis required.

Post-Master's Program

Applying *Required:* RN license, essay, 3 letters of recommendation, transcript of college record, master's in nursing. *Application deadline:* rolling. *Application fee:* $35.

Degree Requirements 24–30 total credit hours dependent upon track.

SEATTLE UNIVERSITY
School of Nursing
Seattle, Washington

Programs • Generic Baccalaureate • RN Baccalaureate • BSN to Master's

The University Independent Roman Catholic comprehensive coed institution. Founded: 1891. *Primary accreditation:* regional. *Setting:* 46-acre urban campus. *Total enrollment:* 5,988.

The School of Nursing Founded in 1934. *Nursing program faculty:* 32 (41% with doctorates).

Academic Facilities *Campus library:* 208,000 volumes (7,259 in health, 2,159 in nursing); 1,575 periodical subscriptions (122 health-care related). *Nursing school resources:* CAI, computer lab, nursing audiovisuals, interactive nursing skills videos, learning resource lab.

Student Life *Student services:* health clinic, child-care facilities, personal counseling, career counseling, institutionally sponsored work-study program, campus safety program, special assistance for disabled students, minority student affairs, campus ministry, learning center, substance abuse prevention program. *International student services:* counseling/support, special assistance for nonnative speakers of English, ESL courses, student development programs. *Nursing student activities:* Sigma Theta Tau, student nurses association.

Calendar Quarters.

NURSING STUDENT PROFILE

Undergraduate **Enrollment:** 281
Women: 87%; **Men:** 13%; **Minority:** 25%; **International:** 0%; **Part-time:** 29%
Graduate **Enrollment:** 17
Women: 88%; **Men:** 12%; **Minority:** 30%; **International:** 0%; **Part-time:** 100%

BACCALAUREATE PROGRAMS

Contact Ms. Diane Kumfferman, Administrative Secretary to the Dean, School of Nursing, Seattle University, Broadway and Madison, Seattle, WA 98122-4460, 206-296-5660. *Fax:* 206-296-5544.

Expenses *Tuition:* $14,265 full-time, $317 per credit part-time. *Full-time mandatory fees:* $495–$818. *Room and board:* $4713–$6465. *Room only:* $3438–$4620. *Books and supplies per academic year:* $2500.

Financial Aid Institutionally sponsored need-based grants/scholarships, institutionally sponsored non-need grants/scholarships, Federal Direct Loans, Federal Nursing Student Loans, Federal Pell Grants, Federal Perkins Loans, Federal Supplemental Educational Opportunity Grants, Federal Work-Study. 80% of undergraduate students in nursing programs received some form of financial aid in 1995–96. *Application deadline:* 3/1.

Generic Baccalaureate Program (BSN)

Applying *Required:* SAT I or ACT, TOEFL for nonnative speakers of English, minimum high school GPA of 2.75, minimum college GPA of 2.75, high school chemistry, high school transcript, 2 letters of recommendation, written essay, transcript of college record. 65 prerequisite credits must be completed before admission to the nursing program. *Options:* Advanced standing available through advanced placement exams. Course work may be accelerated. May apply for transfer of up to 135 total credits. *Application deadlines:* 2/1 (priority financial aid consideration), rolling. *Application fee:* $45.

Degree Requirements 180 total credit hours, 90 in nursing. University core.

RN Baccalaureate Program (BSN)

Applying *Required:* TOEFL for nonnative speakers of English, minimum college GPA of 2.75, high school chemistry, RN license, diploma or AD in nursing, 2 letters of recommendation, written essay, transcript of college record. 75 prerequisite credits must be completed before admission to the nursing program. *Options:* Advanced standing available through the following means: advanced placement exams, credit by exam. Course work may be accelerated. May apply for transfer of up to 135 total credits. *Application deadline:* rolling. *Application fee:* $45.

Degree Requirements 180 total credit hours, 40 in nursing. University core.

MASTER'S PROGRAM

Contact Dr. Janet Quillian, Director of MSN Program, School of Nursing, Seattle University, Broadway and Madison, Seattle, WA 98122-4460, 206-296-5684. *Fax:* 206-296-5544. *E-mail:* jquill@seattlew.edu

Areas of Study Clinical nurse specialist program in community health nursing; nurse practitioner program in family health.

Expenses *Tuition:* $10,290 full-time, $8575 per credits part-time. *Full-time mandatory fees:* $110. *Books and supplies per academic year:* $1000.

Financial Aid Institutionally sponsored loans, institutionally sponsored need-based grants/scholarships. 41% of master's level students in nursing programs received some form of financial aid in 1995-96. *Application deadline:* 7/15.

BSN to Master's Program (MSN)

Applying *Required:* GRE General Test, bachelor's degree in nursing, minimum GPA of 3.0, RN license, 2 years of clinical experience, physical assessment course, statistics course, professional liability/malpractice insurance, essay, letter of recommendation, transcript of college record. *Application deadlines:* 6/1 (fall), 4/1 (spring). *Application fee:* $55.

Degree Requirements 49–62 total credit hours dependent upon track.

UNIVERSITY OF WASHINGTON
School of Nursing
Seattle, Washington

Programs • Generic Baccalaureate • RN Baccalaureate • MN • Master's for Nurses with Non-Nursing Degrees • Master's for Nurses with Non-Nursing Degrees • MN/MPH • Postdoctoral • Continuing Education

The University State-supported coed university. Founded: 1861. *Primary accreditation:* regional. *Setting:* 703-acre urban campus. *Total enrollment:* 33,996.

The School of Nursing Founded in 1918. *Nursing program faculty:* 101 (90% with doctorates).

Academic Facilities *Campus library:* 6.0 million volumes (123,098 in health); 28,561 periodical subscriptions (4,000 health-care related). *Nursing school resources:* CAI, computer lab, nursing audiovisuals, interactive nursing skills videos, learning resource lab.

Student Life *Student services:* health clinic, personal counseling, career counseling, institutionally sponsored work-study program, campus safety program, special assistance for disabled students. *International student services:* counseling/support, special assistance for nonnative speakers of English, ESL courses. *Nursing student activities:* Sigma Theta Tau, student nurses association.

Calendar Quarters.

NURSING STUDENT PROFILE

Undergraduate **Enrollment:** 348
Women: 93%; **Men:** 7%; **Minority:** 25%; **International:** 1%; **Part-time:** 4%
Graduate **Enrollment:** 347
Women: 93%; **Men:** 7%; **Minority:** 11%; **International:** 10%; **Part-time:** 40%

BACCALAUREATE PROGRAMS

Contact Dagmar Jesse, Undergraduate Adviser, Office of Academic Program, T-310 Health Sciences Building, School of Nursing, University of Washington, Box 357260, Seattle, WA 98195, 206-543-8736. *Fax:* 206-685-1613. *E-mail:* sonapo@u.washington.edu

Expenses *State resident tuition:* $1084 per academic year. *Nonresident tuition:* $3289 per academic year. *Room and board:* $5118. *Books and supplies per academic year:* $1200.

Financial Aid Institutionally sponsored need-based grants/scholarships, Federal Nursing Student Loans, Federal Supplemental Educational Opportunity Grants, Federal Work-Study. *Application deadline:* 1/15.

Generic Baccalaureate Program (BSN)

Applying *Required:* TOEFL for nonnative speakers of English, minimum college GPA of 2.5, 3 years of high school math, high school foreign language, high school transcript, letter of recommendation, written essay, transcript of college record. 90 prerequisite credits must be completed

University of Washington (continued)

before admission to the nursing program. *Options:* May apply for transfer of up to 90 total credits. *Application deadline:* 1/15. *Application fee:* $35.

Degree Requirements 180 total credit hours, 88 in nursing.

RN Baccalaureate Program (BSN)

Applying *Required:* ACT-PEP proficiency exam in adult nursing, maternal child nursing, psychiatric mental health nursing, foundations of gerontology, minimum college GPA of 2.0, RN license, high school transcript, 3 letters of recommendation, written essay. 90 prerequisite credits must be completed before admission to the nursing program. *Options:* Advanced standing available through credit by exam. Course work may be accelerated. May apply for transfer of up to 90 total credits. *Application deadline:* 2/1 (summer). *Application fee:* $35.

Degree Requirements 180 total credit hours, 36 in nursing. 10 credits in liberal studies.

MASTER'S PROGRAMS

Contact Ms. Julie Katz, RN, Coordinator, Graduate Recruitment and Admissions, T-304B Health Sciences Building, School of Nursing, University of Washington, Box 357260, Seattle, WA 98195, 206-543-8736. *Fax:* 206-685-1613. *E-mail:* sonapo@u.washington.edu

Areas of Study Clinical nurse specialist programs in cardiovascular nursing, community health nursing, critical care nursing, gerontological nursing, medical-surgical nursing, occupational health nursing, oncology nursing, pediatric nursing, perinatal nursing, psychiatric–mental health nursing, public health nursing, neuroscience nursing, AIDS; nurse midwifery; nursing administration; nursing education; nurse practitioner programs in acute care, adult health, child care/pediatrics, family health, gerontology, neonatal health, primary care, psychiatric–mental health, women's health.

Expenses *State resident tuition:* $1682 full-time, $481 per 2 credits part-time. *Nonresident tuition:* $4159 full-time, $1189 per 2-credits part-time. *Room and board:* $7248. *Books and supplies per academic year:* ranges from $1500 to $2400.

Financial Aid Graduate assistantships, nurse traineeships, fellowships, Federal Nursing Student Loans, institutionally sponsored loans, employment opportunities, institutionally sponsored need-based grants/scholarships, institutionally sponsored non-need-based grants/scholarships. 9% of master's level students in nursing programs received some form of financial aid in 1995-96. *Application deadline:* 2/28.

MN Program

Applying *Required:* GRE General Test, TOEFL for nonnative speakers of English, CGFNS and NCLEX for international applicants, bachelor's degree in nursing, bachelor's degree, minimum GPA of 3.0, RN license, statistics course, essay, 3 letters of recommendation, transcript of college record, criminal history/background check clearance, resume. *Application deadline:* 2/1. *Application fee:* $45.

Degree Requirements 45 total credit hours, 39 in nursing, 6 in other specified areas. Thesis or scholarly project.

Distance learning Courses provided through video. Specific degree requirements include students should be able to reach campus on a weekly basis.

Master's for Nurses with Non-Nursing Degrees Program (MN)

Applying *Required:* GRE General Test, TOEFL for nonnative speakers of English, ACT PEP; CGFNS and NCLEX for international applicants, bachelor's degree, minimum GPA of 3.0, RN license, statistics course, essay, 3 letters of recommendation, transcript of college record, criminal history/background check clearance, resume. *Application deadline:* 2/1. *Application fee:* $45.

Degree Requirements 45 total credit hours, 39 in nursing, 6 in other specified areas. Thesis or scholarly project.

Distance learning Courses provided through video. Specific degree requirements include students should be able to reach campus on a weekly basis.

Master's for Nurses with Non-Nursing Degrees Program (MS)

Applying *Required:* GRE General Test, TOEFL for nonnative speakers of English, ACT PEP, bachelor's degree, minimum GPA of 3.0, statistics course, essay, 3 letters of recommendation, transcript of college record, criminal history/background check clearance, resume. *Application deadline:* 2/1. *Application fee:* $45.

Degree Requirements 49 total credit hours, 43 in nursing, 6 in other specified areas. Thesis required.

MN/MPH Program

Applying *Required:* GRE General Test, TOEFL for nonnative speakers of English, ACT PEP for nurses with non-nursing degrees; CGFNS and NCLEX for international applicants, bachelor's degree in nursing, bachelor's degree, minimum GPA of 3.0, RN license, statistics course, essay, 3 letters of recommendation, transcript of college record, criminal history/background check clearance, resume. *Application deadline:* rolling. *Application fee:* $45.

Degree Requirements 99+ total credit hours dependent upon track, 45+ in nursing. Thesis required.

DOCTORAL PROGRAM

Contact Ms. Julie Katz, RN, Coordinator, Graduate Recruitment and Admissions, T-304B Health Sciences Building, School of Nursing, University of Washington, Box 357260, Seattle, WA 98195, 206-543-8736. *Fax:* 206-685-1613. *E-mail:* sonapo@u.washington.edu

Areas of Study Nursing research.

Expenses *State resident tuition:* $1682 full-time, $481 per 2-credits part-time. *Nonresident tuition:* $4159 full-time, $1189 per 2-credits part-time. *Room and board:* $7248. *Books and supplies per academic year:* ranges from $1500 to $2400.

Financial Aid Graduate assistantships, nurse traineeships, fellowships, dissertation grants, Federal Nursing Student Loans, institutionally sponsored loans, opportunities for employment, institutionally sponsored need-based grants/scholarships, institutionally sponsored non-need-based grants/scholarships. *Application deadline:* 2/28.

Doctorate in Nursing Sciences Program (PhD)

Applying *Required:* GRE General Test, TOEFL for nonnative speakers of English, 1 scholarly paper, statistics course, 3 letters of recommendation, vitae, competitive review by faculty committee, baccalaureate degree, personal statement, criminal history/background check clearance. *Application deadline:* 2/1. *Application fee:* $45.

Degree Requirements 95 total credit hours; 37 credits in theory and domain of knowledge, 31 in research methods and colloquia, 27 in dissertation research; dissertation; oral exam; written exam; defense of dissertation; residency.

POSTDOCTORAL PROGRAM

Contact Office of Academic Programs, T-310 Health Sciences Building, School of Nursing, University of Washington, Box 357260, Seattle, WA 98195, 206-543-8736. *Fax:* 206-685-1613. *E-mail:* sonapo@u.washington.edu

Areas of Study Nursing systems, women's health, psychophysiologic interface, substance abuse, and individualized study.

CONTINUING EDUCATION PROGRAM

Contact Dr. Ruth Craven, Assistant Dean for Continuing Education, T-303 Health Sciences Building, School of Nursing, University of Washington, Box 357260, Seattle, WA 98195, 206-543-1047. *Fax:* 206-543-3624. *E-mail:* cne@u.washington.edu

WALLA WALLA COLLEGE

School of Nursing
Portland, Oregon

Programs • Generic Baccalaureate • RN Baccalaureate

The College Independent Seventh-day Adventist comprehensive coed institution. Founded: 1892. *Primary accreditation:* regional. *Setting:* 77-acre small-town campus. *Total enrollment:* 1,722.

The School of Nursing Founded in 1897. *Nursing program faculty:* 19 (11% with doctorates).

Academic Facilities *Campus library:* 8,000 volumes (500 in health, 7,000 in nursing); 100 periodical subscriptions (95 health-care related). *Nursing school resources:* CAI, computer lab, nursing audiovisuals, learning resource lab.

Student Life *Student services:* health clinic, personal counseling, career counseling, institutionally sponsored work-study program, job placement, campus safety program, special assistance for disabled students. *International student services:* counseling/support, special assistance for nonnative speakers of English, ESL courses. *Nursing student activities:* nursing club, student nurses association.

Calendar Quarters.

NURSING STUDENT PROFILE

Undergraduate **Enrollment:** 125
Women: 80%; **Men:** 20%; **Minority:** 12%; **International:** 2%; **Part-time:** 13%

BACCALAUREATE PROGRAMS

Contact Ms. Lois Whitchurch, Program Adviser, School of Nursing, Walla Walla College, 10345 Southeast Market Street, Portland, OR 97216, 503-251-6115. *Fax:* 503-251-6249.

Expenses *Tuition:* $11,916 full-time, $316 per quarter credit part-time. *Full-time mandatory fees:* $150+. *Part-time mandatory fees:* $0–$150. *Room only:* $1782–$2232. *Books and supplies per academic year:* ranges from $400 to $800.

Financial Aid Institutionally sponsored need-based grants/scholarships, institutionally sponsored non-need grants/scholarships, Federal Direct Loans, Federal Nursing Student Loans, Federal Pell Grants, Federal Perkins Loans, Federal Supplemental Educational Opportunity Grants, Federal Work-Study. 88% of undergraduate students in nursing programs received some form of financial aid in 1995–96. *Application deadline:* 4/1.

Generic Baccalaureate Program (BS)

Applying *Required:* ACT, Michigan English Language Assessment Battery for nonnative speakers of English, Nelson-Denny Reading Test, California Critical Thinking Skills Test, minimum high school GPA of 2.0, minimum college GPA of 2.5, 2 years of high school math, 2 years of high school science, high school transcript, 3 letters of recommendation, written essay, transcript of college record. *Options:* Advanced standing available through credit by exam. May apply for transfer of up to 156 total credits. *Application deadlines:* 2/1 (summer), rolling. *Application fee:* $30.

Degree Requirements 192 total credit hours, 83 in nursing.

RN Baccalaureate Program (BS)

Applying *Required:* ACT, Michigan English Language Assessment Battery for nonnative speakers of English, NLN Mobility Profile II, California Critical Thinking Skills Test, minimum high school GPA of 2.0, minimum college GPA of 2.5, 2 years of high school math, 2 years of high school science, RN license, diploma or AD in nursing, high school transcript, 3 letters of recommendation, written essay, transcript of college record. 48 prerequisite credits must be completed before admission to the nursing program. *Options:* Advanced standing available through credit by exam. Course work may be accelerated. May apply for transfer of up to 145 total credits. *Application deadline:* rolling. *Application fee:* $30.

Degree Requirements 192 total credit hours, 83 in nursing.

WASHINGTON STATE UNIVERSITY

Intercollegiate Center for Nursing Education
Spokane, Washington

Programs • Generic Baccalaureate • RN Baccalaureate • BSN to Master's • Continuing Education

The University State-supported coed university. Founded: 1890. *Primary accreditation:* regional. *Setting:* 656-acre rural campus. *Total enrollment:* 19,571.

The Intercollegiate Center for Nursing Education Founded in 1968. *Nursing program faculty:* 65 (38% with doctorates). *Off-campus program sites:* Vancouver, Richland, Yakima.

Academic Facilities *Campus library:* 1.7 million volumes (12,120 in nursing); 23,386 periodical subscriptions (2,300 health-care related). *Nursing school resources:* CAI, computer lab, nursing audiovisuals, interactive nursing skills videos, learning resource lab, interactive audiovisual telecommunication classrooms, TV production studio, multimedia classroom.

Student Life *Student services:* health clinic, child-care facilities, personal counseling, career counseling, institutionally sponsored work-study program, job placement, campus safety program, special assistance for disabled students, communication disorders clinic, women's resource center, minority counseling service. *International student services:* counseling/support, special assistance for nonnative speakers of English, ESL courses. *Nursing student activities:* Sigma Theta Tau, nursing club, student nurses association, multicultural club, Nurses Christian Fellowship.

Calendar Semesters.

NURSING STUDENT PROFILE

Undergraduate **Enrollment:** 334
Women: 81%; **Men:** 19%; **Minority:** 10%; **International:** 2%; **Part-time:** 24%
Graduate **Enrollment:** 80
Women: 89%; **Men:** 11%; **Minority:** 0%; **International:** 3%; **Part-time:** 78%

BACCALAUREATE PROGRAMS

Contact Ms. Nancy Hoffman, Nursing Recruiter and Adviser, Lighty 260, Washington State University, Pullman, WA 99164-3524, 509-335-2776. *E-mail:* nhoffman@wsu.edu

Expenses *State resident tuition:* $3024 full-time, $151 per semester credit part-time. *Nonresident tuition:* $4264 full-time, $426 per semester credit part-time. *Full-time mandatory fees:* $664–$666. *Part-time mandatory fees:* $540–$542. *Books and supplies per academic year:* ranges from $710 to $935.

Financial Aid Institutionally sponsored need-based grants/scholarships, institutionally sponsored non-need grants/scholarships, Federal Direct Loans, Federal Nursing Student Loans, Federal Perkins Loans, Federal Supplemental Educational Opportunity Grants, Federal Work-Study. 80% of undergraduate students in nursing programs received some form of financial aid in 1995–96. *Application deadline:* 3/1.

Generic Baccalaureate Program (BSN)

Applying *Required:* SAT I or ACT, Washington Pre-College Test (WPCT), 3 years of high school math, 2 years of high school science, high school chemistry, high school biology, high school foreign language, high school transcript, written essay, transcript of college record, immunizations. 60 prerequisite credits must be completed before admission to the nursing program. *Options:* May apply for transfer of up to 60 total credits. *Application deadlines:* 2/15 (fall), 9/1 (spring). *Application fee:* $35.

Degree Requirements 120 total credit hours, 61 in nursing. Writing qualifying exam.

Distance learning Courses provided through two-way audiovisual microwave television.

RN Baccalaureate Program (BSN)

Applying *Required:* SAT I, ACT, minimum college GPA of 2.5, high school transcript, written essay, transcript of college record, immunizations. 60 prerequisite credits must be completed before admission to the nursing program. *Options:* Advanced standing available through credit by exam. May apply for transfer of up to 60 total credits. *Application deadline:* rolling. *Application fee:* $35.

Degree Requirements 120 total credit hours, 61 in nursing.

Distance learning Courses provided through two-way audiovisual microwave television.

MASTER'S PROGRAM

Contact Dr. Marian Sheafor, Associate Dean for Academic Affairs, Intercollegiate Center for Nursing Education, Washington State University, 2917 West Fort George Wright Drive, Spokane, WA 99224-5291, 509-324-7335. *Fax:* 509-324-7336. *E-mail:* sheafor@wsu.edu

Areas of Study Clinical nurse specialist programs in adult health nursing, community health nursing, psychiatric–mental health nursing; nurse practitioner program in family health.

Expenses *State resident tuition:* $4748 full-time, $237 per semester credit part-time. *Nonresident tuition:* $5947 full-time, $595 per semester credit part-time. *Full-time mandatory fees:* $60–$100. *Books and supplies per academic year:* $700.

Financial Aid Graduate assistantships, nurse traineeships, fellowships, Federal Direct Loans, Federal Nursing Student Loans, institutionally sponsored loans, employment opportunities, institutionally sponsored

Washington State University (continued)
need-based grants/scholarships, institutionally sponsored non-need-based grants/scholarships. 33% of master's level students in nursing programs received some form of financial aid in 1995-96. *Application deadline:* 2/15.

BSN to Master's Program (MN)

Applying *Required:* bachelor's degree in nursing, minimum GPA of 3.0, RN license, physical assessment course, statistics course, essay, 3 letters of recommendation, transcript of college record, CPR certification, immunizations, word processing skills; interview for family nurse practitioner track. *Application deadlines:* 3/15 (fall), 11/1 (spring). *Application fee:* $35.

Degree Requirements 39–45 total credit hours dependent upon track, 29–34 in nursing, 10–11 in courses supportive to major and interests. Clinical or other research project or thesis.

Distance learning Courses provided through two-way audiovisual microwave television.

CONTINUING EDUCATION PROGRAM

Contact Dr. Barbara Johnston, Assistant Dean for Continuing Education, Intercollegiate Center for Nursing Education, Washington State University, 2917 West Fort George Wright Drive, Spokane, WA 99204-5291, 509-324-7356. *Fax:* 509-324-7836.

WHITWORTH COLLEGE

Intercollegiate Center for Nursing Education
Spokane, Washington

Programs • Generic Baccalaureate • RN Baccalaureate • BSN to Master's • Continuing Education

The College Independent Presbyterian comprehensive coed institution. Founded: 1890. *Primary accreditation:* regional. *Setting:* 200-acre suburban campus. *Total enrollment:* 2,057.

The Intercollegiate Center for Nursing Education Founded in 1968. *Nursing program faculty:* 65 (38% with doctorates). *Off-campus program sites:* Vancouver, Richland, Yakima.

Academic Facilities *Campus library:* 144,857 volumes (12,120 in nursing); 715 periodical subscriptions (280 health-care related). *Nursing school resources:* CAI, computer lab, nursing audiovisuals, interactive nursing skills videos, learning resource lab, interactive audiovisual telecommunication classrooms, TV production studio, multimedia classroom.

Student Life *Student services:* health clinic, personal counseling, career counseling, institutionally sponsored work-study program, job placement, campus safety program, special assistance for disabled students, tutoring, residence hall programs, spiritual mentoring groups, service learning projects, and internships. *International student services:* counseling/support, special assistance for nonnative speakers of English, ESL courses. *Nursing student activities:* Sigma Theta Tau, nursing club, student nurses association, multicultural club, Nurses Christian Fellowship, student government.

Calendar Semesters.

NURSING STUDENT PROFILE

Undergraduate **Enrollment:** 334
Women: 81%; **Men:** 19%; **Minority:** 10%; **International:** 2%; **Part-time:** 24%
Graduate **Enrollment:** 80
Women: 89%; **Men:** 11%; **Minority:** 0%; **International:** 3%; **Part-time:** 78%

BACCALAUREATE PROGRAMS

Contact Kathleen Kovarik, Nursing Adviser, Intercollegiate Center for Nursing Education, Whitworth College, 2917 West Fort George Wright Drive, Spokane, WA 99224-5291, 509-466-1000. *Fax:* 509-324-7341. *E-mail:* kovarik@wsu.edu

Expenses *Tuition:* ranges from $3024 to $13,410 full-time, ranges from $151 to $550 per semester credit part-time. *Full-time mandatory fees:* $664–$666. *Part-time mandatory fees:* $540–$542. *Books and supplies per academic year:* ranges from $710 to $935.

Financial Aid Institutionally sponsored need-based grants/scholarships, institutionally sponsored non-need grants/scholarships, Federal Nursing Student Loans, Federal Pell Grants, Federal Supplemental Educational Opportunity Grants, Federal Work-Study. 80% of undergraduate students in nursing programs received some form of financial aid in 1995–96. *Application deadline:* 3/1.

Generic Baccalaureate Program (BSN)

Applying *Required:* SAT I, ACT, minimum college GPA of 2.5, high school transcript, written essay, transcript of college record, immunizations. 60 prerequisite credits must be completed before admission to the nursing program. *Application deadlines:* 2/15 (fall), 9/1 (spring). *Application fee:* $30.

Degree Requirements 120 total credit hours, 61 in nursing.

Distance learning Courses provided through two-way audiovisual microwave television.

RN Baccalaureate Program (BSN)

Applying *Required:* SAT I, ACT, minimum college GPA of 2.5, high school transcript, written essay, transcript of college record, immunizations. 60 prerequisite credits must be completed before admission to the nursing program. *Options:* Advanced standing available through credit by exam. May apply for transfer of up to 60 total credits. *Application deadline:* rolling. *Application fee:* $30.

Degree Requirements 120 total credit hours, 61 in nursing.

Distance learning Courses provided through two-way audiovisual microwave television.

MASTER'S PROGRAM

Contact Dr. Marian Sheafor, Associate Dean for Academic Affairs, Intercollegiate Center for Nursing Education, Whitworth College, 2917 West Fort George Wright Drive, Spokane, WA 99224-5291, 509-324-7335. *Fax:* 509-324-7336. *E-mail:* sheafor@wsu.edu

Areas of Study Clinical nurse specialist programs in adult health nursing, community health nursing, psychiatric–mental health nursing; nurse practitioner program in family health.

Expenses *Tuition:* $4748 full-time, $237 per semester credit part-time. *Full-time mandatory fees:* $60–$100. *Books and supplies per academic year:* $700.

Financial Aid Graduate assistantships, nurse traineeships, fellowships, employment opportunities, institutionally sponsored need-based grants/scholarships, institutionally sponsored non-need-based grants/scholarships. 33% of master's level students in nursing programs received some form of financial aid in 1995-96. *Application deadline:* 2/15.

BSN to Master's Program (MN)

Applying *Required:* bachelor's degree in nursing, minimum GPA of 3.0, RN license, physical assessment course, statistics course, essay, 3 letters of recommendation, transcript of college record, CPR certification, immunizations, word processing skills; interview for family nurse practitioner track. *Application deadlines:* 3/15 (fall), 11/1 (spring). *Application fee:* $35.

Degree Requirements 39–45 total credit hours dependent upon track, 29–34 in nursing, 10–11 in courses supportive to major and interests. Clinical or other research project; thesis optional.

Distance learning Courses provided through two-way audiovisual microwave television.

CONTINUING EDUCATION PROGRAM

Contact Dr. Barbara Johnston, Assistant Dean for Continuing Education, Intercollegiate Center for Nursing Education, Whitworth College, 2917 West Fort George Wright Drive, Spokane, WA 99204-5291, 509-324-7356. *Fax:* 509-324-7836.

WEST VIRGINIA

ALDERSON-BROADDUS COLLEGE

Department of Nursing
Philippi, West Virginia

Programs • Generic Baccalaureate • RN Baccalaureate • LPN to RN Baccalaureate

The College Independent comprehensive coed institution, affiliated with Baptist Church. Founded: 1871. *Primary accreditation:* regional. *Setting:* 170-acre rural campus. *Total enrollment:* 851.

The Department of Nursing Founded in 1946.

Academic Facilities *Campus library:* 107,000 volumes (6,000 in health); 600 periodical subscriptions (172 health-care related).

Calendar Semesters.

BACCALAUREATE PROGRAMS

Contact Chairperson, Department of Nursing, Alderson-Broaddus College, Box 246, Philippi, WV 26416, 304-457-1700 Ext. 285. *Fax:* 304-457-6308.

Financial Aid Institutionally sponsored need-based grants/scholarships, institutionally sponsored non-need grants/scholarships, Federal Direct Loans, Federal Pell Grants, Federal Perkins Loans, Federal Supplemental Educational Opportunity Grants, Federal Work-Study, Federal Stafford Loans.

Generic Baccalaureate Program (BS)

Applying *Required:* SAT I or ACT, high school transcript. *Application fee:* $10.

Degree Requirements Comprehensive exam and 2.00 GPA in major.

RN Baccalaureate Program (BS)

Applying *Required:* SAT I or ACT, TOEFL for nonnative speakers of English, NLN Mobility Profile II, RN license, high school transcript, 1 year of experience as an RN. *Application fee:* $10.

Degree Requirements 55 total credit hours in nursing. Comprehensive exam and 2.00 GPA in major.

LPN to RN Baccalaureate Program (BS)

Applying *Required:* SAT I or ACT, TOEFL for nonnative speakers of English, NLN Mobility Profile I, high school transcript, LPN license. *Application fee:* $10.

Degree Requirements 55 total credit hours in nursing.

MARSHALL UNIVERSITY
School of Nursing
Huntington, West Virginia

Programs • Generic Baccalaureate • RN Baccalaureate • MSN

The University State-supported comprehensive coed institution. Part of University System of West Virginia. Founded: 1837. *Primary accreditation:* regional. *Setting:* 70-acre urban campus. *Total enrollment:* 12,468.

The School of Nursing Founded in 1960. *Nursing program faculty:* 24 (33% with doctorates). *Off-campus program sites:* Logan, Williamson, Point Pleasant.

Academic Facilities *Campus library:* 400,000 volumes (20,015 in health, 6,005 in nursing); 2,319 periodical subscriptions (486 health-care related). *Nursing school resources:* CAI, computer lab, nursing audiovisuals, interactive nursing skills videos, learning resource lab.

Student Life *Student services:* health clinic, personal counseling, career counseling, institutionally sponsored work-study program, job placement, campus safety program, special assistance for disabled students. *International student services:* counseling/support, ESL courses. *Nursing student activities:* Sigma Theta Tau, student nurses association, Nurses Christian Fellowship.

Calendar Semesters.

NURSING STUDENT PROFILE

Undergraduate **Enrollment:** 325
Women: 92%; **Men:** 8%; **Minority:** 1%; **International:** 0%; **Part-time:** 9%
Graduate **Enrollment:** 34
Women: 98%; **Men:** 2%; **Minority:** 2%; **International:** 0%; **Part-time:** 66%

BACCALAUREATE PROGRAMS

Contact Dr. Judith Sortet, BSN Program Director, School of Nursing, Marshall University, 400 Hal Greer Boulevard, Huntington, WV 25755-9500, 304-696-6759. *Fax:* 304-696-6739. *E-mail:* sortet@marshall.edu

Expenses *State resident tuition:* $2366 full-time, $99 per credit hour part-time. *Nonresident tuition:* $4548 full-time, $270 per credit hour part-time. *Full-time mandatory fees:* $200. *Part-time mandatory fees:* $99–$270+. *Room and board:* $1750–$2850. *Room only:* $840–$1335. *Books and supplies per academic year:* ranges from $200 to $400.

Financial Aid Institutionally sponsored need-based grants/scholarships, institutionally sponsored non-need grants/scholarships, Federal Nursing Student Loans, Federal Pell Grants, Federal Perkins Loans, Federal Supplemental Educational Opportunity Grants, Federal Work-Study. *Application deadline:* 3/1.

Generic Baccalaureate Program (BSN)

Applying *Required:* ACT, minimum high school GPA of 2.5, minimum college GPA of 2.5, high school transcript, transcript of college record. 12 prerequisite credits must be completed before admission to the nursing program. *Options:* May apply for transfer of up to 72 total credits. *Application deadline:* 1/15. *Application fee:* $30.

Degree Requirements 128 total credit hours, 64 in nursing.

RN Baccalaureate Program (BSN)

Applying *Required:* minimum college GPA of 2.3, RN license, diploma or AD in nursing, transcript of college record. *Options:* May apply for transfer of up to 72 total credits. *Application deadline:* rolling. *Application fee:* $30.

Degree Requirements 128 total credit hours, 35 in nursing.

Distance learning Courses provided through live satellite delivery.

MASTER'S PROGRAM

Contact Dr. Giovanna Morton, Graduate Program Director and Professor, School of Nursing, Marshall University, 400 Hal Greer Boulevard, Huntington, WV 25755-9500, 304-696-2636. *Fax:* 304-696-6739. *E-mail:* mortong@marshall.edu

Areas of Study Nursing administration; nurse practitioner program in family health.

Expenses *State resident tuition:* $1348 full-time, $150 per hour part-time. *Nonresident tuition:* $3700 full-time, $412 per hour part-time. *Full-time mandatory fees:* $200. *Part-time mandatory fees:* $128–$356+. *Books and supplies per academic year:* ranges from $400 to $600.

Financial Aid Graduate assistantships, Federal Nursing Student Loans, tuition waivers. *Application deadline:* 3/1.

MSN Program

Applying *Required:* GRE General Test, bachelor's degree in nursing, minimum GPA of 3.0, RN license, statistics course, transcript of college record. *Application deadlines:* 7/1 (fall), 11/1 (spring). *Application fee:* $10–25.

Degree Requirements 36–42 total credit hours dependent upon track, 36–42 in nursing. Research utilization project.

SHEPHERD COLLEGE
Department of Nursing Education
Shepherdstown, West Virginia

Programs • Generic Baccalaureate • Accelerated RN Baccalaureate

The College State-supported 4-year coed college. Part of State College System of West Virginia. Founded: 1871. *Primary accreditation:* regional. *Setting:* 320-acre small-town campus. *Total enrollment:* 3,602.

The Department of Nursing Education Founded in 1973. *Nursing program faculty:* 10.

Academic Facilities *Nursing school resources:* CAI, computer lab, nursing audiovisuals, learning resource lab.

Student Life *Student services:* health clinic, personal counseling, career counseling, institutionally sponsored work-study program, job placement, campus safety program, special assistance for disabled students. *International student services:* counseling/support. *Nursing student activities:* student nurses association.

Calendar Semesters.

NURSING STUDENT PROFILE

Undergraduate **Enrollment:** 60

BACCALAUREATE PROGRAMS

Contact Dr. Charlotte R. Anderson, Chair, Department of Nursing Education, Shepherd College, Shepherdstown, WV 25443, 304-876-5341. *Fax:* 304-876-3101.

Expenses *State resident tuition:* $2160 full-time, $90 per credit hour part-time. *Nonresident tuition:* $5098 full-time, $213 per credit hour part-time.

Shepherd College (continued)

GENERIC BACCALAUREATE PROGRAM (BSN)

Applying *Required:* SAT I or ACT, minimum college GPA of 2.5, high school transcript, interview, letter of recommendation, transcript of college record. *Application deadline:* 2/1. *Application fee:* $25.

Degree Requirements 128 total credit hours, 63 in nursing.

ACCELERATED RN BACCALAUREATE PROGRAM (BSN)

Applying *Required:* minimum college GPA of 2.5, RN license, diploma or AD in nursing, interview, letter of recommendation, transcript of college record, 1 year of clinical experience. *Application deadline:* 2/1. *Application fee:* $25.

Degree Requirements 128 total credit hours, 63 in nursing.

UNIVERSITY OF CHARLESTON

Department of Nursing
Charleston, West Virginia

Program • Generic Baccalaureate

The University Independent comprehensive coed institution. Founded: 1888. *Primary accreditation:* regional. *Setting:* 40-acre urban campus. *Total enrollment:* 1,322.

The Department of Nursing Founded in 1987. *Nursing program faculty:* 10 (40% with doctorates).

Academic Facilities *Campus library:* 125,000 volumes (3,200 in health, 1,300 in nursing); 565 periodical subscriptions (60 health-care related). *Nursing school resources:* CAI, computer lab, nursing audiovisuals, interactive nursing skills videos, learning resource lab.

Student Life *Student services:* personal counseling, career counseling, institutionally sponsored work-study program, job placement, campus safety program. *International student services:* counseling/support, special assistance for nonnative speakers of English, ESL courses, international student organization. *Nursing student activities:* Sigma Theta Tau, student nurses association, Nursing Honor Society.

Calendar Semesters.

NURSING STUDENT PROFILE

Undergraduate

Women: 94%; **Men:** 6%; **Minority:** 2%; **International:** 0%; **Part-time:** 18%

BACCALAUREATE PROGRAM

Contact Mr. Alan Liebrecht, Director of Admissions, Division of Health Sciences, University of Charleston, 2300 MacCorkle Avenue, SE, Charleston, WV 25304, 304-357-4750. *Fax:* 304-357-4715. *E-mail:* gouc@citynet.net

Expenses *Tuition:* $10,990 per academic year. *Full-time mandatory fees:* $127–$147. *Room and board:* $3720–$4835. *Room only:* $1600–$2450. *Books and supplies per academic year:* ranges from $500 to $750.

Financial Aid Institutionally sponsored need-based grants/scholarships, institutionally sponsored non-need grants/scholarships, Federal Nursing Student Loans, Federal Pell Grants, Federal Perkins Loans, Federal Supplemental Educational Opportunity Grants, Federal Work-Study, Federal PLUS Loans, Federal Stafford Loans. *Application deadline:* 3/1.

GENERIC BACCALAUREATE PROGRAM (BSN)

Applying *Required:* SAT I, ACT, TOEFL for nonnative speakers of English, minimum high school GPA of 2.5, 3 years of high school math, high school chemistry, high school transcript. *Application deadline:* 12/31. *Application fee:* $20.

Degree Requirements 128 total credit hours, 51 in nursing.

WEST LIBERTY STATE COLLEGE

Department of Nursing
West Liberty, West Virginia

Programs • Generic Baccalaureate • Accelerated RN Baccalaureate

The College State-supported 4-year coed college. Part of State College System of West Virginia. Founded: 1837. *Primary accreditation:* regional. *Setting:* 290-acre rural campus. *Total enrollment:* 2,435.

The Department of Nursing Founded in 1988. *Nursing program faculty:* 10 (20% with doctorates). *Off-campus program sites:* Warwood, Weirton.

Academic Facilities *Campus library:* 200,000 volumes; 750 periodical subscriptions. *Nursing school resources:* CAI, computer lab, nursing audiovisuals, learning resource lab.

Student Life *Student services:* health clinic, child-care facilities, personal counseling, career counseling, institutionally sponsored work-study program, job placement, special assistance for disabled students. *International student services:* counseling/support, special assistance for nonnative speakers of English. *Nursing student activities:* student nurses association.

Calendar Semesters.

NURSING STUDENT PROFILE

Undergraduate **Enrollment:** 88

Women: 95%; **Men:** 5%; **Minority:** 2%; **International:** 0%; **Part-time:** 15%

BACCALAUREATE PROGRAMS

Contact Dr. Donna Lukich, Chairperson, Department of Nursing, West Liberty State College, West Liberty, WV 26074, 304-336-8108. *Fax:* 304-336-8285.

Expenses *State resident tuition:* $2200 full-time, $84 per credit hour part-time. *Nonresident tuition:* $5460 full-time, $228 per credit hour part-time. *Full-time mandatory fees:* $100–$150. *Room and board:* $3000. *Books and supplies per academic year:* ranges from $250 to $500.

Financial Aid Institutionally sponsored need-based grants/scholarships, institutionally sponsored non-need grants/scholarships, Federal Nursing Student Loans, Federal Pell Grants, Federal Perkins Loans, Federal Supplemental Educational Opportunity Grants, Federal Work-Study. *Application deadline:* 3/1.

GENERIC BACCALAUREATE PROGRAM (BSN)

Applying *Required:* SAT I, ACT, minimum high school GPA of 3.0, minimum college GPA of 2.5, 2 years of high school math, 2 years of high school science, high school transcript, interview, letter of recommendation, transcript of college record, immunizations, high school transcript or GED certificate, health exam. 28 prerequisite credits must be completed before admission to the nursing program. *Options:* Advanced standing available through the following means: advanced placement exams, credit by exam. May apply for transfer of up to 72 total credits. *Application deadline:* 2/15.

Degree Requirements 128 total credit hours, 64 in nursing.

ACCELERATED RN BACCALAUREATE PROGRAM (BSN)

Applying *Required:* minimum college GPA of 2.0, RN license, diploma or AD in nursing, interview, letter of recommendation, transcript of college record. 28 prerequisite credits must be completed before admission to the nursing program. *Options:* Advanced standing available through credit by exam. Course work may be accelerated. May apply for transfer of up to 72 total credits. *Application deadline:* 2/15.

Degree Requirements 128 total credit hours, 64 in nursing.

WEST VIRGINIA UNIVERSITY

School of Nursing
Morgantown, West Virginia

Programs • Generic Baccalaureate • RN Baccalaureate • MSN • Post-Master's

The University State-supported coed university. Part of University of West Virginia System. Founded: 1867. *Primary accreditation:* regional. *Setting:* 541-acre small-town campus. *Total enrollment:* 21,517.

The School of Nursing Founded in 1960. *Nursing program faculty:* 59 (39% with doctorates). *Off-campus program sites:* Charleston, Parkersburg, Glenville.

NOTEWORTHY

West Virginia University School of Nursing offers revised curricula at undergraduate and graduate levels. Exciting programs in primary care, advanced technology, and rural health prepare graduates for practice in the 21st century. Caring, critical thinking, communication, professional development, and nursing interventions in a variety of clinical settings are curricular themes. The graduate program offers a Master of Science in Nursing in rural primary health care with preparation in advanced practice nursing, nursing administration, or nursing education. The advanced practice track focuses on vulnerable family populations with specialization in family health, child health, elder health, or women's health. Alternative tracks to the BSN and the MSN degrees are available.

Academic Facilities *Campus library:* 1.7 million volumes (205,737 in health, 2,950 in nursing); 11,099 periodical subscriptions (2,055 health-care related). *Nursing school resources:* CAI, computer lab, nursing audiovisuals, learning resource lab.

Student Life *Student services:* health clinic, personal counseling, career counseling, institutionally sponsored work-study program, job placement, campus safety program, special assistance for disabled students. *International student services:* counseling/support, special assistance for nonnative speakers of English, ESL courses. *Nursing student activities:* Sigma Theta Tau, student nurses association.

Calendar Semesters.

NURSING STUDENT PROFILE

Undergraduate **Enrollment:** 360
Women: 84%; **Men:** 16%; **Minority:** 3%; **International:** 0%; **Part-time:** 24%
Graduate **Enrollment:** 125
Women: 99%; **Men:** 1%; **Minority:** 2%; **International:** 0%; **Part-time:** 78%

BACCALAUREATE PROGRAMS

Contact Ms. Jacqueline W. Riley, Assistant Dean, Student and Alumni Affairs, 6702 HSS, School of Nursing, West Virginia University, PO Box 9600, Morgantown, WV 26506-9600, 304-293-1386. *Fax:* 304-293-6826. *E-mail:* jriley@wvu.edu

Expenses *State resident tuition:* $2794 full-time, $119 per credit hour part-time. *Nonresident tuition:* $4351 full-time, $365 per credit hour part-time. *Room and board:* $4108–$5208. *Room only:* $2292–$3054. *Books and supplies per academic year:* ranges from $200 to $900.

Financial Aid Institutionally sponsored need-based grants/scholarships, institutionally sponsored non-need grants/scholarships, Federal Direct Loans, Federal Nursing Student Loans, Federal Pell Grants, Federal Perkins Loans, Federal Supplemental Educational Opportunity Grants, Federal Work-Study, Federal scholarships for disadvantaged students, ROTC scholarships, USPHS Co-Step Program, VA scholarships. 73% of undergraduate students in nursing programs received some form of financial aid in 1995–96. *Application deadline:* 3/1.

Generic Baccalaureate Program (BSN)

Applying *Required:* SAT I or ACT, TOEFL for nonnative speakers of English, minimum college GPA of 2.5, 3 years of high school math, 2 years of high school science, high school biology, high school transcript, written essay, transcript of college record, minimum 3.2 college GPA for nonresidents. 33 prerequisite credits must be completed before admission to the nursing program. *Options:* Advanced standing available through credit by exam. May apply for transfer of up to 72 total credits. *Application deadline:* 2/15. *Application fee:* $10.

Degree Requirements 136 total credit hours, 73 in nursing.

RN Baccalaureate Program (BSN)

Applying *Required:* minimum college GPA of 2.5, RN license, diploma or AD in nursing, written essay, transcript of college record. 3 prerequisite credits must be completed before admission to the nursing program. *Options:* Advanced standing available through the following means: advanced placement exams, credit by exam. Course work may be accelerated. May apply for transfer of up to 72 total credits. *Application deadline:* rolling. *Application fee:* $10.

Degree Requirements 128–129 total credit hours dependent upon track, 84 in nursing.

MASTER'S PROGRAMS

Contact Ms. Jacqueline W. Riley, Assistant Dean, Student and Alumni Affairs, 6702 HSS, School of Nursing, West Virginia University, PO Box 9600, Morgantown, WV 26506-9600, 304-293-1386. *Fax:* 304-293-6826. *E-mail:* jriley@wvu.edu

Areas of Study Nursing administration; nursing education; nurse practitioner programs in adult health, child care/pediatrics, family health, primary care, women's health.

Expenses *State resident tuition:* $3006 full-time, $169 per credit hour part-time. *Nonresident tuition:* $4530 full-time, $506 per credit hour part-time. *Full-time mandatory fees:* $1642–$4718. *Room and board:* $6215–$6445. *Room only:* $2350. *Books and supplies per academic year:* ranges from $250 to $500.

Financial Aid Graduate assistantships, nurse traineeships, fellowships, Federal Direct Loans, Federal Nursing Student Loans, employment opportunities, state-sponsored health sciences scholarships. 44% of master's level students in nursing programs received some form of financial aid in 1995-96. *Application deadline:* 3/1.

MSN Program

Applying *Required:* GRE General Test (minimum combined score of 1250 on three tests), bachelor's degree in nursing, minimum GPA of 3.0, RN license, physical assessment course, statistics course, essay, 3 letters of recommendation, transcript of college record. *Application deadlines:* 6/1 (fall), 10/1 (spring), 3/1 (summer). *Application fee:* $45.

Degree Requirements 44–47 total credit hours dependent upon track, 37–40 in nursing, 7 in advanced physiology, pharmacotherapy. Thesis or master's paper.

Distance learning Courses provided through compressed video. Specific degree requirements include periodic on-campus sessions; MDTV courses available only at approved sites in West Virginia.

Post-Master's Program

Applying *Required:* minimum GPA of 3.0, RN license, physical assessment course, essay, 3 letters of recommendation, transcript of college record, MSN. *Application deadlines:* 6/1 (fall), 10/1 (spring), 3/1 (summer). *Application fee:* $45.

Degree Requirements 26 total credit hours, 19 in nursing, 7 in advanced physiology/pathophysiology; applied pharmacology.

Distance learning Courses provided through compressed video. Specific degree requirements include periodic on-campus sessions; MDTV courses available only at selected sites in West Virginia.

WEST VIRGINIA WESLEYAN COLLEGE

Department of Nursing
Buckhannon, West Virginia

Programs • Generic Baccalaureate • RN Baccalaureate • Baccalaureate for Second Degree

The College Independent comprehensive coed institution, affiliated with United Methodist Church. Founded: 1890. *Primary accreditation:* regional. *Setting:* 80-acre small-town campus. *Total enrollment:* 1,679.

The Department of Nursing Founded in 1961. *Nursing program faculty:* 9 (30% with doctorates).

Academic Facilities *Campus library:* 150,000 volumes (4,000 in health, 600 in nursing); 672 periodical subscriptions (90 health-care related). *Nursing school resources:* CAI, computer lab, nursing audiovisuals, interactive nursing skills videos, learning resource lab, nursing skills lab.

Student Life *Student services:* health clinic, child-care facilities, personal counseling, career counseling, institutionally sponsored work-study program, job placement, campus safety program, special assistance for

West Virginia Wesleyan College (continued)
disabled students. *International student services:* counseling/support, special assistance for nonnative speakers of English, ESL courses. *Nursing student activities:* Sigma Theta Tau, student nurses association.

Calendar Semesters.

NURSING STUDENT PROFILE

Undergraduate **Enrollment:** 154
Women: 97%; **Men:** 3%; **Minority:** 2%; **International:** 1%; **Part-time:** 49%

BACCALAUREATE PROGRAMS

Contact Dr. Nancy Alfred, Chairperson, Nursing Department, West Virginia Wesleyan College, 59 College Avenue, Buckhannon, WV 26201-2995, 304-473-8224. *Fax:* 304-472-2571. *E-mail:* alfred@academ.wvwc.edu

Expenses *Tuition:* $14,975 full-time, $625 per credit hour part-time. *Full-time mandatory fees:* $75–$125. *Room and board:* $3550–$5600. *Room only:* $1450–$3500. *Books and supplies per academic year:* ranges from $250 to $350.

Financial Aid Institutionally sponsored need-based grants/scholarships, institutionally sponsored non-need grants/scholarships, Federal Nursing Student Loans, Federal Pell Grants, Federal Perkins Loans, Federal Supplemental Educational Opportunity Grants, Federal Work-Study. 44% of undergraduate students in nursing programs received some form of financial aid in 1995–96. *Application deadline:* 3/15.

Generic Baccalaureate Program (BSN)

Applying *Required:* SAT I, ACT, TOEFL for nonnative speakers of English, minimum high school GPA of 2.35, minimum college GPA of 2.5, high school transcript, transcript of college record. *Options:* Advanced standing available through credit by exam. May apply for transfer of up to 96 total credits. *Application deadlines:* 8/15 (fall), 1/15 (spring). *Application fee:* $25.

Degree Requirements 128–136 total credit hours dependent upon track, 58 in nursing.

RN Baccalaureate Program (BSN)

Applying *Required:* TOEFL for nonnative speakers of English, minimum college GPA of 2.0, RN license, diploma or AD in nursing, transcript of college record, professional liability/malpractice insurance. *Options:* Advanced standing available through the following means: advanced placement exams, credit by exam. May apply for transfer of up to 96 total credits. *Application deadlines:* 8/15 (fall), 1/15 (spring). *Application fee:* $25.

Degree Requirements 128–136 total credit hours dependent upon track, 58 in nursing.

Baccalaureate for Second Degree Program (BSN)

Applying *Required:* TOEFL for nonnative speakers of English, minimum college GPA of 2.5, transcript of college record. *Options:* Advanced standing available through credit by exam. May apply for transfer of up to 96 total credits. *Application deadlines:* 8/15 (fall), 1/15 (spring). *Application fee:* $25.

Degree Requirements 128–136 total credit hours dependent upon track, 58 in nursing.

WHEELING JESUIT COLLEGE
Department of Nursing
Wheeling, West Virginia

Programs • Generic Baccalaureate • RN Baccalaureate • MSN

The College Independent Roman Catholic (Jesuit) comprehensive coed institution. Founded: 1954. *Primary accreditation:* regional. *Setting:* 70-acre suburban campus. *Total enrollment:* 1,500.

The Department of Nursing Founded in 1976.

Academic Facilities *Campus library:* 9,550 volumes (191 in health, 382 in nursing); 553 periodical subscriptions (83 health-care related).

Student Life *Student services:* health clinic, campus safety program. *Nursing student activities:* student nurses association.

Calendar Semesters.

NURSING STUDENT PROFILE

Undergraduate **Enrollment:** 180
Women: 95%; **Men:** 5%
Graduate **Enrollment:** 20
Women: 95%; **Men:** 5%

BACCALAUREATE PROGRAMS

Contact Admissions Office, Department of Nursing, Wheeling Jesuit College, 316 Washington Avenue, Wheeling, WV 26003-6233, 304-243-2359.

Expenses *Tuition:* $13,000 full-time, ranges from $175 to $360 per credit part-time.

Generic Baccalaureate Program (BSN)

Applying *Required:* SAT I or ACT, TOEFL for nonnative speakers of English, high school transcript. *Options:* Advanced standing available through advanced placement exams. *Application fee:* $25.

Degree Requirements 120 total credit hours, 54 in nursing.

RN Baccalaureate Program (BSN)

Applying *Required:* TOEFL for nonnative speakers of English, RN license, diploma or AD in nursing, high school transcript, transcript of college record. *Application fee:* $25.

Degree Requirements 122 total credit hours, 59 in nursing.

MASTER'S PROGRAM

Contact Assistant for Graduate Programs, Department of Nursing, Wheeling Jesuit College, 316 Washington Avenue, Wheeling, WV 26003-6233, 304-243-2227. *Fax:* 304-243-2243.

Expenses *Tuition:* $330 per credit.

MSN Program

Applying *Required:* GRE General Test, bachelor's degree in nursing, minimum GPA of 3.0, statistics course, 3 letters of recommendation. *Application fee:* $25.

Degree Requirements 41 total credit hours, 29 in nursing, 12 in business administration. Thesis required.

WISCONSIN

ALVERNO COLLEGE
Nursing Division
Milwaukee, Wisconsin

Programs • Generic Baccalaureate • RN Baccalaureate • Continuing Education

The College Independent Roman Catholic 4-year women's college. Founded: 1887. *Primary accreditation:* regional. *Setting:* 46-acre suburban campus. *Total enrollment:* 2,084.

The Nursing Division Founded in 1930. *Nursing program faculty:* 24 (21% with doctorates).

Academic Facilities *Campus library:* 85,279 volumes (1,545 in health, 3,911 in nursing); 1,434 periodical subscriptions (154 health-care related). *Nursing school resources:* CAI, computer lab, nursing audiovisuals, interactive nursing skills videos, learning resource lab, on-line/electronic searching.

Student Life *Student services:* health clinic, child-care facilities, personal counseling, career counseling, institutionally sponsored work-study program, campus safety program, special assistance for disabled students, off-campus learning experiences, international study courses. *International student services:* counseling/support, special assistance for nonnative speakers of English, ESL courses. *Nursing student activities:* student nurses association, Black Students Nurses of Alverno.

Calendar Semesters.

NURSING STUDENT PROFILE

Undergraduate **Enrollment:** 430
Women: 100%; **Minority:** 29%; **International:** 0%; **Part-time:** 42%

BACCALAUREATE PROGRAMS

Contact Dr. Jean E. Bartels, Chairperson, Nursing Division, Alverno College, 3401 South 39th Street, PO Box 343922, Milwaukee, WI 53234-3922, 414-382-6281. *Fax:* 414-382-6279. *E-mail:* jbartels@execpc.com

Expenses *Tuition:* $4992 full-time, $416 per semester hour part-time. *Full-time mandatory fees:* $25–$50. *Room and board:* $1945–$2225. *Books and supplies per academic year:* ranges from $100 to $300.

Financial Aid Institutionally sponsored need-based grants/scholarships, institutionally sponsored non-need grants/scholarships, Federal Pell Grants, Federal Perkins Loans, Federal Supplemental Educational Opportunity Grants, Federal Work-Study, State Minority Retention Grant Program, State Tuition Grant. 96% of undergraduate students in nursing programs received some form of financial aid in 1995–96. *Application deadline:* 4/15.

Generic Baccalaureate Program (BSN)

Applying *Required:* ACT, TOEFL for nonnative speakers of English, Alverno performance assessment, high school chemistry, high school biology, high school transcript, transcript of college record. *Options:* Advanced standing available through the following means: advanced placement exams, credit by exam. *Application deadline:* rolling. *Application fee:* $10.

Degree Requirements 115–120 total credit hours dependent upon track, 45 in nursing. Non-nursing support area/minor of student's choice.

RN Baccalaureate Program (BSN)

Applying *Required:* Alverno performance assessment, RN license, diploma or AD in nursing, high school transcript, transcript of college record, 3 courses each in behavioral and natural science. *Application deadlines:* 8/1 (fall), 12/15 (spring). *Application fee:* $10.

Degree Requirements 115–120 total credit hours dependent upon track, 47 in nursing. Non-nursing support area/minor of student's choice.

CONTINUING EDUCATION PROGRAM

Contact Ms. Debra Pass, Director, Telesis Institute, Nursing Division, Alverno College, 3401 South 39th Street, PO Box 343922, Milwaukee, WI 53234-3922, 414-382-6177. *Fax:* 414-382-6354.

BELLIN COLLEGE OF NURSING
Green Bay, Wisconsin

Programs • Generic Baccalaureate • Continuing Education

The College Independent 4-year specialized primarily women's college. Founded: 1909. *Primary accreditation:* regional. *Total enrollment:* 211. Founded in 1909. *Nursing program faculty:* 24 (4% with doctorates).

Academic Facilities *Campus library:* 2,400 volumes (1,600 in health, 800 in nursing); 200 periodical subscriptions (200 health-care related). *Nursing school resources:* CAI, computer lab, nursing audiovisuals, interactive nursing skills videos, learning resource lab.

Student Life *Student services:* health clinic, personal counseling, institutionally sponsored work-study program, campus safety program. *Nursing student activities:* Sigma Theta Tau, student nurses association.

Calendar Semesters.

NURSING STUDENT PROFILE

Undergraduate **Enrollment:** 218
Women: 88%; **Men:** 12%; **Minority:** 3%; **International:** 0%; **Part-time:** 8%

BACCALAUREATE PROGRAM

Contact Ms. Nancy Norman, Admission Assistant, Bellin College of Nursing, PO Box 23400, 725 South Webster Avenue, Green Bay, WI 54305-3400, 414-433-5803. *Fax:* 414-433-7416. *E-mail:* njnorman@bcon.edu

Expenses *Tuition:* $8025 per academic year. *Full-time mandatory fees:* $166. *Books and supplies per academic year:* $500.

Financial Aid Institutionally sponsored need-based grants/scholarships, institutionally sponsored non-need grants/scholarships, Federal Perkins Loans, Federal Supplemental Educational Opportunity Grants, Federal Work-Study. *Application deadline:* 4/1.

Generic Baccalaureate Program (BSN)

Applying *Required:* ACT, minimum high school GPA of 2.9, minimum college GPA of 2.7, 3 years of high school math, 3 years of high school science, high school chemistry, high school biology, high school transcript, interview, 3 letters of recommendation, transcript of college record, high school class rank: top 33%. *Options:* Advanced standing available through advanced placement exams. Course work may be accelerated. May apply for transfer of up to 98 total credits. *Application deadlines:* 1/1 (summer), rolling. *Application fee:* $20.

Degree Requirements 128 total credit hours, 63 in nursing.

CONTINUING EDUCATION PROGRAM

Contact Ms. JoAnn G. Hanaway, Coordinator, Educational Outreach, Bellin College of Nursing, PO Box 23400, 725 South Webster Avenue, Green Bay, WI 54305-3400, 414-433-7456. *Fax:* 414-433-7416.

CARDINAL STRITCH COLLEGE
Department of Nursing
Milwaukee, Wisconsin

Programs • Generic Baccalaureate • RN Baccalaureate • LPN to Baccalaureate • Accelerated MSN

The College Independent Roman Catholic comprehensive coed institution. Founded: 1937. *Primary accreditation:* regional. *Setting:* 40-acre suburban campus. *Total enrollment:* 5,176.

The Department of Nursing Founded in 1981. *Nursing program faculty:* 25 (12% with doctorates).

Academic Facilities *Campus library:* 115,000 volumes (5,500 in health, 5,000 in nursing); 1,114 periodical subscriptions (74 health-care related). *Nursing school resources:* CAI, computer lab, nursing audiovisuals, interactive nursing skills videos, learning resource lab.

Student Life *Student services:* health clinic, personal counseling, career counseling, institutionally sponsored work-study program, job placement, campus safety program, special assistance for disabled students. *International student services:* counseling/support, ESL courses. *Nursing student activities:* student nurses association, all campus organizations.

Calendar Semesters.

NURSING STUDENT PROFILE

Undergraduate **Enrollment:** 350
Women: 85%; **Men:** 15%; **Minority:** 14%; **International:** 1%; **Part-time:** 28%

BACCALAUREATE PROGRAMS

Contact Ms. Janet Beitz, Nursing Adviser, Department of Nursing, Cardinal Stritch College, 6801 North Yates Road, Milwaukee, WI 53217-3985, 414-352-5400. *Fax:* 414-351-7516.

Expenses *Tuition:* $8960 full-time, $310 per credit hour part-time. *Full-time mandatory fees:* $967. *Part-time mandatory fees:* $30+. *Room and board:* $3880–$3910. *Books and supplies per academic year:* ranges from $300 to $500.

Financial Aid Institutionally sponsored need-based grants/scholarships, institutionally sponsored non-need grants/scholarships, Federal Direct Loans, Federal Nursing Student Loans, Federal Pell Grants, Federal Perkins Loans. 80% of undergraduate students in nursing programs received some form of financial aid in 1995–96. *Application deadline:* 7/1.

Generic Baccalaureate Program (BSN)

Applying *Required:* ACT, TOEFL for nonnative speakers of English, minimum college GPA of 2.25, 3 years of high school math, 3 years of high school science, high school chemistry, high school biology, high school transcript, transcript of college record. *Options:* Advanced standing available through the following means: advanced placement exams, credit by exam. *Application deadlines:* 8/1 (fall), 1/1 (spring). *Application fee:* $20.

Degree Requirements 129 total credit hours, 66 in nursing.

RN Baccalaureate Program (BSN)

Applying *Required:* ACT, TOEFL for nonnative speakers of English, minimum college GPA of 2.25, 3 years of high school math, 3 years of high

Cardinal Stritch College (continued)

school science, high school chemistry, high school biology, RN license, diploma or AD in nursing, high school transcript, transcript of college record. *Options:* Advanced standing available through the following means: advanced placement exams, credit by exam. *Application deadlines:* 8/1 (fall), 1/1 (spring). *Application fee:* $20.

Degree Requirements 129 total credit hours, 66 in nursing.

LPN to Baccalaureate Program (BSN)

Applying *Required:* ACT, TOEFL for nonnative speakers of English, minimum college GPA of 2.25, 3 years of high school math, 3 years of high school science, high school chemistry, high school biology, high school transcript, transcript of college record, LPN transcript. *Options:* Advanced standing available through the following means: advanced placement exams, credit by exam. *Application deadlines:* 8/1 (fall), 1/1 (spring). *Application fee:* $20.

Degree Requirements 129 total credit hours, 66 in nursing.

MASTER'S PROGRAM

Contact Dr. Zaiga Kalnins, Chair and Professor, Department of Nursing, Cardinal Stritch College, 6801 North Yates Road, Milwaukee, WI 53217-3985, 414-352-5400 Ext. 316. *Fax:* 414-351-7516.

Areas of Study Nursing education.

Expenses *Tuition:* $290 per credit.

Accelerated MSN Program

Applying *Required:* Miller Analogies Test, TOEFL for nonnative speakers of English, bachelor's degree in nursing, physical assessment course, statistics course, professional liability/malpractice insurance, essay, 2 letters of recommendation, transcript of college record. *Application deadlines:* 8/1 (fall), 1/1 (spring).

Degree Requirements 66 total credit hours, 66 in nursing. Project.

COLUMBIA COLLEGE OF NURSING
Milwaukee, Wisconsin

Programs • Generic Baccalaureate • RN Baccalaureate • Accelerated RN Baccalaureate

The College Independent 4-year specialized coed college. Founded: 1982. *Primary accreditation:* regional. *Total enrollment:* 395. Founded in 1901. *Nursing program faculty:* 21 (38% with doctorates). *Off-campus program sites:* Moorhead, MN; Sells, AZ.

Academic Facilities *Campus library:* 7,112 volumes (1,132 in health, 5,730 in nursing); 221 periodical subscriptions (198 health-care related). *Nursing school resources:* CAI, computer lab, nursing audiovisuals, interactive nursing skills videos, learning resource lab.

Student Life *Student services:* health clinic, personal counseling, career counseling, institutionally sponsored work-study program. *Nursing student activities:* nursing club, student nurses association.

Calendar Semesters.

NURSING STUDENT PROFILE

Undergraduate **Enrollment:** 373
Women: 92%; **Men:** 8%; **Minority:** 7%; **International:** 1%; **Part-time:** 43%

BACCALAUREATE PROGRAMS

Contact Dr. Marian H. Snyder, Dean and Chief Executive Officer, Columbia College of Nursing, 2121 East Newport Avenue, Milwaukee, WI 53211, 414-961-4202. *Fax:* 414-961-4121.

Expenses *Tuition:* $13,190 full-time, $220 per credit part-time. *Full-time mandatory fees:* $400+. *Room and board:* $2800–$4420. *Room only:* $1980–$3140. *Books and supplies per academic year:* $490.

Financial Aid Institutionally sponsored need-based grants/scholarships, institutionally sponsored non-need grants/scholarships, Federal Nursing Student Loans, Federal Pell Grants, Federal Perkins Loans, Federal Supplemental Educational Opportunity Grants, Federal Work-Study. 63% of undergraduate students in nursing programs received some form of financial aid in 1995–96. *Application deadline:* 3/15.

Generic Baccalaureate Program (BSN)

Applying *Required:* TOEFL for nonnative speakers of English, ACT (minimum score): 20, 2 years of high school science, high school chemistry, high school biology, high school transcript, transcript of college record, personal evaluation by secondary school guidance counselor, high school algebra. *Options:* Advanced standing available through the following means: advanced placement exams, credit by exam. *Application deadline:* rolling.

Degree Requirements 128 total credit hours, 60 in nursing.

RN Baccalaureate Program (BSN)

Applying *Required:* TOEFL for nonnative speakers of English, minimum college GPA of 2.3, RN license, interview, transcript of college record. *Options:* Advanced standing available through the following means: advanced placement exams, credit by exam. May apply for transfer of up to 64 total credits. *Application deadline:* rolling.

Degree Requirements 128 total credit hours, 60 in nursing.

Accelerated RN Baccalaureate Program (BSN)

Applying *Required:* ACT, minimum college GPA of 2.3, RN license, interview, transcript of college record. *Options:* Advanced standing available through advanced placement exams. May apply for transfer of up to 64 total credits. *Application deadline:* rolling.

Degree Requirements 128 total credit hours, 60 in nursing.

CONCORDIA UNIVERSITY WISCONSIN
Nursing Division
Mequon, Wisconsin

Programs • Generic Baccalaureate • RN Baccalaureate • Accelerated RN Baccalaureate • LPN to Baccalaureate • BSN to Master's • Continuing Education

The University Independent comprehensive coed institution, affiliated with Lutheran Church–Missouri Synod. Founded: 1881. *Primary accreditation:* regional. *Setting:* 155-acre suburban campus. *Total enrollment:* 3,719.

The Nursing Division Founded in 1982. *Nursing program faculty:* 17 (18% with doctorates).

Academic Facilities *Campus library:* 88,000 volumes (303 in health, 797 in nursing); 1,177 periodical subscriptions (200 health-care related). *Nursing school resources:* CAI, computer lab, nursing audiovisuals, learning resource lab.

Student Life *Student services:* health clinic, child-care facilities, personal counseling, career counseling, institutionally sponsored work-study program, job placement, campus safety program, special assistance for disabled students. *International student services:* counseling/support, special assistance for nonnative speakers of English, ESL courses. *Nursing student activities:* nursing club, student nurses association.

Calendar Semesters.

NURSING STUDENT PROFILE

Undergraduate **Enrollment:** 200
Women: 95%; **Men:** 5%; **Minority:** 5%
Graduate **Enrollment:** 60
Women: 94%; **Men:** 6%; **Minority:** 3%; **Part-time:** 96%

BACCALAUREATE PROGRAMS

Contact Prof. Grace Peterson, Chairperson, Nursing Division, Concordia University Wisconsin, 12800 North Lake Shore Drive, Mequon, WI 53097, 414-243-4374. *Fax:* 414-243-4351. *E-mail:* gapete@bach.cuw.edu

Expenses *Tuition:* $10,760 full-time, $450 per credit hour part-time. *Room and board:* $3770. *Books and supplies per academic year:* ranges from $150 to $400.

Financial Aid Institutionally sponsored need-based grants/scholarships, institutionally sponsored non-need grants/scholarships, Federal Direct Loans, Federal Pell Grants, Federal Supplemental Educational Opportunity Grants, Federal Work-Study. *Application deadline:* 5/1.

Generic Baccalaureate Program (BSN)

Applying *Required:* SAT I, ACT, TOEFL for nonnative speakers of English, minimum college GPA of 2.5, 3 years of high school math, 3 years of high school science, high school chemistry, high school biology, high school transcript, written essay, transcript of college record. *Options:* Advanced standing available through advanced placement exams. Course work may be accelerated. May apply for transfer of up to 70 total credits. *Application deadline:* rolling. *Application fee:* $25.

Degree Requirements 133 total credit hours, 60 in nursing. Participation in 3 winterims.

RN Baccalaureate Program (BSN)

Applying *Required:* minimum college GPA of 2.5, RN license, diploma or AD in nursing, transcript of college record, 2 years of nursing experience. *Options:* Course work may be accelerated.

Degree Requirements 131 total credit hours, 60 in nursing. Participation in 3 winterims.

Accelerated RN Baccalaureate Program (BSN)

Applying *Required:* minimum college GPA of 2.5, RN license, diploma or AD in nursing, written essay, transcript of college record, 2 years of nursing experience. *Options:* May apply for transfer of up to 90 total credits. *Application deadlines:* 6/1 (fall), 11/1 (spring). *Application fee:* $25.

Degree Requirements 133 total credit hours, 60 in nursing. Participation in 3 winterims.

LPN to Baccalaureate Program (BSN)

Applying *Required:* minimum college GPA of 2.5, diploma or AD in nursing. *Options:* Course work may be accelerated. May apply for transfer of up to 90 total credits. *Application deadlines:* 7/1 (fall), 11/1 (spring). *Application fee:* $25.

Degree Requirements 132 total credit hours, 60 in nursing. Participation in 3 winterims.

MASTER'S PROGRAM

Contact Dr. Ruth Gresley, Director, Graduate Nursing, Nursing Division, Concordia University Wisconsin, 12800 North Lake Shore Drive, Mequon, WI 53097, 414-243-4452. *Fax:* 414-243-4506. *E-mail:* rgresley@bach.cuw.edu

Areas of Study Nursing education; nurse practitioner programs in family health, gerontology.

Expenses *Tuition:* $5400 full-time, $300 per credit part-time. *Full-time mandatory fees:* $0.

Financial Aid Institutionally sponsored loans.

BSN to Master's Program (MSN)

Applying *Required:* TOEFL for nonnative speakers of English, bachelor's degree in nursing, minimum GPA of 3.0, RN license, 2 years of clinical experience, physical assessment course, statistics course, essay, interview, 2 letters of recommendation, transcript of college record. *Application deadline:* rolling. *Application fee:* $50.

Degree Requirements 43 total credit hours, 30 in nursing, 13 in pathophysiology, pharmacotherapeutics, education, counseling, family issues. Clinical project and 3-credit global perspectives course, or thesis.

Distance learning Courses provided through correspondence, video, on-line. Specific degree requirements include residency course in diagnostic modalities (2 credits).

CONTINUING EDUCATION PROGRAM

Contact Prof. Grace Peterson, Chairperson, Nursing Division, Concordia University Wisconsin, 12800 North Lake Shore Drive, Mequon, WI 53097, 414-243-4374. *Fax:* 414-243-4351.

See full description on page 432.

EDGEWOOD COLLEGE
Nursing Department
Madison, Wisconsin

Programs • Generic Baccalaureate • RN Baccalaureate • BSN to Master's

The College Independent Roman Catholic comprehensive coed institution. Founded: 1927. *Primary accreditation:* regional. *Setting:* 55-acre suburban campus. *Total enrollment:* 2,056.

The Nursing Department Founded in 1979. *Nursing program faculty:* 14 (36% with doctorates).

Academic Facilities *Campus library:* 65,050 volumes (1,475 in health, 440 in nursing); 480 periodical subscriptions (35 health-care related). *Nursing school resources:* CAI, computer lab, nursing audiovisuals, learning resource lab.

Student Life *Student services:* health clinic, personal counseling, career counseling, institutionally sponsored work-study program, job placement, campus safety program, special assistance for disabled students. *International student services:* counseling/support, special assistance for nonnative speakers of English. *Nursing student activities:* Sigma Theta Tau, student nurses association.

Calendar Semesters.

NURSING STUDENT PROFILE

Undergraduate **Enrollment:** 174
Women: 88%; **Men:** 12%; **Minority:** 3%; **International:** 3%; **Part-time:** 31%
Graduate **Enrollment:** 17
Women: 100%; **Part-time:** 100%

BACCALAUREATE PROGRAMS

Contact Mr. Kevin Kuchera, Admissions Officer, Nursing Department, Edgewood College, 805 Woodrow Street, Madison, WI 53711, 608-257-4861. *Fax:* 608-257-1455.

Expenses *Tuition:* $9000 full-time, $270 per credit part-time. *Full-time mandatory fees:* $120–$620. *Room and board:* $3850–$4050. *Room only:* $1765–$2500. *Books and supplies per academic year:* ranges from $100 to $200.

Financial Aid Institutionally sponsored need-based grants/scholarships, institutionally sponsored non-need grants/scholarships, Federal Pell Grants, Federal Supplemental Educational Opportunity Grants, Federal Work-Study. *Application deadline:* 3/15.

Generic Baccalaureate Program (BS)

Applying *Required:* ACT (for freshmen), minimum high school GPA of 2.5, minimum college GPA of 2.5, 3 years of high school math, high school chemistry, high school biology, high school transcript, transcript of college record, 2.5 GPA in math and science courses. *Options:* May apply for transfer of up to 60 total credits. *Application deadline:* rolling. *Application fee:* $25.

Degree Requirements 128 total credit hours, 46 in nursing.

RN Baccalaureate Program (BS)

Applying *Required:* minimum college GPA of 2.5, RN license, diploma or AD in nursing, high school transcript, transcript of college record, 2.5 GPA in math and science courses. *Options:* May apply for transfer of up to 60 total credits. *Application deadline:* rolling. *Application fee:* $25.

Degree Requirements 128 total credit hours, 21 in nursing.

MASTER'S PROGRAM

Contact Dr. Virginia H. Wirtz, RN, CNAA, Chair and Professor, 855 Woodrow Street, Madison, WI 53711, 608-257-4861 Ext. 2292. *Fax:* 608-257-1455. *E-mail:* vwirtz@edgewood.edu

Areas of Study Nursing administration.

Expenses *Tuition:* $292 per credit.

BSN to Master's Program (MS)

Applying *Required:* TOEFL for nonnative speakers of English, bachelor's degree in nursing, minimum GPA of 3.0, RN license, 1 year of clinical experience, statistics course, essay, 2 letters of recommendation, transcript of college record. *Application deadline:* rolling. *Application fee:* $25.

Degree Requirements 36 total credit hours, 24 in nursing, 12 in business; ethics; studies in change.

MARIAN COLLEGE OF FOND DU LAC
Division of Nursing Studies
Fond du Lac, Wisconsin

Programs • Generic Baccalaureate • RN Baccalaureate

The College Independent Roman Catholic comprehensive coed institution. Founded: 1936. *Primary accreditation:* regional. *Setting:* 50-acre small-town campus. *Total enrollment:* 2,492.

The Division of Nursing Studies Founded in 1965.

Academic Facilities *Campus library:* 100,000 volumes (6,559 in health, 5,075 in nursing); 790 periodical subscriptions (290 health-care related).

Calendar Semesters.

BACCALAUREATE PROGRAMS

Contact Vice President for Enrollment Services, Division of Nursing Studies, Marian College of Fond du Lac, 45 South National Avenue, Fond du Lac, WI 54935, 414-923-7650. *Fax:* 414-923-7154.

Expenses *Tuition:* $10,560 full-time, ranges from $230 to $320 per credit part-time.

Financial Aid Institutionally sponsored need-based grants/scholarships, institutionally sponsored non-need grants/scholarships, Federal Nursing Student Loans, Federal Perkins Loans, Federal Supplemental Educational Opportunity Grants, Federal Work-Study, Federal PLUS Loans, Federal Stafford Loans. *Application deadline:* 3/1.

Generic Baccalaureate Program (BSN)

Applying *Required:* SAT I or ACT, minimum high school GPA of 2.5, minimum college GPA of 2.6, high school chemistry, high school biology, high school transcript, high school class rank: top 50%. 69 prerequisite credits must be completed before admission to the nursing program. *Application deadline:* rolling. *Application fee:* $15.

Degree Requirements 131–135 total credit hours dependent upon track, 64 in nursing.

RN Baccalaureate Program (BSN)

Applying *Required:* minimum college GPA of 2.6, RN license, diploma or AD in nursing, high school transcript, transcript of college record. *Application deadline:* rolling. *Application fee:* $15.

Degree Requirements 133–135 total credit hours dependent upon track, 66 in nursing.

MARQUETTE UNIVERSITY
College of Nursing
Milwaukee, Wisconsin

Programs • Generic Baccalaureate • RN Baccalaureate • MSN • Accelerated RN to Master's • Post-Master's • Continuing Education

The University Independent Roman Catholic (Jesuit) coed university. Founded: 1881. *Primary accreditation:* regional. *Setting:* 80-acre urban campus. *Total enrollment:* 10,774.

The College of Nursing Founded in 1936. *Nursing program faculty:* 33 (66% with doctorates).

Academic Facilities *Campus library:* 1.0 million volumes (46,400 in health, 5,700 in nursing); 7,000 periodical subscriptions (818 health-care related). *Nursing school resources:* CAI, computer lab, nursing audiovisuals, interactive nursing skills videos, learning resource lab.

Student Life *Student services:* health clinic, child-care facilities, personal counseling, career counseling, institutionally sponsored work-study program, job placement, campus safety program, special assistance for disabled students. *International student services:* counseling/support, special assistance for nonnative speakers of English, ESL courses. *Nursing student activities:* Sigma Theta Tau, nursing club, student nurses association.

Calendar Semesters.

NURSING STUDENT PROFILE

Undergraduate **Enrollment:** 397
Women: 92%; **Men:** 8%; **Minority:** 9%; **Part-time:** 10%
Graduate **Enrollment:** 181
Women: 98%; **Men:** 2%; **Minority:** 4%; **Part-time:** 69%

BACCALAUREATE PROGRAMS

Contact Dr. Ruth Waite, Associate Dean, Clark Hall, College of Nursing, Marquette University, PO Box 1881, Milwaukee, WI 53201-1881, 414-288-3808. *Fax:* 414-288-1597. *E-mail:* waiter@ums.csd.mu.edu

Expenses *Tuition:* $15,530 full-time, $315 per credit hour part-time. *Full-time mandatory fees:* $12. *Room and board:* $5000–$5800. *Room only:* $1970–$3230. *Books and supplies per academic year:* $400.

Financial Aid Institutionally sponsored need-based grants/scholarships, institutionally sponsored non-need grants/scholarships, Federal Direct Loans, Federal Nursing Student Loans, Federal Pell Grants, Federal Supplemental Educational Opportunity Grants, Federal Work-Study. 94% of undergraduate students in nursing programs received some form of financial aid in 1995–96. *Application deadline:* 3/1.

Generic Baccalaureate Program (BSN)

Applying *Required:* SAT I, ACT, TOEFL for nonnative speakers of English, minimum high school GPA of 3.0, minimum college GPA of 2.5, 3 years of high school math, 3 years of high school science, high school chemistry, high school biology, high school transcript, written essay, transcript of college record, high school class rank: top 25%. *Options:* May apply for transfer of up to 90 total credits. *Application deadline:* rolling. *Application fee:* $30.

Degree Requirements 129 total credit hours, 65 in nursing.

RN Baccalaureate Program (BSN)

Applying *Required:* SAT I, ACT, TOEFL for nonnative speakers of English, minimum college GPA of 2.5, RN license, diploma or AD in nursing. *Options:* Course work may be accelerated. May apply for transfer of up to 90 total credits. *Application deadline:* rolling. *Application fee:* $30.

Degree Requirements 129 total credit hours, 70 in nursing.

MASTER'S PROGRAMS

Contact Dr. Ruth Waite, Associate Dean, Clark Hall, College of Nursing, Marquette University, PO Box 1881, Milwaukee, WI 53201-1881, 414-288-3808. *Fax:* 414-288-1597. *E-mail:* waiter@ums.csd.mu.edu

Areas of Study Clinical nurse specialist programs in adult health nursing, gerontological nursing, pediatric nursing; nurse midwifery; nursing administration; nurse practitioner programs in adult health, child care/pediatrics, gerontology, neonatal health.

Expenses *Tuition:* $6510 full-time, $465 part-time. *Room only:* $1880–$3360. *Books and supplies per academic year:* $400.

Financial Aid Graduate assistantships, nurse traineeships, Federal Nursing Student Loans, employment opportunities. 13% of master's level students in nursing programs received some form of financial aid in 1995-96. *Application deadline:* 2/15.

MSN Program

Applying *Required:* GRE General Test, bachelor's degree in nursing, minimum GPA of 3.0, RN license, physical assessment course, statistics course, essay, interview, 3 letters of recommendation, transcript of college record, 1 year of clinical experience required for nurse-midwifery, pediatric, and neonatal tracks. *Application deadlines:* 2/15 (nurse midwifery track), rolling. *Application fee:* $40.

Degree Requirements 36–37 total credit hours dependent upon track, 36–37 in nursing.

Accelerated RN to Master's Program (MSN)

Applying *Required:* GRE General Test, minimum GPA of 3.0, RN license, transcript of college record, 1 year of clinical experience required for nurse-midwifery, pediatric, and neonatal tracks. *Application deadlines:* 2/15 (fall), 2/15 (nurse midwifery track). *Application fee:* $40.

Degree Requirements 36–37 total credit hours dependent upon track.

Post-Master's Program

Applying *Application deadline:* rolling. *Application fee:* $40.

Degree Requirements 19–25 total credit hours dependent upon track, 19–25 in nursing. 19 credit hours for pediatric nurse practitioner track, 21 for adult and geriatric nurse practitioner tracks, 25 for nurse midwifery track.

CONTINUING EDUCATION PROGRAM

Contact Dr. Michelle Malin, Interim Director of Continuing Nursing Education, Clark Hall, College of Nursing, Marquette University, PO Box 1881, Milwaukee, WI 53201-1881, 414-288-3804.

UNIVERSITY OF WISCONSIN–EAU CLAIRE
School of Nursing
Eau Claire, Wisconsin

Programs • Generic Baccalaureate • MSN • Continuing Education

The University State-supported comprehensive coed institution. Part of University of Wisconsin System. Founded: 1916. *Primary accreditation:* regional. *Setting:* 333-acre urban campus. *Total enrollment:* 10,319.

The School of Nursing Founded in 1965. *Nursing program faculty:* 33 (50% with doctorates). *Off-campus program site:* Marshfield.

▶ ***NOTEWORTHY***

The School of Nursing has an excellent reputation for the quality of its educational programs and its graduates. The School offers bachelor's and master's degrees in nursing and participates in a statewide Collaborative Nursing Program for registered nurses to earn a BSN. Master's-level options include adult or family health clinical specialization and advanced clinical practice, education, and administration role preparation. Baccalaureate-level students receive clinical experiences in acute-care facilities, community health agencies, schools, home-care agencies, and the School of Nursing clinic. Through distance technology, bachelor's and master's offerings are fully implemented at a satellite in Marshfield, Wisconsin.

Academic Facilities *Campus library:* 548,034 volumes (65,000 in nursing); 40,984 periodical subscriptions (2,049 health-care related). *Nursing school resources:* CAI, computer lab, nursing audiovisuals, interactive nursing skills videos, learning resource lab.

Student Life *Student services:* health clinic, child-care facilities, personal counseling, career counseling, institutionally sponsored work-study program, job placement, campus safety program, special assistance for disabled students. *International student services:* counseling/support, ESL courses. *Nursing student activities:* Sigma Theta Tau, student nurses association.

Calendar Semesters.

NURSING STUDENT PROFILE

Undergraduate **Enrollment:** 638
Women: 88%; **Men:** 12%; **Minority:** 12%; **International:** 0%; **Part-time:** 10%
Graduate **Enrollment:** 126
Women: 95%; **Men:** 5%; **Minority:** 1%; **International:** 0%; **Part-time:** 85%

BACCALAUREATE PROGRAM

Contact Dr. Marjorie Bottoms, Associate Dean and Educational Administrator, School of Nursing, University of Wisconsin-Eau Claire, Eau Claire, WI 54702-4004, 715-836-5287. *Fax:* 715-836-5971. *E-mail:* mbottoms@uwec.edu

Expenses *State resident tuition:* $1287 full-time, $108 per credit hour part-time. *Nonresident tuition:* $4018 full-time, $336 per credit hour part-time. *Full-time mandatory fees:* $0.

Financial Aid Institutionally sponsored need-based grants/scholarships, institutionally sponsored non-need grants/scholarships, Federal Pell Grants, Federal Perkins Loans, Federal Supplemental Educational Opportunity Grants, Federal Work-Study. *Application deadline:* 4/15.

Generic Baccalaureate Program (BSN)

Applying *Required:* ACT, TOEFL for nonnative speakers of English, minimum high school GPA of 2.0, minimum college GPA of 2.75, high school math, high school science, high school chemistry, high school biology, high school foreign language, high school transcript, written essay, transcript of college record. 30 prerequisite credits must be completed before admission to the nursing program. *Options:* Advanced standing available through credit by exam. May apply for transfer of up to 96 total credits. *Application deadlines:* 12/1 (fall), 5/1 (spring). *Application fee:* $25.

Degree Requirements 120 total credit hours, 60 in nursing.

Distance learning Courses provided through video, audio, computer-based media.

MASTER'S PROGRAM

Contact Dr. Marjorie Bottoms, Associate Dean and Educational Administrator, School of Nursing, University of Wisconsin-Eau Claire, Eau Claire, WI 54702-4004, 715-836-5287. *Fax:* 715-836-5971. *E-mail:* mbottoms@uwec.edu

Areas of Study Clinical nurse specialist programs in adult health nursing, family health nursing; nursing administration; nursing education; nurse practitioner programs in adult health, family health.

Expenses *State resident tuition:* $1611 full-time, $180 per credit part-time. *Nonresident tuition:* $4934 full-time, $550 per credit part-time. *Full-time mandatory fees:* $0.

Financial Aid Graduate assistantships, nurse traineeships, Federal Nursing Student Loans, employment opportunities. 20% of master's level students in nursing programs received some form of financial aid in 1995-96. *Application deadline:* 3/1.

MSN Program

Applying *Required:* bachelor's degree in nursing, minimum GPA of 3.0, RN license, 1 year of clinical experience, physical assessment course, statistics course, professional liability/malpractice insurance, essay, transcript of college record. *Application deadline:* rolling. *Application fee:* $35.

Degree Requirements 38 total credit hours, 32 in nursing. Scholarly project, written exam, oral exam.

CONTINUING EDUCATION PROGRAM

Contact Dr. Rita Kisting Sparks, Assistant Dean for Continuing Education, School of Nursing, University of Wisconsin-Eau Claire, Eau Claire, WI 54702-4004, 715-836-5279. *Fax:* 715-836-5971. *E-mail:* sparksrk@uwec.edu

UNIVERSITY OF WISCONSIN–GREEN BAY
Professional Program in Nursing
Green Bay, Wisconsin

Programs • RN Baccalaureate • Continuing Education

The University State-supported comprehensive coed institution. Part of University of Wisconsin System. Founded: 1968. *Primary accreditation:* regional. *Setting:* 700-acre suburban campus. *Total enrollment:* 5,190.

The Professional Program in Nursing Founded in 1980. *Nursing program faculty:* 4 (75% with doctorates). *Off-campus program site:* Rhinelander.

Academic Facilities *Campus library:* 280,000 volumes (675 in nursing); 1,200 periodical subscriptions. *Nursing school resources:* computer lab, nursing audiovisuals, learning resource lab.

Student Life *Student services:* health clinic, child-care facilities, personal counseling, career counseling, institutionally sponsored work-study program, job placement, campus safety program, special assistance for

University of Wisconsin–Green Bay (continued)
disabled students. *International student services:* counseling/support, special assistance for nonnative speakers of English, ESL courses. *Nursing student activities:* Sigma Theta Tau.

Calendar Semesters.

NURSING STUDENT PROFILE

Undergraduate **Enrollment:** 148
Women: 96%; **Men:** 4%; **Minority:** 1%; **International:** 0%; **Part-time:** 100%

BACCALAUREATE PROGRAM

Contact Dr. V. Jane Muhl, Chair and Associate Professor, Professional Program in Nursing, University of Wisconsin-Green Bay, 2420 Nicolet Drive, Green Bay, WI 54311-7001, 414-465-2365. *Fax:* 414-465-2854. *E-mail:* muhlj@gbms01.uwgb.edu

Expenses *State resident tuition:* $2548 full-time, $108 per semester hour part-time. *Nonresident tuition:* $8012 full-time, $335 per semester hour part-time. *Books and supplies per academic year:* ranges from $300 to $600.

Financial Aid Institutionally sponsored need-based grants/scholarships, institutionally sponsored non-need grants/scholarships, Federal Direct Loans, Federal Nursing Student Loans, Federal Work-Study. 50% of undergraduate students in nursing programs received some form of financial aid in 1995–96. *Application deadline:* 4/15.

RN Baccalaureate Program (BSN)

Applying *Required:* ACT, minimum college GPA of 2.25, RN license, diploma or AD in nursing, transcript of college record. 51 prerequisite credits must be completed before admission to the nursing program. *Options:* Advanced standing available through credit by exam. Course work may be accelerated. May apply for transfer of up to 89 total credits. *Application deadline:* rolling. *Application fee:* $25.

Degree Requirements 120 total credit hours, 30 in nursing.

Distance learning Courses provided through compressed video, audiographics, teleconferencing, public TV. Specific degree requirements include on-campus Capstone nursing course.

CONTINUING EDUCATION PROGRAM

Contact Dr. V. Jane Muhl, Chair and Associate Professor, Professional Program in Nursing, University of Wisconsin-Green Bay, 2420 Nicolet Drive, Green Bay, WI 54311-7001, 414-465-2365. *Fax:* 414-465-2824. *E-mail:* muhlj@gbms01.uwgb.edu

UNIVERSITY OF WISCONSIN–MADISON

School of Nursing
Madison, Wisconsin

Programs • Generic Baccalaureate • RN Baccalaureate • MS • RN to Master's • Post-Master's • PhD • Continuing Education

The University State-supported coed university. Part of University of Wisconsin System. Founded: 1848. *Primary accreditation:* regional. *Setting:* 1,050-acre urban campus. *Total enrollment:* 37,890.

The School of Nursing Founded in 1924. *Nursing program faculty:* 25 (96% with doctorates).

▶ ***NOTEWORTHY***

University of Wisconsin–Madison School of Nursing offers BS, MS, and PhD degrees in nursing. Nurse practitioner programs are offered at the MS level in adult, aging, pediatric, and women's health. Wisconsin's nationally recognized nursing programs offer flexibility, including dual option (BS or MS) programs for RN students, full- or part-time study, distance education, and financial assistance. The Madison area provides an excellent cultural and recreational environment and extensive clinical and research facilities.

Academic Facilities *Campus library:* 5.7 million volumes (316,684 in health); 44,818 periodical subscriptions (4,182 health-care related). *Nursing school resources:* CAI, computer lab, nursing audiovisuals, interactive nursing skills videos, learning resource lab.

Student Life *Student services:* health clinic, child-care facilities, personal counseling, career counseling, institutionally sponsored work-study program, job placement, campus safety program, special assistance for disabled students. *International student services:* counseling/support, special assistance for nonnative speakers of English, ESL courses. *Nursing student activities:* Sigma Theta Tau, student nurses association.

Calendar Semesters.

NURSING STUDENT PROFILE

Undergraduate **Enrollment:** 407
Women: 89%; **Men:** 11%; **Minority:** 8%; **International:** 1%; **Part-time:** 27%
Graduate **Enrollment:** 184
Women: 98%; **Men:** 2%; **Minority:** 3%; **International:** 5%; **Part-time:** 60%

BACCALAUREATE PROGRAMS

Contact Ms. Debra Engelberger, Program Assistant, Room K6/232 Clinical Science Center, School of Nursing, University of Wisconsin-Madison, 600 Highland Avenue, Madison, WI 53792-2455, 608-263-5171. *Fax:* 608-263-5332. *E-mail:* dlengelb@facstaff.wisc.edu

Expenses *State resident tuition:* $3032 full-time, $127 per credit part-time. *Nonresident tuition:* $10,150 full-time, $424 per credit part-time. *Full-time mandatory fees:* $0. *Room and board:* $4520. *Books and supplies per academic year:* ranges from $565 to $1498.

Financial Aid Institutionally sponsored need-based grants/scholarships, institutionally sponsored non-need grants/scholarships, Federal Nursing Student Loans, Federal Pell Grants, Federal Perkins Loans, Federal Supplemental Educational Opportunity Grants, Federal Work-Study. 43% of undergraduate students in nursing programs received some form of financial aid in 1995–96.

Generic Baccalaureate Program (BS)

Applying *Required:* TOEFL for nonnative speakers of English, ACT for Wisconsin residents, ACT or SAT for nonresidents, minimum college GPA of 2.5, 3 years of high school math, 3 years of high school science, high school foreign language, high school transcript, written essay, transcript of college record. 24 prerequisite credits must be completed before admission to the nursing program. *Options:* Advanced standing available through credit by exam. *Application deadline:* 2/1. *Application fee:* $28.

Degree Requirements 124 total credit hours, 53 in nursing.

RN Baccalaureate Program (BS)

Applying *Required:* TOEFL for nonnative speakers of English, minimum college GPA of 2.5, 3 years of high school math, 3 years of high school science, RN license, diploma or AD in nursing, high school foreign language, transcript of college record. 24 prerequisite credits must be completed before admission to the nursing program. *Options:* Advanced standing available through credit by exam. *Application deadlines:* 2/1 (fall), 11/15 (spring). *Application fee:* $28.

Degree Requirements 124 total credit hours, 53 in nursing.

Distance learning Courses provided through correspondence, video, audio, computer-based media, on-line.

MASTER'S PROGRAMS

Contact Ms. Susan Kosharek, Graduate Program Admissions Assistant, Room K6/236 Clinical Science Center, School of Nursing, University of Wisconsin-Madison, 600 Highland Avenue, Madison, WI 53792-2455, 608-263-5180. *Fax:* 608-263-5332. *E-mail:* sjkoshar@facstaff.wisc.edu

Areas of Study Clinical nurse specialist programs in community health nursing, gerontological nursing, maternity-newborn nursing, medical-surgical nursing, pediatric nursing, perinatal nursing, psychiatric–mental health nursing, women's health nursing; nursing education; nurse practitioner programs in adult health, child care/pediatrics, gerontology, women's health.

Expenses *State resident tuition:* $2187 full-time, $273 per credit part-time. *Nonresident tuition:* $6648 full-time, $831 per credit part-time. *Full-time mandatory fees:* $0. *Room and board:* $6756. *Books and supplies per academic year:* $665.

Financial Aid Graduate assistantships, nurse traineeships, fellowships, Federal Nursing Student Loans, institutionally sponsored loans, employment opportunities. 33% of master's level students in nursing programs received some form of financial aid in 1995-96. *Application deadline:* 6/1.

MS Program

Applying *Required:* GRE General Test, TOEFL for nonnative speakers of English, bachelor's degree in nursing, minimum GPA of 3.0, 1 year of clinical experience, statistics course, essay, 3 letters of recommendation, transcript of college record, Wisconsin RN license. *Application deadlines:* 3/1 (fall), 10/1 (spring), 3/1 (summer). *Application fee:* $38.

Degree Requirements 36 total credit hours, 18 in nursing, 12 in clinical work and research.

RN to Master's Program (MS)

Applying *Required:* GRE General Test, minimum GPA of 3.0, RN license, 1 year of clinical experience, statistics course, essay, 3 letters of recommendation, transcript of college record, Wisconsin RN licensure. *Application deadlines:* 3/1 (fall), 10/1 (spring). *Application fee:* $38.

Degree Requirements 21 total credit hours, 18 in nursing, 12 in clinical work and research.

Post-Master's Program

Applying *Required:* minimum GPA of 3.0, 1 year of clinical experience, essay, transcript of college record, Wisconsin RN license. *Application deadlines:* 3/1 (fall), 10/1 (spring), 3/1 (summer). *Application fee:* $38.

Degree Requirements 11+ total credit hours dependent upon track, 11+ in nursing.

DOCTORAL PROGRAM

Contact Ms. Gale Barber, Assistant to the Associate Dean, Room K6/242 Clinical Science Center, School of Nursing, University of Wisconsin-Madison, 600 Highland Avenue, Madison, WI 53792-2455, 608-263-5172. *Fax:* 608-263-5332. *E-mail:* mgbarber@facstaff.wisc.edu

Areas of Study Nursing research.

Expenses *State resident tuition:* $2187 full-time, ranges from $174 to $273 per credit part-time. *Nonresident tuition:* $6648 full-time, ranges from $274 to $831 per credit part-time. *Full-time mandatory fees:* $0. *Room and board:* $6756. *Books and supplies per academic year:* $665.

Financial Aid Graduate assistantships, nurse traineeships, fellowships, institutionally sponsored loans. *Application deadline:* 1/15.

PhD Program

Applying *Required:* GRE General Test, TOEFL for nonnative speakers of English, 2 scholarly papers, 3 letters of recommendation, vitae, competitive review by faculty committee, BSN, minimum 3.0 GPA. *Application deadlines:* 1/15 (fall), 9/15 (spring). *Application fee:* $38.

Degree Requirements 59 total credit hours; 21 credits of nursing course work; 12 credits in secondary concentration; 8 credits of research design, statistical analysis, and philosophy of science; 18 credits participation in research; dissertation; written exam; defense of dissertation; residency.

CONTINUING EDUCATION PROGRAM

Contact Ms. Anne Jozwiak, Program Assistant, Room K6/275 Clinical Science Center, School of Nursing, University of Wisconsin-Madison, 600 Highland Avenue, Madison, WI 53792-2455, 608-262-0566. *Fax:* 608-263-5332. *E-mail:* ajozwiak@facstaff.wisc.edu

UNIVERSITY OF WISCONSIN–MILWAUKEE

School of Nursing
Milwaukee, Wisconsin

Programs • Generic Baccalaureate • RN Baccalaureate • Accelerated Baccalaureate for Second Degree • MS • PhD • Continuing Education

The University State-supported coed university. Part of University of Wisconsin System. Founded: 1956. *Primary accreditation:* regional. *Setting:* 90-acre urban campus. *Total enrollment:* 22,342.

The School of Nursing Founded in 1965. *Nursing program faculty:* 41 (98% with doctorates). *Off-campus program site:* Kenosha.

▶ ***NOTEWORTHY***

The University of Wisconsin–Milwaukee is an urban Research II university. The School of Nursing is nationally recognized for its faculty, programs, and alumni. Faculty members and students are involved in education, research, and service in more than 100 health-care settings. The School has 3 community nursing centers and an Institute for Urban Health Partnerships. Other centers of the School include a cultural center, center for nursing history, center for nursing research and evaluation, nursing learning resource center, and center for continuing education. Students are prepared as nurse leaders at the baccalaureate, master's, and doctoral levels for roles in health care.

Academic Facilities *Campus library:* 1.4 million volumes (126,900 in health, 159,000 in nursing); 8,090 periodical subscriptions (1,248 health-care related). *Nursing school resources:* CAI, computer lab, nursing audiovisuals, interactive nursing skills videos, learning resource lab.

Student Life *Student services:* health clinic, child-care facilities, personal counseling, career counseling, institutionally sponsored work-study program, job placement, special assistance for disabled students. *International student services:* counseling/support, ESL courses. *Nursing student activities:* Sigma Theta Tau, student nurses association.

Calendar Semesters.

NURSING STUDENT PROFILE

Undergraduate **Enrollment:** 938
Women: 86%; **Men:** 14%; **Minority:** 18%; **International:** 1%; **Part-time:** 43%
Graduate **Enrollment:** 193
Women: 95%; **Men:** 5%; **Minority:** 6%; **International:** 2%; **Part-time:** 86%

BACCALAUREATE PROGRAMS

Contact Dr. Mary Mundt, Associate Dean, School of Nursing, University of Wisconsin-Milwaukee, PO Box 413, Milwaukee, WI 53201, 414-229-5464. *Fax:* 414-229-6474. *E-mail:* mundt@csd.uwm.edu

Expenses *State resident tuition:* $1551 per academic year. *Nonresident tuition:* $4982 per academic year. *Full-time mandatory fees:* $231. *Room and board:* $3122–$3502. *Books and supplies per academic year:* ranges from $500 to $700.

Financial Aid Institutionally sponsored need-based grants/scholarships, Federal Nursing Student Loans, Federal Supplemental Educational Opportunity Grants, Federal Work-Study. 43% of undergraduate students in nursing programs received some form of financial aid in 1995–96. *Application deadline:* 5/1.

Generic Baccalaureate Program (BS)

Applying *Required:* ACT, TOEFL for nonnative speakers of English, minimum college GPA of 2.5, 4 years of high school math, 3 years of high school science, high school chemistry, high school biology, high school transcript, transcript of college record, high school class rank: top 50%. 48 prerequisite credits must be completed before admission to the nursing program. *Application deadlines:* 6/30 (fall), 11/15 (spring). *Application fee:* $28.

Degree Requirements 124 total credit hours, 70 in nursing.

RN Baccalaureate Program (BS)

Applying *Required:* TOEFL for nonnative speakers of English, minimum college GPA of 2.5, RN license, diploma or AD in nursing, transcript of college record. *Options:* Advanced standing available through the following means: advanced placement exams, advanced placement without credit, credit by exam. *Application deadlines:* 6/30 (fall), 11/15 (spring). *Application fee:* $28.

Degree Requirements 124 total credit hours, 70 in nursing.

Distance learning Courses provided through correspondence, video, audio, computer-based media.

Accelerated Baccalaureate for Second Degree Program (BS)

Applying *Required:* TOEFL for nonnative speakers of English, minimum college GPA of 2.5, transcript of college record. 48 prerequisite credits must be completed before admission to the nursing program. *Options:* Advanced standing available through credit by exam. Course work may be accelerated. *Application deadlines:* 6/30 (fall), 11/15 (spring). *Application fee:* $28.

Degree Requirements 124 total credit hours, 70 in nursing.

MASTER'S PROGRAM

Contact Dr. Mary Mundt, Associate Dean, School of Nursing, University of Wisconsin-Milwaukee, PO Box 413, Milwaukee, WI 53201, 414-229-5468. *Fax:* 414-229-6474. *E-mail:* mundt@csd.uwm.edu

Areas of Study Clinical nurse specialist programs in adult health nursing, occupational health nursing, parent-child nursing, psychiatric–mental health nursing, women's health nursing; nurse practitioner program in family health.

Expenses *State resident tuition:* $2220 per academic year. *Nonresident tuition:* $6661 per academic year. *Full-time mandatory fees:* $231. *Room and board:*

University of Wisconsin–Milwaukee (continued)
$3122–$3502. *Room only:* $2100. *Books and supplies per academic year:* ranges from $500 to $700.

Financial Aid Graduate assistantships, nurse traineeships, fellowships, Federal Nursing Student Loans, employment opportunities. 18% of master's level students in nursing programs received some form of financial aid in 1995-96. *Application deadline:* 1/15.

MS Program

Applying *Required:* GRE General Test, bachelor's degree in nursing, minimum GPA of 2.75, RN license, statistics course, essay, interview, 3 letters of recommendation, transcript of college record. *Application deadlines:* 3/1 (fall), 10/1 (spring). *Application fee:* $35.

Degree Requirements 36–46 total credit hours dependent upon track, 31–46 in nursing, 5 in 5 elective hours in clinical nurse specialist track. Comprehensive exam.

DOCTORAL PROGRAM

Contact Dr. Mary Mundt, Associate Dean, School of Nursing, University of Wisconsin-Milwaukee, PO Box 413, Milwaukee, WI 53201, 414-229-5468. *Fax:* 414-229-6474. *E-mail:* mundt@csd.uwm.edu

Areas of Study Nursing administration, nursing education, nursing research, nursing policy.

Expenses *State resident tuition:* $2220 per academic year. *Nonresident tuition:* $6661 per academic year. *Full-time mandatory fees:* $231. *Room and board:* $3122–$3502. *Books and supplies per academic year:* ranges from $600 to $700.

Financial Aid Graduate assistantships, nurse traineeships, fellowships, dissertation grants, opportunities for employment. *Application deadline:* 1/15.

PhD Program

Applying *Required:* GRE General Test, master's degree in nursing, 2 scholarly papers, statistics course, interview, 3 letters of recommendation, vitae, writing sample. *Application deadline:* 2/1. *Application fee:* $35.

Degree Requirements 48 total credit hours; dissertation; oral exam; written exam; defense of dissertation; residency.

CONTINUING EDUCATION PROGRAM

Contact Ms. Alice Kuramoto, Director, Continuing Education, School of Nursing, University of Wisconsin-Milwaukee, PO Box 413, Milwaukee, WI 53201, 414-229-5617. *Fax:* 414-229-6474. *E-mail:* alicek@csd.uwm.edu

UNIVERSITY OF WISCONSIN–OSHKOSH
College of Nursing
Oshkosh, Wisconsin

Programs • Generic Baccalaureate • RN Baccalaureate • MSN • Continuing Education

The University State-supported comprehensive coed institution. Part of University of Wisconsin System. Founded: 1871. *Primary accreditation:* regional. *Setting:* 192-acre suburban campus. *Total enrollment:* 10,472.

The College of Nursing Founded in 1966. *Nursing program faculty:* 29 (45% with doctorates). *Off-campus program site:* Wausau.

Academic Facilities *Campus library:* 380,000 volumes; 90,000 periodical subscriptions. *Nursing school resources:* CAI, computer lab, nursing audio-visuals, interactive nursing skills videos, learning resource lab.

Student Life *Student services:* health clinic, child-care facilities, personal counseling, career counseling, institutionally sponsored work-study program, job placement, campus safety program, special assistance for disabled students. *International student services:* counseling/support, special assistance for nonnative speakers of English. *Nursing student activities:* Sigma Theta Tau, nursing club, student nurses association.

Calendar Semesters.

NURSING STUDENT PROFILE

Undergraduate **Enrollment:** 613
Women: 86%; **Men:** 14%; **Minority:** 5%; **Part-time:** 9%
Graduate **Enrollment:** 127
Women: 96%; **Men:** 4%; **Minority:** 9%; **Part-time:** 40%

BACCALAUREATE PROGRAMS

Contact Dr. Rosemary Smith, Director, Undergraduate Program, College of Nursing, University of Wisconsin-Oshkosh, 800 Algoma Boulevard, Oshkosh, WI 54901-8660, 414-424-1028. *Fax:* 414-424-0123. *E-mail:* smith@uwosh.edu

Expenses *State resident tuition:* $2444 full-time, $103 per credit part-time. *Nonresident tuition:* $7988 full-time, $334 per credit part-time. *Full-time mandatory fees:* $0. *Part-time mandatory fees:* $0. *Room and board:* $2752–$3728. *Books and supplies per academic year:* ranges from $300 to $600.

Financial Aid Institutionally sponsored need-based grants/scholarships, institutionally sponsored non-need grants/scholarships, Federal Nursing Student Loans, Federal Work-Study. *Application deadline:* 3/15.

Generic Baccalaureate Program (BSN)

Applying *Required:* SAT I, ACT, minimum college GPA of 2.75, 3 years of high school math, 3 years of high school science, transcript of college record, high school class rank: top 50%. 32 prerequisite credits must be completed before admission to the nursing program. *Options:* Advanced standing available through advanced placement exams. *Application deadlines:* 2/15 (fall), 9/15 (spring). *Application fee:* $28.

Degree Requirements 122 total credit hours, 64 in nursing.

RN Baccalaureate Program (BSN)

Applying *Required:* RN license, diploma or AD in nursing, transcript of college record. 60 prerequisite credits must be completed before admission to the nursing program. *Options:* Advanced standing available through advanced placement exams. May apply for transfer of up to 60 total credits. *Application deadlines:* 3/1 (fall), 10/1 (spring). *Application fee:* $28.

Degree Requirements 122 total credit hours, 57 in nursing.

Distance learning Courses provided through video, audio, computer-based media, on-line.

MASTER'S PROGRAM

Contact Ms. Mary Barker, Director, Graduate Program, College of Nursing, University of Wisconsin-Oshkosh, 800 Algoma Boulevard, Oshkosh, WI 54901-8660, 414-424-2106. *Fax:* 414-424-0123. *E-mail:* barkerm@uwosh.edu

Areas of Study Nursing administration; nursing education; nurse practitioner programs in family health, gerontology.

Expenses *State resident tuition:* $3248 full-time, $181 per credit part-time. *Nonresident tuition:* $10,106 full-time, $562 per credit part-time. *Full-time mandatory fees:* $0. *Part-time mandatory fees:* $0. *Room and board:* $2752–$3728. *Books and supplies per academic year:* ranges from $300 to $700.

Financial Aid Graduate assistantships, nurse traineeships. *Application deadline:* 1/15.

MSN Program

Applying *Required:* bachelor's degree in nursing, minimum GPA of 3.0, RN license, physical assessment course, statistics course, essay, interview, 3 letters of recommendation, transcript of college record. *Application deadline:* 1/15. *Application fee:* $35.

Degree Requirements 36 total credit hours, 36 in nursing. Thesis or clinical paper.

CONTINUING EDUCATION PROGRAM

Contact Ms. Barbara Tungate, Coordinator, Continuing Education, College of Nursing, University of Wisconsin-Oshkosh, 800 Algoma Boulevard, Oshkosh, WI 54901-8660, 414-424-7239. *Fax:* 414-424-0123. *E-mail:* tungate@uwosh.edu

VITERBO COLLEGE
School of Nursing
LaCrosse, Wisconsin

Programs • Generic Baccalaureate • RN Baccalaureate

The College Independent Roman Catholic comprehensive coed institution. Founded: 1890. *Primary accreditation:* regional. *Setting:* 5-acre urban campus. *Total enrollment:* 1,846.

The School of Nursing Founded in 1967.

Academic Facilities *Campus library:* 84,000 volumes (80 in health, 65 in nursing); 725 periodical subscriptions.

Calendar Semesters.

BACCALAUREATE PROGRAMS

Contact Director of Admissions, School of Nursing, Viterbo College, 815 South 9th, La Crosse, WI 54601-4797, 608-791-0420. *Fax:* 608-791-0367.

Expenses *Tuition:* $10,560 full-time, $305 per credit hour part-time. *Full-time mandatory fees:* $80+. *Room and board:* $2810–$4970. *Room only:* $1130–$2720. *Books and supplies per academic year:* $400.

Financial Aid Institutionally sponsored need-based grants/scholarships, institutionally sponsored non-need grants/scholarships, Federal Nursing Student Loans, Federal Pell Grants, Federal Perkins Loans, Federal Supplemental Educational Opportunity Grants, Federal Work-Study, Federal PLUS Loans, Federal Stafford Loans. *Application deadline:* 3/15.

Generic Baccalaureate Program (BSN)

Applying *Required:* SAT I or ACT, minimum college GPA of 2.5, high school transcript, high school class rank: . *Options:* Advanced standing available through advanced placement exams. May apply for transfer of up to 64 total credits. *Application deadline:* rolling. *Application fee:* $15.

Degree Requirements 128 total credit hours, 58 in nursing.

RN Baccalaureate Program (BSN)

Applying *Required:* RN license, diploma or AD in nursing, high school transcript. *Options:* Advanced standing available through credit by exam. *Application deadline:* rolling. *Application fee:* $15.

Degree Requirements 128 total credit hours, 23 in nursing.

WYOMING

UNIVERSITY OF WYOMING
School of Nursing
Laramie, Wyoming

Programs • Generic Baccalaureate • RN Baccalaureate • MS • RN to Master's • Master's for Nurses with Non-Nursing Degrees • Post-Master's • Continuing Education

The University State-supported coed university. Founded: 1886. *Primary accreditation:* regional. *Setting:* 785-acre small-town campus. *Total enrollment:* 11,361.

The School of Nursing Founded in 1951. *Nursing program faculty:* 25 (52% with doctorates). *Off-campus program sites:* Casper, Rock Springs, Cheyenne.

Academic Facilities *Campus library:* 955,391 volumes (88,877 in health, 2,172 in nursing); 11,874 periodical subscriptions (698 health-care related). *Nursing school resources:* CAI, computer lab, nursing audiovisuals, interactive nursing skills videos, learning resource lab, nursing center.

Student Life *Student services:* health clinic, child-care facilities, personal counseling, career counseling, institutionally sponsored work-study program, job placement, campus safety program, special assistance for disabled students, women's center, adult reentry office, minority affairs office. *International student services:* counseling/support, special assistance for nonnative speakers of English, family programs. *Nursing student activities:* Sigma Theta Tau, student nurses association.

Calendar Semesters.

NURSING STUDENT PROFILE

Undergraduate **Enrollment:** 264
Women: 88%; **Men:** 12%; **Minority:** 11%; **International:** 0%; **Part-time:** 25%

Graduate **Enrollment:** 58
Women: 93%; **Men:** 7%; **Minority:** 7%; **International:** 1%; **Part-time:** 64%

BACCALAUREATE PROGRAMS

Contact Dr. Elizabeth Wiest, Assistant to the Dean, School of Nursing, University of Wyoming, PO Box 3065, Laramie, WY 82071-3065, 307-766-4314. *Fax:* 307-766-4294. *E-mail:* betsyw@uwyo.edu

Expenses *State resident tuition:* $2144 full-time, $81 per credit hour part-time. *Nonresident tuition:* $6872 full-time, $278 per credit hour part-time. *Full-time mandatory fees:* $250–$300. *Room and board:* $3520. *Room only:* $1512. *Books and supplies per academic year:* ranges from $300 to $500.

Financial Aid Institutionally sponsored need-based grants/scholarships, institutionally sponsored non-need grants/scholarships, Federal Direct Loans, Federal Pell Grants, Federal Perkins Loans, Federal Supplemental Educational Opportunity Grants, Federal Work-Study. *Application deadline:* 3/1.

Generic Baccalaureate Program (BSN)

Applying *Required:* SAT I, ACT, TOEFL for nonnative speakers of English, minimum high school GPA of 2.75, 3 years of high school math, 3 years of high school science, high school chemistry, high school biology, high school transcript, transcript of college record, minimum 3.0 high school GPA for out-of-state students. 53 prerequisite credits must be completed before admission to the nursing program. *Options:* Advanced standing available through the following means: advanced placement exams, credit by exam. *Application deadlines:* 2/15 (fall), 11/15 (spring). *Application fee:* $30.

Degree Requirements 130 total credit hours, 60 in nursing.

RN Baccalaureate Program (BSN)

Applying *Required:* ACT PEP, minimum high school GPA of 2.0, minimum college GPA of 2.0, RN license, diploma or AD in nursing, high school transcript, letter of recommendation, transcript of college record, minimum 2.3 high school GPA for out-of-state students. *Options:* Advanced standing available through the following means: advanced placement exams, credit by exam. Course work may be accelerated. *Application deadlines:* 2/15 (fall), 11/15 (spring). *Application fee:* $30.

Degree Requirements 130 total credit hours, 25 in nursing.

Distance learning Courses provided through correspondence, video, computer-based media, compressed video. Specific degree requirements include some courses offered at site.

MASTER'S PROGRAMS

Contact Dr. Marcia L. Dale, Dean, School of Nursing, University of Wyoming, PO Box 3065, Laramie, WY 82071-3065, 307-766-6569. *Fax:* 307-766-4294. *E-mail:* marcia@uwyo.edu

Areas of Study Clinical nurse specialist program in community health nursing; nursing education; nurse practitioner program in family health.

Expenses *State resident tuition:* $2591 full-time, $131 per credit hour part-time. *Nonresident tuition:* $7325 full-time, $394 per credit hour part-time. *Full-time mandatory fees:* $250–$300. *Room and board:* $3520. *Room only:* $1512. *Books and supplies per academic year:* ranges from $300 to $600.

Financial Aid Graduate assistantships, nurse traineeships, Federal Direct Loans, employment opportunities, institutionally sponsored need-based grants/scholarships, institutionally sponsored non-need-based grants/scholarships, minority student grants. *Application deadline:* 3/1.

MS Program

Applying *Required:* TOEFL for nonnative speakers of English, GRE General Test (minimum combined score of 900 on two sections), bachelor's degree in nursing, bachelor's degree, minimum GPA of 3.0, RN license, 1 year of clinical experience, professional liability/malpractice insurance, 3 letters of recommendation, transcript of college record, certification as Advanced Practice Nurse. *Application deadlines:* 11/15 (fall), 11/15 (spring).

Degree Requirements 30 total credit hours, 24 in nursing. Thesis required.

RN to Master's Program (MS)

Applying *Required:* TOEFL for nonnative speakers of English, GRE General Test (minimum combined score of 900 on two sections) and SAT,

University of Wyoming (continued)

ACT, or ACT PEP, minimum GPA of 3.0, RN license, professional liability/malpractice insurance, interview, 3 letters of recommendation, transcript of college record, diploma or AD in nursing, high school transcript. *Application deadlines:* 11/15 (fall), 11/15 (spring).

Degree Requirements 163–172 total credit hours dependent upon track, 60–69 in nursing. Thesis required.

Master's for Nurses with Non-Nursing Degrees Program (MS)

Applying *Required:* TOEFL for nonnative speakers of English, GRE General Test (minimum combined score of 900 on two sections), bachelor's degree in nursing, bachelor's degree, minimum GPA, RN license, professional liability/malpractice insurance, interview, 3 letters of recommendation, transcript of college record. *Application deadlines:* 11/15 (fall), 11/15 (spring).

Degree Requirements 41–50 total credit hours dependent upon track, 35–47 in nursing. Thesis required.

Post-Master's Program

Applying *Required:* TOEFL for nonnative speakers of English, bachelor's degree in nursing, bachelor's degree, minimum GPA of 3.0, RN license, professional liability/malpractice insurance, interview, 3 letters of recommendation, transcript of college record, MS in nursing. *Application deadlines:* 11/15 (fall), 11/15 (spring).

Degree Requirements 37 total credit hours, 37 in nursing.

CONTINUING EDUCATION PROGRAM

Contact Dr. Elizabeth Wiest, Director of Off-Campus Programs, School of Nursing, University of Wyoming, PO Box 3065, Laramie, WY 82071-3065, 307-766-4314. *Fax:* 307-766-4294. *E-mail:* betsyw@uwyo.edu

CANADA

ALBERTA

ATHABASCA UNIVERSITY
Centre for Nursing and Health Studies
Athabasca, Alberta

Program • RN Baccalaureate

The University Province-supported comprehensive coed institution. Founded: 1970. *Primary accreditation:* provincial charter. *Setting:* 480-acre small-town campus. *Total enrollment:* 11,591.

The Centre for Nursing and Health Studies Founded in 1990. *Nursing program faculty:* 4 (50% with doctorates).

Academic Facilities *Campus library:* 113,000 volumes (3,000 in nursing); 1,100 periodical subscriptions (50 health-care related). *Nursing school resources:* CAI, computer lab, nursing audiovisuals, interactive nursing skills videos.

Student Life *Student services:* personal counseling, institutionally sponsored work-study program, special assistance for disabled students. *International student services:* counseling/support. *Nursing student activities:* student nurses association, Nursing Network.

Calendar Year-round monthly enrollment.

NURSING STUDENT PROFILE

Undergraduate **Enrollment:** 732
Women: 96%; **Men:** 4%; **International:** 1%; **Part-time:** 90%

BACCALAUREATE PROGRAM

Contact Dr. Roberta Carey, Director, Center for Nursing and Health Studies, Athabasca University, Box 10000, Athabasca, AB T9S 1A1, 403-675-6392. *Fax:* 403-675-6186. *E-mail:* bobbiec@cs.athabascau.ca

Expenses *State resident tuition:* $2613 full-time, $261 per 3- or 4-credit course part-time. *Nonresident tuition:* ranges from $2978 to $3343 full-time, ranges from $298 to $334 per 3- or 4-credit course part-time.

RN Baccalaureate Program (BN)

Applying *Required:* RN license, transcript of college record, 60% average, RN registration with a provincial licensing association. *Options:* Advanced standing available through advanced placement exams. Course work may be accelerated. May apply for transfer of up to 47 total credits. *Application deadline:* rolling. *Application fee:* $50.

Degree Requirements 69 total credit hours, 33 in nursing.

Distance learning Courses provided through correspondence, video, audio, computer-based media, on-line.

UNIVERSITY OF ALBERTA
Faculty of Nursing
Edmonton, Alberta

Programs • Generic Baccalaureate • RN Baccalaureate • MN • PhD • Postdoctoral

The University Province-supported coed university. Founded: 1906. *Primary accreditation:* provincial charter. *Setting:* 154-acre urban campus. *Total enrollment:* 29,238.

The Faculty of Nursing Founded in 1918. *Nursing program faculty:* 61 (67% with doctorates). *Off-campus program sites:* Red Deer, Grande Prairie, Ft. McMurray.

Academic Facilities *Campus library:* 5.0 million volumes; 26,424 periodical subscriptions. *Nursing school resources:* CAI, computer lab, health assessment lab, interviewing lab.

Student Life *Student services:* health clinic, child-care facilities, personal counseling, career counseling, job placement, campus safety program. *International student services:* counseling/support, special assistance for nonnative speakers of English, ESL courses, international center. *Nursing student activities:* Sigma Theta Tau, nursing club, student nurses association.

Calendar Semesters.

NURSING STUDENT PROFILE

Undergraduate **Enrollment:** 959
Women: 94%; **Men:** 6%; **Part-time:** 8%
Graduate **Enrollment:** 144
Women: 98%; **Men:** 2%; **International:** 3%; **Part-time:** 43%

BACCALAUREATE PROGRAMS

Contact Ms. Sharon Bookhalter, Student Adviser, 3-107 Clinical Sciences Building, Faculty of Nursing, University of Alberta, Edmonton, AB T6G 2G3, 403-492-4404. *Fax:* 403-492-2551. *E-mail:* sbookhal@ua-nursing.ualberta.ca

Expenses *State resident tuition:* $4892 full-time, $204 per 3-credit course part-time. *Nonresident tuition:* $9782 full-time, $407 per 3-credit course part-time. *Full-time mandatory fees:* $340. *Part-time mandatory fees:* $90. *Books and supplies per academic year:* ranges from $800 to $1000.

Financial Aid Institutionally sponsored non-need grants/scholarships, Federal Direct Loans, Alberta student finance.

Generic Baccalaureate Program (BScN)

Applying *Required:* TOEFL for nonnative speakers of English, TSE for nonnative speakers of English, minimum high school GPA of 2.0, minimum college GPA of 2.0, high school math, high school science, high school chemistry, high school biology, high school transcript, written essay, transcript of college record. *Options:* Advanced standing available through credit by exam. Course work may be accelerated. May apply for transfer of up to 60 total credits. *Application deadline:* 5/1. *Application fee:* $60.

Degree Requirements 146 total credit hours. CPR certification, up-to-date immunization.

RN Baccalaureate Program (BScN)

Applying *Required:* TOEFL for nonnative speakers of English, TSE for nonnative speakers of English, minimum college GPA of 2.0, RN license, diploma or AD in nursing, high school transcript, 2 letters of recommendation, written essay, transcript of college record, questionnaire, immunizations. 12 prerequisite credits must be completed before admission to the nursing program. *Options:* Course work may be accelerated. May apply for transfer of up to 30 total credits. *Application deadline:* 5/1. *Application fee:* $60.

Degree Requirements 71 total credit hours. CPR certification, up-to-date immunization.

MASTER'S PROGRAM

Contact Dr. Phyllis Giovannetti, Associate Dean, Graduate Education, 3rd Floor, Clinical Sciences Building, Faculty of Nursing, University of Alberta, Edmonton, AB T6G 2G3, 403-492-6764. *Fax:* 403-492-2551. *E-mail:* pgiovann@ua-nursing.ualberta.ca

Areas of Study Clinical nurse specialist programs in cardiovascular nursing, community health nursing, critical care nursing, family health nursing, gerontological nursing, maternity-newborn nursing, medical-surgical nursing, oncology nursing, parent-child nursing, pediatric nursing, perinatal nursing, psychiatric–mental health nursing, public health nursing, women's health nursing, advanced neonatal intensive care nursing.

Expenses *State resident tuition:* $4462 full-time, $301 per 3 credit course part-time. *Nonresident tuition:* $8282 full-time, $539 per 3 credit course part-time. *Full-time mandatory fees:* $435. *Part-time mandatory fees:* $170. *Room and board:* $8500+. *Room only:* $3480. *Books and supplies per academic year:* $900.

Financial Aid Graduate assistantships, fellowships, institutionally sponsored loans, employment opportunities, institutionally sponsored non-need-based grants/scholarships, research grants, travel grants, provincial loans. 25% of master's level students in nursing programs received some form of financial aid in 1995-96.

University of Alberta (continued)

MN Program

Applying *Required:* TOEFL for nonnative speakers of English, bachelor's degree in nursing, minimum GPA of 3.0, RN license, 1 year of clinical experience, physical assessment course, statistics course, 3 letters of recommendation, transcript of college record, CPR certification. *Application deadlines:* 7/31 (fall), 12/31 (spring). *Application fee:* $60.

Degree Requirements 32–35 total credit hours dependent upon track, 23–29 in nursing, 6–9 in statistics, research, and other specified elective areas. 2 terms of thesis or course-based MN.

DOCTORAL PROGRAM

Contact Dr. Phyllis Giovannetti, Associate Dean, Graduate Education and Professor, Faculty of Nursing, University of Alberta, Edmonton, AB T6G 2G3, 403-492-6764. *Fax:* 403-492-2551. *E-mail:* pgiovann@ua-nursing.ualberta.ca

Areas of Study Nursing theory and knowledge.

Expenses *State resident tuition:* $3056 full-time, $412 per 3-credit course part-time. *Nonresident tuition:* $5673 full-time, $739 per 3-credit course part-time. *Full-time mandatory fees:* $435. *Room and board:* $8500+. *Room only:* $3480. *Books and supplies per academic year:* $900.

Financial Aid Graduate assistantships, fellowships, dissertation grants, grants, institutionally sponsored loans, opportunities for employment, institutionally sponsored non-need-based grants/scholarships, research grants, travel grants.

PhD Program

Applying *Required:* TOEFL for nonnative speakers of English, master's degree in nursing, 2 years of clinical experience, year in proposed area of specialization, statistics course, 3 letters of recommendation, vitae, writing sample, competitive review by faculty committee, qualified faculty member to supervise. *Application deadlines:* 7/31 (fall), 12/31 (spring). *Application fee:* $60.

Degree Requirements dissertation; oral exam; written exam; defense of dissertation; residency.

POSTDOCTORAL PROGRAM

Contact Dr. Phyllis Giovannetti, Associate Dean, Graduate Education and Professor, Faculty of Nursing, University of Alberta, Edmonton, AB T6G 2G3, 403-492-6764. *Fax:* 403-492-2551. *E-mail:* pgiovann@ua-nursing.ualberta.ca

Areas of Study Individualized study.

See full description on page 520.

THE UNIVERSITY OF CALGARY
Faculty of Nursing
Calgary, Alberta

Programs • Generic Baccalaureate • Master's • Doctoral

The University Province-supported coed university. Founded: 1945. *Primary accreditation:* provincial charter. *Setting:* 304-acre urban campus. *Total enrollment:* 23,042.

The Faculty of Nursing Founded in 1970.

Academic Facilities *Campus library:* 5.8 million volumes (288,350 in health, 115,340 in nursing).

Calendar Semesters.

BACCALAUREATE PROGRAM

Contact Student Affairs Adviser, Undergraduate Program, Faculty of Nursing, University of Calgary, 2500 University Drive, NW, Calgary, AB T2N 1N4, 403-220-4636. *Fax:* 403-284-4803.

Generic Baccalaureate Program (BN)

Applying *Required:* CPR certification, 3 years of high school English, mathematics.

MASTER'S PROGRAM

Contact Admissions Adviser, Graduate Program, Faculty of Nursing, University of Calgary, 2500 University Drive, NW, Calgary, AB T2N 1N4, 403-220-6241. *Fax:* 403-284-4803.

DOCTORAL PROGRAM

Contact Admissions Adviser, Graduate Program, Faculty of Nursing, University of Calgary, 2500 University Drive, NW, Calgary, AB T2N 1N4, 403-220-6241. *Fax:* 403-284-4803.

UNIVERSITY OF LETHBRIDGE
School of Nursing
Lethbridge, Alberta

Program • Generic Baccalaureate

The University Province-supported comprehensive coed institution. Founded: 1967. *Primary accreditation:* provincial charter. *Setting:* 576-acre urban campus. *Total enrollment:* 4,909.

The School of Nursing Founded in 1979.

Academic Facilities *Campus library:* 472,918 volumes (8,899 in health, 1,577 in nursing); 2,175 periodical subscriptions (75 health-care related).

Calendar Semesters.

BACCALAUREATE PROGRAM

Contact Student Program Adviser, School of Nursing, University of Lethbridge, 4401 University Drive, Lethbridge, AB T1K 3M4, 403-329-2649. *Fax:* 403-329-2668.

BRITISH COLUMBIA

UNIVERSITY OF BRITISH COLUMBIA
School of Nursing
Vancouver, British Columbia

Programs • Generic Baccalaureate • Master's • Doctoral

The University Province-supported coed university. Founded: 1915. *Primary accreditation:* provincial charter. *Setting:* 1,000-acre urban campus. *Total enrollment:* 30,914.

The School of Nursing Founded in 1919.

Calendar Semesters.

BACCALAUREATE PROGRAM

Contact Student Records Office, School of Nursing, University of British Columbia, T206-2211 Wesbrook Mall, Vancouver, BC V6T 2B5, 604-822-7497. *Fax:* 604-822-7466.

Expenses *State resident tuition:* $1703 full-time, $56 per credit part-time. *Nonresident tuition:* $4258 full-time, $140 per credit part-time.

Generic Baccalaureate Program (BSN)

Applying *Required:* English language proficiency, high school mathematics.

MASTER'S PROGRAM

Contact Graduate Adviser, School of Nursing, University of British Columbia, T206-2211 Wesbrook Mall, Vancouver, BC V6T 2B5, 604-822-7446. *Fax:* 604-822-7466.

DOCTORAL PROGRAM

Contact Graduate Adviser, School of Nursing, University of British Columbia, T206-2211 Wesbrook Mall, Vancouver, BC V6T 2B5, 604-822-7446. *Fax:* 604-822-7466.

UNIVERSITY OF VICTORIA
School of Nursing
Victoria, British Columbia

Programs • Generic Baccalaureate • RN Baccalaureate • MN • Master's for Nurses with Non-Nursing Degrees • PhD • Continuing Education

The University Province-supported coed university. Founded: 1963. *Primary accreditation:* provincial charter. *Setting:* 380-acre suburban campus. *Total enrollment:* 17,010.

The School of Nursing Founded in 1976. *Nursing program faculty:* 18 (83% with doctorates). *Off-campus program site:* Vancouver.

Academic Facilities *Campus library:* 1.6 million volumes (1,752 in health, 2,089 in nursing). *Nursing school resources:* computer lab, nursing audiovisuals, interactive nursing skills videos, learning resource lab.

Student Life *Student services:* health clinic, child-care facilities, personal counseling, career counseling, institutionally sponsored work-study program, job placement, campus safety program, special assistance for disabled students, interfaith chaplaincy, athletics and recreation. *International student services:* counseling/support, orientation. *Nursing student activities:* student nurses association.

Calendar Semesters.

NURSING STUDENT PROFILE

Undergraduate **Enrollment:** 625
Women: 96%; **Men:** 4%; **Part-time:** 87%
Graduate **Enrollment:** 22
Women: 94%; **Men:** 6%; **Part-time:** 17%

BACCALAUREATE PROGRAMS

Contact Mr. Richard Toogood, Admissions and Liaison Officer, School of Nursing, University of Victoria, PO Box 1700, Victoria, BC V8W 2Y2, 250-721-6334. *Fax:* 250-721-6231. *E-mail:* rtoogood@hsd.uvic.ca

Expenses *State resident tuition:* ranges from $992 to $1653 full-time, $110 per unit part-time. *Full-time mandatory fees:* $146. *Part-time mandatory fees:* $87. *Room and board:* $3194–$3942. *Books and supplies per academic year:* ranges from $493 to $617.

Financial Aid Institutionally sponsored need-based grants/scholarships, institutionally sponsored non-need grants/scholarships, Federal Nursing Student Loans, Federal Work-Study. *Application deadline:* 6/1.

Generic Baccalaureate Program (BSN)

Applying *Required:* SAT II Writing Test, TOEFL for nonnative speakers of English, minimum high school GPA of 2.5, minimum college GPA of 2.0, 3 years of high school math, 3 years of high school science, high school foreign language, transcript of college record, students complete first two years at a collaborative college, then apply to complete their degree. 23 prerequisite credits must be completed before admission to the nursing program. *Options:* May apply for transfer of up to 9 total credits. *Application deadlines:* 9/30 (spring), 12/31 (summer). *Application fee:* $20.

Degree Requirements 31 total credit hours, 30 in nursing.

Distance learning Courses provided through correspondence, video, teleconference.

RN Baccalaureate Program (BSN)

Applying *Required:* SAT II Writing Test, TOEFL for nonnative speakers of English, minimum high school GPA of 2.5, minimum college GPA of 2.0, 3 years of high school math, 3 years of high school science, RN license, diploma or AD in nursing, high school foreign language, high school transcript, written essay, transcript of college record, completion of basic life support level "C" course. *Options:* Course work may be accelerated. May apply for transfer of up to 9 total credits. *Application deadlines:* 4/1 (fall), 9/30 (spring). *Application fee:* $20.

Degree Requirements 30 total credit hours, 27 in nursing. 21 units of coursework must be completed at the University of Victoria.

Distance learning Courses provided through correspondence, video, teleconference.

MASTER'S PROGRAM

Contact Dr. Laurene Shields, Graduate Adviser, School of Nursing, University of Victoria, PO Box 1700, Victoria, BC V8W 2Y2, 250-721-6467. *Fax:* 250-721-6231. *E-mail:* lshields@hsd.uvic.ca

Expenses *State resident tuition:* $1410 full-time, $705 per academic year part-time. *Full-time mandatory fees:* $49. *Part-time mandatory fees:* $49.

Financial Aid Graduate assistantships, Federal Nursing Student Loans. *Application deadline:* 6/1.

MN Program

Master's for Nurses with Non-Nursing Degrees Program

Applying *Required:* bachelor's degree in nursing, bachelor's degree, RN license, 1 year of clinical experience, statistics course, essay, 2 letters of recommendation, transcript of college record, minimum college GPA (9.0 scale): 6.0. *Application deadline:* 3/15. *Application fee:* $45.

Degree Requirements 21 total credit hours. Thesis required.

DOCTORAL PROGRAM

Contact Dr. Janet Storch, School of Nursing, University of Victoria, PO Box 1700, Victoria, BC V8W 2Y2, 250-721-7953. *Fax:* 250-721-6231. *E-mail:* jstorch@hsd.uvic.ca

Areas of Study Individualized study.

Expenses *State resident tuition:* $1410 full-time, $705 per academic year part-time. *Full-time mandatory fees:* $49. *Part-time mandatory fees:* $49.

Financial Aid Graduate assistantships, fellowships, grants, institutionally sponsored loans, opportunities for employment. *Application deadline:* 2/15.

PhD Program

Applying *Required:* TOEFL for nonnative speakers of English, master's degree in nursing, year of clinical experience, interview, letter of recommendation, vitae, writing sample, competitive review by faculty committee, program plan, approval of supervisory committee. *Application deadline:* 3/15. *Application fee:* $100.

Degree Requirements dissertation; oral exam; written exam; defense of dissertation; residency.

CONTINUING EDUCATION PROGRAM

Contact Dr. Janet Storch, Director, School of Nursing, University of Victoria, PO Box 1700, Victoria, BC V8W 2Y2, 250-721-7955. *Fax:* 250-721-6231. *E-mail:* jstorch@hsd.uvic.ca

MANITOBA

BRANDON UNIVERSITY
Department of Nursing and Health Studies
Brandon, Manitoba

Programs • RN Baccalaureate • RPN to Baccalaureate

The University Province-supported comprehensive coed institution. Founded: 1899. *Primary accreditation:* provincial charter. *Setting:* 30-acre small-town campus. *Total enrollment:* 3,182.

The Department of Nursing and Health Studies Founded in 1995. *Nursing program faculty:* 10.

Academic Facilities *Campus library:* 190,000 volumes; 1,800 periodical subscriptions. *Nursing school resources:* CAI, computer lab, nursing audiovisuals, interactive nursing skills videos, learning resource lab.

Student Life *Student services:* child-care facilities, personal counseling, career counseling, campus safety program. *International student services:*

Brandon University (continued)

counseling/support, special assistance for nonnative speakers of English, ESL courses. *Nursing student activities:* Sigma Theta Tau, nursing club, student nurses association.

Calendar Semesters.

NURSING STUDENT PROFILE

Undergraduate **Enrollment:** 146
Women: 92%; **Men:** 8%; **Minority:** 8%; **International:** 0%; **Part-time:** 80%

BACCALAUREATE PROGRAMS

Contact Prof. Renee Will, Chair, Department of Nursing and Health Studies, Brandon University, 270 18th Street, Brandon, MB R7A 6A9, 204-727-7460. *Fax:* 204-726-5793. *E-mail:* will@brandonu.ca

Expenses *Tuition:* $153 per three credit hours. *Part-time mandatory fees:* $56–$388. *Room and board:* $3897–$4929.

Financial Aid Institutionally sponsored non-need grants/scholarships, Federal Nursing Student Loans. *Application deadline:* 5/1.

RN Baccalaureate Program (BScN)

Applying *Required:* minimum college GPA of 2.0, RN license, diploma or AD in nursing, 2 letters of recommendation, membership or eligibility for membership in Manitoba Association of Registered Nurses, 1 year of nursing experience. *Options:* May apply for transfer of up to 33 total credits. *Application deadline:* rolling. *Application fee:* $25.

Degree Requirements 67 total credit hours, 34 in nursing.

RPN to Baccalaureate Program (BScMH)

Applying *Required:* minimum college GPA of 2.0, diploma or AD in nursing, 2 letters of recommendation, transcript of college record, RPN license, membership or eligibility for membership in Registered Psychiatric Nurses Association of Manitoba, 1 year of practice experience. *Options:* May apply for transfer of up to 33 total credits. *Application deadline:* rolling. *Application fee:* $25.

Degree Requirements 67 total credit hours, 34 in nursing.

UNIVERSITY OF MANITOBA
Faculty of Nursing
Winnipeg, Manitoba

Programs • Generic Baccalaureate • RN Baccalaureate • Master's for Nurses with Non-Nursing Degrees • Continuing Education

The University Province-supported coed university. Founded: 1877. *Primary accreditation:* provincial charter. *Setting:* 685-acre suburban campus. *Total enrollment:* 23,967.

The Faculty of Nursing Founded in 1943. *Nursing program faculty:* 100 (16% with doctorates). *Off-campus program site:* Brandon.

Academic Facilities *Campus library:* 1.6 million volumes (137,100 in health, 5,000 in nursing); 11,532 periodical subscriptions (2,208 health-care related). *Nursing school resources:* CAI, computer lab, nursing audiovisuals, interactive nursing skills videos, learning resource lab, nursing skills lab.

Student Life *Student services:* health clinic, child-care facilities, personal counseling, career counseling, campus safety program, special assistance for disabled students. *International student services:* counseling/support, special assistance for nonnative speakers of English, ESL courses, international student center. *Nursing student activities:* Sigma Theta Tau, student nurses association, Manitoba Association of Nursing Students, Canadian Nursing Students Association.

Calendar Semesters.

NURSING STUDENT PROFILE

Undergraduate **Enrollment:** 789
Women: 90%; **Men:** 10%; **Minority:** 2%; **Part-time:** 39%
Graduate **Enrollment:** 76
Women: 95%; **Men:** 5%; **International:** 0%; **Part-time:** 60%

BACCALAUREATE PROGRAMS

Contact Ms. Loxie Armstrong, Student Adviser, 246 Bison Building, Faculty of Nursing, University of Manitoba, Winnipeg, MB R3T 2N2, 204-474-6217. *Fax:* 204-275-5464. *E-mail:* loxie_armstrong@umanitoba.ca

Expenses *State resident tuition:* $2259 per academic year. *Room and board:* $5112. *Books and supplies per academic year:* ranges from $1035 to $1644.

Financial Aid Institutionally sponsored need-based grants/scholarships, institutionally sponsored non-need grants/scholarships, Federal Direct Loans, provincial student loans. *Application deadline:* 6/30.

Generic Baccalaureate Program (BN)

Applying *Required:* TOEFL for nonnative speakers of English, minimum high school GPA of 2.0, minimum college GPA of 2.0, 3 years of high school math, 3 years of high school science, high school chemistry, high school transcript, transcript of college record, 3 years of high school English. *Options:* Advanced standing available through credit by exam. Course work may be accelerated. May apply for transfer of up to 42 total credits. *Application deadline:* 7/1. *Application fee:* $30.

Degree Requirements 135 total credit hours, 90 in nursing.

RN Baccalaureate Program (BN)

Applying *Required:* RN license, diploma or AD in nursing, practicing member of Canadian RN association/college, minimum 1,125 hours nursing experience defined by Manitoba Association of Registered Nurses. *Options:* Advanced standing available through credit by exam. *Application deadline:* 3/1. *Application fee:* $30.

Degree Requirements 67 total credit hours, 34 in nursing.

Distance learning Courses provided through correspondence, video, audio. Specific degree requirements include 2 workshops and a final test on campus.

MASTER'S PROGRAM

Contact Ms. Darlene McWhirter, Graduate Program Assistant, 246 Bison Building, Faculty of Nursing, University of Manitoba, Winnipeg, MB R3T 2N2, 204-474-6216. *Fax:* 204-275-5464. *E-mail:* darlene_mcwhirter@umanitoba.ca

Areas of Study Nursing administration.

Expenses *State resident tuition:* $2355 per academic year. *Nonresident tuition:* $4122 per academic year. *Full-time mandatory fees:* $153. *Part-time mandatory fees:* $153. *Room only:* $5100–$6300. *Books and supplies per academic year:* ranges from $1140 to $1367.

Financial Aid Graduate assistantships, fellowships, Federal Direct Loans, employment opportunities, institutionally sponsored need-based grants/scholarships, institutionally sponsored non-need-based grants/scholarships. 30% of master's level students in nursing programs received some form of financial aid in 1995-96.

Master's for Nurses with Non-Nursing Degrees Program (MN)

Applying *Required:* TOEFL for nonnative speakers of English, bachelor's degree, minimum GPA of 3.0, RN license, statistics course, 3 letters of recommendation, transcript of college record, research methods course, active practicing nurse registration. *Application deadline:* 2/28. *Application fee:* $50.

Degree Requirements 27 total credit hours, 21 in nursing. Thesis or practicum.

CONTINUING EDUCATION PROGRAM

Contact Ms. Brenda Miller, Secretary, 246 Bison Building, Faculty of Nursing, University of Manitoba, Winnipeg, MB R3T 2N2, 204-474-6266. *Fax:* 204-275-5464.

NEW BRUNSWICK

UNIVERSITÉ DE MONCTON
École des Sciences Infirmières
Moncton, New Brunswick

The Institution Province-supported comprehensive coed institution. Founded: 1963. *Primary accreditation:* provincial charter. *Setting:* 400-acre urban campus. *Total enrollment:* 7,435.

The École des Sciences Infirmières Founded in 1955.

UNIVERSITY OF NEW BRUNSWICK
Faculty of Nursing
Fredericton, New Brunswick

Programs • Generic Baccalaureate • Accelerated Baccalaureate • RN Baccalaureate • BSN to Master's

The University Province-supported coed university. Founded: 1785. *Primary accreditation:* provincial charter. *Setting:* 7,100-acre urban campus. *Total enrollment:* 7,733.

The Faculty of Nursing Founded in 1958. *Nursing program faculty:* 46 (1% with doctorates). *Off-campus program sites:* Saint John, Moncton, Bathurst.

Academic Facilities *Campus library:* 1.1 million volumes (12,547 in health, 1,910 in nursing); 5,032 periodical subscriptions (250 health-care related). *Nursing school resources:* CAI, computer lab, nursing audiovisuals, interactive nursing skills videos, learning resource lab.

Student Life *Student services:* health clinic, child-care facilities, personal counseling, career counseling, job placement, campus safety program, special assistance for disabled students. *International student services:* counseling/support, ESL courses, full-time adviser. *Nursing student activities:* student nurses association, Canadian Nursing Students Association.

Calendar Semesters.

NURSING STUDENT PROFILE

Undergraduate **Enrollment:** 560
Women: 97%; **Men:** 3%; **Minority:** 0%; **International:** 0%; **Part-time:** 14%
Graduate **Enrollment:** 30
Women: 97%; **Men:** 3%; **Minority:** 0%; **International:** 0%; **Part-time:** 77%

BACCALAUREATE PROGRAMS

Contact Prof. Nancy Wiggins, Assistant Dean, Faculty of Nursing, University of New Brunswick, Postal Box 4400, Fredericton, NB E3B 5A3, 506-453-4642. *Fax:* 506-447-3057. *E-mail:* wiggins@unb.ca

Expenses *State resident tuition:* $2073 full-time, $191 per 3 credit course part-time. *Nonresident tuition:* $3752 per academic year. *Full-time mandatory fees:* $162. *Room and board:* $4145. *Room only:* $2200. *Books and supplies per academic year:* $800.

Financial Aid Institutionally sponsored need-based grants/scholarships. 25% of undergraduate students in nursing programs received some form of financial aid in 1995–96. *Application deadline:* 4/15.

Generic Baccalaureate Program (BN)

Applying *Required:* minimum college GPA of 3.0, 2 years of high school math, high school chemistry, high school biology, high school foreign language, high school transcript, written essay, transcript of college record. *Options:* Course work may be accelerated. May apply for transfer of up to 73 total credits. *Application deadline:* 3/31. *Application fee:* $25.

Degree Requirements 146 total credit hours, 96 in nursing.

Accelerated Baccalaureate Program (BN)

Applying *Required:* minimum college GPA of 3.0, 3 years of high school math, high school chemistry, high school biology, high school transcript, written essay, transcript of college record. 60 prerequisite credits must be completed before admission to the nursing program. *Options:* May apply for transfer of up to 60 total credits. *Application deadline:* 3/31. *Application fee:* $25.

Degree Requirements 155 total credit hours, 95 in nursing.

RN Baccalaureate Program (BN)

Applying *Required:* minimum college GPA of 2.0, 2 years of high school math, high school chemistry, high school biology, RN license, diploma or AD in nursing, high school foreign language, high school transcript, letter of recommendation, transcript of college record, 1 year of nursing experience. *Options:* May apply for transfer of up to 48 total credits. *Application deadline:* 3/31. *Application fee:* $25.

Degree Requirements 76 total credit hours, 43 in nursing.

Distance learning Courses provided through video, audio, computer-based media.

MASTER'S PROGRAM

Contact Judith Wuest, Director of Graduate Studies, Faculty of Nursing, University of New Brunswick, PO Box 4400, Fredericton, NB E0H 1TO, 506-453-4642. *Fax:* 506-447-3057.

Expenses *State resident tuition:* $1599 full-time, $1440 per academic year part-time. *Nonresident tuition:* $1599 full-time, $1440 per academic year part-time. *Full-time mandatory fees:* $37–$73. *Room and board:* $2920. *Books and supplies per academic year:* $365.

Financial Aid Graduate assistantships, fellowships. 27% of master's level students in nursing programs received some form of financial aid in 1995-96. *Application deadline:* 2/1.

BSN to Master's Program (MN)

Applying *Required:* GRE General Test, bachelor's degree in nursing, minimum GPA of 3., RN license, 2 years of clinical experience, statistics course, essay, 3 letters of recommendation, transcript of college record, undergraduate research/eligibility for registration in New Brunswick. *Application deadline:* 4/1. *Application fee:* $25.

Degree Requirements 21 total credit hours, 18 in nursing. Electives/statistics. Thesis required.

Distance learning Courses provided through video, audio, computer-based media. Specific degree requirements include travel to university library, as needed; 4 students per site.

NEWFOUNDLAND

MEMORIAL UNIVERSITY OF NEWFOUNDLAND
School of Nursing
St. John's, Newfoundland

Programs • Generic Baccalaureate • RN Baccalaureate • MN

The University Province-supported coed university. Founded: 1925. *Primary accreditation:* provincial charter. *Setting:* 220-acre urban campus. *Total enrollment:* 17,571.

The School of Nursing Founded in 1966. *Nursing program faculty:* 28 (21% with doctorates).

Academic Facilities *Campus library:* 3.8 million volumes (105,086 in health); 10,241 periodical subscriptions (1,656 health-care related). *Nursing school resources:* computer lab, nursing audiovisuals, learning resource lab.

Student Life *Student services:* health clinic, child-care facilities, personal counseling, career counseling, institutionally sponsored work-study program, job placement, campus safety program, special assistance for

Memorial University of Newfoundland (continued)

disabled students. *International student services:* counseling/support, special assistance for nonnative speakers of English, ESL courses. *Nursing student activities:* student nurses association.

Calendar Semesters.

NURSING STUDENT PROFILE
Undergraduate **Enrollment:** 311
Women: 90%; **Men:** 10%; **Minority:** 1%; **International:** 0%; **Part-time:** 35%
Graduate **Enrollment:** 35
Women: 100%; **Minority:** 0%; **International:** 0%; **Part-time:** 20%

BACCALAUREATE PROGRAMS

Contact June Ellis, Admissions Officer, School of Nursing, Memorial University of Newfoundland, St. John's, NF A1B 3V6, 709-737-6695. *Fax:* 709-737-7037. *E-mail:* junee@morgan.ucs.mun.ca

Expenses *State resident tuition:* $2529 full-time, $77 per credit hour part-time. *Nonresident tuition:* $5059 full-time, $153 per credit hour part-time. *Full-time mandatory fees:* $73. *Room and board:* $2847–$3005. *Room only:* $981–$1212. *Books and supplies per academic year:* ranges from $300 to $800.

Financial Aid Canada Student Loans.

Generic Baccalaureate Program (BN)

Applying *Required:* TOEFL for nonnative speakers of English, 3 years of high school math, high school chemistry, high school biology, high school transcript, 2 letters of recommendation, transcript of college record. *Options:* May apply for transfer of up to 64 total credits. *Application deadline:* 3/1. *Application fee:* $30.

Degree Requirements 129 total credit hours, 93 in nursing. 6 credit hours of English, 3 of biochemistry, 3 of microbiology, 3 of psychology, 3 of statistics, 12 of electives.

RN Baccalaureate Program (BN)

Applying *Required:* TOEFL for nonnative speakers of English, RN license, diploma or AD in nursing, transcript of college record. 12 prerequisite credits must be completed before admission to the nursing program. *Options:* Advanced standing available through advanced placement exams. May apply for transfer of up to 60 total credits. *Application deadline:* 3/1. *Application fee:* $30.

Degree Requirements 120 total credit hours, 87 in nursing. 6 credit hours of science plus electives to total 120 credit hours.

Distance learning Courses provided through correspondence. Specific degree requirements include approval of clinical placements and preceptors for clinical courses by school; preceptor for health assessment or attendance at a regional practice; in-province testing location.

MASTER'S PROGRAM

Contact Prof. Shirley Solberg, Associate Director, Graduate Program and Research, School of Nursing, Memorial University of Newfoundland, St. John's, NF A1B 3V6, 709-737-6679. *Fax:* 709-737-7037. *E-mail:* ssolberg@morgan.ucs.mun.ca

Expenses *State resident tuition:* ranges from $798 to $1205 per academic year. *Full-time mandatory fees:* $105.

Financial Aid Graduate assistantships, fellowships, employment opportunities. *Application deadline:* 12/31.

MN Program

Applying *Required:* TOEFL for nonnative speakers of English, bachelor's degree in nursing, minimum GPA of 3.0, RN license, 1 year of clinical experience, statistics course, 3 letters of recommendation, transcript of college record, research course, registration or eligibility for registration in Newfoundland. *Application deadline:* 12/31. *Application fee:* $30.

Degree Requirements Thesis required.

NOVA SCOTIA

DALHOUSIE UNIVERSITY
School of Nursing
Halifax, Nova Scotia

Programs • Generic Baccalaureate • RN Baccalaureate • MN • Master's for Nurses with Non-Nursing Degrees • MN/MHSA

The University Province-supported coed university. Founded: 1818. *Primary accreditation:* provincial charter. *Setting:* 67-acre urban campus. *Total enrollment:* 10,921.

The School of Nursing Founded in 1949. *Nursing program faculty:* 12 (92% with doctorates). *Off-campus program sites:* Saint John, Fredericton, Sydney.

Academic Facilities *Nursing school resources:* CAI, computer lab, nursing audiovisuals, interactive nursing skills videos, learning resource lab.

Student Life *Student services:* health clinic, personal counseling, career counseling, institutionally sponsored work-study program, job placement, campus safety program, special assistance for disabled students. *International student services:* counseling/support, special assistance for nonnative speakers of English. *Nursing student activities:* student nurses association.

Calendar Semesters.

NURSING STUDENT PROFILE
Undergraduate **Enrollment:** 495
Women: 93%; **Men:** 7%; **Minority:** 2%; **International:** 1%; **Part-time:** 32%
Graduate **Enrollment:** 97
Women: 99%; **Men:** 1%; **Minority:** 0%; **International:** 1%; **Part-time:** 71%

BACCALAUREATE PROGRAMS

Contact Barbara McLennan, Undergraduate Programs Secretary, Admissions, School of Nursing, Dalhousie University, Halifax, NS B3H 3J5, 800-500-0912. *Fax:* 902-494-3487. *E-mail:* barbara.mclennan@dal.ca

Expenses *Tuition:* ranges from $3088 to $5059 full-time, $307 per half-credit part-time. *Full-time mandatory fees:* $139. *Part-time mandatory fees:* $44+. *Room and board:* $3416–$3672. *Room only:* $1938–$2194. *Books and supplies per academic year:* $511.

Financial Aid Institutionally sponsored long-term loans, institutionally sponsored non-need grants/scholarships, Federal Nursing Student Loans, provincial student loans. 64% of undergraduate students in nursing programs received some form of financial aid in 1995–96.

Generic Baccalaureate Program (BScN)

Applying *Required:* SAT I for U.S. students, minimum college GPA of 2.5, high school chemistry, high school biology, high school transcript, transcript of college record, 70% average in Grade 12 math, chemistry, biology, and English. *Options:* Course work may be accelerated. May apply for transfer of up to 43 total credits. *Application deadline:* 6/1. *Application fee:* $35.

Degree Requirements 129 total credit hours, 87 in nursing. 33 required non-nursing credit hours, 9 credit hours of electives.

RN Baccalaureate Program (BScN)

Applying *Required:* minimum college GPA of 2.5, RN license, diploma or AD in nursing, high school transcript, transcript of college record, grade 12 math and chemistry. *Options:* May apply for transfer of up to 17 total credits. *Application deadlines:* 8/1 (fall), 11/15 (spring). *Application fee:* $35.

Degree Requirements 78 total credit hours, 36 in nursing. 33 required non-nursing credit hours, 9 credit hours of electives.

MASTER'S PROGRAMS

Contact Dr. Frances Gregor, Associate Director, Graduate Program, School of Nursing, Dalhousie University, Halifax, NS B3H 4H6, 902-494-2391.

Areas of Study Clinical nurse specialist programs in adult health nursing, community health nursing, maternity-newborn nursing, pediatric nursing, psychiatric–mental health nursing, public health nursing; nurse practitioner program in neonatal health.

Expenses *Tuition:* $3390 full-time, $1159 per year part-time. *Books and supplies per academic year:* ranges from $200 to $400.

Financial Aid Graduate assistantships. 22% of master's level students in nursing programs received some form of financial aid in 1995-96. *Application deadline:* 3/31.

MN Program

Master's for Nurses with Non-Nursing Degrees Program

Applying *Required:* GRE General Test, TOEFL for nonnative speakers of English, bachelor's degree, minimum GPA of 3.0, RN license, 1 year of clinical experience, statistics course, professional liability/malpractice insurance, interview, 3 letters of recommendation, transcript of college record. *Application deadline:* 3/31. *Application fee:* $55.

Degree Requirements 48 total credit hours, 39 in nursing, 3 in statistics.

Distance learning Courses provided through audio, on-line.

MN/MHSA Program

Applying *Required:* GRE General Test, TOEFL for nonnative speakers of English, bachelor's degree in nursing, minimum GPA of 3.0, RN license, 1 year of clinical experience, statistics course, interview, letter of recommendation, transcript of college record. *Application deadline:* 3/31. *Application fee:* $55.

Degree Requirements 87 total credit hours, 42 in nursing, 45 in health services administration. Thesis required.

See full description on page 436.

ST. FRANCIS XAVIER UNIVERSITY
Department of Nursing
Antigonish, Nova Scotia

Programs • Generic Baccalaureate • RN Baccalaureate • Continuing Education

The University Independent Roman Catholic comprehensive coed institution. Founded: 1853. *Primary accreditation:* provincial charter. *Setting:* 60-acre small-town campus. *Total enrollment:* 3,785.

The Department of Nursing Founded in 1927. *Nursing program faculty:* 11 (30% with doctorates). *Off-campus program site:* Halifax.

Academic Facilities *Campus library:* 500,000 volumes (3,800 in nursing); 1,494 periodical subscriptions (1,015 health-care related). *Nursing school resources:* CAI, computer lab, nursing audiovisuals, interactive nursing skills videos, learning resource lab.

Student Life *Student services:* health clinic, child-care facilities, personal counseling, career counseling, campus safety program, special assistance for disabled students. *International student services:* counseling/support, special assistance for nonnative speakers of English. *Nursing student activities:* nursing club, student nurses association.

Calendar Semesters.

NURSING STUDENT PROFILE

Undergraduate **Enrollment:** 440

Women: 96%; **Men:** 4%; **Minority:** 3%; **International:** 1%; **Part-time:** 71%

BACCALAUREATE PROGRAMS

Contact Dr. Angela J. Gillis, Chair and Professor, Department of Nursing, St. Francis Xavier University, PO Box 5000, Antigonish, NS B2G 2W5, 902-867-3955. *Fax:* 902-867-2448. *E-mail:* agillis@stfx.ca

Expenses *State resident tuition:* $4636 full-time, $675 per 6-credit course part-time. *Nonresident tuition:* $5877 full-time, $1733 per 6-credit course part-time. *Full-time mandatory fees:* $128. *Books and supplies per academic year:* ranges from $75 to $400.

Financial Aid Institutionally sponsored need-based grants/scholarships, institutionally sponsored non-need grants/scholarships, Federal Nursing Student Loans. *Application deadline:* 1/30.

Generic Baccalaureate Program (BScN)

Applying *Required:* 3 years of high school math, 3 years of high school science, high school chemistry, high school biology, high school transcript. 15 prerequisite credits must be completed before admission to the nursing program. *Options:* May apply for transfer of up to 10 total credits. *Application deadline:* 8/1. *Application fee:* $100.

Degree Requirements 132 total credit hours, 57 in nursing. April-June intersession required during second and third year of program.

Distance learning Courses provided through correspondence. Specific degree requirements include attendance at on-campus orientation (encouraged).

RN Baccalaureate Program (BScN)

Applying *Required:* 3 years of high school math, 3 years of high school science, high school chemistry, high school biology, RN license, diploma or AD in nursing, high school transcript, interview, 3 letters of recommendation, transcript of college record. 15 prerequisite credits must be completed before admission to the nursing program. *Options:* May apply for transfer of up to 10 total credits. *Application deadlines:* 8/30 (fall), 1/30 (spring). *Application fee:* $100.

Degree Requirements 96 total credit hours, 42 in nursing.

Distance learning Courses provided through correspondence. Specific degree requirements include attendance at on-campus orientation (encouraged).

CONTINUING EDUCATION PROGRAM

Contact Dr. Angus Braid, Director, Continuing Education, Department of Nursing, St. Francis Xavier University, PO Box 5000, Antigonish, NS B2G 2W5, 902-867-5190.

ONTARIO

LAKEHEAD UNIVERSITY
School of Nursing
Thunder Bay, Ontario

Program • Generic Baccalaureate

The University Province-supported comprehensive coed institution. Founded: 1965. *Primary accreditation:* provincial charter. *Setting:* 345-acre suburban campus. *Total enrollment:* 7,918.

The School of Nursing Founded in 1965.

Calendar Semesters.

BACCALAUREATE PROGRAM

Contact Director, School of Nursing, Lakehead University, 955 Oliver Road, Thunder Bay, ON P7B 5E1, 807-343-8395. *Fax:* 807-343-8246.

Expenses *State resident tuition:* ranges from $1181 to $1789 per academic year. *Nonresident tuition:* ranges from $6747 to $11,000 per academic year.

Generic Baccalaureate Program (BScN)

Applying *Required:* basic cardiac life support certificate, advanced level mathematics, English.

LAURENTIAN UNIVERSITY
School of Nursing
Sudbury, Ontario

Programs • Generic Baccalaureate • RN Baccalaureate

Laurentian University (continued)

The University Province-supported comprehensive coed institution. Founded: 1960. *Primary accreditation:* provincial charter. *Setting:* 700-acre suburban campus. *Total enrollment:* 7,867.

The School of Nursing Founded in 1967. *Nursing program faculty:* 22 (1% with doctorates).

Academic Facilities *Nursing school resources:* nursing audiovisuals, learning resource lab.

Student Life *Student services:* health clinic, child-care facilities, personal counseling, career counseling, campus safety program, special assistance for disabled students. *Nursing student activities:* student nurses association.

Calendar Semesters.

NURSING STUDENT PROFILE

Undergraduate **Enrollment:** 60
Women: 98%; **Men:** 2%; **Minority:** 5%; **Part-time:** 35%

BACCALAUREATE PROGRAMS

Contact Ms. Sandy Bullock, Clinical and Administrative Supervisor, School of Nursing, Laurentian University, Sudbury, ON P3E 2C6, 705-673-6589. *Fax:* 705-675-4861.

Expenses *State resident tuition:* $2767 full-time, $1384 per course part-time. *Full-time mandatory fees:* $316. *Room and board:* $2440–$2880. *Books and supplies per academic year:* ranges from $600 to $800.

Generic Baccalaureate Program (BScN)

Applying *Required:* senior-level chemistry, biology, English/French. *Application deadline:* rolling.

RN Baccalaureate Program (BScN)

Applying *Required:* RN license, senior-level chemistry, biology, English/French. *Options:* Advanced standing available through credit by exam. *Application deadline:* rolling.

Distance learning Courses provided through correspondence, video, audio.

MCMASTER UNIVERSITY
School of Nursing
Hamilton, Ontario

Programs • Generic Baccalaureate • RN Baccalaureate

The University Province-supported coed university. Founded: 1887. *Primary accreditation:* provincial charter. *Setting:* 300-acre urban campus. *Total enrollment:* 17,527.

The School of Nursing Founded in 1946.

BACCALAUREATE PROGRAMS

Contact Ms. V. Lewis, Admissions Coordinator, Nursing, Health Sciences Center 2E10, School of Nursing, McMaster University, 1200 Main Street West, Hamilton, ON L8N 3Z5.

Expenses *State resident tuition:* $2511 full-time, $81 per unit part-time. *Nonresident tuition:* $12,338 full-time, $409 per unit part-time.

Generic Baccalaureate Program (BScN)

Applying *Required:* high school chemistry, immunizations, high school English, mathematics, and either biology or physics. *Application fee:* $50.

RN Baccalaureate Program (BScN)

Applying *Required:* immunizations, College of Nurses of Ontario registration card. *Application deadline:* 2/15. *Application fee:* $50.

QUEEN'S UNIVERSITY AT KINGSTON
School of Nursing
Kingston, Ontario

Programs • Generic Baccalaureate • Master's

The University Province-supported coed university. Founded: 1841. *Primary accreditation:* provincial charter. *Setting:* 160-acre urban campus. *Total enrollment:* 16,662.

The School of Nursing Founded in 1942.

Academic Facilities *Campus library:* 3.5 million volumes (148,172 in health, 3,900 in nursing); 13,600 periodical subscriptions (1,014 health-care related).

Calendar Semesters.

BACCALAUREATE PROGRAM

Contact Admissions Department, Victoria School, Room 202, School of Nursing, Queen's University at Kingston, Kingston, ON K7L 3N6, 613-545-2218. *Fax:* 613-545-6810.

Expenses *State resident tuition:* $2143 per academic year. *Nonresident tuition:* $10,513 per academic year. *Full-time mandatory fees:* $367. *Room and board:* $4036–$4184. *Room only:* $2208. *Books and supplies per academic year:* $1543.

Generic Baccalaureate Program (BNSc)

Applying *Application deadline:* 3/1.

MASTER'S PROGRAM

Contact Coordinator, Cataraqui Building, School of Nursing, Queen's University at Kingston, 90 Barrie Street, Kingston, ON K7L 3N6, 613-545-2668. *Fax:* 613-545-6770.

RYERSON POLYTECHNIC UNIVERSITY
School of Nursing
Toronto, Ontario

Programs • Generic Baccalaureate • RN Baccalaureate

The University Province-supported 4-year coed college. Founded: 1948. *Primary accreditation:* provincial charter. *Setting:* 20-acre urban campus. *Total enrollment:* 14,241.

The School of Nursing Founded in 1973.

BACCALAUREATE PROGRAMS

Contact Ms. Nancy Pemberthy, Admissions Officer, School of Nursing, Ryerson Polytechnic University, Toronto, ON M5B 2K3, 416-979-5000 Ext. 6001. *Fax:* 416-979-5341.

Expenses *State resident tuition:* $2457 full-time, $231 per course part-time. *Nonresident tuition:* $8030 full-time, $816 per course part-time.

Generic Baccalaureate Program (BAA)

Applying *Required:* high school chemistry, high school transcript, English, eitherbiology or physics, mathematics, basic cardiac life support certification. *Application deadline:* 3/15. *Application fee:* $30.

RN Baccalaureate Program (BAA)

Applying *Required:* RN license, diploma or AD in nursing, letter of recommendation, transcript of college record, psychology, sociology, 2 years of full-time nursing experience. *Application deadline:* 2/1. *Application fee:* $30.

UNIVERSITY OF OTTAWA
School of Nursing
Ottawa, Ontario

Programs • Generic Baccalaureate • RN Baccalaureate • MScN

The University Province-supported coed university. Founded: 1848. *Primary accreditation:* provincial charter. *Setting:* 70-acre urban campus. *Total enrollment:* 23,894.

The School of Nursing *Nursing program faculty:* 77 (6% with doctorates).

Academic Facilities *Nursing school resources:* CAI, computer lab, nursing audiovisuals, interactive nursing skills videos, learning resource lab.

Student Life *Student services:* health clinic, child-care facilities, personal counseling, career counseling, campus safety program, special assistance for disabled students. *Nursing student activities:* student nurses association.

Calendar Semesters.

NURSING STUDENT PROFILE

Undergraduate **Enrollment:** 1017
Women: 85%; **Men:** 15%; **Part-time:** 40%
Graduate **Enrollment:** 42
Women: 100%; **Part-time:** 60%

BACCALAUREATE PROGRAMS

Contact Ms. Yolande Chenier, Academic Administrator, Faculty of Health Sciences, Room 2044, School of Nursing, University of Ottawa, 451 Smyth Road, Ottawa, ON K1H 8M5, 613-562-5800 Ext. 8062. *Fax:* 613-562-5470.

Expenses *State resident tuition:* $2237 full-time, $75 per credit part-time. *Nonresident tuition:* $5313 per academic year. *Full-time mandatory fees:* $248.

Generic Baccalaureate Program (BScN)

Applying *Required:* high school chemistry, high school biology, high school transcript. *Application deadline:* 4/1.

Degree Requirements 139 total credit hours.

RN Baccalaureate Program (BScN)

Applying *Required:* RN license, diploma or AD in nursing, 2 letters of recommendation, transcript of college record. *Options:* Course work may be accelerated. May apply for transfer of up to 42 total credits. *Application deadline:* 5/1.

Degree Requirements 72 total credit hours, 39 in nursing.

Distance learning Courses provided through audio teleconference.

MASTER'S PROGRAM

Contact Ms. Yolande Chenier, Academic Administrator, Faculty of Health Sciences, Room 2044, School of Nursing, University of Ottawa, 451 Smyth Road, Ottawa, ON K1H 8M5, 613-562-5800 Ext. 8062. *Fax:* 613-562-5470.

Areas of Study Clinical nurse specialist program in primary and tertiary care; nurse practitioner program in primary health.

Expenses *State resident tuition:* $2983 full-time, $373 per course part-time. *Nonresident tuition:* $5406 full-time, $373 part-time. *Full-time mandatory fees:* $145.

Financial Aid Graduate assistantships, Ontario graduate scholarships.

MScN Program

Applying *Required:* bachelor's degree in nursing, bachelor's degree, minimum GPA of 3.0, RN license, 2 years of clinical experience, physical assessment course, statistics course, essay, 2 letters of recommendation, transcript of college record. *Application deadline:* 4/1.

Degree Requirements 24 total credit hours, 18 in nursing, 6 in statistics, electives. Thesis required.

Distance learning Courses provided through video.

UNIVERSITY OF TORONTO
Faculty of Nursing
Toronto, Ontario

Programs • Generic Baccalaureate • RN Baccalaureate • Master's • Doctoral

The University Province-supported coed university. Founded: 1827. *Primary accreditation:* provincial charter. *Setting:* 900-acre urban campus. *Total enrollment:* 54,000.

The Faculty of Nursing Founded in 1942.

BACCALAUREATE PROGRAMS

Contact Office of Admissions, Faculty of Nursing, University of Toronto, 50 St. George Street, Toronto, ON M5S 1A1, 416-978-2863.

Expenses *State resident tuition:* $2547 per academic year. *Nonresident tuition:* $8829 per academic year.

Generic Baccalaureate Program (BScN)

Applying *Application deadline:* 3/1.

RN Baccalaureate Program (BSN)

Applying *Application deadline:* 3/1.

MASTER'S PROGRAMS

Contact Graduate Department, Faculty of Nursing, University of Toronto, 50 St. George Street, Toronto, ON M5S 1A1, 416-978-8069.

DOCTORAL PROGRAM

Contact Graduate Department, Faculty of Nursing, University of Toronto, 50 St. George Street, Toronto, ON M5S 1A1, 416-978-8069.

THE UNIVERSITY OF WESTERN ONTARIO
Faculty of Nursing
London, Ontario

Programs • Generic Baccalaureate • RN Baccalaureate • MScN • RN to Master's

The University Province-supported coed university. Founded: 1878. *Primary accreditation:* provincial charter. *Setting:* 402-acre suburban campus. *Total enrollment:* 27,722.

The Faculty of Nursing Founded in 1920. *Nursing program faculty:* 56 (31% with doctorates).

Academic Facilities *Campus library:* 2.1 million volumes (357,263 in health); 12,858 periodical subscriptions (124 health-care related). *Nursing school resources:* CAI, computer lab, nursing audiovisuals, interactive nursing skills videos, learning resource lab.

Student Life *Student services:* health clinic, child-care facilities, personal counseling, career counseling, institutionally sponsored work-study program, job placement, campus safety program, special assistance for disabled students, ombudsperson. *International student services:* counseling/support, special assistance for nonnative speakers of English, ESL courses. *Nursing student activities:* Sigma Theta Tau, student nurses association.

Calendar Semesters.

NURSING STUDENT PROFILE

Undergraduate **Enrollment:** 341
Women: 93%; **Men:** 7%; **International:** 0%; **Part-time:** 20%
Graduate **Enrollment:** 55
Women: 99%; **Men:** 1%; **Minority:** 0%; **International:** 0%; **Part-time:** 47%

BACCALAUREATE PROGRAMS

Contact Ms. Elsie MacMaster, Coordinator, Undergraduate Program, Faculty of Nursing, University of Western Ontario, London, ON N6A 5C1, 519-661-3398. *Fax:* 519-661-3928. *E-mail:* emacmast@nursing.uwo.ca

Expenses *State resident tuition:* $3597 full-time, $701 per course part-time. *Full-time mandatory fees:* $600–$700. *Part-time mandatory fees:* $110–$350. *Room and board:* $4000–$7000. *Books and supplies per academic year:* ranges from $1000 to $1500.

Financial Aid Institutionally sponsored need-based grants/scholarships, institutionally sponsored non-need grants/scholarships, small bursaries,

The University of Western Ontario (continued)

awards for nursing students. 75% of undergraduate students in nursing programs received some form of financial aid in 1995–96. *Application deadline:* 10/15.

Generic Baccalaureate Program (BScN)

Applying *Required:* TOEFL for nonnative speakers of English, minimum high school GPA of 3.2, minimum college GPA of 2.3, high school chemistry, high school biology, high school transcript, transcript of college record, specific level high school math. *Options:* May apply for transfer of up to 10 total credits. *Application deadline:* 2/15. *Application fee:* $125.

Degree Requirements 81 total credit hours.

RN Baccalaureate Program (BScN)

Applying *Required:* TOEFL for nonnative speakers of English, minimum college GPA of 2.3, RN license, diploma or AD in nursing, high school transcript, transcript of college record. *Application deadline:* 2/15. *Application fee:* $125.

Degree Requirements 60 total credit hours.

MASTER'S PROGRAMS

Contact Dr. Carroll L. Iwasiw, Associate Professor and Coordinator, Graduate Program, Faculty of Nursing, University of Western Ontario, London, ON N6A 5C1, 519-661-3398. *Fax:* 519-661-3928.

Areas of Study Nursing administration; nursing education.

Expenses *State resident tuition:* $4400 full-time, $2400 per year part-time. *Full-time mandatory fees:* $237–$669. *Books and supplies per academic year:* ranges from $400 to $1000.

Financial Aid Graduate assistantships, Federal Nursing Student Loans, institutionally sponsored loans, institutionally sponsored need-based grants/scholarships, institutionally sponsored non-need-based grants/scholarships. *Application deadline:* 4/30.

MScN Program

Applying *Required:* TOEFL for nonnative speakers of English, bachelor's degree in nursing, minimum GPA of 3.0, RN license, 1 year of clinical experience, statistics course, essay, interview, 3 letters of recommendation, transcript of college record. *Application deadlines:* 2/1 (fall), 11/15 (spring). *Application fee:* $50.

Degree Requirements 54 total credit hours, 50 in nursing. Thesis or research project.

RN to Master's Program (MScN)

Applying *Required:* TOEFL for nonnative speakers of English, bachelor's degree in nursing, RN license, 1 year of clinical experience, statistics course, interview, letter of recommendation, transcript of college record. *Application deadlines:* 2/1 (fall), 11/15 (spring). *Application fee:* $50.

Degree Requirements 54 total credit hours, 50 in nursing. Research thesis or research project.

UNIVERSITY OF WINDSOR

School of Nursing
Windsor, Ontario

Programs • Generic Baccalaureate • RN Baccalaureate • MSc

The University Province-supported coed university. Founded: 1857. *Primary accreditation:* provincial charter. *Setting:* 125-acre urban campus. *Total enrollment:* 16,600.

The School of Nursing Founded in 1952. *Nursing program faculty:* 37.

Academic Facilities *Nursing school resources:* CAI, computer lab, nursing audiovisuals, interactive nursing skills videos, learning resource lab.

Student Life *Student services:* health clinic, personal counseling, career counseling, institutionally sponsored work-study program, job placement, campus safety program, special assistance for disabled students, academic writing center. *International student services:* counseling/support. *Nursing student activities:* student nurses association, Canadian Nursing Students Association.

Calendar Semesters.

NURSING STUDENT PROFILE

Undergraduate **Enrollment:** 500
Women: 90%; **Men:** 10%; **Minority:** 13%; **Part-time:** 25%

Graduate **Enrollment:** 21
Women: 95%; **Men:** 5%; **Minority:** 0%; **International:** 5%; **Part-time:** 100%

BACCALAUREATE PROGRAMS

Contact Ms. Sharon Klinck, Program and Clinical Coordinator, School of Nursing, University of Windsor, 401 Sunset Avenue, Windsor, ON N9B 3P4, 519-253-4232 Ext. 2266. *Fax:* 519-973-7084. *E-mail:* sklinck@uwindsor.ca

Expenses *State resident tuition:* $3303 full-time, $294 per course part-time. *Full-time mandatory fees:* $124. *Room and board:* $3412. *Room only:* $2712–$4361. *Books and supplies per academic year:* ranges from $500 to $600.

Financial Aid Institutionally sponsored need-based grants/scholarships, institutionally sponsored non-need grants/scholarships, Ontario Student Assistance Program. *Application deadline:* 6/15.

Generic Baccalaureate Program (BScN)

Applying *Required:* TOEFL for nonnative speakers of English, minimum high school GPA, high school chemistry, high school biology, high school transcript. *Application deadline:* 5/1. *Application fee:* $75.

RN Baccalaureate Program (BScN)

Applying *Required:* TOEFL for nonnative speakers of English, minimum college GPA, RN license, diploma or AD in nursing, high school transcript, interview, letter of recommendation, transcript of college record, written essay for primary-care nurse practitioner track. *Options:* Advanced standing available through credit by exam. *Application deadlines:* 2/1 (primary care nurse practitioner track), rolling. *Application fee:* $75.

MASTER'S PROGRAM

Contact Dr. Janet Rosenbaum, Graduate Coordinator, School of Nursing, University of Windsor, 401 Sunset Avenue, Windsor, ON N9B 3P4, 519-253-4232 Ext. 2259. *Fax:* 519-973-7084. *E-mail:* rosenb4@uwindsor.ca

Expenses *State resident tuition:* $350 per course. *Books and supplies per academic year:* ranges from $300 to $500.

Financial Aid Graduate assistantships, institutionally sponsored need-based grants/scholarships, institutionally sponsored non-need-based grants/scholarships. *Application deadline:* 2/1.

MSc Program

Applying *Required:* bachelor's degree in nursing, RN license, physical assessment course, statistics course, essay, interview, 3 letters of recommendation, transcript of college record. *Application deadline:* 2/1. *Application fee:* $75.

Degree Requirements Thesis or project.

YORK UNIVERSITY

Atkinson College Department of Nursing
North York, Ontario

Programs • RN Baccalaureate • Continuing Education

The University Province-supported coed university. Founded: 1959. *Primary accreditation:* provincial charter. *Setting:* 650-acre urban campus. *Total enrollment:* 39,692.

The Atkinson College Department of Nursing Founded in 1993. *Nursing program faculty:* 10 (80% with doctorates). *Off-campus program sites:* Toronto, Brampton, Barrie.

Academic Facilities *Nursing school resources:* CAI, computer lab.

Student Life *Student services:* health clinic, child-care facilities, personal counseling, career counseling, institutionally sponsored work-study program, campus safety program, special assistance for disabled students.

International student services: counseling/support, special assistance for nonnative speakers of English, ESL courses. *Nursing student activities:* student nurses association.

Calendar Trimesters.

NURSING STUDENT PROFILE

Undergraduate **Enrollment:** 300
Women: 99%; **Men:** 1%; **Minority:** 40%; **Part-time:** 90%

BACCALAUREATE PROGRAM

Contact Office of Admissions, Department of Nursing, York University, Atkinson College Room 410, 4700 Keele Street, North York, ON M3J 1P3, 416-736-5000. *Fax:* 416-736-5420.

Expenses *State resident tuition:* $5048 full-time, $84 per credit part-time. *Nonresident tuition:* $15,709 full-time, $262 per credit part-time. *Books and supplies per academic year:* ranges from $146 to $292.

Financial Aid Institutionally sponsored need-based grants/scholarships, institutionally sponsored non-need grants/scholarships, Federal Work-Study, Canadian government loans, professional nursing organization scholarships and grants. 30% of undergraduate students in nursing programs received some form of financial aid in 1995–96.

RN Baccalaureate Program (BScN)

Applying *Required:* TOEFL for nonnative speakers of English, minimum college GPA of 3.0, 4 years of high school math, 4 years of high school science, high school chemistry, high school biology, RN license, diploma or AD in nursing, high school transcript, 2 letters of recommendation, written essay, transcript of college record, 2 years experience within last 5 years in primary care delivery setting for nurse practitioner option. *Options:* Course work may be accelerated. May apply for transfer of up to 10 total credits. *Application deadline:* rolling. *Application fee:* $50–75.

Degree Requirements 120–121 total credit hours dependent upon track, 48–54 in nursing. 6 credits of math (stats), 6 of philosophy, 3 of economics; extensive practicum experiences for nurse practitioner option.

Distance learning Courses provided through correspondence, video, audio, computer-based media, on-line.

CONTINUING EDUCATION PROGRAM

Contact Office of Admissions, Department of Nursing, York University, Atkinson College Room 410, 4700 Keele Street, North York, ON M3J 1P3, 416-736-5000. *Fax:* 416-736-5420.

PRINCE EDWARD ISLAND

UNIVERSITY OF PRINCE EDWARD ISLAND
School of Nursing
Charlottetown, Prince Edward Island

Program • Generic Baccalaureate

The University Province-supported comprehensive coed institution. Founded: 1834. *Primary accreditation:* provincial charter. *Setting:* 130-acre small-town campus. *Total enrollment:* 2,925.

Calendar Semesters.

Financial Aid Institutionally sponsored non-need grants/scholarships.

QUEBEC

MCGILL UNIVERSITY
School of Nursing
Montreal, Quebec

Programs • Generic Baccalaureate • RN Baccalaureate • Baccalaureate for Second Degree • MSc • Master's for Non-Nursing College Graduates • PhD

The University Province-supported coed university. Founded: 1821. *Primary accreditation:* provincial charter. *Setting:* 80-acre urban campus. *Total enrollment:* 31,592.

The School of Nursing Founded in 1920. *Nursing program faculty:* 19 (37% with doctorates).

Academic Facilities *Nursing school resources:* computer lab, nursing audio-visuals, learning resource lab.

Student Life *Student services:* health clinic, child-care facilities, personal counseling, career counseling, institutionally sponsored work-study program, job placement, campus safety program, special assistance for disabled students. *International student services:* counseling/support, special assistance for nonnative speakers of English, ESL courses. *Nursing student activities:* student nurses association.

Calendar Semesters.

NURSING STUDENT PROFILE

Undergraduate **Enrollment:** 105
Women: 96%; **Men:** 4%; **International:** 2%; **Part-time:** 22%
Graduate **Enrollment:** 50
Women: 96%; **Men:** 4%; **International:** 2%; **Part-time:** 24%

BACCALAUREATE PROGRAMS

Contact Ms. Anna Santandréa, Student Affairs Coordinator, School of Nursing, McGill University, 3506 University Street, Montreal, PQ H3A 2A7, 514-398-4151. *Fax:* 514-398-8455. *E-mail:* asantand@wilson.lan.mcgill.ca

Expenses *State resident tuition:* $1218 full-time, $41 per credit part-time. *Nonresident tuition:* $5445 full-time, $181 per credit part-time. *Full-time mandatory fees:* $1095–$1460.

Generic Baccalaureate Program (BScN)

Applying *Required:* TOEFL for nonnative speakers of English, Admissions Testing Program, minimum high school GPA of 3.0, 3 years of high school math, high school chemistry, high school biology, high school transcript, 2 letters of recommendation, transcript of college record. 34 prerequisite credits must be completed before admission to the nursing program. *Application deadlines:* 1/15 (spring), 3/1 (Canadian applicants). *Application fee:* $60.

Degree Requirements 108 total credit hours, 108 in nursing.

RN Baccalaureate Program (BScN)

Applying *Required:* TOEFL for nonnative speakers of English, RN license, diploma or AD in nursing, high school transcript, letter of recommendation, transcript of college record. 30 prerequisite credits must be completed before admission to the nursing program. *Options:* May apply for transfer of up to 30 total credits. *Application deadlines:* 1/15 (spring), 3/1 (Canadian applicants). *Application fee:* $60.

Degree Requirements 104 total credit hours, 104 in nursing.

Baccalaureate for Second Degree Program (BScN)

Applying *Required:* TOEFL for nonnative speakers of English, minimum college GPA of 3.0, high school transcript, letter of recommendation, transcript of college record. 34 prerequisite credits must be completed before admission to the nursing program. *Options:* May apply for transfer of up to 30 total credits. *Application deadlines:* 1/15 (spring), 3/1 (Canadian applicants). *Application fee:* $60.

Degree Requirements 108 total credit hours, 108 in nursing.

McGill University (continued)

MASTER'S PROGRAMS

Contact Ms. Anna Santandréa, Student Affairs Coordinator, School of Nursing, McGill University, 3506 University Street, Montreal, PQ H3A 2A7, 514-398-4151. *Fax:* 514-398-8455. *E-mail:* asantand@wilson.lan.mcgill.ca

Expenses *State resident tuition:* $1218 full-time, $41 per credit part-time. *Nonresident tuition:* $5445 full-time, $181 per credit part-time. *Full-time mandatory fees:* $1827.

Financial Aid Fellowships, institutionally sponsored need-based grants/scholarships. 20% of master's level students in nursing programs received some form of financial aid in 1995-96. *Application deadline:* 2/1.

MSc Program

Applying *Required:* GRE General Test, TOEFL for nonnative speakers of English, bachelor's degree in nursing, minimum GPA of 3.0, RN license, 1 year of clinical experience, statistics course, essay, interview, 3 letters of recommendation, transcript of college record. *Application deadline:* 3/1. *Application fee:* $60.

Degree Requirements Thesis required.

Master's for Non-Nursing College Graduates Program (MSc)

Applying *Required:* GRE General Test, TOEFL for nonnative speakers of English, bachelor's degree, minimum GPA of 3.0, 1 year of clinical experience, statistics course, essay, interview, 2 letters of recommendation, transcript of college record, 30 credits of biological and behavioral sciences. *Application deadline:* 3/1. *Application fee:* $60.

Degree Requirements Thesis required.

DOCTORAL PROGRAM

Contact Ms. Anna Santandréa, Graduate Secretary, School of Nursing, McGill University, 3506 University Street, Montreal, PQ H3A 2A7, 514-398-4151. *Fax:* 514-398-8455. *E-mail:* asantand@wilson.lan.mcgill.ca

Expenses *State resident tuition:* $3654 per academic year.

Financial Aid Fellowships. *Application deadline:* 2/1.

PhD Program

Applying *Required:* TOEFL for nonnative speakers of English, master's degree in nursing, interview, 2 letters of recommendation, vitae, competitive review by faculty committee, acceptance by faculty adviser, knowledge of French and English, demonstrated research ability, statement of goals, statement of proposed research. *Application deadline:* 2/1. *Application fee:* $60.

Degree Requirements dissertation; oral exam; written exam; defense of dissertation.

UNIVERSITÉ DE MONTRÉAL
Faculté des Sciences Infirmières
Montréal, Quebec

Programs • Generic Baccalaureate • RN Baccalaureate • MSc • PhD • Continuing Education

The Institution Province-supported coed university. Founded: 1920. *Primary accreditation:* provincial charter. *Setting:* 150-acre urban campus. *Total enrollment:* 35,438.

The Faculté des Sciences Infirmières Founded in 1962. *Nursing program faculty:* 28 (80% with doctorates).

Academic Facilities *Campus library:* 2.4 million volumes (109,551 in health, 13,500 in nursing); 15,006 periodical subscriptions (2,997 health-care related). *Nursing school resources:* CAI, computer lab, nursing audiovisuals, learning resource lab.

Student Life *Student services:* health clinic, child-care facilities, personal counseling. *International student services:* counseling/support, ESL courses, special assistance for nonnative speakers of French. *Nursing student activities:* nursing club, student nurses association.

Calendar Trimesters.

NURSING STUDENT PROFILE

Undergraduate **Enrollment:** 1000
Women: 82%; **Men:** 18%; **Minority:** 30%; **International:** 5%; **Part-time:** 40%
Graduate **Enrollment:** 121
Women: 85%; **Men:** 15%; **Minority:** 10%; **International:** 5%; **Part-time:** 40%

BACCALAUREATE PROGRAMS

Contact Danielle Fleury, Assistant to the Vice-Dean, Faculté des Sciences Infirmières, Université de Montréal, CP 6128, Succursale Centre-Ville, Montréal, PQ H3C 3J7, 514-343-6436. *E-mail:* fleuryd@ere.umontreal.ca

Expenses *State resident tuition:* $1460 full-time, $46 per credit part-time. *Books and supplies per academic year:* ranges from $219 to $365.

Financial Aid Federal Direct Loans. *Application deadline:* 6/1.

Generic Baccalaureate Program (BScN)

Applying *Required:* minimum college GPA, transcript of college record, Degree in health sciences. *Options:* May apply for transfer of up to 45 total credits. *Application deadline:* 3/1. *Application fee:* $40.

Degree Requirements 102 total credit hours.

RN Baccalaureate Program (BScN)

Applying *Required:* RN license, diploma or AD in nursing, transcript of college record. *Options:* May apply for transfer of up to 45 total credits. *Application deadlines:* 3/1 (fall), 11/1 (spring). *Application fee:* $40.

Degree Requirements 90 total credit hours.

MASTER'S PROGRAM

Contact Ms. Suzanne Kérouac, Dean, Faculté des Sciences Infirmières, Université de Montréal, CP6128, Succursale Centre-Ville, Montréal, PQ H3C 3J7, 514-343-6436. *Fax:* 514-343-2306. *E-mail:* kerouacs@ere.umontreal.ca

Areas of Study Clinical nurse specialist programs in adult health nursing, community health nursing, family health nursing, gerontological nursing, maternity-newborn nursing, oncology nursing, pediatric nursing, perinatal nursing, psychiatric–mental health nursing, rehabilitation nursing, women's health nursing.

Expenses *State resident tuition:* $1971 full-time, $986 per academic year part-time. *Nonresident tuition:* $6570 per academic year. *Books and supplies per academic year:* $365.

Financial Aid Graduate assistantships, fellowships, institutionally sponsored loans. 10% of master's level students in nursing programs received some form of financial aid in 1995-96.

MSc Program

Applying *Required:* bachelor's degree in nursing, RN license, statistics course, proficiency in French. *Application deadline:* 2/1. *Application fee:* $40.

DOCTORAL PROGRAM

Contact Ms. Suzanne Kérouac, Dean, Faculté des Sciences Infirmières, Université de Montreal, CP6128, Succursale Centre-Ville, Montréal, PQ H3C 3J7, 514-343-6436. *Fax:* 514-343-2306. *E-mail:* kerouacs@ere.umontreal.ca

Areas of Study Nursing research.

Expenses *State resident tuition:* $1971 full-time, $986 per academic year part-time. *Nonresident tuition:* $6570 per academic year.

Financial Aid Graduate assistantships, nurse traineeships, fellowships, institutionally sponsored loans, opportunities for employment.

PhD Program

Applying *Required:* interview, 2 letters of recommendation, competitive review by faculty committee. *Application deadline:* 2/1. *Application fee:* $40.

Degree Requirements 90 total credit hours; dissertation; oral exam; written exam; defense of dissertation; residency.

CONTINUING EDUCATION PROGRAM

Contact Ms. Suzanne Kérouac, Dean, Faculté des Sciences Infirmières, Université de Montréal, CP 6128, Succursale Centre-Ville, Montréal, PQ H3C 3J7, 514-343-6436. *E-mail:* kerouacs@ere.umontreal.ca

UNIVERSITÉ DE SHERBROOKE

Département Sciences Infirmières
Sherbrooke, Quebec

Program • RN Baccalaureate

The Institution Independent coed university. Founded: 1954. *Primary accreditation:* provincial charter. *Setting:* 800-acre urban campus. *Total enrollment:* 21,124.

The Département Sciences Infirmières Founded in 1978.

Calendar Trimesters.

BACCALAUREATE PROGRAM

Contact Director, Faculté de Médecine, Département des Sciences Infirmières, Université de Sherbrooke, Sherbrooke, PQ J1H 5N4, 819-564-5354. *Fax:* 819-564-5378.

Expenses *State resident tuition:* $1827 full-time, $41 per credit part-time. *Nonresident tuition:* $8167 per academic year. *Full-time mandatory fees:* $57–$301.

RN Baccalaureate Program (BSN)

Applying *Required:* membership in l'Ordre des infirmières et infirmiers du Québec.

UNIVERSITÉ DU QUÉBEC À HULL

Module des Sciences de la Santé
Hull, Quebec

Program • Generic Baccalaureate

The Institution Province-supported comprehensive coed institution. Part of Université du Québec. Founded: 1981. *Primary accreditation:* provincial charter. *Total enrollment:* 5,438.

The Module des Sciences de la Santé Founded in 1978.

Academic Facilities *Campus library:* 165,411 volumes; 2,057 periodical subscriptions.

Calendar 4-1-4.

BACCALAUREATE PROGRAM

Contact Director, Module des Sciences de la Santé, Université du Québec à Hull, CP 1250, Succursale B, Hull, PQ J8X 3X7, 819-595-2345. *Fax:* 819-595-2212.

UNIVERSITÉ DU QUÉBEC À RIMOUSKI

Module des Sciences de la Santé
Rimouski, Quebec

Program • Generic Baccalaureate

The Institution Province-supported comprehensive coed institution. Part of Université du Québec. Founded: 1973. *Primary accreditation:* provincial charter. *Total enrollment:* 5,393.

The Module des Sciences de la Santé Founded in 1980.

BACCALAUREATE PROGRAM

Contact Director, Module des Sciences de la Santé, Université du Québec à Rimouski, 300 Avenues des Ursulines, Rimouski, PQ G5L 3A1, 418-724-1571. *Fax:* 418-724-1525.

UNIVERSITÉ LAVAL

École des Sciences Infirmières
Québec, Quebec

Programs • Generic Baccalaureate • Master's for Non-Nursing College Graduates

The Institution Independent coed university. Founded: 1852. *Primary accreditation:* provincial charter. *Setting:* 465-acre urban campus. *Total enrollment:* 32,089.

The École des Sciences Infirmières Founded in 1967. *Nursing program faculty:* 22 (50% with doctorates).

Academic Facilities *Campus library:* 3.2 million volumes (95,360 in health, 3,478 in nursing); 948 health-care related periodical subscriptions. *Nursing school resources:* nursing audiovisuals, learning resource lab.

Student Life *Student services:* health clinic, child-care facilities, personal counseling, career counseling, job placement, campus safety program, special assistance for disabled students. *International student services:* counseling/support, special assistance for nonnative speakers of English. *Nursing student activities:* student nurses association.

Calendar Semesters.

NURSING STUDENT PROFILE

Undergraduate **Enrollment:** 512
Women: 90%; **Men:** 10%; **Minority:** 0%; **International:** 0%; **Part-time:** 60%
Graduate **Enrollment:** 59
Women: 97%; **Men:** 3%; **Minority:** 0%; **International:** 0%; **Part-time:** 67%

BACCALAUREATE PROGRAM

Contact Mariette Blais, Responsable de l'Admission, École des Sciences Infirmières, Université Laval, Québec, PQ G1K 7P4, 418-656-7304. *Fax:* 418-656-7747. *E-mail:* mariette.blais@esi.ulaval.ca

Expenses *State resident tuition:* $1600 full-time, $86 per credit part-time. *Nonresident tuition:* $5788 full-time, $193 per credit part-time. *Full-time mandatory fees:* $6–$12. *Books and supplies per academic year:* ranges from $200 to $300.

Generic Baccalaureate Program (BScN)

Applying *Required:* transcript of college record, diplôme d'études collégiales or equivalent. *Options:* Advanced standing available through credit by exam. May apply for transfer of up to 72 total credits. *Application deadline:* 3/1. *Application fee:* $55.

Degree Requirements 96 total credit hours.

MASTER'S PROGRAM

Contact Linda LePage, Program Coordinator, École des Sciences Infirmières, Université Laval, Quebec, PQ G1K 7P4, 418-656-7304. *Fax:* 418-656-7747. *E-mail:* linda.lepage@esi.ulaval.ca

Areas of Study Clinical nurse specialist programs in adult health nursing, community health nursing, family health nursing, gerontological nursing, maternity-newborn nursing, medical-surgical nursing, oncology nursing, parent-child nursing, perinatal nursing, psychiatric–mental health nursing, rehabilitation nursing, women's health nursing.

Expenses *State resident tuition:* $1600 full-time, $86 per credit part-time. *Nonresident tuition:* $5788 full-time, $193 per credit part-time. *Full-time mandatory fees:* $100–$125. *Part-time mandatory fees:* $10–$12.

Master's for Non-Nursing College Graduates Program (MSN)

Applying *Required:* bachelor's degree in nursing, bachelor's degree, statistics course, 3 letters of recommendation, transcript of college record. *Application deadline:* 3/1.

Degree Requirements Thesis required.

SASKATCHEWAN

UNIVERSITY OF SASKATCHEWAN
College of Nursing
Saskatoon, Saskatchewan

Programs • Generic Baccalaureate • RN Baccalaureate • MN • Continuing Education

The University Province-supported coed university. Founded: 1907. *Primary accreditation:* provincial charter. *Setting:* 363-acre urban campus. *Total enrollment:* 17,666.

The College of Nursing Founded in 1938. *Nursing program faculty:* 43 (5% with doctorates).

Academic Facilities *Campus library:* 1.6 million volumes (120,000 in health, 7,000 in nursing); 13,000 periodical subscriptions (1,500 health-care related). *Nursing school resources:* CAI, computer lab, nursing audiovisuals, learning resource lab.

Student Life *Student services:* health clinic, child-care facilities, personal counseling, campus safety program, special assistance for disabled students. *International student services:* counseling/support, ESL courses. *Nursing student activities:* student nurses association.

Calendar Semesters.

NURSING STUDENT PROFILE

Undergraduate **Enrollment:** 443
Women: 90%; **Men:** 10%; **Minority:** 3%; **International:** 0%; **Part-time:** 33%
Graduate **Enrollment:** 35
Women: 97%; **Men:** 3%; **Minority:** 0%; **International:** 0%; **Part-time:** 75%

BACCALAUREATE PROGRAMS

Contact Ms. Eileen McLean, Admissions and Records, A102 Health Sciences Building, College of Nursing, University of Saskatchewan, 107 Wiggins Road, Saskatoon, SK S7N 5E5, 306-966-6231. *Fax:* 306-966-6621. *E-mail:* zagiel@abyss.sask.ca

Expenses *State resident tuition:* $2670 full-time, $89 per credit part-time. *Full-time mandatory fees:* $60–$192. *Room and board:* $3510–$3822. *Room only:* $1459. *Books and supplies per academic year:* ranges from $90 to $800.

Financial Aid Institutionally sponsored need-based grants/scholarships, institutionally sponsored non-need grants/scholarships, Federal Nursing Student Loans.

GENERIC BACCALAUREATE PROGRAM (BSN)

Applying *Required:* TOEFL for nonnative speakers of English, minimum high school GPA of 3.0, high school chemistry, high school biology, high school transcript, English A30, English B30, math at a 30 level. *Application deadline:* 5/15. *Application fee:* $35.

Degree Requirements 126 total credit hours, 102 in nursing.

RN BACCALAUREATE PROGRAM (BSN)

Applying *Required:* RN license, diploma or AD in nursing, 1 year minimum of clinical work following RN completion. *Options:* May apply for transfer of up to 54 total credits. *Application deadline:* 5/15. *Application fee:* $35.

Degree Requirements 84 total credit hours, 33 in nursing.

Distance learning Courses provided through correspondence, video.

MASTER'S PROGRAM

Contact Dr. Karen Wright, Chairperson, Graduate Program, A102 Health Sciences Building, College of Nursing, University of Saskatchewan, 107 Wiggins Road, Saskatoon, SK S7N 5E5, 306-966-6228. *Fax:* 306-966-6703. *E-mail:* wright@skyfox.usask.ca

Areas of Study Clinical nurse specialist programs in adult health nursing, community health nursing, gerontological nursing, psychiatric–mental health nursing, public health nursing; nursing administration; nursing education.

Expenses *State resident tuition:* $3337 full-time, $98 per credit hour part-time. *Full-time mandatory fees:* $88–$200. *Room and board:* $3510–$3822. *Room only:* $1459. *Books and supplies per academic year:* $220+.

Financial Aid Graduate assistantships, institutionally sponsored non-need-based grants/scholarships. 17% of master's level students in nursing programs received some form of financial aid in 1995-96. *Application deadline:* 2/28.

MN PROGRAM

Applying *Required:* TOEFL for nonnative speakers of English, bachelor's degree in nursing, RN license, 1 year of clinical experience, statistics course, essay, 3 letters of recommendation, transcript of college record, minimum college average of 75 percent. *Application deadline:* 2/28.

Degree Requirements 30 total credit hours, 28 in nursing.

CONTINUING EDUCATION PROGRAM

Contact Barbara Smith, Director, Continuing Nursing Education, University of Saskatchewan, Box 60000 RPO - University, Saskatoon, SK S7N 4J8, 306-966-8364. *Fax:* 306-866-8718. *E-mail:* smithb@sask.usask.ca

IN-DEPTH DESCRIPTIONS OF NURSING PROGRAMS

The following two-page descriptions were prepared exclusively by officials of the nursing school or department or of the college of which the nursing school or department is a part. Each description is designed to help give students a better sense of the individuality of the school, in areas that include campus environment, programs of study, affiliations with health-care facilities, academic facilities, location, student group, costs, and the faculty.

The absence from this section of any institution does not constitute an editorial decision on the part of Peterson's. In essence, this section is an open forum for nursing schools or departments, on a voluntary basis, to communicate their particular messages to prospective students. The descriptions are arranged alphabetically by the official name of the institution.

Adelphi University
School of Nursing
Garden City, New York

THE UNIVERSITY

Adelphi University was founded in Brooklyn and chartered by the state of New York in 1896 as Adelphi College. The first degree-granting liberal arts institution of higher education on Long Island, it was granted university status in 1963. It is private, nonsectarian, and coeducational. The University is composed of eight divisions: the College of Arts and Sciences, the Graduate School of Arts and Sciences, the University College, the Schools of Business, the School of Social Work, the School of Nursing, the School of Education, and the Institute of Advanced Psychological Studies. On-campus facilities include a cafeteria, a rathskeller, a nursery school for preschoolers, athletic facilities, a computer center, and a comprehensive library. The student health center is capable of handling emergency health needs and minor health problems and offers counseling and health instruction. Psychological services are available.

Adelphi University has a strong tradition of commitment to liberal education. Today, Adelphi is becoming a distinctive center of national education, with a preeminent reputation for integrating liberal arts and professional education.

THE SCHOOL OF NURSING

The School of Nursing has a history rich in achievement. Founded in 1943 as a cadet nurse corps program, it was the first professional school at Adelphi University and the first collegiate nursing program on Long Island. In 1949, Adelphi became one of a small number of schools to offer a master's degree in nursing. The School offers a post-master's nurse practitioner certificate program as well as other programs designed to meet the needs of practicing nurses in today's health-care environment.

Recognizing the growing complexity of health care and the high cost of nursing education, the School has developed a new curriculum designed to prepare traditional and nontraditional students efficiently and expertly. This curriculum emphasizes self-directed learning, concentrates on case studies, and promotes clinical nursing competence using a wide array of learning resources.

The Adelphi University School of Nursing remains on the cutting edge as it moves into a new era of health care. In keeping with Adelphi University's commitment to intellect, the School of Nursing emphasizes the principles and processes of nursing care through programs that integrate humanistic foundations, theoretical inquiry, and clinical practice. The School believes that only by means of such thorough preparation can the nursing profession respond to the challenges that confront the health-care system as it moves into the next century.

PROGRAMS OF STUDY

The School of Nursing offers a Bachelor of Science program with a major in nursing for basic students whose educational objective is to obtain the degree and become eligible to take the licensing examination for Registered Professional Nurse. The School also offers a program for registered nurses from associate degree or diploma nursing programs who wish to obtain the Bachelor of Science degree. An accelerated B.S./M.S. program is offered for qualified RN students. The Master of Science is offered for nurses seeking advanced education in professional nursing. Post-master's certificate programs are available for clinical specialization and pediatric, family, adult, and gerontological nurse practitioner.

The Bachelor of Science program for basic students is based on a planned progression of courses arranged to build upon previous knowledge and to develop skills and performance at an increasing level of competence. Students are required to complete 35 credits in the University's unique CORE Curriculum, 31 credits in courses supportive to the nursing major, and 57 credits in professional courses. Throughout the curriculum, concepts relating to promotion of health care during illness and rehabilitation in relation to the patient, the family, and the community are developed. Dynamics of practice in the health-care delivery system of the twenty-first century are emphasized.

The focus of the curriculum for registered nurses is on developing an expanded body of knowledge encompassing primary (patients entering the health-care system) and tertiary (patients with long-term illnesses) care. Emphasis is also placed on expanded assessment abilities, strategies for planning for future nursing care delivery modes, and ability to solve complex problems and to effect change.

The accelerated B.S./M.S. program allows qualified RN students to register for 12 credits in the master's program, which are used to fulfill degree requirements in both programs.

The M.S. program prepares nurses for advanced practice as nursing educators, nursing service administrators, clinical specialists, and advanced practice nurses in adult health, parent-child, and psychiatric–mental health nursing. The M.S. is awarded at the completion of 43 credits and a master's project for clinical nurse specialist and 48 credits plus a project for master's level nurse practitioner students.

The Ph.D. program prepares nurses to be knowledgeable, creative critical thinkers who can fill leadership positions in nursing education, administration, and clinical research. The curriculum consists of 40 credits of required and elective courses plus a dissertation. The program is designed for part-time study but easily accommodates full-time study. All required Ph.D. courses meet on Fridays.

The post-master's certificate programs provide an opportunity for nurses who hold master's degrees to refocus and respecialize in another area of concentration.

AFFILIATIONS WITH HEALTH-CARE FACILITIES

The School of Nursing is affiliated with a variety of clinical resources, including Winthrope University Hospital, Long Island Jewish Medical Center, North Shore University Medical Center, Parker Jewish Geriatric Center, Visiting Nurse Service of New York, and Schneider's Children's Hospital. Access to medical centers in New York City allows the School to provide unique and specialized experiences on an individualized basis. Numerous community agencies, such as HMOs, schools, clinics, home health agencies, senior centers, and day-care centers, are used throughout the course of study.

ACADEMIC FACILITIES

The Swirbul Library houses about 624,000 volumes, 37,000 listening and viewing materials, and 625,000 items in microformat and subscribes to 5,000 periodicals. It is fully automated for literature searches and has a computerized catalog.

The Computing Center has workstations throughout the campus, along with a number of printers and plotters and an optical scanner. Software includes a variety of programming languages, color graphics, database management systems, simulations, and models.

The School of Nursing Learning Resource Center includes two learning laboratories and a computer laboratory. The learning laboratories simulate the hospital and home settings with all appropriate and supportive models and supplies.

LOCATION

Garden City, a suburban residential community in Nassau County, Long Island, is less than an hour from midtown Manhattan by car or train. Both the county and nearby New York City offer a wide variety of athletic, cultural, and social resources to meet the many needs of a large and diverse population.

STUDENT SERVICES

School of Nursing Acting for Progress (SNAP) and VISION are the undergraduate student organizations. SNAP is the basic student organization and VISION is the RN student group. These organizations serve to stimulate interest and involvement in professional and social issues and provide a conducive environment for informal socialization among members.

The University provides many resources and service offices to meet student needs. These include the Chaplains' Center, University Center, Barnes & Noble Bookstore, the Rathskeller, Center for Career Placement and Planning, Health Services Center, Hy Weinberg Center for Communication Disorders, Center for Psychological Services, Social Services Center, Office of Alcohol and Substance Abuse Prevention, Child Activity Center, Athletic Center, University Learning Center, Computing Center, Library, and housing and dining services.

THE NURSING STUDENT GROUP

In spring 1996, the School of Nursing enrolled more than 675 undergraduate, graduate, and doctoral students.

COSTS

The 1996–97 tuition for undergraduate students was $395 per credit or $13,400 for full-time study. For graduate students, tuition was $400 per credit or $13,500 for full-time study. University fees were $300 per semester. Other fees and housing costs are determined on an individual basis.

FINANCIAL AID

Adelphi University offers a wide variety of financial assistance programs in addition to the various federal and state programs that exist. The amounts and types of financial assistance that a student receives are determined by the eligibility of the applicant for each program.

APPLYING

Applicants for the basic Bachelor of Science program must meet the general conditions of admission to the University. High school chemistry, physics, and 2½ years of mathematics are recommended. Transfer applicants must have a minimum GPA of 2.8. The acceptable grade in science courses is C+ or better. Transfer applicants must interview. RN applicants must hold a current registered nurse license in one of the fifty states or territories; must meet general University requirements for admission; must have graduated from a National League for Nursing–accredited associate degree program or, if a graduate of a nonaccredited or diploma program, must have completed the Regents College Examinations; and must have a minimum GPA of 2.5.

Applicants to the master's and post-master's programs are required to have a current license as a registered nurse in one of the fifty states or territories, to hold an earned B.S. or M.S. degree in nursing from an NLN-accredited school, to have a minimum GPA of 3.0 on a 4.0 point scale, and provide letters of reference.

Correspondence and Information:

Office of Undergraduate Admissions
Adelphi University
Garden City, New York 11530
Telephone: 516-877-3050

Allegheny University of the Health Sciences
School of Nursing
Philadelphia, Pennsylvania

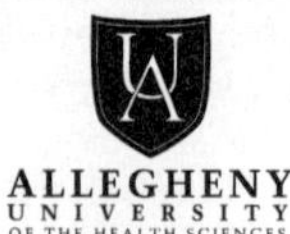

THE UNIVERSITY

Allegheny University of the Health Sciences (AUHS) is an academic health center that includes more than 3,100 students in the Medical College of Pennsylvania•Hahnemann School of Medicine, the School of Health Professions, the School of Nursing, and the School of Public Health. The University grants degrees from the associate through the doctorate in more than forty health sciences programs. The University was formed through the 1993 consolidation of Medical College of Pennsylvania and Hahnemann University, and was given its present name in June 1996.

THE SCHOOL OF NURSING

Allegheny University of the Health Sciences has a 130-year legacy of educating nurses. Hospital-based nursing programs were begun in 1864 at the former Female Medical College of Pennsylvania and in 1890 at the Hahnemann Hospital Training School for Nurses. With the consolidation of Medical College of Pennsylvania and Hahnemann University in 1993, Hahnemann's undergraduate and graduate nursing programs and Medical College of Pennsylvania's nurse anesthesia program were combined into a new School of Nursing.

The continuing education programs are nationally known for their products and design. Major continuing education conferences, such as Trends in Critical Care, Nurse Educator, and Psychiatric Nursing, have been offered in major cities across the United States.

PROGRAMS OF STUDY

The School of Nursing offers both undergraduate and graduate programs. The RN-B.S.N. program builds on the registered nurse student's prior learning to provide a firm foundation for career mobility and graduate study. Nursing courses rest on a strong foundation of liberal arts and science and focus on the workings of managed health-care systems, nursing research and leadership, information and direct care technologies, clinical competencies in health promotion and disease prevention, health assessment, public health, home health nursing, and tertiary nursing care practice. There is a strong emphasis on promoting healthy lifestyles in diverse communities through empowerment processes, understanding and confronting ethical issues, managing information and costs, and coordinating care within the context of accountability.

Graduates of National League for Nursing–accredited associate degree nursing programs or diploma nursing programs may receive credit for up to 30 semester hours of nursing to apply toward program entrance requirements. The State of Pennsylvania Nursing Articulation Model guides advanced placement decisions in the RN-B.S.N. program.

All non-nursing prerequisite courses may be completed prior to matriculation at AUHS. All nursing major requirements are offered at the Center City campus and at a variety of satellite campuses surrounding Philadelphia and across the state. Courses are offered during times and in formats friendly to the practicing nurse.

The School of Nursing offers two graduate programs that lead to the Master of Science in Nursing degree and a third graduate program leading to a post-master's certificate. The graduate nursing program prepares advanced practice nurses who will make important contributions to the health, education, and social and political structures of society. Interdisciplinary opportunities are available to medical students, students of public health, and students in other health professions. The School of Nursing fosters a community of clinical scholars capable of promoting research, creative activities, and leadership for the profession.

The RN-M.S.N. program is designed for registered nurse graduates of diploma and associate degree nursing programs. The program accelerates the student through the RN-B.S.N. program by permitting enrollment in selected graduate-level courses while completing the B.S.N. Specific M.S.N.-level courses are substituted for 9 elective credits of undergraduate work.

The master's program offers the Master of Science in Nursing degree in areas of advanced practice nursing. Among specializations offered in the master's program are the M.S.N. in nurse anesthesia (NA), which prepares nurses for certification as registered nurse anesthetists, and the M.S.N. in nurse practitioner (NP) options, including family nurse practitioner, acute care nurse practitioner, pediatric nurse practitioner, psychiatric–mental health nurse practitioner, and perioperative nurse practitioner. A women's care nurse practitioner option is available through a collaborative arrangement with the Planned Parenthood Federation of America.

Other M.S.N. programs, as well as the M.S.N.-Master of Public Health, are in development.

The post-master's certificate program is designed for individuals who have earned a master's degree in nursing and seek further preparation to qualify for state and/or national certification as a nurse practitioner. The program can be completed in one year of part-time study.

An option is available enabling graduates of certificate (NA and NP) programs to earn the M.S.N. degree.

Graduates of all specializations are eligible for certification by the appropriate professionally designated body. Full- and part-time study are offered in the day and evening.

AFFILIATIONS WITH HEALTH-CARE FACILITIES

AUHS is the academic anchor of Allegheny Health, Education and Research Foundation, a statewide health-care system that also includes Allegheny General Hospital in Pittsburgh, Allegheny University Hospitals and St. Christopher's Hospital for Children in Philadelphia, and Allegheny Integrated Health Group. More than 3,000 nurses in all specialties and arenas of practice are part of Allegheny's statewide health-care system, in which education and research are core components of the mission. In addition, the University is committed to improving health care in a targeted area of the city, and students from all of the schools learn together in community settings.

ACADEMIC FACILITIES

For clinical research, students have ready access to the University's comprehensive system of health care, including two tertiary-care adult hospitals, one specialty children's hospital, two community hospitals, and a large number of practice sites. The University's modern laboratories are well equipped for biomedical research. The libraries and supporting services provide specialized facilities for a variety of research projects, and microcomputer facilities and on-line search capabilities are available to all students. The University's location in Philadelphia provides access to other excellent science and medical libraries.

LOCATION

Nursing students are on the University's Center City campus, where they have easy access to all the attractions of central Philadelphia. The University has a second Philadelphia campus in the East Falls section of the city. The city's historic, cultural, scientific, sports, entertainment, and dining advantages—many within walking distance—are available to students. AUHS is convenient to and accessible by bus, rail, and subway lines. New York City, Atlantic City and other New Jersey shore points, the Pocono Mountains, and Washington, D.C. are but a few of the recreational areas within a 1- to 5-hour commute from the University.

STUDENT SERVICES

AUHS has full-time counselors who provide diagnostic educational services, career counseling, and personal support counseling. For students having academic difficulty, remedial academic counseling, peer tutoring, and group tutoring are available free of charge. Support groups and referral services are available for stress reduction and resolution of more serious personal problems. The Office of Minority Affairs serves as an advocate for the minority applicant and student, while the Office of International Programs and Services coordinates support services for international students.

THE NURSING STUDENT GROUP

The School of Nursing population is a diverse group composed of both traditional and nontraditional students. Because so many of the students remain employed while attending school, programs are offered with a variety of flexible scheduling options, including evening and weekend classes and practice experiences.

COSTS

In 1996–97, the undergraduate tuition for full-time students was $4760 per semester; per-credit-hour tuition for nonmatriculating and part-time matriculating students was $415.

The tuition for graduate nursing programs was $5265 per semester in 1996–97, with a $100–$500 nonrefundable deposit, depending on the program; per-credit-hour tuition for nonmatriculating and part-time matriculating students was $585.

All full-time students must pay a student activity fee of $30 per semester. Students are required to maintain adequate medical insurance. All particulars relating to tuition and fees are subject to change.

FINANCIAL AID

AUHS awards funds to students from loan programs and numerous scholarship and grant programs. Awards are based on financial need, with the neediest students funded first. Some scholarship funds are awarded to students based on a combination of financial need and academic merit. Students must complete the Free Application for Federal Student Aid (FAFSA) to be considered for any aid from the University.

APPLYING

Applicants to the B.S.N. program must have RN licensure, a minimum overall undergraduate GPA of 2.5, 60 hours of college prerequisites, official copies of high school and college transcripts, and have graduated from high school or hold an equivalency certificate. Graduates of associate degree nursing programs or NLN-accredited diploma nursing programs who are clinically current may receive credit for up to 30 semester hours of nursing to apply toward program entrance requirements. No challenge examinations are required. The deadline for applications and supporting credentials is August 1.

Applicants to the master's program must have a B.S.N. degree, RN licensure, official college transcripts, satisfactory scores on the Graduate Record Examinations or Miller Analogy Test, a minimum undergraduate GPA of 3.0, and one or more years of clinical experience in critical care for nurse anesthesia or an area related to the proposed specialization for nurse practitioner. The deadlines for applications and supporting materials are April 1 for nurse anesthesia and May 15 for nurse practitioner.

Applicants to the post-master's certificate program must have an M.S.N. degree with a minimum graduate GPA of 3.5, current Pennsylvania RN licensure, two years' post-master's professional experience, a personal goals statement, and three letters of recommendation.

Applicants to the master's degree completion program must submit a portfolio, including transcripts from their original NP/NA program; undergraduate and graduate transcripts, if applicable; three letters of reference, two of which specifically address NP/NA experience; curriculum vitae, including details of NP/NA work experience; evidence of physiology, pathophysiology, and pharmacology course work; and documentation of certification, if applicable.

There is a nonrefundable application fee of $30 for undergraduate students and $50 for graduate students.

Correspondence and Information:

University Office of Admissions and Recruitment
Allegheny University of the Health Sciences
School of Nursing
Broad and Vine Streets, Mail Stop 472
Philadelphia, Pennsylvania 19102-1192
Telephone: 215-762-8288
World Wide Web: http://www.allegheny.edu/

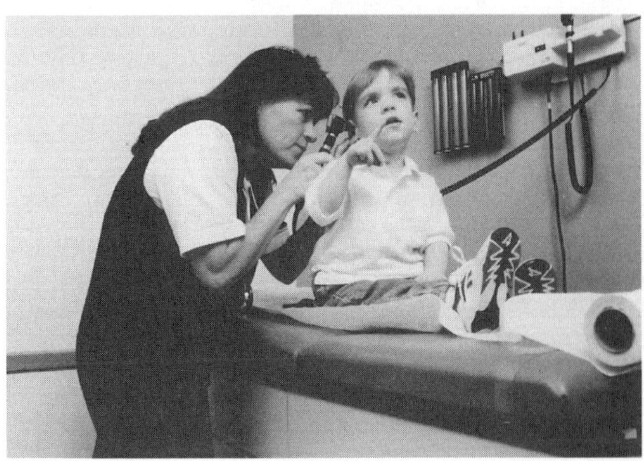

Pediatric nurse practitioner is one of the specializations offered in the master's program.

Bethel College
Department of Nursing
North Newton, Kansas

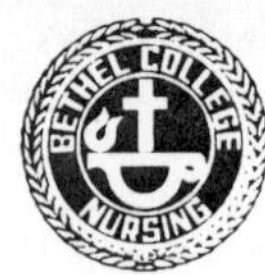

THE COLLEGE

Bethel College is a distinguished liberal arts and sciences undergraduate college affiliated with the General Conference Mennonite Church and known for its special emphasis combining academic excellence with a tradition of biblically based service. As the oldest Mennonite college in North America (founded in 1887), the College identifies with a 450-year-old Anabaptist heritage as evidenced by its commitment to Christ-centered learning, service to others, peacemaking, and conflict resolution. Bethel College is a vibrant community of faculty and students that is recognized as explicitly Christian, unapologetically Mennonite, intentionally open, and academically excellent.

The student body numbers approximately 650, while the teaching faculty consists of approximately 50 full-time equivalents. Because of its small size, Bethel is positioned to provide an individualized program to meet each student's interests and needs. At Bethel, teaching is conducted by professors, not by graduate teaching assistants, so students benefit from the experience and scholarship of the faculty in the classroom. Of the tenured faculty members, approximately 80 percent hold terminal degrees in their academic disciplines. Academic excellence is evidenced by a number of measures, including Bethel's first rank among all colleges and universities in Kansas in the number of graduates moving on to earn doctoral degrees. When this percentage is compared with the most prestigious and productive undergraduate institutions in the entire nation, Bethel ranks thirty-seventh.

THE DEPARTMENT OF NURSING

In 1900, Sister Frieda Kaufman presented herself to Reverend David Goerz, then business manager of Bethel College, and initiated the planning through Bethel College for the development of a school of nursing. In 1903, the Bethel Deaconess Home and Hospital Society was officially incorporated. Between 1908 and 1974, the Bethel Deaconess Hospital School of Nursing provided the diploma nursing education needs of this rural and largely Mennonite area of south-central Kansas. In 1948, the diploma school developed a formal plan of study with Bethel College whereby the students enrolled first at the College in natural and social science courses before taking the nursing course work at the hospital. Thus, diploma graduates electing to finish their baccalaureate degree received nursing credit toward a B.S.N. degree after completing remaining general education requirements through the College. With the closing of the diploma program in 1974, a strong community voice developed, urging the College to continue nursing education by developing a professional program of nursing study on the campus of Bethel College. Based upon the results of a feasibility study conducted in 1977, as well as 1979–80 consultant work, the Bethel College Department of Nursing began on-campus course work in the fall of 1980 with the first professional class graduating in the spring of 1982. The Bethel College Department of Nursing today remains the only professional nursing program available in a Mennonite institution of higher education west of the Mississippi.

PROGRAMS OF STUDY

The Bethel Deaconess–Bethel College Department of Nursing offers the B.S.N. degree for traditional students and adult learners as well as an accelerated B.S.N. degree for nontraditional students with previous college degrees. In addition, Bethel College offers nurses an RN to B.S.N. completion program through its unique RN outreach home-study program and an on-campus LPN to B.S.N. program of study.

Bethel's nursing programs are fully accredited by the Kansas State Board of Nursing and the National League for Nursing. The College is a member of the American Association of Colleges of Nursing.

The Bethel nursing curriculum is unique in that it is based on the totality paradigm. The nursing program is committed to the foundation of a Christian liberal arts college that connects faith and learning into a distinctive nursing educational experience linking theory and practice in a multicultural society. The Department functions to prepare professional graduates as generalists for beginning positions in a wide variety of health-care areas as well as to provide a baccalaureate foundation for currently practicing nurses for expanded roles and study at the graduate level.

AFFILIATIONS WITH HEALTH-CARE FACILITIES

A highlight of the Bethel nursing program is that students have the opportunity to spend each semester in a different clinical facility, giving them increased clinical exposure and flexibility. Over twenty rural and urban environments are available as clinical sites. Exposure to both rural and urban health-care environments is important for the well-rounded and versatile nurse in today's increasingly mobile society. The clinical experience sites for Bethel nursing students range from medical centers such as Via Christi Regional Medical Center, the largest medical center in Kansas, to rural hospitals of less than 100 beds and a large variety of community agencies such as home health agencies, schools, industrial sites, and homeless shelters.

ACADEMIC FACILITIES

Because the Bethel Deaconess–Bethel College Department of Nursing is located on the Bethel College campus, students have access to the academic facilities and libraries on campus. The nursing program has a laboratory that includes a simulated nurse's station as well as private patient hospital rooms and an examination room. The examination room, through the use of a one-way mirror, also serves as an observation room. The nursing practice area also includes a fully equipped audiovisual room and multimedia library with interactive computing network capabilities.

An exciting new addition to the facilities is the nurse-managed clinic, which houses a mini-laboratory, consultation room, and two fully equipped exam rooms for a variety of health restoration, health promotion, and counseling services. Nursing faculty members provide the practitioner skills for the collegewide community and supervise student learning in this innovative environment.

LOCATION

Located in the center of the nation, Bethel College is adjacent to the city of Newton (population 18,000) in the incorporated village of North Newton, a rural region of south-central Kansas. Wichita, the largest city in Kansas (population 320,000), lies 30 minutes to the south and provides a wealth of urban opportunities. This location places the Bethel College Department of Nursing in the unique position of bordering rural

America, where there is an increasing demand for health-care services to the north and west, and also offers the opportunities to the south and east of the largest medical centers in Kansas, some of which are located in Wichita.

STUDENT SERVICES

Because the Bethel Deaconess–Bethel College Department of Nursing is located on the Bethel College campus, students are afforded the same student service opportunities that are available to the entire campus community. Current student services include an academic support center, individualized advising network, individual and group tutoring and testing programs, counseling services for personal and career concerns, campus ministry network, chapel, and a newly developed wellness center. Traditional student services include the bookstore, computer lab, housing, and dining services.

A variety of opportunities are available in the nursing program, including membership in BC-KANS, the Bethel College unit of the National Student Nurses Association; membership opportunities in Nurses Christian Fellowship; and student membership in Sigma Theta Tau, an international nursing honor society. Students can also be active in the nursing student alumni association and numerous other campus clubs and organizations. A number of nursing students participate in Bethel sports such as volleyball, football, basketball, tennis, soccer, and track. Many nursing students also participate in music programs such as choir, bands, and symphony. Others have been active in drama programs and student government.

THE NURSING STUDENT GROUP

The Bethel nursing program has an enrollment of 200 students as of the 1996–97 academic year. Nearly 20 percent of the nursing students are from minority groups, including men and students of different cultures. The graduates of the Bethel nursing program have averaged an overall pass rate of 98 percent on the nursing licensing exam and 90 percent for first-time test takers over the history of the program.

COSTS

Tuition costs for the 1996–97 academic year were $4850 per semester for both in-state and out-of-state students. Fees for all students were $100 per semester. Nursing students are not charged additional tuition fees. Room and board costs vary according to the residence hall selected. Additional fees for nursing students include books, supplies, and uniforms, which vary semester to semester.

FINANCIAL AID

Bethel College offers a full program of financial aid in the form of merit scholarships, performance awards, grants, campus work-study opportunities, and low-interest educational loans. Additional financial aid and work programs are available to nursing students who qualify. For more information about financial aid, prospective students should contact Dick Koontz, Director of Financial Aid, at 800-522-1887 (toll-free).

APPLYING

All students requesting admission to the nursing program at Bethel College are considered through one of two rolling admission options. The guaranteed admission program reserves a seat in the nursing program for students who plan to major in nursing but complete general education requirements at the College prior to entering the nursing program. The competitive admission program allows students who are transferring to Bethel College only to study nursing to compete for admission. Students are selected on the basis of GPA, interview, references, and transcripts. For more information about admission to the nursing program, prospective students are encouraged to contact Dr. Janice Unruh Davidson, Program Director, at 316-284-5307.

Correspondence and Information:

Bethel College
Office of Admissions
300 East 27th Street
North Newton, Kansas 67117
Telephone: 800-5BC-1887 (toll-free)

THE FACULTY

Janlee Blosser, Associate Professor of Nursing; M.N., Wichita State. Maternal-child health.

Janice Unruh Davidson, Program Director and Associate Professor of Nursing; M.N., Wichita State; Ph.D., Texas Woman's; FNP-C, Wisconsin–Oshkosh. Nursing theory, research, and family nurse practitioner.

Verda Deckert, Assistant Professor of Nursing; M.N., Wichita State. Leadership and management.

Rojean DuBois, Assistant Professor of Nursing; M.N., Wichita State; FNP–C, Fort Hays State. Women's health and family nurse practitioner.

Dorothy Goertz, Assistant Professor of Nursing; M.S.N., Wichita State. Mental health nursing.

Dorothy Matthew, Associate Professor of Nursing; M.N., Wichita State. Critical care nursing.

Marie Maugans, Assistant Professor of Nursing; M.N., Wichita State. Mental health nursing.

Katherine Fischer Mick, Assistant Professor of Nursing; M.Ed., Missouri–St. Louis; M.S.N., Wichita State. Community health and mental health nursing.

Carol Moore, Associate Professor of Nursing; M.N., Wichita State; Ph.D., Kansas State. Adult health.

W. Kaye Penner, Assistant Professor of Nursing; M.S.N., Wichita State. Adult health.

Martha J. Morgan Sanders, Associate Professor of Nursing; M.S.N., Clarkson; Ph.D., Kansas State. Childbirth education.

Gregg Schroeder, Assistant Professor of Nursing; M.S.N., Wichita State. Men's health and critical care nursing.

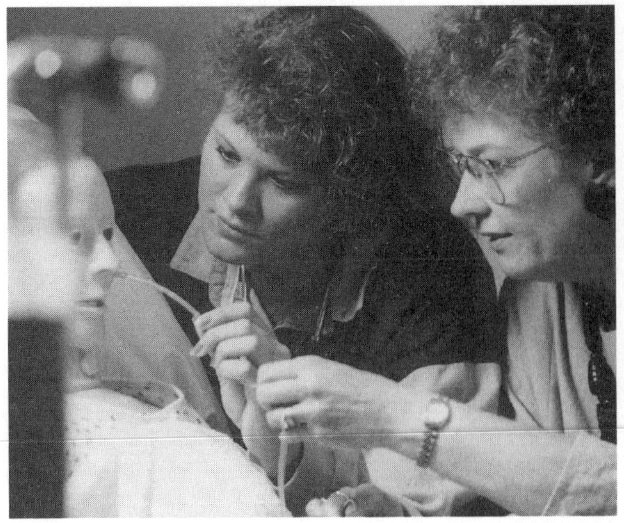

Nursing student and assistant professor practice nasogastric tube insertion in the simulated hospital laboratory at Bethel College.

Boston College
School of Nursing
Chestnut Hill, Massachusetts

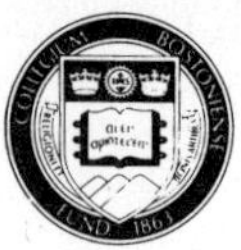

THE COLLEGE

Boston College is a coeducational university with eleven schools, colleges, and institutes that offer thirteen degree programs and one certification program. Founded in 1863, it is one of the oldest Jesuit-affiliated universities in the country and one of the largest private universities in the nation, with an enrollment of over 14,000.

The reputation of the school, securely established after more than a century of proven excellence, continues to gain stature. In recent years, surveys undertaken by periodicals such as *Barron's* and *U.S. News & World Report* have consistently ranked Boston College among the top colleges and universities in the nation.

THE SCHOOL OF NURSING

Founded in 1947, the Boston College School of Nursing is the largest Jesuit school of nursing. Currently, the School of Nursing offers baccalaureate, master's, RN/M.S., M.S./M.B.A., doctoral, and continuing education programs. Graduates of the programs are highly successful in clinical, academic, and administrative careers in nursing. They are widely respected and sought after for positions in the Boston region and throughout the nation.

The School of Nursing has 49 full-time faculty members teaching in both the undergraduate and graduate programs. They are highly qualified, clinically and academically, and many are certified for clinical practice by the American Nurses' Association or by a nursing specialty organization. Ninety-four percent of the faculty members hold an earned doctorate in nursing or in related fields, and all professors are actively engaged in research. The faculty is widely published and includes nursing scholars who are recognized as experts and leaders in their respective fields. A number of faculty members are nationally known; the works of a few are used internationally. Faculty members serve as advisers to each student for the entire program of study.

PROGRAMS OF STUDY

The baccalaureate program spans eight full-time semesters for a total of 121 credits. Course work consists of university core requirements; electives; nursing courses, which include simulated and audiovisual laboratory activities on campus; and clinical learning activities in a vast variety of health-care settings. Courses in the nursing major include theories of wellness, illness, rehabilitation, and health maintenance, which serve as the basis for professional nursing practice. Clinical practice offers experience with people in all age groups and in varied levels of wellness. All programs emphasize ethics for health-care professionals and the research process in nursing care.

The main objective of the master's program is to prepare nurses for advanced practice, including clinical specialist and nurse practitioner. There are four areas of specialization: adult health, community health, maternal/child health, and psychiatric–mental health nursing. In addition, the RN/M.S. plan and the M.S./M.B.A. dual degree offer other pathways to the Master of Science degree in nursing. An Additional Specialty Concentration is available for RNs who have an M.S. in nursing and wish to enhance their educational background in an additional specialty area. The focus in the specialty areas is on human responses to actual or potential health problems. The approach to clients is multifaceted and includes the development of advanced competencies in nursing diagnosis and therapeutic judgment. Numerous community agencies in and around Boston are used for the clinical practicum of the program. Requirements for completion of the master's degree are 45 credits. A thesis is optional. Full-time students can complete the program in 1½ to 2 years, and part-time students may take up to 5 years.

The Ph.D. program in nursing is the first doctoral program in nursing to be offered at a Jesuit university. The focus of the Ph.D. program is the preparation of scholars for leadership positions in clinical nursing research. Areas of research concentration include ethics and ethical judgment, nursing diagnosis and diagnostic-therapeutic judgment, and selected life processes/patterns. Core areas of doctoral study are concepts of nursing science, methods of theory development, and qualitative and quantitative research methods needed to extend nursing knowledge. The three-year plan allows the student to take 10 credits of course work per semester for the first two years of study before entering the dissertation phase of the program. The four-year plan allows the student to take 6 to 7 credits of course work per semester for the first three years of study before entering the dissertation phase of the program. A variety of learning opportunities are available through independent study, interdisciplinary colloquia at the university and health-care agencies, and clinical research practicums with faculty mentors.

ACADEMIC FACILITIES

Boston College's libraries offer a wealth of resources and services to support student research activities. The book collection consists of over 1 million volumes, and the nursing holdings have been characterized by nursing leaders as one of the finest collections in the world. The university's membership in two academic consortia provides students with access to millions of volumes and other services of the member institutions. The nursing resource facilities available to enhance student learning include the Kennedy Audiovisual Center and the Nursing Simulation Laboratory, both housed within the School of Nursing. The university also offers a wide range of other support services, such as audiovisual facilities and computer hardware, applications, and peripherals.

LOCATION

Boston College is located in a beautiful suburban setting just minutes from downtown Boston. Boston is a city that offers an unparalleled combination of history, culture, and vitality, and it is home to a number of the world's most renowned health-care institutions. Students and faculty enjoy the unique advantages of metropolitan Boston in addition to the beauty and tranquility of the suburban campus. The scenic grounds and stately Gothic architecture of the 200-acre campus provide an atmosphere conducive to both study and socializing.

STUDENT SERVICES

Health and counseling services are available to all graduate and undergraduate students, including programs for African-American, Hispanic, Asian, and Native American students through AHANA. A complete recreation complex and career-planning guidance are also available to students.

THE NURSING STUDENT GROUP

Students at Boston College reflect a diversity of interests and backgrounds. The student body is drawn from every race, religion, and economic background as well as from every state in the Union and numerous countries. Currently, the School of Nursing has 420 undergraduate, over 200 full- and part-time master's, and 39 doctoral students. The students' ages range from 18 to 50, and many are employed and/or married with children.

COSTS

For 1996–97, undergraduate tuition was $18,820. Room rates averaged $4685, board was $3330, and health, recreation, and activity fees averaged $600. Books, supplies, and other expenses were estimated at $600.

For 1996–97, graduate tuition was $566 per credit hour. Charges for books, fees, supplies, housing, and transportation are additional.

FINANCIAL AID

Boston College offers a variety of scholarships, grants, loans, and employment to assist students in financing their education. Overall, 83 percent of the undergraduate class of 1995 received some form of financial aid. Financial aid awards are made by the financial aid office to freshmen and transfer students on the basis of academic promise and demonstrated financial need. Notice of such awards made to incoming freshmen and transfer students usually accompanies notification of the students' acceptance by the university. Work-study opportunities are also available.

Graduate students may apply for financial assistance from both the university Financial Aid Office and the School of Nursing. In addition, tuition remission scholarships and university fellowships are available for nursing graduate students. Faculty research grants and Boston health-care agencies offer the student many employment opportunities.

APPLYING

For the undergraduate program, the type of college-preparatory program viewed as the best foundation for college work usually includes at least 4 units of English, 3 units of a foreign language, 3 units of math, and 2 units of a laboratory science. Students applying to the School of Nursing are required to complete at least 2 units of a laboratory science, including 1 unit of chemistry. All applicants must complete the Scholastic Assessment Test (SAT I) and SAT II Subject Tests in writing, mathematics (level I or II), and a third subject of the applicant's choice. In place of the Scholastic Assessment Test, applicants may take American College Testing's ACT Assessment. Students may earn advanced placement at Boston College through the attainment of qualifying scores on Advanced Placement exams and by the successful completion of college courses prior to freshman enrollment.

All candidates for admission to the undergraduate program must complete the Preliminary Admissions Application and submit it with a $45 nonrefundable application fee to the Office of Undergraduate Admissions. Subsequently, the Office of Undergraduate Admissions will mail to the applicant the Secondary Application, which consists of a Personal Data Form, Guidance Counselor Form, Teacher Recommendation Form, and the Boston College Financial Aid Application, which is due prior to February 1. Although an admission interview is not required, students and parents are encouraged to visit the Boston College campus and meet with an admission representative and a School of Nursing faculty member.

Applicants to the master's program should submit GRE scores, three references, and a personal goal statement. A minimum GPA of 3.0, a transcript from an NLN-accredited baccalaureate nursing program, and previous course work in statistics and physical assessment are required. Application deadlines are as follows: for full-time and part-time study during the summer sessions, February 1; and for part-time study during the spring semester, October 15.

Applicants to the doctoral program should submit GRE scores; three references; a career goals statement; evidence of scholarship, including a writing sample; a curriculum vitae; transcripts from NLN-accredited B.S. and M.S. programs in nursing; and previous course work in statistics and nursing research. An interview is required. The deadline is January 31 of the year of admission. The application fee for each program is $40 and is nonrefundable.

Correspondence and Information:

Director of Undergraduate Admissions
Boston College
Devlin Hall, Room 208
Chestnut Hill, Massachusetts 02167
Telephone: 617-552-3100

Associate Dean, Undergraduate Program, or
Associate Dean, Graduate Programs
Boston College
School of Nursing
Chestnut Hill, Massachusetts 02167
Telephone: 617-552-4250

Capital University
School of Nursing
Columbus, Ohio

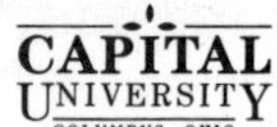

THE UNIVERSITY

With a foundation firmly based in a history and tradition of academic excellence, Capital University's undergraduate and graduate programs are preparing students for lifelong learning in the global environment of the twenty-first century. Since its founding by the Lutheran church in 1830, Capital has been at the forefront of preparing students for the future through a high-quality liberal arts education that is coupled with professional training. Ethical, moral, and religious values essential to leadership in society are an integral part of the Capital experience.

Capital University is composed of three undergraduate colleges—the School of Nursing, College of Arts and Sciences, and Conservatory of Music—and two graduate schools—the Law School and the Graduate School of Administration (M.B.A. program). An Adult Degree Program is available in Columbus, Cleveland, and Dayton. Capital offers six undergraduate degrees and six graduate degrees, with more than forty majors. Of the approximately 4,000 students enrolled at Capital, more than 1,800 are traditional undergraduates. Approximately 70 percent of these students reside on campus in the University's four residence halls.

Through the years, Capital has repeatedly earned recognition as an outstanding university. Capital was included in the most recent issue of *Barron's Best Buys in College Education,* and the School of Nursing was included in a recent edition of *Ruggs Recommendations on the Colleges.*

THE SCHOOL OF NURSING

In 1950, a nursing program was first established at Capital University as a department in the College of Arts and Sciences. In 1965, the School of Nursing was formally established. Capital offers its nursing students a curriculum that blends liberal arts with professional nursing studies. Training goes beyond studies in the clinical, technical, and scientific aspects of health care to include consideration of the emotional, social, cultural, and spiritual needs of patients. At Capital, nursing students' insight into the human experience forms the foundation upon which they build their nursing skills.

Teaching and guiding the approximately 300 students enrolled in the School of Nursing are faculty members who are skilled practitioners and professional educators. Throughout the year, they apply current research findings and state-of-the-art technology to their many clinical specialty areas.

The School of Nursing is approved by the Ohio State Board of Nursing, is accredited by the National League for Nursing, and is a member of the American Association of Colleges of Nursing.

PROGRAMS OF STUDY

Students are admitted as freshmen into the Capital University School of Nursing and are assigned a faculty adviser to help ensure successful progression through the program. During the first year, students complete foundation studies, including biophysical sciences, social sciences, and University Core Curriculum courses. Students begin Level I nursing courses during the second year concurrently with additional School and University requirements. Level II, III, and IV courses are completed during the two years of upper-division study. Students who successfully complete the requirements of the 134-semester-hour nursing curriculum earn a Bachelor of Science in Nursing degree and are eligible to write the licensure examination for practice as professional nurses.

Clinical practice begins in the laboratories of the School of Nursing under direct supervision of the faculty in the sophomore year. In an eight-week required summer school course following the sophomore year, students begin to care for clients in Columbus hospitals and community agencies. Students have access to virtually every major health facility in the area as they learn to care for newborns and families, children, adults, and the elderly who need perinatal, medical-surgical, psychiatric, and home care. The clinical experience is characterized by a low student-faculty ratio (8:1) and individualized teaching approaches. During their senior year, students select an area of clinical practice for an intensive precepted learning experience. The Ohio Board of Nursing has adopted the guidelines for this precepted learning experience for use in all nursing education programs in the state.

Nursing students also may secure part-time positions in area health-care settings, including local long-term-care facilities, which provide students with opportunities to apply classroom learning and clinical skills through paid employment.

In addition to its baccalaureate program for traditional undergraduates, the School of Nursing also offers a bachelor's degree completion program for approximately 100 registered nurses each semester in cooperation with Capital's Adult Degree Program. Since this program began in 1987, more than 200 registered nurses have earned their Bachelor of Science in Nursing degrees, enabling them to assume even greater managerial and leadership roles in their field.

Capital University offers the Master of Science in Nursing degree, designed with an interdisciplinary approach combining nursing with concentrations in family/community health, administration, legal studies, and theological studies. In cooperation with Capital's Graduate School of Administration, its Law School, and Trinity Lutheran Seminary, dual degrees are available in nursing and administration (M.S.N./M.B.A.), nursing and law (M.S.N./J.D.), and nursing and theology (M.S.N./master's in lay ministry).

AFFILIATIONS WITH HEALTH-CARE FACILITIES

Affiliations with almost forty hospitals and community agencies provide nursing students with a wide range of clinical experiences that prepare them for the diversity of employment opportunities they will encounter upon graduation and throughout their careers. In addition, a semester-long study abroad program with The University of the West Indies provides seniors with experience in pediatric and community health nursing in Jamaica.

ACADEMIC FACILITIES

Within the School of Nursing, located in the Battelle Hall of Science and Nursing, are ten hospital beds and five modern examining rooms that provide nursing students with one of the finest skills labs in Ohio. In addition, the Helene Fuld Health Trust Learning Resources Laboratory gives student nurses access to the latest in microcomputers, instructional software, and lab equipment to enhance their studies.

LOCATION

Capital is located in the Columbus suburb of Bexley, which is primarily a residential community with a number of small shops and restaurants. Downtown Columbus is just 4 miles from campus and is easily reached by city buses. As Ohio's capital and the state's largest city, Columbus offers a wealth of cultural, educational, recreational, and social activities. Many of the city's attractions are free or offer substantial student discounts. Popular attractions include performances by the Columbus Symphony Orchestra, BalletMet, Opera Columbus, and the Columbus Jazz Orchestra; the Columbus Zoo; the Columbus Museum of Art; an expansive network of parks and bike trails; and an endless array of theaters, galleries, shops, restaurants, and sporting events.

Capital and Columbus are within a short flying time of many major U.S. cities—Chicago, Atlanta, Nashville, and New York City are within 90 minutes. The campus is approximately a 10-minute drive from Port Columbus International Airport.

STUDENT SERVICES

The School of Nursing recognizes outstanding leadership and scholarship among students through election to the Theta Theta Chapter of Sigma Theta Tau International Honor Society of Nursing.

Capital nursing students can take advantage of an extensive array of University resources to support their academic and personal development, including the University library, the Kline Health Center, a networked computer center with personal computers for student use, exercise rooms with Nautilus equipment, and a campus center that houses the University's bookstore, a theater for student stage productions, mail services, a recreation center, student organizations and publications offices, a Career Services office, the main campus dining room, and the Crusader Club snack bar. The Office of Multicultural Affairs sponsors numerous events promoting cultural awareness and diversity throughout the year. Capital's Office of International Education offers overseas study opportunities.

THE NURSING STUDENT GROUP

Graduates of the program are actively recruited for positions as staff nurses in hospitals with potential for advancement to management, for community and industrial health nursing, and for commission as officers in the armed forces. In fact, one of the largest nursing ROTC programs in the nation is at Capital. The program is one of only forty in the nation that is recognized as a Partner in Nursing Education institution by the U.S. Army.

COSTS

In 1996–97, tuition and fees for traditional undergraduate students were $14,200. Room and board fees were $4000. Additional educational expenses for nursing students include clinical fees, the summer clinical course, a nursing kit, professional liability insurance, and uniforms.

FINANCIAL AID

Part of Capital's tradition includes a commitment to helping students and parents find resources to finance their university experience. Approximately 95 percent of Capital's undergraduate students receive some form of financial assistance. Financial need is met through a combination of scholarships, fellowships, grants, loans, and employment.

By completing the Free Application for Federal Student Aid (FAFSA), a student is considered for all federal, state, and institutional funds administered by Capital.

APPLYING

Students applying for admission into the freshman class must be enrolled in, or a graduate of, a college-preparatory course of study. Students should submit their applications by early January for fall enrollment. Admission is based on a completed application file that includes a first-time student application, a $15 nonrefundable application fee, ACT or SAT I score results, an official high school transcript, and a counselor evaluation (using the form attached to the application).

Transfer students must submit the following: a transfer student application, a $15 nonrefundable application fee, official transcripts from each college or university attended, an official high school transcript, and a College/University Transfer Report (using the form attached to the application). A minimum composite grade point average of 2.5 is recommended.

A separate application procedure is in place for individuals interested in the B.S.N. Completion Program offered through Capital's Adult Degree Program.

Correspondence and Information:

Capital University
Admission Office
Columbus, Ohio 43209-2394
Telephone: 614-236-6101 (in Columbus)
800-289-6289 (toll-free)
Fax: 614-236-6820
E-mail: admissions@capital.edu

B.S.N. Completion Program
Capital University
Columbus, Ohio 43209-2394
Telephone: 614-236-6378
Fax: 614-236-6157

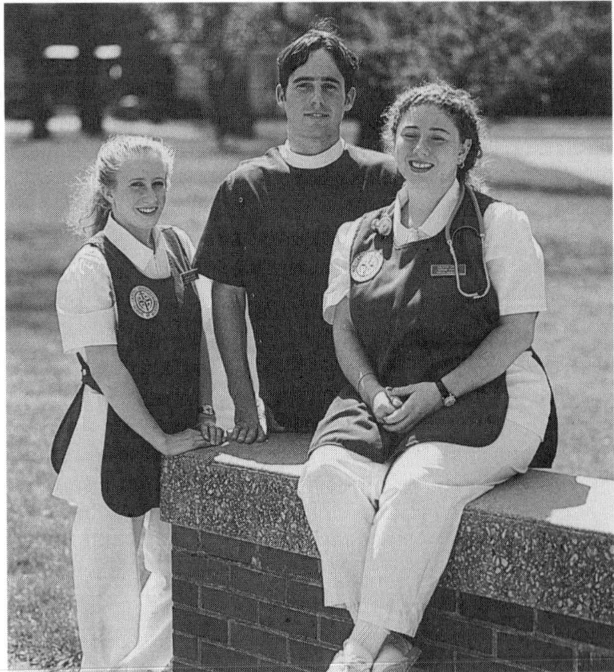

For Capital University nursing students, graduation opens the door to unlimited professional opportunities in a variety of health-care settings.

Case Western Reserve University
The Frances Payne Bolton School of Nursing
Cleveland, Ohio

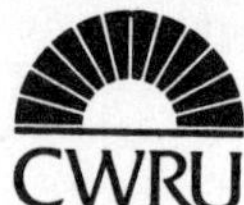

THE UNIVERSITY

Formed in 1967 by the federation of Case Institute of Technology and Western Reserve University, Case Western Reserve University is today one of the nation's major independent universities. Currently, almost 10,000 graduate and undergraduate students are enrolled in programs in the health sciences, engineering, science, management, the arts, humanities, and the social and behavioral sciences.

THE SCHOOL OF NURSING

The Frances Payne Bolton School of Nursing, one of the six professional schools of Case Western Reserve University, traces its heritage to the Lakeside Hospital Training School for Nurses, which was established in 1898. Largely as a result of a generous endowment from Frances Payne Bolton, the School of Nursing as it now exists was established in 1923, on an equal basis with other schools and colleges of the University. In addition to the Bachelor of Science in Nursing (B.S.N.), the School of Nursing offers the Master of Science in Nursing (M.S.N.), the Doctor of Nursing (N.D.), and the Doctor of Philosophy (Ph.D.) in nursing.

The School assumes responsibility for the preparation of individuals committed to excellence and leadership in scholarly inquiry and professional service locally, nationally, and internationally. Locally, the Bolton School has developed the first Nursing Health Center designed to provide both primary health-care and a birthing center in a medically underserved community. Internationally, the Bolton School is participating in projects designed to develop educational programs that will impact health-care delivery in Africa, Europe, Asia, and South America. Designation as a World Health Organization Collaborating Center underscores the School's commitment to share resources with countries throughout the world.

The Bolton School offers innovative options for study, including a large number of courses offered in an intensive semester format. This provides students an opportunity to further their nursing education while continuing to meet their professional and personal obligations.

PROGRAMS OF STUDY

The Bolton School offers the B.S.N. and an accelerated B.S.N. for registered nurses (RN-to-B.S.N.). The B.S.N. curriculum provides education in the humanistic delivery of home health and acute-care nursing in highly technical health-care settings and is a four-year program consisting of sciences, humanities, the arts, and nursing. Computer technology and nursing informatics are integrated throughout the curriculum. The RN-to-B.S.N. program may be completed on a full-time or part-time basis.

The M.S.N. degree is designed for nurses seeking preparation for advanced practice nursing. Nurses from all basic nursing programs accredited by the NLN are eligible to apply. Associate or diploma nurses may also qualify for admission to the program. The M.S.N. requires approximately 40 semester hours of study. Specialization is offered in nurse midwifery; nurse anesthesia; medical-surgical, community health, critical-care, and oncology nursing; and acute care, neonatal, adult, family, gerontological, pediatric, psychiatric–mental health, and women's health nurse practitioner studies. Baccalaureate-prepared, certified advanced practice nurses may qualify to complete the M.S.N. in 18–21 semester hours in the intensive semester format. Two dual-degree programs are also offered: an M.S.N./M.A. in anthropology and an M.S.N./M.B.A. in conjunction with the Weatherhead School of Management of Case Western Reserve University.

The Doctor of Nursing (N.D.) degree is a four-year, entry-level graduate program designed for college graduates with a baccalaureate degree in a discipline other than nursing. The first two years (levels) of the program consist of the prelicensure nursing curriculum and include all course work required to sit for the professional nursing licensing examination (NCLEX-RN). The goal of the postlicensure component of the program is to prepare students for advanced practice and clinical research in nursing. Clinical specialties offered at this level are nurse midwifery and adult, family, gerontological, pediatric, psychiatric–mental health, and women's health nurse practitioner studies. Entry into level III of the program requires a license to practice nursing and is available to graduates of baccalaureate nursing programs. Master's-prepared, nationally certified, advanced practice nurses may qualify for entry to level IV of the N.D. program.

The Ph.D. program is designed for individuals who seek preparation in research and who have completed either an M.S.N. degree with a clinical nursing major or at least 24 semester hours of graduate study, including 12 semester hours of supervised clinical nursing practice. The Ph.D. student concentrates on the organization and development of nursing knowledge.

ACADEMIC FACILITIES

The School of Nursing is located in the University Health Sciences Center, which has modern research and laboratory space, computer and audiovisual facilities, and library resources. The Health Sciences Center is adjacent to the University Hospitals of Cleveland, an aggregate of specialized hospitals with over 900 beds.

LOCATION

The University is located in University Circle, a cultural extension of the campus, which comprises 500 acres of parks, gardens, theaters, schools, hospitals, churches, and human service institutions. The Cleveland Museum of Art, the Cleveland Museum of Natural History, and Severance Hall, home of the Cleveland Orchestra, are within walking distance. Downtown Cleveland is 10 minutes by RTA rapid transit, which also runs from University Circle directly to Cleveland Hopkins International Airport.

STUDENT SERVICES

The University offers students a wide variety of services, including a 24-hour health service whose staff includes nurse practitioners and counselors. Free access to fitness equipment is available to all students, and a full-service fitness center is available for a fee. Three day-care centers in University Circle are used by University faculty, staff, and students. International students receive guidance and assistance from the Office of International Student Services.

THE NURSING STUDENT GROUP

During 1996–97, the Bolton School enrolled 300 undergraduate students and 410 graduate students. Students come from thirty-five states and twelve other countries. Over half of the students are registered nurses, working in hospitals, clinics, academic settings, and research.

COSTS

For the 1996–97 academic year, tuition was $713 per semester hour for students taking 1 to 11 credit hours and $17,100 for students taking 12 to 17 credit hours. Books and supplies cost approximately $700 per year. Undergraduate students are required to live on campus. Housing costs ranged from $2960 to $3850. For graduate students, there are a variety of options available on and off campus. Graduate dormitory costs ranged from $3110 to $3550. University meal plans ranged in cost from $1830 to $2430. The University requires students to have health insurance and offers a policy for approximately $600 per year. This fee may be waived if the student can demonstrate coverage from an outside source.

FINANCIAL AID

Each year, 102 undergraduate applicants identified as Bolton Scholars receive paid awards of 50 percent of tuition. A family financial statement is not required, and the award is not based on need. Additional financial assistance is available through grants, loans, and work-study. Additional information is available from the Office of Financial Aid at Case Western Reserve University.

At the graduate level, financial assistance is awarded through grants, scholarships, loans, and work agreements. Information may be obtained from the Office of Student Services at the School of Nursing.

APPLYING

Applicants to all programs should present appropriate transcripts, letters of recommendation, and testing information as described in the *School of Nursing Bulletin.* The programs of study for the B.S.N., the M.S.N. in nurse anesthesia, and the N.D. prelicensure curriculum begin in the fall term each year. Students in all other programs may begin in the fall, spring, or summer term. The application deadline for the B.S.N. and the M.S.N. in nurse anesthesia is January 15. Applications for all other programs are processed on a rolling basis and must be completed two months before the term begins. It is recommended that students apply at least six months prior to the term in which they intend to enroll. Applicants are encouraged to contact the Department of Student Services with any questions they may have.

Correspondence and Information:

Office of Student Services
Frances Payne Bolton School of Nursing
Case Western Reserve University
10900 Euclid Avenue
Cleveland, Ohio 44106-4904
Telephone: 216-368-2529
800-825-2540 Ext. 2529 (toll-free)
E-mail: emv4@po.cwru.edu (freeNet)

THE FACULTY

Kim Adams-Davis, Assistant Professor; N.D., Case Western Reserve.
Gene C. Anderson, Professor; Ph.D., Wisconsin.
Claire M. Andrews, Associate Professor; Ph.D., Wayne State.
Mary K. Anthony, Assistant Professor; Ph.D., Case Western Reserve.
Susan E. Auvil-Novak, Assistant Professor; Ph.D., Texas at Austin.
Carol E. Blixen, Associate Professor; Ph.D., Brandeis.
Dorothy Brooten, Professor; Ph.D., Pennsylvania.
Barbara Daly, Associate Professor; Ph.D., Bowling Green.
Sara L. Douglas, Assistant Professor; Ph.D., Illinois State.
Donna Dowling, Assistant Professor; M.N., Illinois.
Sue V. Fink, Assistant Professor; Ph.D., Michigan.
Joyce J. Fitzpatrick, Elizabeth Brooks Ford Professor of Nursing and Dean; Ph.D., NYU.
Marion Good, Assistant Professor; Ph.D., Case Western Reserve.
Gloria Harman, Assistant Professor; Ph.D., Case Western Reserve.
Marie R. Haug, Professor Emeritus; Ph.D., Case Western Reserve.
Laura L. Hayman, Professor; Ph.D., Pennsylvania.
Marion M. Hemstrom, Assistant Professor; D.N.Sc., Rush.
Patricia A. Higgins, Assistant Professor; Ph.D., Case Western Reserve.
Hae-Ok Lee, Assistant Professor; D.N.S., California, San Francisco.
Elizabeth A. Madigan, Assistant Professor; Ph.D., Case Western Reserve.
Ida M. Martinson, Carl W. and Margaret Davis Walter Visiting Professor of Pediatric Nursing; Ph.D., Illinois at Chicago.
Patricia E. McDonald, Assistant Professor; Ph.D., Case Western Reserve.
Graham J. McDougall Jr., Assistant Professor; Ph.D., Texas at Austin.
Doris M. Modly, Professor; Ph.D., Case Western Reserve.
Shirley M. Moore, Associate Professor; Ph.D., Case Western Reserve.
Diana Morris, Assistant Professor; Ph.D., Case Western Reserve.
Carol M. Musil, Assistant Professor; Ph.D., Case Western Reserve.
Sandra Fulton Picot, Assistant Professor; Ph.D., Maryland.
Beverly L. Roberts, Associate Professor; Ph.D., Case Western Reserve.
Shyang-Yun Pam Shiao, Assistant Professor; Ph.D., Case Western Reserve.
Theresa S. Standing, Assistant Professor; Ph.D., Case Western Reserve.
Debera J. Thomas, Assistant Professor; D.N.S., SUNY at Buffalo.
Lucille L. Travis, Assistant Professor; Ph.D., Ohio State.
Marie Linda Ann Workman, Associate Professor; Ph.D., Cincinnati.
May L. Wykle, Florence Cellar Professor of Nursing and Associate Dean for Community Affairs; Ph.D., Case Western Reserve.
JoAnne M. Youngblut, Associate Professor; Ph.D., Michigan.
Jaclene A. Zauszniewski, Associate Professor; Ph.D., Case Western Reserve.

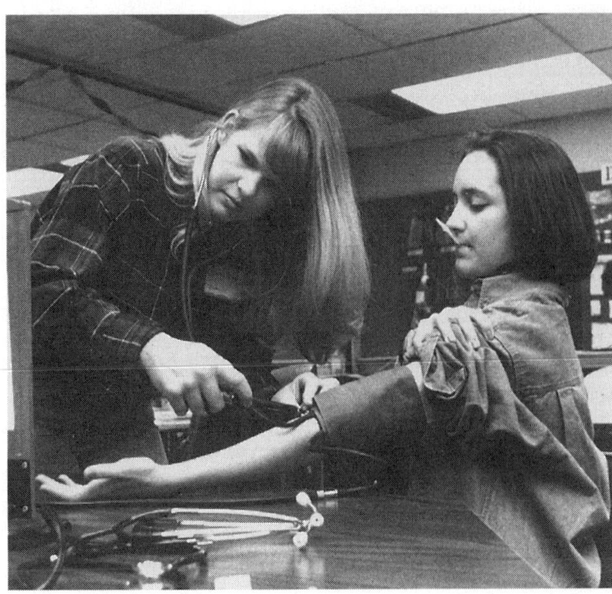

Nursing students develop their clinical skills in the School's multipurpose lab.

Clayton College & State University
School of Health Sciences
Department of Baccalaureate Degree Nursing
Morrow, Georgia

THE UNIVERSITY

Clayton College & State University (CCSU) offers the advantages of an intimate academic setting with small classes and personalized instruction. Students receive excellent preparation for professional practice, including technology and concepts for the twenty-first century.

Founded in 1969, CCSU is a part of the University System of Georgia. More than 5,000 students from Atlanta's "Southern Crescent," every region of the United States, and fifty countries pursue degrees in more than seventy different areas that range from early music to health sciences. The average age of students is 28, with nontraditional students comprising approximately 65 percent of the enrollment. One third of the students are under the age of 22. In addition, 29 percent of the students are members of minority groups. CCSU also facilitates the continuing education goals of 60,000 individuals annually, making the program the second largest in Georgia.

All CCSU students have access to the vigorous, thriving metropolitan area of Atlanta as well as ever-expanding ties to the international community. These ties benefit the growing co-op and internship experiences available to students. CCSU has more than 135 full-time faculty members. Two thirds of the faculty members teaching in programs leading to the baccalaureate degree hold the highest degrees in their field.

Clayton College & State University has a demonstrated commitment of service to its community and region. CCSU incorporates five common elements in all of its programs and services: developing effective communication, recognizing and responding to the increasingly global context of our society, promoting community-based experiential learning to create durable and meaningful connections between education and all other aspects of life, focusing on continuous education and growth, and understanding and developing a facility with modern technology. CCSU's core mission is to provide superior career-oriented studies that will prepare students to succeed in the world of work in the twenty-first century.

The University is accredited by the Southern Association of Colleges and Schools. Health sciences programs are accredited by the Commission on Dental Accreditation of the American Dental Association and the National League for Nursing, and are approved by the Georgia Board of Nursing.

CCSU students can participate in intercollegiate competition in men's basketball, cross-country, golf, and soccer and in women's basketball, cross-country, soccer, and tennis. The Laker athletic programs hold provisional NCAA Division II membership.

THE DEPARTMENT OF NURSING

The goal of the School of Health Sciences Department of Baccalaureate Degree Nursing is to provide educational excellence in nursing and health care through a caring and supportive environment. The Department facilitates student understanding of the complex, changing, and increasingly interprofessional health-care environment. The overall objective of the Department is to educate health-care providers with a broad base of knowledge, so that they are able to care for diverse populations.

Courses are outcome-based and are assessed by a teaching faculty of whom 50 percent hold doctorates. The student-teacher ratio is 20:1 in the classroom and 8:1 in clinical settings. The program gives students great flexibility in terms of class schedules and in course sequencing. Part-time, full-time, evening, day, and year-round classes are available and are geared to the working student.

A new nurse-managed clinic and wellness center (for students and faculty and community members) contribute to the nursing program directly and indirectly.

PROGRAMS OF STUDY

The School of Health Sciences Department of Baccalaureate Degree Nursing offers two tracks—basic licensure and RN/B.S.N.—leading to the Bachelor of Science in Nursing degree, and a dual degree (B.S.N./B.S.) in health-care management.

The basic licensure track is for students seeking entry into the nursing profession who do not currently hold licensure as registered nurses. Students build upon a solid liberal arts background in the upper-division nursing and elective courses. Admission is contingent upon successful completion of the general education core with at least a 2.5 GPA. Accelerated placement into nursing is available for candidates currently holding a baccalaureate or higher degree in another area of study. Students may progress full- or part-time in this track. A weekend study option is also available.

The RN/B.S.N. track provides registered nurses who are graduates of associate degree or diploma nursing programs with the upper-division course work necessary to remain competitive in the ever-changing health-care environment. This track builds upon previously attained knowledge and experiences and recognizes the unique educational needs and abilities of adult learners. CCSU's RN/B.S.N. track participates in the Georgia Statewide Articulation Model. Validation of 37 quarter credits in nursing is provided through this model. Additional advanced standing credit is available through CLEP testing and other validation of prior learning.

The dual degree B.S.N./B.S. in Health Care Management allows students to compete more effectively in a market-driven, competitive health-care environment. Students choosing this option complete an additional 55 quarter hours of prescribed credit in order to receive the second baccalaureate degree. The dual degree graduate will have both the practical skills and leadership qualifications demanded by the industry.

AFFILIATIONS WITH HEALTH-CARE FACILITIES

The CCSU School of Health Sciences has affiliations with a variety of health-care facilities, giving students a choice of working in rural, suburban, or inner-city settings or in private industry or government and a choice of caring for a variety of patients from neonatal to geriatric. The School is affiliated with the following Georgia institutions: Southern Regional Medical Center, Riverdale; DeKalb Medical Center, Decatur; Grady Memorial Hospital, Atlanta; Henry Medical Center, Stockbridge; St. Joseph's Hospital, Atlanta; Scottish Rite Children's Medical Center, Atlanta; Egleston Children's Hospital; South Fulton Medical Center, East Point; Vencor, Atlanta; Wesley Woods Geriatric Center, Atlanta; and numerous city, county, and state health departments.

ACADEMIC FACILITIES
The campus library has a reference and circulating print collection of more than 62,000 volumes, 26,000 pieces of audiovisual software, and a Media Services Division as well as access to on-line computer services and the new University System of Georgia GALILEO on-line library system with 1,100 academic journals and access to 7 million volumes. CCSU also has a Learning Center and a cooperative education program.

Educational program collaboration is a major emphasis at CCSU, the only university in Georgia that collaborates with other schools to create local Centers for Higher Education. The collaborative approach provides educational opportunities close to home/work for potential students in counties where college access would otherwise require a long commute. The Centers in Rockdale and Fayette Counties have been developed in collaboration with DeKalb, DeKalb Tech, and the Rockdale Public Schools and in collaboration with the Fayette County Board of Education, the Board of Commissioners, and Griffin Tech. The Fulton County Center for Lifelong Learning has been developed with the Fulton County School System.

Distance learning via interactive video and computer networks, including GSAMS, Media One Cable, Georgia Public Television, and the Public Broadcasting System, are major initiatives now under way.

LOCATION
CCSU is located on Georgia's Highway 54 North, one mile from I-75 South's exit 76 and 10 minutes south of Atlanta's Hartsfield International Airport. The University is located on 163 acres of parkland; the lakes, trees, and waterfowl make it one of the most beautiful campuses in the South. CCSU provides a peaceful and safe environment that is conducive to learning.

STUDENT SERVICES
CCSU's versatile student services attend to the needs of its diverse student body. These services include career counseling and placement, computer-guided career assistance, counseling, a wellness program, a nurse-managed clinic, a minority advising program, and multicultural and veterans' affairs services.

THE NURSING STUDENT GROUP
The more than 300 CCSU nursing students represent a diverse mix ethnically and professionally and by age. Approximately 15 percent are originally licensed overseas, 45 percent are members of minority groups, and 15 percent are male. The University enrolls 2 percent of all registered nurses nationwide to its upper-division completion track.

Students at CCSU may participate in numerous opportunities designed to enhance professional development. The Baccalaureate Organization for Nursing Development (BOND) is open to RN/B.S.N. students. This group provides mentorship and support for the RN returning student. The CCSU chapter of the Georgia Association of Nursing Students (GANS) is open to all nursing students. GANS is an affiliate of the National Student Nurses Association (NSNA). CCSU also houses the Xi Rho Chapter of Sigma Theta Tau, the international honor society for nursing. Membership is selective and is based on the student's ability to demonstrate scholarship and leadership potential. Students must have a minimum 3.0 GPA and be in the upper third of the B.S.N. class.

CCSU graduates have gone to work for such prestigious health-care-related facilities as the Centers for Disease Control and Prevention and Emory University Hospital, both in Atlanta. Graduates are also employed in health maintenance organizations, private medical practices, clinics, hospitals, home-care agencies, long-term-care facilities, and in private industry. More than 50 percent of CCSU's baccalaureate graduates return to school for a master's degree and, according to their reports, have found themselves well prepared for graduate school.

COSTS
Quarterly tuition and fees for the 1997–98 academic year are $528 for 12 quarter credit hours or more and $44 per quarter hour for fewer than 12 credit hours for Georgia residents. They are $1824 for 12 quarter hours or more and $152 per quarter hour for fewer than 12 quarter credit hours for nonresidents. In addition, each student pays a $66 student activities/athletic fee and a $20 parking/Universal Card fee per quarter. Nursing courses requiring a lab have an additional fee of $15.

FINANCIAL AID
The University offers several federal, state, and private financial aid programs, including loans, grants, scholarships (which include Georgia's HOPE Scholarship), and work-study plans. CCSU also offers State Direct Health Career loans (SDHC). These loans are based on career choice, and students may cancel repayment of SDHC loans by practicing their profession in Georgia for one calendar year.

APPLYING
Applicants to the nursing programs must have completed a minimum of 45 quarter credit hours of prerequisites, hold a baccalaureate or higher degree, or be currently registered nurses. Admission to the basic licensure track is competitive and spaces are limited. Admission to the RN/B.S.N. track is available for each academic term. At the present time, there are no restrictions on the number of enrollees. All applicants to any nursing track must meet application guidelines and deadlines published by CCSU. High school graduates may apply for admission to CCSU; however, meeting the admission standards for the University does not guarantee admission to nursing.

Correspondence and Information:

Admissions Office
Clayton College & State University
5900 North Lee Street
P.O. Box 285
Morrow, Georgia 30260
Telephone: 770-961-3500
770-961-3484 (School of Health Sciences)
E-mail: burley@cc.clayton.edu
World Wide Web: http://www.clayton.edu/

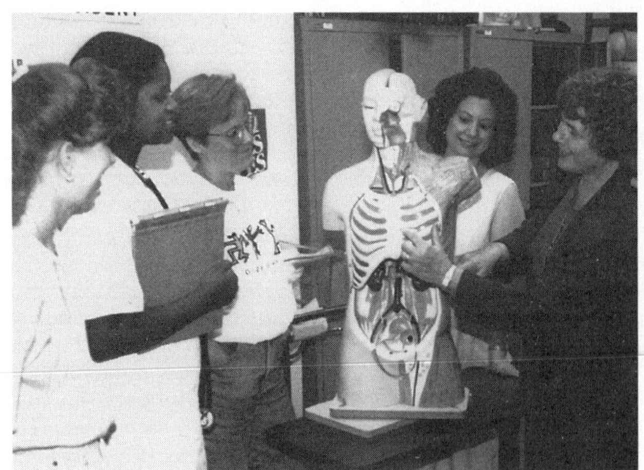

RN/B.S.N. students examine a torso model in nursing assessment class at Clayton College & State University.

Colby-Sawyer College
Department of Nursing
New London, New Hampshire

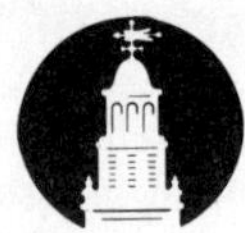

THE COLLEGE

Colby-Sawyer College, a coeducational, residential undergraduate college founded in 1837 and evolving out of the New England academy tradition, has been engaged in higher education since 1928. The College provides programs of study that innovatively integrate the liberal arts and sciences with professional preparation. Through all of its programs, the College encourages students of varied backgrounds and abilities to realize their full intellectual and personal potential so that they may gain understanding about themselves, others, and the major forces shaping today's rapidly changing and pluralistic world. At present, students come from all over the United States and from seven other countries, with 70 percent of the students coming from outside of New Hampshire.

Colby-Sawyer has a distinguished faculty dedicated to undergraduate teaching, and a personalized education is assured by the 14:1 student-faculty ratio and average class size of 18. The College is accredited by the New England Association of Schools and Colleges, and professional programs carry the appropriate accreditations. Colby-Sawyer has repeatedly been recognized by *U.S. News & World Report* as one of the top ten colleges in its category.

THE DEPARTMENT OF NURSING

Nursing students at Colby-Sawyer experience great individual support and guidance in their development as professionals, which results in high achievement rates and measurable success upon graduation.

The Department of Nursing offers students unique opportunities for clinical internships in a variety of settings, from an Ivy League teaching institution such as Dartmouth-Hitchcock Medical Center to acclaimed community health centers like New London Hospital and Lake Sunapee Home Care and Hospice to Concord Hospital, an institution known for its vision and creativity in serving both urban and rural areas.

The faculty members in the Department of Nursing have diverse and extensive experience in both practice and teaching. The College's faculty members are graduates of the finest schools and colleges of nursing in the country. They have practiced in a variety of renowned settings and are known for their scholarship and professional work.

PROGRAM OF STUDY

The Department of Nursing offers the Bachelor of Science degree with a major in nursing. The nursing major emphasizes professional study grounded in the liberal arts. Students are prepared to be knowledgeable, caring, and technologically competent nurses who will independently and collaboratively provide care to the client with a sensitivity to individual needs.

In its students, the program develops accountability and abilities to communicate effectively in a therapeutic situation and to intervene successfully in clinical situations. The Colby-Sawyer program promotes personal and professional growth as well as contributions to society and the nursing profession. Upon completion of the program, graduates are eligible to take the National Council Licensure Examination for Registered Nurses (NCLEX-RN) in New Hampshire, are prepared for professional nursing practice in hospital and community settings, and have been provided with a foundation for graduate study.

Students must take a minimum of 120 credit hours to graduate. The curriculum includes core courses in the liberal arts, mathematics, and science as well as nursing-specific courses. Nursing courses cover a range of topics and issues, including health assessment and skills, pathophysiological concepts, pharmacological therapeutics, health attainment, social health concerns, health enhancement, and health optimization. Clinical internships begin during the sophomore year of the program, continue through graduation, and provide extensive practical experiences. The clinical courses allow students to synthesize the knowledge and skills needed to coordinate and deliver professional nursing care. Students work under the mentorship of a clinical preceptor to achieve competence in providing safe, effective care at a novice level of clinical practice as a graduate nurse.

The Department of Nursing at Colby-Sawyer College offers a flexible and innovative program of study for a registered nurse (RN) who is a graduate of an accredited associate degree program or a diploma program. The B.S. degree assures upward mobility for RNs seeking a baccalaureate education by meeting their unique needs while maintaining the high standards of the College and of the profession of nursing. Faculty members who are experts in the nursing specialties are available as academic advisers to assist in planning a program of study tailored to the student's professional and personal life. The program provides opportunities for new learning in community health, nursing research, and health-care management. Individually designed leadership experiences examine the humanistic, technological, ethical, economic, and legal issues challenging the rapidly changing health-care system.

The nursing program is approved by the New Hampshire Board of Nursing and accredited by the National League for Nursing.

AFFILIATIONS WITH HEALTH-CARE FACILITIES

The nursing program is enriched by its relationship with Dartmouth-Hitchcock Medical Center, one of the most thoroughly equipped and technologically advanced teaching hospitals in North America. The program is also affiliated with Concord and New London hospitals.

ACADEMIC FACILITIES

The College, through its strong commitment to the Department, has provided a state-of-the-art Nursing and Health Laboratory. The laboratory equipment ranges from the finest fundamental instruments to advanced critical-care technology. The Department also has a Computer Assisted Learning Laboratory to support students in their course work and prepare them for the registered nurse licensing examination. Students also have access to an interactive videodisc/CD-ROM computer laboratory that enables them to participate in critical procedures before their first hospital clinical experience in their sophomore year.

The Susan Colgate Cleveland Library/Learning Center has 70,000 volumes, 575 periodical subscriptions, and 118,500 microforms. Access to these materials is provided by a Dynix automated catalog system and by on-line and CD-ROM databases for periodical research. The center also houses a curriculum lab, an audiovisual room, and a networked computer classroom with twenty-four PCs and CD-ROM interactive multimedia teaching equipment. Interlibrary loan service provides access to library holdings throughout New England and beyond.

The Academic Development Center at James House provides one-on-one peer tutorials that range from developmental to honors levels. The staff consists of faculty, peer tutors (student academic counselors), and two learning specialists who assist students with learning differences. Among the services available to students with diagnosed learning differences are classroom modifications, personal counseling, and professional as well as peer tutoring. The Academic Development Center also works with all students to enhance word processing skills, essay composition, and the study skills necessary for successful college time management, note-taking, and exam preparation.

The Colby-Sawyer campus computing environment includes five computer laboratory/classrooms and six mobile multimedia teaching stations, which provide computer graphics and audiovisual capabilities using the latest CD-ROM technology. Computing facilities were recently enhanced by a $250,000 grant to provide 100 brand new IBM-type Model 486 personal computers equipped with the latest Microsoft Windows applications, 30 Macintoshes, and 40 laser and ink-jet printers for student and faculty use. The College now has an 11:1 student-computer ratio. Internet access is available through the Library/Learning Center.

LOCATION

Colby-Sawyer's 80-acre campus is located on the crest of a hill in New London, New Hampshire. Its beautifully maintained grounds and stately Georgian architecture create a picturesque and safe environment that is conducive to learning. Colby-Sawyer is located in the heart of the Dartmouth–Lake Sunapee region, a four-season recreational and cultural community known for the natural beauty of its lakes and mountains. Boston is only 1½ hours away and Montreal is 3½ hours away, so students have access to these major cities by van or bus. The nearby seacoast at Portsmouth and the surrounding lakes, mountains, and state parks provide opportunities for hiking, camping, golf, tennis, canoeing, swimming, ice skating, and Nordic and Alpine skiing. Arts and cultural opportunities can be found in New London as well as in nearby Concord, the state capital, and Hanover, the home of Dartmouth College.

STUDENT SERVICES

There are eight varsity sports for women (NCAA Division III basketball, soccer, tennis, lacrosse, volleyball, and track and field; NCAA Division I Alpine ski racing; and IHSA riding) and seven for men (NCAA Division III basketball, soccer, tennis, baseball, and track and field; NCAA Division I Alpine ski racing; and IHSA riding).

All students are members of the Student Government Association, which is structured to provide considerable interaction among student representatives, faculty, and administration. In addition, there are numerous groups that provide students with leadership possibilities outside of the classroom, which include the Campus Activities Board (CAB), the dance club, Alpha Chi honor society, yearbook, Admissions Key Association, Art Students' League, Film Society, Student Nurses Association, community service, Environmental Action Committee (EAC), AIDS/HIV Educators, radio station, drama club, *The Courier* (newspaper), and other clubs and intramural sports.

The Dan and Kathleen Hogan Sports Center contains a large field house with three multipurpose courts, a suspended walking/jogging track, a six-lane NCAA-size swimming pool, and a fitness center furnished with top-flight equipment.

THE NURSING STUDENT GROUP

There are currently 100 nursing major students at Colby-Sawyer College.

COSTS

For 1996–97, the comprehensive fee, which includes tuition, room, board, and fees, was $21,480. Tuition was $15,530, room was $3270, and board was $2680. Approximately $1700 should be allowed for travel, books, supplies, and personal expenses.

FINANCIAL AID

Through its financial aid program, Colby-Sawyer encourages the attendance of students from a variety of ethnic and cultural backgrounds, economic levels, and geographic regions. Sixty-three percent of the students currently receive some form of financial assistance, and Colby-Sawyer provides more than $3 million a year in grant assistance to its students. Both need-based and merit awards are available, including recently established merit awards for outstanding academic achievement or student leadership. Merit awards are also available for students with special talents in art, music, or creative writing and for students who have been significantly involved in community service. Each applicant must submit the Free Application for Federal Student Aid (FAFSA) and the Colby-Sawyer Application for Financial Aid. Candidates for merit awards must also submit the Application for Merit Awards. Priority will be given to students who complete and postmark all forms on or before the March 1 deadline. A modest amount of financial assistance is available for international students.

APPLYING

The College recommends that prospective students present at least 15 units of college-preparatory work. The usual program includes 4 years of English, 3 years of mathematics, 2 or more years of social studies, and 2 or more years of a laboratory science. Prospective nursing students should have completed courses in biology and chemistry or physics. Colby-Sawyer operates on a rolling admission system. Once they are complete, applications are reviewed beginning in December, and candidates are generally notified within two to three weeks. A completed application includes a transcript of the candidate's high school work (including first-quarter grades for the senior year), SAT I or ACT scores, two letters of recommendation (one from a teacher and one from a guidance professional), a personal statement, and a $40 nonrefundable application fee. While an admissions interview is not required, every applicant is encouraged to visit Colby-Sawyer for a tour and interview. Interviews often play an important part in the final admissions decision.

Correspondence and Information:

Office of Admissions
Colby-Sawyer College
100 Main Street
New London, New Hampshire 03257
Telephone: 603-526-3700
800-272-1015 (toll-free)
Fax: 603-526-3452

Columbia University
School of Nursing
New York, New York

THE UNIVERSITY

By royal charter of King George II of England, Columbia University was founded in 1754 as King's College. It is the oldest institution of higher learning in New York State and the fifth-largest in the nation. A private, nonsectarian institution, Columbia University has, since its inception, addressed the issues of the moment, making important contributions to American life through teaching and research. It is organized into fifteen schools and is associated with more than seventy research and public service institutions and twenty-two scholarly journals. One of its most notable affiliations is with the research-oriented Columbia–Presbyterian Medical Center. The Presbyterian Hospital, together with the Health Science Division of Columbia University, which includes the Schools of Medicine, Dental and Oral Surgery, Nursing, and Public Health and programs in physical therapy, nutrition, and occupational therapy, constitute the University's Health Science Campus. Total enrollment is close to 2,500 at the Health Science Campus and nearly 17,500 at the Morningside Campus.

THE SCHOOL OF NURSING

Founded in 1892 as the Presbyterian Hospital School of Nursing, the School began offering baccalaureate degrees when it joined Columbia University's Faculty of Medicine in 1937. In 1956, it became the first nursing program in the country to award a master's degree in a clinical nursing specialty. The School currently offers educational programs at the graduate, advanced certificate, and doctoral levels. Underlying these programs is the belief that nursing is a practicing art that is dedicated to the health of the people. Acquisition of knowledge of the art and science of nursing and development of skills to implement this knowledge enable the nurse to fulfill the goals of providing comfort with compassion, promoting the optimal level of health, and acting effectively during periods of illness. Curricula are evaluated on a continual basis to maintain high academic standards and to ensure that graduates meet the needs of a dynamic society and advance the profession.

The faculty has substantial experience in curriculum and instructional design, and its members maintain expertise in their areas of teaching responsibility through participation at local, regional, and national conferences; involvement in scholarly presentations and publications; and faculty practice. There are more than 50 full- and part-time faculty members and more than 100 associates.

In addition to its nursing programs, the School sponsors four centers: the Center for Child and Adolescent Health, the Center for Urban Health Policy Studies, the Center for AIDS Research, and the Center for Advanced Practice.

PROGRAMS OF STUDY

The School of Nursing offers four levels of educational programs. The Entry to Practice (ETP) Program is an accelerated combined-degree program (B.S./M.S.) for non-nurse baccalaureate prepared graduates, designed to prepare the student for a career as an advanced practice nurse. Academic studies are closely integrated with clinical experience. Phase I of the program consists of 60 credits that are completed in twelve months of full-time study. Upon completion, the B.S. degree is granted and the graduate is eligible to take the professional nurse licensure examination in any state. In Phase II, the post-licensure M.S. phase, the student follows the curriculum for a clinical specialty, which is described later in this section. Part-time study is available in Phase II.

The Accelerated Master's Program (AMP) is also a combined-degree program (B.S./M.S.), designed to further the educational and career goals of RNs who have a diploma or Associate Degree in Nursing and at least 60 liberal arts credits. Phase I consists of 31 credits of course work and 30 credits granted through the successful completion of the NLN's Nursing Mobility Profile II exams. With full-time study, this B.S./M.S. program can be completed in five semesters; however, part-time study is available for both phases.

The Graduate Program, leading to the M.S. degree, affords baccalaureate-prepared nurses the opportunity to increase their knowledge in advanced nursing practice. The school currently offers ten graduate majors that prepare qualified professionals to function as nurse practitioners. These clinical majors include anesthesia, critical-care, psychiatric–mental health nursing, midwifery, oncology, the primary-care specialties (adult, family, geriatric, and pediatric), and women's health. The credit requirements range from 45 to 51 and are allocated among core, major, and elective courses. Cross-site curricula are available in selected programs. Joint degrees are available with the Schools of Public Health and Business.

The Advanced Certificate Program allows RNs with a master's degree in nursing to pursue an advanced practice program as a nurse practitioner. The credit requirements range from 22 to 34 credits.

The Doctor of Nursing Science Program is designed to prepare clinical nurse scholars to examine, shape, and refine the health-care delivery system. The program consists of 90 credits beyond the baccalaureate degree. Of these, 45 credits are credits earned at the master's level in a clinical specialist/nurse practitioner program. All students are expected to be certified in a clinical specialty.

AFFILIATIONS WITH HEALTH-CARE FACILITIES

The center of clinical activity at the Health Science Campus is the Columbia–Presbyterian Medical Center, which includes a number of world-renowned facilities. Among the most notable are the Neurological Institute, the Eye Institute, Babies Hospital, Sloane Hospital for Women, the Center for Geriatrics and Gerontology, the Organ Transplant Center, and the Center for Health Promotion and Disease Prevention. In addition, approximately 150 other sites in the tristate area are available for clinical education.

ACADEMIC FACILITIES

The Augustus C. Long Library is the fourth-largest academic medical library in the country and is part of the Columbia University Library system, which encompasses approximately forty libraries and over 4 million volumes. The Long Library houses over 400,000 volumes and receives over 4,500 journals, most of which can be accessed through on-line computer search programs. The Media and Computer Center contains over 3,000 audiovisual and computer-assisted instruction programs including slides, videodiscs, tapes, and a wide variety of personal computer applications. Other services include microfilming, interlibrary loans, study and conference facilities, and photocopying services. The Special Collections Section houses several thousand rare works including the Florence Nightingale Collection, which is featured at exhibitions along with rare holdings of Freud and Webster.

The School of Nursing's Technology Learning Center contains seven patient units, which provide a hands-on environment for developing psychomotor skills, as well as state-of-the-art computer-assisted monitoring equipment that simulates a real clinical environment.

LOCATION

The School of Nursing is located on the Health Science Campus, a 20-acre campus overlooking the Hudson River on Manhattan's Upper West Side. Students can avail themselves of the recreational, cultural, and educational events and entertainment that have made New York City famous.

STUDENT SERVICES

The Office of Student Affairs is the hub of all student projects, programs, and services, and it coordinates activities with many other departments. Among the services provided and organizations are housing, dining, health, athletic facilities, a Wellness Program, counseling and advisement, parking, shuttle bus, financial aid, a bookstore, orientation, student records, the Office of Multicultural Affairs, Disability Services, and the International Student Office.

THE NURSING STUDENT GROUP

The over 600 students enrolled in the School of Nursing represent a diverse group of nursing professionals. They come from all over the country, but most are from the tristate area.

COSTS

During the 1996–97 academic year, tuition for undergraduates was $629 per credit. For graduate students, tuition was $629 per didactic credit and $793 per clinical credit. Average housing costs on the Health Science Campus were $5749 for a twelve-month period. Other expenses, including health fees, books, personal expenses, transportation, and uniforms, were estimated at $5018.

FINANCIAL AID

The goal of the School of Nursing financial aid program is to provide as many students as possible with sufficient resources to meet their needs and to distribute funds to eligible students in a fair and equitable manner. Financial aid is met through a combination of scholarships, grants, work, and loans. Students should be able to meet all expenses for the academic year through a combination of these resources.

APPLYING

Applications are accepted throughout the year (please call for deadlines). Admission is based on past academic and professional performance. Admission requirements include an application form with fee, a typed personal statement describing professional goals and aspirations, three letters of reference, official transcripts from all postsecondary schools, official scores on the GRE or MAT, an undergraduate course in statistics, and an interview (by invitation). Applicants to all programs must have a minimum cumulative grade point average of 3.0. Applicants to the ETP program must have 9–12 credits of science (i.e., biology, chemistry, and physics). All RN applicants must submit a copy of their current license and registration and have a course in physical assessment and a minimum of one year of clinical experience in nursing in an area relevant to their chosen clinical major. There are additional requirements for the D.N.Sc. program.

Correspondence and Information:

Dr. Theresa M. Doddato, Ed.D., Associate Dean
Columbia University School of Nursing
630 West 168th Street
New York, New York 10032
Telephone: 212-305-5756
Fax: 212-305-3680

THE FACULTY

The following is a list of full-time faculty members in the School of Nursing.

Joyce Anastasi, Assistant Professor and Director, HIV/AIDS Program; Ph.D., Adelphi. AIDS, HIV symptomology.

Carolyn Auerhahn, Assistant Professor and Director, Geriatric Nurse Practitioner Program; Ed.D., Columbia Teachers College.

Barbara Barnum, Professor of Clinical Nursing; Ph.D., Chicago; RN.

Mary Byrne, Assistant Professor and Director, Women's Health Practitioner Program; Ph.D., Adelphi. High-risk families.

Sarah Sheets Cook, Assistant Professor and Associate Dean of Academic/Clinical Affairs; M.Ed., Columbia.

Renee D'Auita, Assistant Professor of Clinical Nursing and Director, Adult Nurse Practitioner Program; M.S.N., Columbia; ANP.

Theresa M. Doddato, Assistant Professor, Associate Dean of Student Affairs, and Director of Nurse Anesthesia Program; Ed.D., Columbia Teachers College; CRNA. Technology in primary care.

Jennifer Dohrn, Instructor; M.S.N., Columbia; CNM.

Joanne Falletta, Assistant Professor of Clinical Nursing; M.S.N., M.P.H., Columbia.

Mary Ann Feldstein, Assistant Professor and Director of Psychiatric–Mental Health Program; Ed.D., Columbia; Certified Child and Adolescent Psychiatric Specialist. Family therapy and grieving.

Donna A. Gaffney, Assistant Professor and Director, Entry to Practice Program; D.N.Sc., Pennsylvania; Certified Child and Adolescent Psychiatric Clinical Specialist. Children's fears, adolescent suicide.

Richard Garfield, Assistant Professor; Dr.P.H., Columbia. Health policy and community access patterns for health care, epidemiology.

Kristine Gebbie, Assistant Professor of Nursing; Dr.P.H., Michigan.

Marianne Glasel, Instructor and Director, Oncology and Accelerated Master's Program; M.S., CUNY, Hunter.

Barbara Hackley, Assistant Professor of Clinical Nursing; M.S.N., Columbia.

Libby Hall, Assistant Professor of Clinical Nursing; M.S., FNP.

Judy Honig, Instructor and Director, Pediatric Nurse Practitioner Program; Ed.D., Columbia; PNP.

Sherry Ikalowych, Instructor in Clinical Nursing; M.S.N., Columbia; CRNA.

Elizabeth Lenz, Professor of Nursing Research and Associate Dean/Director of Doctoral Program; Ph.D., Delaware.

Ronnie Lichtman, Assistant Professor and Director of Nurse Midwifery Program; M.S., Columbia; CNM.

Mary Jo Manley, Associate Dean of Academic/Clinical Affairs; Ed.D., Columbia.

Marlene McHugh, Assistant Professor of Clinical Nursing; M.S.N., Columbia; FNP.

Mary O. Mundinger, Dean and Professor; Dr.P.H., Columbia. Health policy, family care of the frail elderly, technology assessment in home care.

Patricia Murphy, Assistant Professor; Dr.P.H., Columbia; CNM. Epidemiology of ovarian cancer, risk factors for preterm birth.

Carol Roye, Instructor; Ed.D., Columbia; PNP.

Jo Sapp, Instructor and Director of Continuing Education; M.S., Columbia; Certified Psychiatric Nurse Specialist.

Betty Smith, Instructor and Director of Neonatal Nurse Practitioner Program; Ph.D. candidate, NYU; NNP.

Jan Weingrad Smith, Instructor; M.S./M.P.H., Columbia; CNM.

Edwidge Thomas, Instructor of Clinical Nursing; M.S., ANP.

Joan Valas, Assistant Professor of Clinical Nursing and Director, Critical Care Nurse Practitioner Program; M.S., CCRN, ANP.

Concordia University Wisconsin
Nursing Division
Mequon, Wisconsin

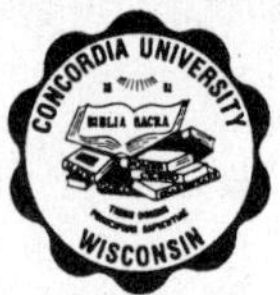

THE UNIVERSITY

Concordia University was founded in 1881 as a school of The Lutheran Church–Missouri Synod and officially became a university on August 27, 1989. Concordia is one of twelve colleges and seminaries maintained by The Lutheran Church–Missouri Synod. In addition to its traditional focus on teacher training (teacher supply for Lutheran parochial schools, lay ministry/preseminary education), innovative programs in the liberal arts, business, nursing, and adult education have been added. A master's program was established in 1988.

Since the move to Mequon in 1983, Concordia has become the fastest growing Lutheran college in the country, growing from 784 students to more than 4,000 to date. It is a four-year, NCA-accredited, coeducational, liberal arts school offering thirty-five majors of study.

THE NURSING DIVISION

Concordia University Wisconsin has offered a baccalaureate degree in nursing since 1982. The National League for Nursing made its initial visit to Concordia and granted NLN accreditation to the nursing program in 1988. Accreditation was granted in 1996 for eight years. The Bachelor of Science in Nursing track for registered nurses was developed, and in May of 1991, the first RN to B.S.N. completion students graduated. The first LPN graduated as a graduate nurse in the summer of 1995. In the fall of 1995, Concordia began a Master of Science in Nursing degree program.

The B.S.N. completion track, the LPN to RN track, and the traditional generic track of nursing are rooted in the same philosophy. The conceptual framework that is utilized is the Betty Neuman Systems Model. The delivery of the courses differs in that the B.S.N. completion program was designed for the adult learner. Modular courses are delivered over three to seven weeks time during day and evening hours to facilitate the working adult. The delivery of the traditional course content is typically over a semester's length.

CUW faculty members are published and are recognized leaders in their fields of expertise. In addition, because of a low student-faculty ratio (13:1), they are able to know their students as individuals.

PROGRAMS OF STUDY

The curriculum in nursing prepares individuals for a beginning practice of professional nursing and is built around the core curriculum and supplemental courses that facilitate the development of a professional nurse. Students will have an opportunity to gain a basis of knowledge from the liberal arts curriculum. The traditional student's nursing experience begins with on-campus instruction in both the classroom and nursing laboratory. The first learning experience with patients begins in the sophomore year. Throughout the program, students are introduced to nursing experiences in both hospitals and community agencies. Upon graduation, the students are eligible to take the NCLEX-RN exam administered by the State Board of Nursing.

LPNs and RNs are admitted to the University as students who have completed one year of the nursing program. Depending upon how classes are scheduled, it may be possible to complete the program in three academic years or less.

The RN seeking a baccalaureate degree is offered a curriculum focusing on the liberal arts and nursing. Classes are offered emphasizing adult education principles with flexible scheduling in the late afternoons and evenings.

The Parish Nurse is the visible symbol of a congregation's pursuit of wellness, which is people's faith response to Jesus Christ, driven by the Holy Spirit. This wholistic health program is based on the belief that health is growth towards well-being of body, soul, mind, and relationships. The Parish Nurse is available to all age levels of the congregation and becomes part of the ministry team, which also includes the pastor and members of the congregation.

The M.S.N. program (seeking accreditation) is designed to prepare nurses for advanced practice nursing as nurse practitioners and nurse educators or in the gerontological field. Nurses from all basic nursing programs accredited by the NLN are eligible to apply. Both an on-campus and a long-distance (50 miles or more away from CUW) course of study are available. The first graduating class is anticipated in 1997. Accreditation procedures will immediately follow. Forty-three to 46 credit hours are required, depending upon the program.

The program's biggest plus is its emphasis on a Christian response in nursing and respect for human life. The professional faculty provides individualized attention and emphasizes "Excellence in Christian Education."

ACADEMIC FACILITIES

Clinicals are held in neighboring hospitals and health-care facilities. Computer literacy is a must on the Concordia campus. The new Health Services building features state-of-the-art labs for physical and occupational therapy along with offices.

LOCATION

Concordia is located just 15 minutes from Milwaukee, which is a modern commercial center with an old European flavor. This metropolitan area of more than 1.5 million people supports an interesting variety of art and culture. Students may choose the world-renowned Milwaukee Symphony or the Great Circus Parade, ballet, or repertory theater. Art lovers can visit the Milwaukee Art Museum.

STUDENT SERVICES

Students have access to the numerous events in Milwaukee. CUW's Student Activities arranges for tickets to some of the events taking place in town.

On campus there are tennis courts, drama and music groups, and plays and concerts. The new Field House is open to all indoor intercollegiate sports, and with its 2,000 seating capacity, hosts many activities. Century Stadium is the place for football and soccer games as well as CUW's 400-meter track. The Falcon's Nest is the campus gathering place. Fast food and open hours that only a collegian world would understand are the mainstay.

THE NURSING STUDENT GROUP

The total enrollment for the 1996–97 academic year is 318. Concordia has an SNA (Student Nurses' Association) that sponsors various events throughout the year, such as a Christmas Tea, health fair, blood banks, and various fund-raisers.

COSTS

All students have an initial application fee and tuition deposit of $25 and $100, respectively. Educational fees per semester are $5350, with room and board at $1750 (fifteen-meal plan) or $1850 (nineteen-meal plan). Costs for the B.S.N., M.S.N., LPN, and Parish Nurse programs, vary depending upon how many credits a student has in the program based on previous transcripts. Average cost per credit averages $200.

FINANCIAL AID

The amount of financial aid awarded is based mainly on the applicant's financial need. As a general rule, the primary financial responsibility lies with the student and parents. Therefore, in order to help determine student need and make it possible to grant aid fairly, the parents of aid applicants are asked to file a confidential statement of the income, assets, expenses, and liabilities. On the basis of this financial information, the University is able to determine the difference between University costs and the amount a student and parents can reasonably be expected to provide. The difference is defined as need. If a student is self-supporting and not dependent on parents, the student should submit a financial statement without parental information. There are various loans, grants, and scholarships available as well as veteran's educational assistance.

APPLYING

Students must submit evidence of adequate preparation for college from a regionally accredited high school. A minimum of 16 units of secondary school work is required, of which at least 11 should be in basic liberal arts areas. A minimum entrance grade point average of 2.5 is required. When entering other than the traditional program, transcripts from previous colleges and universities attended are required.

Correspondence and Information:

Nursing Division
Concordia University Wisconsin
12800 N. Lake Shore Drive
Mequon, Wisconsin 53097
Telephone: 414-243-4374
Fax: 414-243-4351
E-mail: gapete@bach.cuw.edu

Culver-Stockton College
Canton, Missouri

Blessing-Rieman College of Nursing
Quincy, Illinois

THE COLLEGE
Culver-Stockton College is an independent, private college affiliated with the Christian Church (Disciples of Christ). The mission of Culver-Stockton College is to help promising young men and women attain a four-year bachelor's degree and develop the skills and knowledge necessary for productive lives of service. This career development is heightened by a liberal arts curriculum and takes place within a supportive yet challenging environment that emphasizes the formation of examined values.

THE COLLEGE OF NURSING
Blessing-Rieman College is NLN-accredited as a single purpose institution and confers the Bachelor of Science in Nursing (B.S.N.) degree to basic and registered nurse students. Staff and faculty from the campuses of both Culver-Stockton and Blessing-Rieman combine to bring the unique benefits of expertise, resources, and commitment to offer students a highly professional and educationally sound four-year program leading to the B.S.N. degree.

The mission of Blessing-Rieman College of Nursing is to teach persons of diverse backgrounds to acquire the knowledge, skills, attitudes, and values needed for professional nursing practice and lifelong learning. This mission is accomplished in a community of learning dedicated to excellence and caring in professional nursing education.

PROGRAM OF STUDY
Culver-Stockton/Blessing-Rieman College of Nursing offers a four-year B.S.N. degree program. The purposes of the program are to enable students to acquire essential values, attitudes, knowledge, and skills for beginning nurse practitioners and to develop the skills nurses need to make a contribution as leaders and change agents in the nursing profession and health-care delivery systems, both locally and globally.

Nursing classes begin in the freshman year, when students primarily attend Culver-Stockton College. During the sophomore year at Culver-Stockton, a transition to applied nursing is begun as students have clinical experiences at Blessing Hospital and other health-care agencies in and near Quincy, Illinois. In the third and fourth years of nursing study, students attend classes primarily on the Blessing-Rieman campus, and the focus is increasingly on nursing courses and hands-on nursing practice.

Nursing courses are designed to assist students in the systematic acquisition of knowledge, skills, and values derived from nursing and other related science theories for the purpose of caring for human beings in a creative way. The use of self, research, leadership, and the nursing process are recurring and progressive themes.

Students have approximately 1,000 hours of hands-on clinical experience in a wide variety of health-care settings, including acute-care hospitals, extended-care facilities, schools, and a number of community health programs and settings. Upon completion of the program, students will have provided nursing care to patients of all age groups.

Students are taught in the clinical setting by professors who practice the art and science of nursing in a variety of specialty areas. The student-faculty ratio is 8:1.

AFFILIATIONS WITH HEALTH-CARE FACILITIES
Blessing Hospital, in Quincy, Illinois, is a state-of-the-art facility that has continuously attracted some of the finest health-care professionals in the nation since its founding in 1875. Blessing operates as a general hospital and conducts a full range of health and medical-care services for both inpatients and outpatients.

Nursing units within Blessing provide acute medical-surgical care, emergency and trauma care, pediatric care, full maternity services, rehabilitation, intensive and coronary care, renal dialysis, oncology services, and long-term care. Hospice and home health care services are also offered.

Today, in both caseload and scope of care, Blessing Hospital is the largest medical center within a 100-mile radius. A recent acquisition of another health-care facility in the city has increased Blessing's campus to more than six blocks in downtown Quincy.

ACADEMIC FACILITIES
Blessing-Rieman has dedicated significant resources toward its classrooms and equipment. A nursing-dedicated computer lab provides access to the best step-by-step tutorials and NCLEX reviews. The materials greatly enhance the knowledge students gain from regular class work and clinical lab experience.

A complete and detailed library on the Blessing-Rieman campus is devoted to nursing and provides access to monograph collections in nursing, the arts, and the sciences; 179 journal subscriptions; software; and audiovisual equipment and materials. Students also have access to the Blessing Hospital medical library and various networks and consortia. These tools help focus and define student research and provide students with a source of up-to-the-minute information.

The nursing skills laboratory has the latest in ICU technology and abundant teaching stations. Students use state-of-the-art clinical equipment in simulated hospital room settings, so they can practice nursing skills as well as develop the skills of clinical decision making.

Culver-Stockton College also remains in touch with the latest advances in each field. The College is connected to the Internet, and students have access to more than 100 computers on campus, including computers in the residence halls. The library is automated. The integration of computer and writing skills takes place at all levels of the curriculum. The full-service library on campus houses 132,260 periodicals, 4,719 microfilms, 367 periodical subscriptions, and 1,937 records and tapes.

LOCATION
Overlooking the mighty Mississippi River, Culver-Stockton College is situated in Canton, Missouri (population 3,000), and provides students with a safe and secure environment. The quiet, reflective atmosphere is ideal for the development of new ideas and new friendships. Blessing-Rieman College of Nursing is located across the river (approximately 30 minutes) in Quincy, Illinois. Quincy is a charming city (population 45,000) noted for its rich heritage, strong cultural base, architectural significance, and superb quality of life.

STUDENT SERVICES

At Culver-Stockton, forty clubs and organizations provide leadership opportunities for students. The Culver-Stockton social life features an active fraternity and sorority system, nationally ranked NAIA athletic teams for both men and women, dramatics and musical activities open to all students, student publications, and a variety of other special interest clubs and activities. Religious activities, organized by a full-time chaplain, are offered several times each week.

The Student Nurses' Organization (SNO) is open to all Blessing-Rieman College of Nursing students and provides a governance structure through which community and social activities are organized. Among the activities coordinated each year by SNO are a health fair on the Culver-Stockton campus and the Teddy Bear Clinic, where children bring their favorite stuffed animals for "check-ups."

THE NURSING STUDENT GROUP

There are 204 nursing majors at Culver-Stockton College. Ten percent are men; 4 percent are from minority groups.

COSTS

Tuition for the 1996–97 school year was $8800. Room and board at Culver-Stockton College cost $4000; rent for apartments at the Blessing-Rieman campus during the junior and senior years was $1600.

FINANCIAL AID

Culver-Stockton College and Blessing-Rieman College of Nursing have two of the finest financial aid programs available. Approximately 95 percent of all Culver-Stockton and Blessing-Rieman students are receiving some form of financial aid. Scholarships, grants, loans, and student assistantships are available.

Since the freshman and sophomore years are spent primarily on the Culver-Stockton College campus, financial aid is awarded exclusively by Culver-Stockton for those years. The junior and senior years are spent primarily at Blessing-Rieman College of Nursing, and financial aid is awarded exclusively by Blessing-Rieman. Awards are specifically designed to provide a continuity or matching equivalent of funding as long as eligibility criteria are maintained.

APPLYING

Culver-Stockton/Blessing-Rieman College of Nursing gives full consideration to all applicants for admission and financial aid without regard to race, creed, sex, age, national origin, marital status, veteran status, or disability. Applications are required by May 1 for persons wishing to enter in the fall and by December 1 for persons wishing to enter mid-year. Admission is on a rolling basis, and applicants will be notified immediately of acceptance. Entering students must have at least a 3.0 high school grade point average, an ACT score of at least 20, and rank in the upper half of their graduating class. Students who have already completed some college work are accepted on the basis of space availability and scholastic record. Students should contact the Admissions Office at Culver-Stockton/Blessing Rieman College of Nursing for complete admission requirements.

Correspondence and Information:

Culver-Stockton College
One College Hill
Canton, Missouri 63435-1299
Telephone: 800-537-1883 (toll-free)
Fax: 217-231-6611
E-mail: admissions@culver.edu
World Wide Web: http://www.culver.edu

Blessing-Rieman College of Nursing
Broadway at 11th Street
P.O. Box 7005
Quincy, Illinois, 62305-7005
Telephone: 800-877-9140 (toll-free)
Fax: 217-223-6400
E-mail: bradmiss@moses.culver.edu

THE FACULTY

Carole L. Piles, Professor, President, and Dean; M.S.N., Ph.D., Saint Louis.

Brenda Beshears, Instructor; M.S., Southern Illinois–Edwardsville.

Pamela Brown, Assistant Professor and Acting Assistant Dean; M.S., Southern Illinois–Edwardsville.

Sheila Capp, Assistant Professor; M.S., Missouri–Columbia.

Corinne Fessenden, Assistant Professor; M.S., Missouri–Columbia.

Cindy Huang, Associate Professor; Ph.D., Saint Louis; FNP.

Candice Leeper, Instructor; M.S.N., Southern Illinois–Edwardsville.

Karen Mayville, Assistant Professor; M.S.N., Marquette.

Carol Ann Moseley, Assistant Professor; Ph.D. candidate, Texas Woman's.

Ann O'Sullivan, Assistant Professor; M.S.N., Northern Illinois.

Sherry Pomeroy, Assistant Professor; M.S.N., Rochester.

Charlene Romer, Assistant Professor; M.S., Illinois–Peoria.

Debra Walton-Hart, Instructor; M.S., Southern Illinois at Edwardsville.

Margaret Williams, Assistant Professor; M.S., Southern Illinois–Edwardsville.

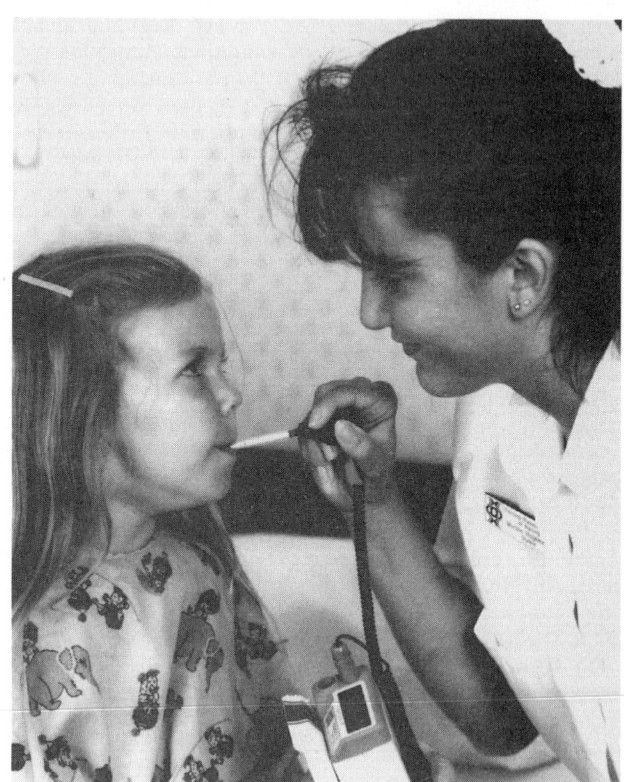

A junior nursing student attends to a pediatric patient at Blessing Hospital.

Dalhousie University
School of Nursing
Halifax, Nova Scotia, Canada

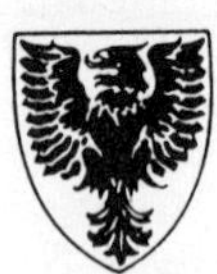

THE UNIVERSITY

One of Canada's top research and teaching institutions, Dalhousie University offers a first-class postsecondary education to nearly 11,000 students in 127 undergraduate and graduate degree programs, including 28 Ph.D. programs. Nursing is one of eight programs in the Faculty of Health Professions at Dalhousie University.

THE SCHOOL OF NURSING

Founded in 1949, the Dalhousie School of Nursing originally offered one-year diplomas in public health nursing and teaching in schools of nursing to registered nurses from Atlantic Canada. E. A. Electa MacLennan served as director of the School from 1949 until 1972. During that time the School inaugurated a baccalaureate program and grew to become a major site for educating nurses in the Atlantic Canadian region.

Currently, there are almost 500 undergraduate nursing students and 103 nurses studying at the graduate level. Dalhousie University prepares nurses for challenging careers in an increasingly diversified field by delivering its B.Sc.N. and B.Sc.N./RN program in collaboration with the Queen Elizabeth II Health Science Center; the IWK/Grace Health Center for Women, Children and Families; the Reproductive Care Program of Nova Scotia; and the Western Regional Health Center. In September 1995, the Yarmouth Regional Hospital and Dalhousie University formed a partnership to allow Dalhousie's top-quality instruction and recognition to also be offered at the Yarmouth site. In September 1991, the master's of nursing program was distanced to faculty in Yarmouth.

Dahousie's teaching and research strengths go hand in hand. The faculty members at the School of Nursing are involved in ongoing research in areas that have an impact on many communities.

PROGRAMS OF STUDY

Dalhousie University's Bachelor of Science in Nursing (B.Sc.N.) program prepares graduates, through four years of full-time study and clinical practice, to work with individuals, families, groups, and communities to promote, maintain, and strengthen health. Advanced standing is available to students who bring sufficient postsecondary education to the program to be able to achieve their B.Sc.N. in only three years.

Postdiploma program options include a modified degree program for diploma nurses who can achieve their Bachelor of Science in Nursing in two years of full-time study plus two spring semesters. Students studying on a part-time basis can work at their own pace over a maximum of ten years.

The Perinatal Education Partnership Project, or PEPP, offers five courses with a perinatal focus from the Dalhousie nursing program with access to innovative distance technology and interactive learning approaches. Following the completion of the five PEPP courses, students exit with a "Certificate of Completion" from the PEPP and with a Dalhousie University transcript indicating the completion of the five courses. Students may then choose to continue in the B.Sc.N./RN program to complete the remaining requirements of the degree program.

Clinical major options similar in design to PEPP are being developed for September 1997 registration. Nurses may choose selected course offerings from the B.Sc.N. curriculum that focus on the areas of clinical practice that interest them most. Interested nurses should contact the admissions office of the School of Nursing to learn what areas of clinical focus are being offered yearly.

The master's of nursing program prepares graduates to be leaders in the professional discipline of nursing with an advanced level of academic and clinical preparation. The graduate has rigorous academic preparation and strong skills in critical inquiry, logical analysis, and decision making that can be applied in educational, clinical, or research positions and in graduate education at the doctoral level. The master's of nursing program at Dalhousie University is a two-year research-oriented program.

AFFILIATIONS WITH HEALTH-CARE FACILITIES

Dalhousie University offers the Bachelor of Science in Nursing degree program in collaboration with the Queen Elizabeth II Health Science Center; the IWK/Grace Health Center for Women, Children and Families; the Reproductive Care Program of Nova Scotia; and the Western Regional Health Center. The collaborative nature of the program allows students to work with faculty and staff members in the largest health-care facilities in the Maritime Provinces and provides valuable links to a large variety of nursing practice settings.

ACADEMIC FACILITIES

The Dalhousie University Library System supports the undergraduate, graduate, and professional teaching programs; research; and public service functions for the University. Its libraries include the Killam Memorial Library (social sciences, humanities, sciences) and the W. K. Kellogg Health Sciences Library (medicine, nursing, dentistry, and other health professions). Library resources can be accessed via the homepages of both the W. K. Kellogg Health Sciences Library and the Killam Memorial Library (arts and humanities and science). These homepages document library services, tutorials, and policies and are continuously updated and expanded. They provide direct access to the Novanet public access catalogue (OPAC) and to forms for on-line requests for articles via the Novanet Express service and provide links to Internet resources in the health sciences in general and to nursing resources in particular. Within the School of Nursing, the skills lab and audiovisual lab offer facilities for nursing students to practice clinical skills and take advantage of course-specific computer software.

LOCATION

Dalhousie University is located in the port city of Halifax, Nova Scotia, on Canada's east coast. The capital of Nova Scotia, Halifax is a city of beauty, tradition, and maritime charm; a city bridging the best of old and new worlds. Atlantic Canada's centre of commerce, learning, technology, and innovation, Halifax offers a community of spirit, diversity, and culture to students from four different universities. The cultural mosaic is made up of more than 100 different ethnic groups represented province-wide, including Lebanese, Filipinos, Scottish, Irish, British, Indian, Vietnamese, Portuguese, Asian, Jamaican, Greek, and Italian.

STUDENT SERVICES

Dalhousie offers many student services, from recruiting programs that help potential students with a path to meet their university goals to academic advising, financial and personal counselling, and health services. Support services for students from black and native communities, for students with disabilities, and for those from outside of Canada are also available. Student employment and volunteer opportunities are provided through a unique on-campus program. The athletic facility, Dalplex, provides an arena for a variety of exciting recreational and varsity activities.

THE NURSING STUDENT GROUP

The Dalhousie University Nursing Society—Canadian Nursing Students' Association (DUNS-CNSA) serves all undergraduate students of the Dalhousie School of Nursing by promoting the activities of the DUNS-CNSA to foster student comradery. The Nursing Society is a leader and a partner in providing support to nursing students. The recently developed Peer Support Network has received national recognition.

COSTS

Full-time tuition fees for the 1996–97 academic year were Can$4420. Individual courses fees were Can$915 for a full credit and Can$480 for a half credit. Books are estimated to cost Can$700 per year. Mantoux testing is available for a Can$5 fee, and Hepatitis-B vaccinations are recommended at an approximate cost of Can$80. A variety of residence facilities are available, ranging from Can$4680 to Can$5030 for traditional dormitory-style accommodations with a meal plan. Apartment-style facilities are offered beginning at Can$2565, and meal plans are available separately for Can$2025 for nineteen meals per week and Can$1955 for fourteen meals per week.

FINANCIAL AID

Students coming directly from high school are considered for scholarships of Can$500 to Can$6000 if they apply by April 1. The Student Employment Assistance program provides job opportunities (experience and cash), and financial assistance is available through the Dalhousie Bursary Program. The Awards Office (Dalhousie University, Halifax, NS, B3H, 4H6) provides information on financial aid. To apply for loans under the Canada Student Loan Programme, students should contact the Student Aid Authority of the province of residence.

APPLYING

Nova Scotia grade 12 or equivalent, including academic grade 12 English, math, chemistry, and biology with a minimum 70 percent final average in each subject and an overall average of at least 70 percent, is the basic requirement for admission. Students with postsecondary education must have a minimum cumulative grade point average of 2.5. Mature students are at least 23 years old, out of full-time school study for at least four years, and have not attended university. Mature applicants must complete GED grade 12 with a university preparatory grade 12 math and chemistry. Applicants whose native language is not English are required to take the TOEFL and receive a minimum score of 580 or take the MELAB exam and earn a minimum score of 90. Official high school transcripts and postsecondary transcripts are necessary. B.Sc.N./RN applicants must include diploma school transcripts and RN exam grades. The application deadline is June 1.

Correspondence and Information:

Barbara McLennan
Undergraduate Program Secretary–Admissions
Dalhousie University School of Nursing
5869 University Avenue
Halifax, Nova Scotia B3H 3J5
Canada
Telephone: 902-494-2603
800-500-0912 (toll-free in Canada during regular business hours)
Fax: 902-494-3487
E-mail: Barbara.McLennan@dal.ca
World Wide Web: http://www2.dal.ca

THE FACULTY

M. Amirault, M.N., Dalhousie; RN.
M. Arklie, B.N., Dalhousie; Ph.D., Texas at Austin; RN.
E. Bethune, B.Sc.N., Mount Saint Vincent; RN.
J. Black, B.N., Dalhousie; Dip.P.H., Dalhousie; Ed.D., British Columbia; RN.
B. Bleasdale, B.N., Dalhousie; RN.
D. Bowes, B.N., Dalhousie; RN.
M. Brennen, M.N., Dalhousie; RN.
S. Cobbett, B.N., Dalhousie; Dip.Ger., Mount Saint Vincent; RN.
K. Cockersell,, B.Pharm., Bradford; Dip.O.P./C.H., Dalhousie; RN.
S. Daniels, M.N., Dalhousie; RN.
D. Denney, M.N., Dalhousie; RN.
B. L. Downe-Wamboldt, B.N., M.Ed., Dip.P.H., Dalhousie; Ph.D., Texas at Austin; RN.
M. L. Ellerton, M.N., McGill; RN.
S. Foster, M.N., Dalhousie; RN.
J. Francis, B.N., Dalhousie; RN.
F. Gregor, M.N., Ph.D., Dalhousie; RN.
H. Hackney, B.Sc.N., Dalhousie; Dip.O.P./C.H., Dalhousie.
G. Hart, M.S.N, British Columbia; RN.
J. Hartigan-Rogers, B.N., Dalhousie; RN.
M. J. Horrocks, B.S.N., British Columbia; M.S. (psych. nursing), M.S. (comm. health nursing), Dip.C.M.H., California, San Francisco.
J. M. Hughes, B.N., Dalhousie; M.S., Boston University; RN.
B. Keddy, B.Sc.N., Mount Saint Vincent; Ph.D., Dalhousie; RN.
A. LeBlanc, B.N., Dalhousie; RN.
R. Martin-Misener, B.Sc.N., Dip.O.P./C.H., Dalhousie; RN.
P. Melanson, M.N., Dalhousie; RN.
L. L. Mensah, B.N., M.A., Dip.P.H., Dalhousie; RN, CNM.
A. Miller, M.N., Calgary; RN, CNM.
C. F. Wight Moffatt, B.N., Memorial of Newfoundland; M.S., Boston College; RN.
M. Muise-Davis, M.N., Dalhousie; RN.
G. Tomblin Murphy, M.N., Dalhousie; RN.
R. A. Pogoda, Cert.C.H., Manitoba; RN.
P. Reid, B.N., New Brunswick; M.Sc., Dalhousie; RN.
J. A. Ritchie, M.N., Ph.D., Pittsburgh; RN.
D. Sheppard-LeMoine, B.N., Dalhousie; RN.
C. L. Smillie, B.Sc.N., British Columbia; M.Sc., Dalhousie; RN.
D. Sommerfeld, M.S.N, British Columbia; RN.
K. Stares, B.N., Dip.O.P./C.H., Dalhousie; RN.
M. Stewart, M.N., Dalhousie; Ph.D., Dalhousie; RN.
D. L. Tamlyn, B.N., McGill; M.Ed., Ottawa; Ph.D., Dalhousie; RN.
P. Thorpe, B.N., M.A., Dalhousie; RN.
A. R. Vukic, B.N., Dalhousie; RN.
A. Ward, B.Sc.N., Ottawa; RN.
L. Wittstock, B.Sc.N., St. Francis Xavier; RN.
J. Wong, M.Sc.N, Western Ontario; Ph.D., Dalhousie; RN.
S. Wong, M.Sc.N, Western Ontario; Ph.D., Dalhousie; RN.
D. Younker, M.N., Western Ontario; RN.
J. Zevenhuizen, M.N., Dalhousie; RN.

Dominican College of Blauvelt
Division of Nursing
Orangeburg, New York

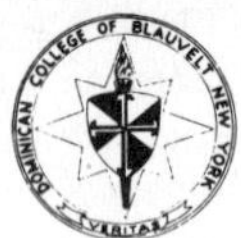

THE COLLEGE

Dominican College is an accredited four-year independent institution for women and men. It was founded by the Dominican Order in 1952 and grants degrees in both the liberal arts and professional areas. Over 1,800 men and women of all ages, races, and religions are enrolled in day, evening, and weekend programs. The student-faculty ratio is 12:1. Classes are small, encouraging open discussion.

The College awards B.A., B.S., B.S.Ed., B.S.N, Accelerated B.S.N., M.S., and M.S.Ed. degrees and offers a wide range of academic divisions and programs: Arts and Sciences, Social Sciences, Social Work, Occupational Therapy, Education, Business, Computers, and Nursing.

Nine buildings make up the present facilities of the College, including three buildings constructed since 1994: a student center, a dining facility, and a residence hall. All buildings are wheelchair-accessible, and assignment of rooms for classes is adjusted to accommodate students with physical limitations. Classroom and study assistance is available for visually impaired and hearing-impaired students.

THE DIVISION OF NURSING

The Division of Nursing offers a program leading to a Bachelor of Science in Nursing degree for students with no prior background in nursing and for graduates of associate degree, diploma, and licensed practical nurse programs. A Weekend College program is available to RNs. In addition, a one-day-per-week upper-division RN option is available to nursing graduates of diploma and associate degree programs. An accelerated option (A.B.S.N.), which permits completion of the nursing requirements in one calendar year, is available to applicants who hold a non-nursing baccalaureate degree.

The nursing curriculum is designed to prepare nurse generalists at the baccalaureate level who will be able to promote health and provide nursing care to people of all ages, across all socioeconomic levels.

The program prepares nurses who will participate collaboratively with health, community, and political institutions in promoting the improvement of health-care delivery in a rapidly changing society. It stimulates the desire for lifelong learning experiences and provides the foundation for graduate education in nursing. All courses are taught by College faculty members, not graduate assistants.

In 1993, the Division again received a laudatory evaluation and reaccreditation by the National League for Nursing.

PROGRAMS OF STUDY

The Office of Admissions determines eligibility to matriculate at Dominican College. Candidates for the four-year baccalaureate program in nursing must first be admitted to the College through the Office of Admissions. Eligibility for admission to the nursing program is established by the Division of Nursing.

Nursing students must complete a minimum of 123 semester hours within a six-year period. Advisement and course approval are provided initially by a liberal arts adviser during the prerequisite general education and liberal arts courses. A nursing adviser is appointed for advisement when nursing courses begin.

Generic program applicants must have a minimum cumulative index of 2.5 in order to be admitted to sophomore-level nursing courses.

Upper-division program applicants must be graduates of diploma or associate degree programs in nursing and have a minimum cumulative index of 2.5. A.B.S.N. applicants must hold a previous baccalaureate degree and have an undergraduate grade point average of 2.5 or higher. Grades lower than C in natural sciences courses are not acceptable. All applicants must complete an essay specified by the Division of Nursing prior to admission to the nursing program.

An English placement examination is required on entry to the College. A mathematics placement examination is required for those who have not previously taken a college-level mathematics course.

To maintain one standard of entry for graduates of associate degree programs and diploma schools of nursing into the RN Completion Program, the upper-division nursing program, advanced standing in nursing at the baccalaureate level is based on a system of credit-by-validation examinations.

Prior to entrance into the junior year, several sets of examinations must be passed. Thirty-one credits for baccalaureate-level knowledge will be awarded for successful completion of the following examinations: the NLN Nursing Mobility Profile II Examinations covering (I) Care of the Adult Client, (II) Care of the Client during Childbearing and Care of the Child, and (III) Care of the Client with Mental Disorder.

The Division of Nursing welcomes applications from licensed practical nurses seeking upward career mobility. LPNs from accredited programs who hold state licensure follow the same course progression as four-year basic baccalaureate students. The faculty recognizes the knowledge of LPNs through award of credit by examinations. Prior to entrance into the nursing sequence, students must pass the NLN Mobility Profile I Examination covering Foundations of Nursing as well as the Division of Nursing Departmental Examination: NR28, Pharmacologic Agents & Nursing Practice. A total of 11 credits is awarded for successful completion of these examinations.

AFFILIATIONS WITH HEALTH-CARE FACILITIES

Dominican's Division of Nursing is affiliated with a variety of clinical agencies in New York and New Jersey. Health promotion is a main focus, and students engage in primary prevention activities at a number of community health agencies. Acute and rehabilitative nursing is also practiced in both suburban and metropolitan settings.

ACADEMIC FACILITIES

The College library, located in Pius X Hall, provides more than 103,000 volumes and approximately 670 periodical titles, with over 14,300 volumes of additional back files on microfilm. The collection includes reference sources, basic indexes, and other bibliographic aids.

Casey Hall contains classrooms, computer labs, and a Learning Resources Center. A mainframe computer is located in Cooke Hall, the administrative building. Doyle Hall, the teacher education building, provides seminar rooms and houses the Instructional Materials Center. Forkel Hall is the location of nursing and science classes and laboratories. Rosary Hall is a classroom building that also houses the library periodical collection and a computer center.

LOCATION

Dominican College is located in Rockland County, New York, 17 miles from Manhattan and just minutes from Bergen,

Orange, and Westchester counties. This convenient setting offers a small suburban environment and access to the outstanding cultural, recreational, and educational resources of New York City. The College can be easily reached by car or public transportation.

STUDENT SERVICES

Dominican directs its efforts and resources toward meeting the needs of its students, enabling them to develop personal, intellectual, moral, and social competencies. College service offices include Campus Ministry, the bookstore, the Residence Center, Career Counseling & Placement, the Learning Resources Center, and the newly constructed Student Life Center, which features a physical fitness center, a suspended track, and a multipurpose room for student activities. The Student Development Office provides social and cultural programs and sponsors student organizations and activities such as the yearbook, College newspaper, drama club, international club, honor societies, and athletic events. The Freshman Directorate pairs each first-year student with an academic adviser and peer and assists in the selection of a personalized learning plan. Nontraditional and transfer students receive one-on-one advisement.

The Weekend College program specifically meets the needs of registered nurses from diploma and associate degree programs. Both clinical experiences and classroom content are taught during the weekend.

THE NURSING STUDENT GROUP

Students come from diverse backgrounds and include registered nurses working full-time and attending Weekend College classes, licensed practical nurses attending part-time, full-time traditional students, and students interested in pursuing a second career. Adult learners and traditional college students are well represented at Dominican and are encouraged to apply.

COSTS

Dominican College offers a fixed tuition rate under which new full-time students registered in the fall or spring semester are guaranteed tuition protected from increase for the entire period of continuous enrollment. The basic expenses for 1996–97 were $9750 per academic year for tuition and $6000 per academic year for room and board. For part-time and weekend students, the tuition was $325 per semester hour.

FINANCIAL AID

Dominican College administers four types of aid: scholarships, loans, grants, and work-study programs. Aid opportunities are available through nursing student loans, nursing scholarships, the New York State Tuition Assistance Program (TAP), various federal grant and loan programs, and private scholarships. Students applying for aid should file the Financial Aid Form with the College Scholarship Service by March 15.

APPLYING

Entering freshmen are expected to have completed a secondary school program or its equivalent. Special consideration is given to nontraditional students whose educational background may vary from the recommended program but who show promise of the ability to do college work. All freshman applicants for admission should have an official high school transcript sent directly to the College from their high schools, in addition to SAT I or ACT scores and any other information they wish to have considered. An interview with an admissions counselor is strongly recommended. Students should contact the Office of Admissions for complete admission requirements and deadlines.

Correspondence and Information:

Colleen O'Connor, Director of Admissions
Dominican College
470 Western Highway
Orangeburg, New York 10962
Telephone: 914-359-7800
201-476-0600
Fax: 914-359-2313

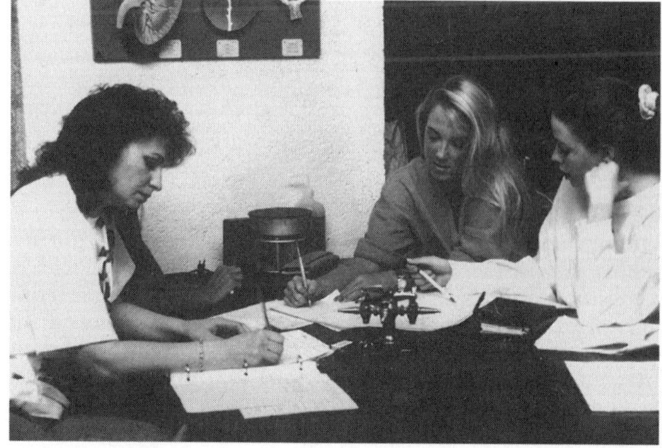

Nursing students at Dominican exchange ideas and information during a laboratory course.

Dominican College of San Rafael
School of Nursing
San Rafael, California

THE COLLEGE
Dominican College of San Rafael is a coeducational, independent, Catholic liberal arts college offering bachelor's and master's degrees in seventeen fields. Dominican has a commitment to interdisciplinary study in the humanities, a global perspective, and the involvement of students in their own intellectual, spiritual, ethical, and social development. The College was founded in 1890 by the Dominican Sisters of San Rafael. It was the first Catholic college in the state of California to offer the baccalaureate degree to women. Today, Dominican College derives no direct financial support from the church or the state.

THE SCHOOL OF NURSING
The School of Nursing strives to support the idea that nursing is a dynamic, interpersonal process based on the premise of individual worth and human dignity and to teach that the goal of nursing is to help individuals, families, and groups achieve and maintain self-care in coping with actual and potential health problems. Nursing is a human service provided when clients' self-care capabilities are inadequate to promote, maintain, and restore health. The School of Nursing faculty members bring deep understanding and rich backgrounds of both clinical and teaching experience to the program. All full-time faculty members are master's prepared, and the majority are also doctorally prepared or are currently engaged in doctoral work.

PROGRAM OF STUDY
Dominican College offers a Bachelor of Science in Nursing (B.S.N.) for women and men wishing to enter the field of professional nursing. Students complete one year of prerequisite courses before beginning the clinical nursing major in the sophomore year. Clinical experiences in the sophomore, junior, and senior years take place at a variety of affiliated agencies. Throughout the four-year program, lecture classes are held on the Dominican campus. Upon satisfactory completion of the nursing curriculum, students are granted the Bachelor of Science in Nursing degree, are eligible to take the State Board Examination for licensure as a registered nurse (RN), and can obtain a California Public Health Nursing Certificate. Advanced placement is available for transfer students from other nursing programs, registered nurses, licensed vocational nurses, and health-care workers who wish to obtain a baccalaureate degree in nursing. Registered nurses can also earn a B.S.N. through the College's evening and weekend program. A 30-unit option is also available for licensed vocational nurses. The nursing program is accredited by the California Board of Registered Nursing and the National League for Nursing.

AFFILIATIONS WITH HEALTH-CARE FACILITIES
The School of Nursing is affiliated with a number of health-care agencies and institutions in the Bay Area, offering students clinical learning opportunities with diverse populations in a wide variety of settings. Agencies include Marin General Hospital, Marin County Health Department, San Francisco General Hospital, and Kaiser Permanente in San Rafael and Santa Rosa, California.

ACADEMIC FACILITIES
The Archbishop Alemany Library houses more than 90,000 volumes in open stacks, over 2,000 reels of microfilm, and subscriptions to nearly 500 periodicals. Almost 1,200 volumes are health- and nursing-related, with nearly 50 periodicals dealing with these topics. Reference services, including access to a variety of computerized database and indexes, and multimedia facilities are provided to assist students with their studies and assignments. Nursing students have access to CINAHL on CD-ROM and to MEDLINE, an on-line health information resource. The library also houses the campus computer center.

Within the School itself, the new E. L. Wiegand Nursing Laboratory offers students the opportunity to acquire nursing skills in a simulated clinical setting. Interactive video programs, computer-assisted instruction, and a number of other audiovisual programs are available for student use in this lab. With the recent addition of the new E. L. Wiegand Nursing Laboratory, Dominican College nursing students are exposed to the latest techniques in teaching nursing skills in a hands-on, simulated clinical environment.

LOCATION
The College is located on 80 wooded acres in a peaceful residential neighborhood of San Rafael, just 15 minutes north of San Francisco and less than an hour's drive from Pacific Ocean beaches. Students at the College enjoy the intimacy of a small college while benefitting from easy access to the resources of Marin County and the broader San Francisco Bay Area. Marin offers hills for hiking, redwood forests, and ocean shoreline for walking, and, in general, an unsurpassed life-style. In addition, students are only a short distance from San Francisco, which offers world-renowned opera, symphonies, ballet, museums, and championship athletic teams. Dominican is also less than an hour's drive from California's wine country and Silicon Valley.

STUDENT SERVICES
The Office of Student Development coordinates many of the services that support the College's educational mission and the personal, social, physical, spiritual, and professional development of students. Services provided include career services, athletics (NAIA basketball, volleyball, soccer, tennis, and cross-country), recreational sports, on-campus housing, campus ministry, the campus health center, counseling services, and student government (ASDC). There are also many student-formed groups and clubs to choose from on campus. The School of Nursing has an active chapter of the California Nurses Students' Association and a newly founded nursing honor society.

THE NURSING STUDENT GROUP
There are currently 271 students enrolled in the undergraduate nursing programs; of these, 89 percent are women, 43 percent are members of minority groups, 1 percent are international, and 36 percent are enrolled as part-time students.

COSTS
The 1997–98 tuition costs for full-time students (12–17 units) are $15,120. Part-time students pay $630 per unit. Room and board are an additional $6624. The registration fee for Dominican students is $304, and there is an additional nursing major fee of $704. Mandatory insurance is also available for $392 per semester for those without health insurance.

Additional expenses for the nursing program include uniforms, books, supplies, a physical examination, annual tuberculosis screening and immunization, and transportation between the College and affiliated clinical agencies.

FINANCIAL AID

The College manages an extensive financial assistance program to ensure that a highly qualified and diverse population is able to matriculate and continue to graduation. The assistance programs take two major forms: merit scholarships and need-based financial aid. In addition to administering federal and state aid programs, Dominican College also awards a number of scholarships and grants annually from income provided by annual gifts and endowed funds as well as from its own general funds. The Financial Aid Office matches the intentions of the donor to the academic and other qualifications of students with need.

APPLYING

The size of clinical nursing classes is limited by the availability of faculty members and health-care facilities used for student clinical experiences. Each year, applicants who are qualified for admission to Dominican College are admitted as nursing majors in the preclinical program. Students are considered for placement in sophomore clinical classes the ensuing fall or spring if the following minimal admission criteria are fulfilled: (1) completion of elementary algebra/math; (2) completion of all prerequisite courses (inorganic and organic chemistry/CHM 10 and 11; human anatomy and physiology/BIO 16a; nutrition/BIO 11; introduction to psychology/PSY 10, sociology/SCS 1, or anthropology/SCS 2; introduction to nursing/NRS 1; and English/ENG 2); and (3) maintenance of an overall GPA of at least 2.5. Advanced placement students can be admitted for either the spring or fall semesters.

Correspondence and Information:

Office of Admissions
Dominican College
50 Acacia Avenue
San Rafael, California 94901-2298
Telephone: 415-485-3204
800-788-3522 (toll-free)
E-mail: enroll@dominican.edu

Dominican College School of Nursing
Telephone: 415-485-3295
E-mail: nursing@dominican.edu

THE FACULTY

Anna Alexander, Clinical Instructor; M.S.N., San Francisco; RN.
Marie Paz T. Bautista, Lecturer; M.S.N., San Francisco State.
Tamara Bolinger, Assistant Professor; M.N., UCLA; RN.
Pamela Bunnell, Assistant Professor; M.S.N., California, San Francisco; RN.
Penny Fairman, Instructor; Ed.D., San Francisco.
Patricia Ferjancsik, Assistant Professor; M.S.N., California, San Francisco; RN.
Sally Fuller, Lecturer; M.S.N., Sonoma State.
Linda Gabriel, Assistant Professor; M.S.N., California, San Francisco.
Mary Ann Haeuser, Assistant Professor; M.S., California, San Francisco; F.N.P. certificate, Sonoma State; RN.
Marilyn Jossens, Instructor; Dr.P.H., Berkeley; RN.
Leonard Kania, Clinical Instructor; M.A., Chapman; RN.
Luanne Linnard-Palmer, Assistant Professor; Ed.D., San Francisco.
Sherry Lynch, Lecturer; M.S., San Francisco State.
Robin Marci, Instructor; M.S., California, San Francisco.
Ron Morrison, Visiting Lecturer; M.S.N., Dallas Baptist.
Bridget Murphy, Lecturer; M.S.N., California, San Francisco.
Dee Ann Naylor, Instructor; M.S.N., Sonoma State.
Martha Nelson, Associate Professor and Dean, School of Nursing; Ph.D., California, San Francisco; RN.
Carol Oleson, Lecturer; M.S.N., Texas Woman's.
Nancy Pullen, Assistant Professor; Ph.D. candidate, Wright Institute; RN.
Lisa Roberts, Lecturer; B.S.N., St. Mary's College.
Vince Salyers, Assistant Professor; M.S.N., San Francisco State; Ed.Dip. candidate, San Francisco; RN.

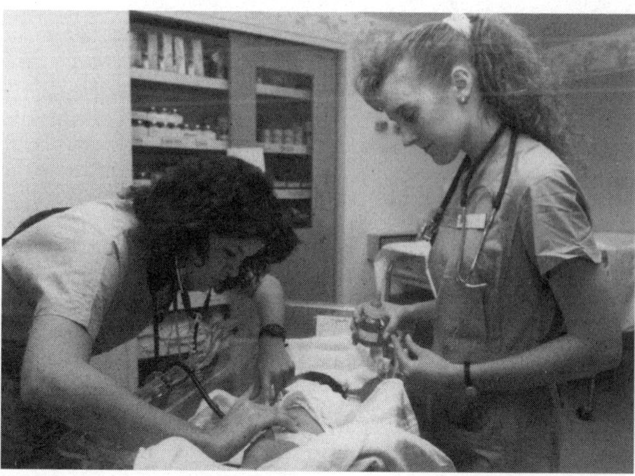

The School of Nursing at Dominican College of San Rafael offers its students a wide variety of clinical experiences.

Drake University
Department of Nursing
Des Moines, Iowa

THE UNIVERSITY
Founded in 1881, Drake University is a private and independent university that provides a student-centered learning environment of exceptional quality and vigor that challenges and prepares students for productive careers, active leadership, and responsible citizenship in the global and diverse community of the twenty-first century. Drake maintains a low 16:1 student-faculty ratio, allowing students to learn from and work with outstanding professors, 93 percent of whom hold the highest degree in their field. Approximately 6,000 students, representing nearly all fifty states and forty-eight countries, are enrolled in the six colleges and schools of the University.

Drake University has been recognized for the last three years by *U.S. News & World Report* as an outstanding teaching institution in the Midwest region. Drake faculty members challenge traditional assumptions, use information technology and other resources imaginatively, and actively involve students in the teaching-learning process.

THE DEPARTMENT OF NURSING
Founded in 1985, the Department of Nursing offers a baccalaureate completion (B.S.N.) program, a Master of Science in Nursing (M.S.N.) program, and a post-master's family nurse practitioner certificate program. All doctorally prepared faculty members teach in both the undergraduate and graduate programs; all courses are taught by full-time members of the teaching faculty. Eighty percent of the nursing faculty members hold doctoral degrees. The majority of nursing students are nontraditional students who hold positions in the health-care arena and attend classes on a part-time basis. The faculty members are innovative and creative educators who have accumulated a vast array of clinical and service experiences throughout their distinguished careers. The Department of Nursing fosters a student-oriented environment that focuses on the teaching-learning process as well as meeting the professional and personal needs of the various student populations.

PROGRAMS OF STUDY
The baccalaureate completion program has been designed for part-time students, with courses offered in the evenings and on the weekends. Fully accredited by the National League for Nursing and the Iowa Board of Nursing, the B.S.N. program is a 124-credit-hour program that consists of 60 credit hours of liberal arts and sciences courses and 64 credit hours in the nursing major. The Department of Nursing is a participant in the Iowa State Board of Nursing Articulation Plan and offers baccalaureate nursing students options for receiving credit for prior education. All of the options are a part of the Department of Nursing's high-quality, flexible program, and each option values previous education and experience by granting as many as 62 credit hours for basic nursing education.

The Master of Science in Nursing program prepares nurses for advanced nursing practice. Students synthesize knowledge from nursing theory, research, and practice to promote innovative, high-quality health care. Students also participate in collaborative, multidisciplinary approaches to health care delivery. Courses in this program emphasize critical analysis of political, legal, and cultural issues affecting health care. Students are prepared to evaluate creative strategies that contribute to improved health care, the advancement of the nursing profession, and the development of health policy. The Master of Science in Nursing program has two options: a role area option in nursing education/nursing administration and a family nurse practitioner option. The core courses, all 3 semester hours of credit and all required of students pursuing a Master of Science in Nursing program, are Introduction to Advanced Nursing Practice, Advanced Nursing Research, Theoretical Bases of Advanced Nursing Practice, Conceptual Models of Advanced Nursing Practice, and Seminar in Advanced Nursing Practice.

The nursing education/nursing administration role area is designed for part-time students, with courses offered in the evenings and on the weekends. Open to registered nurses with baccalaureate degrees in nursing, this 36-credit-hour option includes a thesis or graduate project. Students have five years in which to complete the program.

The family nurse practitioner option in the M.S.N. program is designed for full-time study during a twenty-month period. All courses in this 49-credit-hour option are scheduled on Monday evening, Tuesday during the day, and Tuesday evening, allowing students from diverse areas to attend classes within a compact time frame. The curriculum is structured so that the first year of the program involves didactic classroom experiences, which include the required core courses, a course in ethics, a course in advanced pharmacotherapeutics, and a course in family theory. Clinical learning situations are structured to occur during the first summer and the second academic year of the program. All clinical learning environments are arranged in the student's home area as much as possible. No thesis or graduate project is required in this option.

A post-master's certificate as a family nurse practitioner is also available. Students who hold a master's degree obtain transfer credit based on individual transcripts. The maximum number of hours in the post-master's certificate program is 28, and this may be reduced if the student can demonstrate graduate course work in ethics or advanced pharmacotherapeutics specific to the family nurse practitioner. All post-master's students enroll in full-time graduate study for the final two semesters to allow for the successful completion of the required number of clinical learning experiences.

ACADEMIC FACILITIES
As a computer-intensive university, Drake has many computer laboratories located throughout the campus, some of which are available 24 hours a day for nontraditional students. Drake's computer-based Information Resource Service (IRS), accessible from computers in the residence halls, computer labs, and off campus via a modem, helps students learn about the variety of services available, from getting help with a class topic to exploring career options. Many courses are enhanced by technological initiatives, such as computer bulletin boards and other forms of electronic communication. Cowles Library contains more than twenty-five databases that augment the computerized library resources available for the students in both the undergraduate and graduate nursing programs.

LOCATION
Drake is located in Des Moines, Iowa's capital and largest city. Des Moines is served by six major airlines, and the University is easily accessible by interstate highway. Des Moines offers many amenities available to Drake's students. An extensive network of

skywalks downtown, local bicycle trails, the Des Moines Art Center, Science Center, Living History Farms, and Botanical Center are all within easy access. In addition, Des Moines hosts many dramatic, cultural, and musical events throughout the year.

STUDENT SERVICES
Student services available include two bookstores, a Career Center, computer laboratories, a computer store, counseling center, two libraries, a commuter student lounge, and an on-campus convenience store. A number of child-care facilities are available during the day and during evening and weekend hours and are all located near the campus. All providers are certified by ChildNet. Referrals and information are available on campus. Recreational facilities include a swimming pool, weight room, gym, aerobic dance room, and basketball, volleyball, and badminton courts as well as a Tennis Center, an outdoor running track, and a multipurpose sports facility. The Student Life Center offers a variety of activities and programs for students throughout the year, including a weekly film series.

THE NURSING STUDENT GROUP
All students enrolled in the Department of Nursing must be registered nurses with licenses to practice in Iowa. All students enrolled in the baccalaureate completion program and the nursing education/nursing administration option of the master's program are employed. Students in the family nurse practitioner option of the master's program are pursuing full-time graduate education and, for the most part, are employed on a part-time basis. Because of the nontraditional nature of the nursing student population, the students focus on academic achievement while at Drake and find that interaction with their peers augments their professional network and goals. Exposure to diverse clinical learning opportunities enhances their competencies and comfort in various health-care environments.

COSTS
Tuition in 1996–97 was $225 per credit hour for the baccalaureate completion program and $335 per credit hour for the nursing education/nursing administration option in the master's program. Full-time graduate tuition, appropriate only for those in the family nurse practitioner option of the master's program, was $7590 per semester. Post-master's students pursuing family nurse practitioner certification pay part-time graduate tuition for the first three semesters, assuming all relevant courses receive transfer credit, and full-time graduate tuition for the final two semesters.

FINANCIAL AID
Loan funds and a limited number of need-based scholarships are generally available.

APPLYING
Baccalaureate completion students must have completed basic nursing education with at least a 2.5 GPA and have a license to practice nursing in Iowa. As a participant in the Iowa Articulation Plan, Drake University offers several options for admission to the B.S.N. program, each of which gives credit for previous education and experience; advisers assist applicants in determining which option is most appropriate. Students entering the nursing education/nursing administration option of the M.S.N. program must have a baccalaureate degree in nursing; at least a 2.5 GPA overall; a minimum 3.0 GPA in upper-division nursing course work; completed a statistics course, a course in nursing research, and a course in health assessment at the undergraduate level; and a license to practice nursing in Iowa. A year of work experience, two letters of reference, a statement of personal and professional goals, test scores on the Graduate Record Examinations or the Miller Analogies Test, and a personal and professional biography are also required. Students wishing to enter the family nurse practitioner option of the master's program must submit the same materials required for the nursing education/nursing administration option plus have completed two years of work experience. Students applying to the post-master's family nurse practitioner certification option must submit a transcript from their master's in nursing program in addition to the materials required of other graduate nursing applicants.

Drake University does not unlawfully discriminate on the basis of sex, race, color, religion, creed, national or ethnic origin, age, disability, status in administration of its employment and personnel policies, educational policies, admission policies, scholarship and loan programs, and athletic and other University-administered programs. Further, Drake University reserves the right to take affirmative action in connection with this policy in accordance with applicable law. Drake University admits students without regard to sexual orientation to all rights, privileges, programs, and activities generally accorded to or made available to students at the University and does not discriminate on the basis of sexual orientation in administration of its employment and personnel policies, educational policies, admission policies, scholarship and loan programs, and athletic and other University-administered programs except when such discrimination is required by federal or state law or regulations.

Correspondence and Information:

Department of Nursing
452 Olin Hall
Drake University
2507 University Avenue
Des Moines, Iowa 50311
Telephone: 515-271-2830
Fax: 515-271-4569

Duke University
School of Nursing
Durham, North Carolina

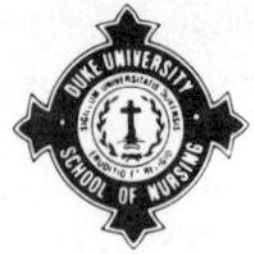

THE UNIVERSITY

Since its founding in 1839 as the Union Institute, and later as Trinity College before incorporating in 1924, the basic principles of Duke University have remained constant. Through changing generations of students, the objective has been to encourage individuals to achieve, to the extent of their capacities, an understanding and appreciation of the world in which they live, their relationship to it, their opportunities, and their responsibilities. Located in Durham, North Carolina, Duke University rests on a spacious sylvan campus. The Gothic architecture of Duke's West Campus is famous the world over, and the culturally diverse population combines with the elegance of Durham's southern charm to make Duke an intellectually stimulating experience. Today, Duke University has more than 11,450 students, of whom 5,250 (400 of whom are part-time) are enrolled in the graduate and professional programs representing nearly every state and many countries. Established in 1930 in association with the School of Medicine and Duke Hospital, the School of Nursing joins the Schools of Medicine, Law, Engineering, Divinity, Business, and Environment in preparing qualified individuals for professional leadership and developing excellence in education for the professions.

By opening the first major outpatient clinics in the region in 1930, Duke recognized its responsibility to provide high-quality care to the people of the Carolinas. The School of Medicine, School of Nursing, and Duke Hospital and Health Network are the core institutions of the Duke University Medical Center and Health System, which ranks among the outstanding health-care centers of the world. Today, the Medical Center at Duke University occupies approximately 140 acres on the West Campus. The goal of the Medical Center is to be a leader in contemporary health care. This involves maintaining superiority in its four primary functions: patient care, dedication to educational programs, national and international distinction in the quality of research, and service to the region, the nation, and the world.

THE SCHOOL OF NURSING

Since the founding of the School in 1930, Duke has prepared outstanding clinicians, educators, and researchers and is continuing this tradition. Drawing on the intellectual and clinical resources of both Duke University Medical Center and Duke University, the School offers a Master of Science in Nursing degree program that balances education, practice, and research.

The School of Nursing is located on the West Campus between Duke Hospital North and Duke Hospital South and is accessible from all other University facilities.

The faculty works closely with students to challenge and nurture them; students not only practice with state-of-the-art science and technology in a great medical center but also have opportunities to work in rural and underserved areas. The program prepares nurses with advanced training in the areas of greatest need for tomorrow.

PROGRAMS OF STUDY

The Master of Science in Nursing program is intended to assist students in developing the expertise necessary for leadership roles in professional nursing practice. Since students have different backgrounds and goals, the program emphasizes flexibility within a basic structure designed to accommodate each student's professional objectives. The purpose of the master's program is to prepare professional nurses for advanced practice either in a clinical specialty or in administration. Clinical specialties offered include nurse practitioner programs in gerontology, pediatrics, family, acute care, and adult oncology/HIV; adult general primary care; and adult cardiovascular care. Clinical nurse specialist programs are offered in oncology/HIV, pediatrics, and gerontology. The nursing systems administration program, designed for those professionals who will function as nursing administrators in complex organizations, offers a nursing informatics sequence. Nursing informatics is designed to integrate nursing, computer, and information sciences. Although this is a minor within the nursing systems administration program, courses may be taken by students in other majors. This sequence is also offered as a post-master's certificate.

The core requirements of the master's program enable students to acquire a framework for advanced nursing practice and research. Five courses constitute the core, with courses in the area of specialization and the research option completing the 39–45-credit course of study. The integration of education, practice, and research is basic to the entire curriculum as well as to the activities of individual students. The School of Nursing offers a post-master's certificate to students who have already earned an M.S.N. degree and are seeking specialized knowledge within a major offered in the School's master's program. The student must successfully complete the required courses in the chosen nursing major; the number of credits required to complete the certificate varies by major. Completion of the certificate program will be documented on the student's academic transcript. Depending on the specialty area, students may meet the qualifications for advanced practice certification. For example, students who complete the post-master's certificate in the nurse practitioner majors are eligible to sit for certification examinations.

Students in the School of Nursing may pursue a graduate certificate in women's studies, a multidisciplinary forum for the study of women's roles and gender differences in various societies, past and present.

AFFILIATIONS WITH HEALTH-CARE FACILITIES

Duke Hospital, one of the largest private hospitals in the South, is part of the Duke University Medical Center and currently is licensed for 1,048 beds. It offers patients modern comprehensive diagnostic and treatment facilities and special acute-care and intensive-care nursing units for seriously ill patients. The clinical faculty members of the Duke University School of Nursing number more than 100 and represent all specialties. Clinical faculty members actively participate in graduate nursing education and practice nursing in hospitals and ambulatory settings. Cooperative teaching and clinical facilities, including health departments, retirement centers, and private practices in both urban and rural settings, are available to students mostly within the state of North Carolina. Occasionally, placements are arranged out-of-state or in other countries to accommodate the student's needs.

ACADEMIC FACILITIES

The goal of the Duke Nursing Research Center is to facilitate the conduct of clinical research by students, faculty, and nursing staff. The center provides support for research through assistance with literature searches, development of research designs, the Institutional Review Board and/or the protection of human subjects consultation, data collection and data management, grant proposal development, and editorial review. In addition to individual consultation, short courses and workshops are offered.

The Duke School of Nursing has a state-of-the-art computer laboratory containing fifteen computer workstations. The computers are connected to the local area network (LAN) as well as the World Wide Web. Students have e-mail accounts that can be accessed either through the computer lab within the School of Nursing or from their modem-equipped home computers. The lab is available to students on a 24-hour basis and is equipped with the most widely used, up-to-date computer applications in word processing, graphics, spreadsheet, database, and statistical entry and analysis.

Nationally recognized centers include the Duke Heart Center, the Center for Aging and Human Development, the Comprehensive Cancer Center, the Comprehensive Sickle Cell Center, Alzheimer's Disease Research Center, Duke Hypertension Center, Duke–VA Center for Cerebrovascular Research, Cystic Fibrosis/Chest Center and Clinic, Sleep Disorders Center, the Eye Center, and the Geriatric Research, Education, and Clinical Center.

The Medical Center Library, located in the Seeley G. Mudd Communications Center and Library Building, provides services and collections necessary to support educational, research, and clinical activities. The library has sizable holdings of nursing books and journals, as well as audiovisual materials. Indexes available include the International Nursing Index, the Cumulative Index to Nursing and Allied Health Literature, and the Nursing Studies Index. MEDLINE, CINAHL, and many other databases are available through computer searches. Additional materials from major medical center libraries are available through interlibrary loans. The uniform borrowing privileges apply to all registered users.

LOCATION

Durham, a city of 130,000, is about 250 miles south of Washington, D.C. Durham and nearby Raleigh and Chapel Hill constitute the three points of the Research Triangle, one of the nation's foremost centers of research-oriented industries and government, research, and regulatory agencies.

STUDENT SERVICES

The University has many resources and activities to offer students. These include the Graduate and Professional Student Council, the Women's Center, the Mary Lou Williams Center for Black Culture, and the International House as well as the full programs of the Office of Cultural Affairs, the Duke University Campus Ministry, the Duke University Union, the Office of Student Activities, and recreational clubs.

THE NURSING STUDENT GROUP

Approximately 220 students are enrolled in the M.S.N. and post-master's certificate programs at Duke. Of these, about 7 percent are men and 11 percent are members of minority groups.

COSTS

Tuition in 1997–98 is $530.50 per credit hour.

FINANCIAL AID

Merit and need-based scholarships, traineeships, and loan funds are generally available.

APPLYING

Admission requirements include a bachelor's degree with an upper-division nursing major from an NLN-accredited program, an undergraduate scholastic average of 3.0 or better on a 4.0 scale, an introductory course in descriptive and inferential statistics, Graduate Record Examinations or Miller Analogies Test scores not more than five years old, and licensure as a registered nurse in North Carolina. One year of clinical experience is recommended but not required. Students lacking clinical experience will be advised to take core courses in the first year and secure employment, which will help them meet the experience recommendation. An interview is requested; if distance prohibits this, a telephone interview may be arranged. Exceptions to any of the above qualifications will be considered on an individual basis.

Duke University does not discriminate on the basis of race, color, national and ethnic origin, handicap, sexual orientation or preference, gender, or age in the administration of educational policies, admission policies, financial aid, employment, or any other University program or activity. It admits qualified students to all the rights, privileges, programs, and activities generally accorded or made available to students.

Correspondence and Information:

Judith K. Carter
Admissions Officer/Financial Aid Specialist
Duke Graduate School of Nursing
Box 3322 Medical Center
Duke University
Durham, North Carolina 27710
Telephone: 919-684-4248
Fax: 919-681-8899
E-mail: carte026@mc.duke.edu
World Wide Web: http://son3.mc.duke.edu

THE FACULTY

Jane Blood-Siegfried, Assistant Professor; RN, D.N.Sc., CPNP, UCLA, 1995. Pediatric nursing.

Dorothy J. Brundage, Associate Professor; Ph.D., Walden, 1980. Critical-care nursing (adult).

Mary T. Champagne, Dean; Ph.D., Texas at Austin, 1981. Critical-care nursing, gerontological nursing.

Susan Denman, Assistant Professor; RN, Ph.D., FNP, North Carolina at Chapel Hill, 1996. Family nurse practitioner.

Bonnie J. Friedman, Associate Clinical Professor; Ph.D., North Carolina at Chapel Hill, 1990. Family nurse practitioner.

Linda K. Goodwin, Assistant Professor; RN, Ph.D., Kansas, 1992. Nursing informatics, research and development of expert systems.

Donna S. Havens, Assistant Professor; Ph.D., Maryland, 1990. Nursing systems administration.

Mary H. Hawthorne, Assistant Professor; Ph.D., Adelphi, 1989. Critical-care nursing, adult and pediatric cardiovascular surgery.

Donna W. Hewitt, Assistant Clinical Professor and Director, Continuing Education; M.N., South Carolina, 1972. Nursing and technology.

Marcia S. Lorimer, Assistant Clinical Professor; M.S.N., CPNP, Virginia, 1988. Pediatric nurse practitioner.

Eleanor S. McConnell, Assistant Professor; RN, Ph.D., North Carolina at Chapel Hill, 1996. Gerontology.

A. Sue McIntire, Associate Professor; Ed.D., North Carolina State, 1985. Oncological nursing, adult education.

Sally Messick, Assistant Clinical Professor; M.S.N., North Carolina at Chapel Hill, 1973. Family nurse practitioner.

Jerri M. Oehler, Associate Professor; Ph.D., Duke, 1985. Nursing care of neonates and children.

Ruth M. Ouimette, Assistant Clinical Professor; M.S.N., Yale, 1975. Gerontological nurse practitioner studies.

Marva Mizell Price, Assistant Clinical Professor; Ph.D. candidate, North Carolina at Chapel Hill, 1996. Women's health.

Barbara S. Turner, Associate Dean and Director of Nursing Research; D.N.Sc., California, San Francisco, 1984. Physiologic and neonatal nursing.

Sharon Wallsten, Assistant Clinical Professor; Ph.D., North Carolina State, 1987. Gerontological nursing.

Margaret J. Wilkman, Assistant Clinical Professor; M.P.H., FNP, North Carolina at Chapel Hill, 1971. Family nurse practitioner.

Fairleigh Dickinson University
Henry P. Becton School of Nursing and Allied Health
Teaneck-Hackensack, New Jersey

FDU

THE UNIVERSITY

Founded in 1942, Fairleigh Dickinson University is an independent nonsectarian institution of higher education offering high-quality, career-oriented undergraduate and graduate programs. FDU is one of New Jersey's leading institutions of private higher education, with nearly 100 career-oriented programs on the undergraduate and graduate levels. The University has two campuses in northern New Jersey—Florham-Madison and Teaneck-Hackensack—and the Wroxton College campus in Oxfordshire, England.

All nursing courses are conducted on the Teaneck-Hackensack Campus and at various clinical sites, although students may take non-nursing courses at FDU's other campuses. The Henry P. Becton School of Nursing and Allied Health is part of FDU's University College: Arts • Sciences • Professional Studies.

THE SCHOOL OF NURSING

The 44-year-old nursing program at Fairleigh Dickinson University features a program of study that is designed for individuals who share a sense of obligation to society and a desire to actively participate in its betterment. This philosophy reflects the educational tradition that has been the hallmark of an FDU education, which has long been recognized for its career-oriented studies enriched by the liberal arts tradition.

The faculty of the School of Nursing and Allied Health is committed to the belief that a basis of scientific knowledge is essential for professional nursing practice. The program views the professional nurse as an independent and interdependent practitioner who functions as a client advocate, change agent, innovator, planner, leader, and consumer of research. The emphasis in the nursing education experience is on the promotion of the professional nurse's efforts to understand the cultures and relationships of human beings and their environment; approach nursing as a humanistic discipline combined with a scientific knowledge base; and articulate and integrate a personal belief system that concerns human beings, environment, health, and nursing as a process.

PROGRAMS OF STUDY

The undergraduate program offers two specific study tracks leading to the Bachelor of Science in Nursing (B.S.N.) degree: basic four-year studies and a choice of accelerated one-year (full-time) or two-year (evening) studies for individuals who already hold a baccalaureate degree.

The basic four-year B.S.N. program offers both full- and part-time study options. All nursing courses are offered during the daytime, although many of the required and elective liberal arts courses for the degree are also available during the evening.

The accelerated B.S.N. program is an intensive, concentrated course of study designed to enable participants to complete their degree in one or two calendar years. Nursing courses for one-year students are offered during the daytime, starting mid-May, five days per week; nursing courses for two-year students are offered during the evening, starting in the fall semester, two to four evenings per week.

The Master of Science in Nursing (M.S.N.) curriculum is designed for individuals who wish to study advanced nursing as a discipline or profession. Special emphasis is given to nursing as a human science, nursing education, and advanced nursing practice. The M.S.N. program consists of 45 credits, which full-time students can complete in two academic years, including the intervening summer. Graduates of the program are eligible to take the American Nurses Association (ANA) certification exams for adult nurse practitioners, community health clinical nurse specialists, and staff development.

AFFILIATIONS WITH HEALTH-CARE FACILITIES

The School of Nursing and Allied Health has built a strong network of participating clinical agencies to provide excellent and diverse clinical experiences for nursing students. These agencies include Bergen Community Health Care, Inc., Westwood; Bergen Pines County Hospital, Paramus; Beth Israel Medical Center, Newark; Children's Specialized Hospital, Mountainside; Chilton Memorial Hospital; Columbus Hospital, Newark; Elizabeth General Medical Center; Fair Oaks Hospital, Summit; General Hospital Center of Passaic; Hackensack Medical Center; Holy Name Hospital, Teaneck; Home Health Agency of Hackensack Medical Center; Morristown Memorial Hospital; Northwest Covenant Healthcare System, Dover; Overlook Hospital, Summit; St. Joseph's Hospital and Medical Center, Paterson; St. Mary's Hospital, Passaic; Tri-Hospital Home Health Program; United Hospitals Medical Center, Newark; University Hospital, UMDNJ, Newark; The Valley Hospital, Ridgewood; Valley Home and Community Health Care, Ridgewood; Visiting Nurse and Health Services, Elizabeth; and Wayne General Hospital.

ACADEMIC FACILITIES

The Teaneck-Hackensack Campus has more than seventy buildings situated on 125 acres. In addition to the computer and laboratory facilities available at any major institution of higher education, FDU provides state-of-the-art equipment specifically for nursing students. In fall 1994, the University completed a $12-million renovation of Dickinson Hall, which houses the School of Nursing and Allied Health. The facilities have been fully modernized to include four special nursing laboratories and a nursing skills lab. The School of Nursing and Allied Health also has bedside computer equipment and interactive video software, giving nursing students access to up-to-date simulated hospital, clinical, and other nursing settings.

LOCATION

FDU's Teaneck-Hackensack Campus is situated along the east and west banks of the Hackensack River about 10 minutes from New York City. The campus is directly accessible from Route 4 and is 6 miles west of the George Washington Bridge. Easy access to New York City enables students and faculty members to take advantage of the city's financial, cultural, and international activities.

STUDENT SERVICES

The University community is a total learning environment shared by students, faculty, and staff. To this end, strong support services are provided to enhance both the classroom and extracurricular experiences. Academic and career advisement and library and computer services are complemented by personal counseling, social and cultural activities, and programs that promote cross-cultural understanding. Lectures, seminars, concerts, performances, and special events are frequently offered to members of the University community.

The Fairleigh Dickinson University Student Nurses Association sponsors a variety of professional and social activities.

Throughout each semester, the association invites guest speakers to address topics of interest as part of their special Lunch & Learn Series. Past discussions have included the role of nursing in the Peace Corps and the expanding roles for nursing professionals. In addition, FDU is home to the Epsilon Ro chapter of Sigma Theta Tau, the international nursing honor society.

THE NURSING STUDENT GROUP

Approximately 200 students are enrolled at the School. Sixteen percent are men, and 40 percent are members of minority groups. More than 90 percent of FDU School of Nursing and Allied Health graduates passed the National Council Licensure Examination for Registered Nurses in 1993.

COSTS

Undergraduate full-time tuition at FDU is based on a flat tuition rate of $12,600; the individual undergraduate credit rate is $409. Total tuition costs for the graduate program are approximately $21,195, based on a 45-credit class load and dependent on fees. Graduate tuition is $471 per credit. Nursing students are also required to pay for nursing lab fees, books, and uniforms. Room and board costs are $6264 annually.

FINANCIAL AID

Each year, FDU awards more than $27 million in financial aid to students from federal, state, and University sources. In addition to its excellent need-based financial aid awards, the University also recognizes outstanding academic performance through its Presidential Scholarships (valued at up to full tuition) and University Scholarships (ranging from $3000 to $8000 in value).

Under Fairleigh Dickinson's Family Plan, if a family has two or more dependent children attending the University simultaneously as full-time undergraduate students, only the first one pays full tuition; the others receive $2500 grants. Similarly, if both a husband and wife are concurrently enrolled as full-time undergraduates, one may receive a $2500 grant. Parents and grandparents of a dependent who is a full-time undergraduate may receive half-tuition grants for undergraduate courses (up to $2500 a year), provided that class space is available.

For information on merit- and need-based financial aid at FDU, students should contact the Office of Financial Aid on the Teaneck-Hackensack Campus at 201-692-2368.

APPLYING

For admission into the basic 128-credit, four-year track leading to the B.S.N. degree, applicants should be graduates of an accredited secondary school with a record indicating potential to succeed in college. Applicants should have completed the following high school studies: 4 units of English, 2 units of history, 1 unit of chemistry with lab, 1 unit of biology with lab, and 2 units of college-preparatory mathematics. In addition, 2 units of foreign language and 1 unit of physics are recommended. A minimum of 16 high school academic units is required for admission. A minimum score of 1010 on the Scholastic Assessment Test (SAT I) is necessary for admission. November, December, or January test scores are preferred. An interview with the nursing faculty is also required.

Applicants to FDU's 54-credit accelerated track leading to the B.S.N. degree should have earned a baccalaureate degree from a regionally accredited college or university with a cumulative GPA of 2.5 or higher (based on a 4.0 scale). The following prerequisites, completed at a college level, are also required for enrollment: human anatomy and physiology (6 credits, with lab), chemistry (6 credits, with lab), microbiology (4 credits, with lab), psychology (3 credits), sociology or anthropology (3 credits), statistics (3 credits), and a pharmacology course comparable to FDU's course Drugs and the Body (2 credits). An interview with the nursing faculty is also required.

To be considered for FDU's M.S.N. program, applicants should be graduates of a National League for Nursing (NLN) accredited B.S.N. program with an undergraduate cumulative GPA of 3.0 or higher. Proof of registered nurse licensure, GRE scores, two essays showing evidence of suitability for graduate study in nursing, and proficiency in spoken and written English also are required. Undergraduate prerequisites include courses in health assessment, introduction to computers, statistics, and nursing research. A personal interview may be necessary on request from the faculty.

Students interested in transferring to FDU's School of Nursing and Allied Health from regionally accredited institutions may be admitted with advanced standing upon presentation of official transcripts to the Office of University Admissions and an interview with a School of Nursing and Allied Health faculty member. To transfer, a student must have grades of C or higher. Students transferring from baccalaureate degree nursing programs accredited by the National League for Nursing may be awarded credit for nursing courses with grades of C+ or higher that are comparable to FDU's courses. A student interview and catalog descriptions and syllabi of previous courses are used to determine comparability.

Correspondence and Information:

Caroline P. Jordet
Director, School of Nursing and Allied Health
Fairleigh Dickinson University
1000 River Road
Teaneck, New Jersey 07666
Telephone: 201-692-2888 (School of Nursing and Allied Health)
800-338-8803 (Office of University Admissions, toll-free)

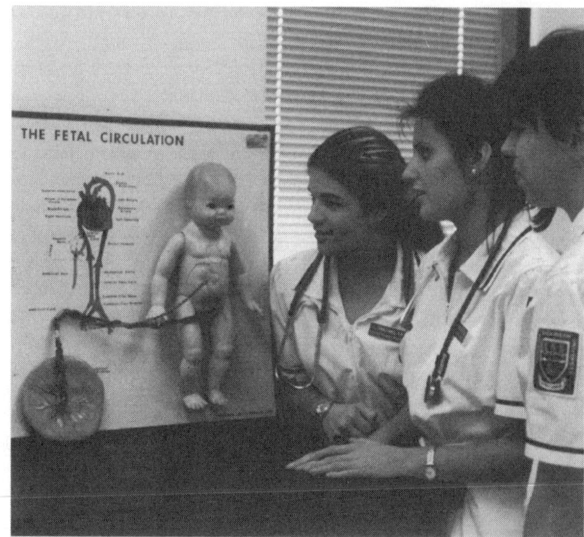

Students examine a student-created learning aid.

Gannon University
Department of Nursing
Erie, Pennsylvania

THE UNIVERSITY

A Catholic, Diocesan, student-centered university, Gannon is dedicated to holistic education in the Judeo-Christian tradition. The University faculty and staff are committed to excellence and continuous improvement in teaching, learning, scholarship, research, and service.

Gannon University is a coeducational institution with approximately 4,000 students, providing a caring environment that fosters inclusiveness and cultural diversity. Gannon's outstanding, values-based education combines the liberal arts with professional specializations to prepare students for leadership roles in their careers, society, and church.

A range of campus organizations and activities encourage academic interests, community service, and moral and spiritual growth. Gannon also offers students a broad program of intramural and intercollegiate athletics.

Gannon University offers associate, bachelor's, master's, and preprofessional degrees.

THE DEPARTMENT OF NURSING

The Department of Nursing offers baccalaureate and master's degree programs. Gannon's nursing curriculum maintains a balance between general education, cognate courses, and professional education in nursing. All programs are accredited by the National League for Nursing. Gannon's nursing faculty members have graduate preparation in their clinical areas of specializations and are skilled clinical practitioners.

The specific purposes of the professional nursing program are to prepare professional nurses who use a systematic methodology in promoting, restoring, and maintaining the client's adaptation in situations of health and illness; to assist students in developing a comprehensive understanding and commitment to human values; to provide opportunities for socialization in the professional role; and to prepare students for future professional and educational goals.

Gannon is able to accommodate an entering class of 60 each year.

PROGRAMS OF STUDY

In the baccalaureate program, the professional nurse's roles are integrated in each clinical nursing course. Emphasis is placed on understanding health in a broad perspective and on understanding modern health-care delivery. The professional nurse's role is developed through a variety of clinical experiences in various areas of specialization, including maternity—home care, labor, delivery, and newborn nursing; hospital pediatrics; hospital medical-surgical units; rehabilitation settings; inpatient mental health units and home care of outpatients from mental health centers; intensive care; step-down units; and care of clients from a variety of community agencies.

In cooperation with the School of Education, Gannon offers a certification program for school nurses. Requirements include successful completion of the B.S.N. program requirements, successful completion of required additional course work, and licensure in the commonwealth of Pennsylvania.

Gannon also offers a graduate program in nursing. The Master of Science in Nursing (M.S.N.) program integrates nursing education, research, and practice and is designed so that the professional nurse can respond to the challenge of unresolved problems in nursing and in health-care systems. Students may choose the Master of Science in Nursing degree program with options in nursing administration, medical-surgical nursing, family nurse practitioner studies, or anesthesia; the RN to M.S.N. admissions option; or the combined M.S.N./M.B.A degree program.

The M.S.N. program requires a total of 42 to 48 credits depending on the specific option. The curriculum plan includes core courses, 6 credits; research component, 9 credits; specialty area, 18 credits; and cognate/support courses, 6 credits. Each graduate student is expected to complete a research thesis or project. The program may be completed by enrolling full-time or part-time, with the exception of the anesthesia option which can be completed only by enrolling full-time.

ACADEMIC FACILITIES

The Nash Learning Resource Center currently has more than 210,000 bound volumes. The library subscribes to more than 1,400 periodicals and has book and periodical materials on microfilm and microcards. The library contains a personal computer lab, a lecture room, a curriculum library, the Founder's Room for fine and rare books, lounges, study rooms, typing rooms, an information-retrieval system, a TV studio, and the latest audiovisual and tape equipment. Students also have access to the Internet. In addition, students may use the facilities and resources of the Erie County Law Library and the Erie City and County Library. For specialized research projects, an efficient interlibrary loan service is available.

The Zurn Science Center has laboratories for research in biology, anatomy, physics, chemistry, and engineering. The building also houses three computer laboratories, including an IBM PC lab. There are two language laboratories, classrooms, and two auditoriums in the building. Other University facilities include a commercial TV and radio station, a theater, and the Career and Counseling Center.

LOCATION

Gannon's campus is located in the heart of downtown Erie. Erie is Pennsylvania's third-largest city and is located in the northwest corner of the state on the shore of Lake Erie. It is approximately 120 miles north of Pittsburgh, Pennsylvania; 90 miles east of Cleveland, Ohio; and 90 miles west of Buffalo, New York. The campus is within 5 miles of Interstates 79 and 90 and 5 miles from Erie International Airport. Erie is also serviced by rail and bus transportation.

STUDENT SERVICES

Gannon prides itself on meeting the personal and professional needs of all students. The Office of Counseling and Career Services helps students in all stages of career preparation, from determining interests and aptitudes to writing a résumé and conducting a job search. Counselors are also available whenever support is needed for personal concerns.

Gannon has a math center, writing center, and advising center that students can visit for additional help on assignments.

THE NURSING STUDENT GROUP

There are currently 141 students in the Bachelor of Science in Nursing program and 76 students in the Master of Science in Nursing program. Ninety percent of the B.S.N. graduates are employed in their field, and more than 90 percent of the M.S.N. students are employed in the nursing profession.

COSTS

In 1997–98, full-time undergraduate tuition is $6050 per semester or $12,100 per academic year. Room and board average $2355 per semester. The total cost for the academic year at Gannon, including books and supplies, is approximately $13,200 for commuting students and $17,910 for resident students.

FINANCIAL AID

In order to bring a Gannon education to qualified students who could not otherwise afford it, the University offers a comprehensive financial aid program of scholarships, loans, and employment. An application for financial aid must be filed with the application for admission. The filing has no effect on the decision of the Committee on Admissions. Gannon's financial aid program is open to all full-time students attending classes during the nine-month period from September to May. All students seeking aid should file the admission and financial aid applications no later than March 1.

APPLYING

To obtain admission into the B.S.N. program, students must have completed work equal to a standard high school curriculum with a minimum of 16 units with a grade of C or better to meet the preprofessional requirements of the State Board of Nursing. Requirements include 4 units of English, 3 units of social studies, 2 units of science in biology and chemistry with labs, and 2 units of college-preparatory math, one of which must be algebra. Additional requirements include a minimum overall GPA of 2.5 (transfer students must also have a 2.5), a combined SAT I score of 1010 or higher with a mathematics score of at least 480, and rank in the top 40 percent of the high school class. All applicants are required to submit scores on either the SAT I or ACT, an up-to-date transcript of the high school record showing rank in class (plus a college transcript for transfer applicants), a completed application form, and a nonrefundable $25 application fee.

Requirements for students applying to graduate programs include a statistics course, competitive scores on the GRE General Test or the Miller Analogies Test (or GMAT scores for M.S.N./M.B.A. program applicants), three letters of recommendation, RN licensure, and an interview with program coordinators.

Correspondence and Information:

Director of Admissions
Gannon University
824 Peach Street
Erie, Pennsylvania 16541
Telephone: 814-871-7240
800-GANNON-U (toll-free)
Fax: 814-871-5803

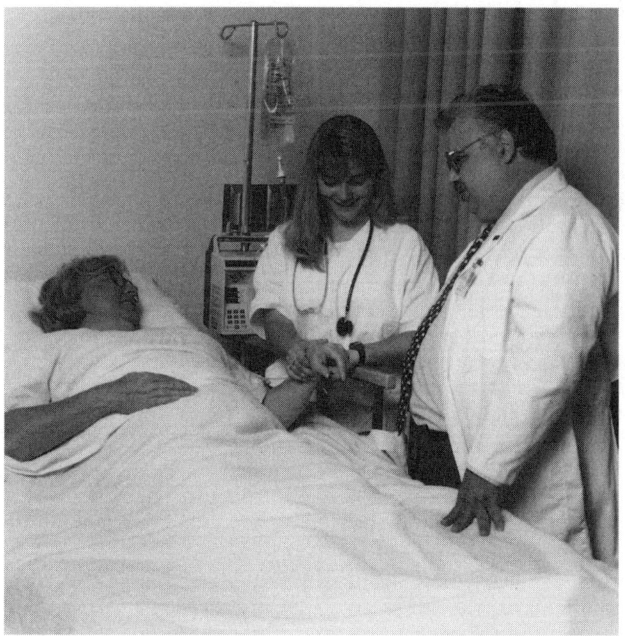

Gannon University nursing students participate in professional clinical rotations offering a variety of specialty areas with patients of different age groups and health conditions.

Georgetown University
School of Nursing
Washington, D.C.

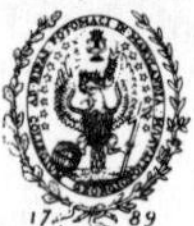

THE UNIVERSITY
Georgetown University was founded in 1789 and is the oldest Catholic, Jesuit institution of higher learning in the United States. Washington, D.C., the nation's capital, is one of the most important cities in the world. Health policy and medical economics decisions are debated daily in many arenas, and decisions are made that shape the delivery of health care in this country and abroad. Cultural and social opportunities are limitless.

The diversity of the student population at Georgetown provides a stimulating environment for student life and study. All fifty states and more than forty countries are represented by the 12,000 men and women currently enrolled in undergraduate, graduate, and professional programs.

THE SCHOOL OF NURSING
The School of Nursing is conveniently located on the Main Campus next to the Georgetown University Medical Center. The Concentrated Care Center, Georgetown University Hospital, Pasquerilla Healthcare Center, Perinatal Center, and Lombardi Cancer Research Center provide access to an abundant patient population, while their proximity to the John Vinton Dahlgren Library yields an ideal coordination of academic, clinical, and research facilities. This physical and functional relationship among nursing, medical, and academic facilities creates an integrated, comprehensive educational environment unavailable at many other universities.

PROGRAMS OF STUDY
The School of Nursing offers baccalaureate and master's degrees in nursing. All programs have been accredited by the National League for Nursing. The Bachelor of Science degree programs enroll traditional undergraduate students and registered nurses and include an accelerated option for college graduates. The nursing component is a balance between a strong theoretical base and clinical skills. Students study the curative and restorative aspects of health care, as well as health maintenance and health education. Clinical practice culminates in the senior practicum. This practicum is designed to ease the transition of the individual from the role of nursing student to that of graduate professional nurse. Students are permitted to choose an area of concentration based on the various clinical settings available to the School of Nursing. In keeping with the University's commitment to international work and study, students have opportunities for intercultural clinical experience; to date, these have included work in Appalachia, Guatemala, England, and Ireland.

The Master of Science degree programs lead to advanced nursing practice in four specialty areas: nurse midwifery, acute-care nurse practitioner, family nurse practitioner, and nurse anesthesia.

AFFILIATIONS WITH HEALTH-CARE FACILITIES
In addition to the Georgetown University Medical Center, the School of Nursing is affiliated with many of the Washington area health institutions. Some of these include Bethesda Naval Medical Center, National Children's Hospital, U.S. Department of Human Services, Walter Reed Hospital, and Hospice of the District of Columbia, to name only a few.

ACADEMIC FACILITIES
The School's classrooms, faculty, and administration are located in St. Mary's Hall. Nursing students also have classes and laboratories on the main campus and in the medical school. The Medical Center's exciting research, innovative techniques, and sophisticated instrumentation provide an exemplary background for student clinical practice. A special clinical emphasis in home health care is included. There are varied educational resources at Georgetown's three campus libraries: the Lauinger Library, the Riggs Bioethics Library, and the Dahlgren Medical Library.

LOCATION
Georgetown is located in a small community of cobblestone streets, trolley tracks, and fine shops and restaurants. Cultural and social opportunities are limitless in Washington, D.C. The Kennedy Center for the Performing Arts and the many museums of the Smithsonian Institution are only a few examples of the resources available to Georgetown students.

STUDENT SERVICES
The Leavey Center serves as a hub of activity for social and academic campus life. The building includes three distinct components, a Conference Center, Guest House, and Student Activities Building. The Leavey Center also contains a 450-seat cafeteria, fast-food shops, a bookstore, the Faculty Club, and the Hoya Restaurant. At Georgetown, athletic activity and physical well-being are integral to the happiness and health of its students, and Yates Field House provides every means necessary to achieve this goal. It is a four-level, 142,300-square-foot structure with facilities for tennis, squash, basketball, racquetball, badminton, handball, swimming, volleyball, weightlifting, and track.

THE NURSING STUDENT GROUP
Approximately 300 undergraduate students are currently enrolled in the B.S.N. program. The M.S.N. program has approximately 150 students.

COSTS
Undergraduate tuition for the 1996–97 academic year was $19,696. Room and board were estimated at $7,462 per year. Full-time graduate program tuition was $16,670 per year. University housing includes apartments, dormitories, town houses, and college houses. Accommodations are also available in apartments and houses in the Georgetown area surrounding the University. Both the University and the public transportation system provide excellent facilities to meet students' needs.

FINANCIAL AID
In cases of economic need, the University makes every effort to provide financial aid in the form of scholarships, grants, loans, and jobs to enable students to come to Georgetown. The amount of financial assistance given varies with the demonstrated financial need of the applicant. Qualified applicants may be admitted to the U.S. Army or Naval ROTC, which supports a unit on the Georgetown campus. Full-tuition scholarship assistance and subsistence allowances are available. An Air Force unit is available at a neighboring institution.

APPLYING

The School of Nursing welcomes applications from men and women, without distinction on the basis of race, sex, or religious beliefs. Transfer students and candidates with degrees in fields other than nursing are encouraged to apply. All candidates are required to take the Scholastic Assessment Test (SAT I) offered by the College Board or the ACT examination offered by American College Testing.

Graduate school admission requirements include a baccalaureate degree in nursing from a school accredited by the National League for Nursing, a minimum undergraduate GPA of 3.0 on a 4.0 scale, RN licensure, three letters of reference, Graduate Record Examinations scores or the Miller Analogies Test scores, completion of an introductory course in statistical methods, and one year's experience as an RN. For a more detailed description of the application process students should contact the admissions office.

Correspondence and Information:

Office of Undergraduate Admissions
White Gravenor, 101
Georgetown University
37th and O Street, NW
Washington, D.C. 20057
Telephone: 202-687-3600

Office of Graduate Admissions
Intercultural Center, 302
Georgetown University
37th and O Street, NW
Washington, D.C. 20057
Telephone: 202-687-5568

Office of Student Affairs
School of Nursing
3700 Reservoir Road, NW
Washington, D.C. 20007
Telephone: 202-687-8439

THE ADMINISTRATION

Elaine L. Larson, Professor and Dean; Ph.D., Washington (Seattle); RN, FAAN.

Denise M. Korniewicz, Associate Dean for Academic Development; D.N.Sc., Catholic University; RN, FAAN.

Judith Baigis-Smith, Associate Dean for Research and Scholarship; Ph.D., NYU; RN, FAAN.

Dorrie Fontaine, Director of Academic Programs; D.N.Sc., Catholic University; RN, FAAN.

Hartwick College
Department of Nursing
Oneonta, New York

THE COLLEGE

Hartwick College is a liberal arts institution whose roots reach back to 1797. The College exists to make a difference in the lives of its students. This means providing a rich and challenging academic program and effective, engaging teachers. It means developing within this community an array of activities and opportunities for expanding interests and sharpening personal skills. Students receive a personal computer notebook and printer at the start of their college career. The campus is networked and students have access from their dorm rooms to informational services worldwide.

The 375-acre hillside campus is located on Oyaron Hill and commands an impressive view of the city of Oneonta and the Susquehanna Valley in the foothills of the Catskills. Hartwick's 914-acre Pine Lake Environmental Center, 8 miles from the main campus, offers a unique setting for classes, independent study, and recreational and residential opportunities.

Total enrollment is approximately 1,500 students. The faculty is teaching oriented. With small classes and close advising relationships, students can come to know the faculty well. The curriculum is designed to assure that students will explore the fundamental components of the kind of liberal education to which Hartwick is committed. Thirty-one majors are available through three divisions: Humanities, Physical and Life Sciences, and Social and Behavioral Sciences.

The College is organized on a 4-1-4 curriculum plan, which requires that students take four courses each semester and one course for in-depth study either on campus or off campus during the four-week January term. A wide variety of learning opportunities enable students to study overseas and pursue independent study or internships.

THE DEPARTMENT OF NURSING

The professional component of the major program requires that each student demonstrate not only mastery of theoretical knowledge but also competence in the application of theory to practice—cognitive, affective, and psychomotor skills. The curriculum and teaching strategies focus on the students' use and application of knowledge more than the acquisition of knowledge, because the faculty understands that nurses need to be competent information processors in order to thrive in the rapidly changing field of health care and the age of information explosion.

All of the Department's full-time, tenure-track faculty members maintain an active clinical practice in their area of specialty and most are either doctorally prepared or are engaged in doctoral study. The College also utilizes the services of a group of well-prepared clinical, administrative, and educational preceptors.

The nursing program has been a part of the College for the past fifty years, and there are over 1,000 nursing alumni. The graduates are reflective practitioners who are well-versed in the use of critical thinking skills to make clinical and personal decisions. They must be excellent communicators and be prepared to assume positions of leadership in patient care and management. Graduates are well respected by their employers, and a high percentage pursue graduate study in nursing after graduation.

PROGRAMS OF STUDY

The Department of Nursing offers a B.S.N. for traditional college-age students, a special Summer Accelerated Program for transfer students with previous college credits and students who wish to spend a semester abroad, and an RN to B.S.N. program for graduates of diploma and associate degree programs in nursing. The course of study is designed to prepare nurses to accept increased responsibility within the health-care system and to assume leadership roles within the nursing profession.

Multicultural perspectives are developed during the January term of the junior year, when nursing majors spend two weeks in large urban medical center hospitals studying inpatient pediatric nursing and two weeks in an off-campus culturally diverse community setting. Experiences have included working with Hurricane Andrew victims in a nurse-run clinic and caring for Native American families in Indian Health Service settings in Arizona and New Mexico. During the January term of the senior year, students select an agency anywhere in the world to complete a four-week independent practicum that serves to perfect technical skills and raise self-confidence prior to graduation.

Nursing courses begin in the freshman year and continue with at least one clinical nursing course throughout the four-year curriculum. The curriculum uses the nursing process as a framework, with the students caring for both healthy and ill clients in a variety of settings. The program of study culminates in a senior thesis in which the student analyzes and evaluates a major nursing theorist. This theory base is then applied as a part of the senior independent practicum.

The liberal arts are seen as essential to the holistic development of the nursing major. Students are required to have a firm foundation in the life and natural sciences, social sciences, and humanities. Students have the opportunity to take one elective each semester throughout their college career.

The Summer Accelerated Program allows transfer students who have met the necessary prerequisites to take the first three nursing courses in a concentrated ten-week summer program. After successfully completing the summer course work these students move into the junior year. The program then can be completed in two years and one summer after the prerequisite course work. This summer program also allows students who wish to double major or to study abroad the ability to finish the program in four years.

The R.N. Mobility Program allows registered nurse students the ability to validate their prior learning and gain advanced standing through the NLN Mobility Profile II exam. After completing the exam and a transition course, the RN students enroll in the eight required senior-level nursing courses.

AFFILIATIONS WITH HEALTH-CARE FACILITIES

The College is affiliated with a wide variety of clinical facilities in New York, including At-Home Care, Oneonta; Albany Medical Center Hospital, Albany; Mary Imogene Bassett Hospital, Cooperstown; Columbia-Presbyterian Medical Center, New York; A. O. Fox Memorial Hospital and Nursing Home, Oneonta; Nader Towers for the Elderly, Oneonta; Otsego County Public Health Nursing Service, Oneonta; and University Hospital, Syracuse. The areas of health promotion and community-based care are addressed by affiliation with a large number of community agencies, including adult homes, schools, ambulatory clinics, and primary care offices.

Recent student internship placements include New York Hospital; Memorial Sloan-Kettering Hospital; Georgetown University Hospital, Washington, D.C.; Johns Hopkins Medical Center, Baltimore, Maryland; Yale–New Haven Hospital, New Haven, Connecticut; Mary Hitchcock Hospital, Hanover, New Hampshire; New England Medical Center; Dana Farber Cancer Institute; Beth Israel Hospital, Boston Children's Hospital, Brigham and Women's Hospital, Boston, Massachusetts; and Baylor University Medical Center, Dallas, Texas.

ACADEMIC FACILITIES

The Stevens-German Library provides a comfortable and effective area for student research and study. Included in the library are over 245,000 books and periodicals and subscriptions to over 1,500 journals and newspapers. These holdings are complemented by access to national and international bibliographic databases and an effective system of interlibrary loan privileges that extend library resources far beyond the confines of the Hartwick campus. Library resources can be accessed via personal computers and terminals in the library and through the campus computer network.

The nursing department utilizes the Godley Learning Laboratory as a place for students to practice skills in simulated settings and to use a wide variety of computer-assisted instructional tools and videotapes, audiotapes, and simulation equipment.

The College provides each student with his or her own personal computer, enabling access via the campus network to both College-owned computer-assisted instructional offerings and a wide variety of offerings that exist on national and international information network systems.

LOCATION

Oneonta, New York, with a population of 17,500, is located in the northern foothills of the Catskills. It is equidistant from Utica, Albany, and Binghamton (approximately 65 miles) and is 190 miles northwest of New York City.

Hartwick benefits from the presence in Oneonta of the State University College at Oneonta. An exchange agreement enables students to cross-register for courses on the other campus and use the library facilities of both institutions.

STUDENT SERVICES

The College has many resources and services designed to meet students' needs. These include the Hartwick College Counseling Center; Multicultural Affairs Office; Trustee Center for Career Planning and Professional Development; Pine Lake Challenge programs and Awakening, an Outward Bound–type orientation program; Greek life, with eight nationally chartered social fraternities and sororities; Perrella Health Center; Fitness Center; and a well-developed interscholastic and intramural athletics program.

THE NURSING STUDENT GROUP

Ninety-three percent of the 132 nursing majors are traditional-age (18–22) students who normally take four years to complete the program. Another 9 percent are transfer students with previous college experience. In recent years, 100 percent of these graduates have practiced for at least a year in an inpatient setting.

The RN students represent about 15 percent of the total nursing student body. These students most often pursue study on a part-time basis and typically take about three years to complete the program. Most of the RNs in the program work full-time in the inpatient settings of local hospitals.

COSTS

The annual tuition charge covers nine courses in the academic year and includes the cost of a personal computer notebook and printer (spread out over four years). Tuition, room, board, and fees are set by the Board of Trustees. For 1996–97 these costs totaled $26,375. The estimated cost of books, uniforms and supplies, personal expenses, and transportation for nursing majors was approximately $1200 per year.

FINANCIAL AID

Financial assistance at Hartwick College is of two types: aid based on financial need and aid based on other criteria, such as academic achievement (non-need-based aid). Financial need is met by a combination of scholarships, grants, student loans, College-sponsored parent loans, and work-study and the minority assistance program, when applicable. Several nursing scholarships are available to eligible students.

APPLYING

Application to the nursing program is through the admission office. The framework of recommended courses of secondary school study for applicants includes 4 years of English; 3 years of a modern or classical foreign language; 3 years of mathematics; 3 years of a laboratory science; and 3 years of history. Transfer students interested in the Summer Accelerated Program and RN students must have completed college-level anatomy and physiology (two courses), general or organic chemistry (one course), microbiology (one course), an introductory course in sociology and psychology; and life span developmental psychology. CLEP and/or ACT and PEP exams may be considered for these college prerequisites. Students should contact the admissions office at the College for complete information about admission requirements and application deadlines.

Correspondence and Information:

Admission Office
Hartwick College
Oneonta, New York 13820
Telephone: 607-431-4150
888-HARTWICK (toll-free)
Fax: 607-431-4154

Dianne M. Miner, Ph.D., RN, CNRN
Associate Professor and Acting Chair, Department of Nursing
Hartwick College
Oneonta, New York 13820
Telephone: 607-431-4780
Fax: 607-431-4850
E-mail: minerd@hartwick.edu

Hawaii Pacific University
Nursing Program
Honolulu, Hawaii

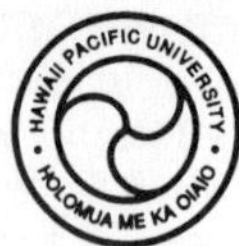

THE UNIVERSITY

Hawaii Pacific University (HPU) is an independent, coeducational, career-oriented, comprehensive university with a foundation in the liberal arts. Undergraduate and graduate degrees are offered in approximately fifty different areas. Hawaii Pacific prides itself on maintaining small class size and individual attention to students.

Students at HPU come from every state in the union and over eighty countries around the world. The diversity of the student body stimulates learning about other cultures firsthand, both in and out of the classroom. There is no majority population at HPU. Students are encouraged to examine the values, customs, traditions, and principles of others to gain a clearer understanding of their own perspectives. HPU students develop friendships with students from throughout the United States and the world and make important connections for success in the global community of the twenty-first century.

THE NURSING PROGRAM

The nursing program began with 36 students in the fall of 1982 as a program designed to facilitate the completion of the baccalaureate degree by registered nurses. In September 1984, the program was expanded to accommodate the educational needs of licensed practical nurses. In the fall of 1987, 24 students were accepted into a newly developed four-year program. The qualities of humanism, caring, and collaboration provide a foundation to the comprehensive study of the art and science of nursing. Students learn in a flexible, multicultural environment and receive high-quality instruction in classrooms consisting of 24 to 35 students and clinical groups consisting of 8 to 10 students.

The education and expertise gained by HPU nursing students allow them to help with the physical, mental, emotional, and spiritual needs of people from varied age groups and multiple ethnic backgrounds.

PROGRAMS OF STUDY

The nursing program offers five pathways toward a Bachelor of Science in Nursing degree. These include a B.S.N. Pathway for the beginning or transfer student with fewer than 45 college credits, a Twenty-Three Month Pathway for transfer students who have at least a 3.0 GPA and are able to complete a degree in twenty-three months, an LPN/B.S.N. Pathway for licensed practical nurses, an RN/B.S.N. Pathway for licensed registered nurses from associate degree or diploma programs, and an International Nurse Pathway for persons who have graduated from a nursing program in another country and are not licensed in the United States.

The goal of the nursing program at Hawaii Pacific University is to prepare a liberally educated professional nurse. The professional nurse has the following attributes: he or she synthesizes knowledge from the humanities, the arts, and the natural, behavioral, and nursing sciences to provide competent nursing services within a multicultural society; incorporates the caring ethic as the foundation of nursing practice; develops a commitment to altruistic service valued by society, is sensitive to the diverse needs of vulnerable groups, and has active involvement in health-care delivery policy; and promotes the integration of body, mind, and spirit through utilizing the nursing process, diagnostic and ethical reasoning, and critical thinking to assist the client in achieving mutually determined health goals. The professional nurse also practices autonomously along the continuum of novice to expert through collaboration and consultation as a member of a multidisciplinary health-care team; applies beginning leadership and management knowledge and skills to nursing practice; participates in the research process, evaluates findings for applicability and utilization in nursing practice, and contributes to the body of nursing practice; and continues to pursue knowledge and expertise commensurate with the evolving professional scope of practice.

AFFILIATIONS WITH HEALTH-CARE FACILITIES

The nursing program chooses facilities that give students the best experience possible. Within these facilities, the choice of clinical units is made based upon the learning needs of the students. The majority of clinical faculty members are currently actively employed in the clinical specialties and facilities where they teach.

ACADEMIC FACILITIES

All nursing classes are held on the suburban and residential Windward campus where life revolves around the Amos N. Starr and Juliette Montague Cooke Academic Center (AC). The AC houses faculty and staff offices, classrooms and nursing laboratories, an art gallery, and the Atherton Learning Resources Center, which includes a library with extensive collections in the areas of Asian studies, marine science, and nursing. The Boyd MacNaughton Pacific Resources Room houses the Hawaiiana and Pacific special collections. The Academic Computer Center provides access to both Macintosh and IBM computers. The Learning Assistance Laboratory includes a collection of automated audio, video, and interactive nursing learning resources. In addition, nursing students utilize the resources of the Hawaii Medical Library, the most comprehensive facility of its type in the state.

LOCATION

With two campuses linked by shuttle, Hawaii Pacific combines the excitement of an urban, downtown campus with the serenity of the Windward residential campus set in the lush foothills of the Koolau Mountains. The main campus is located in downtown Honolulu, the business and financial center of the Pacific. Eight miles away, situated on 135 acres in Kaneohe, the Windward campus is the site of the nursing, environmental science, and marine science programs and a variety of other course offerings. Students may attend classes on either campus. The beautiful weather, for which Hawaii is famous, allows for unlimited recreational opportunities year-round. The emphasis on a career-related curriculum keeps students focused on their academic goals. The economy in Hawaii makes cooperative education and internship experiences hard to beat. Students desiring to expand their horizons in preparation for the changing global economy find Hawaii a working laboratory. The many opportunities available at HPU provide for a healthy combination of school, work, and fun.

STUDENT SERVICES

The University has many services to meet student needs, including a professional staff of advisers who are available throughout the year to assist undergraduate students in advising and counseling matters. Other services include career placement programs; a cooperative education program; international student advising; various student organizations, including the Student Nurses' Association; and numerous honor societies, including Sigma Theta Tau International Nursing Honor Society. A director of student life and a residence life staff are actively involved in all aspects of student life.

HPU competes in NAIA intercollegiate sports. Men's athletic programs include baseball, basketball, cross-country, soccer, and tennis. Women's athletics include cross-country, soccer, softball, tennis, and volleyball.

The Housing Office at HPU offers many services and options for students. Residence halls with cafeteria service are available on the Hawaii Loa campus, while University-sponsored apartments are available in the Waikiki area, near the downtown campus, for those seeking more independent living arrangements.

THE NURSING STUDENT GROUP

The students in the nursing program are representative of the global community in terms of age, ethnicity, citizenship, gender, and professional experience. More than 75 percent of the 600 students are enrolled full-time, with a substantial number of these students choosing to accelerate the completion of their degree by studying during summer sessions. Various nursing courses are offered during summer sessions.

COSTS

Tuition for the 1996–97 academic year was $7100 for freshmen and sophomores and $11,000 for juniors and seniors. Laboratory fees, health insurance, malpractice coverage, books, and other fees may increase the costs by several hundred dollars. Part-time student tuition was $296 per credit for freshmen and sophomores and $460 per credit for juniors and seniors. Residence hall room and board were $6510. University-leased apartments were $3950 for the academic year.

FINANCIAL AID

The University provides financial aid for qualified students through institutional, state, and federal aid programs. Approximately 50 percent of the University's students receive financial aid. Among the forms of aid available are Federal Perkins Loans, Federal Stafford Student Loans, Guaranteed Parental Loans, Federal Pell Grants, and Federal Supplemental Educational Opportunity Grants. To apply for aid, students must submit the Free Application for Federal Student Aid (FAFSA). The FAFSA may be submitted at any time, but the priority deadline is March 1. Several local health-care agencies award low-interest loans to student nurses, which are forgiven for various lengths of service following successful completion of the NCLEX-RN examination.

APPLYING

Candidates are notified of admission decisions on a rolling basis, usually within two weeks of receipt of application materials. Early entrance and deferred entrance are available. HPU accepts the Common Application form.

Correspondence and Information:

Office of Admissions
Hawaii Pacific University
1164 Bishop Street, Suite 200
Honolulu, Hawaii 96813
Telephone: 808-544-0238
800-669-4724 (toll-free)
Fax: 808-544-1136
E-mail: admissions@hpu.edu
World Wide Web: http://www.hpu.edu

THE FACULTY

Dale Allison, Adjunct; Ph.D., Pennsylvania.
Linda Beechinor, Assistant Professor; M.S.N., Hawaii.
Diane DePew, Assistant Professor; M.S.N., Maryland at Baltimore.
Judith Holland, Assistant Professor; Ph.D., Denver.
Barbara Ingwalson, Assistant Professor; M.S., Hawaii.
Holly Kailani, Assistant Professor; M.S., Hawaii.
Betty Kohal, Assistant Professor; M.S.N., Vanderbilt.
Patricia Lange-Otsuka, Assistant Professor; Ed.D., Nova Southeastern.
Carole Meshot, Associate Professor; Ed.D., North Carolina at Greensboro.
Mercy Mott, Assistant Professor; M.N., UCLA.
Patricia Slachta, Associate Professor; Ph.D, Adelphi.
Brenda Smith, Assistant Professor; Ed.D., Hawaii.
Frances Spohn, Assistant Professor; M.S., Hawaii.
John Stepulis, Assistant Professor; M.S.N., Vanderbilt.
Ruth Stepulis, Assistant Professor; M.S.N., Vanderbilt.
Hobie Thomas, Assistant Professor; Tennessee.
Jeanine Tweedie, Assistant Professor; M.S.N., Utah.
Janet Viola, Adjunct; Psy.D., American School of Professional Psychology.
Carol Winters-Maloney, Professor; Ph.D., Pittsburgh.

Holy Family College
Division of Nursing
Philadelphia, Pennsylvania

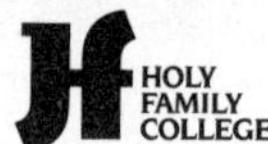

THE COLLEGE

Holy Family College, founded in 1954 by the Congregation of the Sisters of the Holy Family of Nazareth, is a fully accredited, Catholic, private, coeducational, four-year commuter college. It has campuses conveniently located in northeast Philadelphia and in Newtown (Bucks County), Pennsylvania. The College provides liberal arts and professional programs for more than 2,200 full- and part-time undergraduate students in day and evening classes and in summer sessions. Students must take a core curriculum of courses in the humanities and social and natural sciences, which helps them develop ethical and moral values and perspectives.

THE DIVISION OF NURSING

The program in nursing at Holy Family College was inaugurated in 1971 in response to increasing student and public interest and the growing need for qualified health-care professionals. The nursing faculty is committed to a firm liberal arts foundation. The student is expected to assume an active and selective role in the learning experience.

Teaching involves many approaches that are focused on enhancing the student's ability to integrate and use health-related concepts and principles. The faculty members also view their teaching role as one of facilitator and change agent, providing guidance needed for the learning process to proceed. As nurse educators, faculty members also recognize their responsibilities to prepare nursing students to change concurrently with the health-care needs of contemporary society.

The Division of Nursing is the largest of the five academic divisions and occupies the Nursing Education Building, centrally located on campus near the College library, the student College Center, and the administration building.

The Division of Nursing currently offers an educational program at the undergraduate level, including a post-licensure B.S.N. program. A Master of Science in Nursing is also offered.

The Division of Nursing has 22 full-time faculty members, a full-time learning resources coordinator, and 26 part-time faculty members. The student-faculty ratio in the clinical courses is 8:1, maintaining clinical groups at a size that affords each student valuable learning experiences with appropriate instruction, guidance, and supervision.

The nursing division administration consists of a division head, B.S.N. chair, and 4 team leaders in the B.S.N. program. All of the faculty members hold at least a master's degree.

The Division also offers students the services of a full-time student support coordinator as well as faculty members who are available for advising and counseling students about courses, rostering, and student concerns.

PROGRAMS OF STUDY

The baccalaureate nursing program prepares a nursing generalist who possesses the ability to develop selected leadership roles in the delivery of nursing services. The roles of caregiver, client advocate, teacher, and counselor emerge as responsible expectations for baccalaureate graduates. In addition, the ability to propose, critique, and use research studies appropriately is anticipated along with beginning data collection skills. As professional nurses, the graduates accept responsibility for their own professional growth and for the advancement of the profession at large.

Prior to the upper-division clinical nursing courses, a student must have completed a minimum of 60 semester hours in prerequisites and general education. During the third and fourth years, the clinical courses provide the opportunity for students to apply theory to practice in a variety of health-care settings. The diversity of clinical sites affords the student caregiving experiences to clients of various cultural, socioeconomic, and religious backgrounds throughout the life span in both urban teaching tertiary-care centers and smaller community-based settings. In addition to these clinical courses, two seminar courses, which are prepared and presented by the student in a small group environment, focus not only on content but also on group process. The research-related focus helps to prepare the student for practice and for advanced nursing education.

The nursing program may also be completed on a part-time basis. Nursing theory courses are offered in the evening, and clinical experience is offered on Saturday.

The Division of Nursing welcomes and encourages registered nurses to continue their education and to pursue a Bachelor of Science in Nursing degree, as evidenced by the post-licensure B.S.N. curriculum. Recognizing that registered nurses already have a background in clinical nursing, the College respects the students' prior education in order to prevent unnecessary repetition of nursing courses completed in their basic programs. The 126-credit program includes courses designed specifically for RNs, coupled with a plan to accept direct transfer of 32 college nursing credits. Graduates of hospital-based, diploma programs are also eligible for 32 nursing credit acceptances. Registered nurses who graduated eight years or more before admission to Holy Family College have the opportunity to validate prior learning through the ACT-PEP challenge examination process. Applicants' experiences and transcripts are evaluated individually to determine which exams are required. The focus of this curriculum is community-based and includes content in case management and critical pathway design and evaluation.

In 1992, the nursing program once again earned full accreditation from the National League for Nursing. The Division of Nursing is also accredited as a provider of continuing education in nursing by the American Nurses Credentialing Center. Contact hours are awarded by the Pennsylvania Nurses Association (PNA). The Division of Nursing is committed to the ongoing professional development of nurses. Continuing education programs provide the opportunity for the acquisition of new knowledge and skills to meet the ever-changing demands within the health-care arena.

This commitment is very much apparent in the interdenominational Parish Nurse (nondegree) program. The program is designed to educate registered professional nurses (RNs) to function in their communities as members of a ministry team. Through the healing ministry of the church, the parish nurse develops early intervention programs to provide the community with access to health, social, and educational resources and to promote positive changes in lifestyle. The Parish Nurse program focuses on the concepts and principles of holistic nursing practice foundational to the parish nurse's role in the community.

AFFILIATIONS WITH HEALTH-CARE FACILITIES

The Division maintains affiliations with about twenty clinical agencies and is constantly investigating additional settings that will provide effective learning experiences for the students. Large teaching tertiary-care centers, such as St. Christopher's Hospital for Children, Albert Einstein Medical Center, Wills Eye Hospital, Friends Hospital, and Graduate Hospital in urban Philadelphia are used, as well as community-based institutions such as West Jersey Hospital Voorhees Division. Clinical experiences in the community include hospice care, clinics, home care, and generalized service provided by the health department. Nursing care in the community is integrated into each of the clinical courses and provides students with an understanding of nursing's role with the changing health-care policy and practice.

ACADEMIC FACILITIES

The Division of Nursing has its own learning resource center located in the Nursing Education Building. The center includes a clinical skills laboratory with an advanced skills component, a computer lab, and an audiovisual resources center. This learning resources center has its own coordinator, and the facility is available to students for independent study and for the practice of nursing skills.

LOCATION

The College's two locations are easily accessible from Philadelphia, Montgomery, and Bucks counties in Pennsylvania and Burlington, Camden, Gloucester, Hunterdon, and Mercer counties in New Jersey.

The College's 47-acre Philadelphia campus is located in a quiet, residential section of northeast Philadelphia, close to the Philadelphia–Bucks County line and just a mile from two exits of Interstate 95 (I-95). It can be reached easily by automobile or by public and rail transportation. It is ½ mile from Amtrak's major northeast rail line, which also carries commuter traffic between Trenton, New Jersey, and Philadelphia.

The picturesque campus of Newtown sits on 155 acres off Route 332 (Newtown-Yardley Road) approximately 7/10 of a mile from exit 30 of I-95. It can also be reached from Route 413 north to 413 Bypass.

STUDENT SERVICES

On campus, the nursing student can take advantage of the College's Counseling Center; Campus Ministry; The Cabaret, which offers one night a week of music and student entertainment; the Rainbow Connection, a support group for anyone who might feel different because of age, race, or ethnic background; the bookstore; volleyball activities; three racquetball courts; and a weight room and auxiliary gym for personal conditioning. Nursing students can join the Delta Tau Chapter of Sigma Theta Tau, the international nursing honor society, as well as the strong and active Student Nurses Association at Holy Family (SNAHF), which participates in campus activities to promote health. For those so inclined, the College's volunteer services offer opportunities for individuals to help at a variety of charitable agencies within the community.

THE NURSING STUDENT GROUP

Enrollment in the B.S.N. program continues to grow, with traditional and nontraditional students, full-time and part-time students, transfer students, and registered nurses making up the culturally diverse student population.

Upon completion of the program, graduates usually find employment in hospitals and agencies in or near the city of Philadelphia. A number of graduates each year are offered employment in agencies affiliated with the Division of Nursing. Graduate follow-up surveys indicate a growing number of graduates are pursuing advanced nursing education.

COSTS

The College has one of the most competitive tuition structures in the Philadelphia area. For the 1996–97 academic year, tuition, general fees, and clinical fees were $10,550 for full-time junior and senior nursing students; $215 per credit for regular part-time courses; $225 per credit for part-time nursing courses; and $245 per credit for part-time clinical nursing courses, plus a $150 clinical fee per course.

FINANCIAL AID

In addition to Federal Pell Grants and Pennsylvania Higher Education Assistance Agency (PHEAA) grants, the financial aid program includes scholarships, grants-in-aid, loans, and work programs. Of particular interest is the Nursing Student Loan Program, which provides federal and institutional funds to aid eligible students pursing a career in nursing through low interest, long-term loans with repayment period beginning nine months after withdrawal or when a student ceases to study on at least a half-time basis. For details students should call the Financial Aid Office at 215-637-5538.

APPLYING

Holy Family College has a rolling admissions policy but encourages early application. High school students must submit an application form, a nonrefundable $25 fee, a high school transcript, SAT I scores, and a letter of recommendation. Transfer students must submit an application form, a nonrefundable $25 fee, previous college transcripts, high school transcripts (or GED test scores), and a letter of recommendation. Application forms are available from the address given below.

Correspondence and Information:

Director of Admissions
Holy Family College
Grant and Frankford Avenues
Philadelphia, Pennsylvania 19114-2094
Telephone: 215-637-3050

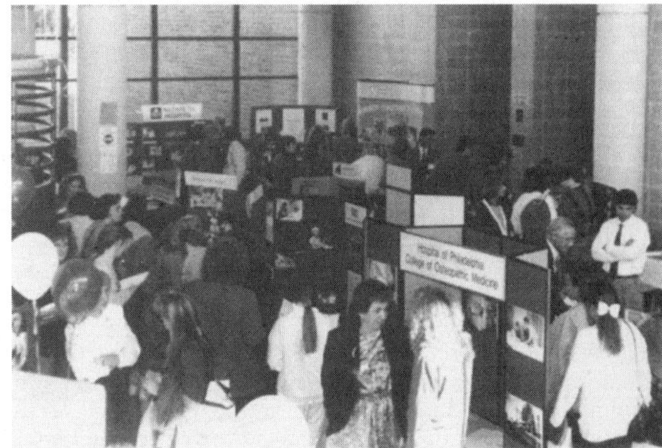

Nurse Recruiting Day at Holy Family College allows nursing students to explore job opportunities as recruiters from hospitals and health-care agencies visit the campus.

Husson College
School of Nursing and Health Professions
Bangor, Maine

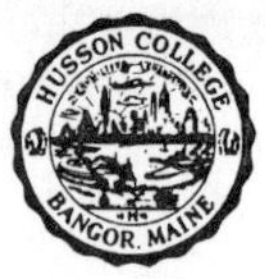

THE COLLEGE

Husson College was founded in 1898 as a college committed to the development of business skills. In 1968, the College moved to its present location, a beautiful 200-acre campus on the edge of the city and approximately a mile from downtown Bangor. Modern residence halls provide comfortable living quarters for students. The total enrollment of 1,832 includes 996 undergraduates.

Campus life accommodates a wide range of interests. Women's intercollegiate sports include basketball, soccer, softball, and volleyball. Men compete in baseball, basketball, and soccer. Golf is a coed intercollegiate sport. There are sororities, fraternities, professional business societies, a student government, a student newspaper, and WHSN, the student radio station. Events at the College include concerts, movies, lectures, and similar activities. Residential life also plays an important role in the education of the students. On-campus housing is guaranteed for four years. Student residence halls are coeducational by floor, and there are no triples. Husson is accredited by the New England Association of Schools and Colleges and the National League for Nursing. The College campus is nearly barrier-free.

THE SCHOOL OF NURSING AND HEALTH PROFESSIONS

Husson College School of Nursing graduates are in high demand. Year after year students achieve job placement prior to graduation. This success is attributed to the fact that Husson offers twice the number of clinical hours as most baccalaureate programs: the wide variety of clinical experiences include hospitals; elementary and secondary schools; prenatal, immunization, oncology, and pediatric clinics; rehabilitation facilities; and health-promotion programs.

Counseling and tutoring are also offered to help students compete scholastically at the college level. Counselors, peer tutors, and outstanding juniors and seniors are all available to work one-to-one with students.

PROGRAMS OF STUDY

Husson offers a graduate course of study leading to a Master of Science in Nursing (M.S.N.) in Family and Community Nurse Practitioner studies. Husson also offers an M.S. in physical therapy (a five-year program). Other programs include a Bachelor of Science in Nursing (B.S.N.) program and RN completion and RN to M.S.N. programs for registered nurses wishing to complete their degrees.

The Family and Community Nurse Practitioner Program is a graduate M.S.N. program that reflects Husson's ongoing commitment to educating nurses for the challenges of the twenty-first century. Admission to the graduate program entails permission for a student to attempt graduate-level work at Husson College. Consistent with Husson College's mission, the Husson College Family and Community Nurse Practitioner Program has been developed to educate advanced-practice nurses at the master's-degree level so they can cost-effectively provide improved access to family health care. This increased access is especially important in areas that are medically underserved. Believing that principles of community assessment are essential in the planning and delivery of high-quality health care, the program is committed to providing course and clinical experiences that promote this perspective. Opportunities to practice in health-care facilities with diverse client populations provide insight into the unique community needs that must be addressed by nurse practitioners in order to deliver realistic and comprehensive health care to those populations.

Graduates are eligible to sit for the ANCC Family Nurse Practitioner Certification Exam. Upon completion of the program, graduates are expected to provide primary health care to clients of all ages within diverse practice settings; utilize community assessment in evaluating client needs and planning health care; incorporate relevant theories and specialized knowledge into their clinical practices; analyze research used for improving health outcomes; contribute to the improvement of family health care by influencing health policy; influence family nursing practices by exhibiting competence in leadership, management, and teaching; and assume responsibility for continued professional growth and development.

The Husson nursing program is carefully designed to equip students for the best and broadest nursing career possible, give them a well-rounded education, and help them to realize their personal potential. It also offers a variety of nursing electives, from a nursing internship earn-while-you-learn program to nursing electives in such specialities as oncology and neuroscience. The program provides a highly personalized education with small class sizes, allowing for one-on-one teaching and attention to individual needs.

Physical therapy is one of the fastest growing health professions, combining rigorous science training with the art of caring for people. The Husson physical therapy program is a five-year combined bachelor's and master's degree. For the first two years, students study mathematics; chemistry; physics; English; statistics; health-related courses such as anatomy, physiology, and human growth and development; and electives of their choice. The professional phase of training occupies years three, four, and five. Both academic and clinical courses are required, with students training in a variety of settings.

AFFILIATIONS WITH HEALTH-CARE FACILITIES

Husson College nursing programs are affiliated with several major hospitals as well as community-based programs throughout the state. Students attain clinical experience in settings that range from the Eastern Maine Medical Center (Maine's second-largest hospital and a leader in Maine nursing education since 1892) to smaller community-based facilities and outreach programs that provide health-care needs to patients on an individual and personalized basis.

ACADEMIC FACILITIES

The College has two microcomputer labs with fifty PCs. The labs provide instructional and operational assistance to users. The library, in addition to its collection of nursing and health-care–related materials, can locate necessary materials in other libraries through interlibrary loan. The School of Nursing and Health Professions has its own skills-competency laboratories and a media lab that provides state-of-the-art interactive video disc programs.

LOCATION

Bangor, a city of 33,000 people, is located on the Penobscot River, about 40 miles from the Atlantic Ocean with famed Bar Harbor and Mt. Desert Island to the south; it is equidistant from the Canadian border on the east and New Hampshire on the west. Mount Katahdin, Baxter State Park, Moosehead Lake, and several well-known ski areas are within a 1- to 3-hour drive of the campus. There are trails for hiking, campsites, and lakes for summer recreation, all within a radius of 50 miles.

STUDENT SERVICES

Husson College offers a variety of services to its students, including personal and academic counseling, assistance for students with disabilities, peer tutoring and mentoring, a writing center where students can go for help with writing assignments, career development services, and a job bank.

THE NURSING STUDENT GROUP

There are approximately 380 students attending classes in the various nursing programs at Husson College, with more than 95 percent passing their licensing exams and acquiring employment upon graduation. The vast majority of Husson students are from the state of Maine. However, students from beyond the state are welcome and strongly encouraged to apply.

COSTS

The basic academic-year expenses in 1996–97 for undergraduate students were $8400 for tuition, $4490 for room and seven-day board, $80 for the health services fee, and $100 for the comprehensive fee. Even though the cost of living in the area is somewhat lower than that in other parts of the country, students should plan to have sufficient funds available for books and personal expenses.

FINANCIAL AID

The majority of Husson students receive some form of financial aid. The dollar amount of financial aid to be offered to the student is determined by the Free Application for Federal Student Aid (FAFSA). On the basis of this review, financial aid is authorized in the form of Federal Pell Grants, Federal Supplemental Educational Opportunity Grants, Federal Perkins Loans, and Federal Work-Study awards. There are several academic scholarships awarded annually on a competitive basis. The College strives to help each student find whatever financial aid is available and appropriate to help reduce the cost of education. Part-time jobs off campus are also available.

APPLYING

Each student is evaluated on an individual basis. Criteria guidelines for the nursing program include combined SAT I scores of at least 850 (or ACT equivalent), two recommendations, and successful completion of 2 years of math (including algebra), 2 years of science, including 1 year of chemistry and 1 year of an acceptable life science (biology preferred). These courses should be completed with a grade of C or better.

To be admitted to the Master's program, an applicant must have received a B.S.N. from an NLN-accredited institution and must show promise of ability and motivation to pursue graduate-level study, as evidenced by achievement of at least a 3.0 GPA and completion of the undergraduate health assessment and statistics courses.

Interested applicants should contact the Office of Admissions (207-941-7100) for further assistance and/or more information about the programs offered by the Husson School of Nursing and Health Professions. For information regarding the Family and Community Nurse Practitioner Program, applicants should call 207-941-7182.

Correspondence and Information:

Office of Admissions
Husson College
One College Circle
Bangor, Maine 04401
Telephone: 207-941-7100

THE FACULTY

Elizabeth A. Burns, Dean, School of Nursing and Health Professions; Ed.D., M.S.N., RN.

Lorrie L. Allen, Assistant Professor, Adult Health/Pulmonary Health; M.S.N.

Donna L. Ault, Assistant Professor, Pediatric/Medical-Surgical; M.S.N.

Monica Collins, Associate Professor, Parental-Child Health; Ed.D., M.S.N.

Sandra L. Curwin, Associate Professor and Director, Physical Therapy Program; Ph.D.

Ann P. Ellis, Professor, Medical/Surgical Adult Health; Ed.D., M.S.N.

Suzanne Gordon, Academic Coordinator for Clinical Education/Physical Therapy; M.A.

Susan Ellis-Hermanson, Assistant Professor, Adult Health/Gerontology; M.S.N.

Katherine M. Hanson, Assistant Professor, Midwifery/Women's Health; M.S.N.

Barbara S. Higgins, Associate Professor and Director, Family and Community Nurse Practitioner Program; Ph.D., M.S.N.

Cathy R. Kessenich, Associate Professor, Adult Health/Research; D.Sc.N.

Mimi Padgett, Assistant Professor, Community Health; M.S.N.

Serina Petrolino-Roche, Assistant Professor, Adult Health/Community Health; M.S.N.

Karen Rich, Assistant Professor, Community Health/Gerontology; M.S.N.

Ben Sidaway, Associate Professor, Physical Therapy; Ph.D.

Ann E. Sossong, Assistant Professor, Medical/Surgical Adult Health; M.Ed., M.S.N.

Teresa Steele, Associate Professor, Psychiatric-Mental Health; M.S.N.

Mary E. Stone, Assistant Professor, Community Health/Medical-Surgical Adult Health; M.S.N.

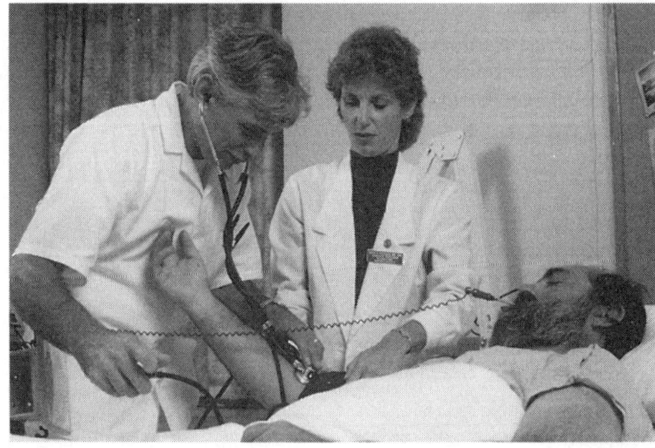

A nursing student gains valuable clinical experience.

Illinois Wesleyan University
School of Nursing
Bloomington, Illinois

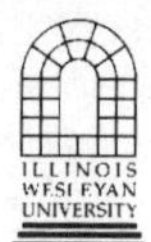

THE UNIVERSITY

Illinois Wesleyan University is a private, coeducational, liberal arts university, founded in 1850, with a 146-year tradition of excellence. The University's enrollment of 1,900 students is planned to provide students with a singular opportunity for intellectual and personal growth and the chance to form close, lifelong friendships. Illinois Wesleyan offers a wealth of academic programs in a small college setting. The College of Liberal Arts, the College of Fine Arts, and the four-year professional School of Nursing provide great diversity to the curriculum. Students have opportunities to explore subjects in each of the schools.

Illinois Wesleyan is situated on 60 acres in Bloomington's northside residential district. The heart of the campus is the central quadrangle. Buildings range in style from gray stone Gothic to modern brick and glass. A $22-million Natural Science Center opened in fall 1995. A new dorm and Center for Liberal Arts open in 1997–98.

THE SCHOOL OF NURSING

Established in 1958, the School of Nursing offers an NLN-accredited program of study leading to the Bachelor of Science in Nursing degree. The School is a model of integration of liberal and professional learning, with students enrolling in liberal arts courses throughout the four years of study. The program emphasizes the development of critical thinking and decision-making skills, communication across disciplines, and preparation for a lifetime of learning. Practicum study begins in the first semester of the sophomore year. An advanced placement program, added in 1980, offers the opportunity for study at the upper division to registered nurses and selected transfer students.

Consistent with the University's mission, the School of Nursing strives for excellence in undergraduate nursing education by preparing practitioners with a strong theoretical foundation, including Orem's Self-Care Deficit Theory of Nursing. Graduates are known and recruited for their clinical abilities and leadership potential. The School also offers health studies that emphasize knowledge of self-care, decision making, and an understanding of health-care issues, including those that are international.

Enhanced by the low faculty-student clinical ratios, the School of Nursing prides itself on the outstanding rapport among the 110 students and the faculty. All full-time faculty members teach in the clinical area; more than 80 percent of the tenure-line faculty members are doctorally prepared, the majority with degrees in nursing.

PROGRAM OF STUDY

The School of Nursing offers one program of study leading to the B.S.N. Students are admitted directly to the School of Nursing as freshmen, completing the prerequisites of anatomy and physiology, chemistry, and human growth and development during the first two semesters. All students who successfully complete these requirements enter the nursing sequence in the first semester, sophomore year, and are guaranteed placement in subsequent clinical courses. Students must complete 32 course units (128 semester hours), 15 course units of which are in nursing. Health promotion across the life span is emphasized during the sophomore year, with a focus on the healthy mother-infant dyads and the well elderly. In the junior year, students study adults and children with stable, acute, and chronic physical and mental health conditions. Seniors have experiences ranging from those in critical-care units, high-risk obstetrics, and home health care to leadership and management and community health study, with emphasis on groups, aggregates, and community assessment. The faculty-student ratios in the intensive care areas are limited to 1:6.

The University's unique calendar, which includes an optional May short term, provides opportunities for travel, internships, and additional classroom and clinical work in the area of the student's interest. Current short-term travel courses include Health Care in the Netherlands, Transcultural Nursing in Hawaii, and Transcultural Nursing with Native Americans in Arizona. A strong research honors program within the University allows exceptional students to conduct undergraduate research with a faculty member during the senior year. Independent study is available in the area of student interest, such as nursing history, trauma care, or nurse-administered anesthesia. Other options include school nurse certification, enhanced science option, enhanced clinical practice option, prelaw option, and two minors, human services management (in conjunction with the Division of Business and Economics) and health.

The advanced placement program for registered nurses allows students to complete the B.S.N. in three semesters of full-time study. After completing challenge examinations, students must complete a minimum of 13 course units at Illinois Wesleyan University.

AFFILIATIONS WITH HEALTH-CARE FACILITIES

The School prides itself on providing students with diverse clinical experiences, including those in local hospitals, large regional medical centers, residential units for the well elderly, community health and home health agencies, clinics, and early childhood centers. Experiences in multiple sites enable students to compare various health-care delivery systems and to learn about care to diverse populations. Transportation is provided to all group clinicals outside of Bloomington.

ACADEMIC FACILITIES

The University's main computer facilities are located in Buck Memorial Library. Computerized classrooms and a central open-access workroom equipped with IBM and Macintosh computers are available for student use. Also available is an interactive learning center with additional computers and interactive videodisc systems. All students have access to the Internet.

The School of Nursing, housed in Stevenson Hall, has a new learning laboratory for skills acquisition at all levels of the program. Selected classrooms are equipped with interactive computer equipment, with projection capabilities, to facilitate group discussion in the classroom.

Sheean Library is the primary educational materials resource center for the University. The library offers numerous on-line and CD-ROM reference materials, including CINAHL (Cumulative Index to Nursing and Allied Health Literature), Lexis/Nexis, First Search, and Current Contents for Science. The University is a member of the Library Computer System, a network of Illinois academic libraries that provides an on-line catalog as well as an extensive bibliographic database of over 21 million volumes throughout the state.

LOCATION

Illinois Wesleyan is located in Bloomington/Normal, Illinois, midway between Chicago and St. Louis. The cities, with a combined population of 100,000, are a center for insurance, manufacturing, agribusiness, and higher education. Bloomington is one of the fastest-growing communities in the country and is listed among the most desirable places to live in the nation. Situated in the center of the state, Bloomington is easily accessible by car, plane, or train.

STUDENT SERVICES

The University has many resources and services to meet the needs of students. About 86 percent of IWU students live in University housing, which provides a variety of living experiences from large halls to small houses. The newly renovated Bertholf Commons provides students several meal plans to meet their needs. The Arnold Health Center provides a comprehensive health program for all University students and staff. The Career Education Center offers various career planning programs and job placement programs to help students start their careers. Additional services available include the Counseling Center, multicultural programs, and more than fifty clubs and organizations.

Students are active in campus life, including athletics such as football, swimming, women's softball, basketball, and tennis. Students often have multiple interests, including language study, music or theater, computer science, and business. Students participate actively in Alpha Tau Delta (national nursing fraternity), the Student Nurses Association, and Sigma Theta Tau (international honor society of nursing).

THE NURSING STUDENT GROUP

The majority of the School's 110 students are traditional undergraduate students.

COSTS

Tuition and fees for the 1997–98 academic year are $17,380, with an additional charge for room and board of $4590. Personal expenses and books are estimated to be about $1100 per year. The University offers an interest-free monthly payment plan to those students who wish to spread the payment out over the entire year.

FINANCIAL AID

The University arranges a financial aid proposal, according to its institutional methodology, to meet the demonstrated need of any student whose application is accepted for admission. Financial need is met through a combination of grants, scholarships, loans, and jobs. All students requesting financial assistance must submit the Financial Aid PROFILE, designating Illinois Wesleyan University as the recipient. Students who receive ROTC nursing scholarships attend with additional support from IWU.

APPLYING

Students should have 15 academic units in the areas of English, foreign language, mathematics, laboratory science, and social science; rank in the top 30 percent of the class; and have SAT I or ACT results showing comparable aptitude. In addition, candidates for admission to the School of Nursing should have completed, upon graduation from high school, a minimum of 1 year each of biology, chemistry, algebra, and geometry. Any RN who graduated from an approved nursing program and who holds a current Illinois license or is eligible for licensure in Illinois may apply for admission to the School of Nursing. A review of previous education and experience will be made to determine placement in the curriculum.

Correspondence and Information:

James R. Ruoti, Dean of Admissions
Illinois Wesleyan University
P.O. Box 2900
Bloomington, Illinois 61702-1900
Telephone: 800-332-2498 (toll-free)

Donna P. Hartweg, Director
School of Nursing
Illinois Wesleyan University
Bloomington, Illinois 61702
Telephone: 309-556-3051
Fax: 309-556-3043
E-mail: nursing@titan.iwu.edu

THE FACULTY

Jane Brue, Associate Professor; M.S.Ed., Illinois; M.S.N., Indiana, 1984; RN. Transcultural nursing in Hawaii and with Native Americans, therapeutic touch, international health.

Connie Dennis, Associate Professor; Ph.D., Illinois State, 1990; RN. Computers in nursing, self-care theory.

Eileen Fowles, Assistant Professor; Ph.D., Loyola, 1993; RN. Maternal and prenatal role attachment, postpartum attachment.

Donna Hartweg, Professor and Director; Ph.D., Wayne State, 1991; RN. Self-care of middle-aged women, self-care theory.

Sheila Jesek-Hale, Assistant Professor; D.N.Sc., Rush, 1994; RN. Self-care of pregnant adolescents.

Sharie Metcalfe, Associate Professor; Ph.D., Wayne State; RN. Self-care of persons with COPD, self-care theory, caring in nursing.

Charla Renner, Associate Professor; M.S., Illinois, 1982; RN. Advocacy; health beliefs and practices in Botswana.

Kathryn Scherck, Associate Professor; D.N.Sc., Rush, 1989; RN. Coping with myocardial infarction, qualitative methods.

Margaret Tennis, Associate Professor; Ed.D., Illinois State, 1993; Certified Pediatric Nurse Practitioner, RN. Pediatric assessment, hyperactivity disorders in children.

Susan Westlake, Assistant Professor; Ph.D., Wisconsin, 1991; RN. Research and public policy; women's responses to breast cancer; pain in cancer patients; decision making by clinicians and patients.

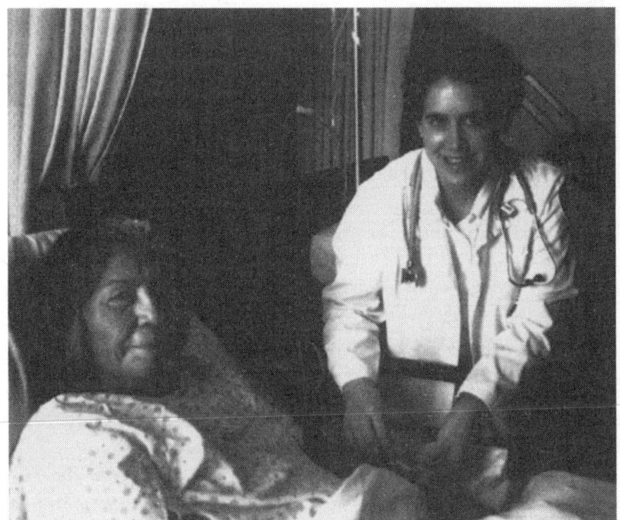

A student explores transcultural nursing with a patient at Phoenix Indian Medical Center.

Indiana University
School of Nursing
Indianapolis, Bloomington, and Columbus, Indiana

THE UNIVERSITY

Founded in 1820, Indiana University (IU) has grown from its modest beginnings into one of the oldest and largest universities in the Midwest and one of the nation's finest educational institutions. Offering 838 degree programs at eight campuses around the state, IU attracts students from every state in the United States and around the world. IU's residential campus at Bloomington and its urban center in Indianapolis form the core of the University. Campuses in Gary, Kokomo, New Albany, Richmond, and South Bend join those in Bloomington, Columbus, and Indianapolis to bring a high-quality education within the reach of any student. IU is accredited by the North Central Association of Colleges and Schools.

THE SCHOOL OF NURSING

Since its inception as The Indiana University Training School for Nurses in 1914, the Indiana University School of Nursing (IUSON) has become one of the largest multipurpose schools of nursing in the United States. Ranked as one of the country's best nursing schools, IUSON offers the following academic degrees, ranging from the associate to the doctoral levels: the Associate of Science in Nursing (A.S.N.), the Bachelor of Science in Nursing (B.S.N.), the Master of Science in Nursing (M.S.N.), and the Ph.D. in nursing science.

The School's A.S.N., B.S.N., and M.S.N. programs are accredited by the National League for Nursing (NLN). A.S.N. and B.S.N. programs are accredited by the Indiana State Board of Nursing, and the School's continuing education department is accredited by the American Nurses Credentialing Center's Commission on Accreditation. IUSON is an agency member of NLN's Council of Associate Degree Programs and the Council of Baccalaureate and Higher Degree Programs as well as the Committee for Institutional Cooperation. The School is also a constituent member of the NLN, the American Association of Colleges of Nursing, and the Midwest Alliance in Nursing.

PROGRAMS OF STUDY

The purpose of IUSON's A.S.N. degree program is to prepare graduates to function in entry-level staff nursing positions. The program is designed to meet the educational needs of students planning to enter the professional field of nursing as their first career as well as students who intend to change their career goals. Students entering the program complete courses in the physical sciences, behavioral sciences, and humanities as well as the nursing discipline. Learning takes place through instruction in structured classrooms, laboratories, and clinical settings. Students use this knowledge to provide direct care to patients of all ages in a variety of health-care environments. The A.S.N. degree program, which requires completion of 65 to 67 semester hours of credit, including concurrent course work in general education and nursing, may be completed on a full-time or part-time basis.

The B.S.N. degree program provides a comprehensive academic foundation in the sciences and humanities essential for preparing students for a generalist practice role. The baccalaureate program appeals to students wishing to combine general education with professional course work and also serves as a foundation for graduate study. (It is recommended that those interested in graduate studies enter nursing education at the B.S.N. level.) The program takes a minimum of four years of full-time study to complete. The program emphasizes health promotion, maintenance, and preventions as well as managing individuals and families coping with acute and chronic illnesses. Indiana University–Purdue University at Columbus offers courses toward the completion of the LPN to A.S.N. mobility option. Indiana University Bloomington offers the first three years of the B.S.N. program along with fourth-year clinical placement options for those students wishing to maximize their time on the Bloomington campus.

The goal of the M.S.N. degree program is to prepare its graduates for leadership roles in advanced nursing practice, clinical specialization, and nursing administration. Majors are offered in ten areas: adult psychiatric/mental health nursing, child/adolescent psychiatric/mental health nursing, community health nursing, nursing administration, nursing of adults, nursing of children at risk, pediatric nurse practitioner, adult nurse practitioner, family nurse practitioner, and OB/GYN nurse practitioner. Post-master's options are available in all clinical areas and in nursing administration and teacher education. Students select a major area of study when they apply for admission. Students may elect to follow a full- or part-time course of study. All degree requirements must be met within six years of initial enrollment.

The Ph.D. in nursing science degree program, which builds on baccalaureate nursing education, is based on the beliefs that professional nursing is a scientific discipline and that it has a unique role and body of knowledge that can be expanded, applied, and validated through recognized methods of scholarly inquiry. The primary goal of the program is the preparation of scholars in one of the following focus areas: environments for health, acute and chronic health problems, health promotion, and family health adaptation. The 90-credit curriculum includes concentrations in theory, research, and statistics; nursing science and research; an external cognate minor; and a dissertation. Thirty credits may be met by course work completed while earning an M.S.N.

Nurses wishing to pursue additional academic education at IUSON can also take advantage of several "mobility options." The LPN to A.S.N. mobility program enables students to apply previous nursing education toward earning an Associate of Science in Nursing degree. Graduates are eligible to take the registered nurse licensure examination. The associate/diploma RN to B.S.N. mobility program facilitates the application of previous course work toward the Bachelor of Science in Nursing degree. Nursing knowledge is substantiated through "bridging courses" rather than through testing. The associate/diploma RN to M.S.N. mobility program offers a unique opportunity for those individuals who have accumulated advanced nursing knowledge and skill through additional experiences. The RN to M.S.N. educational mobility option is available to qualified registered nurses who do not hold a baccalaureate degree in nursing but who have earned academic credit in addition to their initial registered nurse program. Included are those whose highest academic credential is the diploma in nursing, the A.S.N. degree, or the baccalaureate degree in a non-nursing field. Specific mobility courses are offered on the Indianapolis, Bloomington, and Columbus campuses.

AFFILIATIONS WITH HEALTH-CARE FACILITIES

The Indiana University Medical Center (IUMC), located on the Indiana University–Purdue University at Indianapolis (IUPUI) campus, includes the Schools of Nursing, Medicine, Social Work, Allied Health, and Dentistry. IUMC's extensive diagnostic clinics and five teaching hospitals are Indiana's primary referral hospitals and its chief centers for clinical instruction in the health professions. The School's commitment to practice is also reflected in the number of its innovative programs and ongoing cutting-edge research. The Maternity Outreach Mobilization project provides prenatal care to needy women in Indianapolis. The Institute of Action Research in Community Health, dedicated to working in cities across the state to improve community health, has been designated a World Health Organization (WHO) Collaborating Center in Healthy Cities. The WHO Center provides multiple opportunities for student learning experiences, interdisciplinary research, and collaboration with visiting WHO scholars. The Mary Margaret Walther Program for Cancer Care Research Center, located on the IUPUI campus, is a leader in oncology care research.

ACADEMIC FACILITIES

Library facilities for student use are extensive. IUPUI facilities include the University Library, the School of Law Library, the School of Dentistry Library, the Medical Science Library, Herron School of Art Library, and a School of Nursing reference library. The Medical Science Library houses the largest and most complete health science library in Indiana. The new multimillion-dollar University Library employs state-of-the-art electronic information systems technology.

LOCATION

All four academic nursing programs are offered on the IUPUI campus; the A.S.N. is offered at IU East (Richmond), IU Kokomo, IU Northwest (Gary), and IU South Bend; IUPUI's Columbus Center offers the LPN to A.S.N. mobility option and selected courses toward the RN to B.S.N. mobility option; and the B.S.N. degree may be obtained at IU East, IU Kokomo, IU Northwest, IU Southeast (New Albany), and IU South Bend. Prerequisite and selected courses in the nursing major and the RN to B.S.N. mobility option are offered on the Bloomington campus. Graduate programs are offered through the campus of IUPUI in Indianapolis. Selected baccalaureate- and master's-level nursing courses are offered over the Indiana Higher Education Telecommunication System via closed-circuit television.

STUDENT SERVICES

The mission of the student services area of the School of Nursing is to help students attain their academic and professional goals. Support services for disadvantaged students are available; however, services may vary from campus to campus.

THE NURSING STUDENT GROUP

The headquarters of Sigma Theta Tau International, nursing's honor society, is located on the Indianapolis campus, where it was founded in 1922. All prenursing and nursing undergraduates are eligible for membership in the National Student Nurses Association and the Indiana Association of Nursing Students. Chi Eta Phi Sorority is a service organization open to all qualified undergraduate nursing students. The Minority Nursing Student Organization is a peer support group for minority nursing students. Membership in the RN to B.S.N. Organization is open to all registered nurses in the baccalaureate program.

COSTS

Tuition and fees vary by campus. Indiana residents pay approximately $102.15 per credit hour for undergraduate courses and $138.75 per credit hour for graduate courses. Nonresidents pay approximately $315 per credit hour for undergraduate courses and $400 per credit hour for graduate courses. Students may also be responsible for student technology fees, student activity fees, and laboratory and other fees.

FINANCIAL AID

Financial aid, including scholarships, grants, and loans, is provided by the federal government, the state of Indiana, Indiana University, IUSON, and individual donors. Students should contact the Office of Scholarships and Financial Aid at the campus of undergraduate attendance for information.

APPLYING

High school graduates, LPNs, and individuals with prior college credit may seek competitive admission to one of three A.S.N. admission categories after being accepted at Indiana University. Students interested in the B.S.N. degree program must be accepted to and begin studies with required general education course work. Students who meet all admission requirements are eligible to apply for competitive admission to the nursing program.

Requirements for admission to the M.S.N. program are as follows: a B.S.N. from an NLN-accredited program or its equivalent, a minimum 3.0 GPA on a 4.0 scale, a score of 400 or better on two of the three sections of the GRE, a current Indiana registered nurse license (international applicants must submit evidence of passing the Council of Graduates of Foreign Nursing Schools qualifying examination and must receive licensure in Indiana prior to enrollment), a TOEFL score of 550 or above for those whose native language is not English, completion of a 3-credit statistics course within the last three years with at least a grade of B–, verification of ability to use computer technologies, and verification of physical assessment skills.

The criteria for consideration for admission to the Ph.D. program are a baccalaureate degree with a major in nursing from an NLN-accredited program or its equivalent; a baccalaureate cumulative GPA of 3.0 or higher on a 4.0 scale (for those holding a master's degree, a graduate GPA of 3.5 or higher is required); completion of a 3-credit statistics course with a grade of B or higher within three years before the date of proposed enrollment; ability to secure current registered nurse licensure in Indiana; scores of 500 or better on the verbal, quantitative, and analytic sections of the GRE; scores of 550 or better on the TOEFL for students whose first language is not English (a written test of English is also required); a two- to three-page essay; evidence of the capacity for original scholarship and research in nursing; three references; and an interview.

Correspondence and Information:

Office of Educational Services
Indiana University School of Nursing
1111 Middle Drive, NU 122
Indianapolis, Indiana 46202
Telephone: 317-274-2806
Fax: 317-274-2996
E-mail: klynn@wpo.iupui.edu

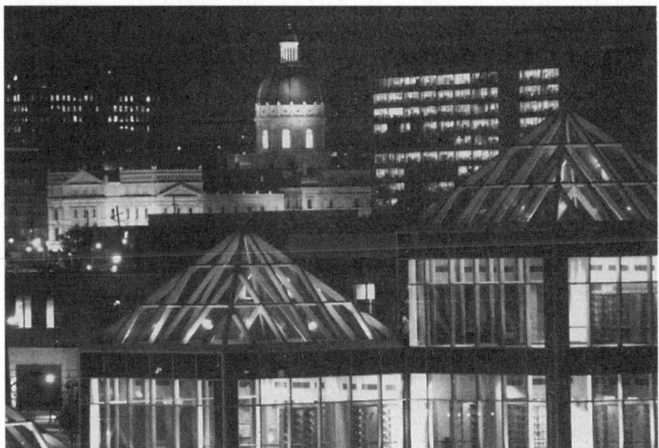

In the foreground is the IUPUI Medical Library. In the background is downtown Indianapolis.

Johns Hopkins University
School of Nursing
Baltimore, Maryland

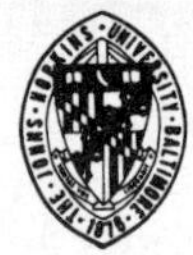

THE UNIVERSITY

Since its founding in 1876, the Johns Hopkins University has been in the forefront of higher education. Originally established as an institution oriented toward graduate study and research, it is often called America's first true university. Today, the Johns Hopkins commitment to academic excellence continues in its eight academic divisions: Nursing, Medicine, Public Health, Arts and Science, Engineering, Continuing Studies, Advanced International Studies, and the Peabody Conservatory of Music. With a full-time enrollment of approximately 7,000 students, it is the smallest of the top-ranked universities in the United States and, by its own choice, remains small.

THE SCHOOL OF NURSING

The School of Nursing was established in 1983 by the Johns Hopkins University, in affiliation with three Baltimore hospitals: Church, Johns Hopkins, and Sinai. Together, these institutions form the Consortium for Nursing Education, Inc., united for innovation and excellence in teaching, research, and patient care.

By choosing to attend the Johns Hopkins University School of Nursing, students become leaders in the nursing profession. A Hopkins education provides a solid foundation on which to base a lifelong career in the ever-growing field of nursing. Hopkins students enjoy the advantages of an education at an institution with a worldwide reputation and an outstanding network of alumni who are willing to serve as guides and mentors. Students at the School of Nursing are given the opportunity to participate in designing an educational program tailored to their individual needs. A rigorous academic curriculum, which includes a strong scientific orientation, gives students the background to understand the health-care decisions they will make as professionals. Students learn in an atmosphere where excellence is expected, valued, and reinforced.

The School of Nursing is one of only a few in the country that emphasizes undergraduate research. Its graduates are prepared for professional practice through an educational process that emphasizes clinical excellence, critical thinking, and intellectual curiosity.

PROGRAMS OF STUDY

The Johns Hopkins University School of Nursing prepares students for professional nursing practice through an educational process that combines a strong academic curriculum with intensive clinical experience. The program is built on the University's commitment to research, teaching, patient service, and educational innovation and the consortium hospitals' commitment to excellence in clinical practice. The School's mission is to prepare its students academically and technologically for challenges of the future and to graduate professional nurses who can participate in all aspects of modern health care.

The School of Nursing offers an NLN-accredited upper-division program leading to a Bachelor of Science degree with a major in nursing. College graduates with a degree in any major other than nursing are eligible to apply to either the thirteen-month accelerated program, which begins annually in June, or to the two-year program.

Undergraduate students who are already registered nurses may enter with 33 credits of the ACT challenge examinations. A minimum of 30 of the 63 credits in the upper division must actually be taken at the Johns Hopkins University.

The Johns Hopkins University School of Nursing has a collaborative program of study that integrates academic study at the Johns Hopkins University and volunteer service in the Peace Corps. The program combines four semesters at the School of Nursing or the thirteen-month accelerated program followed by Peace Corps training and two years of volunteer service. Returned Peace Corps Volunteers are eligible to participate in the Peace Corps Fellows program while enrolled in the school. This provides a unique opportunity for clinical education in community health nursing while meeting the human needs of low-income, underserved, and homeless families through preventive health services. Funding has been obtained for an AmeriCorps Program at the School of Nursing.

The School of Nursing also offers a B.S.-M.S.N. option of study for exceptionally qualified students. The School of Nursing offers an NLN-accredited graduate program leading to the Master of Science in Nursing (M.S.N.) degree. The purpose of the master's program is to prepare nurses for leadership positions in advanced nursing practice and/or health care management in a variety of settings. The master's program emphasizes flexibility and is designed to accommodate individual professional objectives. Johns Hopkins provides unsurpassed opportunities for personal and professional development in advanced clinical practice, the research process, and leadership management of health-care environments. Graduates of the M.S.N. in advanced practice nursing with an adult or pediatric focus are eligible to apply for ANCC certification as an adult or pediatric nurse practitioner and/or clinical specialist. Nurses with master's degrees in nursing are eligible to apply to the 18-credit Post-Master's Nurse Practitioner Program, also with an adult or pediatric focus.

Other majors offered in the M.S.N. degree program are nursing systems and management; a dual master's degree with The School of Continuing Studies in nursing management and business; community health nursing; a joint M.S.N./M.P.H. degree program with the School of Hygiene and Public Health; and an advanced practice nursing clinical specialty in AIDS/HIV, oncology, and adult health.

The goal of the doctoral program is to prepare nurse scholars to conduct research that advances the theoretical foundation of nursing practice and health-care delivery. Graduate study and research opportunities are available in selected areas the correspond with the expertise of the faculty.

Postdoctoral programs are available to prepare nurses with advanced skill and knowledge in a selected area of practice with expertise in the design and conduct of related research. The program includes fellowships in infection prevention and wound care.

AFFILIATIONS WITH HEALTH-CARE FACILITIES

The Johns Hopkins Medical Institutions (JHMI) campus is part of a world-renowned academic health center that includes the Schools of Nursing, Medicine, and Hygiene and Public Health; the Johns Hopkins Hospital; and the William H. Welch Medical Library.

The Johns Hopkins Health System includes, in addition to the Johns Hopkins Hospital, three other hospital campuses, one of which houses the National Institute on Aging Gerontology Center and the National Institute on Drug Abuse Addiction Research Center.

ACADEMIC FACILITIES

The William H. Welch Medical Library is the central resource library serving the Johns Hopkins Medical Institutions. Students gain free 24-hour-a-day access to WELMED. WELMED is a retrieval system that integrates services, such as on-line requests for photocopying and document delivery, with several bibliographic databases. The Nursing Information Resource Center (NIRC), located in the School of Nursing, is managed by the Welch Library. The NIRC maintains a core collection of books to support student course work, a reprint file of material used in the students' courses, a pamphlet file of material from the National League for Nursing, and clinical skills videocassettes. In addition, the facilities and 2 million volumes of the University's Milton S. Eisenhower Library, on the Homewood Campus, are available to the School of Nursing.

A nursing practice lab is available to provide the student with an opportunity to gain experience and confidence in performing a wide variety of nursing technologies. Practice using actual hospital equipment is an integral part of the laboratory experience, and patient simulators are provided to facilitate clinical skill mastery.

Other academic facilities include the Microcomputer Laboratory; the Center for Nursing Research, which houses postdoctoral programs and resources for grant preparation, conduct, and administration; and the School of Nursing Research Lab, located on the Bayview Research Campus, which supports physiological research.

LOCATION

The School of Nursing is located on the campus of the Johns Hopkins Medical Institutions, including the School of Medicine, the School of Hygiene and Public Health, and the Johns Hopkins Hospital. Located 10 minutes away is the Homewood Campus of the Johns Hopkins University, which is accessible to students via a free shuttle service.

Often referred to as "the biggest small town in America," Baltimore has undergone one of the most successful transformations of any city in the nation. Baltimore's famous Inner Harbor and the National Aquarium are focal points of this revitalization. Washington, D.C., is less than an hour away by car or train.

STUDENT SERVICES

There are more than seventy student organizations within the University, including fraternities and sororities and social, religious, and cultural groups. Each class within the School of Nursing has a government board and a president. There is also the Student Government Association (SGA), which includes all divisions of the entire University. Each class has two representatives to the SGA, and anyone may attend the meetings.

THE NURSING STUDENT GROUP

The School of Nursing attracts a national and international student body of 484 students; 293 undergraduate students and 19 RNs are currently enrolled in the baccalaureate program. The graduate programs enroll 191 students.

COSTS

For the 1996–97 academic year, undergraduate and graduate tuition was $15,750. For the M.S.N./M.P.H. and the doctoral programs, tuition for the 1996–97 academic year was $25,924.

FINANCIAL AID

The Johns Hopkins University School of Nursing attempts to provide financial assistance to all eligible accepted students. The School of Nursing assists those students who qualify for need-based aid. Such assistance is usually in the form of loans, grants, scholarships, and work-study programs. While most of the financial aid received by students is based on financial need, many students also benefit from awards based on academic merit and achievement.

APPLYING

The School seeks individuals who will bring to the student body the qualities of scholarship, motivation, and commitment.

A complete undergraduate and graduate application consists of an application form and a nonrefundable $40 application fee. Doctoral applicants pay an application fee of $150.

Applicants to the undergraduate program are required to have three recommendations, official college transcripts, an official high school transcript (unless the applicant has already completed a college degree), and SAT I or ACT scores, if they are not more than five years old and the student does not already hold a bachelor's degree. Registered nurses must send a copy of their Maryland State nursing license. A grade point average of at least 3.0 (on a 4.0 scale) is recommended. Personal interviews may be requested.

Applicants to the graduate program are required to have graduated from a baccalaureate or master's degree program in nursing with a GPA of at least 3.0 (on a 4.0 scale), a current license to practice nursing, preferably a year of nursing practice, competitive scores on the Graduate Record Examinations (GRE), academic and professional references, and official transcripts from all previous schools attended. Personal interviews may be requested. Students interested in the doctoral program should contact the Office of Admissions for individual counseling regarding entrance requirements.

International students whose native language is not English must submit official test score reports of the Test of English as a Foreign Language (TOEFL) with a score of 550 or better. In order to be considered for admission, nonpermanent residents must establish their ability to finance their education in the United States. International students must submit official records of all university-level course work. To be considered for transfer toward a degree, any courses listed on a foreign transcript must be submitted by the student to the World Education Service (WES). Registered nurses must have their foreign transcripts evaluated by the Commission on Graduates of Foreign Nursing Schools (CGFNS). Students should contact the Office of Admissions for additional information regarding the WES and CGFNS evaluation service.

Correspondence and Information:

The Johns Hopkins University
Office of Admissions and Student Services, Suite 200
School of Nursing
1830 East Monument Street
Baltimore, Maryland 21205

THE FACULTY

The following is a list of Deans and Program Directors. A full list of the faculty is available upon request.

Sue K. Donaldson, Dean and Professor; Ph.D., FAAN, RN.

Stella Shiber, Associate Dean for Professional Education Programs and Practice; Ph.D., RN.

Charles I. Stanton, Associate Dean for Finance and Administration; B.S., M.B.A.

Maryann Fralick, Associate Dean for the School of Nursing and Johns Hopkins Hospital Programs; Dr.P.H., RN, FAAN.

Sandra Angell, Associate Dean for Academic Student Support Services; M.L.A., RN.

Ada Davis, Director of Baccalaureate Programs; Ph.D., RN, CANP.

Fannie Gaston-Johansson, Director of Extramural and International Academic Relations; Dr.Med.Sc., RN, FAAN.

Martha Hill, Director of the Center for Nursing Research; Ph.D., RN.

Martha Neff-Smith, Professor and Coordinator of M.S.N./M.P.H. Nursing Program; M.P.H., Ph.D., RNC.

Judith Vessey, Professor and Coordinator of Advanced Practice Nursing Programs; Ph.D., RN.

Kennesaw State University
School of Nursing
Kennesaw, Georgia

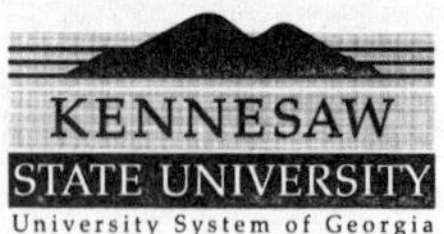

THE UNIVERSITY

Kennesaw State University (KSU) is a public university in the University System of Georgia located in northwest greater metropolitan Atlanta. Chartered in 1963, KSU serves as a rich resource for the region's educational, economic, social, and cultural advancement, offering baccalaureate and professional master's degrees to its 13,000 students in the arts, humanities, sciences, and the professional fields of business, education, social services, and nursing.

KSU offers a high-quality teaching/learning environment that sustains instructional excellence, serves a diverse student body, and promotes high levels of student achievement. It educates the whole person through a supportive campus climate, necessary services, and leadership development opportunities and promotes cultural, ethnic, racial, and gender diversity by practices and programs that embody the ideals of an open, democratic, and global society.

THE SCHOOL OF NURSING

The School of Nursing at KSU began as an associate degree program in 1968. The Department of Baccalaureate Degree Nursing was added in 1985 and included a generic baccalaureate degree option and an RN-B.S.N. completion program. In 1995, the associate degree program was discontinued and an M.S.N. program, to prepare primary-care nurse practitioners, accepted its first class. All programs in the baccalaureate nursing program are accredited by the National League for Nursing. Accreditation is planned for the M.S.N. program in June 1998.

PROGRAMS OF STUDY

The School of Nursing offers baccalaureate and master's degree programs in nursing. The Department of Baccalaureate Degree Nursing offers a generic B.S.N. program and a B.S.N. completion option for registered nurses. The curriculum includes courses in the humanities and the biological and social sciences as well as the theoretical and clinical practice background necessary for the practice of professional nursing. Baccalaureate majors had risen to a total of 639 in the fall of 1996. Generic students are admitted twice annually to maintain smaller classes.

The B.S.N. completion option for registered nurses is based on the statewide articulation plan formulated by nursing programs in the state of Georgia. Upon completion of a bridge course, registered nurse students receive credit for 38 quarter hours of sophomore- and junior-level nursing courses and may enter the senior-level courses. This program admits students twice a year and is planned to provide flexible options for the working nurse. Emphasis at the senior level is on community and family nursing, career development, and professional growth. Clinicals are individually tailored to meet students' needs.

The M.S.N. program prepares experienced registered nurses as primary-care nurse practitioners eligible for national certification as family nurse practitioners. The program is designed for working professional nurses, with all classes scheduled on alternate weekends. Students are admitted to the primary-care nurse practitioner program once a year in the fall.

AFFILIATIONS WITH HEALTH-CARE FACILITIES

The School of Nursing has affiliations with more than sixty health and community agencies in the metropolitan Atlanta area and northwest Georgia. Two of the major reasons cited by students for choosing KSU are location and access to experience in both the major acute-care facilities in Atlanta and a tremendously diverse array of other community-based health and social agencies.

The primary-care nurse practitioner program collaborates with more than 50 nurse practitioners, physicians, and physician assistants in a variety of primary-care settings. These professionals serve as clinical preceptors for the nurse practitioner students.

ACADEMIC FACILITIES

The School of Nursing is located in modern office and classroom facilities approximately a mile from the main campus. Modern classrooms, faculty offices, conference rooms, study areas, a learning resource center, and computer facilities are all located in the same building. The KSU library is housed in a 100,000-square-foot building and is networked with on-line computer databases and document retrieval facilities. Students have access to library resources, e-mail, and the Internet both on campus and from home computers. The School of Nursing has a goal of increasing the use of technology in the classroom and has invested in many computer learning resources that are available to students.

LOCATION

Nestled in the hills just 20 miles north of metropolitan Atlanta, KSU is easily accessible to its 13,000 students. The 182-acre campus is memorable for its beautiful grounds, oak-lined streets, manicured lawns, and colorful flower beds. The University offers a diverse array of cultural enrichment opportunities for the community, including concerts, recitals, art exhibitions, plays, and lectures. It boasts NCAA national baseball and softball championships. Its proximity to Atlanta offers a vast field of cultural and recreational opportunities, from theater productions and major art exhibits to professional football, basketball, and baseball.

STUDENT SERVICES

KSU encourages student involvement through more than forty campus activities, social fraternities and sororities, student government, student publications, and intramural and leisure programs. Support services include career planning and placement, personal counseling, financial aid, an Advisement Center, a Wellness Center, and a special Lifelong Learning Center that caters to the nontraditional age student. There is a limited child-care facility, a well-equipped gym, and a Student Development Center, which concentrates support services for minority, international, and special needs students.

THE NURSING STUDENT GROUP

KSU is a nontraditional, commuter university serving a diverse student body. There are more than 400 students enrolled in the undergraduate and graduate nursing programs. Generic students tend to be slightly older than traditional college-age students, with an average age of 29 years and a range of 20 to 54 years. RN-B.S.N. students average 35 years of age, with a range of 25 to 47 years. Approximately 18 percent of the students are male, and approximately 20 percent have a previous degree in another field. KSU has a growing population of international and historically underrepresented students.

Students in the master's program are professional nurses with a minimum of three years of experience. They work in a variety of settings scattered over the geographic region of northwest Georgia and the metropolitan Atlanta area.

COSTS

Tuition for full-time undergraduate student status is approximately $600 per quarter (based on a four-quarter year). Graduate student tuition is slightly higher. Nonresident fees for out-of-state students add an estimated $1000 per quarter. There are no on-campus quarters.

FINANCIAL AID

The University financial assistance program provides need-based, scholastic, and athletic scholarships. The Office of Student Financial Aid, located in the library, processes need-based scholarships and grants, government-guaranteed loans, and work-study programs. Co-op programs and Army and Air Force ROTC also help defray costs. In addition, KSU participates in the HOPE program for superior students. Nursing students are also eligible for Service Cancellable Loans and various targeted scholarships.

APPLYING

B.S.N. applicants must have full admittance to the University, which requires an official transcript from high school and SAT or ACT scores and/or official transcripts from each university attended, along with a $20 application fee.

Applications are taken spring quarter and summer quarter for acceptance into the following winter or summer B.S.N. class. Completion of seven of the twelve prerequisites with a grade point average of at least 2.5 is the minimum requirement for admission. Admission is competitive.

Registered nurses are admitted during spring quarter to begin the one-year completion program in summer or fall. Students must complete sixteen prerequisite courses with a minimum grade point average of 2.5 and include a letter of reference for consideration.

Applicants to the M.S.N. primary-care nurse practitioner program must have a baccalaureate degree in nursing from an NLN-accredited institution, with a GPA of at least 2.5; a minimum of three years' full-time professional experience within the last five years involving direct patient care documented in a professional résumé; a current license in the state of Georgia; an acceptable score on the GRE; a statement of personal goals for the program; an undergraduate physical assessment course; and full admission into KSU.

Correspondence and Information:

Fran Paul
Administrative Coordinator
School of Nursing
Kennesaw State University
1000 Chastain Road
Kennesaw, Georgia 30144-5591
Telephone: 770-499-3211
770-423-6565
Fax: 770-423-6627

Kent State University
School of Nursing
Kent, Ohio

THE UNIVERSITY

Founded in 1910, Kent State University is today a Carnegie Research II institution and the third largest of Ohio's public universities. The eight-campus system throughout northeastern Ohio enrolls nearly 34,000 students. The Kent campus offers baccalaureate, master's-level, and doctoral study in the Colleges of Arts and Science, Business Administration, Education, and Fine and Professional Arts and the School of Nursing. At the seven regional campuses, associate degrees in technical, business, and health fields are offered as well as lower-division baccalaureate study.

The University's primary concern is the student. There is a commitment to providing the academic atmosphere and curricular and extracurricular activities that stimulate curiosity, broaden perspective, enrich awareness, deepen understanding, establish disciplined habits of thought, prepare for a vocation, and help realize potential as an individual and as a responsible and informed citizen.

THE SCHOOL OF NURSING

The Kent State University School of Nursing, established in 1967, offers the most comprehensive program of study in nursing in Ohio, ranks in the 98th percentile in size in the nation, and enjoys a reputation for excellent academic performance, clinical knowledge, and leadership ability of its students and graduates. All programs in nursing at Kent State are accredited by the National League for Nursing.

Since its founding, nursing at Kent State University has enjoyed continued growth, and today it is the largest school of nursing in Ohio. The mission of Kent State University School of Nursing reflects a commitment to furthering nursing knowledge, to excellence in instruction, and to preparing graduates who are able to address changing societal needs. There exists an academic atmosphere that fosters intellectual curiosity, develops professional and personal values, and facilitates the acquisition, interpretation, utilization, and expansion of nursing knowledge for the discipline and for professional practice.

Kent's faculty, skilled in the scholarship of teaching, discovery, application, and integration, fosters the intellectual life of the University. The School of Nursing's faculty members, who number more than 75, are active, creative contributors to the advancement of nursing knowledge and to the improvement of health-care delivery through teaching, research, and service activities at the local, regional, national, and international levels. The nursing faculty is composed of scholars, researchers, and those with strong clinical skills. Currently, 77 percent of the regular, full-time faculty members are doctorally prepared, and 4 are Fellows in the American Academy of Nursing. Teaching excellence is a hallmark of the School of Nursing faculty.

PROGRAMS OF STUDY

The School of Nursing offers associate, baccalaureate, and master's degree programs in nursing. The baccalaureate degree program accommodates generic as well as second degree, licensed practical nurse, and registered nurse students. The master's degree nursing program offers clinical concentrations in nursing of adults (including gerontology), psychiatric–mental health nursing, and parent-child nursing as well as functional concentrations in nurse practitioner clinical specialization, education, and administration. Post-master's nurse practitioner certificate programs are also available in acute and primary care. In addition, dual-degree M.S.N./M.P.A. and M.S.N./M.B.A. options, as well as an interdisciplinary gerontology concentration, are available. University Board of Trustees approval has been received for establishment of a Ph.D. in nursing program in conjunction with the University of Akron College of Nursing. An associate degree in nursing program is offered on three regional campuses (Ashtabula, East Liverpool, and Tuscarawas), and the lower-division baccalaureate nursing curriculum is offered at the East Liverpool, Stark, and Trumbull regional campuses. The associate degree program is a two-year program of study that leads to the associate degree in nursing. The purpose of this program is to prepare practitioners who can assume responsibility for the provision of technical nursing care. Approximately 450 students are currently enrolled in this program.

The baccalaureate nursing program is a four-year undergraduate program leading to the Bachelor of Science in Nursing degree. The curriculum includes courses in the humanities and biological and social sciences as well as theoretical knowledge and clinical practice in the discipline of nursing. Both generic students and nontraditional students (second degree, RNs, and LPNs) are admitted to the program. There are currently more than 1,000 students enrolled in the baccalaureate program. The first two years of the baccalaureate program are available on several of the regional campuses; select upper division courses and all course requirements for RN students to complete the B.S.N. will be available at regional campuses.

The master's program is a two-year graduate program leading to a Master of Science in Nursing degree. The purpose of this program is to prepare specialists for leadership roles in the practice of professional nursing. Enrollment in the master's program is more than 150, with approximately 65 percent of these students pursuing graduate study on a part-time basis.

A program of continuing nursing education is also offered. The School of Nursing is an Ohio Nurses Association–approved provider of continuing education and awards continuing education units (CEUs) for program offerings.

AFFILIATIONS WITH HEALTH-CARE FACILITIES

The School of Nursing has established affiliations with more than sixty health agencies throughout northeastern Ohio for clinical learning experiences. These range from large urban medical centers, including The Cleveland Clinic Foundation and University Hospitals of Cleveland, to small rural hospitals and clinics as well as a variety of long-term and community health-care agencies. Transportation for student travel to the various clinical sites is provided via the Kent State University campus bus service.

ACADEMIC FACILITIES

The School of Nursing is housed in Henderson Hall, a modern building designed and built specifically to house the nursing programs. It contains classrooms, faculty offices, conference rooms, study areas, nursing multipurpose and computer laboratories, a learning resource center, a nursing research center, and a 250-seat auditorium. In addition, the excellent services and resources of the entire Kent State University are available and include more than 100 buildings on the Kent campus. The twelve-story open stack library is a member of the Association of Research Libraries and holds over 1.5 million volumes, including an extensive collection of nursing and medical references. The basic science complex of the consortium of Northeastern Ohio Universities College of Medicine is located 6 miles from the Kent campus and is an integral part of Kent.

LOCATION

Located in Kent, Ohio (population approximately 30,000), the Kent campus is situated on a beautiful 2,264-acre tree-covered area. Close by are the metropolitan areas of Cleveland (35 miles), Akron (15 miles), Canton (35 miles), and Youngstown (35 miles). The seven regional campuses are located in communities 35–80 miles from the Kent campus. The most populous of Ohio's four quadrants, northeastern Ohio is an area rich with cultural and recreational activities. Among these are Kent's Porthouse Theatre and Blossom Music Center, summer home of the Cleveland Orchestra.

STUDENT SERVICES

A comprehensive array of student services are available through the School of Nursing Office of Student Affairs and the University's Michael Schwartz Student Service Center. In addition to academic services, health services, counseling and guidance, career planning and placement, financial aid, residential service, recreation, and student activities programming are provided. There are more than 200 undergraduate and graduate student organizations on campus that welcome members from throughout the University. Opportunities for participation in a variety of intercollegiate sports also exist.

THE NURSING STUDENT GROUP

Kent serves a talented, culturally rich student body from Ohio and around the world, including historically underrepresented and nontraditional students. Students in nursing reflect a microcosm of the University student body. There are more than 1,000 nursing students enrolled in the B.S.N. and M.S.N. programs on the Kent campus. Several hundred more nursing students are at the regional campuses in the associate degree program or lower-division baccalaureate nursing courses.

Students for Professional Nursing (SPN) is a very active student organization that provides opportunity for development of leadership skills, promoting health-care activities on the campus and facilitating socialization into the professional role. In addition, there is a chapter of the Ohio Nursing Students Association (ONSA) at Kent. Graduate students can take an active role in the University Graduate Student Senate and the Graduate Nurse Student Organization (GNSO).

COSTS

For 1996–97, the tuition for full-time baccalaureate study was $2144 per semester; for graduate study, $2284 per semester. The cost of part-time study was $195 per undergraduate credit and $207.75 per graduate credit. Out-of-state students pay an additional nonresident fee. The cost of University room and board was approximately $2000 per semester. For students enrolled in the B.S.N. program, there was a nursing fee of $735 to cover special laboratory, clinical, and transportation costs.

FINANCIAL AID

Kent State University has developed a financial aid program to assist students who lack the necessary funds for a college education. This program consists of scholarships, loans, grants-in-aid, and part-time employment. In addition to the regular University financial aid, nursing students are eligible for financial assistance that is exclusively for nursing students and includes federal, armed services, and hospital tuition assistance. The School of Nursing also has a short-term emergency loan fund for nursing expenses. Registered nurses may find additional financial assistance through the clinical agencies with whom they are employed. Federal traineeships, graduate assistantships, scholarships, and special awards, such as the Ohio Board of Regents Scholars program, are additional sources of financial assistance for graduate students.

APPLYING

Applicants to the B.S.N. program need to submit a completed Kent State University application; a high school transcript; ACT or SAT I scores (for students under 21 years of age); an official transcript from each college, university, or school attended; and a $25 application fee.

Students completing prenursing requirements with a GPA of 2.5 or higher and a 2.5 average or higher in the first-year science courses make application to the nursing sequence, which begins in the second year of the program. Registered nurses and persons holding a non-nursing degree are admitted directly to the School of Nursing.

Applicants to the master's program must have current Ohio licensure as a registered nurse; have a baccalaureate degree in upper-division nursing with supervised clinical practice from an NLN-accredited program; achieve a grade point average of at least 3.0 on a 4.0 scale from the undergraduate program; and have completed an elementary course in research methodology. In addition to an application form, $25 application fee, and official transcript, prospective students are asked to submit three letters of reference and an essay not exceeding 300 words describing previous education and experience, future professional goals, and reasons for seeking graduate nursing education. A satisfactory score on the Graduate Record Examinations is also required. A preadmission interview is recommended.

Correspondence and Information:

Connie Stopper
Assistant Dean, Student Affairs
Kent State University
School of Nursing
Henderson Hall
P.O. Box 5190
Kent, Ohio 44242-0001
Telephone: 216-672-7930
Fax: 216-672-2433

La Salle University
School of Nursing
Philadelphia, Pennsylvania

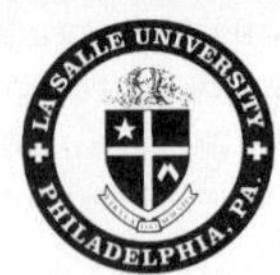

THE UNIVERSITY

La Salle University has evolved over the past decade from a liberal arts college serving the Philadelphia area into a comprehensive university of increasing national prominence. But it has lost none of the warmth, accessibility, and respect for the individual that have characterized the school since it was founded by a Catholic teaching order in 1863. True to the legacy of Saint John Baptist de La Salle and the Christian Brothers order he established 300 years ago, La Salle remains committed to caring, challenging, and inspired teaching.

In recent years, La Salle has enjoyed a growing national reputation for academic excellence and educational value. For example, *U.S. News & World Report* named La Salle one of the country's leading regional universities in recent editions of "America's Best Colleges." The *New York Times, Money* magazine, and *Barron's* all selected La Salle to appear in their guides to the "best buys" in college education.

La Salle's current enrollment of 5,700 men and women includes 2,750 full-time undergraduate students, 1,450 adult students in the School of Continuing Studies, and 1,500 master's degree candidates in the University's ten graduate programs.

THE SCHOOL OF NURSING

La Salle established a nursing department in 1980 for the primary purpose of providing a part-time RN-B.S.N. program for working nurses. Since that time, the University has added a master's program and a full-time bachelor's degree program in nursing. The growth and increasing importance of the nursing programs resulted in the creation of a School of Nursing in 1992, with the assistance of a grant from the Connelly Foundation.

The philosophy of the School of Nursing is to prepare students for the health-care revolution that is under way, in which nurses will take on a more vital and independent role. La Salle is a pioneer in preparing nurses who will provide primary health care in settings outside the hospital. With the growth in jobs expected to be in community health, public health, long-term care, chronic care, and home health care, La Salle has taken a leadership position in producing nurses who are prepared for these new opportunities.

The La Salle faculty consists of professional nurses who have become nationally recognized researchers, published authorities in their fields, and gifted teachers. Eighty-five percent have earned their doctorates. The full-time faculty does all the teaching; La Salle does not use teaching assistants, adjunct professors, or clinical educators. The teaching staff includes 20 full-time faculty members and clinically credentialed professionals.

PROGRAMS OF STUDY

La Salle's School of Nursing offers a full-time B.S.N. program, a B.S.N. completion program for RNs, a Master of Science in Nursing (M.S.N.) program, and an accelerated program for RNs leading to both the B.S.N. and M.S.N. degrees.

The full-time B.S.N. program is designed for students entering from high school who have selected nursing as a career, adult students who are seeking a second undergraduate degree or career change, and transfer students. The program prepares its graduates to qualify for the state board nursing examination to become registered professional nurses and to practice as members of the nursing profession. The four-year program provides the student with a strong foundation in the liberal arts and biological sciences.

La Salle's RN-B.S.N. program has established a national reputation for its unique evening and weekend program for registered nurses. The program is designed for the adult learner—the nurse who is employed and who has family/life obligations and wishes to earn the B.S.N. degree. The goal of the RN-B.S.N. program is to enable the registered nurse to promote health, harmony, and increasing independence in individuals, families, communities, and organizations by expanding the nurse's knowledge and skill in broad-based health and nursing theories and practices.

The program of study leading to the Master of Science in Nursing degree may be completed in any of the following tracks: public health nursing, nursing administration, and adult health and illness nursing (with tracks for clinical nurse specialist and primary care nurse practitioner). The curriculum reflects a balance between liberal and professional education and is designed to foster intellectual inquisitiveness, analytical thinking, critical judgment, creativity, and self-direction under the guidance of a qualified faculty. Students are adult learners from diverse backgrounds who participate in the development of their own agendas for learning within a planned program of studies.

La Salle's RN-M.S.N. program is designed for the registered nurse who is committed to pursuing the Master of Science in Nursing degree. The program accelerates the student through the RN-B.S.N. program by permitting enrollment in selected graduate-level courses while completing the B.S.N. degree. Specific M.S.N.-level courses are substituted for 9 credits of undergraduate work, including one course in the area of specialty at the M.S.N. level.

AFFILIATIONS WITH HEALTH-CARE FACILITIES

La Salle's School of Nursing has established strong ties with a number of hospitals and other health-care facilities in the Philadelphia area. Clinical experiences associated with course work are available at institutions such as Albert Einstein Medical Center, St. Christopher's Hospital for Children, Moss Rehabilitation Center, Chestnut Hill Hospital, Allegheny University Hospital (East Falls), Belmont Psychiatric Institute, and Parkview Hospital. In addition, students have the opportunity to practice at the La Salle University Neighborhood Nursing Center, a nurse-managed public health and primary-care facility.

Four of the health-care institutions and the Neighborhood Nursing Center are within walking distance of La Salle's campus.

ACADEMIC FACILITIES

Considered one of the finest academic libraries on the East Coast, the Connelly Library offers a combination of traditional library services and the latest in information technology. The library features several special departments—including Media Services and Special Collections—and an expanding collection of databases on compact disc.

The University's Computer Center has become an increasingly important resource for the School of Nursing. Efforts to integrate computerized instruction into nursing courses have evolved into a Nursing Informatics Laboratory with state-of-the-art hardware and software and a full-time nursing informatics specialist.

LOCATION

Six miles northwest of Center City Philadelphia, La Salle is bordered by Fairmount Park and the historic residential section of Germantown. The 100-acre campus includes 12 acres of woods and gardens and the restored eighteenth-century home of American portrait painter Charles Willson Peale.

La Salle is surrounded by some of the leading health-care institutions in the Philadelphia area, providing convenient access to a variety of clinical experiences.

La Salle's School of Nursing also offers undergraduate courses and the full M.S.N. program at the La Salle University Bucks County Center in Newtown, Pennsylvania.

STUDENT SERVICES

Among the many resources and services available to students are Career Planning and Placement, Counseling Center, Building Blocks Day Care Center, Sheeky Writing Center, Campus Ministry, Office of Multicultural and International Affairs, Academic Computing and Technology, Honors Program, Financial Aid, Student Affairs, Resident Life, Student Health Services, Fitness Center, Cooperative Education, and Urban Studies and Community Services Center.

There are several organizations for nursing students at La Salle, including the Student Nurses' Association for full-time undergraduates, the Registered Nurses' Organization for RN students, and the Graduate Nurses' Organization for master's candidates. Students also serve on various committees with faculty members and administrators, providing direct input into the School's operations.

THE NURSING STUDENT GROUP

There are 170 full-time students in the B.S.N. program, 375 part-time students in the RN-B.S.N. completion program, and 250 part-time students in the Master of Science in Nursing program. All students in the RN-B.S.N. completion program and M.S.N. program practice as professional nurses in clinical, managerial, and research positions with a variety of health-care organizations in the five-county Philadelphia area, in New Jersey, and in Delaware. More than half of the full-time B.S.N. students participate in paid summer externships in a variety of major health-care centers in Philadelphia.

COSTS

Tuition and fees for the 1996–97 academic year were $14,090 for full-time undergraduate nursing students. Room and board costs for those residing on campus were approximately $6000 for the year. For part-time students, the cost was $256 per credit hour for undergraduate courses and $415 per unit for graduate courses.

FINANCIAL AID

The primary purpose of La Salle's extensive financial aid program is to provide financial assistance to students who, without such aid, would be unable to attend the University. Financial need is met by a combination of scholarships, grants, loans, and other sources. Federal Graduate Nurse Traineeships are offered through the School of Nursing.

Some of the hospitals with which La Salle is affiliated offer paid externships and scholarship programs.

APPLYING

Information on application requirements and deadlines can be obtained by contacting the appropriate office at La Salle University.

Correspondence and Information:

For full-time undergraduate program information:
Christopher P. Lydon
Office of Admission and Financial Aid
La Salle University
Philadelphia, Pennsylvania 19141-1199
Telephone: 215-951-1500

For RN-B.S.N. program information:
Anna Melnyk Allen
Office of Admission and Financial Aid
La Salle University
Philadelphia, Pennsylvania 19141-1199
Telephone: 215-951-1500

For M.S.N. or RN-M.S.N. program information:
Dr. Zane Robinson Wolf
School of Nursing
La Salle University
Philadelphia, Pennsylvania 19141-1199
Telephone: 215-951-1430

THE FACULTY

The following is only a partial listing of the La Salle School of Nursing faculty:

Cynthia F. Capers, Ph.D., RN; Professor and Interim Dean.
Eileen R. Giardino, Ph.D., RN; Associate Professor and Interim Director, Undergraduate Programs.
Katherine K. Kinsey, Ph.D., RN, FAAN; Associate Professor and Director, Neighborhood Nursing Center.
Zane Robinson Wolf, Ph.D., RN, FAAN; Professor and Graduate Director.

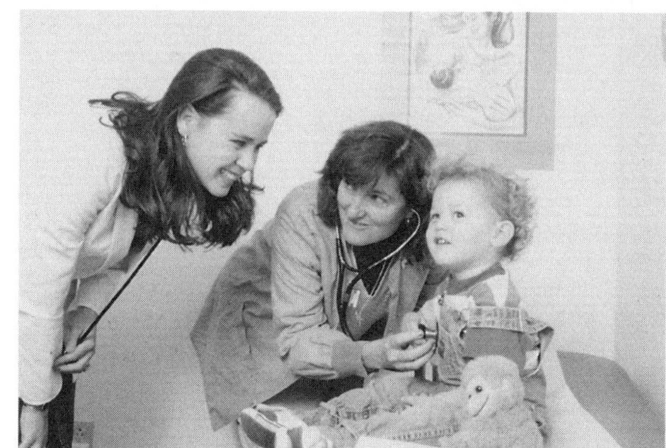

La Salle's School of Nursing operates two nurse-managed public health and primary-care centers in Philadelphia. The La Salle Neighborhood Nursing Center has become a national model, enabling students to work with the faculty in an independent setting.

Loyola University Chicago
Marcella Niehoff School of Nursing
Chicago, Illinois

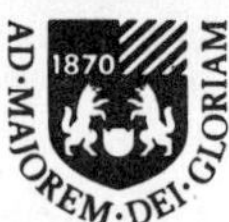

THE UNIVERSITY

Loyola University Chicago, founded in 1870, is an independent, urban, Catholic university with a Jesuit heritage that emphasizes the development of the intellectual, social, and moral values and character of its students. Dedicated to higher education and health care, the University has a regional, national, and international influence. With five campuses, including the Rome Center of Liberal Arts in Italy, Loyola is the largest of the twenty-eight Jesuit colleges and universities in the nation. More than 15,000 students are enrolled in the University's nine schools and colleges. Students come to Loyola from all fifty states and sixty-eight countries.

THE SCHOOL OF NURSING

Loyola's Marcella Niehoff School of Nursing's baccalaureate program is the oldest in Illinois and is considered to be the best in the state. It is an outstanding school of nursing with a sense of history and a vision for the future. The School is committed to providing an environment that reflects the Jesuit tradition of knowledge in the service of mankind.

PROGRAMS OF STUDY

The traditional four-year B.S.N. program attracts the largest number of students. The curriculum builds on the Jesuit core and a science base. B.S.N. students begin at Loyola as freshmen or transfers prior to the second semester of their sophomore year. The program culminates with a transition course designed to facilitate graduates' entry into a clinical area of interest. Loyola B.S.N. graduates practice throughout the world and are often sought after by clinical agencies.

The accelerated program for bachelor's degree students is a program designed for students holding non-nursing bachelor's degrees. The nursing sequence of courses is compressed into a thirteen- or fifteen-month, full-time day program that begins in May or August. Students complete the program the first summer session of the following year.

The RN/B.S.N. Completion Program is designed for students who have been licensed as registered nurses to continue their studies and earn the baccalaureate degree. Nurses who have earned either the Associate Degree in Nursing or a diploma from a hospital school of nursing qualify for the RN/B.S.N. Completion Program.

The RN/M.S.N. Program is designed for students who have been licensed as registered nurses. Nurses who have earned an Associate Degree in Nursing (A.D.N.) or a diploma from a hospital school of nursing qualify for this program. The applicant must also submit a portfolio demonstrating a record of clinical experience and leadership in nursing. In addition to the completion of the required courses for the M.S.N., selected undergraduate courses are also required. The student can choose to study in any one of the majors listed below for the M.S.N Program.

The Marcella Niehoff School of Nursing offers two graduate programs. The Master of Science in Nursing (M.S.N.) prepares nurses to function as a critical care/trauma NP or CNS, oncology CNS or PNP, women's health NP, adult NP, or nursing service administrator (with subfocus areas of long-term-care administration, community/home health administration, and ambulatory care administration). In addition, two dual degrees—M.S.N./M.B.A. and M.S.N./M.Div.—are offered. The second graduate offering is the Ph.D. in nursing, which prepares a nurse scholar, with extensive training in research, to contribute to the body of nursing knowledge. Entry to either graduate program requires a Bachelor of Science in Nursing (B.S.N.) degree from an accredited school of nursing.

AFFILIATIONS WITH HEALTH-CARE FACILITIES

The nursing major is offered at the Lake Shore Campus of Loyola University and at cooperating clinical agencies. These include the Foster G. McGaw Hospital of Loyola University Medical Center, Weiss Memorial Hospital, Humana Hospital–Michael Reese, Hines Hospital, Chicago Department of Health clinics, selected nursing homes, school settings, psychiatric settings, senior citizen centers, and community nursing services of the Marcella Niehoff School of Nursing and the Loyola University of Chicago Medical Center.

ACADEMIC FACILITIES

Loyola's libraries extend to all five campuses. Each library provides a vast array of materials as well as computer access to assist students in their studies.

The Lake Shore campus School of Nursing Learning Resource Center (LRC) is managed by a nurse practitioner and staff to assist students. The LRC is equipped with a bank of simulated nursing unit carrels that allows students to practice their clinical skills. Films, videotapes, interactive videos, and computers, along with demonstrations by the LRC staff, are part of the teaching-learning techniques.

LOCATION

Loyola is located in Chicago, one of the nation's largest, most cosmopolitan cities. Situated on Lake Michigan, Chicago offers many recreational activities. The city is home to well-known museums, including the Museum of Science and Industry, the Art Institute, Shedd Aquarium, and Adler Planetarium. Chicago hosts many events, including the Chicago International Film Festival, jazz and blues festivals, and the annual Taste of Chicago. It is also a center for international theater, ballet, and symphony.

STUDENT SERVICES

Loyola provides a variety of student life experiences that take into account the diversity of the student body. The Offices of Multicultural Affairs, Women's Studies, International Students, and Counseling as well as the Writing Center, Computer Center, and Student Health Center, are among those most used. Residence halls offer a variety of housing options from single rooms to apartment-style living.

Students in the School of Nursing are members of NSNA, the National Student Nurses Association, and SNAIL, the Student Nurses' Association of Illinois. Qualified students are invited to join Sigma Theta Tau, the international nursing honor society, and Alpha Sigma Nu, the Jesuit honor society. Nursing students who qualify may participate in Loyola University Chicago's Honor Program.

THE NURSING STUDENT GROUP

As of fall 1996, there were 455 students enrolled in the undergraduate program and 182 students enrolled in the School of Nursing graduate programs at Loyola. The Jesuit educational setting provides a tradition whereby students may gain knowledge and learn behaviors that support a lifestyle of service to mankind. As a result, Marcella Niehoff School of Nursing graduates are professional nurses whose practice has a humanitarian focus.

COSTS

Tuition costs for the 1996–97 academic year were $14,400 per year for the B.S.N., and $408 per unit for the M.S.N. and Ph.D degree programs.

FINANCIAL AID

The mission of Loyola University Chicago's Office of Student Financial Assistance is to ensure access to and the successful completion of an education by eliminating financial barriers. To fulfill this mission, the Office of Student Financial Assistance provides monetary assistance programs that attempt to meet both the documented and perceived financial needs of the University's students and their families; offers counseling, education, and ombudsman services to students and families; and provides services and programs that enable students and families to better assist themselves.

APPLYING

Applicants to the baccalaureate program must have had 15 high school units, including English, mathematics (algebra and geometry), biology, chemistry, and social science; submit acceptable SAT I or ACT scores; and pass a health examination administered by the School. Applicants to the RN/B.S.N. Completion Program must submit official transcripts from previous schools attended and a copy of a current Illinois nursing license. Requirements for RNs include an overall minimum GPA of 2.5 for all courses attempted at other schools, excluding nursing courses; a minimum grade of C in each science course; and graduation from an NLN-accredited school of nursing. Applicants to graduate programs should contact the Office of Graduate Admissions for specific requirements. Application forms and credentials should be submitted to the admissions office at Loyola.

Correspondence and Information:

Office of Undergraduate Admissions
Loyola University Chicago
820 North Michigan Avenue
Chicago, Illinois 60611
Telephone: 312-915-6500

Office of Graduate Admissions
Marcella Niehoff School of Nursing
Loyola University Chicago
6525 North Sheridan Road
Chicago, Illinois 60626
Telephone: 773-508-3249

THE FACULTY

Shirley Dooling, Dean; Ed.D., Columbia.
Esther Jacobs, Associate Dean; Ph.D., Northwestern.
Anne Jalowiec, Associate Dean; Ph.D., Illinois.
Marcia Maurer, Associate Dean; Ph.D., Loyola Chicago.
Rosemarie R. Parse, Niehoff Chair; Ph.D., Pittsburgh.

Department of Community Mental Health/Administrative Nursing

Sheila Haas, Chairperson; Ph.D., Illinois.
Pamela Andresen, Ph.D., Illinois.
Ida Androwich, Ph.D., Illinois.
Shirley Butler, Ph.D., Loyola Chicago.
Karen Egenes, Ed.D., Northern Illinois.
Carroll Gold, Ph.D., Northwestern.
Diana Hackbarth, Ph.D., Illinois.
Gloria Jacobson, Ph.D., Wisconsin–Milwaukee.
Judy Scully, Ph.D., Illinois.
Elizabeth Tarlov, M.S., Pace.
Marianne Zelewsky, M.S.N., Loyola Chicago.

Department of Maternal Child Health Nursing

Marybeth Young, Chairperson; Ph.D., Loyola Chicago.
Diane Boyer, Ph.D., Northwestern.
Ellen Chiocca, M.S.N., Loyola Chicago.
Linda Janusek, Ph.D., Illinois.
Beverly Kopala, Ph.D., Illinois.
Lucy Martinez-Schallmoser, Ph.D., Illinois.
Mary Ann McDermott, Ed.D., Northern Illinois.
Linda Paskiewicz, Ph.D., Illinois.
Barbara Velsor-Friedrich, Ph.D., Northwestern.
Katherine A. Wiley, Ed.D., Northern Illinois.

Department of Medical-Surgical Nursing

Karyn Holm, Chairperson; Ph.D., Loyola Chicago.
Ardelina A. Baldonado, Ph.D., Loyola Chicago.
Elizabeth Carlson, Ph.D., Loyola Chicago.
Maria Connolly, D.N.Sc., Rush.
Mary Ellen Gulanick, Ph.D., Illinois.
Franklin Hicks, Ph.D., Loyola Chicago.
Judith Jennrich, Ph.D., Illinois.
Vicki Keough, M.S.N., Loyola Chicago.
Diane M. Klein, Ph.D., Illinois.
Mary Koren, D.N.Sc., Rush.
Dorothy Lanuza, Ph.D., Illinois.
Marijo Letizia, Ph.D., Loyola Chicago.
Suling Li, Ph.D. candidate, Loyola Chicago.
Mary Ann Noonan, M.S.N., Loyola Chicago.
Susan M. Penckofer, Ph.D., Illinois.
Nancy Spector, D.N.Sc., Illinois.
Donna Starsiak, M.S.N., Illinois.

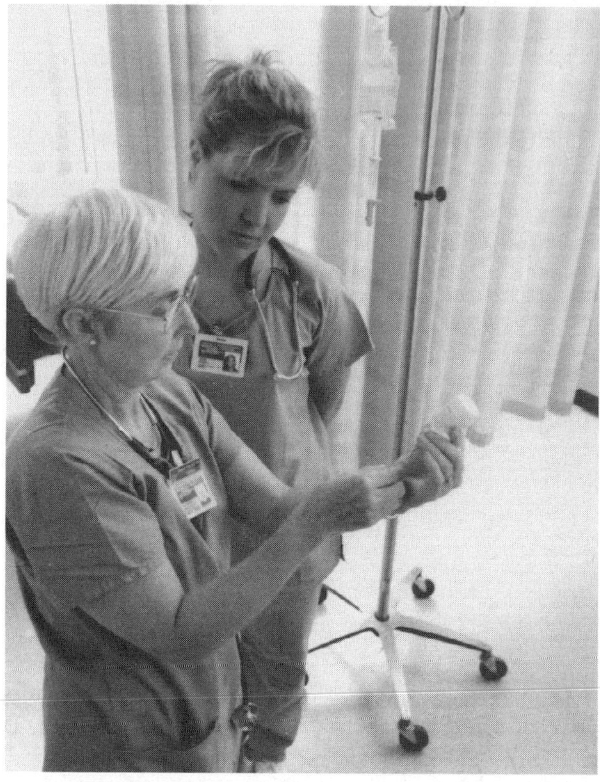

Nursing professor demonstrates clinical practice to a student at Loyola University Medical Center.

Luther College
Department of Nursing
Decorah, Iowa

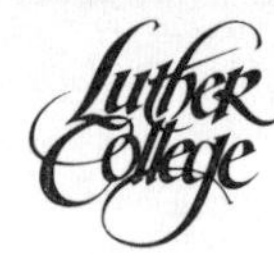

THE COLLEGE

The students and faculty of Luther College are committed to liberal learning in the arts and sciences. Founded in 1861 by Norwegian immigrants, Luther is a college of the Evangelical Lutheran Church in America. While more than thirty-five states and forty countries are represented in the student body of approximately 2,400, most Luther students come from Iowa, Minnesota, Wisconsin, and Illinois. Extensive curricular offerings include sixty majors and preprofessional programs. The College's student-teacher ratio of 13:1 allows for exceptional personal interaction with the faculty.

THE DEPARTMENT OF NURSING

The goals of Luther's nursing program are to prepare nurses to function autonomously and interdependently with individuals, families, groups, and communities to promote, maintain, and restore optimal health in a variety of health-care settings. The nursing major, therefore, offers an integrated program of liberal arts and fourteen professional nursing courses. The program gives students a broad approach to nursing, providing a base for graduate study or immediate entry into the nursing profession. Following graduation with a Bachelor of Arts in nursing, Luther nursing students may write the National Council Licensure Examination for Registered Nurses.

PROGRAM OF STUDY

It is Luther's mission to produce well-rounded and capable students. In the context of a Christian, liberal arts institution, student nurses explore the sciences and the humanities in addition to their nursing courses. The freshman year provides a foundation in the liberal arts. An introductory course in nursing gives the student an overview of the nursing profession. Faculty members advise each student about career opportunities in nursing.

Students entering the nursing program should have a solid background in English, math, biology, and chemistry. They must also take an algebra skills test for appropriate chemistry course placement.

Clinical nursing courses begin in the fall of the sophomore year. Nursing courses at this level emphasize health assessment throughout the life span in a variety of settings. These learning experiences develop new communication and interpersonal skills.

Third-year students engage in a concentrated study of nursing concepts through caring for children and adults with physical and emotional problems. The sites for the clinical experiences include Rochester Methodist Hospital and St. Mary's Hospital, affiliates of the Mayo Medical Center, and the Federal Medical Center as well as a variety of community-based health-care agencies in Rochester, Minnesota.

The senior year provides final preparation for entry into the practice of professional nursing. Courses focus on promoting health and preventing illness in childbearing families and in community groups. One feature of the senior year is the assignment of an expectant mother to each nursing student. The student follows the mother through the entire pregnancy and is present at birth. Following graduation, an NCLEX review course is available to all nursing students.

AFFILIATIONS WITH HEALTH-CARE FACILITIES

Luther College conducts its clinical nursing experiences during the junior year at Mayo Medical Center facilities in Rochester, Minnesota, as well as a variety of community-based facilities. These affiliations afford students the opportunity for exposure to the most recent technical and personal strategies for effective nursing care. Additional clinical experiences occur with Winneshiek County Memorial Hospital, the Oneota Riverview Care Facility, the Winneshiek County Public Health Nursing Service, Minowa Cancer Detection, and a variety of community-based programs in Northeast Iowa.

ACADEMIC FACILITIES

The 800-acre campus includes the Preus Library, housing 316,242 volumes, 1,058 periodicals, and the College art collection. Students have access to an interactive computer program in the nursing computer lab. Modern, well-equipped laboratories in the Valders Hall of Science are supplemented by several other science-teaching facilities on campus. The science facilities also include an extensive field study area and two electron microscopes. Computer facilities include a Hewlett-Packard 9000, an HP 3000/957, 2 HP UNIX workstations, more than 700 microcomputers, connections to the Internet, and a campuswide network connecting classrooms, laboratories, and offices.

LOCATION

Luther is located in Decorah, a city of 8,000 in the scenic bluff country of northeast Iowa. Decorah is a popular recreation area, providing opportunities for spelunking, hiking, fishing, hunting, cross-country and Alpine skiing, camping, cycling, and canoeing. Three airports are located within a 75-mile radius (Rochester, Minnesota; LaCrosse, Wisconsin; and Waterloo, Iowa).

STUDENT SERVICES

Luther provides numerous student services in a setting that includes programming seven days a week. The Regents Center for recreation, the Centennial Union, and the Center for Faith and Life serve as hubs of student life activities. Students are involved in the governance of the College through involvement on college committees and student government organizations. Luther fields nineteen athletic teams and provides more than forty intramural activities. Also, students from every academic department participate in the broad-based music program.

THE NURSING STUDENT GROUP

The Luther College nursing program enrolls approximately 140 students, with 30 to 40 students graduating annually. Since the program was established in 1978, the retention rate of nursing students from sophomore to senior year has typically been 90 percent. Nursing students generally have an average of more than 25 on the ACT and are challenged in a very rigorous program that prepares them well for the profession or for graduate study. Nursing students must achieve a Luther College grade point average of 2.3.

COSTS

For 1997–98, the comprehensive fee is estimated at $19,330, which includes tuition, general fees, facilities fee, room, board, and subscriptions to student publications. A room telephone and health-service program are included.

FINANCIAL AID

Nearly 80 percent of all Luther students receive some financial aid in the form of grants, scholarships from Luther, loans, and jobs on campus. Luther awards significant scholarships to students who demonstrate exceptional academic preparation and provides large amounts of need-based aid. The amount of aid is determined by the analysis of the Free Application for Federal Student Aid. The priority deadline for aid applications is March 1. Students receive notification of their aid awards after their acceptance for admission. All nursing students benefit from the Bernice Fischer Cross and Bert S. Cross Perpetual Endowment for the Luther College Mayo Nursing Program and Health Sciences Program. This endowment is used for equal-share assistance for the Luther College nursing students enrolled in the curriculum provided in the Mayo Medical Center in Rochester, Minnesota. This is not a need-based scholarship.

APPLYING

An application for admission, SAT I or ACT scores, an educator's reference form, and a transcript of previous academic work are required for admission. On-campus interviews are recommended but not required. Luther recommends that students complete the following units in high school: 4 units of English, 3 units of math, 3 units of social science, and 2 units of natural science, including one lab course.

Correspondence and Information:

Admissions Office
Luther College
Decorah, Iowa 52101
Telephone: 319-387-1287
800-458-8437 (toll-free)
Fax: 319-387-2159
E-mail: admissions@luther.edu

THE FACULTY

Donna Kubesh, Department Head; Associate Professor; M.S., Ph.D.; RN.

Associate Professors

Nancy Maloney, M.P.H., Ph.D.; cancer detection nurse specialist certification.

Assistant Professors

Corrine Carlson, M.S.; RN.
Teresa Hansen, M.S.; RN.
Sheryl Juve, M.S.; RN, minister of health certification, long-term-care administration certification.
Janet Kraabel, M.S.N.; RN.
Mary Overvold-Ronningen, M.S., Ph.D. candidate; RN.
Cheryl Pellett, M.S.; RN.

Clinical Instructors

JoEllen Anderson, B.S.N.; RN.
Jean Boyer, B.S.N.; RN.
Sherri Reutlinger, B.A.; RN.

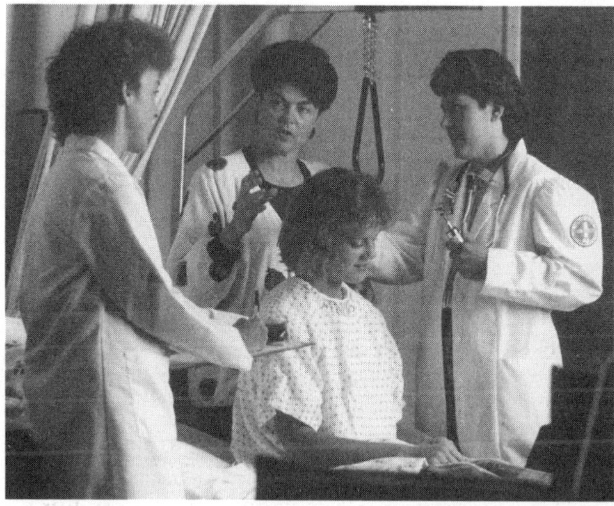

Luther College nursing students gain significant clinical experience in facilities associated with the Mayo Medical Center.

Marywood College
Department of Nursing
Scranton, Pennsylvania

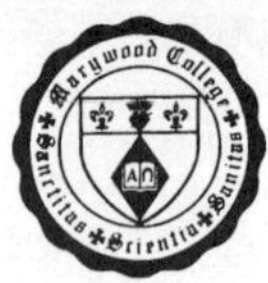

THE COLLEGE

Founded in 1915 by the Congregation of the Sisters, Servants of the Immaculate Heart of Mary, Marywood College is an independent, comprehensive, Catholic College serving men and women representing a variety of backgrounds and religions in myriad academic programs. The College enrolls nearly 3,200 students in an extensive array of undergraduate and graduate programs. Committed to enriching spiritual, ethical, and religious values and a tradition of service and motivated by a pioneering, progressive spirit, Marywood College provides an educational framework that enables students to develop fully as persons and to master professional and leadership skills necessary for meeting human needs on regional and global levels.

The central focus of the undergraduate curriculum is expressed in the phrase "living responsibly in an interdependent world." Students are expected to incorporate this concern for responsible use of resources into their personal and professional lives. The College's historic concern for the enrichment of human life through the honoring of religious values and a tradition of service extends also to the programs at the graduate level.

Marywood's programs are administered through three degree-granting schools. The Undergraduate School offers degrees in nearly fifty academic disciplines including the arts, sciences, music, fine arts, and social work as well as nursing. Opportunities for undergraduates abound through double majors, honors and independent study programs, practicums, internships, and study abroad. Programs leading to master's degrees are offered in the Graduate School of Arts and Science and in the School of Social Work.

THE DEPARTMENT OF NURSING

The nursing program at Marywood College offers a Bachelor of Science in Nursing (B.S.N.) degree program for both RNs and students without a nursing background. The program is fully approved by the State Board of Nursing and is accredited by the National League for Nursing. The baccalaureate program in nursing prepares the graduate to use nursing knowledge and skills to carry out the professional responsibilities of the beginning nurse in a variety of settings. The program also prepares the graduate for advanced study in nursing and for continuing personal and professional development.

Opportunities are provided for the student to apply an academic background in the liberal arts and sciences to the theory and practice of the nursing discipline. Essential human values are emphasized and practical application of the nursing process is stressed. The student applies knowledge of the law and of legislation in caring for the client and learns to communicate effectively with clients, colleagues, and the public.

Skills required to provide nursing care are practiced in a modern, well-equipped laboratory as well as with clients in the clinical setting. The ability to think critically is stressed as are the leadership roles of the nurse as manager of client care, client advocate, educator, and member of the profession. The student is expected to use reports of published research to improve clinical practice. Clinical experiences are designed to provide a wide variety of experiences with clients in many health-care settings.

The faculty members have primarily teaching roles. Fifty percent of the current nursing faculty members have been awarded the doctoral degree. Class sizes are small, providing a significant degree of faculty involvement in each student's education. Clinical groups are small (one faculty member for a maximum of 8 students), permitting personalized instruction while students practice nursing in clinical units.

PROGRAM OF STUDY

Marywood College offers the Bachelor of Science in Nursing degree (B.S.N.) for students who have no prior course work in nursing and for registered nurses who were prepared at a diploma or an associate degree level.

The nursing program consists of 136 credits, 55 of which are nursing credits. At least 28 of the 55 nursing credits must be taken at Marywood College. Completion of the program is accomplished by completing, at Marywood College, the five senior-level required nursing courses and the other requirements of the College.

To be considered for retention, progression, and graduation, students must maintain a 2.5 (C+) grade point average or higher in the cognate courses and in the nursing courses that constitute the nursing major. A minimum 2.0 (C) grade point average is required in the liberal arts courses not designated as cognate courses. In addition, the students must obtain a 2.0 (C) GPA or higher in each course designated as a cognate course and in each nursing course. Students who do not achieve a satisfactory grade in a nursing course may repeat one nursing course one time, space permitting.

Challenge (validation) examinations are available for credit and for advanced placement in certain nursing and other courses. Students should contact the department chairperson for information. In addition, certain college courses may be transferred in order to meet some Marywood College requirements.

AFFILIATIONS WITH HEALTH-CARE FACILITIES

The Department of Nursing maintains affiliations with several local health-care facilities. Students must assume responsibility for transportation to and from facilities used for clinical practice.

ACADEMIC FACILITIES

The Department of Nursing is located in the new Center for Natural and Health Sciences. This center houses general computer labs and a separate nursing computer lab for student and faculty use. The nursing lab provides various word processing programs including APA, CAI software, NCLEX preparation software, and interactive video capabilities. In addition, some of the other support software includes WordPerfect, Lotus 1-2-3, Microsoft Word, StatView, Excel, and many others. These state-of-the-art informational systems and LRC capabilities (noted below) support the organizing framework and program goals of the nursing curriculum; they help to prepare professional nurses who must practice safely and competently as nursing leaders in an interdependent world utilizing effective communication and critical thinking skills.

Marywood's Learning Resources Center (LRC) houses library services, media services, and academic computing services. The library collection includes more than 202,000 volumes of books, 1,800 current journal subscriptions, 233,000 microforms, and more than 41,000 media items. The LRC participates in the interlibrary loan network with 8,000 libraries. The research collection includes many index and abstract services, including Cumulative Index to Nursing and Allied Health Literature, International Nursing Index, and Index Medicus. Index and abstract services in other disciplines are available to supplement these nursing references.

The library catalog has been automated since 1989. The on-line catalog system (MELVIN) is currently available on terminals in the LRC, the Center for Human Services, the Center for Natural and Health Sciences, and from home or office via modem.

The LRC is located near the new Center for Natural and Health Sciences. The collection of books, journals, and nonprint media concerning nursing is continually updated. Computer-assisted instruction in nursing and computer interactive video programs are available for use in the LRC academic computing area, the Nursing Computer Lab, and in general computer labs in the Center for Natural and Health Sciences. The current nursing and medical science holdings number approximately 600 audiovisual materials and twenty-one computer-assisted program tools. The LRC currently subscribes to 134 journals relative to the fields of nursing and medical science. In addition, the LRC subscribes to six CD-ROM databases.

LOCATION

Situated on a hilltop, Marywood's scenic 115-acre campus is part of an attractive residential area of the city of Scranton in northeastern Pennsylvania. With a population of 80,000, Scranton is the fifth-largest city in Pennsylvania and is the county seat of Lackawanna County, whose population is approximately 250,000. Marywood has the advantage of being relatively close to major cities of the Northeast (by automobile, 2½ hours from New York City and Philadelphia, 4 hours from Washington, D.C., and 5½ hours from Boston) and is served by several airlines at the Wilkes-Barre/Scranton International Airport (20 minutes from campus). The Pocono Mountains, offering spectacular scenery and downhill skiing, are only a few minutes from campus.

STUDENT SERVICES

Marywood College and the Division of Student Affairs provide extensive services for students. Seminars are offered through both Students Services and the Department of Continuing Education to support the needs of lifelong learners. The Division of Students Affairs coordinates the operation and services provided by Student Development Services, Career Services, Residential Life, Judicial Affairs, Campus Ministry, Health Services, Student Activities, Collegiate Volunteers, and Athletics and Recreational Services.

Some of the services provided through Student Affairs include a counseling center to help students explore a variety of personal, academic, and career issues. In addition, there is an excellent tutorial program, a learning/writing center, and a math laboratory. Career Services provides counseling, workshops, testing, and a computerized career guidance program. Freshman seminars help students make the transition from high school to college. Older adults are also assisted with their special transitional needs. The Writing Center helps students to strengthen their reading and study skills and to develop specific writing and research skills. Tutorial assistance is also available in various subjects.

THE NURSING STUDENT GROUP

Both commuter and residential students enroll in the nursing program, and they represent great diversity in terms of age and background. In three of the past four years, 100 percent of the graduates of the program were successful in passing the National Council Licensure Exam (NCLEX) on their first attempt.

COSTS

In the 1996–97 academic year, tuition for 32 credit hours was $12,640 ($395 per credit hour), and there was a general fee of $500. Average room and board expenses were $5200. Additional costs include books and supplies (estimated at $600), transportation, and personal expenses.

FINANCIAL AID

More than 84 percent of the undergraduate students receive financial assistance. Marywood College invests its own funds in an extensive scholarship and grant program. In addition, Marywood administers funds of federal and state grant, loan, and employment programs. Marywood applications for financial aid should preferably be submitted no later than February 15. The Free Application for Federal Student Aid (FAFSA) and the state scholarship/grant form should also be submitted to the appropriate agency by February 15.

APPLYING

Marywood welcomes applications for admission from men and women who demonstrate aptitude and academic achievement in a wide range of course work at the secondary school level and/or in a college setting. Either SAT or ACT scores are required for those who wish to enter as freshmen. Personal interviews are highly recommended, and official transcripts and a letter of recommendation are required. Both freshmen and transfer students are accepted in any semester. Admission decisions are announced on a rolling basis. The application fee is $20.

Correspondence and Information:

Fred R. Brooks, Jr.
Director of Admissions
Marywood College
2300 Adams Avenue
Scranton, Pennsylvania 18509
Telephone: 717-348-6234
800-346-5014 (toll-free)
Fax: 717-961-4763
E-mail: ugadm@ac.marywood.edu
World Wide Web: http://www.marywood.edu

Medical College of Georgia
School of Nursing
Augusta, Georgia

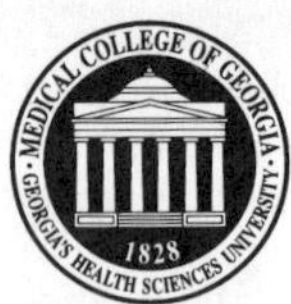

THE COLLEGE

The Medical College of Georgia (MCG), Georgia's health sciences university, is located at Georgia's eastern border on the Savannah River and is the state's primary institution to educate health-care professionals. It is the third-largest of the thirty-two colleges and universities in the state-assisted University System of Georgia, with approximately 2,500 students, interns, and residents. It is the largest single employer in the city of Augusta, with more than 5,000 faculty and staff members. The midtown campus of almost 90 acres includes forty-seven buildings, with construction of new buildings plus expansion and renovation of present buildings continuing the growth trend of the institution.

THE SCHOOL OF NURSING

In response to the wartime need for additional nurses, the University System of Georgia voted August 11, 1943, to offer courses in nursing education. This participation in the U.S. Cadet Nurse Corps paved the way for establishing a department of nursing at the University of Georgia the following fall. The program moved from Athens, Georgia, to Augusta in 1956 and became a part of the Medical College of Georgia. The School of Nursing, with a strong commitment to research, moved forward in its development as a university-based nursing program. In 1974, to meet Georgia's growing need for baccalaureate-prepared nurses, a free-standing, self-contained satellite campus was opened in Athens, Georgia. This campus, for more than twenty years, has consistently prepared one third of the graduates of the baccalaureate program each year. To assist faculty research, an essential component in graduate education, the Center for Nursing Research was established in 1987. In 1994, the Board of Regents approved more than $1 million to renovate the historic Stoney Building, where the School moved in January 1995. In 1996, a second satellite campus was created in cooperation with Gordon College to offer an RN to B.S.N. program using distance learning technology.

The School of Nursing faculty has approximately 60 full-time and 11 part-time members representing many diverse areas of teaching and research. More than 55 percent of the faculty members hold doctoral degrees in nursing or related fields.

PROGRAMS OF STUDY

The School of Nursing is accredited by the National League for Nursing and is a member agency of the Council of Baccalaureate and Higher Degree Programs. Degrees offered are the Bachelor of Science in Nursing (B.S.N.), Master of Science in Nursing (M.S.N.) (clinical nurse specialist program), Master of Nursing (M.N.) (nurse practitioner program and nursing anesthesia), and the Doctor of Philosophy (Ph.D.) in nursing. The baccalaureate program has a community-based curriculum that incorporates a wide variety of clinical experiences in inpatient, outpatient, and community settings. As part of the baccalaureate program, a B.S.N. completion program for registered nurses is offered.

The Master of Science in Nursing program offers specialties in adult nursing, parent-child nursing, mental health–psychiatric nursing, and community health nursing. The Master of Nursing program offers specialties in nursing anesthesia, family nurse practitioner, pediatric nurse practitioner, and neonatal nurse practitioner.

Doctoral program specialties are in health care along the life span and nursing administration.

AFFILIATIONS WITH HEALTH-CARE FACILITIES

Since 1956, MCG has operated the 540-bed teaching hospital, the Medical College of Georgia Hospital and Clinics. The facility is a leading referral center for Georgia and the region. To meet the clinical learning needs of students and the baccalaureate program, more than 165 contracts exist between the School of Nursing and a variety of health-care agencies throughout Georgia and South Carolina.

ACADEMIC FACILITIES

The present five-school campus consists of more than ninety buildings, including a 540-bed teaching hospital, on approximately 90 acres of land. One building and additional acreage comprise the Animal Care Facility at Gracewood State School and Hospital. The university operates community outreach clinics in twenty-eight counties. Telemedicine sites are located across the state. The institution also occupies space in the Georgia cities of Athens and Rome and delivers distance learning to students in Atlanta, Dalton, and Barnesville. The university houses a large multimedia library that participates in the state library system, GALILEO, with MERLIN. GALILEO provides access to more than fifty databases and services pertinent to undergraduate studies. The library also offers an extensive public computing area of Macintosh and IBM-compatible microcomputers and terminals with access to MERLIN and GALILEO and programs for word processing, spreadsheets, graphics, and other services. In addition, students have access to computers within their respective schools.

LOCATION

Due to its location in the Southeast, Augusta provides access to more than just an inland city. In less than 3 hours by automobile, Augustans can visit the mountains, the seashore, or the major metropolitan city of Atlanta, opening many weekend activities. Augusta is the second-largest metropolitan area in Georgia and is a major medical center, with nine local hospitals that serve the Southeast. Students have access to a major art museum, a civic center, malls, annual river activities, Lake Thurmond Reservoir for recreation, and many annual community events, such as Arts in the Hearts of Augusta and the Boshears Memorial Fly-In, attracting pilots nationwide. Air and ground transportation are available. The city is fortunate in having many associations dedicated to the performing and visual arts. Among these are the Augusta Opera Association, the only resident opera company in Georgia; the Augusta Ballet, an "Honor Company" nationally known for the high quality of its performances; the Augusta Players; the Augusta Children's Theatre; the Augusta Symphony; and the Augusta Art Association. The School of Nursing on the Athens campus offers student life in a city that is home to the University of Georgia.

STUDENT SERVICES

MCG's Student Health Services provides primary care for MCG students' medical, dental, and psychological needs. The Minority Academic Advisement Program ensures the recruitment and retention of minority students in schools through the University System of Georgia. The School of Nursing houses the

Learning Resources Center, where students learn psychomotor skills needed to practice nursing. Students also have access to computers, audiovisual materials, nursing journals, and classroom materials.

THE NURSING STUDENT GROUP

Student life at the Medical College of Georgia offers many learning experiences in a variety of settings. There are approximately 200 undergraduate students and 100 graduate students in Augusta and approximately 100 undergraduate students in Athens. The distance learning site in Barnesville houses approximately 20 RN students. Many student organizations are available to enhance the student's career, including the Georgia Association of Nursing Students (GANS); the IMHOTEP-Leadership Honor Society; MCG Student Government Association; Sigma Theta Tau, Beta Omicron Chapter; and Phi Chi Beta of Chi Eta Phi Sorority. The Augusta and Athens chapters of GANS are active on local, state, and national levels. Several students have held national office. More than 90 percent of the graduating class of 1996 were offered employment opportunities at hospitals, outpatient clinics, nursing homes, day-care centers, and physicians' offices immediately upon graduating.

COSTS

Full-time tuition for 1996–97 was $3064 for in-state students, $7545 for out-of-state. Part-time tuition costs ranged from $59 per credit hour to $203 per credit hour. Room and board costs were $1305 to $2169, and activity fee charges were $15 to $83. Students should plan on an additional expenditure of approximately $700 for books, uniforms, equipment, and transportation.

FINANCIAL AID

For a copy of the *Student Financial Aid Bulletin,* students should contact the Financial Aid Office. A limited number of part-time employment opportunities are available through the MCG Personnel Office.

APPLYING

Admission to the Medical College of Georgia School of Nursing is based on high school graduation or its equivalent; scores on the Scholastic Assessment Test (SAT I) or American College Testing's ACT exam; cumulative GPA, with some preference given for outstanding grades in courses supporting nursing; completion of all prerequisite course work; and references. Preference is given to Georgia residents.

Correspondence and Information:

Office of Academic Admissions
AA-170 Kelly Building School of Nursing
Medical College of Georgia
Augusta, Georgia 30912
Telephone: 706-721-2725
Fax: 706-721-0186

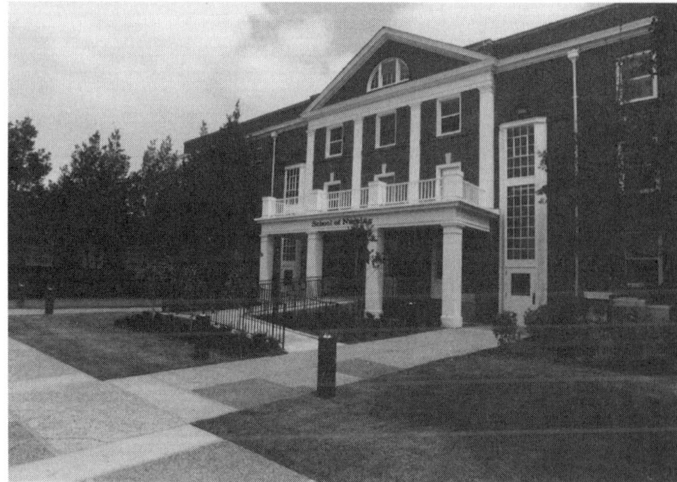

The School of Nursing was founded in 1943 and serves as the University System of Georgia's flagship nursing school, meeting the challenges of an evolving health-care system.

Mennonite College of Nursing

Bloomington, Illinois

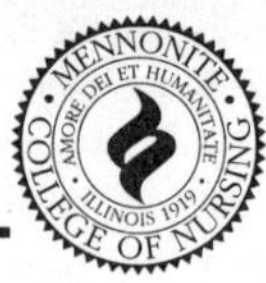

THE COLLEGE OF NURSING

Mennonite College of Nursing was established in 1982 in response to the National Commission on Nursing's 1980 challenge to educational institutions, encouraging them to preserve existing resources and form new high-quality educational programs to meet the needs of a changing society. The College is fully accredited by the North Central Association of Colleges and Schools and by the National League for Nursing.

The College of Nursing is affiliated with BroMenn Healthcare, the multifaceted health-care system formed by the consolidation of Brokaw Health Care Inc. and the Mennonite Hospital Association in 1984.

Chartered in the state of Illinois as an independent, upper-division institution of higher learning, Mennonite College of Nursing provides courses and clinical education for the major in nursing beginning in the junior year for students who transfer from other accredited colleges and universities. The program of study at Mennonite builds upon the liberal arts foundation and prescribed study the students obtain at other institutions.

In the fall of 1995, the first students enrolled in the family nurse practitioner Master of Science in Nursing program. This master's degree program is approved by the Illinois Board of Higher Education and by the Commission on Institutions of Higher Education, North Central Association of Colleges and Schools.

The College maintains cooperative agreements with nine regional postsecondary institutions including Eureka College, Greenville College, Heartland Community College, Illinois College, Illinois State University, Illinois Valley Community College, Lincoln College, Monmouth College, and Springfield College in Illinois.

A small, private institution, Mennonite College made nursing history in 1987 when it became the first independent college of nursing in the United States to be accredited by the National League for Nursing.

PROGRAMS OF STUDY

Mennonite College of Nursing offers the Bachelor of Science in Nursing (B.S.N.) degree for prelicensure nursing students. An RN/B.S.N. track is available to registered nurses who have graduated from an associate degree or diploma program.

The lower-division curriculum consists of required courses that have been specifically selected by the faculty because of their relevance to the upper-division nursing major. The electives enable students to choose subject areas of personal interest to enhance their educational development. A total of 60 semester hours of lower-division courses are required. Academic advisement, including printed transferable course listings, is available to assist students in selecting courses for transfer.

The faculty of the College of Nursing provides an upper-division curriculum that responds to both the nursing needs of society and the learning needs of students. Students are responsible for becoming active participants in the identification of learning needs and in the implementation and evaluation of learning activities. Students also have frequent contact with the faculty members on an individual basis as well as in group settings.

The nursing curriculum extends over a period of four semesters, with an equal number of students admitted in the fall and spring semester. Each semester of the academic year provides for the practice of skills and the application of knowledge through a variety of classroom and laboratory experiences. The curriculum is based upon eight key concepts essential to the practice of nursing: humankind, environment, research, legal/ethical/political dimensions, information processing, teaching-learning, health promotion, and management. These key concepts are organized within four terminal outcome abilities, including caring, critical thinking, communication, and professional practice.

The summer school option is available to all students. A limited number of required and elective courses is offered each summer in order to meet a variety of educational needs. Independent study options are also available, including individual study, clinical experiences, or international transcultural placement.

The Transcultural Nursing Program provides an avenue for personal and professional growth beyond the traditional boundaries of the classroom and clinical practicum. Students are given the opportunity to examine nursing care in a location culturally different from central Illinois.

Students may register for elective credit during summer session in any of the three transcultural nursing study options: N404 Independent Study, N405 International Nursing Study, and N406 Field Nursing Study. Both national and international sites are available for N404 Independent Study, including the Appalachian Regional Hospital System, Harlan and Hazard, Kentucky; Lame Deer Indian Reservation, Lame Deer, Montana; Hospital Albert Schweitzer, Haiti; Kent and Sussex Institute of Nursing, Eastbourne, England; and Red Cross Hospital, Asahikawa, Japan. N405 International Nursing Study provides a tour that includes a survey of health-care systems in several countries.

Mennonite College also offers a family nurse practitioner master's degree. This Master of Science in Nursing degree is designed to prepare nurses to function in advanced practice roles. The program builds on the generalist base of a baccalaureate program, which focuses on nursing practice with individuals, groups, and community systems. Graduates of this program will demonstrate advanced knowledge and skills in an area of nursing practice, excellence in nursing practice by utilizing the processes of scientific inquiry, a commitment to compassionate professional caring through collaborative endeavors with clients and other health-care providers, and the ability to communicate at a level appropriate for public speaking and professional writing. They will also learn to critically evaluate theories and models from nursing and related disciplines for application to nursing practice, provide leadership that reflects an understanding of the health-care delivery system, and respond to the social, economic, political, ethical, and professional issues affecting nursing practice.

The core courses provide foundational knowledge for progression in the program. Support and specialty courses prepare the graduate to function as a family nurse practitioner (FNP). The program features clinical practice in which students are precepted by nurse practitioners or primary-care physicians. Approximately 700 hours of advanced-practice clinical experience are required.

Course 604 Scholarly Project: Advanced Nursing Practice focuses on the conduct of research in an area of interest to the individual student. The course prepares the student to disseminate findings through presentation or publication. The degree requires 43 semester hours of credit distributed among core, support, and nursing specialty courses.

AFFILIATIONS WITH HEALTH-CARE FACILITIES
Throughout the undergraduate curriculum students have the opportunity to work with clients in acute-care and community settings, caring for people of all ages and of all degrees of wellness, from the healthy newborn to the frail elderly. Mennonite's association with over forty clinical agencies, ranging from acute-care hospitals to community health facilities, provides students with a great variety of clinical experiences.

ACADEMIC FACILITIES
Newly remodeled educational facilities include the expanded College library, which has 7,161 holdings, a software collection of 1,751 pieces, and 525 journals. The library currently subscribes to 489 periodicals and houses the computer laboratory and career center. The facilities also include spacious open classrooms and a large nursing laboratory with eight simulated patient-care units. A variety of other resources are available to meet student needs, including a student center with a vending area for relaxing and socializing, a chapel for quiet meditation and reflection, and a fitness room. Administrative and faculty offices are located in Troyer Hall, which also houses conference and reception areas and the residence facility.

LOCATION
Bloomington-Normal, near the geographic and transportation center of the state of Illinois, is located at the crossroads of I-55, I-74, I-39, and Illinois 9, approximately 130 miles from Chicago and 160 miles from St. Louis. Bloomington-Normal, with a population of over 91,000, is easily accessible by all forms of transportation.

STUDENT SERVICES
To facilitate student life, the College provides a broad spectrum of student services, which includes student activities, counseling services, academic advisement, a health-care program, a peer support program, preview and orientation days, registration activities, career development and placement, financial aid, residence housing, and food services. All services support and enrich student life and educational development. Graduate students are invited to participate in student activities of their choosing. In addition, group activities for graduate students are developed to meet the needs and interests of these students.

Being a student at Mennonite College of Nursing means accepting new challenges, expanding awareness of individual potential, utilizing opportunities for involvement in student organizations, forming new relationships, strengthening personal development, and making decisions about future directions.

THE NURSING STUDENT GROUP
Each year, 80 junior students and 10 registered nurse students enroll. Total enrollment in 1996–97 was 241. The average age of enrolled students is 24. The age range is 20 to 50 years. About 14 percent of the students are men. Most students come from within the state of Illinois. In the fall of 1996, thirty-four graduate students were enrolled. Fifteen percent of these students were enrolled full-time.

COSTS
Tuition costs for the 1996–97 academic year were $8834. The room rate was $2046 and the meal plan was $510. The cost of books and supplies was $648, personal expenses ranged from $766 to $1306, and transportation ranged from $555 to $1296. Graduate program tuition was $405 per semester hour.

FINANCIAL AID
A broad program of financial aid enables qualified applicants to obtain a Bachelor of Science in Nursing degree in an educational institution committed to excellence. Funds from federal, state, and private sources are administered and coordinated by the Department of Admissions and Financial Aid. Approximately 85 percent of Mennonite's students receive some form of financial assistance in the form of scholarships, loans, work-study employment, or reimbursement from hospitals and other health-care agencies. A Presidential Scholarship is awarded to an entering junior based on demonstrated academic excellence and leadership qualities or service activities. The benefits of the Presidential Scholarship include full tuition payment for each academic year, providing the student maintains a minimum cumulative GPA of 3.5 while enrolled full-time. Academic scholarships are awarded to entering juniors based on demonstrated academic excellence as indicated by a lower-division GPA of at least 3.5 while enrolled full-time at Mennonite College of Nursing. Other scholarships are awarded on the basis of GPA and financial need.

Financial aid for graduate students is available through employee benefit programs, scholarships, and loans. Federal nurse traineeship funding is available.

APPLYING
Application to the undergraduate program at Mennonite College of Nursing can be made at any time while completing 30 semester hours of the required 60 semester hours of lower-division requirements. Application to the graduate program is on a competitive basis. The application deadline for fall 1998 is February 1.

Correspondence and Information:

Mary Ann Watkins
Director of Admissions and Financial Aid
Mennonite College of Nursing
804 North East Street
Bloomington, Illinois 61701-3078
Telephone: 309-829-0718
Fax: 309-829-0765

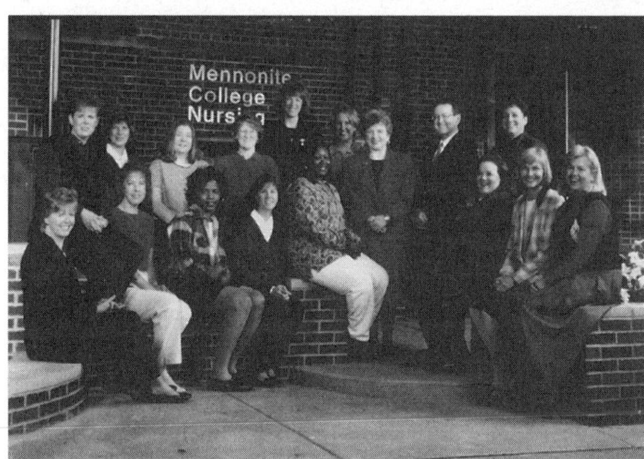

The above photo includes a representative group of the College community, including the President, Academic Dean, staff and faculty, student leaders, and both undergraduate and graduate nursing students.

Mercy College
Department of Nursing
Dobbs Ferry, New York

THE COLLEGE

Mercy College is a private, independent, nonsectarian institution with 156 full-time faculty members and more than 6,000 students. The student-faculty ratio is 17:1. It is a comprehensive college offering curricula in the liberal arts and sciences and in preprofessional and professional fields and granting both undergraduate and graduate degrees. The guiding principles of the College are service to the community through the education of both traditional and nontraditional students, reliance on the liberal arts and sciences as the foundation of education, and dedication to teaching and the advancement of knowledge. Mercy attracts students from Westchester County and the New York/New Jersey/Connecticut metropolitan area as well as throughout the United States and from more than 100 other countires. A 150-room residence hall is located at the main campus in Dobbs Ferry. The Department of Nursing initiated graduate study at the College in 1982. Most recently, graduate programs in physical and occupational therapy and acupuncture and Oriental medicine have been approved.

THE DEPARTMENT OF NURSING

The Department of Nursing offers an upper-division Bachelor of Science program for registered nurses with diploma or associate degree education and a Master of Science degree program in family health nursing. Founded in 1977, the baccalaureate program is designed to advance the education of registered nurses in order to prepare each to be a professional practitioner who is a generalist and who is accountable for the nursing process that promotes and/or restores the health of individuals, families, small groups, and communities. The program also prepares students to collaborate in leadership roles within the changing health-care delivery system, to participate in the inquiry process in nursing, and to pursue graduate study in nursing. Graduate education is built on professionally accredited baccalaureate nursing preparation. The graduate program is organized around the concept of the family as client.

Eighty percent of the Department's full-time faculty members are doctorally prepared. Adjunct faculty members hold at least a master's degree in a clinical specialty area. The program is located in Westchester County in the greater New York City metropolitan area; thus, there is immediate access to outstanding health-care delivery systems. Populations to be served are richly diverse.

Both the B.S. and M.S. programs are accredited by the National League for Nursing.

PROGRAMS OF STUDY

The B.S. program in nursing is designed for RN students, all adults who are returning to school for further professional career preparation. This program has been designed for full- or part-time students. A student may enroll for 2–16 credits per semester. Courses are scheduled for a combination of evenings, days, and weekends. A variety of schedule patterns and teaching-learning methods are utilized.

The undergraduate curriculum is organized around the application of professional nursing process with individuals, families, and communities. Emphasis is placed upon accountability for cognitive and interpersonal nursing process, including research and leadership in the roles of advocate, change agent, and contributor to the profession within the health-care delivery system.

The M.S. program in family health nursing, offered only on a part-time basis, permits registered nurses to continue their professional practice while they seek their second professional degrees. This program prepares advanced clinicians who understand the reciprocal interaction between the health of the family and its members. Graduates of the M.S. program are prepared to work from a family systems perspective in primary, secondary, and tertiary health-care settings. Students are also prepared for the educational and administrative responsibilities inherent in the advanced practice of professional nursing.

In addition to the required course work in the graduate program, students must complete a comprehensive requirement. With the guidance and support of the graduate faculty, students complete either a clinical, educational, administrative, or research project to meet this comprehensive requirement.

AFFILIATIONS WITH HEALTH-CARE FACILITIES

The Department of Nursing is affiliated with a large variety of clinical learning settings. These settings include community and tertiary-care hospitals, long-term-care facilities, public and private community health agencies, senior citizen programs, schools, nursery schools, Head Start programs, day care programs, correctional facilities, and hospice programs.

ACADEMIC FACILITIES

The Department of Nursing is located on the College's main campus at Dobbs Ferry. This campus has five modern, fully equipped air-conditioned buildings housing thirty-eight classrooms, nine science laboratories, a language laboratory, administrative offices, a library, a gymnasium, student activities offices, and a dining hall. Located in the Graduate Center, the Department of Nursing has a nursing lab and a graduate research and resources center. The center provides the faculty and students with computers and software packages for the conduct of their research.

The library provides learning resources to support the College's educational programs. It houses over 293,000 volumes, 1,332 periodicals, a broad range of audiovisual materials, and computer hardware and software. The library's on-line catalog system, MPALS, reflects the holdings of many other academic libraries in the area as well as its own collection. Unlimited searching on several other databases is also offered through MPALS at no cost.

Mercy College installed a powerful new IBM system for academic and administrative computing in 1992. This system runs under the Virtual Machine Enterprise System, which allows students and faculty to use multiple operating systems. Currently, Mercy College is the only college in Westchester offering this advanced system to its faculty and students. Complementing the mainframe facilities, more than 500 microcomputers are distributed throughout Mercy College.

LOCATION

The College's main campus in Dobbs Ferry, where the Department of Nursing is located, overlooks the Hudson River. The village of Dobbs Ferry is located in Westchester County just north of New York City; thus, many business, recreational, and cultural activities of the greater metropolitan area are easily accessible for the College community. The College is accessible by bus, train, or car from Westchester, Rockland, Putnam, Orange, and Dutchess counties, New York City, northern New Jersey, Long Island, and southern Connecticut. Ample parking is available.

STUDENT SERVICES

Students in the nursing programs have full access to many services, including admissions, academic advising, personal counseling, career planning and placement, and many student activities. A health-care service is available. In addition to health care, this service provides the RN students a work-study opportunity. Bookstore and dining services are also available.

Graduates remain engaged with the nursing department through alumni activities and Sigma Theta Tau (the international honor society in nursing) chapter activities.

THE NURSING STUDENT GROUP

Since all of the undergraduate and graduate students are RNs and the majority are practicing full-time, living off campus, serving multiple roles, and meeting several responsibilities, they primarily use the campus facilities and services that are directly associated with their educational programs.

COSTS

Tuition for the undergraduate program for 1996–97 was $285 per credit. Graduate tuition was $350 per credit. There is a $10 parking fee. Full-time students should anticipate other costs such as books (approximately $400 per year) and transportation (approximately $700 per year).

The College permits RNs who have guaranteed reimbursement for their education from their employers to defer tuition (up to the amount reimbursable) until they are compensated.

FINANCIAL AID

Both baccalaureate and master's students have opportunities to apply for a variety of scholarships as well as New York State and federal financial aid programs. The primary purpose of this assistance is to help all eligible matriculated students who would otherwise find it difficult to meet their educational expenses. Financial need is measured by a comprehensive financial statement, the Free Application for Federal Student Aid (FAFSA). Work-study opportunities are also available to RNs in the Health Service. The undergraduate and graduate alumni groups provide scholarships in nursing annually.

APPLYING

Applicants for the B.S. and M.S. programs in nursing must file an application for admission with a $35 application fee, submit official transcripts from all postsecondary educational programs, and provide evidence of licensure as registered nurses.

To matriculate in the B.S. program, a student must be a graduate of a diploma or associate degree program in nursing, have a minimum academic grade point average of 2.5 in both nursing and overall courses, and be licensed to practice as a registered nurse.

Students matriculating in the M.S. program must have a baccalaureate degree with a nursing major from an NLN-accredited program; current RN registration; qualifying scores on either the Miller Analogies Test or the Graduate Record Examinations General Test; a minimum overall and nursing grade point average of 3.0 (on a 4.0 scale) for the undergraduate program; two letters of reference, giving evidence of academic and professional qualifications for graduate study; a year of professional practice; a personal interview; and undergraduate preparation in physical assessment.

Correspondence and Information:

Joy Colelli
Dean for Admissions
Mercy College
555 Broadway
Dobbs Ferry, New York 10522
Telephone: 914-693-7600

THE FACULTY

J. Mae Pepper, Professor and Chairperson; M.A., Ph.D., NYU; RN.

Carolyn Lansberry, Professor and Director of Graduate Program; M.A., Ph.D., NYU; RN.

Alayne Fitzpatrick, Associate Professor; M.S.N., CUNY, Hunter; Ed.D., Columbia; RN.

Honore Fontes, Professor; M.A., Ph.D., NYU; RN.

Mary McGuinness, Assistant Professor; M.S.N., Pennsylvania; RN.

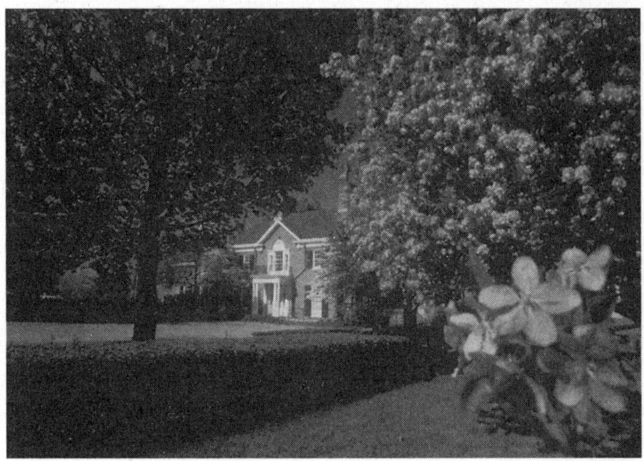

Verrazzano Hall on the Mercy College campus.

New York University
Division of Nursing
New York, New York

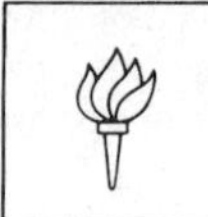

THE UNIVERSITY

New York University (NYU), the largest private university in the country, was founded in 1831. NYU draws top students from every state and from more than 120 countries. The distinguished academic atmosphere attracts a world-famous faculty, and the faculty and the atmosphere together attract students capable of benefiting from both.

The University comprises thirteen schools. As students in NYU's School of Education, nursing students have all the advantages and resources found only at a major research university, yet are part of a small college community that shares a commitment to the health and welfare of humanity. Exchanging ideas with scholars in health, education, and the arts assists growth as professionals and as people.

THE DIVISION OF NURSING

In the late 1940s, Dr. Martha E. Rogers developed nursing's first theoretical model to focus on holistic human beings. Under her leadership, NYU's nursing programs set new standards, and NYU became one of the first universities to treat nursing as a science with a distinct body of knowledge developed through research. Excellence has placed New York University's Division of Nursing among the nation's top nursing programs. The intellectual energies of the faculty and students, the quality of the academic resources, and the rich interaction with a vibrant city provide a learning experience that is unique in its rigor and diversity. All programs—baccalaureate, master's, and doctorate—provide a dynamic balance between nursing theory and practice. These programs prepare graduates for leadership roles in direct care, administration, research, or teaching. They reflect the latest advances in knowledge and technology as well as today's modern health-care environment.

All of the Division's full-time, tenure-track faculty members are doctorally prepared. Part-time faculty members hold at least a master's degree in their clinical specialty area. Faculty members encourage—and expect—students to contribute their own ideas, experience, and research to the learning process. When students graduate, in addition to a wealth of knowledge and skills, they take with them the ability to think analytically—the hallmark of a successful nursing career.

NYU Division of Nursing alumni are in positions of leadership throughout the world, where they practice in diverse clinical, academic, and administrative settings. Many are making their mark through nursing science research. Others have forged new roles as entrepreneurs in private practice or as consultants to health insurers, pharmaceutical companies, and international health organizations.

PROGRAMS OF STUDY

The NYU Division of Nursing offers a four-year, generic B.S. program, which includes a special sequence of courses for registered nurses; a B.S. for college graduates; an M.A. in teaching; an M.A. in delivery of nursing services; an M.A. in advanced practice nursing of adults, the elderly, infants, children, and adolescents or mental health nursing; an M.A. in nurse midwifery; a joint-degree program with the Wagner School of Public Service (M.A. in nursing/M.S. in management); and a Ph.D. in research and theory development in nursing science. The Division of Nursing also offers five post-master's certificate programs in advanced nursing practice: the adult; the elderly; infants, children, and adolescents/pediatric nurse practitioner; mental health nursing; and nurse midwifery.

The B.S. program in nursing prepares students to manage the full scope of nursing care responsibilities in today's complex health-care environment. The innovative nursing science curricula of the Division emphasize a humanistic approach that examines the social, emotional, and environmental context in which wellness and illness occur. Students examine the growth and development of the family structure, patterns of development that characterize different age groups, human behavior in health and illness, and the effects of chronic illness. In the classroom, students learn theories of observation, nursing diagnosis, treatment, and intervention. Students apply these theories in practice through laboratory and clinical study. Students gain experience in all clinical areas, including maternal-child health, adult medical-surgical nursing, community/psychiatric nursing, geriatric nursing, and nursing leadership. Students work with all ages and cultures in a range of settings.

The M.A. programs in advanced education in nursing science prepare students for leadership roles in supervision and management, teaching, and advanced nursing practice. They are unique programs based on the Science of Unitary Human Beings and subscribe to a philosophy and vision of nursing reflecting a commitment to human values and the advancement of nursing as a profession. The programs emphasize critical thinking, the development and use of a theoretical base for advanced practice, the application of systematic methods of inquiry to further nursing practice knowledge, and the promotion of a professional identity. The 45- to 48-point curricula include a core in nursing theory, clinical advanced practice core, an area of concentration, and related cognates and electives. Graduates of the clinical programs are eligible to sit for ANA certification as Nurse Practitioners and/or Clinical Nurse Specialists or are eligible for American College of Nurse-Midwives certification and licensure as a professional midwife in New York State. All advanced practice nursing programs are registered by the state of New York as nurse practitioner programs. The Post-M.A. Advanced Certificate Programs require 27–30 credits.

The Ph.D. program in research and theory development in nursing science prepares nurses for research basic to clinical practice, nursing education, nursing service, and administration. The required course work (approximately 54 points) is taken within the School of Education and in other schools of the University. The curriculum is designed to provide a solid foundation in quantitative and qualitative research methods, theory development in nursing science, methodological approaches to data management, and other aspects of doctoral education.

AFFILIATIONS WITH HEALTH-CARE FACILITIES

The Division of Nursing offers clinical and practicum experience at several of the nation's foremost hospitals, including NYU Medical Center, Bellevue Hospital Center, Mt. Sinai Medical Center, St. Vincent's Hospital, Beth Israel Medical Center, and more than 50 other acute-care hospitals. Students also gain significant experience in community settings, including Visiting Nurse Service, the Midtown Community Court, the Division's school-based health clinics, and other ambulatory and home care settings.

ACADEMIC FACILITIES

NYU's Bobst Library, one of the largest open-stack research libraries in the world, has 38 miles of open stacks housing some 2 million volumes. Bobst is one of seven NYU libraries, including the Medical Center Library, to which nursing students have access. The Division of Nursing provides a Learning Resource Center, which enables students to practice their nursing skills in a simulated hospital setting. The Division also makes use of the latest computer technology, with an interactive computer station located in the Avery Fisher Media Center.

LOCATION

NYU is located in historic Greenwich Village, traditionally a community of artists and intellectuals. NYU's campus is within minutes of off-Broadway drama and dance, Little Italy, Chinatown, and world-renowned museums and libraries. Intellectual stimulation abounds. As an international center of finance, culture, and communications, New York City offers unmatched educational, internship, and social opportunities.

STUDENT SERVICES

The University offers students a variety of services and resources, including the Office of Counseling and Student Services, the Office for African-American Student Services, the University Health Service, the Office of Career Services, the Jerome S. Coles Sports and Recreation Center, the bookstore, mail services, the Academic Computing Facility, the Henry and Lucy Moses Center for Students with Disabilities, and the Loeb Student Center.

THE NURSING STUDENT GROUP

The student body represents most of the fifty states as well as many other countries. This diversification affords opportunities for rich and lasting relationships. The average student is a mature, self-directed individual who assumes both professional and academic responsibilities, often in addition to family commitments.

COSTS

Tuition and fees for 1996–97 were $21,184 (including registration and services fees) for full-time undergraduates or $570 per credit for fewer than 12 credits per term. Graduate students paid $610 per credit.

FINANCIAL AID

Financial aid at NYU comes from many sources. In order to meet an applicant's financial need, the University may offer a package of aid that includes scholarships or grants, loans, or work-study programs. NYU requires the submission of the Free Application for Federal Student Aid (FAFSA).

Nursing students qualify for many Basic Nursing Scholarships, Federal Nursing Student Loans, and a Scholars in Nursing Program available through NYU's School of Education, Phi Theta Kappa Scholarships, and special scholarships for part-time study and for registered nurses who have earned an associate degree. For master's and doctoral candidates, a number of fellowships and assistantships are available. Information on financial aid may be obtained from the Office of Financial Aid by calling 212-998-4444.

APPLYING

As baccalaureate program requirements differ for the generic, RN, and college graduate programs, interested students should contact the Nursing Recruitment Coordinator for specific requirements. For admission to the M.A. program, a candidate must be a graduate of a baccalaureate degree nursing program accredited by the National League for Nursing. A minimum overall GPA of 3.0, RN licensure, two professional letters of reference, a goal statement, and an interview are also required. GRE scores are strongly recommended. TOEFL scores are required for students whose native language is not English. Students who have not met the prerequisites of statistics and nursing research may take them while in the program.

Admission requirements for the post-master's advanced certificate programs are a master's degree in nursing from an NLN-accredited program with a minimum 3.0 GPA. For admission to the Ph.D. program, the applicant must be a nurse with baccalaureate and master's degrees acceptable to NYU, with an upper-division major in nursing. A minimum grade point average of 3.0 on a scale of 4.0 and GRE scores of at least 1000 are required. In addition, the applicant must submit a résumé, demonstration of professional performance/contribution to the nursing profession, two professional reference letters, a three- to five-page goal statement, copies of GRE scores, and transcripts of college-level work. An interview is also required.

Correspondence and Information:

Nursing Recruitment Coordinator
Division of Nursing
School of Education
New York University
50 West Fourth Street, Room 429
New York, New York 10012
Telephone: 212-998-5317

THE FACULTY

Thomas J. Adamski, Clinical Assistant Professor; M.S.N., Hunter; Ed.D., Columbia.
Elizabeth A. Ayello, Clinical Assistant Professor; Ph.D., NYU.
Ellen Baer, Visiting Professor; Ph.D., NYU.
Sonia Baker, Assistant Professor; Ph.D., NYU.
Patricia Burkhardt, Clinical Associate Professor; M.P.H., Dr.P.H., Johns Hopkins.
Cynthia Caroselli, Assistant Professor; Ph.D., NYU.
Barbara Carty, Research Scientist; Ed.D., Columbia.
Terry Fulmer, Professor; Ph.D., Boston College.
Joanne K. Griffin, Associate Professor; Ph.D., NYU.
Judy Haber, Visiting Professor; Ph.D., NYU.
Carol Hoskins, Professor; Ph.D., NYU.
Nancy Jackson, Assistant Clinical Professor; Ed.D., Columbia.
Kathleen Kenney, Research Scientist; M.S.N., SUNY at Stony Brook.
Carl Kirton, Clinical Assistant Professor; M.A., NYU.
Christine Tassone Kovner, Associate Professor; M.S.N., Pennsylvania; Ph.D., NYU.
Phyllis A. Lisanti, Clinical Assistant Professor; M.S.N., Hunter; Ph.D., NYU.
Madeleine Lloyd, Clinical Assistant Professor; M.S., Columbia.
Carla H. Mariano, Associate Professor; M.Ed., Ed.D., Columbia.
Sandra McClowry, Associate Professor; Ph.D., California, San Francisco.
Diane O. McGivern, Professor and Head, Division of Nursing; Ph.D., NYU.
Margaret L. McClure, Clinical Professor; Ed.D., Columbia Teachers College.
Erline P. McGriff, Professor; Ed.D., Columbia.
Mathy Mezey, Independence Foundation Professor of Nursing Education; M.Ed., Ed.D., Columbia.
Madeline A. Naegle, Associate Professor; Ph.D., NYU.
John Phillips, Associate Professor; Ph.D., NYU.
Marianne Roncoli, Clinical Associate Professor; Ph.D., NYU.
Deborah Sherman, Assistant Professor; M.S.N., Pace; Ph.D., NYU.
Margret S. Wolf, Associate Professor; M.Ed., Ed.D., Columbia.
Fay Wright, Associate Research Scientist; M.S., Michigan.

Northeastern University
College of Nursing
Boston, Massachusetts

THE UNIVERSITY

Northeastern University is a private urban university in Boston and a world leader in cooperative education. The University is committed to achieving excellence through high-quality instruction in liberal and professional curricula and providing individuals with opportunities for access to an excellent education. The University has a distinguished, nationally and internationally known faculty who are dedicated teachers, researchers, and scholars.

THE COLLEGE OF NURSING

The primary mission of the College is to prepare nursing leaders for basic and advanced nursing practice that contributes to the health of the nation. The faculty endeavors to achieve this goal by creating a climate of scholarship to maximize the discovery, application, teaching, and integration of knowledge for and with their students, clients, and colleagues.

Northeastern University's College of Nursing was chosen to participate in the community Partnership Project of the W. K. Kellogg Foundation. This initiative refocuses health professionals' education in a multidisciplinary, community-based primary-care mode. The nursing students in the College spend a substantial portion of their clinical time in the neighborhoods of Boston, working and learning with medical students from Boston University.

PROGRAMS OF STUDY

The College offers a five-year cooperative education Bachelor of Science degree program. An RN to B.S.N. track is also available. Transfer students are welcomed, as are students planning a career change who have a degree in another field. A program plan can be developed for some of these students to fulfill degree requirements at an accelerated rate.

The baccalaureate program is designed to prepare students to become professional nurses for practice in a variety of health-care settings, such as communities, hospitals, neighborhood health centers, schools, and homes. In light of the changing health-care scene in the United States, primary care is a key component and focus of the undergraduate nursing education program. Faculty members focus educational efforts on preparing students to learn management of acute and episodic illnesses and complex chronic diseases of clients. Leadership development, case management, discharge planning, and economics of health care are essential components of the curriculum. The College aims to provide all students—including those with diverse backgrounds and changing career goals—with a broadly based education and the stimulus for ongoing personal and professional growth. The curriculum offers instruction in nursing theory and research, the humanities, and the biological, psychological, physical, and social sciences. More than 50 percent of the course work is in sciences and humanities.

The baccalaureate program alternates academic quarters with paid work experience in the student's major field of study. This combination of academic study and co-op assignments produces an overall learning experience that gives greater meaning to the nursing academic program and direction to a student's career choice and development. Working with a Co-op Coordinator, each student develops a plan of co-op experiences that meets individual needs.

Successful completion of the baccalaureate program allows graduates to take the National Council Licensing Examination (NCLEX-RN) to become registered nurses. The program is accredited by the National League for Nursing and approved by the Board of Registration in Nursing of the Commonwealth of Massachusetts.

The Graduate School of Nursing offers a Master of Science degree program that is designed to prepare nurses with a general background for advanced nursing practice as nurse practitioners, clinical specialists, nurse anesthetists, and managers. The master's program includes clinical specializations in administration, anesthesia, community health, critical-care, neonatal-care, primary-care, and psychiatric–mental health nursing. Within the framework of nursing science, the concepts of knowledge, competence, and role provide the foundation for advanced professional practice. The 52-quarter-hour curriculum is designed so that students may pursue either a full-time or part-time program of study. Full-time students may expect to complete the degree requirements in one calendar year. Part-time students may take up to five years to complete the program. Classes are offered in the late afternoon and evening. Some modifications in the curriculum exist to qualify for certification for various specialties. The RN to M.S. degree program is designed for nurses holding a diploma or an associate degree in nursing. This special program offers an innovative pathway to earning a joint B.S.N./M.S. degree. The program requires 85 quarter hours for graduation. The M.S./M.B.A. degree program is an 88 quarter-hour program that prepares nurses for executive-level management in health care.

The Certificate of Advanced Study is a 30-quarter-hour post-master's program. It is designed for nurses with a master's degree in nursing who seek further academic preparation to learn advanced practice skills in another specialization area or to qualify for national certification. Certificates are offered in administration, community health, critical-care, primary-care/nurse practitioner and psychiatric–mental health nursing.

AFFILIATIONS WITH HEALTH-CARE FACILITIES

The University's location in Boston enables the College to collaborate with some of the world's premier health-care organizations. Students have supervised clinical experiences in renowned teaching hospitals and co-op opportunities in a range of acute-care, rehabilitation, and community health facilities. Noted health-care facilities with which the College affiliates include the Massachusetts General Hospital, Brigham and Women's Hospital, Beth Israel Hospital, Boston Medical Center, Dana-Farber Cancer Institute, Children's Hospital, McLean's Hospital, Visiting Nurse Association of Boston, New England Deaconess Hospital, and the New England Medical Center. The College has a partnership with the city of Boston's Commission on Public Health, which oversees all city public health initiatives and its system of neighborhood health centers.

ACADEMIC FACILITIES

Northeastern has several interdisciplinary centers and institutes that engage in research in collaboration with academic departments. The Division of Academic Computing provides students with access to computing resources. A high-speed data network links users and facilities on the central campus and three satellite campuses. In addition, the campus network is connected via the global Internet to computing resources around the world. University libraries contain more than 830,000 volumes, 1.7 million microforms, 150,000 documents, 8,900 serial subscriptions, and 14,000 audio, video, and software titles. A central library contains technologically sophisticated services, including online catalog and circulation systems, a gateway to external networked information resources, and a network of CD-ROM optical disk databases.

LOCATION

Northeastern's 55-acre main Boston campus is in the heart of the Back Bay section of the city, between the Museum of Fine Arts and Symphony Hall and a short walk from Fenway Park. At Northeastern, students discover that part of the adventure of going to college and studying in Boston is exploring the cultural, educational, historical, and recreational offerings of the city. In addition, Cape Cod and the North Shore of Massachusetts are easily reached by car or public transportation for swimming, surfing, and boating. The scenic areas of northern New England are accessible for skiing, hiking, and mountain climbing.

STUDENT SERVICES

The University has many resources and service offices to meet student needs. These include the Lane Health Center, Cabot Physical Education Center, the Marino Recreational Center, campus bookstore, Academic Computing Services, Campus Ministry, housing, dining services, the International Student Office, English Language Center, John D. O'Bryant African-American Institute, and the Counselling and Testing Center. The College of Nursing's Office of Student Affairs offers academic advising and schedules tutorial sessions and other activities.

THE NURSING STUDENT GROUP

There are 880 students in the College of Nursing: 563 undergraduates and 317 graduate students. They represent a wide variety of academic, professional, geographic, and cultural backgrounds. Nursing students include those from Asia, Europe, and Africa as well as students from all across the United States. A significant percentage of the student body are men.

COSTS

In 1996–97, undergraduate tuition was $5015 per quarter for the freshman year, for a total of $15,045 for three quarters. Tuition was $6685 per quarter for upperclass students (after freshman year), for a total of $13,370 for two quarters. The other two quarters of the academic year are scheduled as cooperative education. Costs per quarter hour for freshmen were $418 and for upperclass students were $557. Per-quarter fees included $50 for the use of the student center, a student activity fee of $13.50 per quarter, and a residential activity fee of $15.

Graduate tuition per quarter hour was $390; tuition for full-time students was approximately $14,040. Fees were approximately $506 per academic year, excluding health insurance costs.

On-campus residence room rates for freshman students ranged from $1275 to $1600 per quarter, depending on the number of occupants in a room. A single efficiency apartment was about $2065 per quarter. Per-quarter on-campus residence room rates for upperclass students ranged from $885 for shared living accommodations to $2065 per quarter, depending on the number of occupants. The meal plan prices ranged from $500 to $1240 per quarter, depending upon the number of meals taken per week.

FINANCIAL AID

Approximately 70 percent of all freshmen receive some form of financial aid. Applicants must submit a PROFILE form and a Free Application for Federal Student Aid (FAFSA), available from high school guidance offices, and designate Northeastern as a recipient of the need analysis report. Applicants should file the PROFILE form and the FAFSA by March 1. Northeastern's application for financial aid for return undergraduate and transfer students is due on April 14 to the Financial Aid Office. Further information about financial aid in undergraduate education is available from Northeastern's Office of Financial Aid, 617-373-3190.

Northeastern awards need-based financial aid to graduate students through the Federal Perkins Loan, Federal Work-Study, and Federal Stafford Student Loan programs. The University also offers a limited number of minority fellowships and Martin Luther King, Jr. Scholarships. In addition, the graduate schools offer financial assistance through teaching, research, and administrative assistantship awards that include tuition remission and a stipend of typically about $9000. Funded nurse traineeships are available.

APPLYING

In reviewing undergraduate applications, heavy emphasis is placed on achievement at the secondary school level and on transfer students' college-level performance. Recommendations from high school counselors, official transcripts, and the results of the Scholastic Assessment Test (SAT I) are required for all freshman applicants and for transfer students with less than two years of college work. The application fee is $40 for the undergraduate program. Applications must be submitted before the March 1 priority date.

Applicants to the graduate programs should have an earned baccalaureate degree in nursing from a program accredited by the National League for Nursing. However, the RN to master's degree program allows diploma and A.D. nurses to pursue graduate study. An elementary statistics course is a prerequisite for admission. Additional requirements include a satisfactory scholastic record, an official copy of all college transcripts, satisfactory scores on the General Test of the Graduate Record Examinations, three letters of reference, a personal goal statement, at least one to two years of nursing practice, and current registration to practice nursing in a state or territory. There are some modifications in the requirements for RN-M.S. and international students, including the submission of TOEFL scores by international students whose native language is not English. The application fee is $50 for the graduate programs. Students may be admitted in the fall, winter, spring, or summer quarters, depending on the program of study. However, students interested in full-time study should submit their application by April 1 for admission in the fall quarter.

Correspondence and Information:

Undergraduate Admissions Office
150 Richards Hall
Northeastern University
Boston, Massachusetts 02115-5096
Telephone: 617-373-2200
Fax: 617-373-8780

Graduate School of Nursing
205 Robinson Hall
Northeastern University
Boston, Massachusetts 02115-5096
Telephone: 617-373-3125
Fax: 617-373-8672

THE DEANS

Eileen Zungolo, Dean and Professor; Ed.D., RN.
Carole A. Shea, Associate Dean and Graduate School Director; Ph.D., RN, CS, FAAN.

North Park College
Division of Nursing
Chicago, Illinois

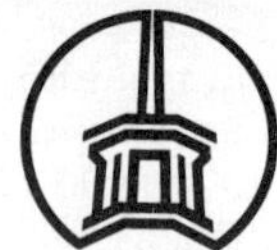

THE COLLEGE

Founded in 1891 by first generation Swedish-Americans, North Park College is a small, private, liberal arts institution affiliated with and supported by the Evangelical Covenant Church. It derives its mission from the traditions of higher education, the tenets of the Christian faith, and the needs of society. The purpose of the College is to provide superior undergraduate and graduate programs in the context of a Christian community to prepare men and women for service in the world. The current undergraduate and graduate enrollment is 1,900 students.

The College comprises five academic units: Social Sciences, Science and Mathematics, Fine Arts, Humanities, and Nursing. Thirty-four undergraduate and seven graduate programs are offered. The denomination also operates North Park Theological Seminary, which offers graduate programs, including the Master of Divinity and Christian Education degree and two doctoral programs.

North Park College is accredited by the North Central Association of Colleges and Schools, with special accreditation by the National League for Nursing (NLN), National Association of Schools of Music, and the state of Illinois for other certification programs.

THE DIVISION OF NURSING

Established in 1964, the Division of Nursing offers a four-year Bachelor of Science degree with a major in nursing. Since 1978, part-time and full-time evening programs for registered nurses seeking a B.S. degree have been offered. The Master of Science degree with a major in nursing was initiated in fall 1993. A post-master's adult nurse practitioner program was initiated in fall 1995.

The Division of Nursing stresses the liberal arts, a vital foundation for professional nursing education. Nursing students are encouraged to develop qualities essential for responsible participation in society and for decision making in the practice of nursing, including critical thinking, synthesis of learning, personal development, and recognition of one's own value system.

The College is affiliated with more than thirty hospital and community-based agencies in metropolitan Chicago, and clinical instruction with direct faculty supervision continues to be a strong component in all nursing courses. All faculty members hold at least a master's degree in their clinical specialty area and teach in that area of specialization. Half of all tenured faculty members are doctorally prepared, and other faculty members are engaged in doctoral study.

PROGRAMS OF STUDY

The Division of Nursing offers a four-year program that leads to a Bachelor of Science degree with a major in nursing. Successful completion of the program qualifies the graduate to apply for the NCLEX-RN, the professional nurse licensing examination.

The purposes of the nursing program at North Park are to prepare a responsible beginning practitioner capable of providing professional nursing care to persons of diverse ages in a variety of settings, foster exploration of a Christian perspective and personal and professional values as they relate to nursing practice, provide the foundation for graduate education in nursing and lifelong personal and professional development, and prepare the graduate to participate in the development of nursing as a profession and in its responses to the changing needs of society, recognizing its past and present roles in the delivery of health care. The curriculum consists of three parts: general education, nursing prerequisites, and courses in the nursing major. The nursing major comprises 49 semester credit hours. The Division offers a part-time or full-time evening program for registered nurses seeking a Bachelor of Science degree. Acceptance into the major is contingent upon successful completion of prerequisite courses with a minimum 2.5 cumulative GPA. Registered nurses must also provide evidence of graduation from an NLN-accredited diploma nursing program or associate degree nursing program and licensure to practice as a registered nurse in the state of Illinois. Credit for upper-division nursing knowledge is awarded after successful completion of specified American College Testing Proficiency Exam Program (ACT PEP) examinations. Registered nurses with diplomas from single-purpose or associate degree programs may enroll in an accelerated registered nurse to Master of Science with a major in nursing track, in which courses may be completed within three years. Many RN degree completion students lack some of the general education requirements; these are offered in the accelerated format (GOAL-Start) and are open to RN degree completion students with the permission of the nursing division. The Bachelor of Science in nursing program for basic and registered nurse students is approved by the Illinois Department of Professional Regulation and is accredited by the NLN.

Designed to prepare graduates for twenty-first-century practice, the Master of Science degree program emphasizes administration, education, and advanced nursing practice. Students are required to have completed introductory courses in college-level mathematics, research, and statistics prior to entrance. Requirements for the M.S. degree include completion of five core courses, two functional role courses in administration or education, two advanced practice courses, and two cognate/elective courses. Each candidate must complete a minimum of 25 semester hours of graduate credit at North Park College with a cumulative GPA of 3.0 or above. No course grade below a C will be counted toward the total for graduation. Courses are offered part-time and full-time on weekday evenings.

North Park also offers M.S./M.B.A. and M.S./M.A.T.S. dual-degree programs and an adult nurse practitioner (ANP) program. The combined M.S./M.B.A. program requires 62 semester hours, and the M.S./M.A.T.S. total is 77 semester hours. The ANP program requirements total 25 semester hours of course work and clinical experiences beyond the master's level. Total practicum hours for the program are 630 (which complies with the American Nurses' Credentialing Center's recommendations for certification). Each semester includes practicum components. Although it is recommended as a full-time course of study, which may be completed in three semesters, the program is also designed to meet the needs of part-time students, who will likely enroll in 3 to 7 semester hours per term and are able to complete the program in five to six semesters. Upon completion of the program, students are eligible to take the American Nurses' Credentialing Center certification examination for adult nurse practitioners.

The Nursing Sweden Exchange Program was established between the Division of Nursing and the College of Health and Care in J"nk"ping, Sweden. Selected nursing students meeting appropriate criteria spend one half to one semester enrolled in required courses for the major, studying and gaining clinical experience in an international health-care system. Participating students may obtain 2 to 4 additional semester credits.

AFFILIATIONS WITH HEALTH-CARE FACILITIES
In addition to the Swedish Covenant Hospital, the Division is affiliated with more than 30 facilities, including Evanston Hospital, Northwestern Memorial Hospital, Children's Memorial Hospital, Lutheran General Hospital, Chicago Board of Health, Korean Self-Help Center, Prentice Women's Center, nursery schools, Chicago-Read Mental Health Center, long-term-care facilities, community clinics, home health agencies, and HMOs.

ACADEMIC FACILITIES
The Division has rich clinical, administrative, and educational resources that enhance all curricular programs. Clinical instruction is enriched by students' experience in the Nursing Learning Resource Center, which includes the Helene Fuld Media Center. Computer and library services support and extend academic instruction.

LOCATION
The College is located in the heart of Chicago, one of the largest and most dynamic cities in the world, providing access to social, cultural, recreational, service, and educational opportunities. The impact of the city on all of North Park's educational programs is significant. Over 300 internship sites have been identified in Chicago for North Park students to test their skills in a faculty-guided vocational experience with such organizations as Hyatt International, the *Journal of the American Medical Association,* and WGN-TV. In addition, certain courses are specifically related to the resources of the city, including certain clinical laboratory courses in nursing and biology.

STUDENT SERVICES
The College has numerous resources and service offices to meet students' needs. These include residence halls and other apartment facilities; a Counseling Center; Student Health Services; Chaplains; a well-equipped Student Center; Campus Bookstore; Academic Advising, which coordinates learning experiences through educational planning and an academic progress review as well as referral for other campus services; Career Planning Services; and International Services.

THE NURSING STUDENT GROUP
Students enrolled in the nursing major are recruited from different cultural and educational backgrounds. They are often older, working parents who may be from disadvantaged, underserved, and/or international backgrounds. Six cultural study centers have been established to foster cultural diversity and enhance recruitment and retention of minority students at North Park. The majority of graduates from the nursing program remain in the Chicago area and find initial employment situations in a health-care agency. However, many graduates practice in other regions of the country and abroad. North Park graduates are aggressively sought after for selected positions nationwide.

COSTS
Tuition for 1996–97 was $495 per semester credit hour on a part-time basis, $6995 per semester full-time for undergraduate programs, $300 per semester hour for RNs in the B.S.N. completion program, and $330 per semester credit hour for graduate courses in the M.S. program. Additional expenses for nursing students in the basic program include uniforms, laboratory fees, yearly health examinations, liability insurance, and travel to clinical sites.

FINANCIAL AID
Financial assistance is available for students who, without aid, would be unable to enroll at the College. The institution seeks to assist students with scholarships, loans, grants, and/or employment through the Placement Office.

APPLYING
Initial application to enroll in the nursing major is made at the end of the first year. Acceptance and advancement in the major are contingent upon academic performance and personal aptitude. Students must have a cumulative grade point average of at least 2.5 and a minimum grade of C in all prerequisite courses in order to enter the nursing major. Transfer students may be accepted into the College at any level prior to the fourth year. Transferring into the nursing major may involve additional course work to comply with North Park College's curriculum. A cumulative GPA of 2.5 or higher is required for all transfer students. Prospective registered nurse students must submit a completed application form, transcripts from all previously attended schools, and scores from the ACT or SAT I, if taken. The nursing office should be contacted to arrange for an interview.

Requirements for admission into the M.S. and ANP programs are a B.S. degree with an upper-division major in nursing from an NLN-accredited program; a minimum grade point average of 3.0 on a 4.0 scale; current licensure in the state of Illinois as a registered nurse; a satisfactory score on the GRE, GMAT, or MAT; a minimum of one year of professional practice; current official record of professional liability insurance; completion of an undergraduate introductory course in nursing research as well as a course in social statistics; a writing sample; three letters of recommendation; and a satisfactory interview. Graduates of nursing schools in other countries must have successfully completed the TOEFL and the Commission on Graduates of Foreign Nursing Schools examinations and be licensed in Illinois. Applications for the M.S. and ANP programs are processed on a continual basis throughout the academic year and the summer term.

Correspondence and Information:

Office of Admissions
Graduate and Special Programs
North Park College
3225 West Foster Avenue
Chicago, Illinois 60625
Telephone: 312-509-5860
800-964-0101 (toll-free)

THE FACULTY

Eugenia Benevich, Assistant Professor; M.S.N., RN. Community health nursing.

Julie Cannon, Associate Professor; M.S., M.S.N., RN. Psychiatric nursing.

Sue Clarren, Visiting Professor; Doctoral candidate, M.S.N., RN. Adult nursing.

Julie Donalek, Visiting Professor; Doctoral candidate, M.S., RN. Psychiatric nursing.

Barbara Coleman, Instructor; M.S.N., RN. Adult nursing.

Linda Duncan, Assistant Professor; N.D., RN. Adult nursing.

Louise Hedstrom, Carlson Professor; D.N.Sc., RN. Maternal-newborn nursing.

Alma J. Labunski, Professor and Chairperson; Ed.D., RN. Adult nursing, aging nursing, graduate nursing.

Elizabeth Ritt, Associate Professor; Ed.D., RN. Adult, graduate nursing.

Virginia Schelbert, Assistant Professor; M.S., RN. Family nursing.

Xavier Smith, Instructor; Doctoral candidate, M.S.N., RN. Adult nursing.

Sandie Soldwisch, Associate Professor; Ph.D., RN. Adult nursing, graduate nursing.

Linda Ungerleider, Assistant Professor; M.S.N., RN. Maternal-child nursing.

Darline Wilke, Professor; Ed.D., RN. Adult nursing.

Janet Nelson Wray, Assistant Professor; Ph.D., RN. RN completion, psychiatric nursing.

Joan Zetterlund, Brandel Professor; Ph.D., RN. Adult nursing, graduate nursing.

Pace University
Lienhard School of Nursing
New York and Westchester, New York

THE UNIVERSITY
Founded in 1906, Pace University is a comprehensive, diversified, coeducational institution with campuses in New York City and Westchester County. Degrees are offered through the Dyson College of Arts and Sciences, the School of Computer Science and Information Systems, the Lubin School of Business, the School of Education, the Lienhard School of Nursing, and the School of Law. Pace University is chartered by the Regents of the State of New York and accredited by the Middle States Association of Colleges and Secondary Schools.

THE SCHOOL OF NURSING
The Lienhard School of Nursing, named for Gustav O. Lienhard, Pace alumnus and honorary trustee of the University, was first established at Pace in 1966 with the introduction of a preprofessional associate degree program at the Pleasantville campus. In 1971, an associate degree program was established at the New York City campus and the undergraduate School of Nursing was founded. Responding to the needs of the registered nurse in the community, the upper-division baccalaureate nursing program was started at the Westchester campus and in 1973 the Graduate School of Nursing, formerly a part of the New York Medical College, became an autonomous school within Pace University. The graduate and undergraduate schools were joined in 1979, forming the Lienhard School of Nursing. The programs of the Lienhard School of Nursing are accredited by the National League for Nursing.

PROGRAMS OF STUDY
The Lienhard School of Nursing offers a four-year Bachelor of Science degree program. This program is designed to prepare students for careers in professional nursing. The graduates are eligible to sit for NCLEX-RN. The Bachelor of Science degree program prepares graduates as generalists in the profession, capable of assuming beginning nursing positions in the community and in all areas of health-care delivery. Nursing courses for this program are offered on the Pleasantville campus in Westchester, although courses from other departments may be taken in Pleasantville or New York City. In addition, a two-year track for RNs with an associate degree or a diploma in nursing that leads to a Bachelor of Science degree is available at both the New York and Pleasantville campuses.

The Department of Graduate Studies offers advanced specialization in nursing. The purpose of the 36-credit master's program (39 credits for family nurse practitioners) is to prepare nurses for clinical specialization in adult nursing, family nurse practitioner, or psychiatric–mental health nursing. The graduate degree program provides students with a foundation for doctoral study in nursing. A combined degree program (B.S.N./M.S.) for college graduates with a baccalaureate degree in an area other than nursing is available at the Pleasantville campus. The Department of Graduate Studies also offers Certificates of Advanced Graduate Study in the clinical majors for nurses with a previous master's in nursing. Additionally, an innovative bridge program for registered nurses with a bachelor's degree in a field other than nursing is available. All clinical specialties are offered at the Pleasantville campus. The family nurse practitioner program is also offered on the New York City campus. Some courses are now available through distance learning.

Designed to prepare students for careers in the health-care system, all the nursing programs combine academic education with supervised clinical experience in hospitals and community agencies. Students are encouraged to take full advantage of the educational opportunities available to them as members of the University community. In addition, the Center for Continuing Education in Nursing and Health Care, with offices in Westchester and Manhattan, is committed to providing a comprehensive, high-quality continuing education program for nurses and other health-care personnel at the local, state, national, and international levels.

Graduate nursing students have the opportunity to complete a master's thesis, a scholarly project, or a research project during their studies at the Lienhard School of Nursing by working on research programs of faculty members and/or researchers in clinical agencies with which the School is affiliated. The students participate in the research by conducting related studies or working directly at the investigator's current stage of research. A contract is negotiated for the activities to be completed during the student's participation.

AFFILIATIONS WITH HEALTH-CARE FACILITIES
Inpatient, outpatient, and community health facilities, including medical teaching centers and community hospitals, are used by the School for clinical experience and fieldwork. Geographically, they include sites in Westchester County, Connecticut, the Bronx, and Manhattan. Master's placements are also available throughout New York, New Jersey, and Connecticut, and are often available in the student's home geographic area.

ACADEMIC FACILITIES
Library facilities are available at the University's New York City, White Plains, and Pleasantville campuses. These provide nursing and medical texts and journals as well as general University holdings. The Center for Nursing Research and Clinical Practice is responsible for facilitating nursing research and clinical practice for the School. Its University Health Care unit, with offices on all campuses, offers high-quality primary health-care services to the University community.

LOCATION
The suburban Westchester campuses are easily accessible by car, bus, and railroad commuter service. They are surrounded by towns and villages that have gifted artisans, musical and theatrical groups, rural museums, retail centers, and corporate headquarters. The New York City campus is located in downtown Manhattan, adjacent to City Hall and close to the historic Wall Street and Battery Park areas.

STUDENT LIFE
Pace offers a wide range of personal and academic support services for its students. Many activities and clubs are also available.

THE NURSING STUDENT GROUP
Students in the entry-level B.S. program are candidates preparing to enter the nursing profession. The RN/B.S. students are practicing RNs seeking baccalaureate degrees. Students in the B.S.N./M.S. Combined Degree Program have diverse educational backgrounds and come from diverse

geographical locations. Students in the master's program are mature, experienced nurses who are seeking advanced knowledge in an area of specialization. Graduates are employed throughout the United States and abroad.

COSTS

Tuition in the Lienhard School of Nursing was $398 per credit for undergraduate courses and $475 per credit for graduate courses in the 1996–97 academic year. Dormitory rooms at the New York City and Westchester campuses of Pace University cost $3900 for the 1996–97 academic year.

FINANCIAL AID

Financial aid includes grants, loans, and scholarships funded by federal, state, and private sources. Undergraduate nursing students may qualify for the following special awards or programs: the Vivian B. Allen Foundation Endowment for Nurse Education Scholarships, the New York State Health Service Corps Scholarship, the Regents Basic Nursing Scholarship, the Regents Professional Opportunity Scholarship, and the Nursing Student Loan. A number of graduate scholarships and assistantships are also available. Grants are made on the basis of outstanding academic performance and demonstrated financial need. Research and administrative assistantships are available for full-time students. Graduate assistants received stipends of up to $5100 in 1996–97 and remission of tuition for up to 24 credits. For further information, students should contact one of the Financial Aid Offices of Pace University. Financial aid applicants should submit the Free Application for Federal Student Aid (FAFSA) to the federal processor by February 8 prior to the following academic year.

APPLYING

Inquiries about admission requirements for undergraduate programs should be directed to the appropriate Office of Undergraduate Admission, listed below. Admission to the B.S.N./M.S. combined degree program requires satisfactory completion of a baccalaureate program at an accredited institution and completion of the GRE General Test or the Miller Analogies Test. Applicants for the master's program must have satisfactorily completed an NLN-approved baccalaureate nursing program and the GRE General Test or the Miller Analogies Test and must have RN licensure. Completion of one year of nursing practice is also recommended. Registered nurses with a bachelor's degree in an area other than nursing are admitted upon satisfactory validation of first-professional-degree knowledge in nursing. Graduate applications should be completed by July 15 (fall), November 15 (spring), and April 15 (summer). Applications for the B.S.N./M.S. degree (June entry) should be submitted to the Office of Graduate Admission by March 1.

Correspondence and Information:

Office of Undergraduate Admission
Pace University
1 Pace Plaza
New York, New York 10038
Telephone: 212-346-1323

Office of Undergraduate Admission
Pace University
861 Bedford Road
Pleasantville, New York 10570
Telephone: 914-773-3746

Office of Graduate Admission
Pace University
1 Pace Plaza
New York, New York 10038
Telephone: 212-346-1531

Office of Graduate Admission
Pace University
1 Martine Avenue
White Plains, New York 10606
Telephone: 914-422-4283

THE FACULTY

Patricia Beaulieu, Assistant Professor (PL); B.S.N., Massachusetts; M.A., Columbia Teachers College.

Patricia Blagman, Associate Professor (PL) and Chairperson, CDP Program; Ed.D., Columbia Teachers College.

Daryle L. Brown, Assistant Professor (PL) and Associate Dean, Department of Undergraduate Studies; Ed.D., Columbia Teachers College.

Susan B. Del Bene, Associate Professor (NY); Ph.D., CUNY Graduate Center.

David Ekstrom, Assistant Professor (PL); Ph.D., NYU.

Harriet R. Feldman, Professor (NY, PL) and Dean; Ph.D., NYU; FAAN.

Frances Fortinash, Assistant Professor (PL); M.S., St. John's (New York); M.S., Pace.

Louise P. Gallagher, Associate Professor (PL); Ed.D., Columbia Teachers College.

Justine Glassman, Assistant Professor (PL); M.S., Yale.

Susan E. Gordon, Professor (NY, PL) and Chairperson, RN/B.S. Program; Ed.D., Columbia Teachers College.

Martha J. Greenberg, Assistant Professor (PL) and Chairperson, B.S. Program; Ph.D., NYU.

Wanda Hiestand, Professor (PL); Ed.D., Columbia Teachers College.

Marilyn Jaffe-Ruiz, Professor and Vice President for Academic Affairs; Ed.D., Columbia Teachers College.

Eileen Karlik, Instructor (PL) and Chairperson, A.D. Program; M.S.N., Adelphi.

Karen Anderson Keith, Assistant Professor (NY, PL) and Chairperson, FNP Program; Ph.D., Adelphi.

Suwersh K. Khanna, Assistant Professor (PL); Ed.D., Columbia Teachers College.

Jeannette A. Landa, Assistant Professor (PL); M.A., NYU.

Sandra Lewenson, Associate Professor (NY, PL); Ed.D., Columbia Teachers College.

Margaret Maher, Assistant Professor (PL); M.S.N., Yale.

Diana J. Mason, Professor (NY, PL) and Associate Dean; Ph.D., NYU.

H. Patricia Neuhs, Professor (NY); Ph.D., NYU.

Jamesetta Newland, Instructor (NY, PL); M.S., Pace.

Mary D. Nurena, Assistant Professor (PL); M.A., NYU.

Alice Irene O'Flynn, Associate Professor (PL) and Chairperson, M.S. Program; M.S.N., Rhode Island; Ph.D., Connecticut.

Ellen Rich, Instructor (NY); M.S., Pace.

Paula F. Scharf, Associate Professor (PL); Ph.D., NYU.

Lillie M. Shortridge-Baggett, Professor (PL) and Director of Center for Nursing Research and Clinical Practice; Ed.D., Columbia Teachers College; FAAN.

Joanne K. Singleton, Assistant Professor (NY); Ph.D., Adelphi.

Barbara Stewart, Professor (PL); Ph.D., NYU.

Shirlee A. Stokes, Professor (PL) and Associate Dean; Ed.D., Columbia Teachers College; FAAN.

Quinnipiac College
Department of Nursing
Hamden, Connecticut

THE COLLEGE

Quinnipiac College, founded in 1929, is an independent coeducational, nonsectarian institution. It is primarily a residential college on an attractive New England campus. Quinnipiac employs a large undergraduate faculty (241 full-time members) relative to the size of its undergraduate student body (3,310), keeping the College-wide student-faculty ratio at 15:1. The full graduate and undergraduate enrollment is 5,200. The College maintains an extensive network of professional associations with the health, business, and education communities through prominent clinical programs and internship placements.

THE DEPARTMENT OF NURSING

From 1970 until 1991, the Department of Nursing had prepared registered nurses with an associate's degree. In 1991, the Associate Degree Program was discontinued, and Quinnipiac began to offer the baccalaureate degree in nursing (B.S.N.). The first class graduated from this program in 1995. The program received full accreditation from the National League for Nursing (NLN) in 1996.

The mission of the Department of Nursing is to provide an academic milieu that fosters intellectual, personal, and professional growth and encourages mutual respect between the teacher and the learner. A humanistic philosophy is the matrix for the teaching and practice of nursing.

The faculty of the Department affirms that professional nursing assists individuals in attaining and maintaining holistic health. Although faculty members see teaching and advising as their main concerns, many are also involved in research. They believe that health occurs on a wellness continuum, is a result of continual person-environment interaction, and is unique to each individual. Each person has the right of access to health care that maximizes his or her potential as an individual, a family member, and a contributing member of a community. Professional nursing may use the political process to influence change in the health-care delivery system and foster support for nursing education, practice, and research.

The nursing curriculum at Quinnipiac seeks to graduate competent, sensitive nursing professionals, willing and able to take on positions of responsibility in the health-care industry. Graduates of the program synthesize theory and nursing practice and build a foundation for graduate study.

PROGRAM OF STUDY

All programs within the School of Health Sciences are based on a comprehensive foundation in the liberal arts and sciences. The Department of Nursing offers the B.S.N. path for basic students and a path within the basic program for registered nurse students. Students may attend on a part-time or full-time basis. Elective courses in gerontologic care and critical care are options in the last semester of the senior year. A state-of-the-art advanced skills laboratory, utilizing resources from other health-related disciplines, is used for teaching advanced skills.

Because nursing demands men and women who can think quickly and act wisely, emphasis is placed on critical thinking based on a broad liberal arts foundation. Nursing students begin with two years of general education courses that prepare them to move ahead in their professional component. Simulated clinical experiences are provided in an on-campus advanced skills laboratory that contains the latest in technologic equipment. A dedicated nursing computer laboratory allows for a multimedia approach to learning. Hands-on learning experiences are carefully selected in the junior year through graduation to support the students' academic and personal growth.

AFFILIATIONS WITH HEALTH-CARE FACILITIES

Classroom and clinical experiences are provided in a wide range of health affiliates. Clinical affiliates exemplify the best in advanced technology and humanistic care. Participating hospitals include Yale–New Haven Hospital, the Hospital of St. Raphael, New Britain General Hospital, Gaylord Hospital, and the Veterans Administration Medical Center. The program offers opportunities in a variety of community-based health services that provide primary care, as well as in more specialized facilities, such as senior centers and homeless shelters.

ACADEMIC FACILITIES

Modern buildings surround 200 acres of rolling fields and streams, adjacent to Sleeping Giant State Park. Library holdings total 304,857 with 4,291 periodicals. The Computer Center holds three laboratory facilities; the main lab is a multipurpose facility on a DEC mainframe. Computer resources include 130 IBM PCs and compatibles, a 15-station teaching lab, and a 20-station IBM PS/2 LAN teaching facility. The Ed McMahon Mass Communications Center features several Macintosh computers linked to scanners and laser printers.

LOCATION

Quinnipiac's campus is located in suburban Hamden, Connecticut, a southern New England town 8 miles from metropolitan New Haven and 25 miles from Hartford. It is easily reached via the Connecticut Turnpike (Interstate 95), Interstate 91, the Wilbur Cross Parkway, and Interstate 84. There are two major airports within 45 minutes of the campus. Area attractions include the Yale Repertory Theater, the Schubert Theatre, the Longwharf Theater, the Peabody Museum, dance clubs, museums, and cinemas.

STUDENT SERVICES

Quinnipiac College has a variety of resources and services to meet the needs of students, including a 28,000-square-foot state-of-the-art recreation and fitness center, the Multicultural Advancement Program, the Learning Center, the International Student Club, and the Counseling and Career Services Center.

THE NURSING STUDENT GROUP

Students in the nursing program come from a wide variety of backgrounds and geographic locations. The majority are resident full-time students. Quinnipiac's low student-faculty ratio of 15:1 ensures that nursing students receive personal attention from their professors. Graduates of the nursing program are employed in large medical centers, community health centers, primary-care facilities, and small community hospitals.

COSTS

Tuition costs for the 1996–97 academic year were $13,440 for 16 credit hours (full-time enrollment). Room and board costs were

$6770 and student fees were $680. Additional expenses include books, lab fees, immunizations, uniforms, malpractice insurance, CPR certification, and travel to and parking at clinical sites.

FINANCIAL AID

Approximately 68 percent of freshmen receive financial aid, with freshman awards averaging $8000 through a combination of grants (which need not be repaid), student loans, and on-campus jobs. The College offers almost 300 merit-based scholarships; the application deadline for these is March 1. Some scholarships recognize diversity or athletic ability. Students should complete and submit Quinnipiac's Financial Aid Form, and the two-part Free Application for Federal Student Aid (FAFSA) to the College Scholarship Service by March 1.

APPLYING

Students may file an application early in their senior year of high school. The results of the SAT I or ACT should be forwarded to Quinnipiac College. The College has a rolling admissions policy. Starting in November, students will be notified about four weeks after the application and required documents are received. Early application is recommended to assure consideration for the program of choice. Freshman students generally have a 2.6 GPA or better average in college-preparatory courses (transfer students have a 3.0 GPA or better), rank in the top 40 percent of their high school class, and have an average combined score of 1050 on the SAT I.

Correspondence and Information:

Joan Isaac Mohr, Vice President and Dean
Carla M. Knowlton, Director
Undergraduate Admissions
Quinnipiac College
275 Mount Carmel Avenue
Hamden, Connecticut 06518
Telephone: 203-281-8600
800-462-1944 (toll-free)
Fax: 203-281-8906

THE FACULTY

E. Jane Bower, Assistant Professor; Ph.D., Adelphi. Maternal and child health nursing.

Joy Ruth Cohen, Assistant Professor; M.S.N., Yale; RN, CNAA, CNM.

Rita Hammer, Associate Professor and Chair, Department of Nursing; Ph.D., Adelphi; Certified Clinical Specialist in Medical/Surgical Nursing. Adult health nursing.

Valerie A. McCarthy, Associate Professor; Ed.D., Massachusetts Amherst; RN, C.

Elizabeth McGann, Assistant Professor of Nursing; M.S.N., CUNY, Hunter. Adult health nursing.

Janice Thompson, Assistant Professor; Ph.D. candidate, Adelphi. Women's health, certified clinical specialist in community health nursing.

Margaret Tufts, Assistant Professor of Nursing; M.S.N., Boston University; Certified Pediatric Nurse. Adult health nursing.

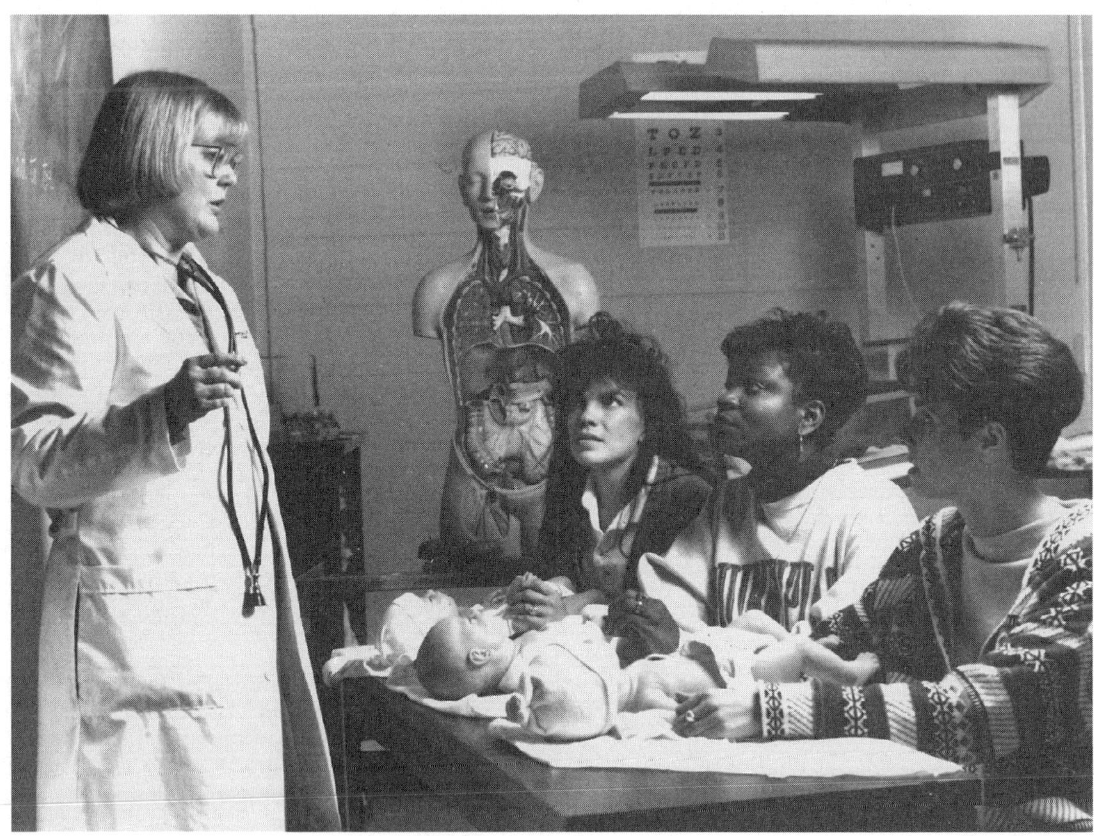

Nursing students utilizing the new critical-care laboratory.

Rivier College
School of Nursing and Health Sciences
Nashua, New Hampshire

THE COLLEGE

Rivier College, a coeducational institution, regards as its mission the education of the whole person. Faithful to the tradition of the Catholic Church and aware of other faiths and philosophies, the College seeks to inspire in its students Judeo-Christian and ethical responsibility in their personal lives and in their careers. As an academic community, Rivier fosters the pursuit of truth by encouraging critical thought and sound judgment and by creating an atmosphere that contributes to the intellectual development of both the faculty and students. Recognizing the value of all branches of knowledge, the College offers a traditional liberal arts curriculum with fields of specialization for undergraduates and advanced professional education on the graduate level.

Rivier College is named in honor of Blessed Anne Marie Rivier, foundress of the Sisters of the Presentation of Mary. Established in 1933, the College was incorporated in 1935 under the laws of the state of New Hampshire and, through two separate charters, was invested with the power to confer both graduate and undergraduate degrees. It is a fully accredited institution that serves its students in four schools; the School of Undergraduate Studies, School of Nursing and Health Sciences, Undergraduate Evening School, and the School of Graduate Studies. Rivier College is a member of the New Hampshire College and University Council (NHCUC), a consortium of institutions of higher learning. Students of member institutions are permitted to register for transfer credit at any of the member colleges. Approximately 2,600 students enroll at Rivier College each semester.

THE SCHOOL OF NURSING AND HEALTH SCIENCES

The School of Nursing and Health Sciences, in accordance with the mission of Rivier College, a Catholic educational institution, regards as its purpose the education of men and women who seek flexibility in the educational process and career mobility in nursing. The School prepares its graduates to care for all persons with respect, valuing their personal worth and dignity. In pursuit of academic excellence, the School bases its curriculum on a strong foundation of sciences and liberal arts, while preparing its graduates for practice at the associate, baccalaureate, and master's degree levels.

The first nursing program at Rivier College, a two-year Associate of Science degree, was started in 1983 as the result of a unique collaborative venture with St. Joseph Hospital. In 1989, a four-year part-time associate degree evening/weekend option was developed. The upper-division baccalaureate program was added in 1987, and the associate, baccalaureate, and master's degree programs are fully accredited by the National League for Nursing.

The graduate program, implemented in 1993, offers a Master of Science degree in primary care in the expanded roles of family nurse practitioner or psychiatric–mental health nurse practitioner.

PROGRAMS OF STUDY

The Associate of Science degree program is designed to prepare graduates to move directly into beginning nursing positions in hospital acute-care facilities, geriatric extended-care facilities, and in other health-care settings. Flexible scheduling is available with courses offered days, evenings, and weekends on a full- or part-time basis.

The program offers several educational options. For individuals seeking an education in technical nursing or choosing to transfer into the program, a two-year daytime curriculum has been established. This curriculum is designed to facilitate mobility opportunities for graduates of approved schools of practical nursing. For these individuals, successful completion of a series of challenge examinations allows entry into the full-time associate degree program with advanced standing. This program is also available in an outreach satellite option in Keene, New Hampshire. The four-year part-time evening/weekend option was established to meet student needs. Advanced placement options are also available on a part-time evening and weekend schedule, providing enrollment is sufficient. Upon completion of the two-year program, graduates are eligible to continue their education in the Rivier College–St. Joseph baccalaureate program or other four-year institutions.

The baccalaureate degree program provides an opportunity for registered nurses who are graduates of diploma or associate degree programs to continue their education in nursing. Students may attend on a full-time basis and complete the program in two years or choose a part-time schedule and have up to six years to complete the program. Day and evening courses are available. Graduates of the baccalaureate program are prepared to function as generalists in structured and unstructured health-care settings and to pursue graduate studies.

The graduate nursing program at Rivier College was developed to prepare registered nurses with baccalaureate degrees in nursing for advanced practice. The program offers both a family nurse practitioner track and a psychiatric–mental health nurse practitioner track. Registered nurses with baccalaureate degrees in fields other than nursing are prepared through specialized course work and achievement on standardized examinations for admission into the master's program. A second purpose of the graduate nursing program is to provide a basis for doctoral study.

The curriculum of the nurse practitioner tracks meet the theoretical and clinical requirements of the state of New Hampshire for the advanced registered nurse practitioner (ARNP) designation. Students may choose a full-time, half-time, or part-time schedule. A full-time study option is completed in two years, a half-time option in three years, and a part-time study option in five years.

AFFILIATIONS WITH HEALTH-CARE FACILITIES

The School of Nursing and Health Sciences is affiliated with a wide variety of clinical facilities, including Massachusetts General Hospital, Brigham and Women's Hospital, Catholic Medical Center, Nashua Memorial Hospital, and St. Joseph Hospital. Because of its focus on health promotion, a variety of community agencies are utilized, including schools, health departments, and community clinics.

ACADEMIC FACILITIES

Learning resources available to students include Regina Library on the Rivier campus; the Health Science Library and the Helene Fuld Media Center, which are located in the Academic Center at St. Joseph Hospital; the Computer Center; and nursing skills simulation labs located on campus.

Regina Library reference and circulating collections, both print and nonprint, are current and adequate to meet the needs of students. Microfilm and microfiche reader/copiers and three coin-operated photocopy machines are available. The library currently subscribes to more than 900 periodicals, including sixty-seven nursing journals.

An integrated library system and a computerized catalog (CD-ROM) provide a database of the library's holdings. Integrated circulation, cataloging, acquisition, and serial modules ensure current information on library holdings and their availability. EBSCO Host gives students access to CINAHL and Healthsource, which contain more than 1,000 nursing and health-related citations.

Access to Internet resources is provided to Rivier College faculty, staff, and students who register for a personal account. Internet pointers provide access to information and are available at the reference desk.

Audiovisual equipment such as televisions, VCRs, video cameras, film and slide projectors, and tape recorders is available through an audiovisual coordinator. Televisions with closed-caption decoders for the hearing impaired are available.

Cooperation between academic institutions enables students to borrow directly from other participating facilities. Through the NHCUC, the library provides access to more than 7 million volumes of print materials and more than 250,000 journals. The New Hampshire State Library offers Article Express, a document delivery service supporting more than 400 titles. In addition, Regina Library is a member of DOCLINE and a user of Carl UnCover document delivery service. These systems provide worldwide access to resources in nursing, medicine, and allied health and to documents of general interest.

The School of Nursing and Health Sciences houses a Helene Fuld learning lab, where audiovisual materials and computerized learning systems are available. Additional facilities include a physical assessment laboratory with examining tables and state-of-the-art equipment and a simulated critical-care unit.

LOCATION

The College is located on a 60-acre campus, 1 mile from downtown Nashua, in a quiet residential area. Easy access to Boston provides students with opportunities for intellectual, cultural, and social enrichment. Proximity to the seacoast and the White Mountains of New Hampshire offers additional recreational advantages. The services of Logan Airport; the airport in Manchester, New Hampshire; and local bus lines allow convenient travel to and from campus.

STUDENT SERVICES

Students are offered a comprehensive guidance program to assist them in academic, personal, and vocational areas. Student services include health services, academic advisement, personal counseling, career development and placement, and services related to spiritual and personal growth.

Students in the School of Nursing and Health Sciences associate degree program are members of the New Hampshire Student Nurses' Association and National Student Nurses Association. Undergraduate students are encouraged to become members of the American Nurses Association.

THE NURSING STUDENT GROUP

There are approximately 600 students enrolled in the School of Nursing and Health Sciences; 3 percent are men and about 3 percent are members of minority groups.

COSTS

In 1996–97, tuition and fees for day programs were $390 per credit (1–11 credits) or $5850 per semester (12–18 credits or a maximum of five courses). Room and board costs were $2625 per semester. For evening programs, tuition was $184 per credit (1–11 credits). A tuition deposit of $25 is required for part-time students, and a deposit of $50 is required for full-time students. A $100 deposit is required to reserve a dorm room.

FINANCIAL AID

The primary purpose of the financial aid program at Rivier College is to provide financial assistance to accepted students who, without aid, would be unable to attend the college. Rivier College uses a uniform method of needs analysis when considering financial aid applicants. When awarding aid, Rivier College places primary emphasis on demonstrated financial need but will also consider the academic standing, character, and future promise of a student.

Financial aid supplements the resources of the student and the student's family. The responsibility for the education of a student rests with the student and the family. Parents are expected to contribute according to their means, taking into account their income, assets, number of dependents, and other relevant information. Students are also expected to contribute from their own assets and earnings, including appropriate borrowing against future earnings.

APPLYING

Applicants for the associate degree program should submit an application form accompanied by a nonrefundable $25 fee; SAT I scores (with a minimum combined score of 800); evidence of rank in graduating high school class; a letter of recommendation from guidance personnel, a teacher, a recent employer, or a member of the health-care profession; evidence of satisfactory completion of high school chemistry and algebra with a grade of 70 percent or higher; a certified high school transcript or GED test scores; official transcripts of any credit earned at institutions of higher education; a statement on the application indicating the applicant's professional goals; and completed health forms. The School's pre–nursing school aptitude examination may be required. International students must also submit TOEFL scores.

Applicants for the baccalaureate program must submit an application with a nonrefundable $25 fee; evidence of completion of an associate degree or hospital-based program in nursing; official transcript(s) of any additional credits earned at institutions of higher learning; and evidence of current RN licensure. Transfer credits for courses with a grade of C or better are accepted for comparable courses at the undergraduate level.

Master's degree program applicants must have a baccalaureate degree from an accredited institution and submit a completed application with a statement of professional goals; two letters of recommendation; official transcripts from an undergraduate program; evidence of RN licensure; satisfactory scores on either the Graduate Record Examinations (GRE) or Miller Analogies Test (MAT); and a nonrefundable $25 fee.

Correspondence and Information:

For graduate program information:
Dr. Joan Lewis
School of Nursing and Health Sciences
Rivier College
420 Main Street
Nashua, New Hampshire 03060-5086

For undergraduate program information:
Maureen Karr
Admissions Office
Rivier College
420 Main Street
Nashua, New Hampshire 03060-5086

Rush University
College of Nursing
Chicago, Illinois

THE UNIVERSITY

Rush University is the academic component of Rush-Presbyterian–St. Luke's Medical Center. Founded in 1972, the University has expanded from one college and fewer than 100 students to four colleges and more than 1,400 students. It includes Rush Medical College, the College of Nursing, the College of Health Sciences, and the Graduate College.

The purpose of Rush University is to educate students as practitioners, scientists, and teachers who will become leaders in advancing health care and to further the advancement of knowledge through research. As a major component of Rush-Presbyterian–St. Luke's Medical Center, the University integrates patient care, education, and research through the practitioner-teacher model. Rush University encourages the growth of its students by committing itself to the pursuit of excellence, to free inquiry, and to the highest intellectual and ethical standards.

THE COLLEGE OF NURSING

The heritage of the College of Nursing dates back to 1885, when the College's first antecedent, St. Luke's Hospital Training School of Nursing, opened to offer diploma education to nurses. In 1903, the Presbyterian Hospital School of Nursing accepted its first students. From 1956 to 1968 nurses were taught at the merged Presbyterian–St. Luke's Hospital School of Nursing. Before the establishment of the College of Nursing in 1972, more than 7,000 nurses had graduated from these three schools. Today, more than 200 baccalaureate, master's, and doctoral nursing students graduate each year.

The mission of the College of Nursing is to set a national standard for excellence in the professional education of nurses, in research programs that contribute to the scientific basis of nursing practice, and in the creation of nursing practice systems that respond to the health needs of society.

Education in the College is facilitated by the unification of the academic and clinical practice components of the health-care system. This unique integration stimulates excellence in education, practice, scholarly activities, and professional leadership by the faculty and the graduates of the College of Nursing.

The faculty of the College of Nursing is currently involved in a variety of funded research studies, including individual and interdisciplinary collaborative projects, that will have an impact on current health practices. Some of the current research areas are: physiological responses in health and illness, behavioral and psychological responses in health and illness, and outcomes of health-care interventions and services.

PROGRAMS OF STUDY

The curriculum allows multiple entry and exit options for students. Previous academic and professional education serves as the foundation for programs of study preparing students for progressive levels of specialization and responsibility as professional nurses. Four exit options are available, depending on the background of the student. They are the Bachelor of Science (B.S.), Master of Science (M.S.), Doctor of Nursing (N.D.), and Doctor of Nursing Science (D.N.Sc.).

Baccalaureate students enter Rush as juniors after completing two years of study at another college or university. The B.S. program is designed to give students a broad perspective on the problems patients face and to establish a foundation for the skills and knowledge needed for a variety of entry-level nursing positions. Six quarters and 90 quarter hours are needed for the baccalaureate degree. Graduates are eligible to take the National Council Licensure Examination (NCLEX). Registered nurses with a diploma or an associate degree may also earn a baccalaureate degree by completing a combination of core and clinical courses and proficiency exams.

The master's degree study option focuses on clinical specialist and nurse practitioner roles with intensive examination of the biological and behavioral sciences and their application within the context of nursing practice, education, and research. Degree requirements include courses in nursing theory, advanced practice role, biostatistics, research, and biological and behavioral sciences. Clinical seminars and practice are required in the area of concentration. Advanced practice options include acute care, adult, anesthesia, cardiopulmonary, critical care, community health, genetic health, gerontology, medical-surgical, neonatal, oncology, pediatric, psychiatric, rehabilitation, transplant, and women's health nursing. A minimum of fifty-five quarter hours of credit is needed for the M.S. degree. Graduates are eligible for certification exams in the various areas of specialization. A dual M.S./M.M. degree is available in conjunction with the Kellogg School of Management at Northwestern University. Post-master's nurse practitioner preparation is available in several areas: acute care, adult, gerontologic, neonatal, and pediatric nursing.

The Doctor of Nursing study option prepares nurses to function as advanced clinical specialists or practitioners, integrating the role of teacher, consultant, and manager of clinical practice. Doctor of Nursing students learn to implement clinical research utilization studies. The same specialty areas available at the master's level are available at the N.D. level. Practitioner preparation in family/community health nursing is available at the N.D. level only. A minimum of 85 postbaccalaureate credits are needed for the N.D. degree.

The Doctor of Nursing Science curriculum prepares expert clinicians with the investigative skills of nurse researchers and the leadership skills necessary to influence health-care systems and develop health policy. Core courses in research, theory, and role development are combined with cognate studies and clinical practica. The clinical practica are tailored to meet the students' learning needs and help them explore their phenomena of interest. The D.N.Sc. degree can be pursued in a summer option. Summer D.N.Sc. students must enroll full-time their first three summers in the College. At least 125 quarter hours of postbaccalaureate graduate study, exclusive of dissertation, are required for the Doctor of Nursing Science degree.

AFFILIATIONS WITH HEALTH-CARE FACILITIES

Rush–Presbyterian–St. Luke's Medical Center is the center of a comprehensive, cooperative health-care system designed to serve some 2 million people through its own resources and in affiliation with other health-care institutions in northern Illinois and Indiana. Today, the Rush System for Health is comprised of ten hospitals, seven occupational health sites, five nursing homes, three outpatient behavioral health sites, and comprehensive home health and hospice programs. Students gain clinical experience at these sites as well as at many other health-care institutions and community agencies throughout the Chicago metropolitan area.

ACADEMIC FACILITIES

The Rush University library has an automated catalog, including MEDLINE, mini-MEDLINE, and a collection of CD-ROM databases. The library has 124,000 bound volumes, with 10 percent in health and 10 percent in nursing. The library subscribes to 2,125 periodicals, 98 percent of which are health-care related. The library also includes the McCormick Learning Resource Center, an audiovisual learning facility that provides media services for faculty and students.

Through Academic Computing Resources (ACR), including the Personal Computer (PC) and Computer-Assisted Instruction (CAI) labs, students have the use of IBM and Macintosh computers and software, including computer-assisted instruction, word processing, spreadsheets, statistics, graphics, and e-mail.

The College of Nursing has a resource laboratory where students learn how to perform nursing skills and procedures. Audiovisual equipment and computers for student use are also available in the resource laboratory.

LOCATION

The main campus of the University/Medical Center is located on the west side of Chicago not far from the Loop, where numerous cultural and recreational opportunities can be found. Rush is in the Medical Center District, which includes the University of Illinois West Campus, Cook County Hospital, Westside Veterans Administration Hospital, and Illinois State Psychiatric Institute. Rush is surrounded by new town homes and condominiums and Taylor Street restaurants and businesses, and offers easy access to public transportation.

STUDENT SERVICES

Rush has a full range of services available to enhance the personal, academic, and professional aspects of student life. University services include the Student Counseling Center, the bookstore, the Laurence Armour Day School, and the offices of international student advising, housing, student financial aid, and student affairs. College support services include new student orientation, faculty advising, and tutoring. A Student Academic Facilitator is available for both graduate and undergraduate students who need academic assistance with course work or to improve their study and learning skills. A Director of Multicultural Affairs works with the College to address issues of cultural diversity, develop recruitment and retention programs, and provide guidance to students and faculty. Recreational facilities at Rush and the University of Illinois are available for students' use.

Students actively participate in College governance by serving on faculty committees. Students also maintain their own organizations and participate in many public service activities, sometimes in collaboration with other University students and outside professional organizations.

THE NURSING STUDENT GROUP

Students in the College are a diverse group in terms of age, ethnic background, and experience. Though most undergraduates study on a full-time basis, a part-time program of study is also available. Most of the graduate students are employed in health-care organizations and attend school on a part-time basis. Enrollment in the College continues to grow. The current enrollment of 650 includes 255 undergraduate and 395 graduate students.

COSTS

Tuition rates for the 1996–97 year were $3860 per quarter or $300 per credit for undergraduate students and $3877 per quarter or $340 per credit for graduate students.

The approximate cost for books at the undergraduate level is $500 per year. The cost for graduate students is approximately $800 per year. Mandatory fees for all students are about $1400 per year.

FINANCIAL AID

Financial aid at Rush is awarded on the basis of demonstrated financial need. Financial aid includes state, federal, institutional, and other funds that may be available. Full- and part-time students may apply for assistance. All seeking aid must complete the Free Application for Federal Student Aid and the College Scholarship Service Financial Aid Form for determination of financial need. Federal Professional Nurse Traineeships and graduate assistantships are available for qualified graduate students. Predoctoral and postdoctoral research fellowships are also available.

APPLYING

Rush is interested in recruiting students from diverse backgrounds who are adult learners. Students should be committed to excellence in the practice of nursing and to lifelong learning as well as dedicated to the concept of working toward improving health promotion and maintenance for all people. B.S. applicants must complete 60 semester or 90 quarter hours at another college or university with a GPA of 2.75 or better to qualify for admission. RN degree-completion students must be licensed prior to matriculation. M.S. applicants must have at least a B.S. with a minimum GPA of 3.0 and acceptable GRE scores. Licensure must be completed prior to matriculation. Post-master's applicants must have a clinical master's degree from an accredited school of nursing. GRE scores are not required. N.D. applicants must have a baccalaureate degree in nursing, a minimum GPA of 3.0, and acceptable GRE scores. Students with a prior master's degree are not required to take the GRE. D.N.Sc. applicants must have a minimum GPA of 3.0 and acceptable GRE scores if post-baccalaureate. Applicants with a master's degree must have a minimum GPA of 3.5, but are not required to take the GRE exam. All degree applicants must submit three references with their applications. M.S. and N.D. applicants have one interview, and D.N.Sc. applicants have two. Applications are accepted every quarter except for B.S. and D.N.Sc. students, who must apply for summer or fall. Some of the nurse practitioner options have pooled review dates (i.e., all applications are reviewed at one time) with specific deadlines for submission of completed applications. Graduate applications should be complete at least six weeks prior to matriculation. Undergraduate applications must be complete by March 1.

All students should contact the College Admission Services Office for complete information about admission requirements and application deadlines.

Correspondence and Information:

Rush University College Admission Services
Schweppe Sprague Hall, Room 119
1743 West Harrison Street
Chicago, Illinois 60612
Telephone: 312-942-7100
Fax: 312-942-2219
World Wide Web: http://www.univ.rush.edu/univ/

Saint Joseph's College
Department of Nursing
Standish, Maine

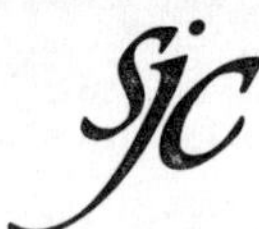

THE COLLEGE

Saint Joseph's College in Maine is a private, Catholic, coeducational liberal arts college founded in 1912 by the Sisters of Mercy. The 1,105 students come from twelve states and three countries. The hallmark of the SJC experience revolves around four principles: small classes, excellent teaching, Catholic values, and a supportive environment. Saint Joe's men and women enjoy a 15:1 student-faculty ratio, with an average class size of only 20. Students enjoy being known by their first names and feel connected with professors, advisers, coaches, and all support staff. The College was recently listed by *Money* magazine as one of the top 100 "best college buys" in the nation.

THE DEPARTMENT OF NURSING

Founded in 1974, the Department of Nursing was established to offer the Bachelor of Science in Nursing degree. Recently, the Department has experienced unprecedented growth and is now the largest academic department at Saint Joseph's College, accounting for 20 percent of full-time enrollment.

The Department's overall goal is to prepare students for a variety of clinical settings as professional nurses or for continuation directly into graduate nursing studies. The ratio of nursing faculty to students is 1:10, with 15 full-time faculty members serving 155 students.

The program is structured as a traditional four-year B.S.N. that emphasizes clinical work as a complement to classroom theory. By the end of the student's four years, he or she will have gained knowledge and experience in nursing concepts and the nursing process to give professional, holistic care to individuals, families, and groups for the purpose of promoting, maintaining, and restoring optimum health. The graduate will also have knowledge and skills in the teaching/learning processes of promoting health; in effective communication; in leadership; in the application of moral, ethical, legal, and Christian humanistic principles; and in the use of published research in planning care for clients.

PROGRAMS OF STUDY

The Department of Nursing offers the Bachelor of Science in Nursing with RN to B.S.N. and LPN to B.S.N. options. The program is fully accredited by the National League for Nursing (NLN).

The Bachelor of Science in Nursing is a traditional four-year program for students without previous nursing experience. Students are accepted into the nursing program in their first year. Courses in nursing and other disciplines are coordinated so students can develop a broad view and understanding of the world and be prepared for professional relationships and service to society. Beginning in the sophomore year, at least 6 hours a week are allocated to clinical studies, with the Roy Model of Nursing and the Nursing Process providing the foundation for all clinical nursing courses.

The RN to B.S.N. and LPN to B.S.N. options are tailored specifically for registered nurses or licensed practical nurses seeking a baccalaureate degree in nursing. In coordination with Distance Education, the RN and LPN to B.S.N. options offer flexibility and accommodate the special needs of adult learners.

AFFILIATIONS WITH HEALTH-CARE FACILITIES

Clinical learning experiences are provided in both large and small hospitals and community health agencies in nearby southern Maine communities. Among the major cooperating agencies are Mercy Hospital; Maine Medical Center; Southern Maine Medical Center; New England Rehab; St. Mary's Hospital; Androscoggin Home Health Care, Inc.; South Portland Health Services; and Community Health and Nursing Services.

Experiences are also provided in day-care centers, nursery and primary schools, and a variety of clinics. These experiences are part of the nursing course work and expose the student to a variety of individuals requiring preventive as well as curative care.

ACADEMIC FACILITIES

The Wellehan Library offers services to students, faculty, alumni, and the neighboring community. It provides a collection of 75,000 print and nonprint materials and more than 400 current periodicals and newspapers. In addition, the library's on-line catalog (WELLCAT) contains title, author, subject heading, and key word access to the library's entire collection. Internet access, including e-mail, is available at several workstations that are located in the library.

The Media Center, a division of the Wellehan Library, provides nonprint services, such as videotapes and audiotapes. Students have access to cassette tape players and recorders; slide, overhead, cassette tape, film loop, and sound film projectors; projection screens; televisions; VCRs; stereos; and Casiotone and Yamaha keyboards.

LOCATION

The 330-acre campus on the shore of Sebago Lake and close to the greater Portland area offers students the advantages of cross-country running, mountain climbing, skiing, and hiking. Favorite haunts include the city of Portland's own symphony orchestra, art museum, theater and dance companies, and athletic teams. Nearby Freeport, Maine, is the home of L.L. Bean, and located 2 hours away is the historic city of Boston. All in all, students have the best of both worlds: a beautiful lakeside campus with easy access to the amenities of southern Maine.

STUDENT SERVICES

The College has many resources to meet student needs. These include the Student Health Service, Bernard P. Currier Gymnasium, Campus Store, Margaret H. Heffernan Center, Campus Ministry, Mercy Hall, housing, dining services, athletic fields, and computer labs. The campus features a small beach by the shore of Sebago Lake.

Nursing majors are encouraged to join the Student Nurses' Association and have the opportunity to become a member of Sigma Theta Tau, the international honor society for nurses. Also available are academic assistance and advising, tutoring, enrollment assistance, and a writing lab equipped with computers and materials.

THE NURSING STUDENT GROUP

There are currently 155 students in the traditional, four-year B.S.N. program and 327 students enrolled in the RN to B.S.N.

and LPN to B.S.N options. In recent years, a majority of students have passed their state boards to become licensed as registered nurses in Maine. Registered nurses have license reciprocity in all fifty states.

COSTS

The College is competitively priced and was recently named one of the top 100 "best college buys" by *Money* magazine. For the 1996–97 year, the comprehensive cost was $16,665. Annual tuition was $10,990 or $190 per credit hour (for part-time students only), fees were $295, and room and board costs were $5380. Students budget between $800 and $1500 for books, travel, and miscellaneous expenses.

FINANCIAL AID

Financial aid is awarded based on demonstrated financial need, scholastic achievement, and other considerations in the form of gift aid (grants and scholarships), employment opportunities, and loans. Students are assisted from the College's own funds and through current federal programs such as the Federal Pell Grant, FSEOG, Federal Work-Study, Federal Perkins Loan, Nursing Student Loan, Federal Stafford Student Loan, Army ROTC, and other loan programs.

APPLYING

Candidates for the B.S.N. degree should have pursued a full college-preparatory high school curriculum including algebra 1 and 2 and geometry as well as lab biology and lab chemistry. Math beyond algebra 2 and a third lab science course are recommended. SAT I or ACT exams are required. Transfer applicants from other colleges are welcome to apply. Early acceptance candidates apply by December 1. A rolling admissions policy is maintained throughout the year, but most students apply before March 1. A counselor recommendation is also required.

Preference is given to students who rank in the top half of their high school class, have SAT I or ACT scores that approximate the national average, and present a solid record of achievement in challenging high school courses. Transfer students must have at least a 2.0 grade point average to be considered.

Correspondence and Information:

Bachelor of Science in Nursing (B.S.N.):
Fredric V. Stone, Director of Admissions
Office of Admissions
Saint Joseph's College
278 White's Bridge Road
Standish, Maine 04084-5263
Telephone: 800-338-7057 Ext. 7746 (toll-free)
RN or LPN to B.S.N. programs:
Dept. 840–Admissions
Saint Joseph's College
278 White's Bridge Road
Standish, Maine 04084-5263
Telephone: 800-752-4723 (toll-free)

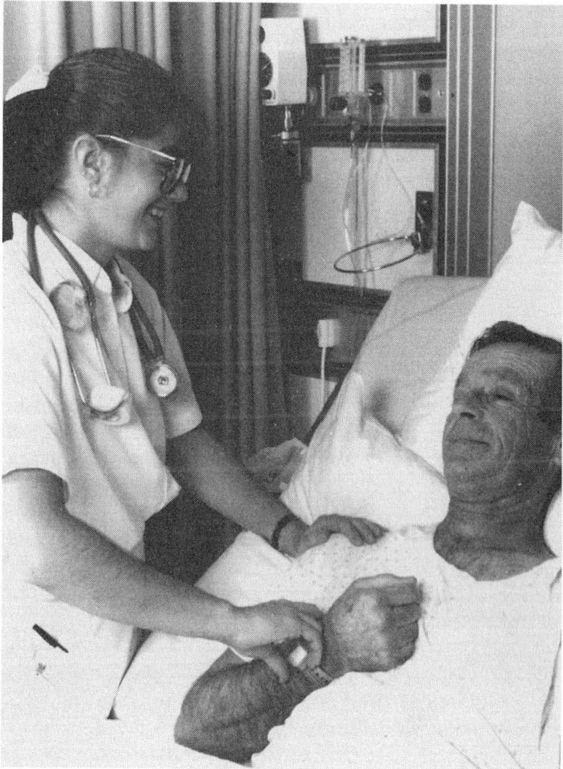

A student nurse attends to one of her patients at Maine Medical Center.

Samuel Merritt College
Intercollegiate Nursing Program
Oakland, California

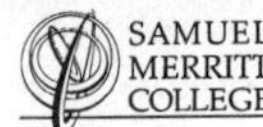

THE COLLEGE

Samuel Merritt College was founded in 1909 as a hospital school of nursing. In 1981, the diploma program was discontinued, and Samuel Merritt College initiated an innovative four-year baccalaureate nursing program with Saint Mary's College of California. The College offers three entry-level graduate degrees—the Master of Occupational Therapy, the Master of Physical Therapy, and the Master of Science in Nursing. Postprofessional degrees include the Master of Science in Nursing, offering programs in certified registered nurse anesthetist and family nurse practitioner, as well as the Master of Science in Physical Therapy.

THE DEPARTMENT OF NURSING

During its seventy years as a school of nursing, Samuel Merritt gained a reputation as a provider of high-quality nursing instruction, graduating over 3,000 well-prepared students. There is an ongoing campus commitment to examine the future of health care, providing programs and courses of study that respond to the educational opportunities tomorrow's professionals will need to meet the industry's constantly changing demands. On both the undergraduate and graduate levels, curricula reflect the need for professionals who are capable of independent and interdisciplinary practice within a variety of health-care settings. The faculty believes that professional nursing practice is characterized by an informed commitment to the uniqueness of the individual, a broad knowledge of the human condition, and the compassionate, skillful, and ethical application of technology.

The College is fully accredited by the Western Association of Schools and Colleges, the Council of Baccalaureate and Higher Degree Programs of the National League for Nursing (M.S.N. program accreditation due to be completed in 1995), and the Council on Accreditation of Nurse Anesthesia Education Programs and is approved by the California Board of Registered Nursing.

PROGRAMS OF STUDY

The Bachelor of Science in Nursing (B.S.N.) degree is a unique, cooperative intercollegiate program that brings together the historical strengths and rich resources of Samuel Merritt College and Saint Mary's College of California. Students are enrolled on both campuses throughout the program. At Saint Mary's the focus is on liberal arts, while at Samuel Merritt the emphasis is on a rigorous professional education. The undergraduate nursing curriculum reflects a community-based education with emphasis on health assessment and the care of clients in a variety of settings. The faculty believes that teaching and learning are shared processes that best occur in an environment that stimulates inquiry, promotes critical and independent thinking, and supports personal and professional development.

The RN/B.S.N. degree completion program is part of the partnership with Saint Mary's and offers two pathways of study, one for the new RN graduate and one for the experienced RN. Courses of study are individually developed with the program's adviser to utilize and build upon previous work and school experience.

The Master of Science in Nursing (M.S.N.) program prepares nurses for advanced practice in the primary care of families (FNP) and nurse anesthesia (CRNA). The family nurse practitioner track requires 49 semester units, earned through either full- or part-time study. The nurse anesthesia track, a joint program with Kaiser Permanente, requires 63 semester units of full-time study. A new track for non-nursing college graduates began in fall 1996. Graduates of the track will have a Master of Science in Nursing with a focus in case management.

AFFILIATIONS WITH HEALTH-CARE FACILITIES

Located within the Summit Medical Center complex, the Department of Nursing is also affiliated with a number of inpatient and community facilities throughout the Bay Area and northern California. The department maintains numerous clinical contracts with health-care agencies, schools, military installations, and housing projects.

ACADEMIC FACILITIES

The John A. Graziano Memorial Library contains one of the largest private health science literature and multimedia collections in the San Francisco Bay Area. It also offers computerized bibliographic searches, 430 active journal subscriptions, private study rooms equipped with VCRs, and interactive computer systems. Personal computers are available to students 24 hours per day in Bechtel Hall. The Nursing Resource Lab is one of many unique facilities on campus and, with the nationally recognized award-winning Studio Three multimedia production facility, serves the entire campus community.

LOCATION

Samuel Merritt College is located in the heart of the Summit Medical Center complex and has unequaled state-of-the-art facilities for learning the art and science of nursing. Oakland has been named one of the United States' "All American Cities" owing to its multicultural spirit. Oakland has ballet, symphony, professional athletics, a multitude of recreational options, and perfect weather—and Samuel Merritt College is in the center of it all. To the east, over the Oakland Hills, lies the Saint Mary's campus in Moraga, California, nestled in an idyllic setting with Spanish-style campus buildings and dormitories. It is the perfect environment for the study of liberal arts in small student-focused seminar classrooms. Saint Mary's was recently named number four in the top fifteen regional universities for the Western Region by *U.S. News & World Report* (September 18, 1995).

STUDENT SERVICES

Samuel Merritt and Saint Mary's College offer many services and activities that support the intellectual, social, and cultural development of each individual. The Dean of Student Affairs coordinates services for students with special needs. The Student Body Association, the California Nursing Students Association, and various associations for graduate students are actively involved in planning educational and social activities throughout the academic year. An active multicultural group encompasses the belief that a high-quality education is enhanced when there is a forum for an exchange of ideas. On-campus housing, a computer center, student lounge, swimming pool, workout room, sundeck, and eating facilities are available to all students. Secured parking is available on campus.

THE NURSING STUDENT GROUP

There are approximately 323 undergraduate and 98 graduate students within the Department of Nursing. Reflective of professional education nationally, students tend to be adult learners, many making career changes within and to nursing. All graduate students in the Master of Science postprofessional program are licensed to practice within California. Many students in the department work part-time while enrolled in the program.

COSTS

In 1996–97, tuition for full-time undergraduate students was $13,865. Part-time undergraduate students (less than 10 units per semester) paid $580 per unit, and graduate students paid $555 per unit. Tuition remained the same for out-of-state and international students. Residence hall charges for a double-occupancy room totaled $3330 for nine months; single-occupancy charges totaled $4410 for nine months. A flat fee is in place for the RN-B.S.N. program. Sample student budgets are available from the Office of Financial Aid.

FINANCIAL AID

Every effort is made to see that no student is denied access to the College because of an inability to pay for educational expenses. Approximately 85 percent of the undergraduate student body and 95 percent of the graduate student body receive financial assistance through scholarships, grants, and loan programs. Excellent student employment opportunities and special payment plans are available. To apply for financial aid, students must complete the Free Application for Federal Student Aid (FAFSA). The priority application filing date is March 2 of each year.

APPLYING

Admission to all programs at Samuel Merritt College is competitive. Freshman candidates are admitted directly into the B.S.N. program for both fall and spring semesters. A minimum academic GPA of 2.5 and an SAT I combined score of 920 (480 verbal, 440 math) are required, along with a strong college-preparatory curriculum with specific prerequisites. Transfer candidates (including those with previous college degrees) are admitted directly into the nursing program for both fall and spring semesters. A minimum academic GPA of 2.5 is required (a 3.0 or higher is highly recommended). Specific prerequisites must be completed or in progress at the time of application. RN-B.S.N. candidates are admitted for fall, spring, and summer semesters. A minimum academic GPA of 2.5 is required. An essay and letter of recommendation are required for admission of all applicants to the undergraduate program. Applicants for whom English is not a native language need a minimum TOEFL score of 550. Application deadlines and prerequisite and specific program information are available by calling the College.

For the M.S.N. program, family nurse practitioner, nurse anesthesia, and entry-level candidates are admitted for fall semester only. All applicants to the postprofessional graduate nursing program must have a B.S.N. (RNs with degrees in other fields will be evaluated individually), a current California RN license, clinical practice experience, and successful completion of statistics prior to entrance. College graduates applying for the entry-level Master of Science in Nursing do not need to meet the admission requirements listed above. All M.S.N. candidates need letters of reference and a goal statement. Applicants for whom English is not a native language need a minimum TOEFL score of 600. Additional admission requirements are applicable to CRNA candidates and include a minimum GPA of 3.0; at least one year of critical care experience as an RN; 6–8 semester units of college chemistry; and competitive GRE scores. An introductory physics course is highly recommended. Students should call the College for information on application deadlines and specific program details.

Correspondence and Information:

John Garten-Shuman
Director of Admission
Samuel Merritt College
370 Hawthorne Avenue
Oakland, California 94609
Telephone: 510-869-6576
800-607-MERRITT (toll-free)
Fax: 510-869-6525

THE FACULTY

The following is only a partial listing of the faculty.

Audrey Berman, Ph.D., RN, OCN.
Jeri Bigbee, Ph.D., RN, FNP, FAAN.
Christine Bolla, D.N.Sc., RN.
Sarah Carroll, Ed.D., RN, FNP.
Linda Chapman, D.N.Sc., RN.
Gail A. DeBoer, M.S.N., RN.
Diana Dunn, M.S.N., RN.
Roberta Durham, Ph.D., RN.
Phylis Easterling, Ed.D., RN.
Scot Foster, Ph.D., CRNA.
Abby Heydman, Ph.D., RN.
Leonard Kaku, M.S.N., RN.
Sarah Keating, Dean of Nursing; Ed.D., RN, C-PNP, FAAN.
Richard C. MacIntyre, Ph.D., RN.
Kate McClure, M.S.N., RN.
Laura Smith McKenna, D.N.Sc., RNC.
Phyllis McKenna, M.S.N., RN.
Marion Mills, M.S.N., RN, PNP.
Patricia Moores, Ph.D., RN.
B. J. Nicholls, M.S.N., RN.
Susan Penner, Ph.D., RN.
Charles Etta Richardsons, M.S.N., RN.
Shirley J. Snyder, Ed.D., RN.
Janice M. Swanson, Ph.D., RN.
Karen VanLeuven, Ph.D., RN.
Celeste Villanueva, M.S.N., CRNA.
Christine Vourakis, D.N.Sc., RN.
Patricia Webb, Ed.D. candidate, RN.
Lisa Wright, M.S.N., RN.

San Diego State University
School of Nursing
San Diego, California

THE UNIVERSITY
San Diego State University was founded in 1897 and in 1971 became part of the California State University and College systems. Today San Diego State University is the largest campus in the CSU system and one of the largest in the western United States. SDSU is a major urban university with strong research programs. Over 29,000 students attend classes in sixty-nine different disciplines on a 271-acre campus. Repeatedly named by college presidents in *U.S. News & World Report* surveys as one of the outstanding comprehensive universities in the western United States, SDSU provides education in a wide variety of humanities, sciences, fine and performing arts, and professional disciplines. The mission-style architecture and broad, flowered walkways give the campus its unique southern California quality.

THE SCHOOL OF NURSING
The School of Nursing is part of the College of Health and Human Services and was established as a baccalaureate program with the University in 1953. Since then, the nursing program has maintained continuous accreditation by the National League for Nursing and the California State Board of Nursing. In 1982, the School of Nursing opened the Master of Science degree program in community health and nursing systems administration. The critical-care concentration began admitting students in 1985, the pediatric specialization began in 1989, and the school nursing program began in 1993. The family nurse practitioner program began in 1994 and the nurse midwifery program in 1995. Both are offered jointly with the University of California, San Diego, School of Medicine. The School admits RNs to the baccalaureate nursing program and offers a health services credential for school nurses. All baccalaureate graduates qualify for the California Public Health Certificate of Nursing.

The tenured faculty members and several lecturers in the School of Nursing are doctorally prepared and conduct research in a wide variety of clinical areas. Some of the research interests of the faculty include stress and coping in children, psychosocial issues of critically ill children, parent-infant relationships, infertility, physiological alterations in the neonate, evoked-potential responses, tissue oxygenation, administrative issues, and cross-cultural nursing. The faculty members are also experts in a variety of research methodologies, including the historical, qualitative, and quantitative methodologies.

PROGRAMS OF STUDY
The baccalaureate program prepares nurses who can function at a beginning level of practice in a wide variety of settings. It also prepares students with the basis for graduate study at the master's and doctoral levels. Undergraduate students are given opportunities to acquire knowledge from the natural and social sciences, to develop critical thinking and professional decision-making abilities, to utilize current research in the application of the nursing process, to develop leadership potential and accountability in professional practice, to become aware of the emerging roles of the professional nurse and of the social forces and trends affecting health and health-care systems, and to balance professional and personal growth and values. Satisfactory completion of 128 credits is required for graduation. Students may sit for the California licensing exam after completing seven semesters of the prescribed program of full-time study. Part-time study is also permitted.

The Master of Science degree in nursing is offered in one of three major concentrations: nursing systems administration, community health nursing, and advanced practice nursing of adults and the elderly. The latter offers specialization in critical care and acute care. Students in community health may specialize in public health or school nursing. Graduates of the program are prepared to function as mid-level and executive-level nursing administrators or clinical nurse specialists. In addition to the clinical or administrative focus, all graduates of the program are prepared for beginning roles as nurse researchers. These roles may involve critical analysis of research, application of research findings to clinical practice, data collection for larger collaborative nursing and medical studies, and acting as principal investigators.

The graduate program requires a minimum of 39 semester units, however some specialties such as NP and midwifery require more. All specialties may be completed in two years of full-time study. Part-time study is also permitted. Students take 12–15 units of core courses that investigate nursing research, theory, professional issues, and organizational systems. The remaining units are devoted to courses supporting the clinical specialty. All students may complete a master's thesis, project, or comprehensive exam. Students receive guided supervision throughout their thesis research.

AFFILIATIONS WITH HEALTH-CARE FACILITIES
The School of Nursing is affiliated with forty-seven different health-care agencies. All the major community hospitals, the Department of Health, the Visiting Nurse Association, schools, HMOs, jails, community clinics, home health agencies, and doctors' offices provide learning experiences for the SDSU nursing students. Patients are also seen in their homes.

ACADEMIC FACILITIES
The School of Nursing has its own media, computer, and skills labs. Students also have access to the College Computer Lab and the University's mainframe and microcomputer facilities. The University Computer Center provides equipment, software, and technical personnel to support student research.

The University library has over 1 million volumes and subscribes to more than 175 periodicals related to nursing and health care. The library provides general reference services and a specific librarian and related services for nursing. The School also has easy access to the Bio-Medical Library of the University of California, San Diego, as well as surrounding hospital libraries.

The SDSU Institute for Nursing was founded in 1988 and includes eight San Diego health-care institutions. The institute promotes collaborative research between service and academia through multisite studies. Its purpose is to promote collaboration in the conduct, dissemination, and utilization of nursing research that contributes to the quality of patient care.

LOCATION
San Diego is the sixth-largest city in the United States. San Diego County is the southernmost county of California, covering 4,255 square miles and ending at the United States–Mexico border. The climate is semi-arid with a mean temperature of 70 degrees year-round. The Pacific Ocean and

the beaches are approximately a 20-minute drive west from the campus. The mountains are 30 miles east and the desert is 80 miles northeast. San Diego offers diverse cultural, athletic, and recreational activities.

STUDENT SERVICES

Services are many and varied. Some examples are Campus Tours, Career Services, Counseling and Psychological Services, Disabled Student Services, Educational Opportunity/Ethnic Affairs, Health Services, On-Campus Housing for Singles, International Student Center, Ombudsmen, Student Athlete Academic Support Services, the Student Resource Center, Leisure Connection, Recreational Sports Office, and Mission Bay Aquatic Center.

THE NURSING STUDENT GROUP

There are currently over 300 undergraduate and over 100 graduate full- and part-time students enrolled in the School of Nursing. The SDSU School of Nursing is the largest supplier of nurses to San Diego and Imperial counties of southern California. The student body is diverse in ethnic background and geographic origin. The University provides many opportunities for students to participate on School and University committees. Graduates of the SDSU nursing programs have been actively recruited for both beginning and advanced practice positions in agencies throughout the United States.

COSTS

Registration fees for California residents in 1997–98 were $618 for 6 or fewer units and $951 for 6.1 or more units. Tuition for nonresidents (U.S. and international) was $246 per unit in addition to the registration fees cited above. Additional academic fees include application fees, thesis binding fees, and graduation charges. Students are also required to have professional liability insurance ($1 million) and transportation.

Although most students choose to live in off-campus housing, University housing is available. The cost of living in San Diego is comparable to that in other large metropolitan areas.

FINANCIAL AID

Financial aid is available in a variety of forms. Information on student loans, grants, and fellowships is available from the Financial Aid Office. Professional nurse traineeships and graduate assistantships are offered to graduate students through the School of Nursing. In addition to the direct student aid offered through the University, employment opportunities with a variety of educational benefits are available in nearby health-care agencies.

APPLYING

The application process has two steps. First an application is made to the University through Admissions and Records; a second application is made to the School of Nursing. For deadlines and criteria, students should contact the School of Nursing office.

Correspondence and Information:

School of Nursing
San Diego State University
San Diego, California 92182-0254
Telephone: 619-594-5357
Fax: 619-594-6527

THE FACULTY

Janet L. Blenner, Professor; Ph.D., NYU; FAAN.
Betty Broom, Associate Professor; Ph.D., Texas at Austin.
Sharon Burt, Lecturer; M.S.N., San Diego.
Carolyn Colwell, Lecturer; M.A., Columbia.
Cynthia Connelly, Lecturer; Ph.D., Rhode Island.
Jo Ann Daugherty, Lecturer; Ph.D., California, San Diego.
Lorraine T. Fitzsimmons, Associate Professor; D.N.S., Indiana.
Joan M. Flagg, Associate Professor; Ph.D., Texas at Austin.
Lorraine Freitas, Associate Professor and Associate Director; Ph.D., Texas at Austin.
Carmen Galang, Lecturer; D.N.S., San Diego.
Kay Gilbert, Lecturer; Ph.D., Texas at Austin.
Sue A. Hadley, Associate Professor; D.N.S., Indiana; NP.
Gail Handysides, Lecturer and HSC Advisor; M.S.N., Boston University.
Janet R. Heineken, Professor; Ph.D., Denver.
Nancy C. Jones, Assistant Professor; Ph.D., George Mason.
John M. Lantz, Professor; Ph.D., Texas A&M.
Nancy Lischke, Lecturer; M.N., UCLA.
Catherine E. Loveridge, Professor; Ph.D., Colorado.
Doris McCarthy, Lecturer; M.S.N., M.A., San Diego State.
Myrna Moffett, Assistant Professor and Undergraduate Advisor; Ph.D., Texas at Austin.
Rita I. Morris, Associate Professor; Ph.D., American.
Jane Rapps, Lecturer; M.S., Maryland.
Richard C. Reed, Associate Professor; Ed.D., Tulsa.
Barbara Riegel, Associate Professor; D.N.Sc., UCLA; F.A.A.N.
Lembi Saarmann, Associate Professor and RN-B.S. Advisor; Ed.D., Columbia.
Martha J. Shively, Professor; Ph.D., Texas at Austin.
Patricia Wahl, Professor and Director; Ph.D., Cincinnati; FAAN.
Carolyn L. Walker, Professor and Graduate Advisor; Ph.D., Utah.
Dolores A. Wozniak, Professor and Dean of the College of Health and Human Services; Ed.D., Columbia.

Simmons College
Department of Nursing
Boston, Massachusetts

THE COLLEGE
Chartered in 1899, Simmons College is a private, nonsectarian comprehensive college. It was one of the first colleges in the nation devoted to the career education of women. Essential to that charge is a curriculum that embodies the principles of a liberal arts and sciences education with the strength of a professional program. Today, Simmons continues this commitment in its rich array of undergraduate programs for women. Simmons College's primary goal is to prepare approximately 1,400 undergraduate students to be well informed, intellectually curious, and sensitive to cultural and social values. Simmons' comprehensive curriculum, excellent faculty, and numerous academic programs consistently rank Simmons as one of the nation's top comprehensive colleges in *U.S. News & World Report* surveys of "America's Best Colleges." In addition, the College's participation in the Colleges of the Fenway Consortium (the five colleges include Emmanuel College, Massachusetts College of Pharmacy and Allied Health Sciences, Simmons College, Wentworth Institute of Technology, and Wheelock College) allows students to cross-register, thus providing a broad range of electives and options from which to choose.

THE DEPARTMENT OF NURSING
Established in 1934, the undergraduate Department of Nursing has been at the forefront of nursing education. Academic excellence is achieved through a rigorous scholastic process. Those students achieving outstanding academic records may be initiated into the Simmons chapter of Sigma Theta Tau, the international nursing honor society. The Department accepts freshmen, transfer students, students seeking a second degree, licensed practical nurses, registered nurses seeking a baccalaureate degree, and Dix Scholars (students ages 23 and older). Graduates are prepared to practice in community health agencies, clinics, acute-care settings, and long-term-care facilities. Simmons College has long been recognized for the excellence of its nursing program, and graduates are recognized nationally and internationally as scholars, researchers, educators, and expert clinicians.

The Department of Nursing faculty members are highly qualified and clinically expert. They are all prepared at the graduate level and most hold earned doctorates in nursing or a related field. All are experts in clinical practice and are certified in their area of specialization. Simmons is a relatively small institution; all classes are taught by the faculty. Similarly, only faculty members supervise students in the clinical practice setting. The student-faculty ratio is generally 8:1 to maximize the students' learning potential. All full-time faculty members serve as advisers to undergraduate students for the duration of their academic program. Individual attention to the students' professional growth and personal development is of prime concern to the nursing faculty.

PROGRAM OF STUDY
The NLN-accredited baccalaureate program is an eight-semester program that can be taken full-time or part-time. Students meet with their faculty advisers to plan their individual course of study. Requirements in the sciences, liberal arts, languages, and the nursing program are identified. Nursing courses consist of both a theory component and a clinical practice component with a senior preceptorship offered in the last semester. Clinical placements are in internationally renowned health-care facilities in the Boston area. An evening/weekend program is offered for students ages 23 and older through the Dix Scholars program.

ACADEMIC FACILITIES
The Simmons College Libraries support the College's academic programs and help provide for the academic research and study needs of the faculty and students. In addition to the traditional library services, they offer support services, including a Media Center for videotape production and microcomputer laboratories and classes. The total library system contains more than 260,000 volumes, more than 2,000 current periodicals and journals, and more than 2,500 media materials. The library has an on-line catalog that provides access to external databases and library collections through the Internet. In addition, databases are available on CD-ROM workstations throughout the library. The libraries belong to the Fenway Library Consortium, which comprises fourteen nearby libraries and is a member of the New England Library Information Network, which links the College to a national bibliographic database of over 27 million titles in 16,000 libraries throughout the world.

LOCATION
Simmons College is located in metropolitan Boston, a city whose rich history and cultural diversity add to the educational experience of the student. The Simmons student has the opportunity to walk next door to the Isabella Stuart Gardner Museum, the Museum of Fine Arts, the Boston Symphony, or Fenway Park. Within a 1-mile radius of the College are some of the world's most recognized health-care, health research, and health education institutions.

STUDENT SERVICES
To enhance the academic experience, Simmons supports a Student Activities Center and numerous student organizations that enrich student life. Health and counseling services are provided through the Health Center with referrals as needed. Simmons actively seeks out the most qualified international students and provides student services to meet their academic goals. A Sports Center is located on the residence campus and is open to all students.

Other services include the Academic Support Center, Office of Financial Aid, the Needham Career Planning and Counseling Center, the Career Services and Student Employment Office, and the Institute on Women: Work, Family, and Social Change.

THE NURSING STUDENT GROUP
The nursing undergraduate student population reflects the Simmons community at large. Students are from geographically diverse areas, cultures, and backgrounds. About one half of the students live on campus and the others choose to live in the local Boston area. There are usually 220–250 undergraduate students in the Department of Nursing programs. Increasingly, a broad range of individuals are returning to school to change careers or to advance their knowledge in the health-care professions.

COSTS
Tuition is based on a charge per semester hour of instruction. The basic tuition charge for 1996–97 was $546 per semester

hour. The residence fee was $7228. Other fees, such as health and student activities, amounted to about $500. Books and supplies were approximately $600 per semester.

FINANCIAL AID

Simmons makes its educational opportunities available to as many capable, promising students as possible. Simmons College offers a number of scholarships, grants, and loans to students seeking financial aid.

APPLYING

For admission, the Simmons application and a nonrefundable fee of $35 should be submitted to the Admissions Office. All applicants must take either the Scholastic Assessment Test (SAT I) or American College Testing's ACT Assessment. TOEFL scores are required for applicants whose first language is not English. A minimum score of 550 is required. All tests should be taken no later than the January testing date of the applicant's senior year. Scores should be reported to Simmons by the College Board. A complete transcript from the secondary school is required. The applicant must submit two official recommendations from the high school, one from a guidance counselor and one from a teacher. It is strongly recommended that each applicant visit the College and have an interview. There are two early decision dates—November 1 and December 15. The regular decision date is February 1 for freshmen and April 1 for transfer students. Advanced placement and a Freshman Honor Program are also available. Transfer students are welcomed. Nursing program applicants' high school course of study should include 4 units of English, 3 units of a foreign language, 2 units of math, and 2 units of a laboratory science.

Correspondence and Information:

Director of Undergraduate Admissions
Simmons College
300 The Fenway
Boston, Massachusetts 02115
Telephone: 617-521-2051

Simmons College
Graduate School for Health Studies
Boston, Massachusetts

THE COLLEGE

Chartered in 1899, Simmons College is a private, nonsectarian comprehensive college. It was one of the first colleges in the nation devoted to the career education of women. Essential to that charge is a curriculum that embodies the principles of a liberal arts and sciences education with the strength of a professional program. Today, Simmons continues this commitment in its rich array of undergraduate programs for women and its distinguished graduate programs for women and men. Simmons College and the Graduate School for Health Studies are first and foremost an academic community whose primary goals are to prepare approximately 1,400 undergraduate students and 2,200 graduate students to be well informed, intellectually curious, and sensitive to cultural and social values. Simmons' comprehensive curriculum, excellent faculty, and numerous academic programs consistently rank Simmons as one of the nation's top comprehensive colleges in *U.S. News & World Report* surveys of "America's Best Colleges."

THE GRADUATE SCHOOL FOR HEALTH STUDIES

The coeducational Graduate School for Health Studies was established in July 1989, underscoring Simmons' commitment to the preparation of students for positions of leadership in the health-care arena. The School's goal is to prepare individuals for clinical and leadership positions in a rapidly changing health-care environment. Its programs are committed to educating students to be sensitive to human needs in terms of access and quality and to also understand the organizational, institutional, and policy constraints that increasingly dominate the health-care system. Since it incorporates both the clinical and administrative programs in one organization, the School is uniquely positioned to respond to the critical need for well-prepared nurse practitioners, to enhance the opportunities for interdisciplinary cooperation, and to expand the resources available.

PROGRAMS OF STUDY

The Graduate Program in Primary Health Care Nursing offers students the opportunity to be active participants in a fully NLN-accredited educational program with an established history of excellence. Simmons' graduate nursing program provides students with specialized education in primary health-care nursing and the foundation necessary for leadership, research, and doctoral study. Graduate education means the exploration and acquisition of knowledge essential to advanced nursing practice. Through systematic inquiry and with an appreciation of the client as a biopsychosocial being, the graduate student obtains the expanded clinical and theoretical knowledge necessary for the critical analysis and synthesis of data. The program prepares adult nurse practitioners with a specialty in occupational health, adult health, and geriatric health; parent-child nurse practitioners with specialties in pediatrics, ob/gyn women's health, and school health; and family nurse practitioners. Dual-degree programs with the Harvard School of Public Health in occupational health (M.S./M.S. in environmental health) and parent-child health (M.S./M.S. in maternal-child health) are available for qualified students. The program also offers a dual degree in primary health-care nursing and health-care administration with the graduate school's Graduate Program in Health Care Administration. An RN/M.S. program for diploma and associate degree graduates, a Certificate of Advanced Graduate Studies program for M.S.N. students who wish to become nurse practitioners, and an M.S. program for practicing nurse practitioners are also available.

The Simmons/Westbrook Partnership in Primary Health Care Nursing offers students the opportunity to complete the M.S. degree in two years of weekend study on the campus of Westbrook College in Portland, Maine. Concentrations in adult, family, and pediatric health are offered.

The Simmons graduate program is also a member of the Dartmouth/Mary Hitchcock Consortium for Graduate Nursing Education. The consortium offers the opportunity for students who live in rural areas of New England to plan an individualized program of study. Students may elect to take four core courses at any of the academic programs in the consortium. They may apply to any of the consortium members before, during, or after completion of the core courses. These core courses will be accepted toward the degree requirements of the participating programs.

Clinical expertise is a major focus of the program. All nursing faculty members are certified nurse practitioners and are currently in practice. Clinical agencies within the New England area are utilized for clinical practicums. Recent completion of a basic statistics course and a course in health assessment are prerequisites.

Forty-four credits are required for the completion of the master's degree. All students must complete a research thesis. Graduate faculty members are actively involved in research studies, and students are encouraged to collaborate with faculty members who are conducting research in the student's area of specialization. Full- and part-time study are available.

ACADEMIC FACILITIES

The Simmons College Libraries support the College's academic programs and help provide for the academic research and study needs of the College's faculty and students. In addition to the traditional library services, they offer support services, including a Media Center for videotape production and microcomputer laboratories and classes. The total library system contains more than 260,000 volumes, over 2,000 current periodicals and journals, and over 2,500 media materials. The library has an on-line catalog that provides access to external databases and library collections through the Internet. In addition, databases are available on CD-ROM workstations throughout the library. The libraries belong to the Fenway Library Consortium, which comprises fourteen nearby libraries and is a member of the New England Library Information Network, which links the College to a national bibliographic database of over 27 million titles in 16,000 libraries throughout the world. Students on the Westbrook campus have access to both Colleges' facilities.

LOCATION

Simmons College is located in metropolitan Boston, a city whose rich history and cultural diversity add to the educational experience of the student. The Simmons student has the opportunity to walk next door to the Isabella Stuart Gardner Museum, the Museum of Fine Arts, the Boston Symphony, or Fenway Park. Within a 1-mile radius of the College are some of the world's most recognized health-care, health research, and health education institutions.

STUDENT SERVICES

To enhance the academic experience Simmons supports a Student Activities Center and numerous student organizations that enrich student life. Health and counseling services are provided through the Health Center with referrals as needed. Simmons actively seeks out the most qualified international students and provides student services to meet their academic goals. A Sports Center is located on the residence campus and is open to all students.

Other services include the Academic Support Center, Office of Financial Aid, the Needham Career Planning and Counseling Center, the Career Services and Student Employment Office, and the Simmons Institute for Leadership and Change.

THE NURSING STUDENT GROUP

The nursing student population reflects the Simmons community at large. Students are from geographically diverse areas, cultures, and backgrounds. There are about 300 nursing students enrolled in the graduate programs. Increasingly, a broad range of individuals are returning to school to change careers or to advance their knowledge in the health-care professions.

COSTS

Tuition is based on a charge per semester hour of instruction. The basic tuition charge for 1996–97 was $546 per semester hour. The residence fee was $8070. Other fees, such as health and student activities, amounted to about $500. Books and supplies were approximately $600 per semester.

FINANCIAL AID

Simmons makes its educational opportunities available to as many capable, promising students as possible. Simmons College offers a number of scholarships, grants, and loans to students seeking financial aid. Graduate students may receive funds from the Department of Health and Human Services Division of Nursing Traineeships when available.

APPLYING

Applicants to the Graduate School for Health Studies should submit the completed application form, an official transcript of all previous college courses, three letters of recommendation, and GRE scores or evidence of successful completion of a Simmons College graduate course in physiology. TOEFL scores are required for applicants whose first language is not English. Students should identify their area of specialization and their preference for part-time or full-time study. The application deadline is January 15. The application fee is $50.

Correspondence and Information:

Assistant Dean
Graduate School for Health Studies
Simmons College
300 The Fenway
Boston, Massachusetts 02115
Telephone: 617-521-2650
E-mail: gshsadm@simmons.edu

State University of New York at Binghamton

BINGHAMTON UNIVERSITY

Decker School of Nursing

Binghamton, New York

THE UNIVERSITY

Binghamton University of the State University of New York, located in the scenic southern tier of New York, enrolls 9,300 undergraduates in five schools and 2,700 graduate students in a variety of programs. Binghamton prides itself on excellent teaching and solid research from a faculty remarkably accessible to students. Teaching and mentoring by faculty members builds upon the strengths students bring, helping them develop their potential to new levels.

In 1996–97, *Money* magazine rated Binghamton the ninth-best buy (quality of educational value) among the 100 top American universities and colleges as well as the very best buy in the Northeast. The 1996–97 *U.S. News & World Report* survey concluded that Binghamton is the third most efficient university in the nation in making the best use of its resources.

THE SCHOOL OF NURSING

Today's complex system of health care, in which people are treated using sophisticated technologies, requires the very best scientific preparation for entry into the professional practice of nursing. Yet a balance must be found between technical skills and humane practice. Nurses must understand mind/body relationships for healing and deliver high-quality comprehensive care. Nurses are assuming expanded roles as respected members of health-care teams, making important decisions and providing essential services to help clients recover. Nurses are expert in health teaching, health counseling, and health promotion and deal with clients of all ages. Nurses attend to persons with a variety of short- and long-term health needs, assessing progress, consulting other team members, administering prescribed treatments, and nurturing with compassion and professionalism. Nurses provide care that hastens recovery and enhances well-being. The Decker School of Nursing offers students the highest quality of academic preparation for professional nursing. Over 320 students pursue a Bachelor of Science in Nursing degree provided by an outstanding nursing faculty in an academic community that values student growth. Graduates are prepared for positions in professional nursing practice in hospitals, community health services, schools, and occupational health services. The program also provides a foundation for graduate study in nursing at Decker or elsewhere to prepare for positions in advanced clinical nursing practice, teaching, administration, or research. Upon graduation from the Decker School, students are eligible to take the licensing examination (NCLEX-RN) required to enter practice. Ninety to ninety-five percent of Decker students typically pass the exam as they graduate. The Decker faculty is known for high-quality research and innovation. The nationally recognized AIDSNET computerized program for homebound AIDS patients reflects an extraordinary blend of compassion and technical expertise.

PROGRAM OF STUDY

Each student is assigned a faculty adviser to help plan an academic program and to lend support as the student moves from classroom to lab to clinical practice settings in the community. The state-of-the-art nursing curriculum is built upon courses offered by the University's Harpur College of Arts and Sciences. From classroom to learning lab to interactive video room, students enjoy the finest learning settings available under the direction of a first-class faculty. Students in the Decker School's undergraduate program complete general education requirements—courses in the humanities and social, behavioral, and natural sciences—during their first two years of study. During the second two years, students take a series of nursing courses that emphasize clinical experiences in local hospitals, nursing homes, psychiatric facilities, and community health centers.

AFFILIATIONS WITH HEALTH-CARE FACILITIES

Over 100 agencies in or near the greater Binghamton area provide clinical training opportunities in the increasingly diversified health-care field. Decker faculty members participate in and oversee the activity of students in the clinical settings, working closely with on-site professionals to ensure the greatest benefit to all.

ACADEMIC FACILITIES

Nursing students enjoy close attention from Decker School faculty while benefiting from Binghamton University's campus resources. The University's libraries house over 3 million items, and the library system's sophisticated computers provide students access, via the Internet, to an extraordinary variety of other libraries around the world. Students may use computers in several instructional centers or connect personal computers to the mainframe from their residence hall rooms by cable. The Center for Academic Excellence provides tutorial services for all students, and a writing center helps students hone their communication skills. Nursing students have access to the many learning resources in the Decker School, including the learning lab, student computer room, multimedia center, and the Helene Fuld Learning Resource Center, which features a variety of hands-on learning models, simulation resources, and equipment. Interactive videodisc workstations bring students closer to actual health-care situations that focus on client care. Modern labs and classrooms of moderate size keep the Binghamton experience personal. The average University class size is under 30 and smaller still for nursing courses. Two new classroom buildings are under construction. One will house the Decker School of Nursing, although the current nursing facility is less than seven years old and very modern.

LOCATION

Binghamton University is located in a suburban setting 10 minutes from Binghamton, a city of 53,000 in a county of 212,000. Binghamton is 200 miles northwest of New York City, 70 miles south of Syracuse, and 150 miles southeast of Rochester. Both bus and air carriers serve the greater Binghamton area.

STUDENT SERVICES

Binghamton students participate in over 150 organized activities, including nineteen NCAA Division III intercollegiate athletic teams for women and men. Students manage the campus television station, FM radio station, ambulance and medical transport service, and bus system. Religious, cultural, athletic, literary, social, and other organizations ensure that Binghamton will never become a "suitcase" campus on weekends. Students develop leadership skills early, and nursing students join campuswide groups as well as some exclusively for them.

Housing is guaranteed for all four undergraduate years. Students live in one of several residential communities on campus. Each community (800 to 1,100 students in four to six low-rise buildings) has a faculty "master" as administrator, plus faculty and staff volunteers who join students for meals and community activities, serving as mentors and friends. Each residential area has its own student government, theater company, library, and special interest housing modules. French and Spanish, computers and robotics, health and wellness, and visual and performing arts as well as African and Asian cultures are active modules.

University apartments house some transfer, upperclass, and married students.

THE NURSING STUDENT GROUP

With over 320 undergraduates and 170 graduate students, the Decker School is full of dedicated and talented women and men. About 15 percent already are registered nurses, and 10 percent are accelerated program members. Undergraduates often participate in programs of the Center for Nursing Research, developing valuable insights for future study. Graduates hold positions in prestigious medical centers such as Columbia Presbyterian Medical Center; Beth Israel Medical Center, Boston; New York Hospital; Yale–New Haven Hospital; Strong Memorial Hospital, Rochester, New York; Duke University Medical Center; Charity Hospital, New Orleans; SUNY Health Science Center, Syracuse, New York; and schools, clinics, and family and community health centers nationwide.

COSTS

State of New York tax dollars keep direct costs to students in the moderate range, while providing a strong resource base for a high-quality education. Expenses are subject to change, but for 1996–97, changes were modest. In 1996–97, for New York residents, tuition was $3400, fees were $626, room and board were $4814, and personal expenses, including books and travel, were $2300, for a total of $11,140. For nonresidents, tuition was $8300; fees, $626; room and board, $4814; and personal expenses, $2500, for a total of $16,240.

FINANCIAL AID

Students should complete the Free Application for Federal Student Aid (FAFSA) and submit it by the annual deadline. New York residents should also file the Tuition Assistance Program (TAP) application. Aid packages prepared by the financial aid staff include resources from federal, state of New York, and Binghamton University Foundation sources. The hope is to enable students to find Binghamton affordable. Financial aid questions may be addressed in writing or by calling 607-777-2428 weekdays from 8:30 a.m. to 5 p.m.

APPLYING

Binghamton is selective and welcomes applications from students who are serious about their futures. The Committee on Admission evaluates each applicant for evidence of academic and other strengths. Quality of courses taken, overall school average, grade trend, class rank if available, and SAT I or ACT scores are weighed. Nursing candidates should have solid work in chemistry and biology. The Supplementary Admission Form, mailed to every candidate upon receipt of the completed initial application, enables students to share achievements as well as hopes and plans. Extracurricular activities and community service are valued and should be described on the supplementary form. Students are admitted as freshmen or transfers each semester. Some new students are already registered nurses; others have a bachelor's degree and pursue the accelerated program. Many enter directly from high school and benefit from close association with older students.

New York residents may obtain an application from local high schools or SUNY campuses. Applications will be mailed to nonresidents and others who cannot obtain one locally. Applicants wishing to review computerized admissions information may contact the admissions office for the easiest mode of connection to the Binghamton campus computer system via BITNET or the Internet.

Visits to Binghamton's lovely 606-acre hillside campus and adjacent 117-acre nature preserve are strongly encouraged. Group information sessions followed by guided walking tours of campus help provide answers to many important questions. Students should call at least one week in advance to arrange a visit. Sessions and tours are scheduled several days weekly, excluding some holiday periods.

Correspondence and Information:

Office of Undergraduate Admissions
Binghamton University
Binghamton, New York 13902-6001
Telephone: 607-777-2171
Fax: 607-777-4445
World Wide Web: http://www.binghamton.edu/

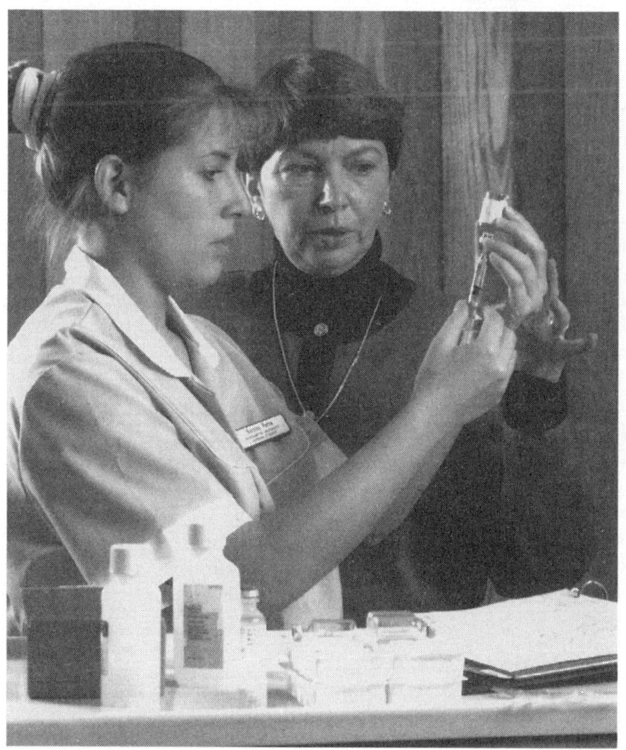

Each student receives individualized attention in a supportive environment.

Syracuse University
College of Nursing
Syracuse, New York

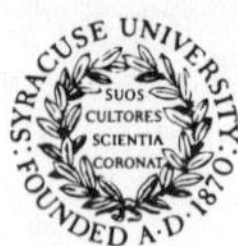

THE UNIVERSITY

Syracuse University (SU) is one of the largest and most comprehensive independent universities in the nation and is a leader in high-quality education. Founded in 1870, Syracuse University is a private residential institution that promotes learning through teaching, research, scholarship, creative accomplishment, and service. It is a member of the Association of American Universities, an agenda-setting body for higher education in the United States and Canada.

The sprawling 200-acre campus of grassy lawns, tall trees, and wide walkways, situated on a hill, overlooks the city and surrounding countryside. It is a blend of contemporary architecture and landmark buildings that reflects SU's rich heritage and the commitment to providing modern technology and research facilities.

The University is organized into fifteen schools and colleges offering a total of 520 degree programs, including 240 undergraduate, 204 master's, and 76 doctoral programs. Total enrollment in the fall 1995 semester was 18,804. Entering students represent forty-one states, twenty-eight other countries, and varied economic and social backgrounds.

THE COLLEGE OF NURSING

The College was founded in 1943 and first offered a master's program in 1948. The nursing program is noted for its individualized approach to the variety of interdisciplinary study available. Programs reflect the signature of the College, "Empowering people for health," which begins with the empowering of students as learners who will have the knowledge and skills to influence major changes in health care.

The mission of the College of Nursing is to prepare leaders in health care who will make an impact by helping reshape health care, health policy, and resource allocation through the generation and transmission of knowledge.

All full-time faculty members of the College are registered nurses with doctoral degrees and have conducted research in their specialties. Together they provide a supportive environment for study.

The College of Nursing occupies its own building on the University campus and houses a learning resource center. A complex of hospitals adjacent to the campus, plus other regional and national health facilities, provide nursing experiences.

PROGRAMS OF STUDY

In the 120-credit B.S. in Nursing (B.S.N.) curriculum, students combine a study of arts and science courses with professional nursing courses throughout their program of study. Freshmen and transfer applicants are admitted directly to the College and begin nursing courses in their first semester. Clinical experiences begin in the first semester of the sophomore year.

Special options available to undergraduate nursing students include the semester away experience. Undergraduate nursing students may also participate in the honors program, study abroad through SU's Division of International Programs Abroad (DIPA), ROTC, and hundreds of professional, social, athletic, and recreational activities available on campus. Students can elect to immediately continue their education in the accelerated M.S. program if they meet the admission criteria.

An accelerated two-year B.S. in Nursing program is available to students who already have a B.S. or B.A. in another discipline. Credits from the student's prior degree are accepted to validate all or the majority of the arts and science component of the B.S. in Nursing, and students immediately enter a concentrated curriculum of nursing theory and clinical studies. Second-degree students may be eligible for special grant incentives and an accelerated M.S.

An accelerated RN-B.S.-M.S. program provides educational opportunity for RNs to continue their education at the baccalaureate and graduate levels in a facilitated pathway. General education components are transferred, and nursing credits are evaluated. Students must meet admission standards for graduate study before continuing. Degrees are awarded separately when requirements are met.

The 45-credit graduate program gives the student, in collaboration with the faculty adviser, the opportunity to design an individualized plan of study based on career goals. Specialties include adult, child, women's, gerontologic, adult and child psychiatric/mental health, family, community, school, and occupational health nursing. Nurse practitioner options are also available in these fields. Joint M.S./M.B.A. and M.S./M.P.A. degree programs are available. Also available is the innovative Summer Limited Residency Independent Study Master's Program. Electives may be in nursing administration, teaching, and informatics, or to enhance the specialty area. A culminating experience is required.

Advanced (post-master's) certificate programs in nurse practitioner studies, nursing administration, teaching, and informatics are programs that qualify students for certification in their chosen focus area.

RN and graduate programs are currently offered at three outreach sites. Programs are designed to meet the needs of working nurses. All programs are NLN-accredited and are offered full-time and part-time.

AFFILIATIONS WITH HEALTH-CARE FACILITIES

Syracuse University students have access to an exceptional variety of hospitals and health agencies representing a full scope of professional nursing practice. Many sites are within a few blocks of campus. Placements are available in nationally recognized facilities.

ACADEMIC FACILITIES

The SU library system is a major academic resource for the region, state, and nation. The collections contain more than 3 million volumes, 11,000 serials, periodicals, and more than 3.4 million microforms. Library services include information and reference, on-line database searching, access to bibliographic information on CD-ROM, interlibrary loans, and library instruction.

The Learning Resource Center at the College of Nursing includes computers with access to University-wide library collections and mainframe computing services, interactive video and video units, and a health assessment laboratory.

LOCATION

Syracuse is located in the geographic center of the state and is approximately 250 miles northwest of New York City. The University's main campus houses 170 academic buildings, libraries, laboratories, and studios. Together they provide all the academic resources and facilities of a major research university.

Metropolitan Syracuse, with a population of 600,000, is large enough to deliver the latest in health care to a diverse population, yet small enough for individual efforts to be recognized.

STUDENT SERVICES

The University has innumerable resources and offices to meet student needs. In addition, undergraduate students at the College of Nursing are encouraged to participate in the National Student Nurses Association (NSNA). Graduate students may take advantage of the Graduate Student Nursing Organization. The College also sponsors the Omicron Chapter of Sigma Theta Tau. ALHANA (African, Latino, Hispanic, Asian, and Native American) Nursing Student Organization represents minority students. Student representation is invited on the College Curriculum Committee, the Student Life Committee, and the Promotion and Tenure Committee.

THE NURSING STUDENT GROUP

There are 848 students in the College of Nursing, 594 at the undergraduate level and 254 at the graduate level. About 80 percent of the graduate students work full-time.

COSTS

Tuition costs for the 1996–97 academic year were $16,710 for full-time undergraduates, $305 per credit for part-time undergraduates, and $503 per credit for graduate and postgraduate students. Rates are the same for in-state and out-of-state students. The undergraduate activity fee, health fees, and books are estimated at $370 per year. Room and board are approximately $7220 per year. Books for graduate students cost $500–$600 per year.

FINANCIAL AID

Approximately 80 percent of all SU students receive financial aid. Many students rely on need-based financial aid to meet the cost of their studies. This may be in the form of loan programs and college work-study. Graduate students may receive merit-based awards and appointments, including fellowships, scholarships, and assistantships. State and federal awards are also available. Nursing employment opportunities are available in the community. Many agencies offer tuition support.

APPLYING

For admission to the B.S.N. program, SAT I or ACT scores, 4 years of science, including 1 year of high school biology and 1 year of high school chemistry, are required. High school seniors must apply by February 1. Transfer and second-degree applications are reviewed on a rolling basis; early application is encouraged. Transfer applicants should have a minimum GPA of 2.5. Second-degree applicants should have a minimum GPA of 2.8.

For the RN-B.S.-M.S. program, a minimum GPA of 2.2 from the A.D. or diploma program is required. The master's and post-master's programs require a B.S.N. or an M.S. in Nursing, respectively, from an NLN-accredited institution. The M.S. requires competence in basic statistics and basic health assessment. The GRE is required. International students must submit TOEFL scores. Students should contact the appropriate nursing office at the College of Nursing for complete information about admission requirements and application deadlines.

Correspondence and Information:

For specific program information:
College of Nursing
Syracuse University
426 Ostrom Avenue
Syracuse, New York 13244-3240
Telephone: 315-443-4266
Fax: 315-443-9807

For an undergraduate application:
Office of Undergraduate Admissions and Financial Aid
201 Tolley Administration Building
Syracuse University
Syracuse, New York 13244-1100
Telephone: 315-443-3611

For a graduate application:
Graduate Admissions Processing
212 Archbold
Syracuse University
Syracuse, New York 13244-1140
Telephone: 315-443-9120

THE FACULTY

Linda Beeber, Associate Professor (Psychiatric–Mental Health Nursing); Ph.D., Rochester, 1987.

Carroll Bouman, Assistant Professor (Medical-Surgical Nursing); Ph.D., Rochester, 1996.

Carol Brooks, Associate Professor (Nursing Administration); D.N.S., Boston University, 1982.

Grace H. Chickadonz, Professor (Community Health Nursing) and Dean; Ph.D., Maryland, 1976.

Denise Cote-Arsenault, Assistant Professor (Child Bearing and Family Nursing); Ph.D., Rochester, 1995.

Irene Di Florio, Assistant Professor (Maternal-Child and Family Nursing); Ph.D., Syracuse, 1995.

Patricia Duncan, Assistant Professor (Community Health Nursing); Ph.D., Syracuse, 1993.

Elizabeth Essman, Associate Professor (Family Nurse Practitioner, Community Health Nursing); Ph.D., Syracuse, 1994.

Barbara Harris, Assistant Professor (Medical-Surgical Nursing); Ph.D., Syracuse, 1990.

Eileen Lantier, Assistant Professor (Medical-Surgical Nursing); Ph.D., Syracuse, 1992.

Rosemary Lape, Associate Professor (Medical-Surgical Nursing); M.S., Syracuse, 1967.

Janet Leeb, Associate Professor (Medical-Surgical Nursing); Ph.D., Syracuse, 1983.

Mary Ann Middlemiss, Associate Professor (Medical-Surgical Nursing); Ph.D., Syracuse, 1987.

Cecilia Mulvey, Associate Professor (Community Health Nursing); Ph.D., Syracuse, 1988.

Bobbie Perdue, Associate Professor (Psychiatric-Child Nursing); Ph.D., NYU, 1993.

Maureen Thompson, Assistant Professor (Child and Family Nursing); Ph.D., Syracuse, 1990.

Barbara VanNoy, Associate Professor (Psychiatric–Mental Health Nursing); Ph.D., Wayne State, 1989.

Kay Wiggins, Professor (Child and Family Nursing); Ph.D., Syracuse, 1983.

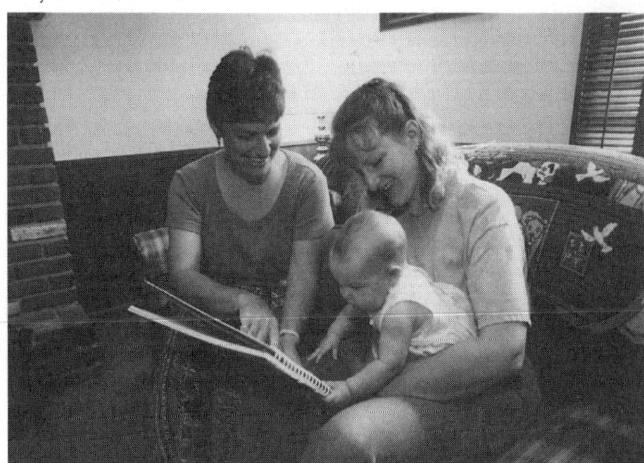

Infant care and parenting skills are taught by a nurse specializing in support for childbearing families.

Texas A&M University–Corpus Christi
Department of Nursing and Health Science
Corpus Christi, Texas

THE UNIVERSITY

Texas A&M University–Corpus Christi is a comprehensive four-year university located on its own 240-acre island just minutes from downtown Corpus Christi. Known as The Island University, A&M–Corpus Christi was one of the fastest growing public institutions in Texas in 1992 and again in 1994. Total enrollment for fall 1996 was 5,678.

In the past five years, student enrollment has grown 45 percent, and faculty levels have increased more than 70 percent. An aggressive building campaign to house this growing student population is in progress. Currently, A&M–Corpus Christi has a faculty-student ratio of 1:14, with 80 percent of the faculty members holding the highest possible degree in their field. Students choose from fifty-one undergraduate and graduate degree programs in the Colleges of Arts and Humanities, Education, Business, and Science and Technology.

THE DEPARTMENT OF NURSING AND HEALTH SCIENCE

Caring is the philosophical foundation upon which A&M–Corpus Christi has built its nursing and health science programs. Here, students are seen as individuals with differing backgrounds, needs, and interests. At A&M–Corpus Christi, students have the freedom and the responsibility to make considered choices.

Almost 2,000 students have graduated from the nursing programs since the introduction of the RN-B.S.N. program in 1974. In 1984, the University began offering the M.S.N. program that has produced 276 master's-prepared nurses over the past twelve years. The generic B.S.N. program was added in 1990, allowing for a complete four-year program through A&M–Corpus Christi. In 1996, A&M–Corpus Christi added an honors track opportunity for RNs to apply for admission directly into the M.S.N. program.

Academic highlights of the A&M–Corpus Christi nursing programs include a 100 percent pass rate for the 1995–96 academic year on the NCLEX exam and a 93 percent pass rate by nursing students on the American Nursing Association's examination for nurse practitioners.

The Department has 20 faculty members. Of those, 60 percent have their doctorates, and 93 percent earned a "superior" performance rating on the annual faculty evaluation.

PROGRAMS OF STUDY

A&M–Corpus Christi offers two program options for a Bachelor of Science in Nursing (B.S.N.) degree. Registered nurses (RNs) with associate degrees or diploma preparation can take advantage of the RN-B.S.N. completion program; high school graduates can apply to the generic baccalaureate program. A&M–Corpus Christi was the first university in the state of Texas to be accredited by the National League for Nursing (NLN) for an RN-B.S.N. program. The University has been accredited by the NLN for all nursing programs through the year 2000.

The Master of Science in Nursing (M.S.N.) program aims to enhance and expand the leadership capabilities of the B.S.N. degree holder and prepare this nurse for role specialization as a nurse administrator, nurse educator, or advanced nurse practitioner (medical-surgical, adult, family, pediatric). A newly created option affords the honors student an opportunity for admission directly to the M.S.N. program as an RN. Then challenge exams and undergraduate course work are completed along with a bridge course before beginning graduate-level course work. Emphasis is placed on facilitating health-care delivery within multicultural and rural communities in both primary- and acute-care settings. Upon program completion, M.S.N. graduates demonstrate responsibility and accountability for providing high-quality nursing care and strengthening the nursing discipline.

In the fall of 1996, A&M–Corpus Christi began serving as a host site for the University of Texas Health Science Center at San Antonio School of Nursing (UTHSC-SA SON) doctoral degree program (Ph.D.). A&M–Corpus Christi faculty members are eligible for appointment as faculty associates to the UTHSC-SA SON and School of Biomedical Sciences. Faculty associates teach and serve on dissertation committees. The doctoral program consists of approximately 60 credit hours. Seven courses are offered on site or televised to the A&M–Corpus Christi campus. Other course requirements are met through the dissertation, cognates, electives, and clinical major courses that may be transferred from any university. The aim of the doctoral program is to educate clinical nurse faculty members who conduct clinical research in collaboration with the biomedical sciences in the specific clinical areas.

AFFILIATIONS WITH HEALTH-CARE FACILITIES

A&M–Corpus Christi undergraduate students begin their clinical education in their junior year. Extensive clinical experiences are a major component of the program. The program utilizes a variety of nearby major medical facilities and community health-care agencies, including Driscoll Children's Hospital, Spohn Memorial Hospital, Spohn South Health Plaza, Columbia Doctor's Regional Hospital, Columbia North Bay, Columbia Rehabilitation Hospital, and Columbia Bay Area Hospital. Outreach programs include clinical settings at Scott & White Hospital in Temple and local hospitals in Victoria.

ACADEMIC FACILITIES

A&M–Corpus Christi's Bell Library houses more than 350,000 volumes of books, periodicals, and state and federal documents. In 1994, the library was fully automated, incorporating the latest information technology, enabling students to communicate with the world via library computers. The Bell Library has more than fifty library information databases and other on-line catalogs from across the globe and continues to add databases to broaden both its scope and reach. The nursing program has its own computer lab, interactive nursing skills videos, a learning resource lab, and nursing audiovisuals to assist students in mastering information and skills.

LOCATION

Situated on the Texas Gulf Coast, A&M–Corpus Christi is the only university in the nation located on its very own island. This beautiful 240-acre island campus blends palm-lined lanes and tropical landscaping with coastal architecture and natural wetlands. The campus is minutes from downtown Corpus Christi and the Padre Island National Seashore.

Corpus Christi is a major tourist destination. This bay community enjoys a subtropical setting that combines a year-round sunny climate with abundant outdoor recreational activities. Visitors and residents alike can touch a stingray at the Texas State Aquarium, sail back in time aboard replicas of Christopher Columbus' fleet, walk the beaches of the Gulf Coast, and sail the waters of the bay and gulf. Cultural opportunities include the Art Museum of South Texas, various theatrical productions, and the Corpus Christi Symphony.

STUDENT SERVICES

The Student Nurse Association meets monthly to provide opportunities for the exchange of ideas among those students who are interested and involved in national, state, and local issues relevant to nursing and health care. Academic support services include freshman academic advising, an academic testing center, a tutoring and learning center, health clinic, personal counseling, and career counseling.

The Student Life and Recreational Sports Offices together provide a variety of services and opportunities for students to get involved in extracurricular activities, from sports to cultural events. On-campus housing provides students with apartment-style residences located at the water's edge. Recreational, cultural, and educational activities are provided as an integrated part of on-campus housing.

THE NURSING STUDENT GROUP

Of the 312 nursing students enrolled in the Department of Nursing and Health Science for the spring of 1996, 104 were in the prenursing program, 70 were in the generic B.S.N. program, 43 were in the RN-B.S.N. program, and 95 were enrolled in the M.S.N. program.

COSTS

Tuition costs for Texas residents for the 1996–97 academic year were $1120 for full-time students with an average annual load of 34 semester credit hours; tuition was $32 per semester credit hour. Mandatory fees for the same average annual load were $1370 per year, with books and supplies costing about $500. Housing and food costs are estimated $5100 annually. Undergraduate and graduate costs are the same. Nonresident tuition was $8364 per year for full-time students with an average annual load of 34 semester credit hours. Nonresident tuition was $246 per semester credit hour.

FINANCIAL AID

In 1995, more than 80 percent of all A&M–Corpus Christi students received financial aid in the form of grants, loans, and scholarships. Some was specifically for nursing majors. Eligibility for aid is based on need as well as academic merit.

APPLYING

Admission is competitive. Applicants are evaluated individually to determine their potential for academic success. A&M–Corpus Christi bases its decisions on the strength of academic preparation, achievement, recommendations, extracurricular activities, personal qualifications, and the pattern of testing on various standardized tests.

Admission into the generic baccalaureate program requires a minimum GPA of 3.0, two letters of recommendation, and a written essay. The application deadline is February 15.

Admission into the RN-B.S.N. program requires a minimum college GPA of 2.5, an RN license, graduation from a diploma or A.D. nursing program, two letters of recommendation, and a written essay. The application deadline is rolling.

Admission into the M.S.N. program requires a B.S.N. degree from an NLN-accredited school of nursing (applicants from nonaccredited programs are considered on an individual basis), a minimum college GPA of 3.0 for the last 60 semester hours of college and at least a 3.0 GPA in nursing courses, a minimum GRE score of 1000, two letters of recommendation, and a written essay. The application deadline is rolling.

Correspondence and Information:

Dr. Rebecca A. Jones, Director
Department of Nursing and Health Science
Texas A&M University–Corpus Christi
6300 Ocean Drive
Corpus Christi, Texas 78412
Telephone: 512-994-2648
Fax: 512-994-2484
WWW: http://www.sci.tamucc.edu/nursing/welcome/html

THE FACULTY

Rebecca A. Patronis Jones, Director and Associate Professor; D.N.Sc.; RN, CNAA.
Violeta Berbiglia, Associate Professor; Ed.D; RN.
Whitney R. Bischoff, Assistant Professor; Dr.P.H.; RN.
Christell O. Bray, Associate Professor; M.S.N.; RN, FNP.
Frances H. D. "Bunny" Forgione, Assistant Professor; M.S.N.; RN, CSN.
Mary Jane Hamilton, Coordinator of Undergraduate Programs and Professor; Ph.D.; RNC.
Claudia L. Johnston, Coordinator of Graduate Programs and Associate Professor; Ph.D.; RN.
Esperanza V. Joyce, Associate Professor; Ed.D; RN, CNS.
Kenn M. Kirksey, Associate Professor; Ph.D.; RN, CS.
Chris M. Kucinkas, Visiting Assistant Professor; M.A.; RN, PNP, CS.
Mary Ellen Miller, Assistant Professor; M.S.N.; RN.
Karen K. Olson, Project Director Family Nurse Practitioner Program and Associate Professor; Ph.D.; RN, FNP.
Sally Preski, Associate Professor; Ph.D.; RN, CNS.
Doris J. Rosenow, Associate Professor; Ph.D.; CCRN, CNS.
Elizabeth Sefcik, Associate Professor; Ph.D.; RN, CS.
Carolyn Flemming Troupe, Associate Professor; Ed.D.; RN.
Julia Whitehurst, Associate Professor; M.S.N.; RN, CS.

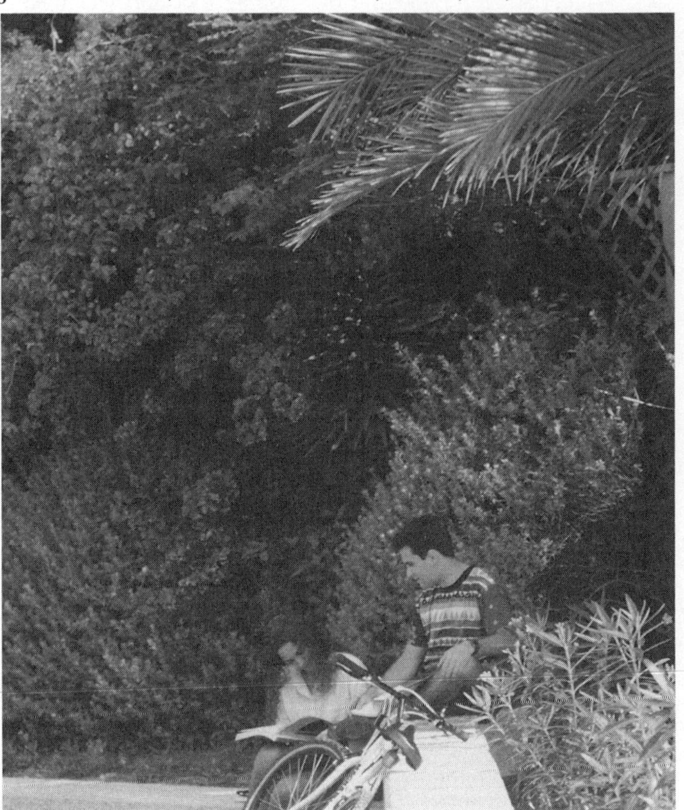

Students study in the surroundings of the tropical university.

Thiel College
Department of Nursing
Greenville, Pennsylvania

THE COLLEGE

Thiel College was founded in 1866 as one of the first coeducational institutions of higher education in the United States. Located in Greenville, Pennsylvania, in the northwestern corner of the commonwealth, Thiel has become known for the quality of its educational offerings and its blending of liberal arts, cutting-edge technology, and experiential learning through extensive cooperative education and internship opportunities.

Affiliated with the Evangelical Lutheran Church in America, the College enrolls a little more than 1,000 women and men. Most students come from Pennsylvania, Ohio, and the Middle Atlantic States. Seven percent of the students are members of minority groups, and 3 percent are from fourteen other countries.

The College is situated on 135 acres. Facilities include historic Greenville Hall, a classroom complex; Roth Hall, which houses the College theater; the Academic/Science Center complex; Beeghly-Rissel Gymnasia; the Howard Miller Center student union; Livingston Hall, for music and the arts; the Respiratory Care building; and the Passavant Center, which contains Burgess Chapel and a 2,000-seat auditorium and convocation center. Six student residence halls and a fraternity housing complex provide attractive on-campus living options.

Thiel has been ranked in the "top tier" of northern liberal arts colleges by *U.S. News & World Report,* and its sciences and mathematics programs are included in *Peterson's Top Colleges for Science.* Thiel's nursing program is accredited by the National League for Nursing and approved by the Pennsylvania State Board of Nursing.

THE DEPARTMENT OF NURSING

The Thiel baccalaureate nursing program is responsive to the holistic health-care needs of society. In keeping with the College's purpose to offer a value-centered liberal arts education, the nursing program prepares beginning professional nurses as generalists who demonstrate clinical competency in a variety of settings. Graduates are trained to become managers of health care and to deliver care to individuals, families, and communities.

The baccalaureate degree program is well suited to prepare graduates for the changing role of the nursing professional in the coming twenty-first century. Classes utilize the wealth of information now available through interactive media, and students are encouraged to actively develop their computer and technology interests through self-directed and faculty-supervised learning experiences.

The nursing faculty members are directly involved in the education of the students within the department. The 8 faculty members in the program are supplemented by a Nursing Learning Resource Center (NLRC) coordinator who assists them through teaching, student practice and skill validation, and recommending and procuring resource materials. All faculty members and the NLRC coordinator hold the minimum of a master's degree, with all but one having the M.S.N. degree. The director of the program and one full-time nursing faculty member have earned doctorates. No graduate students are employed by Thiel.

Currently, 65 students are enrolled in the baccalaureate nursing program. The faculty-student ratio in clinical settings varies from 1:7 to 1:9.

PROGRAM OF STUDY

The nursing curriculum is centered on the philosophies of the Department of Nursing and of Thiel College. The College's major focus is to instill in students an integrated world view or holism. Holism is the underlying theoretical base of the nursing program. It includes the realization that the whole is greater than the sum of its parts and that the part and the whole exist in a dynamic relationship. Holism considers the interrelationship of humans individually and collectively and takes into consideration the factors that affect societies as well as the world community.

Self-directed inquiry with modular learning is the primary method of instruction in the Thiel nursing program. Under the careful mentoring of the nursing faculty, student learners take the initiative to diagnose their learning needs, develop goals, identify human and material resources, choose and implement appropriate learning strategies, and evaluate their learning outcomes. Self-directed inquiry takes place in association with various kinds of facilitators, including professors, tutors, resource people, and peers. Under this model, the Thiel nursing faculty members help students to accept the responsibility for continuing learning throughout their professional careers and beyond.

There are 124 credits required for graduation in the Bachelor of Science degree program in nursing. First-year students are encouraged to build a liberal arts foundation that will prepare them for a better understanding of the world around them and set the stage for later professional courses. English composition, public speaking, chemistry, health, microbiology, psychology, sociology, and the History of Western Humanities I and II are typical first-year classes.

Science and Our Global Heritage I and II, human anatomy, human physiology, and language I and II are the liberal arts components of the second year. In this second year, students move into the clinical setting, with courses in the Fundamentals of Professional Nursing, Health Assessment, Techniques of Clinical Nursing, and Skills of Health Assessment.

By the third year of the program, nursing students are very involved in clinical experiences and nursing courses. Typical courses include psychiatric/mental health, Care of the Childbearing Family, Health and Disease in an Open System, Nursing Care of the Adult, Nursing Care of Children, and statistics as well as professional electives.

The fourth year reinforces the concept of the nursing professional's role in the management of patient care and focuses on the areas of nursing management, adult/clinical health, research methodology, and nursing in the community. This year also includes a senior seminar and special projects.

AFFILIATIONS WITH HEALTH-CARE FACILITIES

Clinical experiences are offered in cooperation with hospitals and community health facilities in Greenville, Grove City, and Farrell in Pennsylvania and in Youngstown and Warren in Ohio. Sites include Horizon Hospital System, Hillside Rehabilitation Hospital, United Community Hospital, Western Reserve Care System, the Community Counseling Center, Mercer County Area Agency on Aging, and the Greenville School system.

Students have the advantage of learning in a number of different clinical settings, which allows for a breadth of experiences and the opportunity to learn from a broad segment of the nursing professional community.

ACADEMIC FACILITIES

The Department of Nursing is headquartered in the Phillips Nursing Center at Thiel. Part of the five-level Academic Center, the nursing department houses faculty offices, classrooms, and the Nursing Learning Resource Center.

The Nursing Learning Resource Center (NLRC) is the hub of the nursing department and is utilized by nursing students at all levels. The NLRC contains three patient care units for students to practice basic nursing skills and a medication area for student practice. Housed in the NLRC is a computer testing and computer-assisted instruction area as well as a word processing section. The NLRC also provides audiovisual access and an audiovisual library that supplements classroom instruction. Individual and group study areas round out the facilities housed in the NLRC.

Nursing students are encouraged to use the Langenheim Memorial Library, which houses more than 130,000 volumes, 921 periodical titles, 7,000 microfilm reels, and 15,000 microfiche items. Thiel is also a federal government document depository for more than 213,000 federal documents.

LOCATION

Thiel College enjoys the advantages of small-town life and easy access to metropolitan Pittsburgh and Cleveland as well as the smaller cities of Erie, Pennsylvania, and Youngstown, Ohio. Greenville is a small town of nearly 10,000 people in northwestern Pennsylvania.

STUDENT SERVICES

A full range of services is available to students at Thiel. A wellness center provides many programs and exercise facilities. The student services office coordinates residence life, minority student services, intramural and intercollegiate athletics, and student government programs. The campus ministry program provides spiritual and personal advice and coordinates religious worship opportunities for students of all faiths. Referral services are available at a nearby health center for personal and psychological counseling.

The Career Services center coordinates job placement, career counseling, and cooperative/internship programs.

The Academic Resource Center provides testing, tutoring, time management, and study skills assistance for all students.

THE NURSING STUDENT GROUP

In 1995–96, 81 percent of the students enrolled in the program were women; 19 percent were men. Out of this group, 96 percent were Caucasian, 3 percent were African-American, and 1 percent were Asian-American. Fifty-seven percent of the students commuted or lived off campus, and 71 percent were younger than 24 years of age.

COSTS

Tuition for 1997–98 is $12,800. Room and board (double-occupancy residence hall room, nineteen meals per week plan) is $5200 per year. Fees and books total an additional $1000 to $1200 per year. Part-time tuition is $394 per credit hour.

FINANCIAL AID

Each student is urged to file the Free Application for Federal Student Aid (FAFSA) or renewal FAFSA each January. Thiel students may be considered for state financial aid programs and for the Federal Pell Grant, FSEOG, Federal Perkins Loan, Federal Work-Study Program, and Federal Stafford Student Loan and Federal PLUS Programs.

Academic, talent, leadership, and nursing program scholarship funds are available from Thiel in amounts up to full tuition and room and board. Special endowed funds are available to children of Lutheran clergy and children of alumni. Family grants are awarded if more than one student is enrolled at Thiel at a time.

Financial aid notification for fall classes begins in late February each year.

APPLYING

Applicants to the baccalaureate program in nursing should complete an application for admission and provide official high school and, if appropriate, college transcripts.

Admission to Thiel College is a highly personalized process, and each application is carefully reviewed by the Admissions Committee. In general, unconditionally admitted students who come to Thiel directly from high school have earned a minimum grade point average of 2.4 (on a 4.0 scale), a rank in class in the upper 60th percentile, an SAT I score of at least 920 or an ACT score of 18, and passing grades in a college prep program that includes 4 years of English, 2 years of mathematics (algebra I and II as a minimum), 2 years of laboratory science, 3 years of social science, and 2 years of a language other than English.

Additional consideration is given for teacher or counselor recommendations and for leadership or participation in school, church, or community activities. An interview prior to application is highly recommended.

Application review is on a rolling basis. Decisions are made within seven to ten days.

Correspondence and Information:

Office of Admissions
Thiel College
75 College Avenue
Greenville, Pennsylvania 16125
Telephone: 412-589-2345
800-248-4435 (toll-free)
Fax: 412-589-2013

University of Akron
College of Nursing
Akron, Ohio

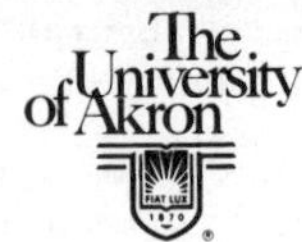

THE UNIVERSITY

The University of Akron is the forty-sixth-largest university in the nation and boasts the third-largest main campus enrollment of any public university in Ohio. The University offers a comprehensive academic package with more than 28,000 students from forty-three states and eighty-three countries enrolled in its ten colleges. The University has a long tradition of serving the needs of part-time and full-time students through day and evening classes and attracts traditional-age students and adult "new majority" students of all economic, social, and ethnic backgrounds. Committed to a diverse campus population, the University is at the forefront of all Ohio universities in recruiting and retaining minority students.

The 170-acre main campus with seventy-nine modern buildings is within walking distance of downtown Akron and is located in a metropolitan area of 1.5 million people. Joining the Mid-American Conference in 1991, the University participates in the NCAA Division I in seventeen sports.

The University comprises ten academic units: University College, Buchtel College of Arts and Sciences, Community and Technical College, College of Business Administration, College of Education, College of Engineering, College of Fine and Applied Arts, College of Nursing, Wayne College, and the nation's only College of Polymer Science and Polymer Engineering. In addition to the degree-granting Colleges, educational opportunities exist within Centers for Economic Education, Environmental Studies, Family Studies, Peace Studies, Urban Studies, and Women's Studies and Institutes for Future Studies, Biomedical Engineering Research, Life-Span Development and Gerontology, and Polymer Engineering.

The University has a Division of Continuing Education that provides lifelong educational opportunities for the northeast Ohio community. A Division of Cooperative Education provides work-study options for many students. The University Honors Program, a Weekend Program, Army ROTC, and Air Force ROTC serve the special educational needs of students. Many student organizations exist on campus including fraternities, sororities, and the marching band.

THE COLLEGE OF NURSING

Founded in 1967, the College has a long tradition of excellence. The College offers multiple educational programs designed to meet the needs of both students aspiring to become professional nurses and practicing professional nurses seeking career advancement.

Located on the campus of the University in Mary Gladwin Hall, the College offers the basic baccalaureate program (B.S.N.), an RN/B.S.N. Sequence for registered nurse graduates of associate degree and diploma programs, an LPN/B.S.N. Sequence for licensed practical nurses aspiring to become professional nurses, the Master of Science in Nursing degree (M.S.N.), and the RN/M.S.N. Sequence for registered nurse graduates of associate degree and diploma programs who meet graduate admission standards. The College is currently developing a joint Ph.D. in nursing program with Kent State University.

There are 54 full-time and 24 part-time faculty members. Twenty-one full-time faculty members (39 percent) hold doctoral degrees. The remainder have master's degrees in nursing, with many having earned advanced certification in clinical specialty areas.

The College offers clinical experiences for students in a wide variety of settings with a diverse patient population, including care of adults in hospitals, community agencies, and homes; care of well and ill elderly; care of newborns and children; care of persons with mental health problems in hospitals and community agencies; critical care; and extended care and rehabilitation.

The College is approved by the Ohio Board of Nursing and accredited by the Council of Baccalaureate and Higher Degree Programs of the National League for Nursing.

International study in nursing through a summer elective course in Norway is available.

PROGRAMS OF STUDY

The basic baccalaureate program leading to the B.S.N. degree and RN licensure is a four-year program that is balanced between nursing courses and University courses. Students enter the program after completing one year of prerequisite University courses. The nursing courses span three years, with clinical experiences in each semester of the program. The senior year features a senior practicum that is designed to give the student greater depth in an area of the student's choosing. The student-faculty ratio does not exceed 10:1.

The RN/B.S.N. Sequence has been serving the educational needs of registered nurses since 1980. The sequence features learning contracts to allow flexible hours for clinical requirements and classroom time scheduled one day per week. Once students are admitted to the College, they can complete the sequence in one calendar year. There is no testing required for admission.

The LPN/B.S.N. Sequence was begun in 1990. The College was one of the first baccalaureate programs in the country to offer a sequence for LPNs. This sequence features testing for advanced placement and credit for prior learning. The LPN can finish the baccalaureate program in four semesters if advanced placement is earned.

The master's program leading to an M.S.N. degree prepares graduates for the role of educator, administrator, or advanced practitioner. Within the advanced practice option the students may elect clinical nurse specialization in adult health, community liaison/community mental health, and gerontology; nurse anesthesia; or primary care in child and adolescent health, gerontology, and adult health, leading to practitioner certification. Each student takes a common core of courses along with advanced clinical and role preparation courses.

The RN/M.S.N. Sequence is designed for RN graduates of associate degree and diploma programs who meet graduate admission criteria. Students take three years to complete the sequence, which includes baccalaureate and master's course work. At the completion of the program, the student receives both the B.S.N. and M.S.N. degrees. This is an accelerated option for those persons whose career goals include a graduate degree.

ACADEMIC FACILITIES

The College has a state-of-the-art learning resources center that includes simulated patient care areas and a computer laboratory. The College also has a Center for Nursing, which links the

College to the community and is used by clients for health-care services and by the faculty and students as a practice and research site. The nursing library holdings are contained in the Science and Technology Library of the University. Nursing students have full access to all the facilities and services of the entire University.

LOCATION

Located in the northeast region of Ohio, Akron offers a wide variety of recreational, business, and cultural activities. The area is perfect for recreational activities that encompass all seasons. The University's presence in northeast Ohio provides numerous opportunities in major collegiate, amateur, and professional sports, concerts, cultural events, and commerce, all within easy driving distance and many accessible via public transportation. On campus, the Ohio Ballet, Emily Davis Art Gallery, University Orchestra, Opera/Musical Theatre, concerts, recitals, choral programs, Touring Arts Program, University Theatre, Repertory Dance Company, and professional artists performing at Edwin J. Thomas Performing Arts Hall contribute to the University's rich cultural environment.

Blossom Music Center, summer home of the Cleveland Orchestra, is located 20 minutes north of the campus. The city of Cleveland with all its fine recreational, sports, and cultural offerings is just 40 minutes from the University.

STUDENT SERVICES

The University has many resource and service offices to meet student needs. Campus resources include the Academic Advisement Center, Adult Resource Center, Sixty Plus Program, Chemical Abuse Resource Education Center, Placement Service and Student Employment, Career Development Service, Student Volunteer Program, Counseling and Testing Center, Financial Aid Office, Student Health Service, Black Cultural Center, Office of International Student Advising and Programming, Office of Minority Student Service, Peer Counseling Program, Service for Students with Disabilities, Campus Ministry, and writing, reading, and math developmental laboratories.

Undergraduate and graduate student organizations exist to involve students in the governance of the College. The Delta Omega chapter of Sigma Theta Tau, the international honor society of nursing, is housed within the College. The Collegiate Nursing Club, which is open to all undergraduate students, is affiliated with the National Student Nurses Association.

A campus natatorium, indoor track, and fitness rooms are all open to nursing students.

THE NURSING STUDENT GROUP

Enrollment in the undergraduate program is 550 and is 300 in the graduate program. Full-time and part-time students are represented in both programs. Postbaccalaureate students, RNs, LPNs, transfer students, and new high school graduates are represented in the College. About 25 percent of each entering class in the undergraduate program are men.

COSTS

Undergraduate tuition for the 1996–97 academic year for Ohio residents was $122.05 per credit up to 12 credits or a $1576.50 flat fee per semester for 13–16 credits. Tuition costs for nonresidents were $308.35 per credit up to 12 credits and a range of $3996.95 for 13 credits up to $4516.60 for 16 credits.

Graduate tuition costs for the 1996–97 academic year were $158.50 per credit for Ohio residents and $301.95 per credit for nonresidents.

Additional costs include housing, transportation, books, course laboratory fees, immunizations, CPR certification, uniforms, and liability insurance.

FINANCIAL AID

Financial aid is available through the University as well as the College of Nursing. The University offers a variety of scholarships, grants, loans, student assistantships, work-study opportunities, and graduate assistantships. The College offers a variety of scholarships, graduate assistantships, and Federal Graduate Nurse Traineeships.

APPLYING

Students applying for the baccalaureate program must have completed one year of prerequisite college/university courses and have earned at least a 2.5 grade point average. Applicants must be enrolled at the University of Akron for the spring semester prior to admission and are ranked according to grade point average after completion of the spring semester. Each year, 160–200 students are admitted into the undergraduate program. Course work begins in the fall.

Students applying to the LPN/B.S.N. Sequence must have completed one year of prerequisite college/university courses with a minimum grade point average of 2.5. Applicants are ranked with the basic baccalaureate students. Once admitted, students take the NLN Mobility Profile I examination to establish credit for prior learning and advanced placement. Course work begins in the summer.

Requirements for the RN/B.S.N. Sequence include completion of prerequisite courses and current Ohio RN licensure. Course work begins in the summer.

Students applying to the M.S.N. program must hold a baccalaureate degree in nursing from an NLN-accredited nursing program; complete prerequisite courses; submit scores from the GRE or Miller Analogies Test taken within the last five years, an essay, and three letters of reference; and hold a current Ohio RN license. Students enrolling in the RN/M.S.N. Sequence prepare a portfolio.

Correspondence and Information:

Office of Undergraduate Admissions
The University of Akron
Akron, Ohio 44325-2001
Telephone: 330-972-7100

Office of Graduate Admissions
Polsky Building, Room 469
The University of Akron
Akron, Ohio 44325-2101
Telephone: 330-972-7663

Financial Aid Office
Spicer Hall 119
The University of Akron
Akron, Ohio 44325-6211
Telephone: 330-972-7032

College of Nursing Information
Student Affairs Office
The University of Akron
College of Nursing
209 Carroll Street
Akron, Ohio 44325-3701
Telephone: 888-477-7887 (toll-free)

University of Alabama in Huntsville
College of Nursing
Huntsville, Alabama

THE UNIVERSITY

The University of Alabama in Huntsville (UAH), one of the three campuses comprising the University of Alabama System, became an autonomous campus in 1968 and is accredited by the Commission on Colleges of the Southern Association of Colleges and Schools to award bachelor's, master's, and doctoral degrees. Nestled in the rolling foothills of north central Alabama, Huntsville is internationally renowned for its high technology industry and its ties to the U.S. space program. UAH was one of the original group of colleges and universities to be designated a Space Grant College. UAH is the only institution offering both undergraduate and graduate nursing programs in north Alabama and is committed to becoming the regional center for research activities in nursing.

The modern 350-acre UAH campus has thirty-one major buildings, including the College of Nursing. UAH has more than 6,500 students and more than 300 full-time faculty members, 88 percent with terminal degrees. The student-faculty ratio is 10:1.

THE COLLEGE OF NURSING

The College of Nursing offers a Bachelor of Science in Nursing (B.S.N.) degree and the Master of Science in Nursing (M.S.N.) degree. The undergraduate and graduate programs are designed to give students the theoretical and experiential bases for current and future practice. The College of Nursing is accredited by the National League for Nursing and is approved by the Alabama Board of Nursing.

Although nursing is becoming highly specialized, it remains, fundamentally, a caring profession. UAH took both of these aspects into consideration when designing its curriculum in nursing. In addition to focusing on essentials of nursing in hospitals, the curriculum also emphasizes community-based practice and primary care. When the revised curriculum for the College of Nursing was submitted for approval, the Alabama Board of Nursing applauded the efforts of the UAH College of Nursing in developing an innovative and forward-looking program for preparing students to function in the rapidly changing nursing field.

The 33 faculty members in the College of Nursing place a high priority on teaching and individual attention to students. The undergraduate student-faculty ratio in clinical areas is generally less than 10:1. The professors have an ongoing concern with some of the most significant issues in nursing today, including AIDS research, nursing ethics, health care to underserved rural populations, and opportunities for nurses in space research.

PROGRAMS OF STUDY

The Bachelor of Science in Nursing (B.S.N.) degree provides the nursing theory, science, humanities, and behavioral science preparation necessary for the full scope of professional nursing responsibilities and provides the knowledge base necessary for advanced education in specialized clinical practice. Building on the foundation provided by 60 semester hours of general education requirements, the baccalaureate curriculum provides extensive clinical opportunities in the context of a holistic, family-centered, community-based approach. Computer technology is integrated throughout the curriculum. A minimum of 128 semester hours are required for the B.S.N.; 66 semester hours must be in nursing.

The UAH College of Nursing also offers a specialized B.S.N. curriculum designed for registered nurses. This program recognizes the unique abilities and needs of registered nurse students and builds on students' existing knowledge and experience. Classes for registered nurses meet only one day a week to accommodate work schedules as much as possible. This twelve-month program offers both full- and part-time attendance options. The students in the RN/B.S.N. program must also earn 128 semester hours of credit. Registered nurse students receive 30 semester hours of validated nursing credit for previous nursing knowledge and take an additional 39 semester hours of nursing at UAH.

The graduate program in nursing leads to the Master of Science in Nursing degree. This program focuses on preparation for advanced nursing practice. It prepares graduates to assume leadership roles in the direct delivery of care as nurse practitioners in primary care (family nurse practitioners) and in acute care (acute-care nurse practitioners) or in the administration of health-care delivery systems (nursing administration). The M.S.N. program can be completed in four semesters, although other options are also available for students who prefer a slower pace. Graduate courses are taught one day a week to accommodate the majority of students who continue to practice while pursuing the M.S.N. Each specialty requires 45 semester hours to earn the degree. Both thesis and nonthesis options are available. Nurse practitioner students complete 588 clinical hours; nursing administration students complete 336 clinical hours.

One of the College's newest offerings is the Post-Master's Family Nurse Practitioner program. The Post-M.S.N. FNP program is designed for individuals who have already earned a master's degree in nursing and who desire additional preparation for family nurse practitioner certification. The program is three semesters in length, and courses are taught on Saturdays. A total of 588 clinical hours are also required in the post-master's option.

ACADEMIC FACILITIES

Located in the center of the UAH main campus, the Nursing Building is a spacious, four-story structure that houses state-of-the-art equipment, lecture rooms, and laboratories for teaching nursing. The building also contains faculty and administrative offices. A Learning Resource Center, equipped with a comprehensive selection of audio-visual materials, is available to students for independent study and group learning activities. A well-equipped computer lab in the Learning Resource Center is available for use by all nursing students.

Located adjacent to the Nursing Building, the UAH library has a collection of 412,571 volumes and receives some 2,766 periodicals. The library houses both monographs and journals useful to nursing students. Students are also eligible to use the Medical Library at the University of Alabama School of Medicine–Huntsville Program, which is located in the heart of the city's medical district.

Clinical experiences are arranged in a variety of appropriate settings within the Huntsville area, which serves as a regional center for state-of-the-art health care. With three major hospitals in Huntsville and a wide variety of health-care facilities located close by, adequate resources are available to offer students a broad array of clinical nursing experiences.

LOCATION

The University is located in Huntsville, Alabama, adjacent to Cummings Research Park and close to Redstone Arsenal and NASA's Marshall Space Flight Center. A wonderful mix of modern amenities and old Southern charm, Huntsville is a regional center for arts, entertainment, industry, and medicine. Located in the foothills of the Appalachian mountain chain, Huntsville is 4 hours from Memphis and Atlanta and approximately 2 hours from Birmingham and Nashville.

STUDENT SERVICES

UAH provides a full-range of student services for all members of the student body. These services include the student counseling center, wellness center, tutorial services, academic advisement center, and office of multicultural affairs.

The College of Nursing funds and supports its own Office of Student Affairs to meet the needs of all students enrolled in the College. Located in the Nursing Building and staffed by education professionals, the Office of Student Affairs provides assistance with admissions, academic advisement and registration services, information on financial aid, and referral services.

The University also provides a rich and varied extracurricular program. There are more than 100 student clubs and organizations on campus, including dozens of honor societies, preprofessional clubs, and sororities and fraternities. Cabarets, films, dances, concerts, and lectures are offered throughout the year. In addition to a full slate of intramural activities, UAH fields varsity teams in eight sports.

THE NURSING STUDENT GROUP

The students in the College of Nursing form a diverse student body representing a wide variety of ages, ethnic backgrounds, and experiences. There are currently 280 students in the clinical component baccalaureate program and 160 students in the graduate program. In addition, there are approximately 170 students enrolled in lower-division courses and another 50 students taking graduate courses in a nondegree status, bringing total enrollment to 660.

COSTS

Tuition and fees for the 1996–97 academic year were approximately $1900 per semester for baccalaureate students. Graduate tuition and fees were approximately $2200 per semester. Uniforms, liability insurance, physical examinations, CPR certification, and Hepatitis B immunizations are required upon admission. For RN/B.S.N. students, additional expenses may include fees for "Credit by Validation."

FINANCIAL AID

Various types of financial aid are available based on scholastic performance and financial need. While some institutional scholarships are awarded solely on a student's academic record, many require demonstration of financial need. Interested students should contact the Office of Financial Aid and complete both a UAH scholarship application and the Free Application for Federal Student Aid.

Federal Professional Nurse Traineeships are available to eligible graduate students. Applications are provided to students after they accept their offer of admission. Some graduate assistantships are also available each academic year.

APPLYING

All applicants for admission to the B.S.N. degree program of the College of Nursing must complete UAH admission requirements, be admitted as regular degree-seeking students, and declare nursing as their major. Students are admitted to the upper division once a year for fall semester. Admission to the upper-division nursing major is competitive. A separate application for the upper-division nursing major must be completed on forms provided by the College of Nursing and received by March 1 preceding the fall semester for which admission is sought. All lower-division course requirements for the nursing major must be completed with a minimum grade of C prior to admission to the upper division.

RN/B.S.N. students are admitted once a year for the summer semester. Registered nurse students must submit proof of current licensure in the state of Alabama. Recent graduates of associate degree or diploma nursing programs who are not yet licensed may be admitted to complete lower-division course work, but they will not be admitted to the upper-division clinical component of the program until they are licensed. All lower-division requirements must be completed with at least a grade of C prior to admission to the RN/B.S.N. program. Deadline for applications is April 1 preceding the summer semester for which admission is sought.

M.S.N. students are admitted once a year for fall semester. The application deadline for priority consideration is April 15 preceding the fall semester for which admission is sought. Applicants must have a B.S.N. from an accredited program, a minimum GPA of 3.0, current GRE or MAT scores, three references, satisfactory completion of a basic statistics course, and an Alabama nursing licence.

Post-master's students are admitted once a year for spring semester. The application deadline is November 1. Applicants must have an M.S.N., credit for graduate-level health assessment and pathophysiology, two references, and completed an applicant's statement.

Prior to admission to any program, students are advised through the College of Nursing Office of Student Affairs. All interested students should contact the Office of Student Affairs for detailed program information, admission requirements, and application deadlines.

Correspondence and Information:

Office of Student Affairs
NB 207
UAH College of Nursing
Huntsville, Alabama 35899
Telephone: 205-890-6742
Fax: 205-890-6026
E-mail: magathm@email.uah.edu

University of Alberta
Faculty of Nursing
Edmonton, Alberta

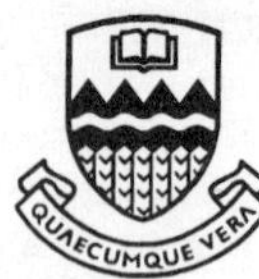

THE UNIVERSITY

The University of Alberta (U of A) is Canada's fourth-largest university. Founded in 1908 in Edmonton, the capital of the province of Alberta, the U of A is a national leader in research and teaching. It is a publicly funded, nondenominational, coeducational institution. In 1996, enrollment stood at more than 29,000 students, academic staff numbered 2,226, and support staff totaled 2,791. Besides the Faculty of Nursing (FON), other health science faculties at the U of A include Medicine and Oral Health, Pharmacy and Pharmaceutical Sciences, Physical Education and Recreation, and Rehabilitation Medicine. The Walter C. Mackenzie Health Sciences Centre, an acute-care teaching hospital with approximately 550 beds, is affiliated with the U of A. The U of A is also home to the Alberta Centre for Well-Being, Centre for Gerontology, Health Law Institute, Healthcare Quality and Outcomes Research Centre, Perinatal Research Centre, and Bioethics Centre.

THE FACULTY OF NURSING

The FON, established in 1923, has a noteworthy history. It offered the first graduate nursing program in Alberta in 1975 and Canada's first funded Ph.D. program in nursing in 1991. Also in 1991, the FON established a successful baccalaureate program in collaboration with four nursing diploma programs in northern Alberta. Each of the U of A's collaborative partners (Grande Prairie Regional College, Grande Prairie; Grant MacEwan Community College, Edmonton; Keyano College, Fort McMurray; and Red Deer Community College, Red Deer) delivers a common curriculum to students.

Through the teaching, research, and public service activities of faculty members, the FON strives to fulfill its mission to be a centre of excellence for the advancement, dissemination, and application of nursing knowledge. Its faculty members are among the best prepared in Canada; a greater percentage have doctoral degrees than at any other Canadian nursing school. Students learn through a variety of mediums, including lectures and seminars, clinical and laboratory experiences, and computer-assisted learning.

The Substance Abusology Research Unit, the Institute for Philosophical Nursing Research, the TELEHEALTH Centre (providing consultation through telemetry equipment that allows the transmission of diagnostic measurements, audio, and video between distant sites), and the FON Health Centre (serving several client groups and fully equipped with examination rooms and demonstration labs) are all located within the FON.

PROGRAMS OF STUDY

The aim of the undergraduate program is to prepare professional nurses who are able to provide and coordinate high-quality care to individuals, families, groups, and communities in many settings. The program provides the necessary background for the national licensure examinations for registered nurses (RNs). In the four-year B.Sc.N. program, context-based learning is the method of instruction. Students, working in small groups with a tutor, explore a series of scenarios that integrate content from nursing, physical sciences, medical sciences, social sciences, and humanities. Each scenario is designed as a narrative that provides information about a patient, his or her life situation, and various health issues or problems, which the group, using academic, laboratory, and clinical resources, works together to understand. Clinical experience in a variety of settings is included in each term of the program. Opportunities for international clinical experiences are available in a number of countries. A two-year Post-RN degree program designed for graduates of diploma nursing programs and a two-year RPN (Registered Psychiatric Nurse) to B.Sc.N. program for graduates from psychiatric nursing programs are also offered.

The two-year Master of Nursing program aims to prepare nurses to function as advanced-level practitioners in acute, community, and continuing health-care settings. Students may choose a thesis or a course-based (nonthesis) route to complete their M.N. Qualified students may be able to accelerate into the Ph.D. program. Students may enroll on a full- or part-time basis.

The goal of the Ph.D. program is to prepare nurses for leadership roles in practice, education, and research and to advance nursing knowledge through identification of issues and the development and testing of theory. The courses vary in number and type according to the student's academic background, experience, and career goals. All doctoral students must complete a dissertation. Two academic years must be served in full-time residency, and students must complete the program within six years. The possibility of offering a flexible Ph.D. program for those residing outside of Edmonton is currently being explored.

ACADEMIC FACILITIES

The U of A houses one of the largest library collections in Canada. The library has an on-line system that enables students to perform literature searches using a variety of commercial databases. The John Scott Health Sciences Library is connected to the FON by a walkway and provides ample study space for undergraduate students. Individual study and research space is available for graduate students.

A well-equipped student computer lab is located in the FON. The FON also has state-of-the-art videoconferencing equipment, used for distance education and communication purposes. Simulated clinical settings are available for learning and practising health assessment and other nursing skills.

LOCATION

Edmonton is a dynamic city with approximately 700,000 residents. Cultural festivals, professional sports and University athletic events, fine restaurants, riverfront parks and walkways, theatres, concerts, museums, and art galleries are among Edmonton's diverse entertainment opportunities. A visit to West Edmonton Mall, the world's largest indoor shopping mall, is a must. Edmonton has an excellent public transportation system, and the Edmonton International Airport offers flights throughout the world. Edmonton has cold, but sunshine-filled, winters and pleasant summers. It is located a few hours' drive from Banff and Jasper National Parks, which offer excellent skiing in winter and hiking and sightseeing in summer.

STUDENT SERVICES

Student services include Career and Placement Services, the International Centre, Native Student Services, Personal and Academic Resources, Services for Students with Disabilities, the Sexual Assault Centre, Student Counselling Services, Student Financial Aid and Information Centre, University Health Services, and several bookstores. Housing is available for 2,600 on campus, with additional units available for families. The Van Vliet Physical Education and Recreation Centre is one of the best-equipped recreational facilities in Canada.

THE NURSING STUDENT GROUP

The undergraduate population of more than 1,000 is a diverse group in terms of ethnicity, age, and gender; about 75 percent are full-time. The graduate program has approximately 120 M.N. students and 30 Ph.D. students; 60 percent are full-time.

COSTS

Tuition fees for a full course load in 1996–97 differed by program and year but ranged from Can$2500 to Can$3700. Students who are not Canadian citizens or permanent residents must pay an additional 100 percent of tuition fees. The cost of books and supplies per year is approximately Can$800. Cost of living, including room and board, transportation, insurance, and other living expenses, is estimated at Can$12,000 per year.

FINANCIAL AID

Financial aid programs include employment opportunities and national, provincial, and institutionally sponsored loans, scholarships, awards, and grants. Graduate students are also eligible for research and travel grants, fellowships, and teaching and research assistantships.

APPLYING

For detailed information about requirements, deadlines, and application procedures for each specific program, students should contact the appropriate office by mail, phone, fax, or e-mail as listed below.

Correspondence and Information:

Office of the Associate Dean, Undergraduate Education
3rd Floor Clinical Sciences Building
Faculty of Nursing, University of Alberta
Edmonton, Alberta T6G 2G3
Canada
Telephone: 403-492-8089
Fax: 403-492-2551
E-mail: leona.laird@ualberta.ca

Office of the Associate Dean, Graduate Education
3rd Floor Clinical Sciences Building
Faculty of Nursing, University of Alberta
Edmonton, Alberta T6G 2G3
Canada
Telephone: 403-492-6251
Fax: 403-492-2551
E-mail: elaine.carswell@ualberta.ca

THE FACULTY

Professors

M. Allen, Ph.D., Case Western Reserve, 1985. Visual impairment.
V. Bergum, Ph.D., Alberta, 1986. Ethics, women's health.
P. J. Brink, Ph.D., Boston, 1969. Transcultural nursing.
T. Davis, Ph.D., Alberta, 1977. Depressive/anxiety disorders.
R. A. Day, Ph.D., Alberta, 1986. Computer instruction, psychomotor skills.
M. R. Elliott, Ph.D., Simon Fraser, 1987. Family/child nursing.
P. Giovannetti, Sc.D., Johns Hopkins, 1981. Quality of care, research methods.
M. J. Harrison, Ph.D., Alberta, 1987. Social support, family nursing.
J. M. Hibberd, Ph.D., Alberta, 1986. Nursing administration.
J. F. Kikuchi, Ph.D., Pittsburgh, 1979. Nursing philosophy, maternal-child nursing.
J. A. Lander, Associate Dean of Research; Ph.D., Manitoba, 1981. Pain, research methods.
J. Morse, Ph.D., Utah, 1981. Qualitative health research methodologies.
A. Neufeld, Ph.D., Saskatchewan, 1987. Community health, gerontology.
A. M. Pagliaro, M.S.N., California, San Francisco, 1976. Nursing history, substance abuse.
J. C. Ross Kerr, Ph.D., Michigan, 1978. Gerontology, history of nursing.
M. Wood, Dean; Dr.P.H., UCLA, 1971. Gerontology.
O. Yonge, Ph.D., Alberta, 1994. Mental health.

Associate Professors

A. M. Anderson, Ph.D., Utah, 1993. Community/family nursing.
L. Douglass, Ph.D., Arizona, 1990. Oncology.
E. J. Drummond, Ph.D., British Columbia, 1992. Infant colic, family health.
P. Hayes, M.H.S.A., Alberta, 1974. Risk perception, nursing theories.
L. A. Jensen, Ph.D., Alberta, 1989. Theories of health and illness, cardiovascular nursing.
J. Norris, Ph.D. candidate, Toronto. Distance education, educational computer-mediated communication.
B. A. C. O'Brien, D.N.S., Rush, 1990. Maternal-child nursing, midwifery.
J. K. Olson, Ph.D., Wayne State, 1993. Community health.
L. I. Reutter, Ph.D., Alberta, 1991. Remarried families, community health nursing.
S. L. Richardson, Ph.D., Alberta, 1988. Nursing history, public policy analysis.
C. Ross, Ph.D., Alberta, 1993. Coping strategies.
D. L. Skillen, Ph.D., Alberta, 1992. Computer-managed instruction.
V. Strang, Ph.D., Alberta, 1991. Community health.
P. Valentine, Ph.D., Alberta, 1988. Mental health, feminism.

Assistant Professors

M. C. Anderson, Ph.D., Alberta, 1993. Gerontology, computer-managed instruction.
W. J. Austin, M.Ed., Alberta, 1986. Counselling.
J. Boman, M.A., Alberta, 1982. Community development.
G. Boschma, Ph.D. candidate, Pennsylvania. History of nursing.
B. Cameron, M.Sc.N., Wales, 1988. Medical-surgical nursing.
E. M. Jackson, Ph.D., Missouri, 1991. Gender differences, mental health and community.
P. Koop, Ph.D., Alberta, 1994. Family theory, stress and coping.
C. Newburn-Cook, Ph.D., British Columbia, 1995. Research methods, epidemiology.
L. D. Ogilvie, Ph.D., Alberta, 1993. Children with respiratory problems, international/intercultural nursing.
P. Paul, Ph.D., Alberta, 1994. Nursing history, orthopaedics.
K. Peters, Ph.D., Washington (Seattle), 1995. Infant responses to the NICU environment.
L. Ray, Ph.D. candidate, Washington (Seattle). Children with chronic health challenges.
M. A. Wales, M.S.N., British Columbia, 1983. Computer-managed instruction, cardiovascular nursing.
D. Williamson, Ph.D., Alberta, 1995. Poverty status, health behavior, and health.
D. Wilson, Ph.D., Alberta, 1993. Gerontology, tube-feeding.

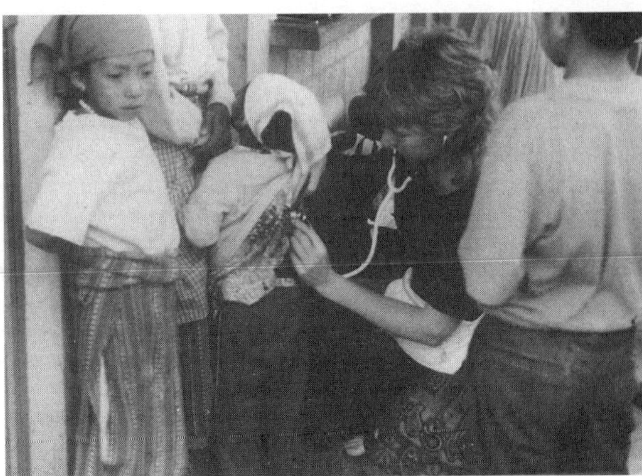

A small child's health is assessed by a University of Alberta nursing student in a clinic in rural Guatemala.

University of Arizona
College of Nursing
Tucson, Arizona

THE UNIVERSITY

The University of Arizona is among the nation's top twenty public research institutions. Established in 1885, it is the oldest university in Arizona, with a student enrollment of nearly 35,000. The University of Arizona is a Research I educational institution that offers graduate programs in more than 100 departments and fields. Doctoral degrees are offered in eighty-four fields, including nursing. The excellence of graduate education and research at the University of Arizona is reflected in its funding record. In fiscal year 1996, $169,612,202 was competitively awarded to the University of Arizona from the federal government. Additional funds from foundations, grants, and contracts from private industry yielded more than $268 million awarded to the University.

The College is a component of the Arizona Health Sciences Center, known nationally for its contributions to health care and research. The Arizona Health Sciences Center includes the University of Arizona Colleges of Medicine, Pharmacy, and Nursing; the School of Health Professions; University Medical Center; and the University Physicians. The Arizona Health Sciences Center and the University of Arizona have a number of strong interdisciplinary programs, including neuroscience, gerontology, public health, and rural health.

THE COLLEGE OF NURSING

The University of Arizona College of Nursing was ranked sixth of 491 nursing programs in the United States and is accredited by the National League for Nursing. In 1996, extramural funds awarded to the College of Nursing totaled $2 million. In 1995 it was listed among the top ten graduate programs in the United States in *U.S. News & World Report.* The mission of the College is to generate and expand the knowledge base of nursing through the education of practitioners, the development and testing of knowledge, and service to the community. The College offers a Bachelor of Science in Nursing degree for generic students, second-degree students, and RN-completion students. In conjunction with the University of Arizona Graduate College, it also offers a Master of Science (M.S.) degree with a major in nursing and a Doctor of Philosophy (Ph.D.) degree with a major in nursing. A minor in clinical nursing research at the doctoral level and opportunities for postdoctoral work in nursing are also offered by the College.

The College of Nursing faculty is diverse in clinical and research expertise. The approximately 65 faculty members are highly qualified and productive. The College maintains both tenure and clinical tracks for the faculty. Tenure-track faculty members are recognized within the University and nationally for their leadership in nursing education and research. The faculty is strongly committed to research and scholarship. Approximately 65 percent of the tenure-track faculty members are recipients of extramural funding. Twenty College of Nursing faculty or adjunct faculty members are members of the American Academy of Nursing. The clinical-track faculty focuses on clinical teaching, clinical scholarship, and professional service. A number of clinical-track faculty members are certified either as specialists in their area of clinical expertise or as nurse practitioners.

The student body is diverse, and College of Nursing students continue to distinguish themselves within the College and University. All students are encouraged to participate fully in the University community. In addition, graduate students are mentored to present research at local, regional, and national meetings and to publish. Doctoral students are encouraged to and assisted to apply for National Research Service Awards through the National Institutes of Health. After graduation, employment opportunities for graduate students in academia and service throughout the world are many.

PROGRAMS OF STUDY

The 129-credit baccalaureate program comprises three semesters of prenursing courses and five semesters of the professional nursing major. General education courses are required in each year. Students who meet University admission requirements are admitted to the College of Arts and Sciences for the prenursing general education portion of the nursing program.

Those who elect to complete a Master of Science degree, which requires a thesis, may select from four options. The Nurse Case Management option is designed to provide advanced nursing preparation and the skills needed to perform as a nurse case manager. The didactic course content of the Nurse Case Management option is applicable to the care of a variety of clients in a variety of settings. Assignments within the courses and clinical experiences allow students to develop unique skills and abilities in the role of nurse case manager, according to individual goals and interests. The Systems Management option is designed to prepare nurses with advanced preparation to use clinical knowledge; knowledge of health policies, regulations, and standards; knowledge of data management, manipulation, analysis, and interpretation; and clinical and cost data to plan, administer, and evaluate a variety of institutional programs. Systems managers are able to assess and analyze clinical situations and organizations, conduct program evaluations, and use research findings and technology to formulate decisions in areas such as case-mix/staff-mix, patient acuity, information management and transfer, and organizational restructuring/renewal. The role blends evaluation and analysis skills with knowledge about computer technologies and nursing. The M.S./M.B.A. option prepares students to identify and formulate business problems, specify and locate the information needed to solve them, and develop and implement practical solutions. These are the keys to success in business and health-care organizations. The Nurse Practitioner option is designed to provide nurses with advanced preparation to function as adult nurse practitioners (ANP), family nurse practitioners (FNP), geriatric nurse practitioners (GNP), or psychiatric–mental health nurse practitioners (P-MH-NP). Each of these focuses on health assessment, primary prevention, health maintenance, clinical decision making, and illness management.

Those who receive a doctoral degree at the University of Arizona College of Nursing are scholars and clinical nurse researchers. The doctoral curriculum is planned as a four-year postbaccalaureate program. Course work in nursing and the sciences occupies a major portion of the first two years of study. During the last two years, the student's time is increasingly devoted to research under the supervision of a faculty researcher. All requirements of the Graduate College with respect to admission, examinations, residency, major and minor fields, and dissertation are followed.

Students may enter the Ph.D. level in two ways. First, they may enter directly from the master's level of the graduate program at the University of Arizona College of Nursing. Second, applicants who have a master's degree with a major in nursing earned at another institution may be admitted. Course content deals with metatheoretical issues, theory development, middle-range nursing theory, clinical nursing research, and advanced content in the clinical area of the student's choice. Three credits of graduate-level social science and 3 credits of graduate level human physiology are prerequisite to the doctoral level of study.

Dissertation topics and substantive clinical courses closely follow the strengths and active funding of the College of Nursing research faculty. As a consequence, special emphasis is given to prevention and management of chronic conditions, nursing systems, and community-based interventions. Students may choose a minor area of study from the behavioral or biological sciences, including anthropology, philosophy, physiology, psychology, management and policy, and sociology. In addition to a major in nursing, students enrolled in a variety of other doctoral programs at the University of Arizona may select clinical nursing research as a doctoral minor.

A variety of opportunities for postdoctoral education are available. There can be a special emphasis at the postdoctoral level on clinical nursing research methodologies, including instrumentation.

AFFILIATIONS WITH HEALTH-CARE FACILITIES

There are over 100 clinical facilities throughout the city of Tucson and surrounding areas currently available to students and faculty. The facilities include acute-care mental health and crisis centers, nursing homes, health departments, adult day health care, hospice, multidisciplinary and nurse-managed clinics, home health agencies, health maintenance organizations, physician practices, and retirement centers.

ACADEMIC FACILITIES

The University library system, which consists of three large but separate library facilities and several departmental libraries, contains almost 7 million items, including books, periodicals, microforms, maps, government publications, manuscripts, and nonbook media. The library offers reference services, on-line searching of computerized databases, and bibliographic course-related instruction.

Facilities for student learning and research in the College include an Instructional Resource Center, Patient Care Learning Center, Office of Research, Computer Laboratory, Behavioral Studies Laboratory, and Biological Studies Laboratory. A local area network allows for in-house statistical processing as well as links to the campus Ethernet.

LOCATION

The University of Arizona College of Nursing is located in Tucson, Arizona, 60 miles north of Mexico. Tucson, a city of almost 700,000 people, is located in southern Arizona's Sonoran Desert. Tucson has a rich western history and culture influenced by Native Americans and Spanish, Mexican, and American pioneers. The desert climate and wealth of educational, cultural, and recreational opportunities attract visitors and students from throughout the world, many of whom eventually relocate to this area.

STUDENT SERVICES

The University provides various services and opportunities to promote students' social and intellectual growth and physical health. These include recreational facilities, student organizations, honor societies, and student programs. There is an active student governing organization as well as specialized support and clinical services. In the College of Nursing, student organizations at the graduate and undergraduate levels are quite active.

THE NURSING STUDENT GROUP

The College of Nursing maintains an enrollment of approximately 250 at the baccalaureate level. Approximately 200 students are enrolled at the graduate level, including about 50 doctoral students. The faculty members are committed to assisting students in achieving their professional career goals, and student advising is an integral part of the educational programs for all students. The College attracts students from Arizona, other U.S. states, and many other countries.

COSTS

In 1996–97, registration fees for Arizona residents were approximately $1000 per semester for full-time study. For nonresidents, registration fees and tuition were estimated at $4189 per semester for full-time study. Living expenses for a single student were approximately $4500 per academic year.

FINANCIAL AID

The University of Arizona provides access to a range of federal, state, and privately donated financial aid funds to students through the Office of Student Financial Aid. Assistance is available to students based on financial need, academic merit, and program of study. In addition, the University of Arizona College of Nursing oversees the distribution of a variety of merit-based and need-based financial awards.

APPLYING

Students seeking admission to the undergraduate nursing program must apply for admission to the College of Arts and Sciences as a pre-nursing major. Special application is then made to the College of Nursing through the Office of Student Affairs. Students must have a grade point average of 2.75 or better to be eligible for admission. An admission grade point average above 3.0 is normally required. The number of applicants admitted is limited, and admission preference is given to Arizona residents. For admission in the fall semester, application to the College must be filed by February 1. Students requesting entry in the spring semester must file the application by August 1 of the previous year.

Nurses are considered for admission to the graduate program when they have fulfilled the general requirements for admission to the Graduate College and, in addition, have presented the following credentials for evaluation: completion of an undergraduate nursing program substantially equivalent to the baccalaureate program at the University of Arizona; current licensure to practice as a registered nurse in Arizona; references attesting to professional competence; satisfactory completion of a course in elementary statistics; Graduate Record Examinations scores: verbal, quantitative, and analytical; evidence of physical assessment skills; evidence of computer literacy; and a statement of academic and professional goals and research interests. Completed application materials must be received by March 15 for fall admission and October 1 for spring admission. For admission to the doctoral level, similar credentials are required. In addition, a personal interview is required after all credentials are available.

Correspondence and Information:

Coordinator, Undergraduate Student Affairs or
Coordinator, Graduate Student Affairs
College of Nursing
University of Arizona
P.O. Box 210203
Tucson, Arizona 85721-0203
Telephone: 520-626-6154
E-mail: info@con.nursing.arizona.edu
World Wide Web: http://www.nursing.arizona.edu

University of California, San Francisco
School of Nursing
San Francisco, California

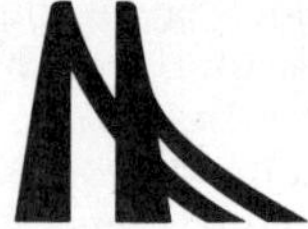

THE UNIVERSITY

The University of California, San Francisco is one of the nine campuses of the University of California and the only one devoted solely to the health sciences. Founded in 1868, it today consists of four top-ranked professional schools: Dentistry, Medicine, Nursing, and Pharmacy; a graduate program in basic and behavioral sciences; two health-policy institutes; a medical center with three hospitals; and one of the largest ambulatory-care programs in the state.

The mission of UCSF is to attract the nation's most promising students and health-care professionals to future careers in the health sciences, with continuing emphasis on open access and diversity; to bring patients the best in health-care service, from primary care to the most advanced technologies available; to encourage and support research and scholarly activities to improve the basic understanding of the mechanisms of disease and the social interactions related to human health; and to serve the community at large through educational and service programs that take advantage of the knowledge and skills of UCSF faculty and staff members and students.

THE SCHOOL OF NURSING

The nationally recognized excellence of the School of Nursing reflects a long history of innovation in nursing education. The School works cooperatively with other health professionals on campus, nationally and internationally, in its search for excellence in teaching, research, practice, and public service. The School of Nursing mission encompasses the following: preparation of students from culturally diverse backgrounds to assume leadership roles in nursing clinical practice, administration, teaching, and research; provision of education and research training in the social, behavioral, and biological sciences focused on health, illness, and health care; advancement of knowledge and theory through research; design and evaluation of the organization, financing, and delivery of health care; generation and testing of innovative professional educational models; promotion and demonstration of excellence in professional nursing practice; and benefiting the public, the profession, and the University through active individual and group involvement in service activities.

The School is composed of four departments of instruction and research: the Department of Family Health Care Nursing; Department of Community Health Systems; Department of Physiological Nursing; and the Department of Social and Behavioral Sciences which, together, offer seventeen areas of specialization. In addition, the Institute for Health and Aging, an organized research unit, focuses on policy research.

A wide range of nursing specialties are offered, including pediatric advanced practice nursing, perinatal clinical nurse specialist, nurse midwifery, family nurse practitioner, adult psychiatric–mental health clinical nurse specialist and nurse practitioner, community-based care systems, adult nurse practitioner, occupational health nurse practitioner and occupational health nurse administrator, cardiovascular clinical nurse specialist, critical care–trauma clinical nurse specialist, gerontological nurse practitioner and clinical nurse specialist, nurse anesthetist, and oncology clinical nurse specialist.

PROGRAMS OF STUDY

The UCSF School of Nursing offers the Master of Science (M.S.) and Ph.D. degrees for those with a nursing background. All applicable programs are accredited by the National League for Nursing.

The Master of Science program prepares leaders in the advanced practice roles of clinical nurse specialist, nurse practitioner, nurse-midwife, nurse-anesthetist, administrator, teacher, and consultant. Courses from nursing and other disciplines provide advanced theoretical knowledge, assessment skills, role/leadership development, advanced clinical practice in a selected specialization, and opportunity to critique and apply nursing theory and research as a scientific base for nursing practice. The program is typically completed in two academic years, usually consisting of two to three days per week in classes and clinical work.

The Doctor of Philosophy in nursing (Ph.D.) program prepares scientists to conduct research in nursing and to contribute to the body of knowledge in nursing. Graduates of this program focus their careers on generating the knowledge base of the nursing discipline through positions as academic or clinical researchers. The curriculum is built around three core areas: research, nursing science, and theory development.

AFFILIATIONS WITH HEALTH-CARE FACILITIES

The School of Nursing is affiliated with a wide variety of clinical resources, including UCSF Medical Center, San Francisco General Hospital Medical Center, San Francisco Veterans Affairs Medical Center, and many others throughout the state. Students are placed in tertiary care or primary care agencies appropriate to the chosen area of specialization.

ACADEMIC FACILITIES

The UCSF library, one of the world's preeminent health sciences libraries, supports the teaching, research, patient care, and community service programs of the UCSF campus. A rapidly expanding training program supports the use of technology in managing information. The library schedules more than thirty seminars each quarter, ranging from instruction on how to use the MEDLINE database and other on-line catalogs to presentations of file management software and computer networks. Through its instructional resources facility, the library works with faculty members who choose to supplement their course work with computer software, videotapes, and other nonprint resources.

The School of Nursing building provides research, office, and classroom space for the nursing faculty and students. There are student lounges, and seminar and study rooms, as well as laboratories for computer self-instruction, human subjects research and observation, and skills development. The Learning Resources Center (LRC) has resource materials for both students and faculty to assist in assignments, research, and publication. References and study materials on nursing practice, administration, research, and education are available, as well as an extensive collection of nursing journals, texts, and audiovisuals. Classes and tutorials on information retrieval, writing skills, and computer applications in nursing are also offered through the LRC.

LOCATION

The UCSF campus is located high on a hill overlooking the Pacific Ocean, the Golden Gate Bridge, and San Francisco Bay.

Golden Gate Park is a short walk from the campus, and Ocean Beach is within easy reach by bus, streetcar, automobile, or bike. The city of San Francisco is noted for its physical beauty, cultural attractions, fine restaurants, and cosmopolitan atmosphere.

STUDENT SERVICES

The University has many resources and service offices to meet student needs. These include the Marilyn Reed Lucia Child Care Study Center; the Student Health Service; a legal assistance clinic; a student placement office; offices providing services to international students and scholars and to students with disabilities; and the Guy S. Millberry Union, which houses a conference center, a fitness center, a housing office, restaurants, and the Millberry Union Bookstore.

THE NURSING STUDENT GROUP

The Master of Science program enrolls approximately 350 students. The doctoral program in nursing enrolls approximately 100. The majority of students attend school full-time and work part-time.

COSTS

Educational and registration fees for the 1996–97 academic year were $5800 for California residents and $14,200 for nonresidents. Living expenses for a single student were approximately $1100 per month.

FINANCIAL AID

The San Francisco campus administers several financial aid programs offering loans, scholarships, grants, and work-study programs. Funds are awarded to students who demonstrate need. In addition, the School of Nursing oversees the distribution of Professional Nurse Traineeships and a variety of need-based and merit-based scholarships.

APPLYING

Admission requirements for the Master of Science program include a baccalaureate degree from an NLN-accredited program in nursing or its equivalent, licensure or eligibility for licensure as a registered nurse in California, completion of an introductory course in statistics, completion of the Graduate Record Examinations (GRE) General Test, and evidence of personal qualification and capacity for graduate study as reflected in the application.

Admission requirements for the Doctor of Philosophy in nursing program include a B.S.N. or M.S. from an NLN-accredited college or university with an undergraduate GPA of 3.2 or graduate GPA of 3.5 or higher, completion of the GRE, a statistics course, an introductory research course, evidence of capacity for original scholarship and research, congruence of the applicant's goals with the program's goals, evidence of ability to communicate in a scholarly manner, licensure as a registered nurse, and a minimum of one year of professional nursing experience.

Correspondence and Information:

Office of Student Affairs
School of Nursing
University of California
San Francisco, California 94143-0602
Telephone: 415-476-1435

THE FACULTY

The following is only a partial listing of the faculty (tenured and tenure-track).

Patricia Benner, Professor, Ph.D., RN, FAAN.
Virginia Carrieri-Kohlman, Professor, D.N.S., RN.
Linda Chafetz, Associate Professor, D.N.S., RN.
Catherine Chesla, Assistant Professor, D.N.S., RN.
Adele Clarke, Associate Professor, Ph.D.
Anne Davis, Professor, Ph.D., RN, FAAN.
Jeanne De Joseph, Associate Professor, Ph.D., RN, FAAN.
Marylin Dodd, Professor, Ph.D., RN, FAAN.
Barbara Drew, Assistant Professor, Ph.D., RN.
Marguerite Engler, Associate Professor, Ph.D., RN.
Mary Engler, Assistant Professor, Ph.D., RN.
Carroll Estes, Professor, Ph.D.
Julia Faucett, Assistant Professor, Ph.D., RN.
Erika Froelicher, Professor, Ph.D., RN, FAAN.
Catherine Gilliss, Professor, D.N.S., RN, FAAN.
Nanny Green, Assistant Professor, Ph.D., RN.
Charlene Harrington, Professor, Ph.D., RN, FAAN.
Suzanne Henry, Assistant Professor, D.N.S., RN.
William Holzemer, Professor, Ph.D., RN, FAAN.
Susan Janson, Professor, D.N.S., RN, FAAN.
Virgene Kayser-Jones, Professor, Ph.D., RN, FAAN.
Christine Kennedy, Assistant Professor, M.S.N, RN.
Patricia Larson, Associate Professor, D.N.S., RN, FAAN.
Kathryn Lee, Associate Professor, Ph.D., RN.
Juliene Lipson, Associate Professor, Ph.D., RN, FAAN.
Afaf Meleis, Professor, Ph.D., RN, FAAN.
Christine Miaskowski, Associate Professor, Ph.D., RN, FAAN.
Robert Newcomer, Professor, Ph.D.
Jane Norbeck, Professor, D.N.S., RN, FAAN.
Carmen Portillo, Assistant Professor, Ph.D., RN.
Kathleen Puntillo, Acting Assistant Professor, D.N.S., RN.
Laura Reif, Associate Professor, Ph.D., RN.
Marilyn Savedra, Professor, D.N.S., RN, FAAN.
Nancy Stotts, Associate Professor, Ed.D., RN.
Diana Taylor, Assistant Professor, Ph.D., RN, FAAN.
Margaret Wallhagen, Assistant Professor, Ph.D., RN.
Sandra Weiss, Professor, D.N.S., Ph.D., RN, FAAN.
Mary White, Assistant Professor, Ph.D., RN.
Holly Wilson, Professor, Ph.D., RN, FAAN.

University of Cincinnati
College of Nursing and Health
Cincinnati, Ohio

THE UNIVERSITY

The University of Cincinnati, founded in 1879, is a multifaceted learning and research center. As a large, urban, state university it represents a diverse community with many opportunities. The University's mission is to function as a model for freedom of intellectual exchange and to provide the highest quality learning environment, world-renowned scholarship, and innovation. The University's campus features the best of both worlds—it is large enough to offer vast educational opportunities, yet small enough to feel cozy.

THE COLLEGE OF NURSING AND HEALTH

The College of Nursing and Health has a long history of excellence in nursing education. In 1916 it became one of the first two baccalaureate programs in nursing in the United States. In addition to the Bachelor of Science in Nursing (B.S.N.), the College offers Master of Science in Nursing (M.S.N.) and Doctor of Philosophy (Ph.D.) in nursing programs. The College prepares beginning and advanced practitioners of professional nursing to function in a variety of settings with diverse populations; provides opportunities for advancing nursing science; educates practicing nurses to maintain, improve, and expand their competencies; and provides services and expertise to health-care consumers.

The College is an integral part of the University and its Medical Center. Cooperative relations among the units of the University, a myriad of health-care settings, and the diversity of the greater Cincinnati community facilitate creative approaches for leadership and excellence in nursing. Some of the College's unique endeavors include a Wellness Center in the Cincinnati Public Schools and a nursing clinic that provides comprehensive services for underserved populations. In addition, the College is a World Health Organization Collaborating Center Affiliate.

The Institute for Nursing Research, a collaborative effort with Patient Care Services at University Hospital, fosters research on phenomena of interest to the nursing profession using both interdisciplinary and multidisciplinary approaches. The institute houses a Center of Gerontological Nursing Excellence and a Center for Addiction. Services of the institute include expert consultation on various aspects of grant proposal preparation, secretarial and graduate assistant support, and help in the preparation of presentations.

PROGRAMS OF STUDY

The College offers several options for those wishing to earn a B.S.N. The options include a traditional track, RN/B.S.N. and RN/M.S.N. tracks, and an accelerated track for individuals holding baccalaureate degrees in other fields who wish to pursue an M.S.N. degree. The B.S.N. curriculum provides a foundation for community-focused professional practice with individuals and families having a variety of health-care needs. Emphasis is placed on clinical competence in multiple environments of care, critical thinking, professional roles, participation in multidisciplinary teams, and a commitment to continued learning. Full- or part-time study is possible.

The master's program in designed to prepare nurses for advanced practice. The M.S.N. degree requires 60–80 quarter credits, depending upon the student's area of specialization and goals. The curriculum consists of a set of core courses plus courses in the student's selected area of clinical focus. A scholarly project is required for degree completion. Full- and part-time options are available for most majors. Specialization is offered in adult health (with acute and chronic care options), community health, genetics, occupational health, and psychiatric nursing; nurse anesthesia; nurse midwifery; nursing service administration; and family, neonatal, and pediatric nurse practitioner studies. An M.S.N./M.B.A. option in conjunction with the College of Business Administration is also offered.

The doctoral program focuses on the preparation of nurses for positions of leadership in academic and health services institutions and health policy agencies. The curriculum is designed with a core of required courses and a cognate area of the student's choosing to support preparation for research in a defined area. Students may enter the doctoral program upon completion of a B.S.N. or M.S.N. degree. Doctoral students are required to be in residence for full-time study during three of five consecutive quarters, excluding those for a dissertation.

AFFILIATIONS WITH HEALTH-CARE FACILITIES

The Medical Center and main University campuses are contiguous. Units in the Medical Center in addition to the College of Nursing and Health include the University Hospital, the Colleges of Pharmacy and Medicine, and the Center for Health Related Programs. Some affiliated institutions adjacent to the Medical Center are the Veterans Affairs Medical Center, the Cincinnati Children's Hospital Medical Center, the Shriners Burns Institute, the Cincinnati Center for Developmental Disorders, and the Cincinnati Health Department. The College affiliates with multiple hospitals, home care services, community agencies, and health service providers. Cooperative relationships provide rich educational, clinical, and research resources.

ACADEMIC FACILITIES

The College is a unit in a Class I research institution and therefore has multiple academic resources. The resources include libraries, computer services, multiple teaching methods, and research support.

The College's Solomon P. Levi Library affords connection to all the University libraries and OhioLINK, the statewide on-line catalogue. These connections provide students with access to the second-largest library system in the country. The system is accessible via home computer. The College's library is one of the best nursing libraries and houses more than 300 journals relevant to nursing.

Computer resources within the College and University are also plentiful. The College has an equipped classroom for interactive television, with multiple off-campus sites and computer connections in all large classrooms. The Learning Resource Center provides a laboratory setting that supports student learning through services such as interactive video and computer-assisted instruction, a staffed computer workroom, audiovisual materials, and clinical practice laboratories.

LOCATION

The University is only 10 minutes from downtown Cincinnati, so students can easily benefit from city activities. The city is big enough to have nationally renowned arts organizations and major-league sports, yet small enough to take pride in its neighborhood cafés and scenic parks. Cincinnati is known for its restaurants, riverfront recreation areas, and festivals such as

Oktoberfest and the Appalachian Fair. Cincinnati is accessible by various modes of transportation and is the hub of a network of interstate highways.

STUDENT SERVICES
Education does not stop at the academic doors. The University is a place where students are continually learning, sharing, and growing. Students may choose to live in residence halls or take part in a variety of clubs. Diversity is an important part of the University community, with a variety of ethnic organizations, services, and events. Students take part in intramural sports, attend College Conservatory of Music concerts and plays, or sometimes just hang out.

THE NURSING STUDENT GROUP
The students in all programs in the College of Nursing and Health represent diverse backgrounds in age, gender, ethnicity, nationality, and experience. The undergraduate program enrollment comprises approximately 650 students, about a third of whom are registered nurses returning for baccalaureate degrees. The master's program enrollment averages 250 students, about 45 percent of whom are enrolled full-time. The doctoral program enrollment is 42 students, two thirds of whom are enrolled full-time. Graduates of the College are sought by local, state, and national employers.

COSTS
Tuition for the 1996–97 three-quarter academic year was $4152 (undergraduate) and $5445 (graduate) for full-time Ohio residents. Full-time, nonresident student tuition was $10,464 (undergraduate) and $10,383 (graduate) per year. Tuition per credit hour was $115 (undergraduate, Ohio resident), $290 (undergraduate, nonresident), $182 (graduate, Ohio resident) and $347 (graduate, nonresident). Fees and other expenses such as health insurance and parking (but excluding housing) range from $90 to $900, depending on the student's status.

University housing costs average $5100 per year for residence hall room and board and $383 to $534 per month for apartments. For those who wish to live off campus, Cincinnati offers reasonable, suitable housing for rent.

FINANCIAL AID
Financial assistance for students derives from a variety of sources such as University scholarships, low-interest loans, University Graduate Assistantships, and Professional Nurse Traineeship funds. Scholarships, assistantships, and traineeships are awarded on a competitive basis.

APPLYING
Applicants to all programs should present appropriate application forms, transcripts, recommendations, and testing information as described in the *College of Nursing and Health Bulletin.* Applicants seeking priority consideration for admission should apply no later than January 1. Acceptance of applicants after this date depends upon the space available. Applicants are encouraged to contact the Office of Student Affairs with questions.

Correspondence and Information:

Office of Student Affairs
College of Nursing and Health
University of Cincinnati
P.O. Box 210038
Cincinnati, Ohio 45221-0038
Telephone: 513-558-3600
Fax: 513-558-7523
E-mail: cnhsa@uc.edu
World Wide Web: http://www.uc.edu/www/nursing

THE FACULTY
Jo-Ann Bryson Adelsperger, Assistant Professor, Ed.D.
Linda Baas, Assistant Professor, Ph.D.
Elizabeth Betemps, Assistant Professor, Ph.D.
Ruth M. Bunyan, Professor, Ed.D.
Helen Clark, Associate Professor, Ph.D.
Doris B. Clement-Burton, Assistant Professor, Ed.D.
Karen D'Apolito, Assistant Professor, Ph.D.
Linda Sue Davis, Associate Professor, Ph.D.
Carol Deets, Professor, Ed.D.
Carolyn DeVore, Assistant Professor, Ph.D.
Kathleen Driscoll, Associate Professor, J.D.
Maureen Dwyer, Assistant Professor, D.N.Sc.
Janice Dyehouse, Professor, Ph.D.
Lou Ann Emerson, Associate Professor, D.N.S.
Dianne Felblinger, Associate Professor, Ed.D.
Evelyn Fitzwater, Associate Professor of Clinical Nursing, Ph.D.
Joyce Fontana, Assistant Professor, Ph.D.
Donna Gates, Assistant Professor, Ed.D.
Barbara Gilman, Assistant Professor, M.N.S.
Marcia Hern, Associate Professor, Ed.D.
Phyllis W. Juett, Assistant Professor, M.S.N.
Carole Kenner, Professor, D.N.S.
Susan Kennerly, Associate Professor, Ph.D.
Linda LaCharity, Instructor, Ph.D.
Adrianne Lane, Assistant Professor, Ed.D.
Andrea R. Lindell, Schmidlapp Professor, D.N.Sc.
Mary Ann Madewell, Assistant Professor of Clinical Nursing, D.N.S.
Madeleine T. Martin, Professor, Ed.D.
Ann McCracken, Professor, Ph.D.
Elaine Miller, Professor, D.N.S.
Margaret Miller, Associate Professor, Ed.D.
Amy Pettigrew, Associate Professor, D.N.S.
Cornelia Ragiel, Associate Professor, Ed.D.
Fay Carol Reed, Associate Professor, Ph.D.
Jo Ann Ruiz-Bueno, Associate Professor of Clinical Nursing, Ph.D.
Nancy Savage, Associate Professor, Ph.D.
Barbara L. Schare, Professor, Ed.D.
Marilyn Sommers, Associate Professor, Ph.D.
Jeannette R. Spero, Professor, Ph.D.
Joan Tiessen, Associate Professor, Ed.D.
Patricia Trangenstein, Associate Professor, Ph.D.
Elizabeth Weiner, Professor, Ph.D.
Mary K. Wolterman, Associate Professor, Ed.D.
Judith A. Wood, Associate Professor, Ph.D.
Linda L. Workman, Associate Professor, Ph.D.

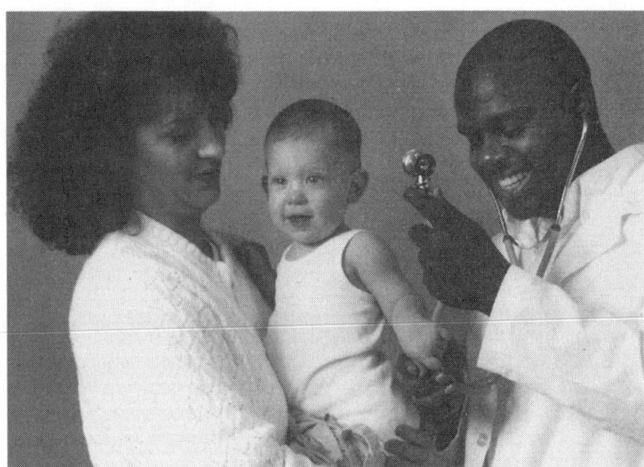

Students in a clinic evaluating a child's health status.

University of Connecticut
School of Nursing
Storrs, Connecticut

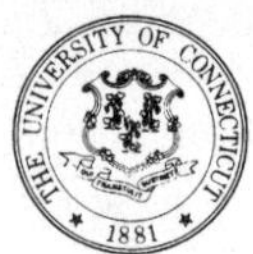

THE UNIVERSITY

The University of Connecticut is a modern, multifaceted institution with more than 24,000 students, 95,000 alumni, 120 major buildings on 3,100 acres at the main campus in Storrs, three professional schools and five regional campuses in other parts of the state, and a library of more than two million volumes. The University Health Center, which houses the Schools of Medicine and Dental Medicine and the University hospital, is located in Farmington, about 40 miles from the main campus in Storrs. Since its founding in 1881, the University has grown steadily and dramatically to fulfill its mandated objectives as a provider of high-quality public education and service and as a contributor to society through research. The University is the land-grant institution in the state and is the only public institution in New England to be designated a Research I institution by the Carnegie Foundation.

THE SCHOOL OF NURSING

The School of Nursing was founded in 1942 and graduated its first baccalaureate nursing students in 1947. During its more than 50-year history, the School has grown in size and stature. In addition to the baccalaureate program, which now has an enrollment of over 450, the School offers a master's program with seven subspecialty areas of study. The master's program has an enrollment of 175. An accelerated RN to M.S. program is offered, and a Ph.D. program in nursing was initiated in fall 1994. The programs are accredited by the Connecticut State Board of Examiners for Nursing and the National League for Nursing. The programs are supported by 37 full-time and 13 part-time faculty members, all of whom have at least a master's degree in a clinical specialty. Eighty percent of the full-time faculty members are prepared at the doctoral level. In addition, the School has access to over 100 adjunct clinical faculty members from a wide variety of agencies in the state to serve as preceptors for graduate students.

PROGRAMS OF STUDY

The undergraduate program provides an opportunity to combine a general education with professional preparation in nursing. The curriculum requires four academic years. Courses in the social, behavioral, and biological sciences and the humanities serve as a foundation for the nursing major. The nursing major is concentrated in the junior and senior years. Upon successful completion of the 130-credit program, students receive the Bachelor of Science degree and are eligible for examination for licensure as registered nurses.

Graduates of a baccalaureate program with a major in nursing may prepare for professional careers in nursing administration, acute-care nursing, community health/community mental health nursing, or perioperative, gerontological, neonatal/perinatal, or primary-care nursing within the School's master's program. In addition, dual-degree options are available in public health in combination with the community health nursing program (M.S./M.P.H.) and in business administration in combination with the nursing administration program (M.S./M.B.A.). Upon successful completion of the 39–42 credits of the three-semester master's program, students receive the Master of Science degree.

Registered nurses may enroll in a modified sequence of courses leading to the master's degree in nursing. Individuals who have completed the 65-credit undergraduate general education requirement are eligible for admission to the upper-division nursing major. Registered nurses who meet the eligibility criteria may earn 30 transfer credits in nursing under the Connecticut Articulation Model for Nurse Educational Mobility. Those who do not meet the articulation criteria may earn 30 nursing credits upon successful completion of a battery of advanced placement examinations. Those enrolled in the RN to B.S. option complete a 35-credit sequence of undergraduate nursing courses to earn the Bachelor of Science degree. Students enrolled in the RN to M.S. option complete a 35-credit sequence of undergraduate and master's nursing courses to earn the Bachelor of Science degree and then go on to complete the remaining credits of the master's program to earn the Master of Science degree.

The Doctor of Philosophy (Ph.D.) program in nursing prepares nurse leaders who will advance the scientific body of knowledge that is unique to professional nursing practice. Educational experiences are offered in nursing theory development, in philosophy of nursing science, in qualitative and quantitative research methods, and in advanced statistics. Study in specialty areas further supports the individual's area of clinical interest. Doctoral students entering the program are mentored by a faculty member with expertise and ongoing research activities in the clinical specialty of interest to the student.

AFFILIATIONS WITH HEALTH-CARE FACILITIES

Students receive their clinical experiences in a wide variety of settings, in both rural and urban areas. The School of Nursing is affiliated with approximately forty health-care agencies within a 30- to 35-mile radius of the Storrs campus. These include not only hospitals but also schools, day care centers, housing for the elderly, private homes, extended care facilities, community health agencies, ambulatory centers, physicians' offices, industry, mental health clinics, inpatient facilities, well-child and obstetrical clinics, and other related settings such as Alcoholics Anonymous, Lamaze, and LeLeche meetings.

ACADEMIC FACILITIES

The University's Homer Babbidge Library is a rich storehouse of valuable information. Ranked among the country's top thirty for research resources, it has a strong book collection in nursing and the physical and social sciences. The journal collection includes more than 500 titles devoted to nursing. With seating for 3,000, the library provides access to data with a 24-hour on-line catalog computer system.

The University Computer Center provides access to the mainframe system nearly 24 hours a day from any of the 1,700 terminals throughout the campus, from PCs attached to the campus network, or via modem. The Computer Center personal computing facilities include in-house IBM and Macintosh labs as well as several labs in both dorms and academic buildings.

Nursing laboratories have been provided for the undergraduate students to facilitate the transfer of knowledge from theory to actual practice. Students practice newly acquired skills in the simulated laboratory before performing them on actual patients in the clinical setting.

LOCATION

The School of Nursing is located on the main campus of the University in Storrs, Connecticut, which is 35 miles east of

Hartford, approximately midway between New York and Boston. Storrs is a small community with the clean air and quiet rural atmosphere of eastern Connecticut, yet the bustling and fast-growing city of Hartford is only 30 minutes away and Boston is less than 2 hours away. Cultural and sports activities abound in the area. The University sponsors numerous theater and musical activities throughout the year, and the cultural activities available in Hartford, New Haven, Boston, and New York City are all close enough to attend on a regular basis. The University has numerous facilities for the active sports enthusiast. For the sports fan, the very competitive Big East basketball season highlights the full slate of intercollegiate sports events.

STUDENT SERVICES

The University offers many services to meet student needs. These include career counseling and placement, student health and personal counseling, tutoring and other academic support services, services for students with physical and learning disabilities, and a number of centers offering students the opportunity to meet and socialize with other students from similar backgrounds. There are centers for African-American, Puerto Rican, Latino, Slavic, Jewish, and women students. Each has an active schedule of social and educational events usually highlighting events and studies important in its culture.

THE NURSING STUDENT GROUP

The population is diverse with respect to age, sex, and ethnicity. The majority of the undergraduate students live on campus and attend full-time. However, an increasing number of students are older, working adults who attend part-time while maintaining either full-time or part-time employment. The majority of graduate students attend part-time; however, within the past several years the number attending full-time has increased substantially.

COSTS

Tuition and fees for the 1997–98 academic year are $5040 for in-state undergraduate students and $13,558 for out-of-state undergraduate students. The room and board costs for those who live on campus average $5124, bringing the total to $10,164 for in-state and $18,682 for out-of-state undergraduate students. In addition, undergraduate students incur an additional one-time cost of $500 for uniforms, equipment, and books. For full-time graduate students the in-state tuition and fees are $6000 and out-of-state tuition and fees are $14,180. The average room and board fees in graduate student housing are similar to those for undergraduate students.

FINANCIAL AID

All students who estimate that they will be unable to defray the cost of their education from their own resources are encouraged to apply for financial assistance. This assistance, in the form of scholarships, grants, loans, and part-time employment, is administered by the Student Financial Aid Office. The application deadline is February 15. In addition to this need-based assistance, graduate students may be awarded graduate assistantships, fellowships, and traineeships.

APPLYING

Undergraduate students apply to the Undergraduate Admissions Office. They must submit an application, a secondary school record, SAT I scores, official transcripts of all postsecondary work completed, and a completed residence affidavit. Upon receipt of all information necessary to complete the application, the admissions office notifies the applicant of the decision by mail.

Graduate students submit two applications, one to the Graduate School and one to the School of Nursing. Students must submit an application, letters of reference, a personal statement, and transcripts of all postsecondary work to the Graduate School Admissions Office. Students must have a GPA of 3.0 or better to be considered for regular admission. In addition to those of the Graduate School, requirements for admission to the School of Nursing include a baccalaureate degree in nursing from an NLN-accredited nursing program or completion of the specially designed course sequence for upper-division nursing content, current nurse licensure in Connecticut, skills in health assessment, and, for some programs, specific work experience and a personal interview. In addition, admission to the doctoral program requires a minimum GPA of 3.25, submission of GRE scores, completion of a graduate-level course in inferential statistics, and submission of any published works or scholarly papers. Admission recommendations are made to the Graduate School by the School of Nursing admissions committees. Notification of a decision is by mail from the Graduate School.

Correspondence and Information:

Academic Advisory Center
University of Connecticut
School of Nursing
231 Glenbrook Road U-26
Storrs, Connecticut 06269-2026
Telephone: 203-486-4730

University of Delaware
Department of Nursing
Newark, Delaware

THE UNIVERSITY

The University of Delaware has marked its 250th year as an educational institution. A private university with public support, the University strives for an atmosphere in which all people feel welcome to learn and one that embraces creativity, critical thinking, and free inquiry and respects the views and values of an increasingly diverse population.

The University of Delaware faculty is committed to academic excellence with high-quality teaching as its primary emphasis. Many members of the faculty, including distinguished professors, teach freshman courses, ensuring that students have early contact with eminent scholars.

The University comprises seven colleges: Agricultural Sciences; Arts and Science; Business and Economics; Engineering; Health and Nursing Sciences; Human Resources, Education, and Public Policy; and Marine Studies. Together, the colleges offer more than 100 majors. Enrollment in the fall 1996 semester was 20,681 students, including 14,829 undergraduates, 3,286 graduate students, and 2,566 continuing education students.

THE DEPARTMENT OF NURSING

The Department of Nursing is housed within the College of Health and Nursing Sciences. It offers curricula leading to the Bachelor of Science in Nursing degree and the Master of Science in Nursing degree. Both degree programs are fully accredited by the National League for Nursing (NLN).

The basic undergraduate program is available to beginning students of nursing, including new high school graduates, transfer students, change of major students, and adults who have previously earned a baccalaureate degree in another discipline. This latter group may choose to pursue an accelerated program of study whereby they complete all their nursing requirements in a thirteen-month period.

A distance education option is available for registered nurses who wish to further their education but are unable to attend traditional campus classes. This program requires only three 1-credit weekend courses on the Newark campus; all other nursing courses are available in a distance learning format.

The graduate program is designed to prepare clinical nurse specialists (CNS), family nurse practitioners (FNP), nursing administrators, and specialized nurse practitioners who also have the knowledge of a clinical nurse specialist. Clinical specialization in the CNS concentration is offered in gerontology, adult cardiopulmonary, oncology/immune deficiency, pediatrics, and mothers and newborns. The nursing administration concentration prepares nurses for leadership positions as nurse managers at a variety of levels. The family nurse practitioner concentration prepares nurses to provide primary health care to clients of all ages.

The combined CNS/NP option combines the above specialty areas with their related practitioner status: adult nurse practitioner, pediatric nurse practitioner, geriatric nurse practitioner, and women's health nurse practitioner. Post-Master's Certificates are available in all areas for students who already hold a Master of Science in Nursing degree. All practitioner graduates are qualified to sit for the national certifying examinations.

PROGRAMS OF STUDY

The Department of Nursing offers two undergraduate majors: basic nursing and the baccalaureate for the registered nurse (BRN). The basic nursing major requires 126 credits for program completion. The first two years of the program include foundation courses in the natural, social, and behavioral sciences. The third and fourth year include clinical and nonclinical nursing courses as well as elective courses. Students who choose to pursue the Accelerated Degree Option must have completed all of their prerequisite courses and have earned a GPI of 3.0 or higher prior to beginning any nursing courses. This option allows adults who have previously earned a baccalaureate degree in another field to complete 58 credits in nursing in an intense thirteen-month period.

The BRN major is an innovative program designed for RNs who are graduates of associate degree or diploma programs. Didactic courses are taught in state-of-the-art instructional TV studios on campus. Videotapes are then sent to participating worksites, including hospitals, clinics, visiting nurse associations, and industry wellness centers. Textbooks and course syllabi are ordered and delivered by mail. Students view the tapes on site or at home; examinations are administered by the site coordinator and returned to the faculty for grading and feedback. Most nursing courses and many support courses are offered in the distance delivery mode. This delivery mode makes most courses available in both academic semesters and summer session. The BRN major requires 125 credits for program completion. All RN students are required to attend three 1-credit on-campus courses offered in a weekend format. Graduates of NLN-accredited associate degree programs may directly transfer up to 30 credits in nursing as evidence of their basic nursing knowledge. Graduates of diploma programs and non-NLN-accredited associate degree programs must successfully complete the NLN Mobility Profile II examinations to be awarded 30 credits for basic nursing knowledge. State-of-the-art technologies are used to facilitate frequent communication, advisement, and course work among and between students and faculty members. A Special Programs Information Line (voice processing), e-mail, and fax communication augment campus and site meetings.

The graduate program includes core concepts in advanced nursing practice as well as concepts specific to the areas of specialization. The curriculum is built on the theories and professional practice students have obtained at the baccalaureate level of nursing education and provides a foundation for future doctoral study. Research is a major emphasis in graduate study. Students may elect to complete either a thesis or nonthesis scholarly project to satisfy the research requirements for graduation. Students in the CNS and nursing administration concentrations must complete 34 credit hours, while students pursuing the FNP or combined CNS/NP concentrations must complete 43 credit hours.

ACADEMIC FACILITIES

University Libraries contain more than 2 million volumes of books and journals, more than 390,000 government publications, and more than 2.3 million items in microtext and subscribe to more than 21,000 periodicals. Collections are broad-based and comprehensive. DELCAT is the UD on-line catalog that contains information for more than 1 million materials. DELCAT may be accessed via the campus network, the Internet, and by telephone and computer modem from anywhere in the world. DELCAT provides access to four databases at no fee to the user. Computerized information services, which are fee-based, provide on-line access to more than 900 additional databases.

The University of Delaware offers a variety of centrally supported computing systems and services. These include microcomputer laboratories for instruction and general purpose, UNIX multiworkstation and timesharing facilities typically used for scientific instruction and research, and an IBM vector processing timesharing service offering a wide range of instructional and research services. An experienced staff of professionals provides consulting, documentation, training, and self-guided tutorials to students and faculty members.

The Department of Nursing has a microcomputer laboratory that includes twenty-four PC stations and ten interactive videodisc stations. The College also houses a large state-of-the-art instructional TV studio where nursing courses and support courses are taught and videotaped for use in the distance delivery system. In addition, some graduate courses are broadcast to selected sites via satellite. Faculty members are committed to the development and integration of technologies in the teaching/learning process.

LOCATION

Situated in the small, picturesque town of Newark, the University's main campus is less than 2½ hours from the metropolitan bustle of New York City, Baltimore, Philadelphia, and Washington, D.C. The campus is convenient to an impressive array of major clinical facilities as well as cultural and recreational resources. Courses are also offered at several satellite campuses throughout the state.

STUDENT SERVICES

The University has many resources and services to meet individual student needs. These include the Student Support Services Program, the University Writing Center, the Center for Counseling and Student Development, the Mathematical Sciences Teaching and Learning Center, the English Language Institute, and the Career Planning and Placement Office.

Nursing students are encouraged to participate in the College Chapter of the National Student Nurses Association. Registered nurse students have their own support group that meets on campus once each semester or as a specific need arises. All returning adult students are invited to join RASA, the University-supported Returning Adult Student Association.

THE NURSING STUDENT GROUP

Approximately 436 students are enrolled in the basic undergraduate program, including 30 adult students pursuing the Accelerated Degree Option. Additionally, 300 matriculated RN students are enrolled in the BRN major. There are more than 200 additional RNs who are taking BRN support courses in a nonmatriculated status. Most of the RN students pursue the B.S.N. degree through the distance delivery system. Enrollment in the graduate program is 152.

COSTS

For the 1996–97 academic year, tuition was $3990 for Delaware residents and $11,250 for nonresidents. Tuition covers registration for 12–17 credits per semester. Students taking less than 12 credits were charged $166 per credit hour for Delaware residents and $469 per credit hour for nonresidents. Registered nurse students enrolled in distance education courses at participating worksites were charged $195 per credit regardless of place of residence. Room and board costs were $4420. All costs are subject to change for the 1997–98 year.

FINANCIAL AID

In most cases, the University awards aid on the basis of need. Financial aid may include grants, loans, and employment opportunities. The University also offers a number of scholarships based on academic proficiency alone. Students have been able to successfully obtain nurse traineeships, National Student Nurses Association scholarships, and other specialty scholarships.

APPLYING

Applicants to both degree programs should request application packets from the College of Health and Nursing Sciences. The application deadlines for 1997–98 are March 1 for fall 1997 admission and November 15 for spring 1998 admission. For information regarding specific requirements, students should contact the appropriate unit in the College.

Correspondence and Information:

For information about the basic nursing program and graduate program:

Department of Nursing
University of Delaware
Newark, Delaware 19716
Telephone: 302-831-2381

For information about the BRN major and the Accelerated Degree Option:

Division of Special Programs
College of Health and Nursing Sciences
University of Delaware
Newark, Delaware 19716
Telephone: 800-UOD-NURS (toll-free)
E-mail: dsp@mvs.udel.edu
WWW: http://www.udel.edu/nursing/udnursing.html

University of Florida
College of Nursing
Gainesville, Florida

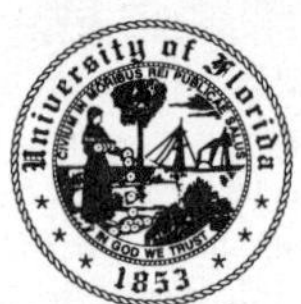

THE UNIVERSITY

The University of Florida is one of the nation's largest and most comprehensive public, land-grant research universities. It is the oldest and largest of Florida's ten universities and is a member of the Association of American Universities (AAU). The University of Florida ranks among the nation's top twenty AAU research universities and among the top five public universities in admission of Merit and Achievement Scholars. Currently almost 40,000 graduate and undergraduate students attend the University. Students come from every state in the nation and more than 100 other countries.

THE COLLEGE OF NURSING

The College of Nursing is one of six professional colleges within the Health Science Center of the University of Florida (UF) campus in Gainesville. In addition to the Gainesville campus, College of Nursing campuses in Orlando and Jacksonville provide urban access for graduate students. The colleges of the Health Science Center and their associated health-care delivery network provide students access to an integrated system of community hospitals and clinics, statewide home health care, and quaternary care at Shands Hospital.

The College of Nursing offers the undergraduate Bachelor of Science in Nursing (B.S.N.) degree and, in conjunction with the University of Florida Graduate School, the graduate degrees of Master of Science in Nursing (M.S.N.) and the Doctor of Philosophy (Ph.D.) with a major in nursing. A post-master's program is also offered. Students in the College have an opportunity to learn and work with students from other Health Science Center colleges in collaborative health-care teams. The College of Nursing maintains and participates in nursing and interdisciplinary clinics for women, children, adults, and the elderly in a variety of settings, with special emphasis on medically underserved and rural areas. Nurse midwifery clinics include urban and rural settings, with clinics focused on comprehensive perinatal care and the prevention of teen pregnancy.

The College offers innovative options for study, including videoteleconferencing among campuses and clinical placements in a wide variety of settings. The College has recently been selected as a national site for the pilot testing of portable computers to link students, faculty members, and client homes for purposes of assessment, planning, and health education.

The approximately 60 faculty members are involved in regional and national research and in faculty practice throughout the state. The majority of faculty members are prepared at the doctoral level, and there are many expert clinicians holding national certification. The College's endowed chair, the Thomas and Irene Kirbo Eminent Scholar Chair, enables the College to develop a unique leadership role in cancer prevention.

PROGRAMS OF STUDY

All College of Nursing programs are State Board approved and nationally accredited. The College of Nursing offers the B.S.N. and an accelerated B.S.N. option for registered nurses. The B.S.N. curriculum is a four-year program, including the physical and social sciences, humanities, and nursing. The program requires 60 credits of general education and preprofessional course work and 64 credits of nursing studies. Computer technology provides simulated clinical situations to extend students' opportunities for clinical decision making. Clinical learning for baccalaureate students is balanced between community-based experiences and the high-technology, acute-care focus of a major health science center. Students have clinical experiences ranging from rural ambulatory clinics to intensive care units for adults and neonates.

The goal of the UF master's degree program is to prepare nurses for advanced practice and leadership roles. Each student completes the graduate nursing core, including nursing theory, research process, statistics, health policy, financing, and health promotion. There is also an advanced practice core with specific clinical content and experiences relevant to the advanced practice area of study. The College currently offers preparation for nurse midwifery and the following nurse practitioner (NP) roles: adult, family, pediatric, and women's health. Students in the adult NP track may elect to add an emphasis in oncology or gerontology. Graduates are eligible for state (Florida) and national certification as nurse practitioners or nurse midwives. The master's degree requires four semesters of full-time study; a part-time plan of study is also available.

Students with a master's degree in nursing may seek admission to post-master's NP study. These students develop individual curriculum plans to meet the certification requirements of nurse practitioner practice areas. Study time varies from one to three semesters, depending upon each student's background and goals. Most post-master's students enroll part-time.

The goal of the College's doctoral program is to prepare scientists, scholars, and leaders in the field of nursing. The College offers comprehensive and intensive research preparation by pairing student interest with the expertise of the faculty. In addition to the research foci of the College of Nursing faculty members, students have access to the rich faculty resources of the entire University of Florida for interdisciplinary study and research. Doctoral students complete a core curriculum in the areas of knowledge development and nursing theory, nursing practice concentration, a selected non-nursing minor, advanced research, and quantitative and qualitative research. Individually directed dissertation research hours are a major aspect of the Ph.D. program. Students have access to exceptional interdisciplinary research facilities in the Health Science Center, including an internationally recognized Brain and Spine Institute, a Cancer Institute, and national centers of study for diabetes, genetics, geriatrics, and rural health. The doctoral curriculum is three years in length for full-time students. Courses in nursing and sciences occupy a major portion of the first half of the program, with increasing time in research under the supervision of a faculty researcher for the latter half.

ACADEMIC FACILITIES

The College of Nursing is located in the Health Science Center, situated on the main University of Florida campus in Gainesville. UF offers the diversity of a broad arts and sciences campus, an institute of agricultural sciences, and an academic health science center all located together in an attractive, exciting campus environment. The UF Health Science Center is the region's most comprehensive academic health center, distinguished by a broad scope of educational programs in which more than 4,500 students are enrolled, a research enterprise attracting close to $100 million per year in external funding, and an innovative health-care delivery system serving residents throughout Florida and the Southeast. The University library system consists of eight separate libraries that contain more than 3 million volumes. The libraries offer state-of-the-art reference services, including on-line searching of national and international computerized databases.

LOCATION

The University of Florida is situated on a 2,000-acre campus in Gainesville, a city of approximately 100,000. Gainesville is located in a lovely semirural area on the rolling plains of North Central Florida. It is approximately two hours north of Disney World, two hours south of the Georgia border, and an hour from the beach in either direction. Over the past five years, Gainesville has consistently been ranked as one of the nation's "most livable" and "best value" small cities. The climate is remarkably pleasant year-round. While there are characteristic Florida palm trees, the area also includes pines and live oaks; flowers bloom all year.

STUDENT SERVICES

The University provides a wide variety of services and opportunities to promote students' social, intellectual, and physical health. The diversity of a large student body is represented in the variety of social organizations on campus. The University has active athletic, academic, and cultural student organizations as well as honors societies, professional organizations, and chapters of national sororities and fraternities. Student Government brings music and cultural events as well as nationally influential guest speakers to campus. The new student recreation and fitness center and a lake for recreational water activities are available to students free of charge. UF is ranked third in the nation for combined women's and men's athletic programs. The UF environment stimulates and supports athletic participation by the majority of students and faculty members. Student Health Services provides a variety of health clinics and counseling services. Baby Gator Child Care is located on campus for students' and faculty members' children.

THE NURSING STUDENT GROUP

The College of Nursing maintains an enrollment of approximately 300 undergraduate students and 350 graduate students, including about 40 doctoral students. Academic advisement is an integral component of each faculty member's responsibilities. Undergraduate advisement can begin prior to admission to UF. Graduate students are advised by expert advanced practice nurses in their clinical track, and doctoral students interview and select a faculty adviser and research mentor on admission.

COSTS

UF is generally regarded as one of the "best buys" in the nation for both undergraduate and graduate students. In 1996–97, the undergraduate in-state tuition and required fees were $1830 for the academic year (two semesters). The undergraduate out-of-state tuition and required fees were $7038 for the academic year. The estimated total budget for an in-state, undergraduate student living on campus for two semesters was approximately $8500.

In 1996–97, full-time graduate in-state tuition and fees were $1400 per semester. The full-time graduate out-of-state tuition and required fees were $4650 per semester. Graduate student and family housing is available on campus.

FINANCIAL AID

The University of Florida provides access to a range of federal, state, and privately donated financial aid funds to students through the University of Florida Office of Student Financial Aid. Assistance is available to students based on financial need, academic merit, and program of study. In addition, the University of Florida College of Nursing oversees the distribution of a variety of merit-based and need-based financial awards. Assistantships in teaching and research provide tuition and stipend support for selected doctoral students each year.

APPLYING

Students seeking admission to the baccalaureate nursing program apply for admission to the University of Florida. Students majoring in nursing who remain on track in the prescribed academic program begin upper-division nursing studies on completion of 60 credits of general education and preprofessional course work. Students may also apply to UF and the College of Nursing to transfer from other colleges into upper-division nursing studies on the completion of the equivalent general education and preprofessional course work. Such admissions are on a competitive basis. An admission grade point average above 3.0 is normally required. The number of students admitted is limited, and preference is given to Florida residents.

The undergraduate and graduate nursing programs admit students each fall semester only. All application materials should be received by the University of Florida Admissions Office no later than February 1 of the calendar year in which one seeks admission.

All international students seeking admission to the Graduate School for study in nursing are required to meet admission requirements for the University of Florida and the College of Nursing as well as submit a score of at least 600 on the TOEFL (Test of English as a Foreign Language).

Applicants are considered for admission to the master's degree program when they have fulfilled the general requirements for admission to the Graduate School and, in addition, have presented the following credentials for evaluation: completion of an undergraduate nursing program substantially equivalent to the baccalaureate program at the University of Florida; eligibility for licensure to practice as a registered nurse in Florida; references attesting to professional competence; Graduate Record Examinations scores in verbal, quantitative, and analytical areas; evidence of computer literacy; and a statement of academic and professional goals. Usually a minimum of one year of clinical practice related to the preferred area of study is required prior to beginning clinical course work.

Nurses are considered for admission to the doctoral program when they have fulfilled the general requirements for admission to the Graduate School and, in addition, have presented the following credentials for evaluation: completion of a master's degree in nursing from a nationally accredited program, eligibility for licensure to practice as a registered nurse in Florida, references attesting to the applicants' potential for doctoral studies; Graduate Record Examinations scores of approximately 500 or above in verbal, quantitative, and analytic areas; a curriculum vitae; and a statement of professional goals and area of research focus. A personal interview is required to establish a faculty mentor who will work with the student to individualize the academic program and structure each student's research focus.

Correspondence and Information:

Office of Admissions/Records
University of Florida
College of Nursing
Health Science Center
Box 100197
Gainesville, Florida 32610-0197
Telephone: 352-392-3518
Fax: 352-392-8100

University of Illinois at Chicago
College of Nursing
Chicago, Illinois

THE UNIVERSITY

The University of Illinois at Chicago serves approximately 25,000 students, who reflect the ethnic and racial diversity of Chicago itself. Seventy-five percent of these students come from Cook County and 48 percent are residents of Chicago. The Colleges of Nursing, Medicine, Pharmacy, Dentistry, and Associated Health Professions and the School of Public Health are located within the 305-acre west side Medical Center District about 2 miles west of downtown Chicago. The district has the world's largest concentration of public and private health-care facilities and includes the University of Illinois at Chicago Medical Center, Cook County Hospital, Rush-Presbyterian-St. Luke's Medical Center, West Side Veterans Administration Medical Center, Institute for Juvenile Research, Illinois State Psychiatric Institute, and Illinois State Pediatric Institute.

THE COLLEGE OF NURSING

The UIC College of Nursing is consistently recognized as one of the top ten nursing programs in the United States. The mission of the College includes the triad of university functions—teaching, research, and service—providing university education in nursing to meet the present and future needs of society. Fully accredited by the National League for Nursing (NLN), the College offers programs leading to the degrees of Bachelor of Science in Nursing, Master of Science in nursing sciences, and Doctor of Philosophy in nursing sciences. The College, which has provided high-quality education for more than forty years, is currently designated as a WHO Collaborating Centre for International Nursing Development in Primary Health Care and is also involved in local projects such as the "I'M READY" program, which goes into the city's junior and senior high schools to interest minority students in a nursing career and prepare them for the University nursing program. The College of Nursing's main Chicago campus building, an eleven-story structure completed in 1969, provides teaching-learning and research facilities and laboratories and offices for the faculty and students.

PROGRAMS OF STUDY

Freshmen and transfer students are admitted to the generic baccalaureate program in Chicago and Urbana-Champaign. The program, which prepares beginning nurses to function in a variety of settings, requires 55 liberal arts and sciences semester hours and 78 nursing semester hours for graduation. Students entering as freshmen may complete the program in 4 years including two required summer terms. Transfer students may complete the program in 2½ years including two required summers. RN-B.S.N. students applying to the program offered in Chicago, Quad Cities, and Urbana-Champaign must meet the transfer admission requirements, which include 55 semester hours of liberal arts and sciences course work and a cumulative GPA of at least 3.5 (A=5.0). Completion of three NLN Mobility Profile II examinations and three transition courses determines credit by exemption for up to 43 semester hours of nursing course work, leaving 35 semester hours of nursing course work, which may be completed in four semesters.

The master's program prepares nurses for advanced practice roles with emphasis on basic, clinical, and nursing sciences; knowledge of health systems and environment; and understanding of professional issues of advanced practice roles, while a research focus is maintained. The roles are clinical nurse specialist, which utilizes advanced information within a specialty to manage complex health problems, and nurse practitioner, which emphasizes the comprehensive care of patients as well as the ability to manage the complex problems addressed by the specialty.

Within each specialty and option, there are several concentrations of study. These include administrative studies in nursing (alone or combined as a dual-degree option with an M.B.A.), medical-surgical nursing (critical care, oncology, cardiopulmonary, neuro-cognitive/musculo-skeletal), maternal-child nursing (nurse midwifery, women's health, pediatric [including PNP], perinatal), public health nursing (dual-degree option with an M.P.H., school health, community nurse specialist, family nurse practitioner, home health-care administration, occupational health nursing), and psychiatric–mental health nursing (child/adolescent, adult).

All courses of study are offered in Chicago. Selected medical-surgical and public health nursing options and concentrations are offered in Peoria, Quad Cities, and Urbana-Champaign; administrative studies, psychiatric–mental health nursing, and selected public health nursing options and concentrations are offered in Rockford. The 36 required semester hours include statistics, nursing inquiry I & II, health environment and systems, and issues of advanced practice in nursing (10 semester hours); advanced nursing courses (23–36 semester hours); electives (2–3 semester hours); a thesis (5 semester hours) or research project (3 semester hours); and a final examination. More than 36 semester hours are required to complete most of the specialty concentrations.

Post-master's programs are available in the women's health and nurse midwifery, pediatric, and family and critical-care nurse practitioner study options, which prepare individuals to sit for examinations for certification in these fields.

The Ph.D. program develops leaders in nursing who influence the provision of health care through systematic investigation, education, policy development and implementation, and expert professional practice. Major areas of research include administration, physiological and psychological studies related to the care of the acutely and chronically ill, health promotion and maintenance, stress and coping, narcolepsy, quality of life, community health nursing, women's health, family, and gerontological nursing. The Ph.D. degree requires 96 semester hours, including nursing theory (6 semester hours), statistics (6 semester hours), research methods (6 semester hours), advanced nursing and non-nursing courses (15 semester hours), independent research (31 semester hours), and a previously completed M.S. program (32 semester hours). A preliminary oral examination, dissertation, and final oral examination are required to earn the Ph.D. in nursing sciences.

Through the CIC, a consortium of the Midwest's "Big Ten" universities plus the University of Chicago, doctoral students may register for course work or independent study in the other universities of the CIC and work with experts in their research areas.

ACADEMIC FACILITIES

UIC libraries hold more than 5.7 million items, including over 6,000 current periodicals and more than 500,000 bound periodical volumes, books, government documents, and audio-visual items housed in the Library of the Health Sciences, which is the regional medical library for 2,700 medical libraries in ten states from Ohio to the Dakotas. The Interlibrary Loan Service is offered to faculty, students, and staff, and the libraries of two other Chicago institutions, the University of Chicago and Northwestern University, are available for use by graduate students. The Academic Computer Center provides computing and network support for instructional and research needs of the University's faculty, students, and staff.

LOCATION

Situated 2 miles west of Chicago's downtown, UIC is surrounded by world-renowned architecture, theater, art, music, and sports activities. Easily accessible from both airports by public transportation and the Eisenhower Expressway, the College is located in a historic neighborhood, currently the center of a new, rapidly growing residential and professional community.

STUDENT SERVICES

The Academic Center for Excellence provides an array of services from career counseling and academic skills courses to personal counseling and assistance for disabled students. Other services include two fitness/recreation centers, a child-care center, the Office of International Studies, and support organizations such as African American Academic Network, Latin American Recruitment and Education Services, and the Native American Support Program for members of minority groups.

THE NURSING STUDENT GROUP

Students reflect the ethnic and racial diversity of Chicago itself. UIC has long provided solid academic training for first-generation college students from the city's numerous ethnic groups and currently provides opportunities to students returning to school following a significant absence due to other career or family responsibilities. About 18 percent of those enrolled in the undergraduate program are men. Even though University housing is available, 85 percent of Chicago students commute or live in apartments near the campus. Enrollment for fall 1996 at the Chicago and regional campuses—Peoria, Quad Cities, Rockford, and Urbana-Champaign—was 641 undergraduate and 588 graduate students.

COSTS

For 1996–97, full-time tuition and fees per semester for undergraduates were $2094 for Illinois residents and $4964 for nonresidents. For full-time graduate students, tuition and fees were $2374 for Illinois residents and $5267 for nonresidents. Part-time undergraduate tuition ranged from $1068 to $1616 for Illinois residents and from $1953 to $3397 for nonresidents; part-time graduate study ranged from $1156 to $1802 for Illinois residents and from $2198 to $3887 for nonresidents. Single student housing was available in Chicago for $5061 for an 11½-month contract; multistudent housing suites cost $4290.

FINANCIAL AID

Several financial assistance programs are available through the Office of Student Financial Aid. Applications for financial aid in the form of research or training assistantships, fellowships, traineeships, and tuition waivers are submitted to the College of Nursing. These financial aid awards are made from the College's resources. The College of Nursing makes recommendations to the Graduate College for such awards as University Fellowships and the Abraham Lincoln Graduate Fellowship.

APPLYING

Applicants for the B.S. degree must be either graduating high school seniors who will complete a strong high school science and math curriculum or transfer students who have completed the following liberal arts and sciences requirements: English composition I and II, general biology, microbiology, general and organic chemistry, anatomy, physiology, psychology, sociology, logic or reasoning, and ethics. For transfer students, a minimum cumulative GPA of 3.5 (A=5.0) and a minimum GPA of 3.0 in natural science courses are required. Freshman applicants must provide either ACT or SAT I scores. All applicants must submit two letters of recommendation, a personal statement, and a writing sample. The applicant to the RN-B.S.N. program must have a current RN license or be scheduled to take the NCLEX at the first opportunity after graduation from an NLN-accredited diploma or associate degree nursing program.

M.S. applicants must have a current RN license (several specialty concentrations require an Illinois license) and either a B.S.N. degree from an NLN-accredited program or a B.S. degree from an accredited institution in a field other than nursing; a minimum GPA of 4.0 (A=5.0); introductory courses in statistics and research methods or their equivalent; GRE General Test scores (or GMAT scores for the M.S.-M.B.A. dual-degree option) and, for international students, TOEFL scores; a statement of career goals; a curriculum vitae; three letters of reference; and a faculty interview.

Ph.D. applicants must meet the requirements for entry into the M.S. program, possess an M.S. degree from an NLN-accredited program, and present evidence of potential for advanced scholarship. The applicant who has a B.S. degree from an accredited nursing program and an M.S. degree in a field other than nursing is eligible for consideration for admission.

Applications for each program are considered as soon as all elements of the application are received; admission decisions are made on a rolling basis. Early application is encouraged; programs may be filled prior to final application deadlines. Students should contact the College of Nursing Office of Academic Affairs for specific application deadlines and priority application dates for the undergraduate program. Applications for the B.S., selected M.S., and the Ph.D. programs are accepted for fall only. Admission to several of the M.S. options is for any term.

Correspondence and Information:

Office of Academic Affairs
College of Nursing (M/C 802)
University of Illinois at Chicago
845 South Damen Avenue
Chicago, Illinois 60612-7350
Telephone: 312-996-7800
Fax: 312-413-4399
World Wide Web: http://www.uic.edu/depts/nadm

University of Kentucky
College of Nursing
Lexington, Kentucky

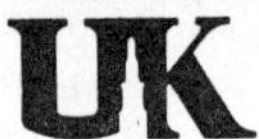

THE UNIVERSITY
The University of Kentucky (UK) was founded in 1865 and is committed to quality higher education. In 1956, the Medical Center was created with the establishment of the Colleges of Nursing, Medicine, and Dentistry and the University Hospital. In 1964, the development of a statewide system of community colleges was initiated as part of the University. In 1982, the University was reorganized into its current three chancellor sectors (the community colleges, the Medical Center, and the Lexington campus) with a central administration. UK is committed to providing excellent instruction at the undergraduate and graduate levels, cutting-edge research, and public service. The University ranks among the top research-intensive universities in the nation (Carnegie classification Research University I) with more than $113 million in research funding in 1995. Students have an opportunity for specialization and the pursuit of a particular interest in seventeen colleges, including the College of Nursing. The University has 24,322 students on the Lexington campus.

THE COLLEGE OF NURSING
The Chandler Medical Center, located on the Lexington campus, is composed of the Colleges of Nursing, Medicine, Dentistry, Pharmacy, and Allied Health; the University Hospital; the Kentucky Clinic (an ambulatory-care facility); and the Veterans Affairs Hospital, all of which provide exceptional learning experiences for nursing students. UK centers of excellence in cancer, aging, rural health (located in Hazard, Kentucky), and in pharmaceutical science and technology also provide educational, research, and service opportunities for faculty and students.

Since the first B.S.N. degrees were awarded in 1964, more than 3,676 nursing students have graduated. In 1971, the College of Nursing instituted a master's degree program designed to provide skills in advanced practice for supervising and managing patient care. In 1988, the Ph.D. program was initiated, and the first graduates completed their program of study in 1992.

The faculty members conduct research on women's and children's health (low birthweight infants, single mother families, and women's mental health), coping with potential threats to health and well-being (injury prevention, pain management, substance abuse prevention, symptom management, and chronic airflow limitations), rural health, care in rural areas, and health services.

One of the College's most exciting efforts is its participation in UK's Center for Rural Health located in Hazard, Kentucky, in the mountains of central Appalachia. The mission of the Center for Rural Health includes health professions education, health policy research, and consultative public service. Through a partnership with this center, the College of Nursing offers master's-level study in Hazard.

Another important component of the College is the Faculty Practice Program through which many faculty members are able to include clinical practice as part of their faculty role. This provides opportunities for students to work with faculty role models.

The College maintains a faculty-student ratio that is conducive to learning and scholarship and that allows the faculty to provide high-quality research and clinical guidance, instruction, and mentorship for students. The undergraduate student-faculty ratio is approximately 10:1.

PROGRAMS OF STUDY
The baccalaureate degree program provides students with the experience and knowledge necessary to take the licensing examination and to assume beginning positions in all areas of nursing practice. In addition to taking core courses in natural sciences, students acquire a background in the humanities, learn clinical and first-level management skills, and receive many hours of supervised clinical preparation. The program emphasizes nursing theory and practice and prepares students to think critically, make independent judgments, and work cooperatively as professional members of the health-care team. The baccalaureate program is offered to four-year students and upper-division registered nurse students.

The Master of Science in Nursing degree program prepares nurses for the advanced practice of nursing in a particular clinical specialty. The program is designed to build on the first professional degree and focuses on nursing theory, research, and practice. Students may specialize in adult nursing (adult client, gerontology, critical care, oncology, ER/trauma, nurse case manager, or acute care nurse practitioner), psychiatric nursing (adult client, geropsychiatry, or substance abuse), parent-child nursing (children, adolescents, and families; pediatric nurse practitioner; neonatal-perinatal; or nurse midwifery), or community health (community health administration, family nurse practitioner, geriatric nurse practitioner, community nursing clinical specialist, or nurse case manager). Many nursing students continue to pursue their nursing careers while working toward a graduate degree through flexible scheduling and selected evening courses.

The RN to M.S.N. program provides the upper-division RN student who enters the program at the junior level an opportunity to attain baccalaureate and master's degrees after five to six years of part-time study. The purpose of the program is to provide experienced RNs with an accelerated approach to career advancement from the associate degree or the hospital diploma in nursing to the Master of Science degree.

The Doctor of Philosophy degree in nursing prepares nurse scholars to assume roles as researchers, educators, and administrators. Doctoral course work is interdisciplinary. It provides a foundation for the development of nursing knowledge through the conduct of clinical research significant to nursing practice. Graduate education at the doctoral level is an immersion into a community of scholars. It requires a commitment to the advancement of nursing knowledge through research. Mentoring by faculty members and collegial interactions among doctoral students support the development of nurse scholars. Students' dissertation research has focused on topics such as pain in the preterm neonate, rehabilitation of amputee farmers, coping of women with breast cancer, caregivers of the chronically mentally ill, and the effectiveness of critical pathways in providing nursing care.

AFFILIATIONS WITH HEALTH-CARE FACILITIES
The College of Nursing has affiliations with a wide variety of clinical agencies that provide primary, secondary, and tertiary

levels of care. Students may complete required clinical experiences within the Lexington–Fayette County area. In addition, there are opportunities for clinical study in settings across the state and nation.

ACADEMIC FACILITIES

The College of Nursing, located in a modern, six-story facility, has research and computer facilities staffed with support personnel. Information and consultation services are available for students and faculty members for developing research efforts. A learning resource center provides audiovisual and computer-generated learning aids, as well as individual and group study space. A central library and a Medical Center library offer periodicals, journals, reference materials, and computer-assisted bibliographic searches through network links with other institutions. Two large teaching hospitals (University of Kentucky Hospital and the Lexington Veterans Affairs Hospital), five community hospitals, and more than 200 other health-care agencies in the central Kentucky area offer rich teaching and research opportunities for all nursing students.

LOCATION

The University is located in Lexington, the heart of the Kentucky Bluegrass country. More than 400 horse farms span a 20-mile radius around the city, which has a population of approximately 250,000. Kentucky's scenic Cumberland Mountains are 30 miles east of Lexington, and the metropolitan areas of both Louisville and Cincinnati are within a 2-hour drive of the campus. Kentucky's forty state and national parks include some of the finest in the nation. Lexington has four seasons and an average annual temperature of 55 degrees.

STUDENT SERVICES

The Medical Center's location on UK's main campus allows nursing students to enjoy the benefits of a major university, including an outstanding athletic program and a full range of cultural activities. Individual student needs are met by student-oriented offices such as the Central Advising Center for undergraduate students, Learning Services Center for Minority Students, Office of African-American Affairs, Office of International Affairs, Campus Ministry, Counseling and Testing Center, Career Center, Campus Recreation, student organizations, Disabilities Resource Center, and the residential fraternities and sororities units.

The College of Nursing also provides funding and support for its own Office of Student Services. This office, located in the College of Nursing, is staffed by professionals who offer assistance with student admissions and registration and to provide ongoing information, support, and referral services to nursing students.

THE NURSING STUDENT GROUP

The College of Nursing currently has 444 B.S.N. students, 168 M.S.N. students, and 29 Ph.D. students.

COSTS

In 1996–97, full-time undergraduate registration fees were $1338 per semester for Kentucky residents and $3678 per semester for nonresidents. Graduate registration fees were $144 per semester hour up to a maximum of $1290 for Kentucky residents and $430 per semester hour up to a maximum of $3870 for nonresidents. A $168 mandatory registration fee was charged to all full-time students, and a $6 registration fee per credit hour was charged to all part-time students. The cost of on-campus room and board in 1996–97 ranged from $3198 to $3898 for undergraduates. The cost of an on-campus food plan for single students was $650 per semester in 1996–97. On-campus apartment housing, which includes adequate furnishings, utilities, and maintenance, costs an estimated $322 per month for an efficiency, $403 for one bedroom, and $420–$520 for two bedrooms.

FINANCIAL AID

More than 50 percent of UK undergraduate students receive some form of financial aid through federal and state grants, loans, work-study opportunities, and University scholarships. Also, undergraduate nursing scholarships are available through the College of Nursing for admitted students.

For graduate students, a limited number of Professional Nurse Traineeships from the Division of Nursing, the Health Resources and Services Administration, and the Public Health Service are available. A limited number of graduate fellowships and assistantships are also available. The assistantships provide wages for helping faculty members with research and teaching; tuition grants may be awarded for meritorious scholars. Doctoral students are assisted in applying for National Research Service Awards from the National Institute for Nursing Research of the National Institutes of Health. UK is a member of the Academic Common Market.

APPLYING

Undergraduate applications are accepted until February 1 for the fall semester. High school seniors must have a minimum cumulative grade point average of 2.5 and meet University standards for automatic admission. Transfer students must have a minimum cumulative grade point average of 2.35 on all previous college work attempted. Decisions are made based on space availability, and students are selected based on grade point average and application date. Admission to UK does not guarantee admission to the College of Nursing.

The B.S.N. upper-division RN program requires a minimum college grade point average of 2.5, RN licensure, and an Associate Degree in Nursing from an accredited program or a diploma with a minimum of 60 college credits in specified course work.

For the RN to M.S.N. program, applicants must meet the same requirements of the B.S.N. upper-division RN program but with one year of clinical work experience and satisfactory references and faculty interviews. The application deadline for admission to the B.S.N. upper-division RN program and the RN to M.S.N. program is February 1.

Applications for admission to the master's program should be completed by March 1. After this date, applicants are considered based on space availability. Applications for admission to the doctoral program should be completed by September 15 for spring admission and February 15 for fall admission. Criteria for entry include, but are not limited to, graduation from a B.S.N. program accredited by the NLN, a postbaccalaureate grade point average of at least 2.5 or a post-master's grade point average of at least 3.3, nursing licensure, and completion of the General Test of the Graduate Record Examinations. Admission is based upon qualifications as evidenced in the application, transcripts, professional references, and interviews.

Students should contact the College of Nursing Office of Student Services for complete information about admission requirements, application deadlines, and scholarships.

Correspondence and Information:

Office of Student Services
College of Nursing
University of Kentucky
Lexington, Kentucky 40536-0232
Telephone: 606-323-5108
World Wide Web: http://www.uky.edu/nursing/

University of Maryland at Baltimore
School of Nursing
Baltimore, Maryland

THE UNIVERSITY

The University of Maryland at Baltimore (UMAB), established in 1807, is the founding campus of the University of Maryland, one of the largest public universities in the United States. The campus includes six professional schools: Nursing, Medicine, Dentistry, Pharmacy, Social Work, and Law; the graduate school; the Maryland Institute for Emergency Medical Systems; the University of Maryland Medical Center; and the Veterans Affairs Medical Center. The University enrolls more than 5,000 students and has nearly 5,000 faculty and staff members.

UMAB is one of the fastest growing biomedical research centers in the United States and maintains more than $100 million in sponsored-program support. Its unique composition enables it to address health care, public policy, and social issues through multidisciplinary research, scholarship, and community action. UMAB's location in the Baltimore-Washington-Annapolis triangle maximizes opportunities for student placements and collaboration with government agencies, health-care institutions, and life science industries.

THE SCHOOL OF NURSING

The School of Nursing, established in 1889 by Louisa Parsons, has been instrumental in strengthening nursing education and shaping the profession. Its mission is to provide leadership through undergraduate, graduate, and continuing education programs as well as research and service of the highest quality.

Maryland consistently ranks among the top ten schools of nursing in the United States. The School awarded its first M.S. degree in 1954 and its first Ph.D. degree in 1984. Alumni include more than 18,500 nurses, and current enrollment is more than 1,600. Eighty-three percent of the School's 115 faculty members are doctorally prepared. The faculty is successful in obtaining research funding, and the School is one of only a few that repeatedly qualifies for Biomedical Research Support Grants from the National Institutes of Health. Faculty research and scholarship are well recognized in the nursing literature. (Senior faculty and administrators are listed in the faculty section.)

The School is organized into four departments—Psychiatric, Community Health, and Adult Primary Care; Acute and Long Term Care; Maternal and Child Health; and Education, Administration, Informatics, and Health Policy. Graduate specialties in nursing informatics and nursing health policy were the first of their kind and remain among the few in the nation. Outreach programs provide access for RN to B.S.N. and M.S. students across the state. Flexible and combined programs of study that accelerate degree completion are in place. The School operates a variety of nurse-managed clinics that serve as practicum sites for students. These include Open Gates, a community health center serving the underinsured. It is a mobile health clinic that provides screening, treatment, and referral for women, children, the homeless, and seven school-linked nurse-managed health centers.

PROGRAMS OF STUDY

The B.S.N. program is an upper-division, professional program accredited by the National League for Nursing. It is based on prerequisite courses that provide a liberal education and support the study of nursing. Two flexible undergraduate tracks that may be completed on a full- or part-time basis are available—basic baccalaureate and registered nurse. The basic baccalaureate track requires students to complete 59 prerequisite credits before matriculation. An accelerated option in the basic track for students who hold a non-nursing bachelor's degree requires 22 prerequisite credits before matriculation. The registered nurse track includes RN to B.S.N. and RN to M.S. options. Students must complete 89 prerequisite credits through three advanced placement choices before matriculating as seniors. The accelerated RN to M.S. option is designed for nurses with baccalaureate degrees in other disciplines or for RNs who do not have baccalaureate degrees but have the interest and ability to pursue leadership and specialty preparation at the master's level.

The NLN-accredited M.S. program focuses on specialization and a commitment to and involvement in the development and refinement of nursing knowledge. The program prepares graduates in more than twenty specialty areas as acute care nurse practitioners, clinical nurse specialists, nurses, primary care nurse practitioners, educators, and administrators. An M.S./M.B.A. joint degree is also offered.

The Ph.D. program is designed for nurses who are committed to leadership in the discovery and refinement of nursing knowledge through research. The curriculum includes 1) core courses that address the technical and empirical basis for nursing and the techniques of theory building and research and 2) specialty courses in either the direct or indirect spheres of nursing. Direct nursing focuses on the health needs of and nursing action provided to clients/patients in a variety of settings; research emphasizes clinical nursing. Indirect nursing focuses on nursing systems and education and nursing action that facilitates clinical nursing practice; research emphasizes health and nursing service organization, administration, health policy, education, and informatics. A Ph.D./M.B.A. joint degree is also offered. Most students enter the doctoral program after earning a master's degree; however, a postbaccalaureate entry option is available.

AFFILIATIONS WITH HEALTH-CARE FACILITIES

The School is affiliated with the University of Maryland Medical System composed of University Hospital, Maryland Cancer Center, R Adams Cowley Shock Trauma Center, James Lawrence Kernan Hospital, and Montebello Rehabilitation Center. Affiliations also include the Veterans Affairs Medical Center and more than 200 additional hospitals, community health centers, health maintenance organizations, health departments, private practices, community clinics, and schools.

ACADEMIC FACILITIES

The University's Health Sciences Library is the regional medical library for the Southeastern states and is part of the National Library of Medicine's biomedical information network. It houses more than 175,000 volumes and 2,000 current journal subscriptions. Campus computer resources include mainframe and microcomputer support for faculty, staff, and students. Electronic mail enables faculty, staff, and students to exchange information on and off campus.

The School's media center includes local area network–driven student computer labs that provide access to innovative software and an interactive video laboratory that utilizes state-of-the-art computerized clinical simulations and decision-making models that enable students to practice clinical skills and critical decision making at their own pace. Clinical simulation laboratories allow students to practice nursing skills using equipment designed to replicate patient care situations. Distance learning technology provides interactive classes involving students from across the state.

LOCATION

Baltimore combines the attractions of contemporary urban living with the advantages of a location within an educational hub composed of thirty colleges and universities. UMAB is part of a district called UniversityCenter; several blocks from campus are Oriole Park at Camden Yards and the Inner Harbor, which includes the National Aquarium and the Maryland Science Center. UMAB is easily accessible; Baltimore-Washington International Airport is nearby, the Baltimore Metro and Light Rail System connects the campus to neighboring counties, the University operates a shuttle service, and student parking is available.

STUDENT SERVICES

The School provides programs that support the academic experience. It conducts seminars to improve writing skills, test taking, study habits, and time management; maintains a peer tutoring program; and offers individual assistance for test taking. The School also conducts career placement and development seminars and advises student governmental and professional organizations. The University's student resources include student health, counseling, athletic facilities, residence life, student development, the student union, records and registration, and financial aid.

THE NURSING STUDENT GROUP

Approximately 820 students are enrolled in the B.S.N. program, 680 in the M.S. program, and 100 in the Ph.D. program. Of the undergraduates, 40 percent are enrolled in the RN to B.S.N. option and most are part-time. Nearly 25 percent of the basic students are enrolled in the accelerated second degree option. More than 90 percent enrolled in the basic baccalaureate option attend full-time. Most graduate students attend part-time.

COSTS

Tuition for the 1996–97 B.S.N. program was $3857 for full-time in-state students, $168 per credit for part-time in-state students, $9787 for full-time out-of-state students, and $252 per credit for part-time out-of-state students. Graduate tuition is on a per credit basis. In-state graduate tuition was $231 per credit, and out-of-state graduate tuition was $416 per credit. Additional educational expenses, including books, insurance, immunizations, and fees for full-time students average $2500 per year.

FINANCIAL AID

The School's financial aid program is available to students who demonstrate need. Students may receive assistance in meeting educational expenses through grants, scholarships, loans, and part-time employment. Federal Graduate Nurse Traineeships are available for qualified full-time students. All enrolled and newly admitted students can use the School's computerized financial aid database to assist them in applying for aid.

APPLYING

Basic B.S.N. applicants must have a minimum 2.0 GPA. Accelerated second degree B.S.N. applicants must have a minimum 3.0 GPA and submit letters of recommendation. Admission to the basic baccalaureate program is competitive; the mean GPA of accepted students is usually above 3.0. Applications for the basic B.S.N. must be submitted by December 1 for early review and by April 15 for regular review. Applications are considered after April 15 as long as space remains in the entering class. Applicants for the RN to B.S.N. or RN to M.S. options must file for admission for spring semester by December 1 and for fall semester by July 1.

M.S. applicants must have a minimum 3.0 GPA and a B.S.N. from an NLN-accredited program.

All Ph.D. applicants, except those in the accelerated B.S.N. to Ph.D. option, must have a minimum 3.0 GPA and a master's degree in nursing from an NLN-accredited program. The GRE is required for all graduate applicants. Students should contact the Office of Admissions and Enrollment Management for complete information on admission requirements.

Correspondence and Information:

Office of Admissions and Enrollment Management
School of Nursing
University of Maryland at Baltimore
655 West Lombard Street
Baltimore, Maryland 21201
Telephone: 410-706-7503
800-328-8346 (toll-free)

THE FACULTY

Carol Easley Allen, Visiting Associate Professor and Acting Assistant Dean, Professional Development and Services; Ph.D., NYU; RN.

Barker Bausell, Professor; Ph.D., Delaware.

Anne Belcher, Associate Professor and Chair, Acute and Long Term Care; Ph.D., Florida State; RN.

Regina Cusson, Associate Professor and Chair, Maternal and Child Health Nursing; Ph.D., Maryland; RN.

Karen Dennis, Professor, Director of Research, and Co-Director, Center for Health Promotion and Disease Prevention; M.S.N., Kentucky; Ph.D., Maryland; RN, FAAN.

Florence Downs, Visiting Professor and Interim Associate Dean for Graduate Studies, Research, and Evaluation; Ed.D., NYU; RN, FAAN.

Barbara Heller, Professor and Dean; Ed.M., Ed.D., Columbia Teachers College; RN, FAAN.

Susan Ludington, Professor; Ph.D., Texas Woman's; RN, CNM, FAAN.

Mary Etta Mills, Associate Professor and Chair, Education, Administration, Health Policy, and Informatics; Sc.D., Johns Hopkins; RN.

Lesley Perry, Associate Professor and Associate Dean, Undergraduate Studies, Outreach, and Instruction; Ph.D., Maryland; RN.

Patricia Prescott, Professor; Ph.D., Denver; RN, FAAN.

Joseph Proulx, Professor; M.S.N., Pennsylvania; Ed.D., Columbia Teachers College; RN.

Sara Torres, Associate Professor and Chair, Psychiatric, Community Health, and Adult Primary Care; Ph.D., Texas at Austin; RN, FAAN.

Carolyn Waltz, Professor and Director, Doctoral Program and Evaluation; Ph.D., Delaware; RN, FAAN.

Susan Wozenski, Assistant Professor and Assistant Dean, Student Affairs; M.P.H., Michigan; J.D., Connecticut.

University of Medicine and Dentistry of New Jersey
School of Nursing
Newark, New Jersey

THE UNIVERSITY

The University of Medicine and Dentistry of New Jersey (UMDNJ) is a national leader in health education and research. Created to consolidate and unify all of the state of New Jersey's public programs in medical and dental education, UMDNJ was founded in 1970 by an act of the State Legislature as the College of Medicine and Dentistry of New Jersey. In 1981, it was granted status as a freestanding university in recognition of its growth and development as a statewide system for the health professions' education and health care.

UMDNJ is dedicated to the pursuit of excellence in the undergraduate, graduate, postgraduate, and continuing education of health professionals and scientists; the conduct of basic biomedical, psychosocial, clinical, and public health research; health promotion, disease prevention, and the delivery of health care; and service to communities and the entire state. The University is the state's university of the health sciences, with programs throughout New Jersey.

THE SCHOOL OF NURSING

The School of Nursing (SN), established as programs in 1990, has quickly been recognized as a driving force in the advancement of nursing education, science, and research. A dynamic institution, the School champions program review and refinement as it prepares its students to meet the health-care challenges of the twenty-first century. The mission of the UMDNJ–SN is to provide innovative leadership in nursing through excellence in scholarship and service and freedom of inquiry. The School has developed a system of articulated nursing education programs throughout the state. The mission of SN is consistent with the University's commitment to excellence in education, research, practice, and service. The nursing faculty members have embraced the constructs of knowledge, clinical competence, teaching and learning, leadership and management, continuous change, scientific research, and professionalism as the essential matrix of the School's curricula. These constructs reflect the faculty's belief in the values of high-quality patient care, professional competence, ethical behavior, interdisciplinary collaboration, and lifelong learning.

The philosophy of nursing education at UMDNJ is based on the conceptual model that humans cannot be understood, studied, or treated apart from the environment. The faculty's beliefs about humans, the environment, nursing, health, and nursing education influence all aspects of the curricula, in both the undergraduate and graduate programs. One mission of nursing education at the School of Nursing is to graduate competent, caring, and accountable nurses at all three degree levels to assume critical roles in today's health-care delivery system. The faculty members believe that nursing provides a spectrum of health care, spanning both generalist, comprehensive care as well as specialty care based on educational preparation and clinical experience.

PROGRAMS OF STUDY

Graduates of the Associate of Science in Nursing program, offered in collaboration with Middlesex County College in Edison, New Jersey, as the partner institution for the general education component, are prepared to practice in today's health-care delivery system and to be contributing citizens of society. Consistent with this mission, the program prepares individuals for nursing roles as providers of care, coordinators of care, and members of the discipline of nursing; graduates individuals who are eligible to take the licensing examination to become registered nurses in New Jersey; and provides educational opportunities for self-awareness and personal growth. Graduates of this program can provide nursing care in a variety of structured health-care settings in which policies and procedures are established. The associate degree program nursing faculty members ascribe to the associate degree nursing competencies as delineated by the National League for Nursing. Graduates can articulate into the joint Bachelor of Science in Nursing degree program.

The School of Nursing's Bachelor of Science in Nursing (B.S.N.) program, in collaboration with Ramapo College of New Jersey in Ramapo and the New Jersey Institute of Technology in Mount Laurel as partner institutions for general education, offers an upper-division curriculum for the registered nurse seeking to complete a baccalaureate program. UMDNJ and Ramapo College also offer a generic curriculum for the individual wishing to become licensed as a registered nurse. This generic track is offered in collaboration with Englewood Hospital and Medical Center. The B.S.N. program's mission is to provide the state of New Jersey with professional registered nurses prepared to assume critical roles in the complex health-care delivery system and to contribute as members of society. Graduates of this program have the knowledge and skills necessary to provide care in collaboration with other health-care providers within complex health-care systems. These graduates practice professional nursing as generalists in a variety of health-care settings.

The University's graduate curriculum leads to the Master of Science in Nursing (M.S.N.) degree. Located on campuses in Newark and Stratford, New Jersey, the program offers some of the most progressive advanced practice nursing programs in the United States. Graduate nursing education is based upon a foundation of undergraduate education that incorporates knowledge from nursing science, basic sciences, social sciences, and humanities. The graduate curriculum emphasizes interdisciplinary education among students in the health sciences. These graduates benefit people through advanced education in nursing and health sciences and via role specialization as advanced practice nurses. Tracks within the M.S.N. program include adult health nurse practitioner, psychiatric–mental health nurse practitioner, adult nurse practitioner with clinical emphasis in occupational health, family health nurse practitioner, nursing informatics, and nurse anesthesia. In addition, a "Transition Program" provides an opportunity for RNs with a bachelor's degree in an area other than nursing to gain matriculation to the M.S.N. program. Graduates provide primary health care in diverse settings in collaboration with other members of the health team. Through advanced preparation in clinical specialties, they also provide expert care in diverse areas.

ACADEMIC FACILITIES

Academic facilities vary by campus. At Middlesex County College, the library houses more than 75,000 bound volumes and holds issues of more than 750 periodicals and newspapers. The twenty-five well-maintained buildings of the campus are of modern design and contain state-of-the-art equipment to meet the needs of students. Ramapo College of New Jersey offers four academic buildings, a library, administration building, and the International Telecommunications Center. At the University of Medicine and Dentistry of New Jersey in Newark, the George F. Smith Library of the Health Sciences collection includes more than 190,000 bound volumes, 2,607 current journal titles, and more than 2,700 audiovisual programs. The UMDNJ School of Nursing Stratford students share the campus with the UMDNJ School of Osteopathic Medicine. Students make full use of the Health Sciences Library located in the academic center. Students also have access to the Educational Media and Resources Department, whose goal is to extend the effectiveness of education through the use of media to communicate ideas, research, and technical information.

STUDENT SERVICES
On-site child care is available at Middlesex County College, Ramapo College of New Jersey, and UMDNJ, Newark. The facilities at Ramapo College of New Jersey also include the student center, gymnasium and playing fields, and housing for 1,200 students. At the UMDNJ campuses in Newark and Stratford, students have access to a fully equipped wellness center.

LOCATION
Middlesex County College, in Edison, New Jersey, is home of the associate degree program. The 200-acre campus is located within easy reach of the state's major highways. Ramapo College of New Jersey is in Mahwah, New Jersey. It is the center of the Northern Region B.S.N. Programs and is located on a 315-acre campus situated in the Ramapo Mountains of Bergen County. The New Jersey Institute of Technology in Mount Laurel, New Jersey, and Burlington County College (BCC) co-own a Technology Engineering Center (TEC) building in Mount Laurel. This building houses the NJIT–UMDNJ joint B.S.N. Program along with NJIT technology engineering programs. The TEC building is strategically located in southern New Jersey close to major highways. UMDNJ, Newark, located in the University Heights section of New Jersey's Renaissance City, is also easily accessed from New Jersey's major highways. The University of Medicine and Dentistry of New Jersey in Stratford, New Jersey, is in a quiet suburban community neighboring Camden and within 10 miles of downtown Philadelphia and 40 miles of Atlantic City.

THE NURSING STUDENT GROUP
There are approximately 400 students enrolled in the School at the undergraduate level and 200 at the graduate level. Ten percent are men, and 22 percent are members of minority groups. Ninety-six percent of UMDNJ School of Nursing graduates passed the National Council Licensure Examination for Registered Nurses in 1996.

COSTS
Students enrolled in joint UMDNJ–SN programs should refer to the catalog and/or handbook of the academic partner institution for information regarding student tuition and fees. Students enrolled in the Master of Science in Nursing program who are New Jersey residents pay $242 per credit; nonresidents pay $322 per credit. There is an administrative fee of $20 per course.

FINANCIAL AID
Students enrolled in joint UMDNJ–SN programs should refer to the catalog and/or handbook of the academic partner institution for information regarding financial aid for their program of study. For students enrolled in the M.S.N. program, a completed application for financial aid consists of the Free Application for Federal Student Aid (FAFSA); a copy of Federal Income Tax forms from parents, spouse, and self; and a Statement of Educational Purpose/Draft Registration Card. No action will be taken on the application until all forms are received. Students who would like further information should contact the UMDNJ Student Financial Aid Office, Administrative Complex, Room 1208, 100 Bergen Street, Newark, New Jersey, 201-982-4376.

APPLYING
Students enrolled in joint UMDNJ–SN programs should refer to the catalog and/or handbook of the academic partner institution for information regarding admission requirements for their program of study. Admission is competitive and dependent upon the availability of openings in each UMDNJ–SN program. Candidates for admission are individually evaluated in accordance with the criteria established for each academic nursing program. Prior to submitting an application for admission, prospective students are encouraged to consult with faculty members of the program in which they wish to matriculate. Students applying to the Master of Science in Nursing program should complete an application in full and return it with a $30 nonrefundable application fee by April 15, 1997. The requirements for admission to the M.S.N. program are a completed UMDNJ–SN application for admission with a $30 fee; transcripts documenting graduation from a National League for Nursing (NLN) accredited baccalaureate degree nursing program or transcripts documenting graduation from an NLN-accredited diploma or associate degree nursing program and a non-nursing baccalaureate degree and all transcripts of all colleges/universities previously attended; evidence of successful completion of the UMDNJ–SN Transition Program for applications with non-nursing baccalaureate degrees; transcripts documenting a minimum 3.0 cumulative grade point average on all undergraduate nursing content; current licensure/reciprocity as a registered nurse in New Jersey; evidence of completion of a basic statistics course, including inferential and descriptive statistics, with a minimum grade of C; evidence of completion of a basic health assessment course within the last five years and completion of a proficiency examination prior to taking the first UMDNJ–SN clinical course; evidence of current Basic Life Support (BLS) certification; three letters of recommendation supporting the applicant's potential success in the M.S.N. program; documentation of the Test of English as a Foreign Language (TOEFL) with a minimum score of 550 for all applicants who are not graduates of a U.S. college/university; evidence of one year's recent experience as a generalist registered nurse prior to entry into the clinical practicum courses; the Admissions Evaluation Essay as administered by UMDNJ-SN; and current physical examination and required immunizations. Applications are reviewed on an individual basis.

Correspondence and Information:

Office of Enrollment and Student Services
Administrative Complex, Room 118
30 Bergen Street
Newark, New Jersey 07107-3000
Telephone: 201-982-6012

University of Michigan
School of Nursing
Ann Arbor, Michigan

THE UNIVERSITY

The University of Michigan, located in Ann Arbor, Michigan, has more than 510,000 alumni worldwide. Graduates of the University have made substantial contributions to intellectual, scientific, and cultural growth. Its internationally ranked faculty, supported by the most advanced research programs, prepares students to teach, lead, heal, and innovate in the global society of the twenty-first century. The University of Michigan is consistently ranked among the nation's top ten universities.

THE SCHOOL OF NURSING

The University of Michigan School of Nursing has held an unsurpassed reputation of excellence for more than 100 years, because it has kept pace with advances in knowledge and technology and trends in health care. The School of Nursing is also unparalleled in terms of its distinguished faculty, with 90 percent of all tenure-track faculty members doctorally prepared. This caliber of faculty preparation enhances the balance between clinical and theoretical experiences for students.

The School of Nursing has extended its vision of leadership to nursing research and pursuing ideas that strengthen nursing practice. The School houses the Center for Nursing Research (CNR). The center provides a general setting for helping scholars undertake and sustain their research efforts. The support of research, as well as the expectation that the faculty will engage in research, contributes to an atmosphere that enhances and encourages productivity.

PROGRAMS OF STUDY

Nursing education is an investment in the future of health care, in terms of both the individual nurse and the overall health-care delivery system. The School of Nursing is strongly committed to the concept that nurses must continue to be challenged educationally in order to meet the rigors of a highly complex, diverse profession. The baccalaureate degree is the basis for a career in nursing. The School of Nursing's B.S.N. four-year program offers applicants direct admission as freshmen. Transfer students may be admitted to the second-year levels of the program. Recently, the School introduced a second career nursing program (concurrent B.S.N./M.S. degrees) for people with bachelor's degrees in other fields. Second career students are able to complete a B.S.N. degree and prepare for the registered nurse NCLEX exam and licensing in nineteen months. A University of Michigan School of Nursing Master of Science degree may then be completed in an additional two to four terms.

In addition to a B.S.N.-completion program in Ann Arbor, the School offers B.S.N.-completion programs in Traverse City and Kalamazoo for the A.D.N. or diploma nurse. There is a three-year RN to M.S. program in Ann Arbor, Michigan. This program combines undergraduate and graduate studies for highly motivated RNs.

At the master's level, the School of Nursing, through the University's's graduate school, offers advanced study in clinical specialist, nurse practitioner, or manager roles in the following programs: adult acute care; adult primary care; community care; family nurse; gerontology; home health care; infant, child, and adolescent health; medical-surgical; nurse midwifery, nursing administration; occupational health; pediatric acute care; psychiatric-mental health; women's health; and M.S./M.B.A. dual degree. Some programs offer post-master's options, and some programs are available through On Job/On Campus.

The On Job/On Campus Program is flexible, offering students an opportunity to learn while maintaining work and family responsibilities. Classes are scheduled for one long weekend a month for twenty to twenty-two months. The emphasis of the program is on home health-care nursing, occupational health nursing, and community care nursing.

The curriculum plan of the master's programs is implemented through four major components: core courses, specialization courses, cognates, and a master's project. Core courses, which are required in all master's-level programs, fall into three subject categories: theory development, leadership, and research. Nursing specialization courses are designed to prepare students for advanced nursing practice in their respective areas of study. Two cognate courses related to a student's program are selected from other University of Michigan graduate areas. All master's degree students are required to complete a master's project that involves participation in research or that is practice- or policy-oriented.

The School's doctoral program is widely regarded as one of the best in the world. The contributions made to nursing research by doctoral alumni add significantly to the increasing body of research that substantiates and influences nursing practice.

The School of Nursing has offered postdoctoral study opportunities since 1987. Currently, this training is offered in health promotion and risk reduction and in neurobehavior, with support from the National Institutes of Health. The goal of the health promotion and risk reduction training program is to develop scientists capable of sustaining independent research careers focused on generating knowledge about health promotion and risk reduction within the theoretical perspective of nursing science. The goal of the neurobehavior training program is to develop scientists capable of sustaining independent research careers focused on generating knowledge about human responses and behaviors associated with altered brain functioning.

ACADEMIC FACILITIES

There are more than 6 million volumes in the twenty-three libraries on the University's campus. Also on campus are nine museums, seven hospitals, hundreds of laboratories and institutes, and more than 12,000 microcomputers.

LOCATION

The University of Michigan is located in Ann Arbor, a city well-known for its parks, rivers, and historical heritage. Ann Arbor's designation as an "All-America City" complements its well-earned title, "Research Center of the Midwest."

STUDENT SERVICES

The University of Michigan has many services available to students, including the Affirmative Action Office, Career Planning and Placement, Center for the Education of Women, Services for Students with Disabilities, the International Center, Lesbian-Gay Male Programs Office, Minority Student Services, Office of Multicultural Affairs, Office of the Ombudsman, Sexual Assault Prevention and Awareness Center, Student Legal Services, Student Organization Development Center, University Health Center, and a multitude of academic and personal counseling services.

THE NURSING STUDENT GROUP

Of the 874 students registered at the School, 573 are undergraduates. The total student body includes 13 percent students of color (African Americans, Native Americans, Asians, and Hispanics). The University of Michigan School of Nursing is proud of its continued commitment to a diverse student body.

COSTS

For 1996–97, full-time tuition costs for resident undergraduate lower-division courses were $2766; for nonresidents, $8869. Tuition costs for resident undergraduate upper-division courses were $3130; for nonresidents, $9500. For resident graduate students, full-time tuition costs were $4661; for nonresidents, $9470.

FINANCIAL AID

Financial assistance based on need is available through the Office of Financial Aid. It may consist of a combination of grants, scholarships, and loans, including Nursing Student Loans and work-study opportunities. A limited number of need-based grants and loans are available after enrollment directly through the School of Nursing. Graduate assistance can be obtained from various sources. Some Graduate Student Teaching and Graduate Student Research Assistantships are available within the School of Nursing. Fellowships and scholarships are available through the Horace H. Rackham School of Graduate Studies.

APPLYING

Applications to the B.S.N. program, RN/B.S.N. program, and master's programs must arrive at the University by February 1; applications to the Second Career Nursing Program are due May 1. The deadline for applications to the doctoral program is December 1. For all current admission information, students should call the University of Michigan School of Nursing at 800-458-8689 (toll-free).

Correspondence and Information:

Office of Undergraduate Admissions
1220 Student Activities Building
The University of Michigan
Ann Arbor, Michigan 48109-1316

Graduate Admissions
Horace H. Rackham School of Graduate Studies
The University of Michigan
Ann Arbor, Michigan 48109-1070

University of Minnesota, Twin Cities Campus
School of Nursing
Minneapolis, Minnesota

THE UNIVERSITY
The University of Minnesota, with its four campuses, ranks among the top twenty universities in the United States. It is both a state land-grant university, with a strong tradition of education and public service, and a major research institution with scholars of national and international reputation. The Academic Health Center on the Minneapolis campus comprises the Medical School, School of Dentistry, School of Nursing, School of Public Health, College of Pharmacy, and the world-acclaimed University of Minnesota Hospital and Clinic.

THE SCHOOL OF NURSING
Established in 1909, the School of Nursing holds the distinction of being the first nursing program on a university campus. In 1989, a new baccalaureate curriculum was implemented and the School established a program for RNs seeking baccalaureate and Master of Science degrees in nursing. The Master of Science graduate program, which offers fifteen areas of study, was established in 1951. The Ph.D. program was established in 1983.

PROGRAMS OF STUDY
The School of Nursing offers three degrees: the Bachelor of Science in Nursing, the Master of Science with a major in nursing, and the Doctor of Philosophy with a major in nursing. The baccalaureate and master's programs are accredited by the National League for Nursing (the NLN does not accredit doctoral programs).

The baccalaureate program is a two-year upper-division major admitting students who have completed 90 credits of transferable prerequisites and liberal arts credits. Ninety-six students are admitted each fall.

The RN/B.S.N./M.S. program is for highly qualified RNs who are seeking a baccalaureate and master's degree. Selected applicants are admitted into the program without specified prerequisite course work.

The Graduate School offers the Master of Science degree with a major in nursing under two plans: Plan A, requiring a thesis, and Plan B, which substitutes additional course work and special projects for the thesis. The M.S. program offers fifteen areas of study, including child and family nursing, family nurse practitioner, gerontological clinical nurse specialist, gerontological nurse practitioner, adult health nursing, nursing administration, nursing education, nurse midwifery, oncology nursing, pediatric nurse practitioner, children with special health-care needs nurse practitioner, psychiatric–mental health nursing, women's health nurse practitioner, and public health nursing with optional emphases in administration; adolescent health; older adult, especially women; parent, child, and family; and school health. An M.P.H./M.S. dual degree is available. The program can be completed in four to six quarters, approximately two years of full-time study.

The Ph.D. program is research-oriented and is designed to prepare creative and productive scholars in nursing. Five areas of study and research are available: development and modification of health-related behaviors, human responses to environmental and life process events disruptive to health, phenomenon of health, organization and system of delivery of nursing care, and organization and system of delivery of nursing knowledge. Students are required to select a minor area of study outside of nursing.

ACADEMIC FACILITIES
The University library system is the fifteenth largest in North America (third in the Big Ten), lending more books and journal articles to other libraries than any other in the nation. Students have access to more than 20,000 computer workstations as well as the clinics and laboratories of the University of Minnesota Hospital and Clinic.

LOCATION
The Twin Cities area, with more than 2 million people, is the metropolitan and cultural center of the upper Midwest. The Minnesota Orchestra, the Tyrone Guthrie Theater, and a rich array of art galleries, museums, and small theaters provide extensive cultural opportunities. Outdoor recreation is exceptional. Numerous lakes within the metropolitan area offer various sports activities throughout the year.

STUDENT SERVICES
The University provides a host of support services for students, including Boynton Health Service, disability services, International Study and Travel Center, student unions, Minnesota Women's Center, Sexual Violence Program, Student Diversity Institute, University Counseling & Consulting Service, student cultural centers, and more.

THE NURSING STUDENT GROUP
The School of Nursing enrollment is about 595 students. The B.S.N. program has approximately 220 students, the master's program has approximately 330 students, and the Ph.D. program has approximately 40 students.

COSTS
Tuition in 1996–97 for the B.S.N. program was $90.45 per credit for residents and $266.80 per credit for nonresidents. For full-time graduate students, tuition (for 7–12 credits) was $1560 for residents and $3130 for nonresidents; it was $275 per credit for students taking fewer than 7 credits or more than 12 credits. Student services fees totaled $156.71.

FINANCIAL AID
Financial aid resources include graduate fellowships, graduate teaching and research assistantships, scholarships from the School of Nursing Foundation, traineeship grants, and loans from the Office of Student Financial Services.

APPLYING
Requirements for B.S.N. program applicants include 90 credits of prerequisites, a preferred minimum grade point average of 2.8 on a 4.0 scale, and a profile statement. The application deadline is April 1.

Applicants to the RN/B.S.N./M.S. program should have a minimum GPA of 2.8 and RN licensure and submit three references and a profile statement. The application deadline is April 1.

M.S. program applicants must have an RN license and a bachelor's degree with a major in nursing or, if the degree is not in nursing, evidence of ability in health promotion, community health nursing, leadership, teaching, and systematic investigation. Applicants must submit three letters of reference and a profile statement. Applications are reviewed October 15 for winter or spring quarter, December 15 for winter or spring quarter, and April 15 for summer or fall quarter. The application deadline for nurse-midwifery and nurse practitioner areas of study is December 15.

Applicants to the Ph.D. program must have a master's degree and a strong background in the physical or behavioral sciences or a bachelor's degree with an exceptionally strong record and submit GRE scores, two letters of reference, and a profile statement. Applications must be received by December 20 to be considered for a Graduate School Fellowship or by January 25 for the fall quarter.

Correspondence and Information:

UMTC School of Nursing
6-101 Weaver-Densford Hall
308 Harvard Street Southeast
Minneapolis, Minnesota 55455
Telephone: 612-624-4454

THE FACULTY

Melissa D. Avery, Assistant Professor; Ph.D. (nursing), Minnesota. Exercise as a therapeutic intervention for women with gestational diabetes, maternal nutrition and other antenatal factors influencing infant birth weight, outcomes of nurse-midwifery care.

Linda H. Bearinger, Assistant Professor; Ph.D. (educational psychology), Minnesota. Public health issues and interventions among adolescents, health decision-making among at-risk populations, adolescent health nursing education.

Donna Z. Bliss, Assistant Professor; Ph.D. (nursing), Pennsylvania. Effects of dietary fiber on the colon.

Derryl E. Block, Assistant Professor; Ph.D. (nursing), Pennsylvania. Child passenger safety, public health nursing, health policy.

Margaret J. Bull, Associate Professor; Ph.D. (urban social institutions), Wisconsin–Milwaukee. Community health nursing, continuity of care, long-term care, outcomes following hospitalization.

Sheila Corcoran-Perry, Professor; Ph.D. (educational psychology), Minnesota. Clinical decision making, expert-novice differences, client decision making.

Patricia Crisham, Associate Professor; Ph.D. (developmental psychology), Minnesota. Moral and ethical issues in health care, nurses' resolution of ethical dilemmas.

Sara S. DeHart, Associate Professor; Ph.D. (developmental psychology), Case Western Reserve. Alcoholism identification and treatment outcomes for women and older adults.

Laura J. Duckett, Associate Professor; Ph.D. (educational psychology), Minnesota. Maternal employment and breastfeeding.

Sandra R. Edwardson, Professor; Ph.D. (hospital and health-care administration), Minnesota. Cost-quality tradeoffs in nursing services, elderly self-care behavior.

Ellen C. Egan, Associate Professor; Ph.D. (nursing), NYU. Instrument development; stress appraisal: challenge and threat; stress interventions: therapeutic touch, hand massage, and relaxation.

Bernadine Feldman, Associate Professor; Ph.D. (educational psychology), Minnesota. Educational research, policy analysis.

Helen E. Hansen, Assistant Professor; Ph.D. (nursing), Kansas. Nursing administration, health-care delivery systems, health team collaboration, leadership.

LaVohn E. Josten, Associate Professor; Ph.D. (hospital and health-care administration), Minnesota. Public health nursing, community health promotion, compliance with health recommendations, not-kept home visit appointments, family violence.

Merrie J. Kaas, Assistant Professor; D.N.Sc. (nursing), California, San Francisco. Older women's mental health, mental health/illness in long-term care.

Kathleen E. Krichbaum, Assistant Professor; Ph.D. (education), Minnesota. Factors contributing to quality of care for the elderly in nursing homes, clinical teaching effectiveness, evaluating clinical learning.

Barbara J. Leonard, Associate Professor; Ph.D. (hospital and health-care administration), Minnesota. Child health care, care of children with special health-care needs.

Marsha L. Lewis, Assistant Professor; Ph.D. (curriculum and instructional systems), Minnesota. Clinical and client decision making, quality of life for the chronically mentally ill.

Betty Lia-Hoagberg, Associate Professor; Ph.D. (higher education), Minnesota. Prenatal care, psychosocial factors and access to care, nursing interventions with high-risk beginning families.

Linda L. Lindeke, Assistant Professor; Ph.D. (educational administration), Minnesota. Advanced nursing practice, high-risk infants.

Ruth D. Lindquist, Associate Professor; Ph.D. (social and administrative pharmacy), Minnesota. Risks of and response to cardiovascular disease, personal control and quality of life in health care, alterations in homeostatic function in elderly, critical care.

Carol J. Pederson, Assistant Professor; Ph.D. (educational psychology), Minnesota. Nonpharmacological interventions with children undergoing painful procedures.

Janice Post-White, Assistant Professor; Ph.D. (nursing), Minnesota. Oncology, psychoneuroimmunology, mental imagery.

Muriel B. Ryden, Professor; Ph.D. (educational psychology), Minnesota. Autonomy and morale in institutionalized aged, aggressive behavior in dementia.

A. Marilyn Sime, Professor; Ph.D. (educational psychology), Minnesota. Cognitive interventions and psychological distress, personal control as a coping strategy in health-care situations.

Mariah Snyder, Professor; Ph.D. (education), Minnesota. Determining efficacy of nursing interventions, management of aggressive behaviors in persons with dementia, coping with chronic health problems, testing impact of advanced practice nurses on health outcomes in elders.

Patricia Short Tomlinson, Professor; Ph.D. (family relations and human development), Oregon State. Family health theory development, parent-child interaction, family stress and adaptation in acute and long-term care.

Barbara A. Vellenga, Associate Professor; Ph.D. (nursing), Texas at Austin. Temperament and self-esteem in children and mothers, perceptions of coping in the chronically mentally ill and in Vietnam veterans.

Mary G. Weisensee, Assistant Professor; Ph.D. (higher education), Michigan State. Caregivers' perceptions.

University of New England
Nursing Programs
Biddeford and Portland, Maine

THE COLLEGE

The University of New England (UNE) is a small, independent, coeducational university that has chosen as its primary fields of education the biological sciences and health (both mental and physical). Related programs in psychology, education, and business management are also important parts of the University's educational plan. The University of New England's philosophy of education and student life places emphasis on the quality of instruction and on the practical application of academic material.

Each program includes the opportunity for learning in a community-based setting. Internships, co-ops, clinicals, and student teaching all add up to the practical experience that allows students at UNE to apply the skills learned in the classroom to real job situations.

The University of New England has two campuses. The University Campus is located on the southern coast of Maine in Biddeford, 90 miles north of Boston and 20 miles south of Portland, Maine's largest city. The campus has a total population of 2,100 students. The Westbrook College Campus is located in Portland, Maine, and has a population of 300 students. As both campuses are geographically placed in areas that afford a high-quality lifestyle, it is only natural that the University of New England consistently engages itself in providing its students with high-quality programming and high-quality education.

The men and women who teach at the University of New England are an experienced group of people whose average age is 40. More than 85 percent have earned the highest degree in their field, and they bring to the University varied backgrounds as teachers and practitioners of their disciplines. They are highly competent, demanding, concerned, accessible, and willing to give individual attention to students. Most important, they have come to the University for many of the same reasons that prompt their students to attend. The match between what the faculty has to offer and what the students need and expect is the key to the rare educational environment at the University of New England. UNE's most recent accreditation report stated that "while many small institutions believe in individual attention, UNE does it."

THE NURSING PROGRAM

The University of New England offers five nursing programs that enroll a total of 307 nursing students. The University of New England's University Campus offers a two-year Associate Degree in Nursing (A.D.N.), a two-year Bachelor of Science in Nursing (B.S.N.) completion program, and a Master of Science-Nurse Anesthesia program. The University's Westbrook College Campus offers a four-year Bachelor of Science in Nursing (B.S.N.) program and a Master of Science Nurse Practitioner program in partnership with Simmons College.

PROGRAM OF STUDY

On the University Campus, students are challenged with a rigorous two-plus-two nursing curriculum that places the students in clinical work and nursing course work during the first year. Clinical work continues through the month of June. At the end of year two, students receive an Associate Degree in Nursing and take their N-Clex-RN exam. After passing this exam students, who are now registered nurses, may opt to work as an RN and continue school part-time to complete their B.S.N. or work as an RN and not return to school. The B.S.N. completion program, the last two years of study, places a great deal of emphasis on community health experience. In addition to the traditional nursing courses, B.S.N. students take advanced courses in professional nursing, physical assessment, clinical decision making, research, clinical theory and practice, and leadership and management.

The Westbrook College Campus of the University of New England offers a more traditional B.S.N. program and is a meaningful combination of two areas of study: a liberal arts education with a focus in the physical and social sciences and a classic nursing education that includes the development of clinical skills. Under the supervision of an on-site faculty member, freshman nursing students work in local hospitals and nursing homes to begin learning and observing clinical skills. Development of on-the-job clinical skills extends beyond the academic year to include three summers of nursing employment, and students are paid at the CNA (certified nursing assistant) rate for their summer co-op experiences. University of New England nursing students on both campuses are awarded a CNA certificate after successful completion of the freshman year. Registered nurses wishing to enter a B.S.N. program may do so at either campus.

Both campuses of the University of New England offer master's degree programs in nursing. The University Campus has a Master of Science-Nurse Anesthesia program. Under the integrated M.S.-Nurse Anesthesia Program, the University awards the Master of Science-Nurse Anesthesia degree to students who satisfactorily complete a 50-credit schedule of classes over a twenty-seven–month period. Successful completion of the program qualifies the student to take the National Certifying Examination. The on-campus didactic portion consists of graduate courses taught by the UNE graduate science faculty and the clinical faculty from the affiliated hospitals. This segment is offered primarily over a nine-month period of study and is followed by the eighteen-month clinical portion that includes continuing lectures, seminars, and independent research courses taught by UNE and hospital faculty members. The University also offers the didactic portion of the program for some hospital-based schools of anesthesia.

The Nurse Practitioner program on the University's Westbrook College Campus is offered in partnership with Simmons College of Boston, Massachusetts. The program has concentrations in adult health, family health, and pediatrics.

AFFILIATIONS WITH HEALTH-CARE FACILITIES

The University uses a wide range of settings for the clinical portion of the nursing programs it offers. These may include but are not limited to: community programs for the homeless or victims of family violence, extended and long-term–care centers, health maintenance organizations, elementary schools, the Department of Health, and hospitals and the more traditional centers and community health agencies. The University also has agreements with a number of hospitals and health-care agencies in New England whereby students may work during their summer co-ops. These agreements have included the Indian Health Service, summer camps for children, and home-care situations.

ACADEMIC FACILITIES
The Josephine S. Abplanalp Library, located on the University's Westbrook Campus, and the Jack S. Ketchum Library on the University Campus provide the students with more than 140,000 volumes and 1,300 periodicals. Students on both campuses have access to computer support that includes IBM and Macintosh along with a full range of software packages. The University Campus also has a computer store that offers educational discounts and services all equipment sold through the store. The Blewett Science Center services the nursing programs on the University's Westbrook College Campus and includes classrooms and science and nursing laboratories. Supporting facilities on the University Campus include the Petts Health Center (nursing classroom), Marcil Hall (nurse anesthesia classroom), and the Harold Alfond Center for Health Sciences, a $20-million state-of-the-art science facility.

LOCATION
The University of New England's Westbrook College Campus is located in a quiet residential area just outside Portland, Maine. Portland is a vibrant city that offers a great variety of entertainment options for the students. Portland's International Jetport allows easy access to the city, which is only a 2-hour drive north of Boston, Massachusetts. The University Campus is located on the banks of the Saco River and the shores of the Atlantic Ocean in Biddeford, Maine. This 425-acre campus is between the towns of Old Orchard Beach and Kennebunkport and is 20 miles south of Portland, Maine, and 90 miles north of Boston, Massachusetts.

STUDENT SERVICES
The University of New England offers a wide range of services on both campuses. Special features include a full health clinic, a dental hygiene clinic, a children's center that operates a kindergarten, career counseling, personal counseling, learning support services, and an extensive student leadership development program.

Both campuses offer a variety of cultural and social events. The Campus Center on the University Campus and the Finley Recreation Center on the Westbrook College Campus provide settings for many recreational and sports activities. The University of New England Athletic Department operates an NCAA Division III varsity athletics program and also holds membership in the NAIA.

THE NURSING STUDENT GROUP
The student population in the four-year B.S.N. program is characterized by the more traditional student entering from high school. The two-year A.D.N. program has a relatively even mix of traditional students and adult learners. Many of the students in the A.D.N. program who complete the B.S.N. portion of the B.S.N. completion program are from the traditional student group. Those students entering the two-year B.S.N. completion program from outside the University are practicing registered nurses.

COSTS
Tuition for 1996–97 was $13,050; room and board was $5495. The A.D.N. program has one 6-credit summer session with an additional $2610 tuition fee. Graduate program costs are per credit hour—the nurse anesthesia program 1996–97 cost per credit hour was $315; the nurse practitioner program (in affiliation with Simmons College) 1996–97 cost per credit hour was $546.

FINANCIAL AID
Every effort is made to provide financial assistance to qualified students who enroll at the University of New England. Approximately 90 percent of matriculated students receive some form of financial aid. Financial aid is based on need as determined by the Free Application for Federal Student Aid (FAFSA). The University also awards scholarships based on academic achievement. Students wishing to receive financial assistance should submit their financial aid materials by April 1. While this is not an absolute deadline, it is a priority date.

APPLYING
Successful applicants to the University Campus associate degree nursing program will have received a high school diploma or GED that includes course work in biology and chemistry (both with labs) and two years of math (including algebra). Competitive candidates will have a C+ average or above and a combined SAT I score of 800 or higher. Students seeking to enroll in the two-year B.S.N. completion program must have a nursing diploma or have completed an A.D.N. program, achieved a minimum cumulative GPA of 2.5, and hold a current RN license.

Applicants to the University's Westbrook College Campus B.S.N. program should have a high school diploma or GED with course work including algebra I and II, geometry, and biology and chemistry with labs. Competitive candidates will have a C+ average or better and SAT I scores totaling 800 or higher.

Admission to the University of New England A.D.N. and B.S.N. programs is somewhat competitive. Decisions are made with particular attention paid to school course work, grades received for this course work, recommendations, and the student's expressed reasons for wishing to enter the nursing profession (this is done in the essay and interview). All applicants are encouraged to visit the campus that offers the program to which they are seeking admission. Admissions are granted on a rolling basis; however, because there generally is a waiting list students are encouraged to apply before March 1.

Correspondence and Information:

University of New England
Office of Admissions
Hills Beach Road
Biddeford, Maine 04005
Telephone: 207-283-0171
Fax: 207-286-3678
World Wide Web: http://www.une.edu/

University of Pennsylvania
School of Nursing
Philadelphia, Pennsylvania

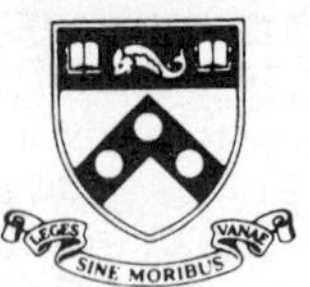

THE UNIVERSITY

The University of Pennsylvania is an independent, nonsectarian institution. As one of the finest universities in the country, it offers an outstanding array of resources for both undergraduate and graduate students. The excellence of its many schools offers students the opportunity to take elective courses across the campus in a wide range of subjects, making it one of the major centers for learning and research in the nation. Penn will be graduating the student of the twenty-first century from a seamless academic community. This concept provides a framework that fosters student and faculty collaboration across the University and enhances opportunities for a diversified approach to education and research.

THE SCHOOL OF NURSING

The University of Pennsylvania is the only Ivy League institution that offers a baccalaureate nursing program that begins day one, master's programs in nursing, and doctoral nursing study. The University of Pennsylvania Medical Center began training professional nurses in 1886. Today the School of Nursing at Penn offers one of the most progressive, flexible, and highly regarded programs in the country.

Recently the University of Pennsylvania School of Nursing was ranked among the nation's top graduate schools of nursing in a major survey conducted by *U.S. News & World Report.* In determining its rankings, the criteria considered were the School's reputation for scholarship, curriculum, research, and the quality of the faculty and students. The undergraduate nursing program is listed in *Ruggs Book of Colleges* as high school guidance counselors' first choice for nursing.

The University has virtually all of its undergraduate and graduate facilities—including its hospitals, libraries, and laboratories—on one campus, giving nursing students access to people, ideas, and information on a multitude of subjects. Nursing students have matchless opportunities for clinical experience at the world-renowned University of Pennsylvania Medical Center, the Children's Hospital of Philadelphia, and Children's Seashore House in addition to many other clinical agencies and health-care institutions in the Philadelphia area.

At Penn, nursing students are taught and advised by a faculty that is nationally and internationally recognized for its leadership in education, practice, and research. Undergraduate and graduate students often take advantage of the opportunity to participate in faculty research and scholarly publications. The Penn faculty members have a deep commitment to their role as teachers as well as to the development of professional and personal alliances between students and faculty.

PROGRAMS OF STUDY

The School of Nursing offers a Bachelor of Science in Nursing (B.S.N.) degree with a program that balances the liberal arts, science, and professional nursing preparation. Courses in the nursing major emphasize interpersonal communication, clinical competence, decision-making skills, and research. Special opportunities include nursing specific study abroad programs; dual-degree programs and minors in Penn's College of Arts and Sciences, Wharton School, or School of Engineering and Applied Science; and submatriculation (initiating pursuit of the M.S.N. degree while working toward the completion of the B.S.N.).

Beginning in fall 1997, the University will initiate a formalized undergraduate dual-degree program offered jointly by the School of Nursing and the Wharton Business School in nursing and health-care management. Additional new programs include a direct entry B.S.N./Ph.D. program and an M.S.N. to Ph.D. program. New programs under development include joint curricular initiatives between the School of Nursing and the University's School of Arts and Sciences and the School of Engineering and Applied Science.

Penn offers a program allowing students already holding a baccalaureate degree to complete a B.S.N. degree. The second degree program builds on an individual's present level of education so that students need only complete required nursing-specific courses.

The RN Return Program is designed to educate hospital diploma and associate degree RNs for an increased leadership role in nursing through the earning of a B.S.N. degree. Previous college and university courses are evaluated for transfer credit, and many clinical nursing courses may be challenged by examination.

The School also offers an accelerated program (B.S.N./M.S.N. Direct Entry Program) for highly motivated, academically talented registered nurses and students already holding a degree in a field other than nursing. Students apply concurrently for admission to the undergraduate program and to one of the School's graduate program offerings. The program is individualized according to the past educational experience of the student.

The School of Nursing offers the Master of Science in Nursing (M.S.N.) degree in over twenty different areas, including adult/acute tertiary nurse practitioner; adult critical-care nurse practitioner; oncology advanced practice nurse specialist; oncology adult and pediatric nurse practitioner; gerontological nurse practitioner; health care of women nurse practitioner; nurse midwifery; perinatal advanced practice nurse specialist; perinatal nurse practitioner; neonatal nurse practitioner; adult, home-care, and pediatric primary care; pediatric acute-/chronic-care nurse practitioner; pediatric critical-care nurse practitioner; occupational health nurse practitioner; occupational health administration/consultation; nursing administration; and psychiatric–mental health advanced practice nurse specialist for adult and special populations, child and family, or geropsychiatric care. An M.S.N. in nursing administration/M.B.A. is also offered in conjunction with the Wharton School.

The School of Nursing recognizes the evolving nature of health care and the desire on the part of many nurses to expand or alter current roles and responsibilities. Two programs of advanced study available are the Post-Master's and dual-major options. The Post-Master's Option is designed for those who already possess a master's degree in nursing and are interested in extending their knowledge and skill in their current area of practice or changing to a new area of nursing practice. The dual-major option is for individuals who would like to pursue two programs of interest.

The Doctor of Philosophy Program provides learning opportunities that emphasize the scholarship and research demands of the discipline of nursing and the doctoral degree. The program can be constructed from either the baccalaureate or the master's degree. The program is flexibly structured into four parts: a clinical field, a required core, a related field, and the doctoral dissertation. The curriculum for the degree is organized to provide a general structure within which students participate in developing their own programs of study based on their nursing backgrounds and their research interests.

ACADEMIC FACILITIES

The University of Pennsylvania libraries house over 4,209,747 bound volumes and 33,384 periodical subscriptions. The Biomedical Library, adjacent to the School of Nursing, houses over 175,980 books and journals in the nursing, medical, and biological sciences. Students may access CD-ROM databases and nine other major information databases, including MEDLINE and nursing data bases.

The School of Nursing has, for student use, a computer lab, a TV studio, a multimedia production center, photography services, learning laboratories, and Pennet with access to Internet.

Specialized centers at the School of Nursing include the Center for Urban Health; International Center of Research for Women, Children and Families; the Center for Health Services and Policy Research; the Center for the Study of the History of Nursing; and the Center for Advancing Care in Serious Illness.

LOCATION

Philadelphia is the fourth-largest city in the United States. The four undergraduate schools and twelve graduate schools of the University are located on a 260-acre tract on the west side of the Schuylkill River. Unified by a network of pedestrian walkways and almost entirely closed off to cars, the campus contributes to the sense of community that is characteristic of Penn. Although situated in a major urban setting just across the river and less than 2 miles from the center of Philadelphia, the University is surrounded by a largely residential community known as University City. Adjacent to the School of Nursing is the Philadelphia Center for Health Care Sciences and two major teaching hospitals, the University of Pennsylvania Medical Center and the Children's Hospital of Philadelphia.

STUDENT SERVICES

The University campus has many resources and services available to meet the needs of the Penn student. These include cultural centers, religious organizations, academic advising, counseling, housing, dining, student health, tutoring, day care, athletic facilities, and computing services.

THE NURSING STUDENT GROUP

The School of Nursing population is a diverse group composed of traditional undergraduates, transfer students, students holding degrees in other fields (second degree students), RN returning students, B.S.N./M.S.N. students, and master's and doctoral students. The School of Nursing is an intimate niche within the University enabling students to receive personalized attention from the faculty and staff. School of Nursing faculty members advise nursing students, further enhancing student-faculty interaction.

COSTS

Tuition for full-time B.S.N. students for the 1996–97 academic year was $18,964. Part-time tuition was $2423 per course. Tuition for full-time M.S.N. students was $19,226; $2581 per course. Ph.D. tuition was $20,644 for full-time students and $2769 per course.

FINANCIAL AID

The University of Pennsylvania is committed to meeting the financial needs of all of its students. Many different sources of aid are available. Scholarships, grants, low-interest student loans, and teaching and research assistantships are awarded appropriately, based on a student's need and level of study. A School of Nursing full-time financial aid counselor is available for individual consultation and support. Students are encouraged to work directly with the School to help them develop the means to support their education.

APPLYING

Freshman applicants to the B.S.N. program should be completing a general college-preparatory program in high school. They must also take the Scholastic Assessment Test (SAT I) and three SAT II Subject Tests, including one in a science and one in writing, or the ACT exams of American College Testing.

Prospective freshman students can apply under one of two admissions plans. The Early Decision Plan is for those applicants who have decided that the University of Pennsylvania School of Nursing is their first-choice college and agree to attend if accepted. Applications are due by November 1, with decisions mailed in mid-December. Regular decision applicants to the School of Nursing are reviewed on a rolling admissions basis. Applications are due by January 1, and students are notified beginning in the middle of February.

Transfer students are admitted in both the fall and spring semesters. The application deadline is October 15 with notification in December for the spring semester and April 1 for the fall semester, with notification beginning by the end of April.

B.S.N./M.S.N. applicants must apply by December 1 for September admission and will hear by late February. The Graduate Record Examinations (GRE) are required for all applicants. Nursing administration/M.B.A. applicants must also take the Graduate Management Admission Test (GMAT).

It is important that applicants to all of the baccalaureate options arrange a personal interview with an admissions counselor in the School of Nursing. This interview will afford students an opportunity to learn more about the specific program they are considering and to better understand the course work required to complete the B.S.N. degree.

All master's and doctoral applicants must have completed an NLN-approved baccalaureate program, a course in basic statistics, and have nursing licensure. Applicants must schedule an interview with the appropriate program director and must submit, along with the completed application form, GRE General Test scores (and GMAT scores, if appropriate), transcripts, and references. Students from other countries must submit the results of the TOEFL. The application deadline for fall entrance is February 15 for master's programs and January 1 for doctoral programs.

Students can access the School of Nursing's World Wide Web address (listed below) to see a photograph of a nurse treating a baby in an infant intensive care unit and can use six clickable buttons that lead to information about the nursing school and other health-care resources.

Correspondence and Information:

University of Pennsylvania
School of Nursing
Nursing Education Building
Philadelphia, Pennsylvania 19104-6096
Telephone: 215-898-4271
Fax: 215-573-8439
E-mail: smithmar@pobox.upenn.edu
WWW: http://www.upenn.edu/nursing/index.html

University of Pittsburgh
School of Nursing
Pittsburgh, Pennsylvania

THE UNIVERSITY

Founded in 1787, the University of Pittsburgh is the oldest institution of higher education west of the Allegheny Mountains. It is an independent, state-related, nonsectarian coeducational institution offering a variety of undergraduate and graduate programs. Total enrollment at the Pittsburgh campus is approximately 29,000, including nearly 10,000 graduate and professional students. In recognition of the strength of its graduate programs, the University was elected in 1974 to the Association of American Universities, an organization of the fifty-eight most respected graduate and research institutions in North America.

THE SCHOOL OF NURSING

Founded in 1939 as an independent school of the University, the School of Nursing strives to have a positive impact on the quality of health care for all segments of the population through its teaching, research, and service. It offers educational programs that anticipate and reflect the health-care needs of the region, state, and nation, resulting in the awarding of almost 5,900 baccalaureate degrees, more than 2,100 master's degrees, and over 100 doctoral degrees to nursing students. With a total student body of fewer than 900, nursing students benefit from the low student-faculty ratio and small class sizes of the School of Nursing, as well as from the extensive resources and enrichment opportunities of a major research university and medical center.

The School is known nationally for the strengths of its clinical and research programs. Students benefit from the variety and excellence of available clinical sites, including three nurse-managed nurse practitioner clinics. Faculty members who teach clinical courses have their own clinical practice in order to share their knowledge and enhance their skills. Current faculty and student research programs reflect the breadth of patient populations and health-care problems that are under investigation.

PROGRAMS OF STUDY

Three study options are available at the undergraduate level: the baccalaureate program, an accelerated B.S.N. program, and programs designed especially for registered nurses (RNs). Baccalaureate students typically enter as freshmen unless they have completed all required freshman courses and are accepted into the sophomore class. The 127-credit curriculum emphasizes the basic liberal arts and sciences the first year and initiates the clinical phase the second year. The last two years include a variety of clinical experiences culminating in a leadership/transition course where seniors work closely with nurse preceptors. Students with a baccalaureate degree in another field can apply to the fast-paced, four-term accelerated B.S.N. program. Graduates of both programs are eligible to take the National Council Licensure Examination (NCLEX) to become RNs. Registered nurse options are the RN-B.S.N. or RN-M.S.N. programs, where the B.S.N. can be earned in one year of full-time study or longer for part-time study.

Graduate programs of study lead to the M.S.N. or Ph.D. degrees. The master's program prepares students for the advanced practice roles of nurse anesthetist or nurse practitioner through the following majors: nurse anesthesia; acute-care nurse practitioner with concentration in cardiopulmonary, critical care, or oncology; and primary care nurse practitioner options in family, pediatrics, psychiatric, or women's health. Minors in nursing education or nursing systems (administration) are also available.

The master's program is five to seven terms in length and varies from 49 to 52 credits. The curriculum consists of core courses, advanced nursing practice specialty courses, role development courses, and electives. Core courses include health promotion, pathophysiology, physical diagnosis, pharmacology, nursing theory and research, and research practicum. A second master's option is also available, and a thesis is optional.

The Ph.D. program prepares scholars to extend scientific knowledge that advances the science and practice of nursing and to contribute to the scientific base of other disciplines. The curriculum includes courses in the history and philosophy of science, nursing theory development, the structure of nursing knowledge, issues influencing leadership and public policy in nursing and health, advanced statistics, quantitative research methods, research methodologies, instrumentation, and a research practicum with an experienced researcher. An area of research emphasis, which matches a faculty member's research emphasis, is selected by the student early in the program. Current faculty research initiatives include adolescent health, chronic disorders, critical care, health promotion, and mental health. The culminating requirement is a dissertation.

Completing the doctoral program full-time requires eight terms of study (60 credits minimum) depending upon the nature and complexity of the dissertation, and part-time study takes four to six years. A one-term full-time residency is required of all doctoral students.

ACADEMIC FACILITIES

Nursing students have access to the Maurice and Laura Falk Library of the Health Sciences, with 2,578 journals and 258,896 volumes, and to the University Library System, with 2,789,302 items. The School of Nursing Learning Resources Center (LRC) provides reference services, a nursing skills practice laboratory, computer laboratory, small television studio, graphics laboratory, and a print collection of 150 journals and 9,050 volumes. The LRC computer laboratory is open 60 hours per week and provides microcomputer capability and access to the University mainframe computer system and to the Internet. Students also use the University's computer labs, which are located around the campus.

LOCATION

The University's 125-acre campus is situated in Oakland, the heart of Pittsburgh's educational, medical, and cultural center. Within walking distance of the campus are theaters, art galleries, museums, libraries, and concert halls.

Pittsburgh has consistently been named one of the nation's most livable cities in various national surveys. Most students and many faculty members live within walking distance of the University, either in Oakland, Squirrel Hill, or Shadyside. These areas abound in ethnic restaurants and in shops of all varieties, reflecting the cosmopolitan background of the residents. Most people find that Pittsburgh is a friendly, warm, active, exciting, and comfortable city in which to live.

STUDENT SERVICES

The University offers students a wide variety of services, including outpatient health care at the Student Health Service;

career development, learning skills, and psychological services; veterans and disabled student services; numerous student activities; and child care.

THE NURSING STUDENT GROUP

In 1995–96, the School of Nursing enrolled 527 undergraduate students and 349 graduate students. More than 50 percent were already registered nurses who were working toward B.S.N., M.S.N., or Ph.D. degrees in order to improve their career mobility, assume a new role, or increase their personal satisfaction.

COSTS

Undergraduate tuition per term in 1996–97 for full-time study was $3484 for in-state and $7524 for out-of-state students. Tuition per credit for part-time study was $238 for in-state and $500 for out-of-state students. Full-time student fees were $262, and part-time student fees were $75 per term. On-campus housing costs ranged from $1065 to $1735 per term. Available meal plan options varied from $700 to $975 per term.

Graduate tuition per term in 1996–97 for full-time study was $4327 for in-state and $8829 for out-of-state students. Tuition per credit for part-time study was $358 for in-state and $729 for out-of-state students. Full-time student fees were $232, and part-time student fees were $68 per term.

FINANCIAL AID

The University awards financial assistance to both undergraduate and graduate students through scholarships, loans, and part-time employment. Freshman applicants apply by March 1 and continuing students by April 1.

Master's students receive a variety of financial aid through the School of Nursing, including Professional Nurse Traineeships for full-time study, University tuition aid for part-time study, specified scholarships, and loans.

Doctoral students also receive aid from the School. Out-of-state full-time students pay in-state tuition rates due to school-based scholarships. Many full-time doctoral students have graduate assistant, researcher, or teaching fellow positions, which are primarily merit-based, pay a stipend, and include a tuition scholarship and individual health insurance. These students work 10–20 hours per week, and many have excellent experiences on faculty research projects or teaching. Workshops on applying for predoctoral and postdoctoral training grant fellowships are provided. In addition, other scholarships and part-time tuition aid are available. Students should apply for all School-based aid by June 1 and should contact the Student Affairs Office for further information.

APPLYING

Applicants to all programs should present appropriate transcripts, admission test scores, and other required material by the deadline date. For the latest and most complete admission information, applicants should contact the Student Affairs Office. In addition, undergraduate applicants should contact the University Office of Admissions and Financial Aid at 412-624-PITT to receive information and an application. Admission decisions are made on a rolling basis, but applicants should apply as early as possible or by February 1. Accelerated B.S.N. program applicants apply through the School of Nursing by December 1. Registered nurse applicants are admitted on a rolling basis for all terms.

Undergraduate applicants are evaluated primarily on the basis of their high school or previous college-level academic work, with an emphasis on performance in science courses. For high school applicants or transfer applicants with fewer than 24 credits, SAT I scores are also considered.

Master's applicants must have a baccalaureate degree in nursing, a current license to practice, and one to two years of experience (for full-time study). Admission decisions are based upon a faculty interview, professional goals, previous academic performance, and GRE or MAT scores. Applications are considered on a rolling basis.

Doctoral applicants must have a baccalaureate degree in nursing, documentation of academic success in an appropriate master's program, evidence of competence in scholarly research and the ability to communicate in writing, and satisfactory GRE scores. Admission decisions are based upon previous academic performance, faculty interviews, professional and research goals, a match between the applicant's research interest and those of available faculty members, and GRE scores. Applications should be received by April 1 for fall term and October 1 for spring term.

Correspondence and Information:

Student Affairs Office
School of Nursing
University of Pittsburgh
3500 Victoria Street
Pittsburgh, Pennsylvania 15261
Telephone: 412-624-2407
Fax: 412-624-2401
E-mail: nursao+@pitt.edu

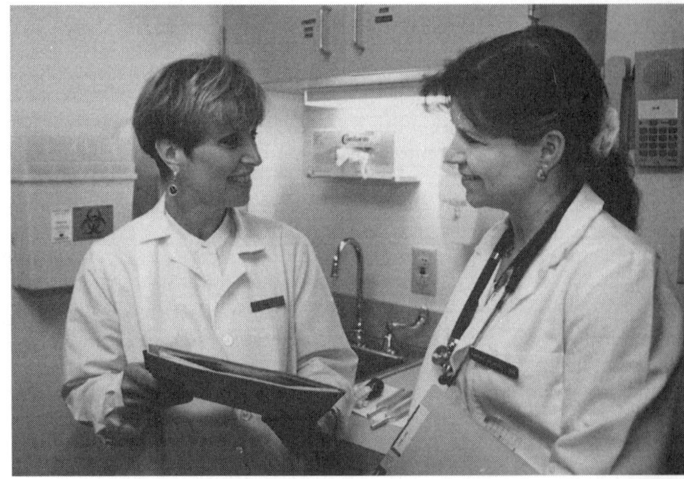

The master's program prepares students for advanced practice roles in six areas.

University of San Diego
Philip Y. Hahn School of Nursing
San Diego, California

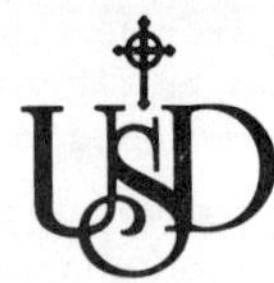

THE UNIVERSITY

The University of San Diego (USD) is an independent, Roman Catholic university founded in 1949. With a holistic philosophy, USD seeks to foster competence, international and cultural sensitivity, professional responsibility, and a spirit of volunteerism in each student. The University places a special emphasis on the exploration of human values and welcomes non-Catholics as well as Catholic students and faculty members.

The 180-acre hilltop campus, known for its Spanish Renaissance architecture, overlooks Mission Bay with breathtaking views of the Pacific Ocean and San Diego Bay. USD's central location offers students easy access to the San Diego area.

The University comprises five academic units: the College of Arts and Sciences and the Schools of Business Administration, Education, Law, and Nursing. Total enrollment in the fall 1996 semester was 6,603 (4,299 undergraduates, 1,080 law students, and 1,224 graduate students).

THE SCHOOL OF NURSING

Founded in 1974 through an endowment by the late Philip Y. Hahn, the School of Nursing was established to offer the Bachelor of Science in Nursing (B.S.N.) for registered nurses. Following the graduation of the first class in 1976, the Master of Science in Nursing (M.S.N.) program was established. The Doctor of Nursing Science (D.N.Sc.) program was approved in 1985, and the first D.N.Sc. degree was awarded in May 1989.

The mission of the Hahn School of Nursing is to be at the forefront of the discipline of nursing by providing excellence in the quality of the School's baccalaureate and graduate programs through its teaching, by strengthening the knowledge base for nursing practice through research, and by providing leadership for the discipline through its faculty and graduates.

All of the School's full-time, tenure-track faculty members are doctorally prepared. Part-time faculty members hold at least a master's degree in their clinical specialty area. The School also has the services of a rich cadre of clinical, administrative, and educational preceptors.

The School of Nursing is centrally located and occupies a beautifully appointed building constructed in 1978 through federal funds and matching funds from Murial Hahn, the widow of Philip Y. Hahn. The youngest and smallest of the five academic units of the University, the School of Nursing offers educational programs at the undergraduate, master's, and doctoral levels.

PROGRAMS OF STUDY

The Philip Y. Hahn School of Nursing offers the B.S.N. for RNs, the Accelerated RN to M.S.N., the M.S.N., a joint M.B.A./M.S.N. with the School of Business Administration, and the D.N.Sc. A School Nurse Health Services Credential and Post-M.S.N. Family and Adult Nurse Practitioner Certificates are also offered. The B.S.N. and the M.S.N. programs are accredited by the National League for Nursing (NLN). The Master of Business Administration (M.B.A.) is accredited by the American Assembly of Collegiate Schools of Business (AACSB).

All the degree programs are designed for RN students—adult learners who reenter the educational setting with a wide variety of personal and professional backgrounds. Classroom and clinical experiences are tailored to meet their unique needs. All programs are designed to prepare nurses to accept increased responsibility within the health-care system and to assume leadership roles within the nursing profession.

The B.S.N. program with an upper-division major in nursing is structured for graduates of hospital diploma and associate degree programs who have met the specified prerequisite admission requirements.

The M.S.N. program is built upon the baccalaureate degree in nursing and emphasizes research, theory, and practice. The M.S.N. program prepares adult nurse practitioners with a subspecialty in gerontology, family health nurse practitioners, school health nurse practitioners, and nurse administrators for leadership and managerial roles in client-care services administration in health-care organizations. The program also prepares advanced-practice nurse case managers for specific client groups in acute care, long-term care, community, and home health settings. Latino health-care and pediatric options are available within the family health nurse practitioner track. Each of the options shares a common core of knowledge and each one is designed to prepare an advanced practice nurse in the respective area.

The Accelerated RN to M.S.N. program is designed for nurses holding a diploma or an associate degree who want to pursue the M.S.N. degree. The program of study leads to the awarding of the B.S.N. degree and eligibility for certification as a public health nurse in the state of California, as well as the M.S.N. degree. The program offers the same specialty options as the M.S.N.

The D.N.Sc. program is designed to prepare nurse scholars who will advance knowledge in the discipline through the extension of the theoretical base of nursing, the generation of new knowledge, and the application of knowledge to professional practice. The program provides learning opportunities that emphasize theory development, research, and leadership ability in response to social, political, and ethical issues in health care.

AFFILIATIONS WITH HEALTH-CARE FACILITIES

The School is affiliated with a wide variety of clinical resources including UCSD Medical Center, Sharp Health Care (Hospitals and Clinics), Children's Hospital, Veterans Administration Hospital, and Balboa Naval Hospital. Because of its focus on health promotion, a large number of community agencies are utilized, including schools, home health agencies, the San Diego Department of Health Services, HMOs, and community clinics.

ACADEMIC FACILITIES

The Helen K. and James C. Copley Library houses more than 300,000 books and bound periodicals and also includes subscriptions to 1,700 journals, collections of reference works, government documents, pamphlets, newspapers in many languages, and rare books. In addition to its own collection, Copley Library has network connections with most academic and large public libraries in North America and with major national bibliographic and information databases available to USD students and faculty. The Media Center, a division of Copley Center, supports the instructional function of the University by providing nonprint information services such as videotapes and audiotapes.

The School of Nursing houses a learning resource center. The center is provided for the student to listen to and view selected instructional media software such as videotapes, audiotapes, and sound/slide presentations. The center also produces audiovisual software and overhead transparencies for faculty and student use.

LOCATION

Located on the southern tip of California, San Diego offers a wide variety of recreational, business, science, art, and cultural activities. With an average temperature of 64 degrees in February and 76 degrees in August, the area is perfect for biking, jogging, tennis, softball, and all aquatic sports. San Diego is also noted for a world-famous zoo, museums, Spanish missions, Sea World, and major sports programs. The proximity to Mexico provides an excellent opportunity for gaining firsthand insights into Mexican culture. The International Airport, downtown, Mission Bay, and the Aquatic Center are just a few minutes from the campus.

STUDENT SERVICES

The University has many resources and services designed to meet student needs. These include the Manchester Family Child Development Center (child care and development), Health Center, Sports and Recreation Center, bookstore, post office, Academic Computing Services, Campus Ministry, housing, dining services, and the Hahn University Center and its facilities, including the new Multicultural Center. The International Resource Center and International Student Association offer personal and academic advising and activities.

THE NURSING STUDENT GROUP

All students in the Hahn School of Nursing are registered nurses and most are practicing, at least part-time. Depending on their experience and the level of program being pursued, students are employed in positions as varied as beginning-level practitioner to nurse educator to middle- or top-level health-care administrator.

COSTS

Tuition costs for the 1996–97 academic year were $510 per unit for the B.S.N., $525 per unit for the M.S.N., and $540 per unit for the D.N.Sc. Since all students are registered nurses, they seldom live in campus housing. However, living expenses, including room and board, transportation, and personal expenses, are estimated at approximately $9000. Other educational expenses, including books, immunizations, instruments, insurance, travel to clinical sites, and student fees, total approximately $4500.

FINANCIAL AID

The primary purpose of the financial aid program at USD is to provide financial assistance to students who, without such aid, would be unable to attend the University. Financial need is met by a combination of scholarships, grants, graduate fellowships, loans, and graduate assistantships. Federal Graduate Nurse Traineeships are offered through the School of Nursing.

APPLYING

Applicants to all degree programs must have California nursing licensure as an RN and professional liability and malpractice insurance. Both the B.S.N. and Accelerated RN to M.S.N. programs require completion of all nursing program prerequisites prior to application and a GPA of 3.0 on a 4.0 scale. The RN to M.S.N. program also requires a minimum of one year's experience as an RN. The master's and post-master's programs further require a B.S.N. or an M.S.N., respectively, from an NLN-accredited institution; a minimum GPA of 3.0 on a 4.0 scale; a 3-unit course in statistics; and one year of professional nursing practice. Additional requirements for the doctoral program include a minimum of one year's experience in clinical nursing beyond the B.S.N. and a minimum graduate school GPA of 3.5 on a 4.0 scale. Applicants with non-nursing baccalaureate or master's degrees may be considered for admission to the M.S.N. and D.N.Sc. programs, respectively. Students should contact the appropriate office at the University for complete information about admission requirements and application deadlines.

Correspondence and Information:

Office of Undergraduate Admissions
University of San Diego
5998 Alcala Park
San Diego, California 92110-2492
Telephone: 619-260-4506

Office of Graduate Admissions
University of San Diego
5998 Alcala Park
San Diego, California 92110-2492
Telephone: 619-260-4524

THE FACULTY

Cheryl Ahern-Lehmann, Instructor; M.S., California, San Francisco; RN.
Mary Jo Clark, Associate Dean and Associate Professor; M.S.N., Texas Woman's; Ph.D., Texas at Austin; RN.
Patricia M. Garver, Assistant Professor; D.N.Sc., Catholic University; RN.
Jane M. Georges, Assistant Professor; M.S.N., California, San Francisco; Ph.D., Washington (Seattle); RN.
Janet K. Harrison, Professor; M.S.N., Maryland; Ed.D., USC; RN.
Diane C. Hatton, Associate Professor; D.N.Sc., California, San Francisco; RN.
Mary Ann Hautman, Professor; M.S.N., Wayne State; Ph.D., Texas at Austin; RN.
Susan Instone, Assistant Professor; D.N.Sc., San Diego; RN.
Kathleen S. James, Assistant Professor; D.N.Sc., San Diego; RN.
L. Colette Jones, Professor; M.S.N., Catholic University; Ph.D., Maryland; RN, FAAN.
Gwen G. Morse, Assistant Professor; M.S.N., California State, Dominguez Hills; Ph.D., Arizona; RN.
Patricia Quinn, Instructor; M.S., California, San Francisco; RN.
Louise Rauckhorst, Associate Professor; M.S.N., Catholic University; Ed.D., Columbia; RN, FAAN.
Janet A. Rodgers, Professor and Dean; Ph.D., NYU; RN, FAAN.
Patricia Roth, Professor; M.S.N., Arizona; Ed.D., USC; RN.
Nancy Jex Sabin, Instructor; M.S., California, San Francisco; RN.
Mary Ann Thurkettle, Associate Professor; Ph.D., Case Western Reserve; RN.

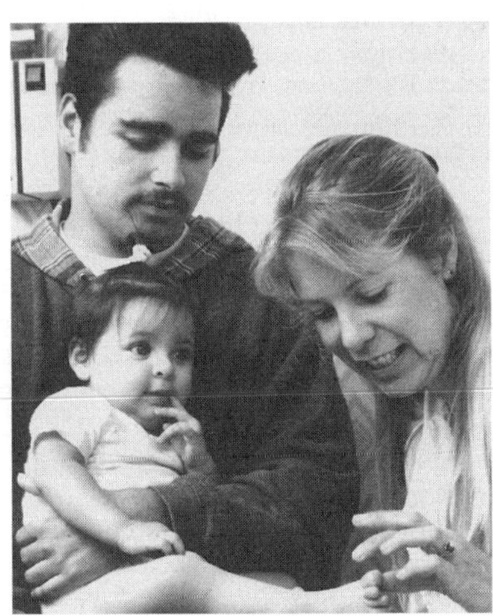

Nurse practitioner student examining a child in a migrant community clinic.

University of San Francisco
School of Nursing
San Francisco, California

THE UNIVERSITY

Established by the Jesuit Fathers in 1855, the University of San Francisco (USF) is a private institution accredited by the Western Association of Schools and Colleges. In addition, the School of Nursing is accredited by the California State Board of Registered Nursing and the National League for Nursing (NLN). There are six schools and colleges within the University: the Schools of Business, Law, Nursing, and Education and the Colleges of Professional Studies and Arts and Sciences. The University has approximately 5,000 undergraduate and 3,000 graduate students.

THE SCHOOL OF NURSING

The School of Nursing at the University of San Francisco has a long history of preparing professional nurses within the Jesuit academic tradition. The first private nursing program in California, the School has been accredited since its first class graduated in 1958. The School of Nursing is the largest private baccalaureate nursing program in the state, enrolling a diverse student body and serving both traditional and nontraditional students. The School offers a four-year program leading to the Bachelor of Science in Nursing (B.S.N.) degree as well as a Master of Science in Nursing (M.S.N.) degree program.

PROGRAMS OF STUDY

The undergraduate curriculum has undergone a major revision in order to better prepare graduates to meet future needs in the health-care delivery system. The curriculum requires that students become more active learners, and the three areas of critical thinking, communication, and therapeutic interventions are basic outcomes of the program. The revised curriculum also prepares graduates for a professional practice in the community as the number of community-based opportunities increases. The mission and goals of the University are reinforced and channeled professionally by the nursing faculty members, who see the liberalizing influence of the humanities as a distinctive feature of the baccalaureate program in nursing for effecting personal fulfillment and professional enrichment. The new nursing curriculum provides both the necessary nursing competencies in the areas of specialization defined by the Board of Registered Nursing and the essential content as mandated by law. In the last semester, a capstone clinical course is provided in the student's specific area of interest. It is a four-year program, and students must complete a minimum of 128 units to graduate. The program is fully accredited, and graduates are eligible for licensure as RNs in California and to receive the Public Health Nursing Certificate.

The School of Nursing also offers an M.S.N. program designed for the practicing registered nurse. Most classes are scheduled in the evening one or two days a week. The program can be completed on either a part-time or full-time basis. Consistent with the national trend in nursing education and practice, the M.S.N. program prepares graduates for maximum career mobility with tracks for adult health advanced practice nursing, family nurse practitioner, and management of clinical systems. Completion of the adult health advanced practice nursing track makes the student eligible for certification as an adult health or family nursing practitioner and/or clinical nurse specialist. Completion of the management of clinical systems track prepares the student for a leadership position in clinical systems throughout the continuum of care and in managed-care organizations. In addition, the School of Nursing and the McLaren School of Business offer a joint M.S.N./M.B.A. program. Graduates of this program are prepared for executive administration positions. Each of the master's in nursing program tracks requires 15 units of core course work and then major course work as follows: 36 units for the adult health advanced practice nursing track, 38 units for the family nurse practitioner track, and 21 units for the management of clinical systems track. The joint M.S.N./M.B.A. program requires either 69 or 71 units, depending on the student's choice of courses. Each program culminates in a comprehensive exam.

AFFILIATIONS WITH HEALTH-CARE FACILITIES

The School of Nursing is affiliated with a wide variety of clinical resources, including UCSF Medical Center, San Francisco General Hospital, St. Mary's Medical Center, and San Francisco Veterans Affairs Hospital. In addition, a large number of community agencies are utilized, including schools, home health agencies, local departments of health, HMOs, and community clinics.

ACADEMIC FACILITIES

USF's Gleeson Library houses more than 1.6 million books, periodicals, microfilms, newspapers, pamphlets, and recordings as well as a special collection of rare books. In addition to the above, students have access to the San Francisco interlibrary loan program.

LOCATION

Situated on a hill rising above Golden Gate Park, USF lies at the heart of a multiethnic and diverse international city. San Francisco is scenic and the climate is temperate, making it the ideal urban campus for graduate study.

STUDENT SERVICES

The student body of USF is very diverse and is reflective of the larger community in which it resides. General student resources include academic support services, the Learning and Writing Center, information technology services, campus ministry, residence life, student health services, Counseling Center, disability-related services, Career Services Center, the Department of Student Leadership and Outreach Services, the Office of Service Learning and Community Service, student government organizations, media and publications, performing arts, clubs and organizations, multicultural student services, recreational sports, and intercollegiate athletics.

THE NURSING STUDENT GROUP

Like the city of San Francisco and its patient population, the School's student body is diverse. Women and men with a wide age range from many ethnic, cultural, religious, and experiential backgrounds enrich the student experience. There are approximately 650 students in the undergraduate and graduate programs. The School's graduates are highly sought, and many of its alumni practice in widely differing settings throughout the Bay Area, California, and the rest of the country.

COSTS

Tuition for undergraduates for the 1997–98 school year is $7923 per semester. Freshman and sophomore students under the age of 21 are required to live in the USF residence halls.

Exemptions are granted to students living with parents who reside at a permanent residence within a 20-mile radius of the USF campus. The Office of Residence Life oversees four residence halls on the University campus. A variety of living options are available to accommodate the diverse student population at USF. For example, residents can live on specialty floors, such as the Freshman Experience Floor, Multicultural Floor, Quiet Floor, and Substance-Free Floor. The cost per semester for housing is $2198 (double room), and meal plans range from $1236 to $1630 per semester.

Tuition for the 1997–98 school year for the graduate nursing program is $627 per unit. Most students in the program either live in the area or find housing in one of the many unique neighborhoods in the city. A few students have stayed in Lone Mountain, where on-campus graduate housing is available. This graduate residence hall is a good interim choice for students who are coming in from out of town. A single room costs $2836 per semester and a double room is $2198 per semester. Meal plans range from $1236 to $1630 per semester.

Information on housing is available from the Office of Residence Life (415-422-6824).

FINANCIAL AID

A number of options are available for students in the B.S.N. program. Students are eligible for scholarships from various sources and loans and grants through USF's Office of Financial Aid. Students in the M.S.N. program are eligible for financial assistance through Federal Nursing Traineeships, scholarships from various sources, and loans and grants through USF's Office of Financial Aid. Information on financial aid is available from the University of San Francisco Office of Financial Aid (415-422-6303).

APPLYING

For admission to the B.S.N. program, all candidates applying for freshman standing should secure an undergraduate admission form from the Office of Admissions and return the completed application form and essay to the Office of Admissions with a nonrefundable application fee of $35, request that their high school counselor or an appropriate teacher complete the letter of recommendation form and mail it directly to the Office of Admissions, request that their high school send an official up-to-date transcript of all previous academic work directly to the Office of Admissions (at the end of the high school year, a final transcript is required to complete the applicant's file), and arrange for SAT I or ACT scores to be sent to the Office of Admissions. In addition, applicants who are not residents of the United States must observe the admission standards and procedures for international students.

For admission to the M.S.N. program, the School of Nursing requires a baccalaureate degree in nursing from an NLN-accredited program or its equivalent (international graduates); RNs with a non-nursing baccalaureate degree are evaluated on an individual basis. Undergraduate courses in nursing research and statistics are required. In addition, applicants should have an undergraduate GPA of at least 3.0 (on a 4.0 scale) in the last 58 upper-division units of earned credit, evidence of licensure to practice nursing in California, Graduate Record Examinations (GRE) scores, one year of clinical practice as a registered nurse (preferred), and a personal interview. A score of at least 600 on the Test of English as a Foreign Language (TOEFL) is required of international students. For other admission requirements for international students, applicants should contact the graduate nursing office.

Correspondence and Information:

B.S.N. program:
Office of Admissions
University of San Francisco
2130 Fulton Street
San Francisco, California 94117-1080
Telephone: 415-422-6563
800-Call-USF (toll-free outside California)
Fax: 415-422-2217

School of Nursing
Cliff Morrison, Assistant Dean for Student Services
Cowell Hall 102
University of San Francisco
2130 Fulton Street
San Francisco, California 94117-1080
Telephone: 415-422-6694
E-mail: morrisonc@usfca.edu

M.S.N. program:
Office of Graduate Admissions
University of San Francisco
2130 Fulton Street
San Francisco, California 94117-1080
Telephone: 415-422-GRAD
800-Call-USF (toll-free outside California)
Fax: 415-422-2217
E-mail: graduate@usfca.edu

Dr. Gay Goss, Director
Graduate Nursing Program
School of Nursing
Cowell Hall 102
University of San Francisco
2130 Fulton Street
San Francisco, California 94117-1080
Telephone: 415-422-6596
E-mail: goss@usfca.edu

THE FACULTY

Professors

Betty J. Carmack, Ed.D., San Francisco, 1981.
Norma Chaska, Ph.D., Boston University, 1975; FAAN.
Jane Corbett, Ed.D., San Francisco, 1985.
Louise Trygstad, D.N.Sc., California, San Francisco, 1984.

Associate Professors

Robin Buccheri, D.N.Sc., California, San Francisco, 1984.
Marsha Fonteyn, Ph.D., Texas at Austin, 1991.
Sister Mary Brian Kelber, D.N.Sc., Catholic University, 1976.
Betsy Stetson, Ed.D., San Francisco, 1989.

Assistant Professors

Sarah Abrams, Ph.D., California, San Francisco, 1992.
Lou Ellen Barnes, D.N.Sc., California, San Francisco, 1991.
Marjorie Barter, Ed.D., San Francisco, 1990.
Mary Lou DeNatale, Ed.D., San Francisco, 1988.
Sister Mary Ellene Egan, Ed.D., San Francisco, 1989.
Gay Goss, Ph.D., California, San Francisco, 1995.
Judith Harr, Ed.D., San Francisco, 1996.
Sally Higgins, Ph.D., California, San Francisco, 1991; FAAN.
Catherine Juve, Ph.D., Minnesota, 1996.
Catherine Kenney, Ed.D., San Francisco, 1979.
Roberta Romeo, Ph.D., Maryland, 1991.
Diane Torkelson, Ph.D., Texas at Austin, 1992.

University of South Alabama
College of Nursing
Mobile, Alabama

THE UNIVERSITY

The University of South Alabama is a highly progressive and rapidly growing state-supported institution. First opened to 264 students in 1964, the University now has an enrollment of more than 12,000 students representing the rich cultural diversity of forty-three states and sixty-six countries.

The University is committed to developing and maintaining programs of excellence in teaching, research, and public service. There are seven colleges and three schools within the University offering a wide range of curricula at both the graduate and undergraduate levels.

THE COLLEGE OF NURSING

Ranked by a 1991 survey in *USA Today* as seventh in enrollment in the United States, the College has a current total enrollment of more than 1,300 students. Fully accredited by the National League for Nursing, the College is an integral part of the University of South Alabama and the academic health-care community, one of the most modern and diversified educational, research, and patient-care facilities in the southeast region of the United States.

The academic health-care community includes the University of South Alabama Hospitals and Clinics, which comprise the Medical Center, the Women's and Children's Hospital, Knollwood Park Hospital, and multiple primary and ambulatory care outpatient clinics.

PROGRAMS OF STUDY

The University of South Alabama College of Nursing offers the Bachelor of Science in Nursing (B.S.N.) and Master of Science in Nursing (M.S.N.) degrees. The B.S.N. program is designed to give professional nurses the knowledge and skills necessary to meet current and emerging needs of a changing society and to provide students a foundation for graduate study and professional continuing education. The B.S.N. program has two tracks, one for generic students and one for registered nurse students who hold an associate degree or diploma in nursing.

Registered nurses (RNs) who are associate degree or diploma graduates are admitted to a special track pending completion of prerequisite cognate courses. Class schedules for RN students are offered every other weekend to accommodate the working student.

The B.S.N. program prepares graduates to (1) deliver professional nursing care that assists individuals, families, and communities with changing needs across the life span for health promotion and maintenance, illness care, and rehabilitation; (2) use theoretical and empirical knowledge from nursing and related disciplines in providing professional nursing care; (3) assume responsibility and accountability for one's own nursing practice; (4) evaluate research findings for use in nursing practice; (5) participate in the improvement of the nursing profession, the health-care delivery system, and the formulation of health policy through leadership, management, and teaching skills; (6) collaborate with health-care providers and consumers to promote the health of individuals, families, and communities; and (7) incorporate ethical, moral, and legal values into professional nursing roles designed to meet the current and emerging health needs of a changing society.

The M.S.N. program builds on the bachelor's degree in nursing. The development of leaders with specialized knowledge and skill in the practice of advanced nursing is a primary emphasis in the program. The M.S.N. program offers the following options for advanced preparation in nursing: neonatal nurse practitioner, adult acute-care nurse practitioner, family nurse practitioner, nursing education, mid-level nursing administration, executive-level nursing administration, clinical nurse specialization in adult health nursing, community/mental health nursing, and woman/child health nursing. The M.S.N. program also has an alternative track for registered nurse students with bachelor's degrees in a field outside of nursing.

The M.S.N. program prepares graduates to (1) integrate advanced knowledge and theories from nursing and related disciplines into nursing practice; (2) demonstrate competence in an advanced nursing practice role; (3) use scientific inquiry to identify researchable problems and participate in nursing research; (4) apply advanced knowledge of leadership, management, and teaching to improve nursing practice; (5) influence the improvement of health-care delivery and the formulation of health policy; and (6) contribute to the focus and direction of the nursing profession.

AFFILIATIONS WITH HEALTH-CARE FACILITIES

In addition to the extensive clinical facilities available through the University of South Alabama Hospitals and Clinics, the College has clinical affiliation agreements with over seventy agencies located in the upper Gulf Coast region. A wide variety of clinical experience in urban and rural areas and with multicultural populations is also available.

ACADEMIC FACILITIES

The College of Nursing building is a modern five-story structure with adequate and attractive space for student instruction. The College has a Computer Resource Center and a Learning Resource Center, which enables the faculty to extend learning supports through simulated practice experiences for students.

The University of South Alabama libraries provide information and access to materials needed to fulfill the teaching, scholarship, and service goals of the University. A multimillion-dollar building project has been completed recently to enhance services and offerings of the libraries.

LOCATION

The University of South Alabama is located in Mobile, Alabama, a port city and metropolitan area with a population of 476,000. While summers are warm, the overall climate is pleasantly mild. The nearby Gulf of Mexico beaches and extensive water resources of Mobile Bay at its tributaries provide outstanding recreational opportunities as well as award-winning cuisine.

STUDENT SERVICES

The University of South Alabama is concerned with the total growth and development of its students. The University has a University Center for students, two bookstores, a campus recreation program, counseling services, international student services, disabled student services, minority student services, health services, and other support services. Over 100 professional and special interest clubs, religious groups, and honor societies are active at the University.

THE NURSING STUDENT GROUP

Of the more than 1,300 students comprising the nursing student group, 289 are graduate students and 1,080 are undergraduate students. Approximately 19 percent of the student group are men and 20 percent are members of ethnic/minority groups. Students are attracted to the College's strong emphasis on teaching and other "user-friendly" characteristics of the nursing program. Graduates of the program are actively recruited by health-care agencies and hold significant leadership positions in the health-care system throughout the Gulf Coast area.

Membership in the College's Nursing Students Association is open to all undergraduate students. The College of Nursing also sponsors a chapter of Sigma Theta Tau International. Membership is by invitation to outstanding nursing students, faculty members, and community leaders.

COSTS

Tuition for the 1996–97 academic year was $52 per credit for undergraduate courses and $68 per credit for graduate courses. University fees per quarter average $66 for full-time in-state students and $475 for full-time out-of-state students. All College theory courses carry a $15 course fee. Clinical practicum course fees are $40.

Residence halls and meal plans are available. Estimated expenses for tuition, fees, and room and board for undergraduate students total $6000 per year. Graduate students spend approximately $7000 per year for these items. Other expenses include travel to clinical sites, books, uniforms, immunizations, malpractice insurance, and health assessment equipment.

FINANCIAL AID

The University of South Alabama subscribes to the principle that the purpose of financial aid is to provide assistance to students who, for lack of funds, would otherwise be unable to attend college. Inquiries about financial aid should be addressed to the Office of Financial Aid, Administration Building, Room 260, University of South Alabama, Mobile, Alabama 36688-0002; telephone: 205-460-6231.

The Graduate School at the University has a limited number of graduate assistantships to assist qualified graduate students. The College of Nursing also receives Federal Professional Traineeships funds to assist a limited number of graduate students with their master's-level study.

APPLYING

While students are admitted to the College every quarter, admission to the B.S.N. program is selective and competitive. When the number of qualified applicants exceeds the number that can be accommodated in clinical courses, priority is based on grade point average.

Applications are reviewed to determine that students have satisfied prenursing requirements in conduct, health, scholastic achievement, and aptitude for nursing. Students are selected based on the following factors: (1) submission of an application; (2) a minimum 2.5 cumulative grade point average on all prerequisite courses (A = 4.0); (3) a minimum grade of C in all science, preprofessional nursing, and health science courses; (4) completion of all remedial work recommended by the student's adviser; (5) submission of a health record and required immunizations; (6) one letter of professional reference; (7) satisfactory completion of the College of Nursing dosage calculation tests; and (8) evidence of CPR certification.

Students are admitted to the M.S.N. program each quarter with regular or provisional status. Admission to the nurse practitioner tracks is selective and competitive. The criteria for regular admission to the program are as follows: (1) graduation from an approved bachelor's degree program with a major in nursing; (2) verification of one course or the equivalent in research and health assessment; (3) a score of at least 45 on the Miller Analogies Test; (4) current registered nurse licensure; (5) two letters of professional reference, preferably one from a faculty member and one from an employer; and (6) a minimum grade point average of 3.0 on all undergraduate work (A = 4.0). An earned graduate degree from any accredited institution of higher education may qualify the applicant for regular standing. Provisional admission requires a score of at least 30 on the Miller Analogies Test. Other criteria remain the same.

Correspondence and Information:

General admissions inquiries:
University Office of Admissions
Administration Building, Room 182
University of South Alabama
Mobile, Alabama 36688-0002
Telephone: 205-460-6141
800-872-5247 (toll-free)

Admission to B.S.N. and M.S.N. programs:
University of South Alabama College of Nursing
Office of Admissions and Advisement
USA Springhill
Mobile, Alabama 36688-0002
Telephone: 205-434-3410

THE FACULTY

The following is a list of graduate faculty members in the College of Nursing.

Amanda S. Baker, Professor and Dean; Ph.D., Florida, 1974.
Alice S. Bohannon, Assistant Professor; Ph.D., Miami (Florida), 1995.
Sandra Britten, Adjunct Clinical Assistant Professor; M.S.N., Florida, 1990.
Cheryl Buchholz, Clinical Assistant Professor; M.S., Colorado, 1994.
Joy H. Carlson, Professor; Ed.D., Florida, 1975.
Carol A. Clements, Professor; D.S.N., Alabama at Birmingham, 1985.
Sherry Daniels, Assistant Professor; M.S.N., Alabama at Birmingham, 1980.
Debra C. Davis, Professor and Associate Dean; D.S.N., Alabama at Birmingham, 1984.
Frank deGruy, Associate Professor of Medicine; M.D., South Alabama, 1977; M.S.F.M., Case Western Reserve, 1985.
Norma O. Doolittle, Professor; Ed.D., Auburn, 1992.
Josephine L. Ercums, Clinical Assistant Professor; M.S.N., Vanderbilt, 1977.
Sharon Fruh, Assistant Professor; Ph.D., Illinois at Chicago, 1995.
Alice J. Godfrey, Assistant Professor; M.P.H., North Carolina, 1971.
Patricia Gropp, Clinical Assistant Professor; M.S.N., South Alabama, 1990.
Brenda J. Holloway, Clinical Assistant Professor; M.S.N., Mississippi University for Women, 1982.
Jane A. Hulett, Clinical Assistant Professor; M.S.N., Mississippi University for Women, 1987.
Jason Jones, Assistant Professor; Ed.D., American, 1991.
Mary Jo Morrissey, Clinical Assistant Professor; D.N.S., LSU, 1996.
Charlene Myers, Clinical Assistant Professor; M.S.N., South Alabama, 1994.
Elizabeth Ramsey, Adjunct Clinical Assistant Professor; M.S.N., Texas at Galveston, 1990.
Rosemary Rhodes, Professor; D.N.S., LSU, 1994.
Candice Ross, Associate Professor; Ph.D., Texas at Arlington, 1983.
Martha N. Surline, Clinical Assistant Professor; M.S., Cornell, 1966.
Elizabeth A. Vande Waa, Assistant Professor; Ph.D., Michigan State, 1986.
Alice Ward, Professor; Ed.D., Florida State, 1982.
Stephanie D. Wiggins, Associate Professor; D.S.N., Alabama at Birmingham, 1990.

University of Southern California
Department of Nursing
Los Angeles, California

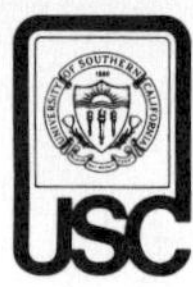

THE UNIVERSITY

Located in the heart of Los Angeles, the University of Southern California (USC) is the oldest independent research university in the western United States. The University is fully accredited by the Accrediting Commission for Senior Colleges and Universities of the Western Association of Schools and Colleges. Since 1960, USC has been a member of the Association of American Universities, an elective body that unites the fifty-eight strongest research universities in the United States and Canada. USC is an international center for research and scholarship. According to the National Science Foundation, USC ranks eighth among private universities receiving federal funds for research and eighteenth among all universities.

Since its establishment in 1880, USC has conferred degrees on more than 250,000 students. It currently offers nearly 500 major/degree combinations in seventy-six fields of study—including bachelor's, master's, and doctoral levels—and boasts eighteen professional schools. The University houses a nationally recognized Center for Health Professions, composed of the independent Departments of Nursing, Occupational Therapy, and Biokinesiology and Physical Therapy as well as the Schools of Medicine, Dentistry, and Pharmacy.

The University enrollment for 1996–97 was 14,690 undergraduate students and 12,980 graduate students. The student body is exceptionally diverse, and USC has the largest number of international students of any major private university.

THE DEPARTMENT OF NURSING

The Department of Nursing was established in 1981 and has grown from a baccalaureate-only program to an academic unit offering both Bachelor of Science in Nursing (B.S.N.) and Master of Science in Nursing (M.S.N.) degrees.

The mission of the Department is to enhance the health of a diverse community by providing excellence in nursing education to develop professional nurses who represent and serve diverse communities, by creating an environment of closeness and willingness to help others, by advancing research-based nursing, and by advocating for continuous improvement in the health-care system and the profession of nursing.

Nursing faculty members are chosen from experts in the field. As a commitment to its mission of creating an environment of closeness and willingness to help others, the Department emphasizes a student-centered approach befitting a private university. Faculty and support staff are responsive to student concerns and suggestions.

PROGRAMS OF STUDY

Baccalaureate nursing education at USC is a combination of supporting sciences, nursing sciences, and humanities. Freshmen admitted as declared nursing majors follow the carefully planned sequence of study for the first two years. Nursing course work begins during the junior year.

USC also offers a Bachelor of Science in Nursing for the Registered Nurse (B.S.N. for the RN). This is a program that provides advanced placement for the registered nurse student while simultaneously providing the full benefits of the Bachelor of Science in Nursing curriculum that generic nursing majors enjoy.

Registered nurses begin the nursing major with upper-division course work designed to build on past nursing experience and knowledge. The registered nurse program offers flexibility and the opportunity for new knowledge growth with elective course work. Registered nurse students may complete the nursing curriculum for the B.S.N. degree in three semesters by attending classes full-time. The curriculum may also be completed on a part-time basis.

For students who know that they want an M.S.N. degree at the time of registration, the Department's Multiple Entry Options program provides a flexible and accelerated pathway to achieve a Master of Science in Nursing degree. By eliminating duplication and organizing the course work, generic bachelor's students, second degree students, and A.D.N. students can progress easily and in a shorter period of time from a bachelor's degree to a Master of Science in Nursing. Detailed information is available from the Department.

The Master of Science program in nursing offers specialty options in nurse midwifery, family nurse practitioner studies, enterostomal therapy, and nursing administration. A dual degree program for students pursuing the nursing administrator role combines nursing with business administration for the dual M.S.N./M.B.A. degree.

The graduate program consists of a three-semester, 40–41 unit course of study that is completed in one academic year. The program includes research, nursing theory, health-care delivery system, seminar on integration into the health-care system, an advanced practicum residency, and a series of courses in the specialty. A comprehensive examination is required. Graduates are eligible for certification by the American Nurses Association, the American College of Nurse-Midwifery, or the International Association of Enterostomal Therapists.

AFFILIATIONS WITH HEALTH-CARE FACILITIES

The Department of Nursing is affiliated with a broad range of clinical facilities in the Los Angeles area. Clinical practice sites in diverse communities include public teaching and private community hospitals, clinics, and home health agencies, large and small. These facilities include the Los Angeles County and USC Medical Center, Huntington Memorial Hospital, Cedars-Sinai Medical Center, California Medical Center Los Angeles, Hollywood Presbyterian–Queen of Angeles Medical Center, Memorial Hospital of Long Beach, Hospital of the Good Samaritan, San Gabriel Valley Community Hospital, Santa Monica Hospital, the Visiting Nurse Association, the Inglewood Health Department, and the Venice Free Clinic.

ACADEMIC FACILITIES

The University of Southern California provides its students and faculty with a full range of physical facilities: a state-of-the-art library system; computer labs providing students and faculty with terminals, dozens of programs and databases, and trained support staff; learning support services for a variety of needs and populations; hundreds of classrooms, many equipped with audiovisual and other learning-support equipment; and auditoriums for academic and community functions.

The Department of Nursing houses a learning resources center where students can listen to and view video and audio tapes. In addition to the numerous campus computer support centers, the Department's learning resources center also houses computers for student use.

LOCATION

The University is located in one of the world's most dynamic cities. For more than 100 years it has enjoyed a rewarding relationship with the Los Angeles community, whose cultural diversity provides a unique environment to learn from and experience urban America. Invaluable educational, cultural, and entertainment opportunities include numerous museums, theaters, cultural events, recreational facilities, theme parks, and sports events. In addition, the city is just an hour's drive from beaches, mountains, and deserts.

STUDENT SERVICES

The University offers a variety of events and involvement opportunities open to all students. Free or inexpensive concerts, stage productions, screenings, lectures, and athletic events are plentiful. Numerous student organizations, devoted to a wide variety of interests and activities, offer students opportunities for community involvement, leadership, and friendship.

The Department of Nursing also offers involvement and leadership opportunities. Members of the Nursing Student Association (NSA), Chi Eta Phi, and Sigma Theta Tau (the nursing honor society) work to meet academic, service, and social needs of nursing students and the community.

THE NURSING STUDENT GROUP

The undergraduate student body enrolled in nursing course work is 232 students. Of these, 10 percent are men and about 67 percent are from minority groups. Graduate students number approximately 90.

COSTS

Tuition costs for the 1996–97 academic year were $645 per unit for part-time students or $13,115 per semester for full-time enrollment. Other educational expenses, including books, immunizations, uniforms, insurance, and student fees for the two years of nursing course work total approximately $2000 per year.

FINANCIAL AID

The generous financial aid program at USC enables students to attend who, without such assistance, would not consider a private baccalaureate nursing education. Financial need is met by a combination of scholarships, grants, loans, work-study programs, and traineeships. Awards are based on both merit and need. The deadline for submission of financial aid applications is February 15 preceding the fall semester of course work.

APPLYING

For entering freshmen, Scholastic Assessment Test (SAT I) scores or American College Testing (ACT) scores are required. In addition to the regular USC freshman admission requirements, two years of high school science courses (including one year of chemistry with lab) must be completed. The Department considers applicants with a minimum grade point average of 3.0 (A=4.0) and acceptable SAT scores.

The equivalent of USC freshman and sophomore course work must be completed prior to beginning the nursing sequence. This course work includes anatomy, physiology, chemistry, microbiology, statistics, sociology, psychology, developmental psychology, adult development and aging, two semesters of English composition, cultural anthropology, and three general education courses. All required science courses must include laboratory work. A list of specific transferable courses may be obtained by contacting the Department of Nursing directly. Transfer students need a cumulative grade point average of 2.75 or higher in college work to be considered competitive. Students within the University of Southern California who wish to change their major to nursing should have a minimum cumulative GPA of 2.5.

General requirements for admission to the Master of Science in Nursing degree program in nursing include a minimum 3.0 undergraduate grade point average; acceptable scores on the verbal and quantitative sections of the Graduate Record Examinations; current licensure as a registered nurse; a bachelor's degree in nursing or a related field; submission of an essay describing the applicant's career goals; completion of an acceptable statistics course; and three letters of reference. Complete information about applications and deadlines can be obtained from the Department.

Correspondence and Information:

Admissions and Student Affairs
Department of Nursing
University of Southern California
1540 Alcazar Street, Room 222
Los Angeles, California 90033
Telephone: 213-342-2001
Fax: 213-342-2091

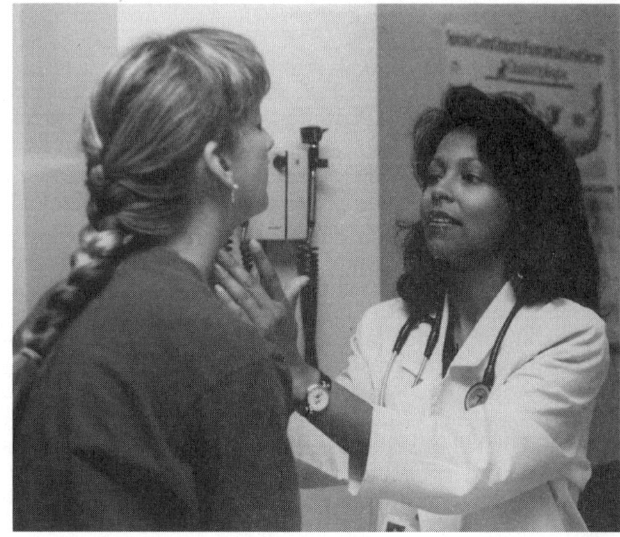

USC Department of Nursing provides education for the future of health care.

The University of the State of New York, Regents College
Nursing Program
Albany, New York

THE COLLEGE

A recognized leader in the field of nontraditional college education for twenty-five years, Regents College of the University of the State of New York has enabled more than 76,000 individuals—primarily working adults—to earn fully accredited associate and bachelor's degrees in liberal arts, business, nursing, and technology. Believing that what individuals know is more valuable than where or how they learned it, the College pioneered the process of assessment and evaluation of knowledge and competence. The College has no residency requirement, and its programs are available worldwide. Most Regents College students are returning to college to complete an education begun elsewhere. The College accepts a broad array of prior college-level credit in transfer, including classroom and distance courses from accredited colleges, proficiency examinations, and accredited on-the-job or military training. Although the College itself does not offer courses, Regents College faculty, drawn from other colleges and universities, designs the curriculum and determines how credit may be earned. Professional academic advisers help students design an individualized study plan using college courses, examinations, and other sources of credit to complete their degree requirements. Students work at their own pace while maintaining a full-time work schedule and family and civic responsibilities.

Regents College is accredited by the Commission on Higher Education of the Middle States Association of Colleges and Schools (3624 Market Street, Philadelphia, Pennsylvania 19104, 215-662-5606). The Commission on Higher Education is an institutional accrediting agency recognized by the U.S. Secretary of Education and the Commission on Recognition of Postsecondary Accreditation. The associate and baccalaureate degree programs in nursing at Regents College are accredited by the National League for Nursing, a specialized accrediting agency recognized by the U.S. Secretary of Education and/or Commission on Recognition of Postsecondary Education. All academic programs are registered (i.e., approved) by the New York State Education Department.

Regents College Examinations are recognized by the American Council on Education, Commission on Educational Credit and Credentials, for the award of college-level credit. They are also endorsed by the American Assembly of Collegiate Schools of Business.

THE NURSING PROGRAM

The Regents College Nursing Program began in 1972 with the Associate in Applied Science in Nursing degree program. The Associate in Science in Nursing was introduced in 1975 and the Bachelor of Science in Nursing degree in 1976. The B.S.N. program graduated its first class in 1979, the same year the College established the Regional Performance Assessment Centers. These centers permit the testing of nursing competencies at different locations across the United States. The Regents College nursing programs were the first nontraditional distance nursing programs in the United States. Regents College offers the largest assessment-based nursing program in the nation, and its programs have served as a model for the development of other nontraditional programs. A certificate program in home health nursing is also available.

PROGRAMS OF STUDY

The purpose of the baccalaureate nursing program is to offer an alternative educational approach to earning a degree in nursing. The student's ability to perform as an educated member of society and a competent professional are documented through an objective assessment program of general and professional education designed to promote an awareness of the human experience, an appreciation of the contributions of individuals from diverse cultures, and a sense of social responsibility as well as provide proficiency in the practice of professional nursing and a foundation for graduate specialization.

The baccalaureate degree program is divided into two components: general education (72 semester hours) and nursing (48 semester hours). Students may elect a minor in human resource management, biology, psychology, or sociology. The general education component is very flexible so that adult students may build the degree to meet their interests and needs. It includes requirements in anatomy, physiology, microbiology, psychology, sociology, and statistics. Students can meet these requirements through classroom or distance courses from regionally accredited colleges or through proficiency examinations. The nursing component comprises five written Regents College Examinations and four performance examinations. To test the clinical competencies of its nursing students, Regents College pioneered the creation of rigorous performance examinations. The program is self-paced, and students can take the performance examinations at the Regional Performance Assessment Center of their choice.

Northeastern Performance Assessment Center locations include Albany Medical Center Hospital, St. Peter's Hospital, and Regents College in Albany, New York; Flushing Medical Center Hospital in Flushing, New York; Ellis Hospital in Schenectady, New York; University Hospital in Syracuse, New York; and St. Joseph's Hospital in Syracuse, New York.

Southern Performance Assessment Center locations include Grady Memorial Hospital, Southern Regional Medical Center, St. Joseph's Medical Center, and Georgia Nurses' Association in Atlanta, Georgia; Medical City Dallas Hospital in Dallas, Texas; and Gwinnett Regional Medical Center Hospital in Lawrenceville, Georgia.

Midatlantic Performance Assessment Center locations include St. Francis Hospital and Thomas Edison State College in Trenton, New Jersey.

Midwestern Performance Assessment Center locations include St. Mary's Hospital in Racine, Wisconsin; Meriter Hospital and Midwestern Performance Assessment Center, Inc., in Madison, Wisconsin; and Ohio State University Medical Center, Children's Hospital, in Columbus, Ohio.

Western Performance Assessment Center locations include Long Beach Memorial Medical Center, Long Beach, California; San Francisco General Hospital, San Francisco, California; and Maricopa Medical Center, Phoenix, Arizona.

College courses in nursing and nursing performance examinations must be completed within five years of enrollment.

ACADEMIC FACILITIES

As a distance education program, Regents College provides a variety of guided learning services to students, such as study guides, learning modules, performance examination workshops, a bookstore, teleconferences, computer conference groups, and a computer bulletin board service. The College maintains DistanceLearn, a database of more than 7,000 courses and examinations available at a distance. Academic advisers and nurse educators are available to provide services to students by telephone, fax, computer, and mail.

LOCATION

Regents College is located wherever students seek a degree. Because its programs are totally portable, the College moves with students whenever and wherever they move. The administrative offices of Regents College are located in Albany, New York, the capital of New York State. Each year the College holds a formal commencement ceremony to recognize all who have completed a degree that year. Proud of their accomplishment, many students travel great distances to attend.

THE NURSING STUDENT GROUP

The 2,900 adult students enrolled in the Bachelor of Science in Nursing program represent diverse backgrounds in terms of age, ethnicity, nationality, and professional experience. Most are registered nurses, while others are paramedics, military service corpsmen, LPNs/LVNs, and respiratory therapists. The average student has ten years of health-care experience. Students come from every state and several countries. Graduates of the College are employed in various health-care settings and are accepted in most graduate programs.

COSTS

Regents College charges a $595 fee for enrollment (which covers initial evaluation and academic advisement services for one year), a $280 annual advisement fee (for each year after the first), and a $375 (associate degree programs) or $400 (baccalaureate degree programs) fee for program completion and graduation. Additional costs depend on the amount of credit that students need to earn and what credit sources they choose. Proficiency examinations are the least expensive mode of earning credit. Students should also figure in costs for books, travel (if necessary), and communication with the College.

FINANCIAL AID

Some financial aid is available, particularly the College's own Chancellor's Scholarships and aid connected with Veterans Affairs benefits. The College participates in the PLATO and TERI supplemental loan programs. Because of the nontraditional nature of Regents College, students seeking financial aid should contact the Regents College Financial Aid Office before enrolling.

APPLYING

Students may enroll in Regents College at any time. The Regents College nursing degrees are specifically designed to serve individuals with significant background or experience in a clinically oriented health-care discipline. Therefore, admission to the program is open to registered nurses, licensed practical/vocational nurses, paramedics, emergency medical technicians, military service corpsmen, individuals who hold a degree in a clinically oriented health-care field in which they have had the opportunity to provide direct patient care (i.e., physicians, respiratory therapists, chiropractors, and physicians' assistants), or individuals who have completed 50 percent or more of the clinical nursing courses in a registered nursing education program. Exceptions may be made for individuals who do not meet these qualifications but who can document significant clinical background.

Correspondence and Information:

Nursing Programs
Regents College
7 Columbia Circle, Box N
Albany, New York 12203-5159
Telephone: 518-464-8500
Fax: 518-464-8777

THE FACULTY

Elizabeth A. Ayello, Ph.D. (nursing), NYU; RN; Clinical Assistant Professor of Nursing, New York University.

Susan B. Bastable, Ed.D. (curriculum and instruction), Columbia Teachers College; RN; Associate Professor of Nursing, SUNY Health Science Center at Syracuse.

Frances Donovan Monahan, Ph.D. (research/theory in nursing), NYU; RN; Professor and Chair, Department of Nursing, Rockland Community College, Suffern, New York.

Gloria R. Gelmann, Ed.D. (family and community education), Columbia Teachers College; RN; Associate Professor of Nursing, Seton Hall University.

C. Alicia Georges, M.A. (community health nursing), NYU; RN; Lecturer, Department of Nursing, Lehman College of the City University of New York.

Linnea L. Jatulis, Ed.D. (program development and evaluation), SUNY at Albany; RN; Associate Professor and Chair, Department of Nursing, Russell Sage College.

Beverly K. Johnson, Ph.D. (nursing), Texas; RN; Assistant Professor, University of Washington (Seattle).

Barbara Marcx, M.S. (psychiatric–mental health nursing), Syracuse, (medical surgical nursing), Colorado; RN; Associate Professor, Nursing, Broome Community College, Binghamton, New York.

Elaine A. Muller, Ed.D. (higher education), Columbia Teachers College; RN; Professor of Nursing, Queensborough Community College, Bayside, New York.

Dicey A. O'Malley, Ph.D. (program development and evaluation), SUNY at Albany; RN; Associate Professor and Chair, Nursing Department, Hudson Valley Community College, Troy, New York.

Dennis G. Ross, Ph.D. (nursing), Case Western Reserve; RN; Professor, Nursing Department, Castleton State College, Vermont.

Robert J. Schaffner Jr., M.S. (cardiac/pulmonary critical care), Rochester; M.B.A. (market and finance), William E. Simon Graduate School of Business Administration; RN; Clinical Nurse Specialist, Strong Memorial Hospital, Rochester, New York.

Margaret F. Warshaw, M.A. (medical surgical nursing), NYU; RN; Professor and Chair, Department of Nursing and Allied Health, County College of Morris, New Jersey.

University of Virginia
School of Nursing
Charlottesville, Virginia

THE UNIVERSITY

The University of Virginia was founded in 1819 by Thomas Jefferson. When the University opened for classes in 1825, there were 68 students and 8 faculty members. The design of Mr. Jefferson's original "academical village" remains widely acclaimed for its architectural achievement.

Today, the University comprises ten independent schools, and the enrollment has grown to nearly 18,000 students. Although a public institution, the University remains highly competitive and is consistently ranked among the very best institutions of higher education in the nation.

There are well over 300 student groups at the University, from Greek organizations and academic societies to Madison House, a community service organization of more than 1,600 student volunteers. The University is particularly well known for its completely student-run honor system.

THE SCHOOL OF NURSING

Nursing was first initiated as a professional discipline at the University of Virginia in 1901. At that time, nursing was a three-year diploma program administered jointly by the University of Virginia Hospital and the Department of Medicine. The first baccalaureate degree in nursing was awarded in 1928. The School of Nursing was established as an independent school of the University in 1956. In 1972, the Master of Science in Nursing program was established. The Ph.D. in nursing program was begun in 1982. Today, the School has 55 faculty members and a total enrollment of approximately 500 students.

The School of Nursing is a member of the Council of Baccalaureate and Higher Degree Programs of the National League for Nursing, the American Association of Colleges of Nursing, and the Southern Council on Collegiate Education for Nursing of the Southern Regional Board; it is accredited by the National League for Nursing and by the Virginia Board of Nursing.

PROGRAMS OF STUDY

The traditional baccalaureate program leading to the B.S.N. degree is a four-year program consisting of 120 semester hours of credit. The program combines a strong liberal arts curriculum with core and interprofessional courses in nursing. During the fourth year, students select a clinical area of focus. Students may transfer into the second year of the program if they have 30 semester hours of previously earned college credit.

Two tracks are offered for nontraditional students wishing to pursue the B.S.N. degree. The Second Degree Program allows students who have a baccalaureate degree to complete the requirements for the B.S.N. in two academic years. The RN to B.S.N. Program permits registered nurses to obtain the B.S.N. degree in one academic year if they have 52 semester hours of transferable credit. The Second Degree Program allows students to progress to specific graduate programs of study if they have maintained at least a 3.0 GPA in the baccalaureate program. The M.S.N. degree can be completed in one additional year of full-time study.

The M.S.N. clinical nurse specialist program consists of 36 semester hours of course work, including core courses in nursing theory, research, role preparation, and health policy, as well as a clinical area. Elective hours complement and expand the program. Part-time study is available. Also offered is an M.S.N. program in health systems management. This program consists of 41 semester hours and prepares nurses to manage the delivery of nursing and health services across multiple settings and specialty areas. A joint M.S.N./M.B.A. program is offered in conjunction with the Colgate Darden Graduate School of Business Administration. This program is designed to prepare top-level managers of health-care agencies who possess a unique blend of clinical and administrative skills. The joint program may be completed in 2½ years of full-time study.

Students may pursue preparation for nurse practitioner certification in several ways. The M.S.N. Primary Care Nurse Practitioner Program, designed for experienced nurses with baccalaureate degrees, offers three tracks: family, pediatrics, and women's health. Nurses with master's degrees can pursue nurse practitioner certification through the Post-Master's NP Program. The M.S.N. primary care program consists of 55 semester hours of course work; the post-master's program can be completed in 29 semester hours. A key element of both tracks is the clinical preceptorship that follows the didactic/clinical portion of the program. In addition, programs to prepare nurses as acute-care nurse practitioners are available at both the master's and post-master's levels.

The Ph.D. in nursing program is a postbaccalaureate program designed to prepare scholars and researchers committed to expanding the base of nursing knowledge. Major components of the program include the nursing field, research, cognates, and electives. The Ph.D. program is administered through the Graduate School of Arts and Sciences.

AFFILIATIONS WITH HEALTH-CARE FACILITIES

The School of Nursing is a part of the University of Virginia Health Sciences Center with its numerous research facilities, the School of Medicine, and inpatient and outpatient care facilities. The University Hospital, Kluge Children's Rehabilitation Center, and Blue Ridge Hospital Division comprise a tertiary-care teaching facility with more than 650 beds. These facilities, along with various state and local agencies, provide a wide range of clinical experiences for students.

ACADEMIC FACILITIES

Nursing students have full access to the University's academic resources. These include the Alderman Library system, which consists of more than 3 million volumes and extensive computing facilities located throughout the grounds. Students may draw upon the resources of the twenty-five academic departments of the College of Arts and Sciences, the facilities of the Schools of Education and Medicine, and the clinical facilities of the Health Sciences Center. Of particular note to nursing students is the Claude Moore Health Sciences Library, with more than 100,000 volumes dedicated to the health-care field.

The School of Nursing is located in a modern five-story building fully equipped with classrooms, videotaping facilities, seminar rooms, audiovisual study carrels, and its own computer laboratory. The School also has clinical laboratories in which students can engage in both independent and assisted practice of nursing skills.

LOCATION

Charlottesville is located in the foothills of the Blue Ridge Mountains in central Virginia. The city is approximately 1 hour from Richmond and 2 hours from Washington, D.C., by automobile. The area is also serviced by bus, rail, and direct air flights from several major U.S. cities.

Charlottesville and surrounding Albemarle County attract thousands of tourists annually to such historic attractions as Monticello and Ash Lawn–Highland, the homes of Thomas Jefferson and James Monroe, respectively. In addition, Charlottesville's proximity to the mountains and Skyline Drive makes the area a favorite stop for those interested in the outdoors. Charlottesville also boasts a wide variety of dining experiences and is home to such annual events as the Dogwood Festival, Foxfield Steeplechase Races, and the Virginia Festival of American Film.

STUDENT SERVICES

The University offers a wide range of resources and services to its students. A variety of housing is available for both undergraduate and graduate students, and dining and recreational facilities are located throughout the grounds. In addition, there are numerous offices designed to meet specific needs. These include the Department of Student Health, the Counseling Center, the Office of Career Planning and Placement, the Office of African-American Affairs, and the International Center.

THE NURSING STUDENT GROUP

Of the nearly 500 students currently enrolled in the School of Nursing, approximately 300 are at the undergraduate level. Because of the many different programs offered by the School, students come with a wide variety of educational and employment experiences. More than 40 percent are already nurses.

COSTS

Full-time tuition and fees for the 1996–97 academic year were $4652 for Virginia residents and $14,438 for nonresidents. Living expenses were about $5000 per year for undergraduate students and $8560 for graduate students. Books and supplies were approximately $600 per year.

FINANCIAL AID

Financial assistance is provided through a combination of scholarships, fellowships, grants, and loans. More than fifty nursing scholarships are awarded each year directly through the School of Nursing. Graduate students are also eligible for teaching and research assistantships and Federal Professional Nurse Traineeships. Individuals requesting financial aid must submit an application directly to the School of Nursing in addition to completing the Free Application for Federal Student Aid (FAFSA). The application deadline for financial aid is March 31.

APPLYING

Applicants to the traditional baccalaureate program must submit an application, a high school transcript, SAT I and II scores, and a recommendation from a high school guidance counselor by January 2 to be considered for the following academic year. The nontraditional baccalaureate programs have an application deadline of March 1. Applicants to the Second Degree Program must submit an application, high school and college transcripts, SAT and GRE scores, and three letters of recommendation. The RN to B.S.N. Program requires 52 general education credits and a copy of a current nursing license.

Applicants to graduate programs must submit an application, college transcripts, GRE scores, three letters of recommendation, validation of health assessment skills, and a copy of a current nursing license. In addition, applicants to the Ph.D. program must provide at least one example of scholarly writing. The application deadline for all graduate programs is April 1, with the exceptions of the post-master's nurse practitioner program and the acute-care nurse practitioner master's program. Those programs have an application deadline of March 1.

Correspondence and Information:

Office of Student Affairs
School of Nursing
McLeod Hall
University of Virginia
Charlottesville, Virginia 22903-3395
Telephone: 888-283-8703 (toll-free)
E-mail: nur-osa@virginia.edu
WWW: http://www.med.virginia.edu/nursing/nursehom.html
Office of Undergraduate Admissions
University of Virginia
P.O. Box 9017
Charlottesville, Virginia 22906
Telephone: 804-982-3200

THE FACULTY

Ivo Abraham, Professor; Ph.D., Michigan.
Sara Arneson, Associate Professor; Ph.D., Iowa.
Kathryn Ballenger, Instructor; M.S.N., Virginia.
Judy Bancroft, Associate Professor; Ph.D., Wisconsin.
Valentina Brashers, Assistant Professor; M.D., Virginia.
Barbara Brodie, Professor; Ph.D., Michigan State.
Josephine Brucia, Assistant Professor; Ph.D., Case Western Reserve.
Suzanne Burns, Associate Professor; M.S.N., Virginia.
Sarah Cargile, Assistant Professor; Ph.D., Virginia.
Barrie Carveth, Instructor; M.S.N., Virginia.
Reba Childress, Instructor; M.S.N., Virginia.
Linda Davies, Assistant Professor; M.S.N., Virginia.
Emily Drake, Instructor; M.S.N., Virginia.
Carolyn Eddins, Assistant Professor; M.S.N., Emory.
Sarah Farrell, Assistant Professor; Ph.D., Medical College of Virginia.
Jeanne Fox, Professor; Ph.D., Nebraska.
Carol Gleit, Associate Professor; Ed.D., North Carolina State.
Doris Glick, Assistant Professor; Ph.D., Penn State.
Doris Greiner, Associate Professor and Associate Dean for Academic Programs; Ph.D., Georgia State.
Patty Hale, Assistant Professor; Ph.D., Maryland.
Emily Hauenstein, Associate Professor; Ph.D., Virginia.
Kathryn Haugh, Instructor; M.S.N., Catholic University.
Shelley Huffstutler, Assistant Professor; D.S.N., Alabama.
Cheryl Jones, Assistant Professor; Ph.D., South Carolina.
Ralph Kahlan, Lecturer and Assistant Dean; M.Ed., North Georgia.
Catherine Kane, Associate Professor; Ph.D., Rochester.
Arlene Keeling, Assistant Professor; Ph.D., Virginia.
Susan Kennel, Assistant Professor and Director of Undergraduate Student Services; M.S.N., Pennsylvania.
John Kirchgessner, Assistant Professor; M.S.N., Virginia.
Pamela Kulbok, Associate Professor; D.N.Sc., Boston University.
B. Jeanette Lancaster, Professor and Dean; Ph.D., Oklahoma.
Sharon Lock, Assistant Professor; Ph.D., South Carolina.
Carol Lynn Maxwell-Thompson, Instructor; M.S.N., Virginia.
Elizabeth Merwin, Associate Professor; Ph.D., Virginia Commonwealth.
Gregg Newschwander, Assistant Professor and Assistant Dean; Ph.D., Marquette.
Lynn Noland, Assistant Professor; Ph.D., Virginia.
Julie Novak, Professor; D.N.Sc., San Diego.
Judy Ozbolt, Professor; Ph.D., Michigan.
Barbara Parker, Professor; Ph.D., Maryland.
JoAnne Peach, Assistant Professor; M.S.N., Virginia.
Sally Reel, Assistant Professor; Ph.D., Virginia.
Judith Sands, Associate Professor; Ed.D., American.
Esther Seibold, Instructor; M.S.N., Pennsylvania.
Joan Shettig, Assistant Professor; M.S.N., Virginia Commonwealth.
Richard Steeves, Associate Professor; Ph.D., Washington (Seattle).
Ann Taylor, Professor; Ed.D., Virginia.
Jean Turner, Associate Professor; Ph.D., Virginia Commonwealth.
Sharon Utz, Associate Professor; Ph.D., Toledo.
Sherry Weinstein, Instructor; M.N., Emory.
Cynthia Westley, Instructor; M.S.N., Virginia.

Vanderbilt University
School of Nursing
Nashville, Tennessee

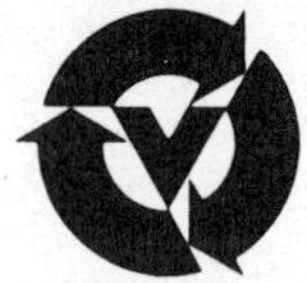

THE UNIVERSITY

Vanderbilt University was established in 1873 through a $1-million donation by Commodore Cornelius Vanderbilt. Vanderbilt University offers a full range of undergraduate programs as well as thirty-nine master's degree programs and thirty-eight Ph.D. programs. There are more than 1,600 full-time faculty members and a diverse student population of almost 10,000.

THE SCHOOL OF NURSING

For nearly ninety years, Vanderbilt University School of Nursing (VUSN) has been providing innovative educational opportunities for its students. The School's proudest tradition is educating nurses who are impassioned professionals capable of meeting—and exceeding—the demands of a constantly evolving profession. By 1926, the School had grown from its initiation as the Vanderbilt Hospital Training School (1909) to a school of nursing, offering a diploma in nursing combined with studies in arts and sciences, leading to a B.S. degree. In 1933, VUSN offered the first B.S.N. in Tennessee and became a charter member of the Association of Collegiate Schools of Nursing (ACSN), which later became the National League for Nursing (NLN), under which the program is currently accredited. The nurse-midwifery program has been preaccredited by the American College of Nurse-Midwives. In 1985, VUSN introduced the Bridge to the Master's program, replacing the B.S.N. degree program. The Bridge offers multiple entry options for students seeking to become advanced practice nurses, including those with 72 hours of college credit, an associate degree or diploma in nursing, or a B.S.N. Recognizing that some nurses who may have earned master's degrees in nursing would like additional or different specialties, VUSN included a Post-Master's Option. In 1993, the Ph.D. in Nursing Science program was established.

PROGRAMS OF STUDY

VUSN, through University Community Health Services, operates two free-standing primary-care sites and a number of physician-nurse practice partnerships. The first primary-care practice, Vine Hill Community Clinic, opened in January 1991. The clinic meets the needs of an average of 400 patients per month and also serves as the primary care provider for 5,100 covered lives. The clinic offers a full range of services, which include management of chronic disease, women's health, treatment of uncomplicated illness, and mental health. The clinic is staffed by full-time and part-time School of Nursing faculty members.

In August 1996, VUSN opened another community-based nurse-practitioner-operated practice, Primary Services at Madison. A state-of-the-art, free-standing primary-care site, the practice offers a full range of preventative and primary-care services to adults and children. The practice currently sees an average of 200 patients per month and has 900 assigned primary-care lives.

Vanderbilt University School of Nursing offers a Master of Science in Nursing (M.S.N.) with multiple entry options. Applicants with a Bachelor of Science in Nursing, an associate degree in nursing, a diploma in nursing and 72 semester hours of college, a bachelor's degree in another field, or at least 72 semester hours of college are eligible to apply to the program.

The M.S.N. degree is offered with the following specialties: acute care adult nurse practitioner; behavioral health nurse practitioner; community systems management; family nurse practitioner; gerontological nurse practitioner; nurse-midwifery; neonatal/infancy, parent/child–adolescent nursing; women's health nurse practitioner; and a joint management and Master of Business Administration concentration (M.S.N/M.B.A dual degree).

Direct admission to the M.S.N. program requires graduation from an NLN-accredited baccalaureate program with an upper-division major in nursing (B.S.N. degree). Applicants from unaccredited nursing programs will be considered on an individual basis.

Admission to the School of Nursing without a B.S.N. degree is possible via the generalist nursing Bridge/M.S.N. program. Students with an associate degree in nursing, a diploma in nursing and at least 72 semester hours of college, a baccalaureate degree in another field, or at least 72 semester hours of college may enter the program and earn the Master of Science in Nursing degree.

The Ph.D. in Nursing Science program is designed for individuals who hold graduate degrees in nursing and wish to pursue academic careers in nursing. The focus of the program is the study of individual, family, and community responses to health and illness across the lifespan and outcomes of care delivery. Students receive intensive research training on faculty research projects related to their major field of study.

Students are strongly encouraged to enroll in full-time study for the first six semesters (two calendar years) of the program. Part-time study is negotiable.

The curriculum is organized into three broad areas: phenomena of concern in nursing science, research and theory, and a minor field (including health policy, psychology and human development, and sociology). Doctoral students have intensive research activities at VUSN as a part of the learning process. Thus, doctoral students are strongly encouraged to plan to be on campus a minimum of three days a week for the first two years of study to complete course work and research experiences. The third year of the program is likely to be more flexible in terms of scheduled time on campus as students complete their dissertation research.

Doctoral students have research access to the facilities of Vanderbilt University Hospital and Clinic, Veterans' Administration Hospital, and a model nurse-managed primary care center and community development project, as well as a variety of clinical agencies affiliated with the School of Nursing.

AFFILIATIONS WITH HEALTH-CARE FACILITIES

Vanderbilt University School of Nursing offers its students opportunities to complete clinical courses, conduct inquiry, and learn in diverse settings. The School maintains more than 600 contracts with clinical practices in hospitals, communities, health departments, private practices, clinics, outpatient facilities, home-health agencies, skilled-care facilities, nursing homes, schools, and industries. Many of these sites are in rural as well as urban settings in Nashville, Tennessee, and several other states. The Vanderbilt University Medical Center itself maintains a reputation for excellence in teaching, practice, and research and provides students with a tertiary academic setting, where patients receive exemplary care from creative health-care teachers and scholars.

ACADEMIC FACILITIES

The Jean and Alexander Heard Library is the collective name for all of the libraries at Vanderbilt, which have a combined collection of more than 2 million volumes. In addition to the Central library, the Biomedical, Divinity, Education, Law, Management, and Science libraries serve their respective schools and disciplines. The General Library Building houses the University Archives and Special Collections. The facilities, resources, and services of these divisions are available to all Vanderbilt students and personnel. An integrated automated system lists the holdings of the libraries and gives up-to-the-minute information on the status of material on order, in process, or on loan. Enhancements of the system allow searching of periodical literature.

Vanderbilt has a sophisticated campuswide computer network. The central computer is the CTRVAX. The Computer Center provides a full range of computing resources to Vanderbilt faculty, staff, and students. The support services include consulting, training, documentation, facilities management, site licensing, software access, and hardware maintenance. VUSN's Helene Fuld Instructional Media Center (HFIMC) provides all nursing students with a CTRVAX account with full Internet connectivity.

LOCATION

Vanderbilt is located on a 333-acre parklike campus approximately 1½ from downtown Nashville, providing a peaceful setting within an urban environment. Long known as a center of banking, finance, and publishing, this capital city of Tennessee is a unique blend of Southern hospitality and cosmopolitan diversity that ranks high in the "quality of life" surveys. Nashville has an international airport and is easily accessible from interstate highways.

STUDENT SERVICES

Vanderbilt provides its students with a comprehensive list of services, including the Career Center, Psychological and Counseling Services, Student Health Center, the Office of International Services, the Child Care Center, the Bishop Joseph Johnson Black Cultural Center, and the Margaret Cuninggim Women's Center, as well as security escort services, shuttle bus services, and graduate and married student housing.

THE NURSING STUDENT GROUP

Vanderbilt University School of Nursing has been successful in attracting students from diverse educational backgrounds and work experiences. Sixty percent of the class began the program in the 1996 academic year without a background in nursing. These individuals will enter the nursing profession in advanced practice after two full calendar years of study. Ages of class members range from 21 to 51, and 13 percent of the students are male. The School's diverse student body includes Asian Americans, African Americans, American Indians, and Hispanic students in addition to international students.

COSTS

Tuition for the Bridge and M.S.N. programs for the 1997–98 academic year is a flat rate of $7716 per semester for full-time students or $643 per semester hour for part-time students. Tuition for the Ph.D. program is $786 per credit hour.

The Master of Science in Nursing (for B.S.N.'s only) is a three-semester program. The Bridge/M.S.N. program is six semesters. Full-time Bridge and M.S.N. students attend fall, spring, and summer sessions and carry 12–18 semester hours. Students enrolled for fewer than 12 hours are considered part-time students and are charged per credit hour.

Expenses for books and supplies vary according to specialty. Equipment such as tape recorders and diagnostic tools is required for certain specialties. Other charges include laboratory fees, student activities and recreation fees, liability insurance coverage, and hospitalization insurance.

FINANCIAL AID

Financial aid is available from several sources for full-time students. All students who wish to apply for financial aid and scholarships must apply to the School of Nursing no later than May 1 for the next academic year.

For information regarding financial aid for the Ph.D. in Nursing Science program, students should contact the Graduate School at 615-322-3938 or write to Graduate School, 411 Kirkland Hall, Vanderbilt University, Nashville, Tennessee 37240.

APPLYING

Admission requirements for applicants to the Bridge/M.S.N. and M.S.N. programs include a minimum 3.0 GPA, three letters of recommendation, an interview, and a minimum GRE score of 1000 (verbal and quantitative only), a Miller Analogies Test score of at least 50, or, for the M.S.N./M.B.A. program, a GMAT score of 550 or better.

Applicants to the Ph.D. program are required to have a personal interview and submit official transcripts, three letters of recommendation, and GRE scores for tests taken within five years of the application date.

Correspondence and Information:

For information on the Bridge/M.S.N. program:
Admissions Office
Vanderbilt University School of Nursing
101 Godchaux Hall
21st Avenue South
Nashville, Tennessee 37240
Telephone: 615-322-3800
Fax: 615-343-0333
E-mail: vusn-admissions@mcmail.vanderbilt.edu
World Wide Web: http://www.mc.vanderbilt.edu/nursing/

For information on the Ph.D. in Nursing Science program:
Graduate School
411 Kirkland Hall
Vanderbilt University
Nashville, Tennessee 37240
Telephone: 615-322-3938

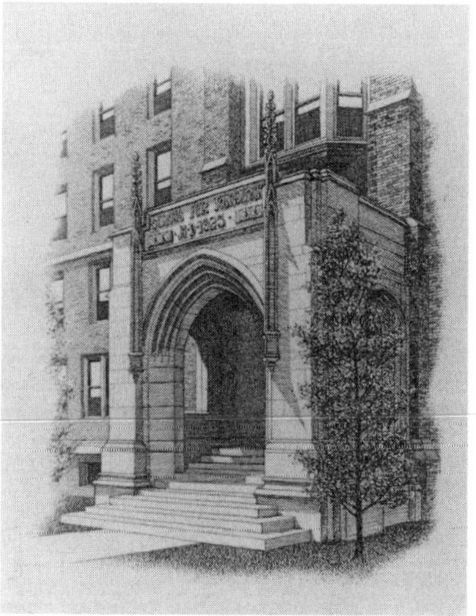

Vanderbilt University School of Nursing.

Villanova University
College of Nursing
Villanova, Pennsylvania

THE UNIVERSITY

Villanova University is an independent coeducational institution of higher learning founded by the Augustinians, one of the oldest teaching orders in the Catholic Church. Since its beginning in 1842, the University's Augustinian character has been evident in its devotion to the principles of scholarship, community, and the relationship between mind and heart as well as in its commitment to producing graduates with strong moral values and proficient skills.

Villanova is a comprehensive university with undergraduate academic colleges in the areas of commerce and finance, engineering, liberal arts and sciences, and nursing. The University offers selected master's and doctoral degrees, including the M.S.N., and maintains a highly regarded School of Law. Villanova has grown to an enrollment today of more than 10,000 students.

Villanova's student body represents almost every state in the nation as well as 44 countries. Approximately 51 percent of its undergraduates are men and 49 percent are women.

THE COLLEGE OF NURSING

The College of Nursing, founded in 1953, has the distinction of being the first collegiate nursing program under Catholic auspices in Pennsylvania, the largest nursing college in the commonwealth within a private university, and the only nursing program in the country under Augustinian sponsorship. All of the programs offered by the College—baccalaureate, master's, and continuing education—are fully accredited. There are approximately 4,000 alumni of the degree-granting programs, and the College currently enrolls approximately 400 undergraduates, the majority of whom are full-time, and 200 graduate students, most of whom enroll on a part-time basis.

The faculty believes that education provides students with opportunities to develop habits of critical, constructive thought so that they may make discriminating judgments in their search for the truth. This type of intellectual development can best be attained in a teaching-learning environment that fosters sharing of knowledge, skills, and attitudes as well as inquiry toward the development of new knowledge. The faculty and students comprise a community of learners and teacher-scholars.

Seventy percent of the full-time faculty members in the College hold an earned doctorate, and many are actively engaged in research. The faculty, however, has teaching as its primary commitment, and most of the teaching is carried out by full-time faculty members.

The College, in conjunction with the University's Office of International Studies, offers a sophomore year abroad in the baccalaureate program at King's College, London. There are a growing number of students sponsored by international organizations who are attending the master's program, and the College is exploring opportunities to expand international experiences for its students.

The continuing education program offers a variety of workshops, seminars, conferences, self-study activities, and short courses and a post-master's certificate in nursing administration. All of these options are designed to assist practicing nurses to advance, maintain, and provide quality health care.

PROGRAMS OF STUDY

Villanova awards the B.S.N. after completion of 136 credits, 72 of which are in nursing; the remaining 64 are in arts and science. The program integrates a liberal education with the ideals, knowledge, and skills of professional nursing practice under the direction of a qualified faculty. Baccalaureate education prepares individuals for professional nursing practice in variety of health-care settings and for continuous personal and educational growth, including entrance into graduate education in nursing. The College welcomes applications from adults who wish to begin preparation for a career in nursing. These include individuals who possess undergraduate and/or graduate degrees in other fields as well as adults entering college for the first time. Part-time study is possible during the introductory level of the program. Full-time study is required during the clinical portion of the program.

Graduates from diploma and associate degree nursing programs are eligible for admission to the baccalaureate program. Through a series of nursing examinations and clinical validation, a registered nurse student may demonstrate current nursing knowledge, earning 45 credits in nursing. A maximum of 50 percent of the credits from the total curriculum may be transferred by either adult learners or registered nurse students.

The M.S.N. program at Villanova University requires the completion of 45 credits and prepares nurses for roles as nurse practitioners; nurse anesthetists; clinical case managers; staff development educators; nurse administrators in acute-care, long-term-care, or community/home-health agencies; or faculty members in schools of nursing. The curriculum includes core courses (including research, theory, and leadership), clinical courses (including a theory and practicum in adult, community, gerontology, parent-child, or psychiatric–mental health nursing), free electives, an independent study course, and role-related courses (including a practicum). No thesis is required; however, students who wish to work with faculty members who are conducting research or who wish to engage in a research-oriented independent study project are encouraged to do so and are assisted in the endeavor.

AFFILIATIONS WITH HEALTH-CARE FACILITIES

The College of Nursing is affiliated with more than seventy health-care agencies in the Greater Philadelphia area that provide clinical settings for undergraduate and graduate student clinical experiences. These facilities include hospitals in large medical centers, community hospitals, extended care facilities, home-health agencies, schools, industrial health settings, senior citizen and community health centers, HMOs, insurance companies, and managed-care agencies.

ACADEMIC FACILITIES

The Falvey Memorial Library provides resources and facilities for study and research by graduate and undergraduate students, faculty members, and visiting scholars. It houses more than 560,000 volumes, of which more than 22,000 are nursing or nursing-related. The library has an extensive periodicals section with 150 nursing and nursing-related holdings. Library services include computerized literature searches with direct access to the National Library of Medicine databases and extensive instructional media services, including a professionally staffed video studio for the production of sophisticated video materials. In addition to the general University library and extensive interlibrary loan access, students in the College of Nursing have access to the Law Library and that of the College of Commerce and Finance.

The computing services available to the University community are extensive, with computer stations located throughout the campus. In addition to those available in the primary computing center, the College of Nursing Learning Resource Center houses computers and interactive video systems that are available for the exclusive use of its students and faculty. The Learning Resource Center also maintains extensive holdings of a wide variety of audiovisual materials, training models, computer software programs, and simulations to support the teaching enterprise. Students and faculty members have access to the fully staffed Center during extended weekday and selected weekend hours.

LOCATION

With its more than 220 landscaped acres in one of the most beautiful residential areas in America, the Villanova campus is among the showplaces in the suburban Philadelphia area. Located on the prestigious Main Line, with a station on its campus, Villanova is easily accessible by train from Philadelphia. It also lies in proximity to several major highways that make the Philadelphia airport as well as the New York and Washington, D.C., areas easily accessible. Such a location provides students with safe and easy access to the cultural and recreational opportunities available in Philadelphia and makes those of New York and Washington, D.C., readily available as well.

STUDENT SERVICES

Villanova University offers a wide variety of student services. Campus Ministry promotes a sense of community through the coordination of a variety of programs that are of a religious and human service character with a view to aiding students with their spiritual and personal growth. A full array of student activities, including a theater, Greek system, music activities, intramural and intercollegiate sports, and a fitness center, are available. Such opportunities facilitate the total development of students, promote a spirit of community, provide opportunities for students to interact with other individuals who have varied interests, and provide the supports necessary to succeed academically. In addition, student health services, a counseling center, career planning and placement services, a writing center, and study skills resources are available to all students in the University.

THE NURSING STUDENT GROUP

Most of the individuals enrolled in the undergraduate program are full-time students who began their nursing studies directly after completing high school. Approximately 20 percent of the B.S.N. population are registered nurses or adult learners. Graduates of this program are employed in major health-care facilities, universities, or other settings throughout the country, and approximately 30 percent have completed or are enrolled in graduate programs.

Approximately 90 percent of the individuals enrolled in the M.S.N. program are part-time students with several years experience as nurses. Students in the program received their undergraduate education in a wide variety of institutions, and the number of international students enrolled in the master's program is increasing steadily. Graduates of this program hold major leadership positions in professional associations, as faculty members in colleges and universities, and as administrators, case managers, and clinical educators in some of the most prestigious health-care institutions in the country. Approximately 20 percent of the M.S.N. graduates have completed or are enrolled in doctoral programs.

COSTS

Full-time tuition for the undergraduate program in the 1996–97 academic year was $18,010. The per credit rate for part-time undergraduate courses was $425, and general fees were $260. For the 1996–97 academic year, tuition for the graduate program was $410 a credit, with a general university fee of $60 per semester.

FINANCIAL AID

Undergraduate financial aid is granted on the basis of need and scholastic ability and includes Villanova University scholastic grants, student loans, federal grants, state grants, and scholarships from outside sources such as corporations, unions, charitable trusts, and service clubs. The University financial aid office assists applicants in this process.

Financial assistance is available to graduate students in the form of graduate assistantships, professional nurse traineeships, scholarships, and loans.

APPLYING

Admission to the undergraduate program is based on evaluation of high school grade point average, SAT I scores, rank in class, participation in extracurricular activities, and recommendations of teachers and counselors. Applications must be submitted by January 15, and applicants are notified of their admission decision on an ongoing basis.

For transfer students, adult learners, and registered nurses, applications must be received no later than November 15 (for January entrance) or April 15 (for September entrance). Criteria used to evaluate these applicants include complete transcripts from previous schools, quality point average at a previously attended institution, and evidence of honorable withdrawal from previously attended institution(s). Transcripts from a secondary school are required if the applicant has never attended an institution of higher learning.

Applications to the M.S.N. program are accepted on an ongoing basis, and students may begin the program in the fall, spring, or summer terms. Admission requirements include the B.S.N., a minimum of one year recent clinical practice in nursing, scores on the MAT or GRE, undergraduate statistics, physical assessment, three letters of reference from professional nurses, and a personal statement of career goals.

Correspondence and Information:

Office of Undergraduate Admissions
Austin Hall
Villanova University
800 East Lancaster Avenue
Villanova, Pennsylvania 19085
Telephone: 610-519-4453
Fax: 610-519-6450

Graduate Nursing Program
College of Nursing
Villanova University
800 East Lancaster Avenue
Villanova, Pennsylvania 19085-1690
Telephone: 610-519-4934
Fax: 610-519-7997

Washburn University of Topeka
School of Nursing
Topeka, Kansas

THE UNIVERSITY

Washburn University was founded in 1865 as a small church school known as Lincoln College. In 1868, the name was changed to Washburn College, in recognition of the financial support of New England philanthropist, Dean Ichabod Washburn. The citizens of Topeka voted in 1941 to make Washburn a municipal university, which it remains today. The University is supported in part by the city and governed by a local Board of Regents. Steeped in a tradition of more than 125 years, Washburn has evolved into a modern, comprehensive public urban university located in the heart of the capital city and principally serving the diverse educational and cultural needs of the residents of Topeka, Shawnee County, and northeast Kansas. The University comprises five major academic units: the College of Arts and Sciences and the Schools of Law, Business, Nursing, and Applied Studies. The University enrollment is approximately 6,400.

THE SCHOOL OF NURSING

The baccalaureate nursing program was established in 1974 in response to a local and statewide need for more nurses and strong community-based support for baccalaureate nursing education. The nursing program maintains both state and national accreditation. It was the first baccalaureate nursing program in the city of Topeka and Shawnee County. The program began as a department within the College of Arts and Sciences and in 1982 was granted School of Nursing status through an act of the Kansas legislature. The program in nursing is designed to prepare women and men for careers in professional nursing. The focus of the program is the study of the individual and family life process from conception through aging in varying stages of health within the context of community and a variety of settings. The baccalaureate nursing program is based on the belief that each human being is a unitary, living, open system and is continuously engaged in a mutual dynamic process with the environment. The Science of Unitary Human Beings is the conceptual framework upon which the nursing program is based and is derived from the work of nursing theorist Martha E. Rogers. The principles of helicy, resonancy, and integrality provide the basis for understanding the mutual process between human beings and the environment and provide for the organization of knowledge essential to the science and practice of nursing. A nursing curriculum is implemented to assist the learner in viewing the person as a unified whole.

PROGRAMS OF STUDY

The School of Nursing has an enrollment of approximately 250 generic and RN undergraduate students majoring in nursing. This population includes beginning college students, college transfer students, second career students, and adult learners. Both lower- and upper-division nursing courses are offered in the major. Lower-division nursing courses may begin at the sophomore level and may be taken concurrently with some general education courses. The upper-division nursing curriculum builds upon the lower-division nursing courses and augments courses in the humanities and the natural and social sciences. Students enter the nursing major with a foundation of life experiences and education. Nursing courses are designed to facilitate the professional development of students and the integration of knowledge. The general education component and supporting courses for the major comprise a total of 65 credit hours and the major in nursing is 59 credit hours, with a total of 124 hours required for the B.S.N. degree. The curriculum is designed to be completed in four academic years, with four or five semesters of nursing courses. Provisions are made for students to extend or shorten their length of study by granting of credit for college work already completed, full-time or part-time study, enrollment in summer sessions or intersessions, or the use of proficiency examinations for obtaining credit. Prenursing students preparing to enter the major are advised by the School of Nursing. An articulation program for registered nurses from associate degree and hospital diploma programs is offered for those seeking the B.S.N. degree. Registered nurse students meet the same general education requirements as generic nursing students. Following admission to the School of Nursing, however, advanced standing and transfer credit allowance is determined for RN students, and they pursue a separate track of nursing major courses. An LPN to B.S.N. program is offered whereby licensed practical nurses may obtain advanced standing lower-division credit in the nursing major upon evaluation of their practical nurse curriculum and determination of equivalence. In addition to the baccalaureate program, the School of Nursing offers continuing education programs for registered nurses, practical nurses, and mental health technicians; a Certification Program for School Nurses in conjunction with the Department of Education and the State Board of Education; and a Re-Entry Into Nursing course (RN refresher) for nurses seeking re-licensure or a career change.

AFFILIATIONS WITH HEALTH-CARE FACILITIES

An advantage of the School is its urban focus and access to Topeka's extensive mental health and medical-care complex, which provides excellent facilities for clinical learning experiences. Clinical laboratory takes place in a variety of community clinics, hospitals, public health agencies, nursery schools, Head Start programs, physicians' offices, youth centers, mental health centers, senior centers, and private homes. The normal developmental processes and health needs of individuals, families, and groups form the basis for the selection of student learning experiences throughout Topeka and in surrounding communities. Students have opportunities to work with persons of all ages and diverse cultural backgrounds.

ACADEMIC FACILITIES

The School of Nursing is located in the Kelsey H. and Edna B. Petro Allied Health Center, a 126,000-square-foot modern facility that also houses the Department of Health and Physical Education and the Athletic Department. The School provides a well-equipped nursing skills laboratory, a health assessment clinic, and a computer laboratory within the Petro building.

Students in the School of Nursing have easy access to Mabee Library, Bennett Computer Center, the Henderson Learning Resources and Instructional Media Center, Memorial Union and Bookstore, and the Administration Building. Students are provided open parking spaces on campus.

The University owns and operates an educational television station, KTWU, in a new facility on campus. Semester course offerings are available over the KTWU network, reaching several areas of the state. KTWU-ETV provides both local and PBS programming and frequent national satellite teleconferences. The University's libraries provide automated on-line catalog and circulation services.

LOCATION

Located in the center of the United States and the heart of the Midwest, Washburn University is also in the geographical center of Topeka. The capital city of Topeka radiates a Midwestern friendliness and provides regional shopping, cultural events, and entertainment. The University cooperates with local businesses, health-care organizations, social agencies, educational institutions, and labor and government entities to bring the highest quality educational and recreational opportunities to Washburn students and the citizens of northeast Kansas. Topeka is known for its world-renowned Menninger Clinic and Hospital, its zoo, civic symphony, civic theater, and art museums as well as for its proximity to Kansas City and major sports programs.

STUDENT SERVICES

A wide variety of student services are offered to complement the academic programs and provide for the students' well-rounded education. Some of the services available to students include the University Child Development Center and Day Care Program; the Center for Learning and Academic Support Services (CLASS), which includes academic advising, counseling, placement, and study skills programs; International Student Center; Disabled Student Services; Veteran Affairs; Minority Affairs; Health Services; Campus Ministry; Office of Student Life and Campus Activities; and Computer Services. Student organizations, including Student Nurses of Washburn (SNOW), Sigma Theta Tau honor society for nursing, Phi Kappa Phi, and other honor societies are available to Washburn students. Student publications, intercollegiate athletics, and fraternities and sororities offer extracurricular activities for students.

THE NURSING STUDENT GROUP

In the fall 1996 admission class, 54 percent of the Washburn nursing students were from Topeka or the state of Kansas. Forty-one percent were admitted from out of state. The average age was 24. Thirty-seven percent of the nursing students are married and 16 percent have dependents. Most students commute to campus from areas within the city, some come from as far as 130 miles, and a few students live on campus. Seventeen percent of enrolled nursing students at Washburn are men; 6 percent are registered nurses. Nine percent have previous baccalaureate degrees and are pursuing second careers. Eighty-six percent of nursing majors are enrolled full-time. Approximately 13 percent are part-time students carrying less than 12 hours per semester. The School of Nursing has a 12 percent minority and international student enrollment.

COSTS

Tuition for the 1996–97 academic year was $96 per credit hour with a $32 student fee for undergraduate Kansas resident students ($2912 for enrollment in 15 hours per semester). For nonresidents, tuition was $211 per credit hour with a student fee of $32 for the academic year ($6362 for one academic year). The tuition and fee structure includes parking, the student newspaper and yearbook, admission to all athletic events, and Washburn Student Health Service. Other costs include books, immunizations and laboratory tests required for the health physical, personal health insurance, liability insurance (currently paid by Washburn University for all nursing students), CPR certification, uniforms, laboratory supplies, health assessment equipment, travel to clinical sites, graduation costs (invitations, caps, gowns), photo for School composite, and RN licensure application fees. These additional costs are estimated at $2000 per year.

FINANCIAL AID

Nursing students with above-average academic records and/or a demonstrated financial need may apply for scholarships, grants-in-aid, or loans through the University Financial Aid Office. The School of Nursing has a number of substantial nursing scholarship endowments that are awarded annually to nursing students through the School of Nursing.

APPLYING

Students may apply for admission to the nursing major following completion of at least 30 hours of specified prerequisite college course work with a minimum cumulative grade point average of 2.7 on a 4.0 scale. Students must apply to the School of Nursing and file the required School of Nursing application form and college transcripts with the nursing office by February 15 for consideration for fall admission and by October 15 for spring admission.

Admission to the nursing major is generally in the second semester of the sophomore year for completion of a five-semester sequence of nursing course work. Students who have completed all general education course work may apply for a four-semester sequence. The number of students admitted to the major each year is determined by an enrollment management plan and is based on adequacy of clinical placements, availability of teaching faculty, and University resources. Students are selected for admission without discrimination on the basis of sex, race, color, national origin, religion, ancestry, age, disability, or sexual preference.

Correspondence and Information:

Washburn University School of Nursing
1700 College Avenue
Topeka, Kansas 66621
Telephone: 913-231-1010 Ext. 1525
Fax: 913-231-1089

THE FACULTY

Alice Adam Young, RN, Ph.D.; Professor and Dean.
Lois M. Rimmer, RN, Ph.D.; Professor and Assistant Dean.
Jane Carpenter, RN, M.S.N.; Assistant Professor.
Barbara Clark, RN, M.N., CCRN, ARNP; Assistant Professor.
Nora K. Clark, RN, M.N.; Assistant Professor.
Janice Dunwell, RN, Ed.D.; Associate Professor.
Cynthia Hornberger, RN, M.S., M.B.A., ARNP; Assistant Professor.
Susan J. W. Hsia, RN, M.N.; Associate Professor.
Patricia Joyce, RN, M.S., SNC; Assistant Professor.
Maryellen McBride, RN, M.N., ARNP; Assistant Professor.
Carolyn Middendorf, RN, M.N., ARNP; Assistant Professor.
Susan M. Pfister, RN, Ph.D.; Assistant Professor.
Rita V. Tracy, RN, M.S., M.N., ARNP; Assistant Professor.
Margaret Anschutz, RN, M.N.; PT Instructor.
Roberta Beller, RN, M.S.N., ANP; PT Assistant Professor.
Joan Denny, RN, M.S., CNM, ARNP; PT Instructor.
William Mach, RN, M.S.; PT Instructor.
Janice Melland, RN, M.S.W.; PT Instructor.
Kathryn Nelick, RN, M.S., ARNP; PT Instructor.
Alleene Pingenot, RN, M.A.; PT Instructor.
Judith Schultz, RN, M.S.; PT Instructor.

Wayne State University
College of Nursing
Detroit, Michigan

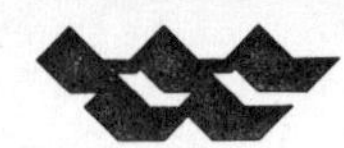

THE UNIVERSITY

Wayne State University (WSU) is among the nation's eighty-eight public and private universities with the distinguished Carnegie Research University I classification. The University is accredited by the North Central Association of Colleges and Schools. High-quality educational programs are offered in more than 600 fields of study leading to more than 300 different degrees at the bachelor's, master's, and doctoral levels. WSU's main campus encompasses 184 acres of landscaped, tree-lined pedestrian malls and ninety-eight research and educational buildings of classic and contemporary design. The multicultural urban context of the University provides a rich environment for student learning.

THE COLLEGE OF NURSING

The College of Nursing is regionally, nationally, and internationally recognized for educating graduate and undergraduate students as practitioners and scholars who provide leadership for the profession and discipline of nursing. The College is committed to research and scholarly activity that contributes to the body of knowledge of care and the human health experience in diverse environmental contexts. Moreover, the College excels in the development, application, and dissemination of knowledge to promote the health and well-being of society through teaching, research, and public service.

The College of Nursing, established in 1945 as an autonomous academic unit within the University, is accredited by the National League for Nursing. Innovative program options at the undergraduate, master's, and doctoral levels are available for learners from diverse backgrounds. The focal areas of research excellence at the College are self-care and caring, transcultural care, urban health, adaptation to acute and chronic illness, and health-care systems.

The Richard Cohn Memorial Building, which is centrally located on the main campus of the University, houses the College of Nursing, the Center for Health Research, the Learning Resource Center, and the Assessment Learning Laboratory.

PROGRAMS OF STUDY

The College of Nursing offers programs leading to B.S.N., M.S.N., and Ph.D. in nursing degrees. The College offers a graduate certificate practitioner program in neonatal nursing and graduate certificates in transcultural nursing and nursing education. Interdisciplinary graduate certificates in gerontology and infant mental health are also available. Within the baccalaureate program, options are available for applicants with diverse academic experience, including a traditional option for high school graduates, an accelerated option for college graduates with degrees in disciplines other than nursing, and an option for registered nurses. Graduates of the baccalaureate program are prepared for entry into professional practice. For academically talented registered nurses, an accelerated A.D.N.-M.S.N. program is available. The M.S.N. program is designed to prepare nurses for advanced nursing practice in the care of culturally diverse individuals, families, groups, and communities within a variety of health-care settings. The program educates nurses to assume leadership roles as nurse practitioners, clinical nurse specialists, and nurse managers. The course experiences are designed to enhance the ability of students to think critically and creatively, engage in scientific inquiry, and use knowledge to direct nursing practice. Within the M.S.N. program, students may study within the following areas of specialization: adult primary care nursing; gerontological nurse practitioner studies; adult acute care nursing; adult critical care nursing; nursing, parenting and families; community health nursing; psychiatric–mental health nursing; and nursing care administration.

The College of Nursing offers a program leading to the Doctor of Philosophy in nursing. Designed to prepare researchers and scholars who will provide leadership to the profession and discipline of nursing, the program emphasizes the development of the student's capacity to make significant, original contributions to nursing knowledge. The curriculum focuses on scientific inquiry and consists of a series of nursing seminars that address research methods, knowledge development, and the substantive domains of the discipline. The courses are designed to enhance the ability of students to construct and test new or extant nursing theories, and acquire skill in the use of both qualitative and quantitative research methods. Three optional paths toward the Ph.D. degree in nursing are offered: two paths for students entering the program post-B.S.N. and one path for those entering post-M.S.N.

AFFILIATIONS WITH HEALTH-CARE FACILITIES

The College of Nursing is affiliated with a wide variety of health-care agencies (approximately 100) within and outside metropolitan Detroit. These include major health-care agencies such as the Detroit Medical Center, Henry Ford Hospital, and the Detroit Health Department as well as primary-care settings, ambulatory practice sites, schools, and community health centers.

ACADEMIC FACILITIES

The University library facilities include Purdy/Kresge, Science and Engineering, and Shiffman Medical libraries. Together these campus libraries provide approximately 2,200,000 books, with 400,000 covering health topics. Periodical subscriptions number 12,500, of which 2,500 are health-care related. CINAHL and MEDLINE are available.

Through the Learning Resource Center (LRC), the College of Nursing provides computer-assisted instruction programs, interactive video programs, videotapes, and audiotapes for group or individualized student instruction. Auxiliary to the LRC is the Assessment Learning Laboratory, which provides the facilities for students to acquire and master knowledge and skills in assessment and nursing technology. The Center for Health Research provides services to the faculty and graduate students in the form of consultation services and technical assistance.

LOCATION

Wayne State University is located in the cultural center of Detroit, within walking distance of the Detroit Institute of Arts, the Detroit Historical Museum, Science Museum, International Institute, Museum of African American History, Detroit Medical Center, and the main branch of the Detroit Public Library. With easy access to numerous facilities by car or bus, students can enjoy the Detroit Symphony Orchestra at Orchestra Hall, Broadway shows, and performances by well-known entertainers at the Fisher theater, the Fox theater, and the Masonic Temple. Historic Bricktown, lively Greektown, and the renowned Renaissance Center are also nearby.

STUDENT SERVICES

The College of Nursing has a full array of student services at both the undergraduate and graduate levels. These include academic advising by professional staff and faculty, academic support services within the College and within the University, placement services, services for students with disabilities, housing, personal counseling, and student activities.

THE NURSING STUDENT GROUP

The College of Nursing enrolls approximately 500 undergraduates, 250 master's students, and 70 doctoral students. The College's undergraduate student population is predominantly from the greater metropolitan area. The graduate programs represent a culturally diverse student population with representation from throughout North America, South America, Europe, and Africa. Graduates of master's and doctoral programs in nursing are in great demand, and employment opportunities are excellent throughout the nation.

COSTS

Undergraduate tuition during the 1996–97 academic year was $124 per credit hour for state residents and $278 per credit hour for nonresidents. These rates reflect junior/senior, upper-division status. Graduate tuition was $153 per credit hour for state residents and $329 per credit hour for nonresidents. A $72 registration fee is also required.

FINANCIAL AID

Opportunities for assistance with educational expenses are available to students through the University's Office of Scholarship and Financial Aid and the College of Nursing. Federal, state, and institutional funds are available based on financial need and academic merit. Assistance for both full- and part-time study is available through scholarships and fellowships, teaching and research assistantships, professional nurse traineeships, and nursing loans. Early application is essential.

APPLYING

All students must apply to both the University and the College of Nursing. To be considered for admission, undergraduate applicants must complete a minimum of 30 credits with a minimum honor point average of 2.5 in prerequisite courses. Students must file a B.S.N. application for admission, including transcripts, by March 31 for fall term admission. Selection is based on scholarship in prerequisite course work. To qualify for admission, applicants for graduate study must have completed an NLN-accredited baccalaureate program in nursing or the equivalent and must have current RN licensure. Selection is based on GRE General Test scores, an autobiographical and goals statement, scholastic achievement, and professional references. Application deadlines for admission to the Master of Science in Nursing program are two months prior to the term of admission. The Ph.D. application deadline is December 1 of the year prior to admission.

Correspondence and Information:

Office for Student Affairs
College of Nursing
Wayne State University
Detroit, Michigan 48202
Telephone: 313-577-4082
800-544-3890 (toll-free)
Fax: 313-577-6949

THE FACULTY

Adult Health and Administration

Nancy Artinian, Associate Professor; Ph.D., Wayne State, 1988. Stress in spouses and families of coronary bypass surgery patients.

Stephen Cavanagh, Associate Professor and Assistant Dean Designee; Ph.D., Texas at Austin, 1987. Stress in nursing students and critical thinking in nursing practice.

A. Dawn Hameister, Associate Professor and Assistant Dean; Ph.D., Michigan, 1989. Career development: nurse practitioner job satisfaction.

Marjorie Isenberg, Professor and Associate Dean; D.N.Sc., Boston University, 1978. Testing Orem's self-care deficit theory with chronically ill populations.

Ada Jacox, Professor and Associate Dean; Ph.D., Case Western Reserve, 1969. Pain management and nursing-sensitive patient outcomes.

Mary Jirovec, Associate Professor; Ph.D., Michigan, 1985. Urinary incontinence in the elderly and measurement of self-care agency in older adults.

Carolyn Lindgren, Associate Professor; Ph.D., Texas at Austin, 1985. Family caregivers of adult chronically ill patients.

Kathleen Moore, Assistant Professor; Ph.D., Illinois at Chicago, 1992. Personal expenditure of women with breast cancer.

Marilyn Oberst, Professor and Interim Dean; Ed.D., Columbia, 1975. Stress and coping in acute and chronic illness.

Nancy O'Connor, Assistant Professor; Ph.D., Wayne State, 1995. Measurement of motivation for self-care and ethnic identity in self-care motivation.

Marilyn Oermann, Professor; Ph.D., Pittsburgh, 1980. Clinical teaching and evaluation in nursing education.

Barbara Pieper, Associate Professor; Ph.D., Wayne State, 1980. Management of pressure ulcers.

Virginia Rice, Associate Professor; Ph.D., Michigan, 1982. Health promotion and smoking cessation.

Frances Wimbush, Assistant Professor (Clinical); Ph.D., Maryland, 1990. Cardiovascular and psychophysiological aspects of nursing.

Family, Community and Mental Health

R. Frances Board, Assistant Professor (Clinical); Ph.D., Michigan, 1988. Instrument development and high-risk pregnancy.

Chandice Covington, Associate Professor; Ph.D., Michigan, 1990. Parental physiological response to infant cry.

Mary J. Denyes, Associate Professor; Ph.D., Michigan, 1980. Self-care nursing research in children's pain.

Judith Floyd, Associate Professor; Ph.D., Wayne State, 1982. Management of sleep problems across the life span.

Hertha Gast, Assistant Professor (Clinical); Ph.D., Texas Woman's, 1983. Child and adolescent mental health.

Effie Hanchett, Associate Professor; Ph.D., NYU, 1974. Philosophical analyses of caring, self-care, and integrality.

Ann Horgas, Assistant Professor; Ph.D., Penn State, 1992. Mental health and aging, nursing home intervention.

Edythe Ellison Hough, Professor; Ed.D., UCLA, 1979. Coping with HIV/AIDS and motherhood, children of HIV/AIDS–infected mothers.

Paulette Hoyer, Associate Professor; Ph.D., Wayne State, 1984. Health promotion of the pregnant adolescent.

Kathleen Huttlinger, Associate Professor and Assistant Dean; Ph.D., Arizona, 1988. Diabetes mellitus in Navajo and Hopi cultures and hypertension in African-Americans.

Karen Labuhn, Associate Professor; Ph.D., Michigan, 1984. Health and occupational exposure to anticancer drugs.

Madeleine Leininger, Professor Emerita; Ph.D., Washington (Seattle), 1965. Transcultural nursing.

Darleen Mood, Professor; Ph.D., Wayne State, 1983. Psychosocial interventions in radiation therapy, measurement of cultural and ethnic affiliation.

Laurel Northouse, Associate Professor; Ph.D., Michigan, 1985. Couples' psychosocial adjustment to breast cancer.

Jeannette O. Poindexter, Associate Professor; Ph.D., Michigan, 1982. Predicting teenage pregnancy.

Fredericka Shea, Associate Professor; Ph.D., Michigan, 1986. HIV prevention and symptom management.

Feleta Wilson, Assistant Professor; Ph.D., Wayne State, 1991. Patients' literacy levels and patient education.

Widener University
School of Nursing
Chester, Pennsylvania

THE UNIVERSITY

Founded in 1821, Widener University is today a multicampus, comprehensive teaching institution located in the commonwealth of Pennsylvania and the state of Delaware. The University serves the educational needs of its students through degree programs ranging from the associate to the doctorate and through other credit and noncredit offerings. The University is recognized both nationally and internationally as a distinguished private educational institution.

Widener is composed of eight schools and colleges offering liberal arts and sciences, professional, and preprofessional curricula. The University's schools include the College of Arts and Sciences, School of Engineering, School of Hotel and Restaurant Management, School of Human Service Professions, School of Management, School of Nursing, University College, and the Widener University School of Law.

Total enrollment in the fall 1996 semester was approximately 8,150 (2,250 day undergraduates, 1,600 evening undergraduates, 2,300 graduate students, and 2,000 students in the School of Law).

THE SCHOOL OF NURSING

Widener's School of Nursing has a long and rich tradition. It has its origins in the Crozer Foundation of Chester, Pennsylvania. The College of Nursing of the Crozer Foundation was established in the early 1960s and became part of Widener in 1970. The School is currently headquartered in the Old Main building on the main campus. The undergraduate program has been continuously accredited by the National League for Nursing (NLN) since 1972. The School chapter (Eta Beta) of Sigma Theta Tau, the international nursing honor society, was chartered in 1983. The RN/B.S.N. program was initiated in 1977 as an evening program. It was expanded in 1982 with the addition of a weekend option. In 1990, the School began offering an accelerated B.S.N./M.S.N. program. The Doctor of Nursing Science (D.N.Sc.) program began in the early 1980s and graduated its first student in 1988. This program prepares leaders in the education of professional nurses who meet the public's need for health care.

PROGRAMS OF STUDY

The School of Nursing offers a variety of baccalaureate programs: a full-time day program, a part-time evening program, and an evening and weekend program for registered nurses. The curriculum is designed to prepare graduates who have a broad education in liberal arts and sciences as well as depth of professional knowledge and skills. Students concentrate on courses in biological and behavioral sciences, humanities, and electives in the first two years of the program. There is a strong emphasis on opportunity for practice in on-campus simulated clinical laboratory settings to prepare students for actual hands-on patient experiences. Nursing courses start in the freshman year. Students earn 63 credits in nursing, 9 credits in electives, 49 credits in liberal arts, and 1 credit in physical education, for a total of 122 credits.

Graduate programs lead to the Master of Science in Nursing and the Doctor of Nursing Science degrees. Within the master's program, tracks are available in community-based nursing, emergency critical-care nursing, and family nurse practitioner studies. Students in the family nurse practitioner track may earn the master's degree or a post-master's certificate. Candidates for the master's program must have a bachelor's degree in nursing from an NLN-accredited program and satisfactory GRE scores from an exam taken within the past five years. To earn a master's degree, students must have a final GPA of at least 3.0 and must have completed 38 semester hours for the adult nursing, community-based, and emergency critical care programs. The family nurse practitioner program requires 44 semester hours.

The Doctor of Nursing Science program prepares leaders in nursing education. The program is designed to meet the special needs and interests of nursing faculty in institutions of higher learning. Those in the program have clinical expertise in nursing at the master's level. Requirements for graduation include completion of at least 48 credits of approved doctoral course work in nursing beyond the master's degree as well as a minimum of 15 credits of dissertation advisement and a dissertation.

A post-master's certificate in nursing education is also offered for students who choose not to earn the doctorate.

AFFILIATIONS WITH HEALTH-CARE FACILITIES

Widener undergraduate students begin their clinical education in the junior year. Extensive clinical experience is a major component of the program. The program utilizes a variety of nearby major medical facilities and excellent community health-care agencies in Pennsylvania, New Jersey, and Delaware, including Liberty Home Health System, Crozer-Chester Medical Center, Mercy Catholic Medical Center, Delaware County Memorial, Riddle Memorial, Community Hospital of Chester, Hospital of the University of Pennsylvania, Children's Hospital of Philadelphia, A. I. Du Pont, and others. Most are within a 15-mile radius of the campus.

ACADEMIC FACILITIES

Widener's Wolfgram Library houses close to 240,000 volumes of books and periodicals, including microfilm, audiovisual, and other nonprint media. Of these, approximately 10,000 are nursing related, and 14,300 are health related. The University also provides several laboratories equipped with IBM microcomputers, printers, and a wide range of software. The CDC Cyber 932, available to all students, supports many high-level programming languages. The CD-ROM database is available for CINAHL, MEDLINE, PSYELIT, and ERIE.

Individualized assistance in improving writing and reading skills is provided at the Academic Skills Center. There is also a Math Center. The Nursing Learning Resource Center includes a wide variety of videotapes, computer-assisted instruction, models, films, and hospital-simulated practice units. There is a strong emphasis on opportunity for practice in simulated clinical settings to prepare students for actual hands-on patient experiences.

LOCATION

Rolling, green lawns, graceful trees, and an eclectic mixture of architecture characterize Widener's spacious suburban campus in Chester, Pennsylvania. The University is ideally located at the intersection of Route 320 and I-95, near Philadelphia's International Airport, with direct access from I-476. It is just 10 miles south of Philadelphia in historic Delaware County, 75 miles from New York, 80 miles from Baltimore, and 100 miles from Washington, D.C. Nearby are both the New Jersey beaches and the famous Brandywine River Valley.

STUDENT SERVICES

The Student Nurses Association meets monthly to provide opportunities for exchange of ideas and the pursuit of educational interests. Officers are elected from the ranks of all classes. Representatives attend the national convention.

Additional opportunities are provided by the Eta Beta chapter of Sigma Theta Tau. Candidates are selected each fall from students in both undergraduate and graduate programs and are welcomed in a formal ceremony.

Academic support services include freshman academic advising, an academic skills program, and an early-warning program for incoming freshmen. On-campus housing is guaranteed to students for all four years. The Career Advising and Placement Office houses an extensive career library and assists students with career development, including résumé development and on-campus job fairs. More than sixty student organizations include a Black Student Union, Commuter Student Organization, Student Government, International Club, and Rotaract Club. In addition, NCAA Division III varsity sports in twenty-two areas and intramural and individual recreational opportunities are available for all students.

THE NURSING STUDENT GROUP

Of the 839 students in the School of Nursing, 615 are in the undergraduate program, and 88 percent of these are women. The remaining 224 students are in graduate programs, and 96 percent of these are women.

COSTS

Tuition costs for the 1996–97 academic year were $13,900 for full-time undergraduate study. Graduate tuition was $395 per credit for master's programs and $420 per credit for doctoral programs. Room and board cost from $5910 to $6730, depending on the accommodations selected.

FINANCIAL AID

In 1995, 81 percent of Widener nursing undergraduates received financial aid in the form of grants, loans, and scholarships—some specifically for nursing majors—and employment. Eligibility for aid is based on need as well as academic merit.

APPLYING

Admission is competitive. Applicants are evaluated individually to determine their potential for academic success. Widener bases its decisions on the strength of academic preparation, achievement, recommendations, extracurricular activities, personal qualifications, and the pattern of testing on various standardized tests. Since the University has a rolling admissions policy, students are notified of the admission decision soon after their application is completed. Admission into the master's program requires a bachelor's degree in nursing from an NLN-accredited program, a minimum GPA of 3.0 in the B.S.N. program, GRE scores from an exam taken in the last five years, and a current license as a registered nurse. Admission into the doctoral program requires a minimum GPA of 3.5 in the M.S.N. program, a graduate statistics course with a grade of at least C, and a graduate course in nursing theories and conceptional models.

Correspondence and Information:

Jane Brennan, Acting Assistant Dean
Undergraduate Program of Study
School of Nursing
Widener University
One University Place
Chester, Pennsylvania 19013-5792
Telephone: 610-499-4210
Fax: 610-499-4216

Mary Walker, Assistant Dean
Graduate Program of Study
School of Nursing
One University Place
Chester, Pennsylvania 19013-5792
Telephone: 610-499-4208
Fax: 610-499-4216

Ann Birney, Director of Special Programs
RN-B.S.N.-M.S.N. Programs
School of Nursing
One University Place
Chester, PA 19013-5792
Telephone: 610-499-4209
Fax: 610-499-4216

THE FACULTY

Marguerite M. Barbiere, Dean and Associate Professor of Nursing; M.S.N., Widener; Ed.D., Temple.
Jane Brennan, Acting Assistant Dean, Undergraduate Studies, and Assistant Professor of Nursing; D.N.Sc., Widener.
Mary Walker, Assistant Dean, Graduate Studies, and Associate Professor of Nursing; M.S.N., Ed.D., Pennsylvania.
Lois Allen, Ph.D., Professor.
Elizabeth W. Bayley, Ph.D., Professor.
Normajean Colby, M.S.N., Lecturer.
Nancy E. Conrad, Ed.D., Assistant Professor.
Norma Dawson, Ph.D., Professor.
Elizabeth L. Dickason, Ed.D., Assistant Professor.
Joan Dresh, M.S.N., Lecturer.
Martha A. From, Ed.D., Assistant Professor.
Jeanne S. Gelman, M.S.N., Associate Professor.
Lynn E. Kelly, Ph.D., Associate Professor.
Judith Kilpatrick, M.S.N., Lecturer.
Lynne E. Leach, Ed.D., Assistant Professor.
Susan Leddy, Ph.D., Professor.
Margaret A. Miller, Ph.D., Assistant Professor.
Karen H. Morin, D.S.N., Associate Professor.
Laurie Murray, D.N.S., Assistant Professor.
Ann Nichols, M.S.N., C.R.N.P., Lecturer; Coordinator, Family Nurse Practitioner Program.
Janette L. Packer, Ed.D., Professor.
Barbara J. Patterson, Ph.D., Assistant Professor.
Janice Reilley, M.S.N., Lecturer.
Eileen M. Roche, D.N.Sc., Assistant Professor.
Mary K. Sienty, Ed.D., Assistant Professor.
Andrea Wolfe, M.S.N., C.R.N.P., Interim Director, Nurse Practitioner Program.
Doris Young, M.S.N., Assistant Professor.

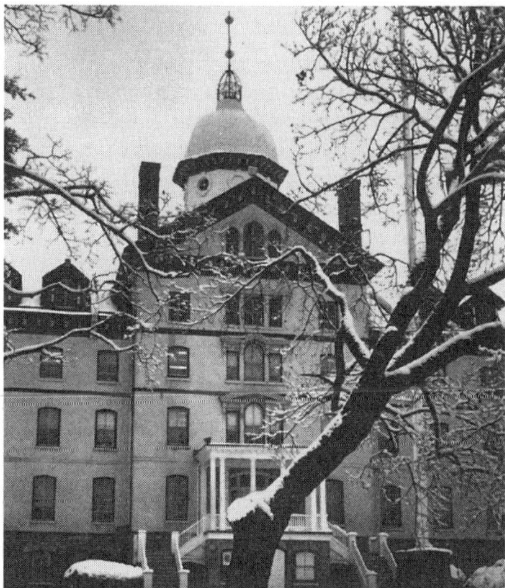

The dome atop Widener's Old Main building.

Wright State University
College of Nursing and Health
Dayton, Ohio

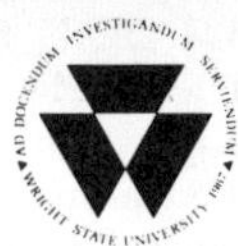

THE UNIVERSITY

Wright State University is a comprehensive, state-assisted institution that was founded in 1964 and was granted full university status in 1967. It serves more than 17,500 students in 100 undergraduate programs, more than 30 master's degree programs, and advanced programs leading to the Ed.S., M.D., Ph.D., and Psy.D. degrees. The University comprises eight academic units: Business and Administration, Education and Human Services, Engineering and Computer Science, Liberal Arts, Medicine, Nursing and Health, Professional Psychology, and Science and Mathematics.

Wright State is a metropolitan university. It is committed to providing leadership in addressing the educational, social, and cultural needs of the Greater Miami Valley and to promoting the economic and technological development of the region through a strong program of basic and applied research and professional service. Wright State is dedicated to excellence in teaching, research, and service.

Wright State seeks to enroll achievement-oriented traditional and nontraditional students and maintains an open admissions policy for undergraduates.

THE COLLEGE OF NURSING AND HEALTH

The College of Nursing and Health's baccalaureate program began in 1973, and the first students were admitted to the master's program in 1978. The College currently enrolls approximately 550 undergraduate and 250 graduate students.

In 1984, the College entered into a collaborative agreement with the Division of Nursing at Miami Valley Hospital to form a Center for Excellence in Nursing. Through collaboration with nursing staff members, this agreement affords unique opportunities for research, clinical practice, and education for students and the faculty.

The College of Nursing and Health reflects the broader mission of the University by providing excellent educational programs that prepare nurses for a dynamic health-care environment. As part of a metropolitan university, the College accepts the obligation to extend its resources to the surrounding region. It provides leadership to address regional health needs and forms partnerships with other disciplines, institutions, and organizations to cooperatively address health-related community problems. The clinical education programs are structured to provide students with a solid foundation in health assessment, health promotion, community-based practice, and primary health-care concepts.

Most of the College's full-time tenure-track faculty members are doctorally prepared. Faculty members teaching in the B.S.N. and M.S. programs have a wealth of clinical expertise. In addition, students gain a breadth and depth of knowledge from nurses serving as preceptors for clinical practicum courses.

PROGRAMS OF STUDY

The College of Nursing and Health offers the B.S.N. degree, the M.S. degree, a joint M.S./M.B.A. degree in conjunction with the College of Business and Administration, and a school nurse certificate program in collaboration with the College of Education and Human Services. For RNs with a baccalaureate degree in a traditional discipline area other than nursing, there is a bridge program that allows students to earn the master's degree after completion of a limited number of undergraduate nursing courses. The B.S.N. and M.S. programs are accredited by the National League for Nursing (NLN), and the M.B.A. program is accredited by the American Association of Collegiate Schools of Business (AACSB).

The baccalaureate program emphasizes health and well-being across the life span and prepares graduates for entry into professional practice as generalists. The program provides entry options for both basic students and RN students who have completed an associate degree or diploma program in nursing. RNs are offered a program that includes transition courses that integrate their previous learning with the new knowledge provided in a baccalaureate program. Courses for RNs are offered on campus in the late afternoon and evening or on designated days at the outreach off-campus sites. The program may be completed in two calendar years of full-time study by RNs with an associate degree. The baccalaureate program accommodates both full-time and part-time students.

The master's program educates nurses for advanced leadership roles in practice, education, and administration, as well as for doctoral study in nursing. The curriculum offers students the opportunity to prepare for roles as clinical nurse specialists in adult health and illness, child and adolescent health, or community health; family nurse practitioners in the Family Nurse Practitioner Program, which has an option for post-master's study; nurse administrators in the Nurse Administration Track or the dual-degree (N.A./M.B.A.) program; or nurse educators with a focus in a clinical specialty.

The master's program accommodates both full-time and part-time students, with most classes offered in the late afternoon and evening. The sequence of course offerings is flexible. Full-time students may complete the program within one calendar year; part-time students must complete all requirements for the degree within five years.

ACADEMIC FACILITIES

The College of Nursing and Health is housed in Allyn Hall. Clinical instructional facilities are abundant and varied. The College has contracts with more than 200 agencies in the area, including hospitals, rehabilitation centers, county health departments, nursing homes, school systems, senior citizen centers, day-care centers, and other community-based settings, which can be used for clinical experiences and research.

For research, both the University Library and the Fordham Health Sciences Library provide abundant resources. The University Library also provides media production services and facilities. The University's Statistical Consulting Center and the College's Center for Nursing and Health Research provide support for research design and data analysis. The College also has a computer laboratory that includes interactive video programs for classroom and independent learning.

LOCATION

The campus is located in a rural-suburban setting 10 miles east of Dayton, a business and manufacturing center with a metropolitan population approaching one million. The University is adjacent to Wright Patterson Air Force Base, which is a center for Air Force research and procurement. A variety of recreational, cultural, art, science, and business activities are available in the metropolitan area. Transportation to the campus via RTA is available from throughout the Miami Valley. The International Airport and downtown are less than 25 miles from campus.

STUDENT SERVICES
The University has many resources and a variety of services for both undergraduate and graduate students. Since Wright State is a leader in providing support and accessibility to students with disabilities, a broad range of physical and academic services are available. In addition, Wright State has an International Student Program, a Childhood Development Center, an on-campus bookstore, Campus Ministry, five housing communities, dining services, Bolinga Cultural Resources Center, Student Health Services, Counseling Services, and the Nutter Center for sports and recreation.

THE NURSING STUDENT GROUP
There are more than 600 undergraduate students and 250 graduate students in the College of Nursing and Health. Many of the undergraduate students are employed at least part-time and attend school full-time. Most graduate students are employed full-time in area health-care agencies in a variety of clinical and administrative positions and pursue the part-time plan.

COSTS
Tuition for undergraduate students in 1996–97 was $112 per credit hour (in-state) and $224 per credit hour (out-of-state); full-time tuition for 11–18 credit hours was $1200 per quarter (in-state) and $2400 per quarter (out-of-state). Tuition for graduate students was $143 per credit hour (in-state) and $255 per credit hour (out-of-state); full-time tuition for 11–18 credit hours was $1517 per quarter (in-state) and $2717 per quarter (out-of-state). Other expenses include books, immunizations, uniforms, insurance, and travel to clinical sites.

FINANCIAL AID
A number of scholarships based on academic excellence, as well as grants based on financial need, are available for undergraduate students. Graduate assistantships and Professional Nurse Traineeships are available for students who meet the criteria. Graduate academic fellowships, awarded on the basis of academic merit, are also available. Need-based Federal Perkins and Federal Stafford Student loans are available to students who qualify.

APPLYING
To be eligible for admission, undergraduate students must be matriculated at the University, complete all designated prerequisite courses with a grade of C or better, and have a cumulative GPA of at least 2.5.

Graduate applicants must have an overall undergraduate GPA of at least 3.0 or an overall GPA of 2.7 with a 3.0 or better in the last 90 quarter hours (60 semester hours); have a B.S.N. degree from an NLN-accredited college or university or a bachelor's degree in a field other than nursing and be a registered nurse with selected support and professional nursing bridge courses; and have an Ohio RN license. All application materials for fall quarter should be submitted by April 15. Applications received after that date are considered on a space-available basis.

Correspondence and Information:

Office of Admissions
E148 Student Union
Wright State University
3640 Colonel Glenn Highway
Dayton, Ohio 45435
Telephone: 513-873-5700

School of Graduate Studies
106 Oelman Hall
Wright State University
3640 Colonel Glenn Highway
Dayton, Ohio 45435
Telephone: 513-873-2975

THE FACULTY

Barbara Bogan, Assistant Professor; M.S., Ohio State (nursing).

Jean Budding, Instructor; M.S., Wright State (nursing administration); M.S., Dayton (education).

Joy Burgess, Instructor; M.S.N., Texas at San Antonio (community health nursing, nursing education).

Donna Miles Curry, Associate Professor; M.S.N., Saint Louis (nursing of children); Ph.D., Ohio State (family relations and human development).

Jane Doorley, Instructor; M.S., Wright State (rehabilitation/community health nursing).

Barbara Fowler, Associate Professor; M.S.N., Cincinnati (parent/child nursing); Ed.D., Cincinnati (curriculum and instruction, nursing education).

Janet S. Fulton, Assistant Professor; M.S.N., Cincinnati (oncology nursing); Ph.D., Ohio State (nursing).

Margaret Clark Graham, Associate Professor; M.S.N., Vanderbilt (family nurse practitioner); Ph.D., Ohio State (community health education).

Kimberly Hickok, Instructor; M.S., Indiana Wesleyan (community health).

Elizabeth Lipp, Associate Professor; Ph.D., Ohio State (nursing).

Patricia Martin, Associate Professor; M.S., Wright State (rehabilitation/community health nursing); Ph.D., Case Western Reserve (nursing).

Virginia Nehring, Associate Professor; M.S.N., Yale (community health); Ph.D., Walden (nursing research, education).

Barbara O'Brien, Assistant Professor and Associate Dean; M.S.N., Cincinnati (child psychiatric nursing); Ph.D., Ohio State (nursing).

Susan Praeger, Professor; M.S., New York Medical College (nursing); Ed.D., Northern Colorado (humanistic nursing education).

Kristine A. Scordo, Assistant Professor; M.S., Ohio State (cardiovascular nursing); Ph.D., Ohio State, (cardiac physiology).

Brenda Stevenson, Assistant Professor; Ph.D., Case Western Reserve (nursing).

Mary L. Stoeckle, Assistant Professor; M.S.N., Cincinnati (burn/trauma); Ph.D., Cincinnati (nursing).

Jane Swart, Professor and Dean; M.A., Columbia Teachers College (psychiatric nursing, education); M.A., Ph.D., Washington, Seattle (sociology).

Patricia Thornburg, Assistant Professor; M.S., Ohio State (nursing); Ph.D., Cincinnati (nursing research).

Celesta Warner, Instructor; M.S., Ball State (maternal/child nursing, education).

Barbara Wise, Instructor; M.S.N., North Carolina (family nurse practitioner).

Yale University
School of Nursing
New Haven, Connecticut

THE UNIVERSITY

Yale University was chartered in 1701. The central mission of the University is to preserve, disseminate, and advance knowledge through teaching and research.

The institution that became Yale was founded as the Collegiate School by 10 congregational ministers in Branford, Connecticut. The small collegiate school moved to New Haven in 1716 and today is nondenominational. The educational mission of Yale University is carried out in its undergraduate school, Yale College, and its eleven graduate and professional schools: Architecture (1972), Art (1865), Divinity (1822), Drama (1955), Forestry and Environmental Studies (1900), Graduate School of Arts and Sciences (1847), Law (1824), Medicine (1813), Music (1894), Nursing (1923), and Organization and Management (1975).

THE SCHOOL OF NURSING

The Yale School of Nursing (YSN) was started in 1923. Under the direction of its first dean, Annie W. Goodrich, the School established a new pattern for nursing education with student instruction and experience based upon an educational plan rather than an apprenticeship system.

Because of an increasing realization that a college education was essential in the profession of nursing, YSN admitted only college graduates after 1934. Fifteen years later, an advanced program in mental health nursing was added to the basic program as a first step in postgraduate education. The basic program was discontinued in 1956, and the curriculum of the advanced program was expanded. A Master of Science in Nursing (M.S.N.) degree was awarded. By the late 1960s and early 1970s, new clinical specialty programs were developed. In 1974, YSN again opened its door to college graduates who were not yet nurses and instituted the Graduate Entry Program in Nursing. In 1994 a doctoral program was established and the first class was admitted.

PROGRAMS OF STUDY

The Yale School of Nursing offers the M.S.N. and D.N.Sc. (Doctor of Nursing Science) degrees and post-master's certificates. The School of Nursing admits both registered nurses who have a baccalaureate degree and college graduates with no previous nursing education who move directly into a chosen area of clinical specialization. The full-time student is expected to complete the requirements for the M.S.N. degree in two academic years. Scheduled part-time study is also available. The Graduate Entry Program in Nursing requires two terms and one summer session in addition to the two-year specialization sequence. The curriculum places emphasis on clinical competence and nursing research. Each student is educated to function in an expanded role in the clinical areas of his or her choice.

The M.S.N. program emphasizes clinical specialization. The programs of study are adult/family nurse practitioner studies, adult and child psychiatric–mental health nursing, nurse-midwifery, adult advanced-practice nursing, pediatric nurse practitioner (chronic illness) and pediatric nurse practitioner (primary care) studies, and nursing management and policy.

The D.N.Sc. degree program is designed to prepare nurse scientists who are expert in clinical research to advance knowledge development for the discipline of nursing by conducting research on nursing phenomena. Graduates of the program will assume major leadership roles in extending the theoretical base of nursing, including shaping responses to political, economic, ethical, and other health-care issues.

AFFILIATIONS WITH HEALTH-CARE FACILITIES

The combined facilities of the Yale School of Medicine, the Yale–New Haven Hospital, the Yale Child Study Center, the Yale School of Nursing, and the Yale Psychiatric Institute constitute the Yale–New Haven Medical Center. The Connecticut Mental Health Center is closely affiliated with this complex. In addition, a large number of community agencies are utilized, including schools, visiting nurses' associations, private practices, and community clinics.

ACADEMIC FACILITIES

The major collection of the Yale School of Nursing is in the Yale Medical Library, which serves the entire Yale–New Haven Medical Center as well as others in the University. The collections, covering nursing, clinical medicine and its specialties, public health, and related fields, number more than 380,000 volumes. About 90,000 or more are source materials or supporting works in the historical collections. More than 2,500 current journals are received regularly. Yale's main library, the Sterling Memorial Library, along with the Beincke Rare Book and Manuscript Library, the Cross Campus Library, and Seeley Mudd Library, contains about 5.6 million volumes.

LOCATION

Yale's effort to help students feel at home in the University is reflected by its central location. The Yale University Art Gallery, Peabody Museum of Natural History, Yale Center for British Art, and Payne Whitney Gymnasium are all accessible to YSN students. In addition, the city of New Haven has long been known for its theater life, music, art, and a range of other cultural activities. An entertainment district adjacent to Yale's Old Campus includes the renovated Shubert and Palace theaters.

STUDENT SERVICES

A distinctive feature of life at Yale is the unusually wide variety of events and activities on the Daily Calendar—plays, exhibits, concerts, films, workshops, lectures, sports events, and seminars. In addition, the Graduate-Professional Student Senate (GPSS) is the student government organization for graduate and professional students.

THE NURSING STUDENT GROUP

The Yale School of Nursing currently enrolls 268 students, of whom 191 are full-time students and 77 are part-time. Approximately three quarters of YSN graduates seek a first position in the advanced clinical practice specialty for which they were educated. Graduates of YSN have gone on to distinguished positions in clinical practice, health service administration, the federal government, and academia.

COSTS

In 1996–97, tuition was $8800 per term for fall and spring terms. Tuition for students in the first year of the Graduate Entry Program in Nursing was $12,275 per term, including the twelve-week summer term. Room and board and other personal expenses were about $11,400. Other educational expenses, including books, health insurance, and student fees, totaled approximately $2100.

FINANCIAL AID

Financial aid is not a consideration in the admissions process. The School of Nursing accepts applications for financial aid from candidates seeking admission in order to expedite the award process. An application for financial aid, provided by the Educational Testing Service, is sent to all active applicants. Financial need is met by a combination of scholarships, nurse traineeships, graduate assistantships, and federal loans.

APPLYING

Students are admitted to the graduate program in nursing once a year in September. The minimum requirement for admission to the Graduate Entry Program in Nursing is a baccalaureate degree from a recognized college or university. No specific major is required. Collegiate courses in biological and social sciences are recommended, and a prerequisite course in undergraduate-level statistics is required. The minimum requirement for the master's program for RNs is a baccalaureate degree from a recognized college or university and graduation from a school of nursing. Personal experience is desirable but not required. Applicants must be licensed to practice nursing in at least one state. An undergraduate course in statistics is required. All students must submit official transcripts of all previous college records; an official transcript of GRE test scores; personal references from three individuals; and an admission essay. Qualified candidates are asked to come to the School for an interview. Students should contact the Student Affairs Office for application deadlines.

Correspondence and Information:

Yale University School of Nursing
Office of Student Affairs
100 Church Street South
P.O. Box 9740
New Haven, Connecticut 06536-0740
Telephone: 203-785-2389

THE FACULTY

Ivy Alexander, Program Instructor; M.S., Northeastern, 1992.
Ann Ameling, Professor; M.S.N., Yale, 1967.
Susan Andrews, Associate Professor; M.S.N., Yale, 1983; CNM.
Patricia Polgar Bailey, Program Instructor; M.S.N., Simmons, 1991.
Margaret Beal, Associate Professor; Ph.D., Union Institute, 1995; CNM.
Clarice M. Begemann, Program Instructor; M.S.N., M.P.P.M., Yale, 1990.
Helen Varney Burst, Professor; M.S.N., Yale, 1963; CNM.
Deborah Chyun, Lecturer; M.S.N., Yale, 1982.
Sally Solomon Cohen, Assistant Professor; Ph.D., Columbia, 1993; FAAN.
Susan M. Cohen, Associate Professor; D.S.N., Alabama, 1983.
Jessica Shank Coviello, Lecturer; M.S.N., Yale, 1983.
Angela Crowley, Associate Professor; M.S.N., NYU, 1975.
Barbara Decker, Associate Professor; Ed.D., Columbia Teachers College, 1989; CNM.
Susan E. Devine, Lecturer; M.S.N., Yale, 1991.
Donna Diers, Professor; M.S.N., Yale, 1964; FAAN.
Linda DiPalma, Assistant Professor; M.S.N., Yale, 1989.
Jane Dixon, Professor; Ph.D., Connecticut, 1973.
Neil F. Ead, Assistant Professor; M.S.N., Yale, 1990.
Deborah Ferholt, Lecturer; M.D., Rochester, 1966.
Marjorie Funk, Associate Professor; Ph.D., Yale, 1992.
Geriann Gallagher, Lecturer; M.S.N., Rush, 1992; ND.
Margaret Grey, Professor and Associate Dean for Research and Doctoral Studies; Dr.P.H., Columbia, 1984; FAAN.
Elaine Gustafson, Program Instructor; M.S.N., Yale, 1986.
Wendy Holmes, Associate Professor; M.S.N., Boston University, 1976.
Carrie S. Klima, Program Instructor; M.S., Illinois, 1983; CNM.
Mary Kathryn Knobf, Associate Professor; M.S.N., Yale, 1982; FAAN.
Judith Krauss, Professor and Dean; M.S.N., Yale, 1970; FAAN.
Melva D. Kravitz, Associate Professor; Ph.D., Utah, 1984.
Jerilynn A. Lamb-Pagone, Lecturer; M.S.N., Hunter, 1980.
Robin Leger, Assistant Professor; M.S., Syracuse, 1984.
Monteen Lucas, Associate Professor; Ph.D., Texas A&M, 1987.
Courtney H. Lyder, Assistant Professor; N.D., Rush, 1990.
Donna M. Mahrenholz, Associate Professor; Ph.D., Maryland, 1990.
Janet Makeover, Lecturer; M.A., NYU, 1979.
Gail Melkus, Associate Professor; Ed.D., Columbia Teachers College, 1989.
Paula Milone-Nuzzo, Assistant Professor; Ph.D., Connecticut, 1989.
Pamela Minarik, Associate Professor; M.S., California, San Francisco, 1981.
Catharine Moffett, Program Instructor; M.S.N., Yale, 1982.
Alison Moriarty, Program Instructor; M.S.N., Yale, 1994.
Beth L. Muller, Program Instructor; M.S.N., Yale, 1987.
Deborah Dornon Navedo, Program Instructor; M.S.N., Columbia, 1986.
Leslie Nield-Anderson, Associate Professor; Ph.D., NYU, 1991.
Douglas P. Olsen, Assistant Professor; Ph.D., Boston College, 1994.
Carole Passarelli, Associate Professor; M.S., Connecticut, 1977.
Linda Honan Pellico, Lecturer; M.S.N., Yale, 1989.
Cassy D. Pollack, Assistant Professor and Associate Dean for Students and Master's Studies; M.S.N., M.P.P.M., Yale, 1983.
Veronica Pollack, Assistant Professor; M.S.N., Pennsylvania, 1986.
Ann Powers, Program Instructor; M.S., Connecticut, 1984.
Elisabeth Reilly, Program Instructor; M.S.N., Yale, 1990.
Heather Reynolds, Associate Professor; M.S.N., Yale, 1980; CNM.
Leslie Robinson, Lecturer; M.S.N., Yale, 1981; CNM.
Mary Ellen Rousseau, Associate Professor; M.S.N., Columbia, 1975; CNM.
Lois Sadler, Lecturer; M.S.N., Yale, 1979.
Lynne Schilling, Research Scientist; Ph.D., Syracuse, 1977.
Dorothy Sexton, Professor; Ed.D., Boston University, 1974.
Gail Simonson, Lecturer; M.S.N., Rochester, 1982.
Geralyn Spollett, Assistant Professor; M.S.N., Boston College, 1982.
Martha Swartz, Associate Professor; M.S., Michigan, 1981.
Ann Williams, Associate Professor; Ed.D., Columbia Teachers College, 1989; FAAN.
Walter Zawalich, Research Scientist; Ph.D., Florida State, 1971.

INDEXES

There are three indexes in this section. The first, *Concentrations Within Master's Degree Programs,* lists schools by the specific areas of study available within their master's programs. The second is an index that sorts the schools by specific program type. The third, *Institution Index,* gives page references for all colleges and universities listed in this guide. If there is an in-depth description for the school, it appears in boldface type.

Concentrations Within Master's Degree Programs

Clinical Nurse Specialist Programs

Andrews University, MI
California State University, Fresno, CA
Carlow College, PA
College of New Rochelle, NY
Gonzaga University, WA
Northern Arizona University, AZ
Northern Kentucky University, KY
Pacific Lutheran University, WA
St. John Fisher College, NY
Samuel Merritt College, CA
Southwest Missouri State University, MO
University of Arizona, AZ
University of Arkansas, AR
University of Mississippi Medical Center, MS
University of Northern Colorado, CO
University of Ottawa, ON
University of San Francisco, CA
University of Southern California, CA
Vanderbilt University, TN

Adult Health Nursing

Adelphi University, NY
Arizona State University, AZ
Arkansas State University, AR
Armstrong Atlantic State University, GA
Azusa Pacific University, CA
Ball State University, IN
Bloomsburg University of Pennsylvania, PA
California State University, Chico, CA
California State University, Los Angeles, CA
California State University, Sacramento, CA
Cedar Crest College, PA
Clemson University, SC
College Misericordia, PA
College of Mount Saint Vincent, NY
College of St. Scholastica, MN
Creighton University, NE
Dalhousie University, NS
East Carolina University, NC
Eastern Michigan University, MI
Eastern Washington University, WA
Emory University, GA
Fort Hays State University, KS
Georgia College, GA
Georgia State University, GA
Grand Valley State University, MI
Hampton University, VA
Incarnate Word College, TX
Indiana State University, IN
Indiana University–Purdue University Indianapolis, IN
Johns Hopkins University, MD
Kent State University, OH
La Salle University, PA
Lehman College of the City University of New York, NY
Loma Linda University, CA
Long Island University, C.W. Post Campus, NY
Louisiana State University Medical Center, LA
Madonna University, MI
Marquette University, WI
Medical College of Georgia, GA
Medical College of Ohio, OH
Medical University of South Carolina, SC
Molloy College, NY
Mount Saint Mary College, NY
Murray State University, KY
New York University, NY
Northeastern University, MA
Northern Illinois University, IL
Northern Michigan University, MI
Northwestern State University of Louisiana, LA
Oakland University, MI
Ohio State University, OH
Oregon Health Sciences University, OR
Otterbein College, OH
Pace University, NY
Pennsylvania State University, University Park Campus, PA
Purdue University Calumet, IN
Radford University, VA
Rutgers, The State University of New Jersey, Camden College of Arts and Sciences, NJ
Rutgers, The State University of New Jersey, College of Nursing, NJ
Saginaw Valley State University, MI
State University of New York at Stony Brook, NY
Syracuse University, NY
Temple University, PA
Texas Woman's University, TX
Thomas Jefferson University, PA
Troy State University, AL
Université de Montréal, PQ
Université Laval, PQ
University of Akron, OH
University of Arkansas for Medical Sciences, AR
University of Central Arkansas, AR
University of Cincinnati, OH
University of Colorado Health Sciences Center, CO
University of Evansville, IN
University of Florida, FL
University of Hawaii at Manoa, HI
University of Iowa, IA
University of Kansas, KS
University of Kentucky, KY
University of Massachusetts Dartmouth, MA
University of Minnesota, Twin Cities Campus, MN
University of Missouri–Columbia, MO
University of Missouri–Kansas City, MO
University of Missouri–St. Louis, MO
University of Mobile, AL
University of Nebraska Medical Center, NE
University of New Hampshire, NH
University of North Carolina at Charlotte, NC
University of North Dakota, ND
University of Saskatchewan, SK
University of South Alabama, AL
University of Southern Maine, ME
University of Southern Mississippi, MS
University of South Florida, FL
University of Tennessee at Chattanooga, TN
University of Tennessee, Knoxville, TN
University of Texas at Austin, TX
University of Texas at El Paso, TX
University of Texas Health Science Center at San Antonio, TX
University of Texas–Pan American, TX
University of Utah, UT
University of Vermont, VT
University of Virginia, VA
University of Wisconsin–Eau Claire, WI
University of Wisconsin–Milwaukee, WI
Valparaiso University, IN
Virginia Commonwealth University, VA
Washington State University, WA
Western Connecticut State University, CT
Whitworth College, WA
Wichita State University, KS
Widener University, PA
Winona State University, MN
Wright State University, OH

Cardiovascular Nursing

Catholic University of America, DC
Indiana University–Purdue University Indianapolis, IN
McNeese State University, LA
Rush University, IL
Saginaw Valley State University, MI
Syracuse University, NY
University of Alberta, AB
University of California, San Francisco, CA
University of Delaware, DE
University of Illinois at Chicago, IL
University of Washington, WA
Yale University, CT

Child Care/Pediatric Nursing

Adelphi University, NY
Arizona State University, AZ
Clemson University, SC
Dalhousie University, NS
Duke University, NC
East Carolina University, NC
Emory University, GA
Grand Valley State University, MI
Gwynedd-Mercy College, PA
Lehman College of the City University of New York, NY

Loma Linda University, CA
Marquette University, WI
Molloy College, NY
New York University, NY
Northeastern University, MA
Ohio State University, OH
Oregon Health Sciences University, OR
Rush University, IL
Rutgers, The State University of New Jersey, College of Nursing, NJ
Saginaw Valley State University, MI
State University of New York at Buffalo, NY
State University of New York at Stony Brook, NY
Syracuse University, NY
Texas Woman's University, TX
Université de Montréal, PQ
University of Akron, OH
University of Alberta, AB
University of Arkansas for Medical Sciences, AR
University of Cincinnati, OH
University of Delaware, DE
University of Florida, FL
University of Illinois at Chicago, IL
University of Iowa, IA
University of Kansas, KS
University of Kentucky, KY
University of Michigan, MI
University of Minnesota, Twin Cities Campus, MN
University of Missouri–Kansas City, MO
University of Missouri–St. Louis, MO
University of Nebraska Medical Center, NE
University of North Carolina at Chapel Hill, NC
University of Oklahoma Health Sciences Center, OK
University of South Alabama, AL
University of South Florida, FL
University of Tennessee, Knoxville, TN
University of Utah, UT
University of Washington, WA
University of Wisconsin–Madison, WI
Valparaiso University, IN
Virginia Commonwealth University, VA
Wichita State University, KS
Wright State University, OH

Community Health Nursing

Albany State College, GA
Allentown College of St. Francis de Sales, PA
Arizona State University, AZ
Augustana College, SD
Azusa Pacific University, CA
Bloomsburg University of Pennsylvania, PA
Boston College, MA
California State University, Sacramento, CA
Capital University, OH
Case Western Reserve University, OH
College Misericordia, PA
Dalhousie University, NS
DePaul University, IL
D'Youville College, NY
Eastern Washington University, WA
Georgia Southern University, GA
Hampton University, VA
Holy Family College, PA
Hunter College of the City University of New York, NY
Indiana State University, IN
Indiana University–Purdue University Indianapolis, IN
Indiana Wesleyan University, IN
Johns Hopkins University, MD
La Roche College, PA
La Salle University, PA
Lewis University, IL
Louisiana State University Medical Center, LA
Medical College of Georgia, GA
Metropolitan State University, MN
New Mexico State University, NM
Northeastern University, MA
Northern Illinois University, IL
Ohio State University, OH
Old Dominion University, VA
Oregon Health Sciences University, OR
Pennsylvania State University, University Park Campus, PA
Rush University, IL
Russell Sage College, NY
Rutgers, The State University of New Jersey, Camden College of Arts and Sciences, NJ
Rutgers, The State University of New Jersey, College of Nursing, NJ
Saginaw Valley State University, MI
Saint Xavier University, IL
San Diego State University, CA
Seattle University, WA
Southeastern Louisiana University, LA
Southern Illinois University at Edwardsville, IL
State University of New York at Binghamton, NY
Syracuse University, NY
Texas Tech University Health Sciences Center, TX
Texas Woman's University, TX
Thomas Jefferson University, PA
Université de Montréal, PQ
Université Laval, PQ
University of Alaska Anchorage, AK
University of Alberta, AB
University of California, San Francisco, CA
University of Central Arkansas, AR
University of Cincinnati, OH
University of Colorado Health Sciences Center, CO
University of Connecticut, CT
University of Florida, FL
University of Illinois at Chicago, IL
University of Iowa, IA
University of Kansas, KS
University of Kentucky, KY
University of Maryland at Baltimore, MD
University of Massachusetts Dartmouth, MA
University of Michigan, MI
University of Nebraska Medical Center, NE
University of Nevada, Reno, NV
University of New Mexico, NM
University of North Carolina at Charlotte, NC
University of Oklahoma Health Sciences Center, OK
University of Portland, OR
University of Saskatchewan, SK
University of South Alabama, AL
University of South Carolina, SC
University of Southern Maine, ME
University of Southern Mississippi, MS
University of South Florida, FL
University of Texas at Austin, TX
University of Utah, UT
University of Vermont, VT
University of Virginia, VA
University of Washington, WA
University of Wisconsin–Madison, WI
University of Wyoming, WY
Valparaiso University, IN
Washington State University, WA
Wayne State University, MI
West Chester University of Pennsylvania, PA
Whitworth College, WA
Wichita State University, KS
Widener University, PA
William Paterson College of New Jersey, NJ
Wright State University, OH

Critical Care Nursing

Boston College, MA
Case Western Reserve University, OH
Columbia University, NY
Emory University, GA
Governors State University, IL
Indiana University–Purdue University Indianapolis, IN
La Roche College, PA
Loma Linda University, CA
Loyola University Chicago, IL
Medical University of South Carolina, SC
Northeastern University, MA
Northwestern State University of Louisiana, LA
Old Dominion University, VA
Purdue University Calumet, IN
Rush University, IL
Rutgers, The State University of New Jersey, College of Nursing, NJ
San Diego State University, CA
Seton Hall University, NJ
State University of New York at Stony Brook, NY
Syracuse University, NY
Thomas Jefferson University, PA
University of Alberta, AB
University of California, San Francisco, CA
University of Cincinnati, OH
University of Colorado Health Sciences Center, CO
University of Florida, FL
University of Illinois at Chicago, IL
University of Kentucky, KY
University of Massachusetts Boston, MA
University of Nebraska Medical Center, NE

University of Puerto Rico, Medical Sciences Campus, PR
University of Rhode Island, RI
University of South Florida, FL
University of Tennessee, Memphis, TN
University of Virginia, VA
University of Washington, WA
Widener University, PA

Family Health Nursing

California State University, Sacramento, CA
Capital University, OH
College of New Jersey, NJ
Creighton University, NE
Georgia College, GA
Graceland College, IA
Mankato State University, MN
Medical University of South Carolina, SC
Mercy College, NY
Northeastern University, MA
Saginaw Valley State University, MI
Saint Joseph College, CT
Salisbury State University, MD
Southeast Missouri State University, MO
State University of New York at Binghamton, NY
State University of New York at New Paltz, NY
Syracuse University, NY
Université de Montréal, PQ
Université Laval, PQ
University of Alberta, AB
University of Florida, FL
University of Illinois at Chicago, IL
University of Kentucky, KY
University of Massachusetts Boston, MA
University of Minnesota, Twin Cities Campus, MN
University of Oklahoma Health Sciences Center, OK
University of Southern Indiana, IN
University of South Florida, FL
University of Wisconsin–Eau Claire, WI
Virginia Commonwealth University, VA
Webster University, MO

Gerontological Nursing

California State University, Dominguez Hills, CA
Cedar Crest College, PA
Clemson University, SC
College of Mount Saint Vincent, NY
Duke University, NC
Duquesne University, PA
Grand Valley State University, MI
Gwynedd-Mercy College, PA
Indiana University–Purdue University Indianapolis, IN
Kent State University, OH
La Roche College, PA
Lehman College of the City University of New York, NY
Marquette University, WI
McNeese State University, LA
Medical University of South Carolina, SC
Neumann College, PA
New York University, NY
Northern Illinois University, IL
Oregon Health Sciences University, OR
Rush University, IL
Saginaw Valley State University, MI
San Jose State University, CA
South Dakota State University, SD
State University of New York at Binghamton, NY
State University of New York at New Paltz, NY
Syracuse University, NY
Temple University, PA
Texas Tech University Health Sciences Center, TX
Université de Montréal, PQ
Université Laval, PQ
University of Akron, OH
University of Alberta, AB
University of California, Los Angeles, CA
University of California, San Francisco, CA
University of Delaware, DE
University of Evansville, IN
University of Florida, FL
University of Hawaii at Manoa, HI
University of Iowa, IA
University of Kentucky, KY
University of Maryland at Baltimore, MD
University of Massachusetts Amherst, MA
University of Massachusetts Boston, MA
University of Michigan, MI
University of Minnesota, Twin Cities Campus, MN
University of Nebraska Medical Center, NE
University of New Mexico, NM
University of Oklahoma Health Sciences Center, OK
University of Rhode Island, RI
University of Saskatchewan, SK
University of South Florida, FL
University of Texas–Houston Health Science Center, TX
University of Washington, WA
University of Wisconsin–Madison, WI
Wichita State University, KS
Wilkes University, PA

Maternity-Newborn Nursing

Adelphi University, NY
Albany State College, GA
California State University, Dominguez Hills, CA
Clemson University, SC
Dalhousie University, NS
East Carolina University, NC
Emory University, GA
Medical University of South Carolina, SC
Northern Illinois University, IL
Northwestern State University of Louisiana, LA
Ohio State University, OH
Rush University, IL
State University of New York at Stony Brook, NY
Syracuse University, NY
Temple University, PA
Texas Woman's University, TX
Troy State University, AL
Université de Montréal, PQ
Université Laval, PQ
University of Alberta, AB
University of Delaware, DE
University of Florida, FL
University of Illinois at Chicago, IL
University of North Carolina at Chapel Hill, NC
University of Oklahoma Health Sciences Center, OK
University of Rhode Island, RI
University of South Alabama, AL
University of Tennessee, Knoxville, TN
University of Wisconsin–Madison, WI
Valparaiso University, IN
Wichita State University, KS

Medical-Surgical Nursing

Angelo State University, TX
Case Western Reserve University, OH
East Carolina University, NC
Emory University, GA
Gannon University, PA
Hunter College of the City University of New York, NY
New Mexico State University, NM
Oregon Health Sciences University, OR
Pontifical Catholic University of Puerto Rico, PR
Rush University, IL
Russell Sage College, NY
Saginaw Valley State University, MI
Saint Xavier University, IL
South Dakota State University, SD
Southern Illinois University at Edwardsville, IL
State University of New York at Stony Brook, NY
Syracuse University, NY
Thomas Jefferson University, PA
Université Laval, PQ
University of Alberta, AB
University of Delaware, DE
University of Illinois at Chicago, IL
University of Maryland at Baltimore, MD
University of Michigan, MI
University of Minnesota, Twin Cities Campus, MN
University of New Mexico, NM
University of North Carolina at Charlotte, NC
University of Oklahoma Health Sciences Center, OK
University of Washington, WA
University of Wisconsin–Madison, WI
Western Connecticut State University, CT
Wichita State University, KS

Occupational Health Nursing

Syracuse University, NY
University of California, San Francisco, CA
University of Cincinnati, OH
University of Illinois at Chicago, IL
University of Michigan, MI

University of Washington, WA
University of Wisconsin–Milwaukee, WI

Oncology Nursing

Case Western Reserve University, OH
Columbia University, NY
Duke University, NC
Emory University, GA
Gwynedd-Mercy College, PA
Indiana University–Purdue University Indianapolis, IN
Johns Hopkins University, MD
Loyola University Chicago, IL
McNeese State University, LA
Rush University, IL
Syracuse University, NY
Université de Montréal, PQ
Université Laval, PQ
University of Alberta, AB
University of California, Los Angeles, CA
University of California, San Francisco, CA
University of Colorado Health Sciences Center, CO
University of Delaware, DE
University of Florida, FL
University of Illinois at Chicago, IL
University of Kentucky, KY
University of Maryland at Baltimore, MD
University of Minnesota, Twin Cities Campus, MN
University of Nebraska Medical Center, NE
University of Pennsylvania, PA
University of South Florida, FL
University of Texas–Houston Health Science Center, TX
University of Utah, UT
University of Washington, WA
Yale University, CT

Parent-Child Nursing

Angelo State University, TX
California State University, Los Angeles, CA
College Misericordia, PA
Hunter College of the City University of New York, NY
Kent State University, OH
Louisiana State University Medical Center, LA
Medical College of Georgia, GA
Medical College of Ohio, OH
Medical University of South Carolina, SC
Ohio State University, OH
South Dakota State University, SD
Syracuse University, NY
Université Laval, PQ
University of Alberta, AB
University of Kentucky, KY
University of New Mexico, NM
University of North Dakota, ND
University of Texas at Austin, TX
University of Texas at El Paso, TX
University of Wisconsin–Milwaukee, WI
Vanderbilt University, TN

Pediatric Nursing (see Child Care...)

Perinatal Nursing

Adelphi University, NY
Emory University, GA
Medical University of South Carolina, SC
Ohio State University, OH
Old Dominion University, VA
State University of New York at Stony Brook, NY
Syracuse University, NY
Université de Montréal, PQ
Université Laval, PQ
University of Alberta, AB
University of California, San Francisco, CA
University of Cincinnati, OH
University of Connecticut, CT
University of Illinois at Chicago, IL
University of Kentucky, KY
University of Pennsylvania, PA
University of Texas–Houston Health Science Center, TX
University of Washington, WA
University of Wisconsin–Madison, WI

Psychiatric–Mental Health Nursing

Adelphi University, NY
Arizona State University, AZ
Boston College, MA
Columbia University, NY
Dalhousie University, NS
East Carolina University, NC
Eastern Washington University, WA
Emory University, GA
Georgia State University, GA
Grand Valley State University, MI
Hampton University, VA
Hunter College of the City University of New York, NY
Indiana University–Purdue University Indianapolis, IN
Kent State University, OH
Louisiana State University Medical Center, LA
Medical College of Georgia, GA
Medical College of Ohio, OH
Medical University of South Carolina, SC
New Mexico State University, NM
New York University, NY
Northeastern University, MA
Northwestern State University of Louisiana, LA
Ohio State University, OH
Oregon Health Sciences University, OR
Pace University, NY
Pontifical Catholic University of Puerto Rico, PR
Rush University, IL
Russell Sage College, NY
Rutgers, The State University of New Jersey, College of Nursing, NJ
Saginaw Valley State University, MI
Saint Joseph College, CT
Saint Xavier University, IL
Southeastern Louisiana University, LA
Southern Illinois University at Edwardsville, IL
State University of New York at Stony Brook, NY
Syracuse University, NY
Temple University, PA
Texas Woman's University, TX
Université de Montréal, PQ
Université Laval, PQ
University of Akron, OH
University of Alaska Anchorage, AK
University of Alberta, AB
University of California, San Francisco, CA
University of Central Arkansas, AR
University of Cincinnati, OH
University of Colorado Health Sciences Center, CO
University of Connecticut, CT
University of Florida, FL
University of Hawaii at Manoa, HI
University of Illinois at Chicago, IL
University of Kansas, KS
University of Kentucky, KY
University of Louisville, KY
University of Maryland at Baltimore, MD
University of Massachusetts Amherst, MA
University of Michigan, MI
University of Minnesota, Twin Cities Campus, MN
University of Missouri–Columbia, MO
University of Nebraska Medical Center, NE
University of New Mexico, NM
University of North Carolina at Chapel Hill, NC
University of North Carolina at Charlotte, NC
University of Oklahoma Health Sciences Center, OK
University of Pennsylvania, PA
University of Rhode Island, RI
University of Rochester, NY
University of Saskatchewan, SK
University of South Alabama, AL
University of South Carolina, SC
University of Southern Maine, ME
University of Southern Mississippi, MS
University of South Florida, FL
University of Tennessee, Knoxville, TN
University of Texas at Austin, TX
University of Texas at El Paso, TX
University of Texas–Houston Health Science Center, TX
University of Utah, UT
University of Virginia, VA
University of Washington, WA
University of Wisconsin–Madison, WI
University of Wisconsin–Milwaukee, WI
Valparaiso University, IN
Virginia Commonwealth University, VA
Washington State University, WA
Wayne State University, MI
Whitworth College, WA
Wichita State University, KS
Yale University, CT

Public Health Nursing

Boston College, MA
Dalhousie University, NS

Louisiana State University Medical Center, LA
Northeastern University, MA
Oregon Health Sciences University, OR
Syracuse University, NY
Thomas Jefferson University, PA
University of Alberta, AB
University of Illinois at Chicago, IL
University of Minnesota, Twin Cities Campus, MN
University of Missouri–Columbia, MO
University of Saskatchewan, SK
University of Tennessee, Memphis, TN
University of Washington, WA

Rehabilitation Nursing

Indiana University–Purdue University Indianapolis, IN
Neumann College, PA
Rush University, IL
Syracuse University, NY
Thomas Jefferson University, PA
Université de Montréal, PQ
Université Laval, PQ
University of Illinois at Chicago, IL

Women's Health Nursing

Arizona State University, AZ
Cedar Crest College, PA
Indiana University–Purdue University Indianapolis, IN
Medical University of South Carolina, SC
Ohio State University, OH
Oregon Health Sciences University, OR
Rush University, IL
State University of New York at Stony Brook, NY
Syracuse University, NY
Université de Montréal, PQ
Université Laval, PQ
University of Alberta, AB
University of Florida, FL
University of Illinois at Chicago, IL
University of Maryland at Baltimore, MD
University of Missouri–Kansas City, MO
University of Missouri–St. Louis, MO
University of Nebraska Medical Center, NE
University of North Carolina at Chapel Hill, NC
University of South Alabama, AL
University of Tennessee, Knoxville, TN
University of Texas at El Paso, TX
University of Texas–Houston Health Science Center, TX
University of Wisconsin–Madison, WI
University of Wisconsin–Milwaukee, WI
Virginia Commonwealth University, VA

Nurse Anesthesia

Allegheny University of the Health Sciences, PA
Bradley University, IL
Case Western Reserve University, OH
Columbia University, NY
DePaul University, IL
Gannon University, PA
Georgetown University, DC
Lehman College of the City University of New York, NY
Medical College of Georgia, GA
Medical University of South Carolina, SC
Murray State University, KY
Northeastern University, MA
Oakland University, MI
Old Dominion University, VA
Rush University, IL
Samuel Merritt College, CA
Southern Illinois University at Edwardsville, IL
State University of New York at Buffalo, NY
University of Akron, OH
University of California, San Francisco, CA
University of Cincinnati, OH
University of Iowa, IA
University of Medicine and Dentistry of New Jersey, NJ
University of New England–University Campus, ME
University of North Carolina at Charlotte, NC
University of North Carolina at Greensboro, NC
University of North Dakota, ND
University of Pittsburgh, PA
University of Puerto Rico, Medical Sciences Campus, PR
University of Southern California, CA
University of Tennessee at Chattanooga, TN
University of Tennessee, Memphis, TN
University of Texas–Houston Health Science Center, TX
Villanova University, PA
Wilkes University, PA

Nurse Midwifery

Arizona State University, AZ
Case Western Reserve University, OH
Columbia University, NY
East Carolina University, NC
Emory University, GA
Georgetown University, DC
Marquette University, WI
Medical University of South Carolina, SC
New York University, NY
Ohio State University, OH
Oregon Health Sciences University, OR
San Diego State University, CA
State University of New York at Stony Brook, NY
University of California, Los Angeles, CA
University of California, San Francisco, CA
University of Cincinnati, OH
University of Colorado Health Sciences Center, CO
University of Florida, FL
University of Illinois at Chicago, IL
University of Kentucky, KY
University of Minnesota, Twin Cities Campus, MN
University of Missouri–Columbia, MO
University of New Mexico, NM
University of Pennsylvania, PA
University of Rhode Island, RI
University of Rochester, NY
University of Southern California, CA
University of Texas at El Paso, TX
University of Texas at Tyler, TX
University of Texas Medical Branch at Galveston, TX
University of Utah, UT
University of Washington, WA
Vanderbilt University, TN
Yale University, CT

Nurse Administration

Abilene Christian University, TX
Adelphi University, NY
Allentown College of St. Francis de Sales, PA
Andrews University, MI
Arizona State University, AZ
Armstrong Atlantic State University, GA
Azusa Pacific University, CA
Ball State University, IN
Barry University, FL
Bellarmine College, KY
Bowie State University, MD
Bradley University, IL
Brigham Young University, UT
California State University, Bakersfield, CA
California State University, Dominguez Hills, CA
California State University, Los Angeles, CA
California State University, Sacramento, CA
Capital University, OH
Case Western Reserve University, OH
Catholic University of America, DC
Cedar Crest College, PA
Clarkson College, NE
Clemson University, SC
College Misericordia, PA
College of Mount Saint Vincent, NY
College of New Jersey, NJ
College of New Rochelle, NY
Creighton University, NE
Delta State University, MS
DePaul University, IL
Drake University, IA
Duke University, NC
Duquesne University, PA
East Carolina University, NC
Eastern Kentucky University, KY
Eastern Michigan University, MI
Edgewood College, WI
Fairleigh Dickinson University, Teaneck-Hackensack Campus, NJ
Florida Atlantic University, FL
Florida International University, FL
Fort Hays State University, KS
Gannon University, PA
George Mason University, VA
Georgia College, GA
Gonzaga University, WA
Governors State University, IL
Graceland College, IA
Grand Valley State University, MI
Hampton University, VA

Hunter College of the City University of New York, NY
Idaho State University, ID
Indiana State University, IN
Indiana University of Pennsylvania, PA
Indiana University–Purdue University Fort Wayne, IN
Indiana University–Purdue University Indianapolis, IN
Johns Hopkins University, MD
Kean College of New Jersey, NJ
Kent State University, OH
La Roche College, PA
La Salle University, PA
Lehman College of the City University of New York, NY
Lewis University, IL
Loma Linda University, CA
Louisiana State University Medical Center, LA
Loyola University Chicago, IL
Madonna University, MI
Marquette University, WI
Marshall University, WV
Marymount University, VA
McNeese State University, LA
Medical University of South Carolina, SC
Molloy College, NY
Montana State University–Bozeman, MT
New Mexico State University, NM
New York University, NY
Northeastern University, MA
Northern Kentucky University, KY
Northern Michigan University, MI
North Park College, IL
Oakland University, MI
Old Dominion University, VA
Otterbein College, OH
Pacific Lutheran University, WA
Pennsylvania State University, University Park Campus, PA
Pittsburg State University, KS
Pontifical Catholic University of Puerto Rico, PR
Regis University, CO
Russell Sage College, NY
Sacred Heart University, CT
Saginaw Valley State University, MI
Saint Francis College, IN
St. John Fisher College, NY
Saint Joseph's College, ME
Saint Xavier University, IL
Salisbury State University, MD
Samford University, AL
San Diego State University, CA
San Francisco State University, CA
San Jose State University, CA
Seattle Pacific University, WA
Seton Hall University, NJ
Sonoma State University, CA
South Dakota State University, SD
Southeastern Louisiana University, LA
Southeast Missouri State University, MO
Southern Connecticut State University, CT
State University of New York at Binghamton, NY
State University of New York Institute of Technology at Utica/Rome, NY
Syracuse University, NY
Texas Tech University Health Sciences Center, TX
Troy State University, AL
University of Akron, OH
University of Alabama in Huntsville, AL
University of Alaska Anchorage, AK
University of Arkansas, AR
University of Arkansas for Medical Sciences, AR
University of California, Los Angeles, CA
University of California, San Francisco, CA
University of Central Florida, FL
University of Cincinnati, OH
University of Colorado Health Sciences Center, CO
University of Connecticut, CT
University of Delaware, DE
University of Florida, FL
University of Hartford, CT
University of Hawaii at Manoa, HI
University of Illinois at Chicago, IL
University of Iowa, IA
University of Kansas, KS
University of Kentucky, KY
University of Manitoba, MB
University of Maryland at Baltimore, MD
University of Massachusetts Boston, MA
University of Michigan, MI
University of Minnesota, Twin Cities Campus, MN
University of Mississippi Medical Center, MS
University of Missouri–Columbia, MO
University of Missouri–Kansas City, MO
University of Missouri–St. Louis, MO
University of Mobile, AL
University of Nebraska Medical Center, NE
University of Nevada, Reno, NV
University of New Hampshire, NH
University of New Mexico, NM
University of North Carolina at Chapel Hill, NC
University of North Carolina at Greensboro, NC
University of Oklahoma Health Sciences Center, OK
University of Pennsylvania, PA
University of Phoenix, AZ
University of Pittsburgh, PA
University of Puerto Rico, Medical Sciences Campus, PR
University of Rhode Island, RI
University of San Diego, CA
University of San Francisco, CA
University of Saskatchewan, SK
University of South Alabama, AL
University of South Carolina, SC
University of Southern California, CA
University of Southern Maine, ME
University of Southern Mississippi, MS
University of Tennessee at Chattanooga, TN
University of Tennessee, Knoxville, TN
University of Tennessee, Memphis, TN
University of Texas at Arlington, TX
University of Texas at El Paso, TX
University of Texas Health Science Center at San Antonio, TX
University of Texas–Houston Health Science Center, TX
University of Texas Medical Branch at Galveston, TX
University of Texas–Pan American, TX
University of Utah, UT
University of Washington, WA
University of Western Ontario, ON
University of Wisconsin–Eau Claire, WI
University of Wisconsin–Oshkosh, WI
Valparaiso University, IN
Vanderbilt University, TN
Villanova University, PA
Virginia Commonwealth University, VA
Wagner College, NY
Wayne State University, MI
West Chester University of Pennsylvania, PA
Western Connecticut State University, CT
West Texas A&M University, TX
West Virginia University, WV
Wichita State University, KS
William Paterson College of New Jersey, NJ
Winona State University, MN
Wright State University, OH
Xavier University, OH

Nurse Education

Adelphi University, NY
Arizona State University, AZ
Azusa Pacific University, CA
Ball State University, IN
Barry University, FL
Bellarmine College, KY
Bowie State University, MD
California State University, Bakersfield, CA
California State University, Chico, CA
California State University, Dominguez Hills, CA
California State University, Los Angeles, CA
California State University, Sacramento, CA
Cardinal Stritch College, WI
Case Western Reserve University, OH
Catholic University of America, DC
Clarkson College, NE
Clemson University, SC
College Misericordia, PA
Concordia University Wisconsin, WI
Creighton University, NE
Delta State University, MS
DePaul University, IL
Drake University, IA
Duquesne University, PA
Eastern Michigan University, MI
Fairleigh Dickinson University, Teaneck-Hackensack Campus, NJ
Florida International University, FL
Fort Hays State University, KS
Gonzaga University, WA
Governors State University, IL

Grand Valley State University, MI
Hampton University, VA
Idaho State University, ID
Indiana State University, IN
Indiana University of Pennsylvania, PA
Kent State University, OH
Lehman College of the City University of New York, NY
Lewis University, IL
Marymount University, VA
McNeese State University, LA
Medical College of Ohio, OH
Midwestern State University, TX
Molloy College, NY
New Mexico State University, NM
New York University, NY
North Park College, IL
Pennsylvania State University, University Park Campus, PA
Pittsburg State University, KS
Pontifical Catholic University of Puerto Rico, PR
Russell Sage College, NY
Saginaw Valley State University, MI
Saint Joseph's College, ME
Samford University, AL
San Francisco State University, CA
San Jose State University, CA
Seattle Pacific University, WA
Seton Hall University, NJ
South Dakota State University, SD
Southeastern Louisiana University, LA
Southeast Missouri State University, MO
Southern Connecticut State University, CT
Southwest Missouri State University, MO
State University of New York at Binghamton, NY
Syracuse University, NY
Teachers College, Columbia University, NY
Texas Tech University Health Sciences Center, TX
Troy State University, AL
University of Akron, OH
University of Arkansas, AR
University of Central Arkansas, AR
University of Hartford, CT
University of Iowa, IA
University of Maryland at Baltimore, MD
University of Massachusetts Amherst, MA
University of Massachusetts Boston, MA
University of Minnesota, Twin Cities Campus, MN
University of Mississippi Medical Center, MS
University of Missouri–Columbia, MO
University of Missouri–Kansas City, MO
University of Missouri–St. Louis, MO
University of Nebraska Medical Center, NE
University of North Carolina at Charlotte, NC
University of North Carolina at Greensboro, NC
University of Northern Colorado, CO
University of Oklahoma Health Sciences Center, OK
University of Phoenix, AZ
University of Pittsburgh, PA
University of Puerto Rico, Medical Sciences Campus, PR
University of Rhode Island, RI
University of Saskatchewan, SK
University of South Alabama, AL
University of Southern Mississippi, MS
University of Tennessee at Chattanooga, TN
University of Texas at Arlington, TX
University of Texas Health Science Center at San Antonio, TX
University of Texas–Houston Health Science Center, TX
University of Texas Medical Branch at Galveston, TX
University of Texas–Pan American, TX
University of Utah, UT
University of Washington, WA
University of Western Ontario, ON
University of Wisconsin–Eau Claire, WI
University of Wisconsin–Madison, WI
University of Wisconsin–Oshkosh, WI
University of Wyoming, WY
Villanova University, PA
Wagner College, NY
Wayne State University, MI
Webster University, MO
West Chester University of Pennsylvania, PA
Western Kentucky University, KY
West Texas A&M University, TX
West Virginia University, WV
Wichita State University, KS
William Paterson College of New Jersey, NJ
Winona State University, MN
Wright State University, OH

Nurse Practitioner Programs

Albany State College, GA
Kent State University, OH
La Salle University, PA
Temple University, PA
Tennessee State University, TN
University of Ottawa, ON

Acute Care

Allegheny University of the Health Sciences, PA
Barry University, FL
Case Western Reserve University, OH
College of New Rochelle, NY
Emory University, GA
Florida State University, FL
Georgetown University, DC
Johns Hopkins University, MD
Monmouth University, NJ
New York University, NY
Northeastern University, MA
Pace University, NY
Rush University, IL
Russell Sage College, NY
Rutgers, The State University of New Jersey, College of Nursing, NJ
State University of New York at Stony Brook, NY
University of Akron, OH
University of Alabama at Birmingham, AL
University of Alabama in Huntsville, AL
University of Arkansas for Medical Sciences, AR
University of California, Los Angeles, CA
University of California, San Francisco, CA
University of Connecticut, CT
University of Illinois at Chicago, IL
University of Kentucky, KY
University of Maryland at Baltimore, MD
University of Massachusetts Worcester, MA
University of Michigan, MI
University of Pennsylvania, PA
University of Pittsburgh, PA
University of Rochester, NY
University of South Carolina, SC
University of South Florida, FL
University of Texas at Arlington, TX
University of Texas–Houston Health Science Center, TX
University of Texas Medical Branch at Galveston, TX
University of Utah, UT
University of Virginia, VA
University of Washington, WA
Vanderbilt University, TN
Virginia Commonwealth University, VA
Wayne State University, MI

Adult Health

Adelphi University, NY
Andrews University, MI
Arizona State University, AZ
Ball State University, IN
Barry University, FL
Bloomsburg University of Pennsylvania, PA
Boston College, MA
Case Western Reserve University, OH
Catholic University of America, DC
College of Mount Saint Vincent, NY
College of St. Catherine, MN
Columbia University, NY
Creighton University, NE
Duke University, NC
East Tennessee State University, TN
Emory University, GA
Fairleigh Dickinson University, Teaneck-Hackensack Campus, NJ
Florida Atlantic University, FL
Florida International University, FL
Florida State University, FL
George Mason University, VA
Grand Valley State University, MI
Gwynedd-Mercy College, PA
Indiana University–Purdue University Indianapolis, IN
Indiana Wesleyan University, IN
Johns Hopkins University, MD
Loma Linda University, CA
Long Island University, Brooklyn Campus, NY
Louisiana State University Medical Center, LA

Loyola University Chicago, IL
Marquette University, WI
McNeese State University, LA
Medical University of South Carolina, SC
MGH Institute of Health Professions, MA
Molloy College, NY
Monmouth University, NJ
New York University, NY
Northeastern University, MA
Northern Kentucky University, KY
Ohio State University, OH
Oregon Health Sciences University, OR
Rush University, IL
Russell Sage College, NY
Rutgers, The State University of New Jersey, Camden College of Arts and Sciences, NJ
Rutgers, The State University of New Jersey, College of Nursing, NJ
San Diego State University, CA
Seattle Pacific University, WA
Seton Hall University, NJ
Simmons College, MA
Southern Illinois University at Edwardsville, IL
State University of New York at Buffalo, NY
State University of New York at Stony Brook, NY
State University of New York Health Science Center at Syracuse, NY
State University of New York Institute of Technology at Utica/Rome, NY
Texas Woman's University, TX
University of Alabama at Birmingham, AL
University of Arizona, AZ
University of California, San Francisco, CA
University of Central Arkansas, AR
University of Colorado Health Sciences Center, CO
University of Connecticut, CT
University of Delaware, DE
University of Hawaii at Manoa, HI
University of Kansas, KS
University of Kentucky, KY
University of Louisville, KY
University of Maryland at Baltimore, MD
University of Massachusetts Boston, MA
University of Massachusetts Dartmouth, MA
University of Massachusetts Worcester, MA
University of Medicine and Dentistry of New Jersey, NJ
University of Michigan, MI
University of Mississippi Medical Center, MS
University of Missouri–Kansas City, MO
University of Missouri–St. Louis, MO
University of Nebraska Medical Center, NE
University of New England–Westbrook College Campus, ME
University of New Hampshire, NH
University of North Carolina at Chapel Hill, NC
University of Pennsylvania, PA
University of Portland, OR
University of Rochester, NY
University of San Diego, CA
University of South Carolina, SC
University of Southern Maine, ME
University of South Florida, FL
University of Texas at Arlington, TX
University of Texas at El Paso, TX
University of Texas–Houston Health Science Center, TX
University of Texas Medical Branch at Galveston, TX
University of Utah, UT
University of Washington, WA
University of Wisconsin–Eau Claire, WI
University of Wisconsin–Madison, WI
Vanderbilt University, TN
Villanova University, PA
Virginia Commonwealth University, VA
Western Connecticut State University, CT
West Virginia University, WV
William Paterson College of New Jersey, NJ
Winona State University, MN
Yale University, CT

Child Care/Pediatrics

Adelphi University, NY
Allegheny University of the Health Sciences, PA
Arizona State University, AZ
Boston College, MA
California State University, Fresno, CA
California State University, Los Angeles, CA
Case Western Reserve University, OH
Catholic University of America, DC
College of St. Catherine, MN
Columbia University, NY
Duke University, NC
Emory University, GA
Florida International University, FL
Florida State University, FL
Georgia State University, GA
Grand Valley State University, MI
Gwynedd-Mercy College, PA
Hunter College of the City University of New York, NY
Indiana University–Purdue University Indianapolis, IN
Johns Hopkins University, MD
Lehman College of the City University of New York, NY
Loma Linda University, CA
Loyola University Chicago, IL
Marquette University, WI
Medical College of Georgia, GA
Medical University of South Carolina, SC
MGH Institute of Health Professions, MA
Mississippi University for Women, MS
Molloy College, NY
New York University, NY
Northeastern University, MA
Ohio State University, OH
Old Dominion University, VA
Oregon Health Sciences University, OR
Regis College, MA
Rush University, IL
Rutgers, The State University of New Jersey, College of Nursing, NJ
Seton Hall University, NJ
Simmons College, MA
State University of New York at Buffalo, NY
State University of New York at Stony Brook, NY
State University of New York Health Science Center at Syracuse, NY
Syracuse University, NY
Texas Woman's University, TX
University of Akron, OH
University of Alabama at Birmingham, AL
University of Arkansas for Medical Sciences, AR
University of California, Los Angeles, CA
University of California, San Francisco, CA
University of Cincinnati, OH
University of Colorado Health Sciences Center, CO
University of Delaware, DE
University of Florida, FL
University of Hawaii at Manoa, HI
University of Illinois at Chicago, IL
University of Iowa, IA
University of Kentucky, KY
University of Massachusetts Amherst, MA
University of Minnesota, Twin Cities Campus, MN
University of Missouri–Kansas City, MO
University of Missouri–St. Louis, MO
University of Nebraska Medical Center, NE
University of New England–Westbrook College Campus, ME
University of North Carolina at Chapel Hill, NC
University of Oklahoma Health Sciences Center, OK
University of Pennsylvania, PA
University of Pittsburgh, PA
University of Rochester, NY
University of San Diego, CA
University of South Carolina, SC
University of South Florida, FL
University of Tennessee, Knoxville, TN
University of Tennessee, Memphis, TN
University of Texas at Arlington, TX
University of Texas at El Paso, TX
University of Texas–Houston Health Science Center, TX
University of Texas Medical Branch at Galveston, TX
University of Utah, UT
University of Virginia, VA
University of Washington, WA
University of Wisconsin–Madison, WI
Virginia Commonwealth University, VA
Wayne State University, MI
West Virginia University, WV
Wichita State University, KS

Yale University, CT

Community Health

Barry University, FL
Boston College, MA
Eastern Kentucky University, KY
Georgia State University, GA
Holy Names College, CA
Northeastern University, MA
Pace University, NY
Rush University, IL
Rutgers, The State University of New Jersey, Camden College of Arts and Sciences, NJ
State University of New York at Binghamton, NY
Syracuse University, NY
University of Pennsylvania, PA
University of Texas at El Paso, TX
University of Utah, UT

Emergency Care

Columbia University, NY
University of Texas–Houston Health Science Center, TX

Family Health

Adelphi University, NY
Allegheny University of the Health Sciences, PA
Arizona State University, AZ
Azusa Pacific University, CA
Ball State University, IN
Barry University, FL
Boston College, MA
Bowie State University, MD
Brenau University, GA
Brigham Young University, UT
California State University, Bakersfield, CA
California State University, Dominguez Hills, CA
California State University, Fresno, CA
Case Western Reserve University, OH
Catholic University of America, DC
Clarion University of Pennsylvania, PA
Clarkson College, NE
Clemson University, SC
College Misericordia, PA
College of New Jersey, NJ
College of New Rochelle, NY
College of St. Scholastica, MN
Columbia University, NY
Concordia University Wisconsin, WI
Creighton University, NE
Delta State University, MS
Drake University, IA
Duke University, NC
Duquesne University, PA
Eastern Washington University, WA
East Tennessee State University, TN
Edinboro University of Pennsylvania, PA
Emory University, GA
Fairfield University, CT
Florida Atlantic University, FL
Florida State University, FL
Fort Hays State University, KS
Gannon University, PA
George Mason University, VA
Georgetown University, DC
Georgia College, GA
Georgia Southern University, GA
Gonzaga University, WA
Graceland College, IA
Grand Valley State University, MI
Hampton University, VA
Hardin-Simmons University, TX
Holy Names College, CA
Houston Baptist University, TX
Howard University, DC
Idaho State University, ID
Indiana State University, IN
Indiana University–Purdue University Indianapolis, IN
Indiana Wesleyan University, IN
Kennesaw State University, GA
La Roche College, PA
Loma Linda University, CA
Long Island University, C.W. Post Campus, NY
Loyola University, New Orleans, LA
Mankato State University, MN
Marshall University, WV
Marymount University, VA
Medical College of Georgia, GA
Medical College of Ohio, OH
Medical University of South Carolina, SC
Mennonite College of Nursing, IL
Metropolitan State University, MN
MGH Institute of Health Professions, MA
Michigan State University, MI
Midwestern State University, TX
Millersville University of Pennsylvania, PA
Mississippi University for Women, MS
Monmouth University, NJ
Montana State University–Bozeman, MT
Murray State University, KY
Niagara University, NY
Northeastern University, MA
Northern Arizona University, AZ
Northern Illinois University, IL
Northern Kentucky University, KY
Northern Michigan University, MI
Oakland University, MI
Old Dominion University, VA
Oregon Health Sciences University, OR
Pace University, NY
Pacific Lutheran University, WA
Pennsylvania State University, University Park Campus, PA
Pittsburg State University, KS
Purdue University Calumet, IN
Radford University, VA
Regis College, MA
Regis University, CO
Research College of Nursing–Rockhurst College, MO
Rivier College, NH
Rush University, IL
Russell Sage College, NY
Rutgers, The State University of New Jersey, College of Nursing, NJ
Sacred Heart University, CT
Saginaw Valley State University, MI
Saint Francis College, IN
St. John Fisher College, NY
Saint Joseph College, CT
Saint Martin's College, WA
Saint Xavier University, IL
Salisbury State University, MD
Samford University, AL
Samuel Merritt College, CA
San Diego State University, CA
San Francisco State University, CA
Seattle Pacific University, WA
Seattle University, WA
Simmons College, MA
Slippery Rock University of Pennsylvania, PA
Sonoma State University, CA
South Dakota State University, SD
Southern Connecticut State University, CT
Southern Illinois University at Edwardsville, IL
Southern University and Agricultural and Mechanical College, LA
Southwest Missouri State University, MO
Spalding University, KY
State University of New York at Binghamton, NY
State University of New York at Buffalo, NY
State University of New York Health Science Center at Syracuse, NY
Syracuse University, NY
Texas Tech University Health Sciences Center, TX
Texas Woman's University, TX
Thomas Jefferson University, PA
Troy State University, AL
University of Alabama at Birmingham, AL
University of Alabama in Huntsville, AL
University of Alaska Anchorage, AK
University of Arizona, AZ
University of Arkansas for Medical Sciences, AR
University of California, Los Angeles, CA
University of California, San Francisco, CA
University of Central Florida, FL
University of Cincinnati, OH
University of Colorado Health Sciences Center, CO
University of Delaware, DE
University of Florida, FL
University of Hawaii at Manoa, HI
University of Illinois at Chicago, IL
University of Indianapolis, IN
University of Kansas, KS
University of Kentucky, KY
University of Maine, ME
University of Maryland at Baltimore, MD
University of Massachusetts Amherst, MA
University of Massachusetts Boston, MA
University of Massachusetts Lowell, MA
University of Medicine and Dentistry of New Jersey, NJ
University of Michigan, MI

University of Minnesota, Twin Cities Campus, MN
University of Mississippi Medical Center, MS
University of Missouri–Columbia, MO
University of Missouri–Kansas City, MO
University of Missouri–St. Louis, MO
University of Mobile, AL
University of Nebraska Medical Center, NE
University of Nevada, Las Vegas, NV
University of Nevada, Reno, NV
University of New England–Westbrook College Campus, ME
University of New Hampshire, NH
University of New Mexico, NM
University of North Carolina at Chapel Hill, NC
University of North Carolina at Charlotte, NC
University of North Dakota, ND
University of Northern Colorado, CO
University of Oklahoma Health Sciences Center, OK
University of Pennsylvania, PA
University of Pittsburgh, PA
University of Rhode Island, RI
University of Rochester, NY
University of San Diego, CA
University of Scranton, PA
University of South Alabama, AL
University of South Carolina, SC
University of Southern California, CA
University of Southern Indiana, IN
University of Southern Maine, ME
University of Southern Mississippi, MS
University of South Florida, FL
University of Tennessee at Chattanooga, TN
University of Tennessee, Knoxville, TN
University of Tennessee, Memphis, TN
University of Texas at Arlington, TX
University of Texas at El Paso, TX
University of Texas at Tyler, TX
University of Texas Health Science Center at San Antonio, TX
University of Texas–Houston Health Science Center, TX
University of Texas Medical Branch at Galveston, TX
University of Utah, UT
University of Virginia, VA
University of Washington, WA
University of Wisconsin–Eau Claire, WI
University of Wisconsin–Milwaukee, WI
University of Wisconsin–Oshkosh, WI
University of Wyoming, WY
Valparaiso University, IN
Vanderbilt University, TN
Virginia Commonwealth University, VA
Wagner College, NY
Washington State University, WA
Westminster College of Salt Lake City, UT
West Texas A&M University, TX
West Virginia University, WV
Whitworth College, WA
Wichita State University, KS
Widener University, PA
Wilmington College, DE
Winona State University, MN
Wright State University, OH
Yale University, CT

Gerontology

Adelphi University, NY
Boston College, MA
California State University, Fresno, CA
Carlow College, PA
Case Western Reserve University, OH
Catholic University of America, DC
College of St. Catherine, MN
Columbia University, NY
Concordia University Wisconsin, WI
Creighton University, NE
Duke University, NC
Emory University, GA
Florida State University, FL
George Mason University, VA
Grand Valley State University, MI
Hampton University, VA
Hunter College of the City University of New York, NY
Indiana University–Purdue University Indianapolis, IN
Indiana Wesleyan University, IN
Marquette University, WI
Medical University of South Carolina, SC
MGH Institute of Health Professions, MA
Michigan State University, MI
Mississippi University for Women, MS
Monmouth University, NJ
Nazareth College of Rochester, NY
New York University, NY
Northeastern University, MA
Pacific Lutheran University, WA
Pittsburg State University, KS
Rush University, IL
Russell Sage College, NY
San Diego State University, CA
Seattle Pacific University, WA
Seton Hall University, NJ
Simmons College, MA
Southwest Missouri State University, MO
State University of New York at Binghamton, NY
Syracuse University, NY
University of Alabama at Birmingham, AL
University of Arizona, AZ
University of Arkansas for Medical Sciences, AR
University of California, Los Angeles, CA
University of California, San Francisco, CA
University of Colorado Health Sciences Center, CO
University of Connecticut, CT
University of Delaware, DE
University of Florida, FL
University of Hawaii at Manoa, HI
University of Iowa, IA
University of Kentucky, KY
University of Louisville, KY
University of Maryland at Baltimore, MD
University of Massachusetts Boston, MA
University of Massachusetts Lowell, MA
University of Massachusetts Worcester, MA
University of Michigan, MI
University of Minnesota, Twin Cities Campus, MN
University of Missouri–Columbia, MO
University of Nebraska Medical Center, NE
University of North Carolina at Greensboro, NC
University of Pennsylvania, PA
University of Rochester, NY
University of San Diego, CA
University of South Carolina, SC
University of Southern California, CA
University of South Florida, FL
University of Tennessee, Memphis, TN
University of Texas at Arlington, TX
University of Texas–Houston Health Science Center, TX
University of Texas Medical Branch at Galveston, TX
University of Utah, UT
University of Washington, WA
University of Wisconsin–Madison, WI
University of Wisconsin–Oshkosh, WI
Vanderbilt University, TN
Wayne State University, MI
Yale University, CT

Neonatal Health

Case Western Reserve University, OH
College of St. Catherine, MN
Dalhousie University, NS
Emory University, GA
Loma Linda University, CA
Louisiana State University Medical Center, LA
Marquette University, WI
Medical College of Georgia, GA
Medical University of South Carolina, SC
Northeastern University, MA
Ohio State University, OH
Old Dominion University, VA
Pennsylvania State University, University Park Campus, PA
Rush University, IL
State University of New York at Stony Brook, NY
University of Alabama at Birmingham, AL
University of California, San Francisco, CA
University of Cincinnati, OH
University of Connecticut, CT
University of Kentucky, KY
University of Louisville, KY
University of Maryland at Baltimore, MD
University of Mississippi Medical Center, MS
University of Pennsylvania, PA
University of South Alabama, AL
University of Tennessee, Knoxville, TN
University of Tennessee, Memphis, TN
University of Texas–Houston Health Science Center, TX

University of Texas Medical Branch at Galveston, TX
University of Utah, UT
University of Washington, WA
Vanderbilt University, TN
Wayne State University, MI

Occupational Health
Simmons College, MA
Syracuse University, NY
University of Alabama at Birmingham, AL
University of California, Los Angeles, CA
University of California, San Francisco, CA
University of Illinois at Chicago, IL
University of Medicine and Dentistry of New Jersey, NJ
University of Pennsylvania, PA
University of Utah, UT
Vanderbilt University, TN

Pediatrics (see Child Care/ Pediatrics)

Primary Care
California State University, Fresno, CA
California State University, Sacramento, CA
DePaul University, IL
Duke University, NC
East Carolina University, NC
Florida State University, FL
George Mason University, VA
Johns Hopkins University, MD
Louisiana State University Medical Center, LA
Marymount University, VA
MGH Institute of Health Professions, MA
New York University, NY
Northeastern University, MA
Oregon Health Sciences University, OR
Pace University, NY
Rush University, IL
Rutgers, The State University of New Jersey, College of Nursing, NJ
San Francisco State University, CA
Southeastern Louisiana University, LA
State University of New York at Binghamton, NY
Syracuse University, NY
University of Akron, OH
University of Alabama at Birmingham, AL
University of Central Arkansas, AR
University of Connecticut, CT
University of Kentucky, KY
University of Massachusetts Amherst, MA
University of Michigan, MI
University of Nebraska Medical Center, NE
University of New Mexico, NM
University of North Carolina at Chapel Hill, NC
University of Pennsylvania, PA
University of Pittsburgh, PA
University of Rochester, NY
University of Tennessee, Knoxville, TN
University of Vermont, VT
University of Virginia, VA
University of Washington, WA
Vanderbilt University, TN
Wayne State University, MI
Western Kentucky University, KY
West Virginia University, WV

Psychiatric–Mental Health
Adelphi University, NY
Arizona State University, AZ
Case Western Reserve University, OH
Catholic University of America, DC
DePaul University, IL
Emory University, GA
Fairfield University, CT
Florida International University, FL
Grand Valley State University, MI
Medical University of South Carolina, SC
New York University, NY
Ohio State University, OH
Oregon Health Sciences University, OR
Rivier College, NH
Rush University, IL
Russell Sage College, NY
State University of New York at Stony Brook, NY
University of Arizona, AZ
University of California, San Francisco, CA
University of Hawaii at Manoa, HI
University of Kansas, KS
University of Massachusetts Lowell, MA
University of Medicine and Dentistry of New Jersey, NJ
University of Michigan, MI
University of North Carolina at Chapel Hill, NC
University of South Carolina, SC
University of Tennessee, Memphis, TN
University of Texas at Arlington, TX
University of Texas–Houston Health Science Center, TX
University of Utah, UT
University of Washington, WA
Vanderbilt University, TN

School Health
California State University, Fresno, CA
Catholic University of America, DC
Seton Hall University, NJ
Simmons College, MA
State University of New York at Buffalo, NY
Syracuse University, NY
University of California, San Francisco, CA
University of Illinois at Chicago, IL
University of San Diego, CA
Yale University, CT

Women's Health
Allegheny University of the Health Sciences, PA
Arizona State University, AZ
Boston College, MA
California State University, Los Angeles, CA
Case Western Reserve University, OH
Columbia University, NY
Florida State University, FL
Georgia State University, GA
Grand Valley State University, MI
Indiana University–Purdue University Indianapolis, IN
Loyola University Chicago, IL
MGH Institute of Health Professions, MA
Ohio State University, OH
Oregon Health Sciences University, OR
Pacific Lutheran University, WA
Seton Hall University, NJ
Simmons College, MA
State University of New York at Buffalo, NY
State University of New York at Stony Brook, NY
Syracuse University, NY
Texas Woman's University, TX
University of Alabama at Birmingham, AL
University of Arkansas for Medical Sciences, AR
University of California, San Francisco, CA
University of Colorado Health Sciences Center, CO
University of Delaware, DE
University of Hawaii at Manoa, HI
University of Illinois at Chicago, IL
University of Kansas, KS
University of Louisville, KY
University of Maryland at Baltimore, MD
University of Medicine and Dentistry of New Jersey, NJ
University of Michigan, MI
University of Minnesota, Twin Cities Campus, MN
University of Missouri–Kansas City, MO
University of Missouri–St. Louis, MO
University of Nebraska Medical Center, NE
University of North Carolina at Chapel Hill, NC
University of Pennsylvania, PA
University of Phoenix, AZ
University of Pittsburgh, PA
University of Rochester, NY
University of South Carolina, SC
University of Tennessee, Knoxville, TN
University of Texas at El Paso, TX
University of Texas–Houston Health Science Center, TX
University of Texas Medical Branch at Galveston, TX
University of Utah, UT
University of Virginia, VA
University of Washington, WA
University of Wisconsin–Madison, WI
Vanderbilt University, TN
Virginia Commonwealth University, VA
Wayne State University, MI
West Virginia University, WV

PROGRAM INDEX

This index categorizes degree and continuing education programs offered by the nursing schools profiled in this guide. Definitions of the programs are provided on page 12. To easily locate programs of interest and the schools where they are offered, refer to the following list.

BACCALAUREATE PROGRAMS

Generic Baccalaureate programs

Accelerated Baccalaureate programs

RN Baccalaureate programs

Accelerated RN Baccalaureate programs

Baccalaureate for Second Degree programs

Accelerated Baccalaureate for Second Degree programs

ADN to Baccalaureate programs

LPN to Baccalaureate programs

Wisconsin
Cardinal Stritch College, Department of Nursing, *Milwaukee* (BSN)
Concordia University Wisconsin, Nursing Division, *Mequon* (BSN)

Accelerated LPN to Baccalaureate programs

North Dakota
Medcenter One College of Nursing, *Bismarck* (BSN)
Minot State University, College of Nursing, *Minot* (BSN)

LPN to RN Baccalaureate programs

West Virginia
Alderson-Broaddus College, Department of Nursing, *Philippi* (BS)

RPN to Baccalaureate programs

Manitoba
Brandon University, Department of Nursing and Health Studies, *Brandon* (BScMH)

International Nurse to Baccalaureate programs

New York
Molloy College, Department of Nursing, *Rockville Centre* (BS)

MASTER'S PROGRAMS

Master's

Alabama
Troy State University, School of Nursing, *Troy* (MSN)
University of Alabama at Birmingham, School of Nursing, *Birmingham* (MSN)
University of Mobile, School of Nursing, *Mobile* (MSN)

Alaska
University of Alaska Anchorage, School of Nursing and Health Sciences, *Anchorage* (MS)

Arizona
Arizona State University, College of Nursing, *Tempe* (MS)
Northern Arizona University, Department of Nursing, *Flagstaff* (MS)
University of Phoenix, Department of Health Care Professions, *Phoenix* (MN)

Arkansas
Arkansas State University, Department of Nursing, *State University* (MSN)
University of Arkansas, Department of Nursing, *Fayetteville* (MNSc)
University of Arkansas for Medical Sciences, College of Nursing, *Little Rock* (MNSc)
University of Central Arkansas, Department of Nursing, *Conway* (MSN)

California
Azusa Pacific University, School of Nursing, *Azusa* (MSN)
California State University, Bakersfield, Department of Nursing, *Bakersfield* (MSN)
California State University, Chico, School of Nursing, *Chico* (MSN)
California State University, Dominguez Hills, Division of Nursing, *Carson* (MSN)
California State University, Fresno, Department of Nursing, *Fresno* (MSN)
California State University, Long Beach, Department of Nursing, *Long Beach* (MS)
California State University, Los Angeles, Department of Nursing, *Los Angeles* (MSN)
California State University, Sacramento, Division of Nursing, *Sacramento* (MSN)
Loma Linda University, School of Nursing, *Loma Linda* (MS)
Samuel Merritt College, Intercollegiate Nursing Program, *Oakland* (MSN)
San Diego State University, School of Nursing, *San Diego* (MSN)
San Francisco State University, School of Nursing, *San Francisco* (MSN)
San Jose State University, School of Nursing, *San Jose* (MS)
Sonoma State University, Department of Nursing, *Rohnert Park* (MSN)
University of California, Los Angeles, School of Nursing, *Los Angeles* (MSN)
University of California, San Francisco, School of Nursing, *San Francisco* (MSN)
University of San Francisco, School of Nursing, *San Francisco* (MSN)
University of Southern California, Department of Nursing, *Los Angeles* (MSN)

Colorado
Beth-El College of Nursing and Health Sciences, Beth-El College of Nursing, *Colorado Springs*
Regis University, Department of Nursing, *Denver* (MSN)
University of Colorado Health Sciences Center, School of Nursing, *Denver* (MS)
University of Northern Colorado, School of Nursing, *Greeley* (MS)

Connecticut
Fairfield University, School of Nursing, *Fairfield* (MSN)
Saint Joseph College, Division of Nursing, *West Hartford* (MS)
Southern Connecticut State University, Department of Nursing, *New Haven* (MSN)
University of Connecticut, School of Nursing, *Storrs* (MS)
University of Hartford, Division of Nursing, *West Hartford* (MSN)
Yale University, School of Nursing, *New Haven* (MSN)

Delaware
University of Delaware, College of Health and Nursing Sciences, *Newark* (MSN)

District of Columbia
Catholic University of America, School of Nursing, *Washington* (MSN)
Georgetown University, School of Nursing, *Washington* (MSN)
Howard University, College of Nursing, *Washington* (MSN)

Florida
Barry University, School of Nursing, *Miami Shores* (MSN)
Florida Atlantic University, College of Nursing, *Boca Raton* (MSN)
Florida International University, School of Nursing, *Miami* (MSN)
Florida State University, School of Nursing, *Tallahassee* (MSN)
University of Central Florida, School of Nursing, *Orlando* (MSN)
University of Florida, College of Nursing, *Gainesville* (MSN)
University of Florida, College of Nursing, *Gainesville* (MN)
University of Miami, School of Nursing, *Coral Gables*
University of South Florida, College of Nursing, *Tampa* (MS)
University of Tampa, Nursing Department, *Tampa* (MSN)

Georgia
Albany State College, School of Nursing and Allied Health, *Albany* (MS)
Armstrong Atlantic State University, Division of Nursing, *Savannah* (MSN)
Brenau University, Department of Nursing, *Gainesville* (MS)
Emory University, Nell Hodgson Woodruff School of Nursing, *Atlanta* (MSN)
Georgia College, School of Nursing, *Milledgeville* (MSN)
Georgia Southern University, Department of Nursing, *Statesboro* (MSN)
Georgia State University, School of Nursing, *Atlanta* (MS)
Kennesaw State University, School of Nursing, *Kennesaw* (MSN)
Medical College of Georgia, School of Nursing, *Augusta* (MN)
Medical College of Georgia, School of Nursing, *Augusta* (MSN)
Valdosta State University, School of Nursing, *Valdosta* (MSN)

Hawaii
University of Hawaii at Manoa, School of Nursing, *Honolulu* (MS)

Accelerated Master's programs

RN to Master's programs

Accelerated RN to Master's programs

Accelerated AD/RN to Master's program

Master's for Nurses with Non-Nursing Degrees

Accelerated Master's for Nurses with Non-Nursing Degrees programs

Master's for Non-Nursing College Graduates programs

Accelerated Master's for Non-Nursing College Graduates programs

Master's for Second Degree programs

Master of Education program

MSN/MBA Programs

MS/MBA Programs

MSN/MS in Business

MSN/MSA Program

MN/MHSA Program

MS/MHSA Program

MSN/MHA (Health Administration) Program

MS/MHA (Hospital Administration) Program

MSN/MPA Programs

MS/MM Program

MA/MSM Program

MSN/Master's in Health Service Managment Program

MSN/MOM Program

MSN/JD Program

MN/MPH Programs

MS/MPH Programs

MSN/MPH Programs

MS or MN/MPH Program

MS/MPS Program

MSN/MSOB Program

MSN/MDiv Programs

MSN/MPPM Program

MS/MA Program

MSN/Master's in Latin American studies program

Post-Master's Programs

DOCTORAL PROGRAMS

Doctoral

Postbaccalaureate Doctoral Programs

Doctoral Program for Nurses with Non-Nursing Degrees

Doctor of Education programs

PhD/MBA Programs

POSTDOCTORAL PROGRAMS

CONTINUING EDUCATION PROGRAMS

Institution Index